Estimated Safe and Adequate Daily Dietary Intakes of Additional Selected Vitamins and Minerals (United States)[a]

AGE (years)	VITAMINS	
	Biotin (µg)	Pantothenic Acid (mg)
Infants		
0–0.5	10	2
0.5–1	15	3
Children		
1–3	20	3
4–6	25	3–4
7–10	30	4–5
11+	30–100	4–7
Adults	30–100	4–7

Age (years)	TRACE ELEMENTS[b]				
	Chromium (µg)	Molybdenum (µg)	Copper (mg)	Manganese (mg)	Fluoride (mg)
Infants					
0–0.5	10–40	15–30	0.4–0.6	0.3–0.6	0.1–0.5
0.5–1	20–60	20–40	0.6–0.7	0.6–1.0	0.2–1.0
Children					
1–3	20–80	25–50	0.7–1.0	1.0–1.5	0.5–1.5
4–6	30–120	30–75	1.0–1.5	1.5–2.0	1.0–2.5
7–10	50–200	50–150	1.0–2.0	2.0–3.0	1.5–2.5
11+	50–200	75–250	1.5–2.5	2.0–5.0	1.5–2.5
Adults	50–200	75–250	1.5–3.0	2.0–5.0	1.5–4.0

[a]Because there is less information on which to base allowances, these figures are not given in the main table of the RDA and are provided here in the form of ranges of recommended intakes.

[b]Because the toxic levels for many trace elements may be only several times usual intakes, the upper levels for the trace elements given in this table should not be habitually exceeded.

SOURCE: *Recommended Dietary Allowances*, © 1989 by the National Academy of Sciences, National Academy Press, Washington, D.C.

Estimated Minimum Requirements of Sodium, Chloride, and Potassium

Age (years)	Sodium[a] (mg)	Chloride (mg)	Potassium[b] (mg)
Infants			
0.0–0.5	120	180	500
0.5–1.0	200	300	700
Children			
1	225	350	1,000
2–5	300	500	1,400
6–9	400	600	1,600
Adolescents	500	750	2,000
Adults	500	750	2,000

[a]Sodium requirements are based on estimates for growth and for replacement of obligatory losses. They cover a wide variation of physical activity patterns and climatic exposure but do not provide for large, prolonged losses from the skin through sweat.

[b]Dietary potassium may benefit the prevention and treatment of hypertension and recommendations to include many servings of fruits and vegetables would raise potassium intakes to about 3,500 mg/day.

SOURCE: *Recommended Dietary Allowances*, © 1989 by the National Academy of Sciences, National Academy Press, Washington, D.C.

Median Heights and Weights and Recommended Energy Intakes (United States)

AGE (years)	WEIGHT		HEIGHT		AVERAGE ENERGY ALLOWANCE	
	kg	lb	cm	inches	cal per kg	cal per day[a]
Infants						
0.0–0.5	6	13	60	24	108	650
0.5–1.0	9	20	71	28	98	850
Children						
1–3	13	29	90	35	102	1,300
4–6	20	44	112	44	90	1,800
7–10	28	62	132	52	70	2,000
Males						
11–14	45	99	157	62	55	2,500
15–18	66	145	176	69	45	3,000
19–24	72	160	177	70	40	2,900
25–50	79	174	176	70	37	2,900
51+	77	170	173	68	30	2,300
Females						
11–14	46	101	157	62	47	2,200
15–18	55	120	163	64	40	2,200
19–24	58	128	164	65	38	2,200
25–50	63	138	163	64	36	2,200
51+	65	143	160	63	30	1,900
Pregnant (2nd and 3rd trimesters)						+ 300
Lactating						+ 500

[a]Average energy allowances have been rounded.

SOURCE: *Recommended Dietary Allowances*, © 1989 by the National Academy of Sciences, National Academy Press, Washington, D.C.

Daily Values (used on food labels)

Daily Reference Values (DRV)		Reference Daily Intakes (RDI)			
Food Component	**DRV**	**Nutrient**	**Amount**	**Nutrient**	**Amount**
protein[c]	50 g	Thiamin	1.5 mg	Vitamin K	80 µg
fat	65 g[d]	Riboflavin	1.7 mg	Calcium	1,000 mg
saturated fatty acids	20 g	Niacin	20 mg	Iron	18 mg
cholesterol	300 mg[e]	Biotin	300 µg	Zinc	15 mg
total carbohydrate	300 g	Pantothenic Acid	10 mg	Iodine	150 µg
fiber	25 g			Copper	2 mg
sodium	2,400 mg	Vitamin B_6	2 mg	Chromium	120 µg
potassium	3,500 mg	Folate	400 µg	Selenium	70 µg
		Vitamin B_{12}	6 µg[f]	Molybdenum	75 µg
		Vitamin C	60 mg	Manganese	2 mg
		Vitamin A	5,000 IU[g]	Chloride	3,400 mg
		Vitamin D	400 IU[g]	Magnesium	400 mg
		Vitamin E	30 IU[g]	Phosphorus	1 g

[a]Based on 2,000 calories a day for adults and children over 4 years old.

[b]Formerly the U.S. RDA, based on National Academy of Sciences' 1968 Recommended Dietary Allowances.

[c]DRV for protein does not apply to certain populations; Reference Daily Intake (RDI) for protein has been established for these groups: children 1 to 4 years: 16 g; infants under 1 year: 14 g; pregnant women: 60 g; nursing mothers: 65 g.

[d](g) grams

[e](mg) milligrams

[f](µg) micrograms

[g]Equivalent values for the three RDI nutrients expressed as IU are: vitamin A, 875 RE; vitamin D, 6.5 µg; vitamin E, 9 mg.

C

NUTRITION
CONCEPTS AND CONTROVERSIES

Seventh Edition

Frances Sienkiewicz Sizer

Eleanor Noss Whitney

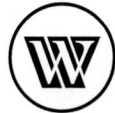

West/Wadsworth
I(T)P® An International Thomson Publishing Company

Belmont, CA • Albany, NY • Bonn • Boston • Cincinnati • Detroit • Johannesburg •
London • Los Angeles • Madrid • Melbourne • Mexico City • Minneapolis/St. Paul •
New York • Paris • San Francisco • Singapore • Tokyo • Toronto • Washington

Publisher: Peter Marshall
Development Editor: Jane Bass
Marketing Manager: Becky Tollerson
Production Editors: Christine Hurney; Lisa Gunderman
Text Designer: Janet Bollow
Copy Editor: Pat Lewis
Dummy Artist: Kristen M. Weber
Illustrators: J/B Woolsey Associates; Randy Miyake
Indexer: Pam McMurry
Cover Designer: Carol Castro
Cover Image: Paul Gauguin 1848–1903, French, *Spring of Miracles*, Hermitage Museum, St. Petersburg, Russia, © SuperStock.
Compositor: Parkwood Composition Service, Inc.

Photo credits follow the index.

Printed in Canada
 3 4 5 6 7 8 9 10

For more information, contact Wadsworth Publishing Company, 10 Davis Drive, Belmont, CA 94002, or electronically at
http://www.thomson.com/wadsworth.html

International Thomson Publishing Europe
Berkshire House 168-173
High Holborn
London, WC1V 7AA, England

Thomas Nelson Australia
102 Dodds Street
South Melbourne 3205
Victoria, Australia

Nelson Canada
1120 Birchmount Road
Scarborough, Ontario
Canada M1K 5G4

International Thomson Publishing GmbH
Königswinterer Strasse 418
53227 Bonn, Germany

International Thomson Editores
Campos Eliseos 385, Piso 7
Col. Polanco
11560 México D.F. México

International Thomson Publishing Asia
221 Henderson Road
#05-10 Henderson Building
Singapore 0315

International Thomson Publishing Japan
Hirakawacho Kyowa Building, 3F
2-2-1 Hirakawacho
Chiyoda-ku, Tokyo 102, Japan

International Thomson Publishing Southern Africa
Building 18, Constantia Park
240 Old Pretoria Road
Halfway House, 1685 South Africa

Library of Congress Cataloging-in-Publication Data
Sizer, Frances Sienkiewicz.
    Nutrition : concepts and controversies. / Frances Sienkiewicz
Sizer, Eleanor Noss Whitney. — 7th ed.
        p. cm.
    Some earlier eds. m.e. under Hamilton, Eva May Nunnalley.
    Includes index.
    ISBN 0-314-09635-3 (soft : alk. paper) (Student version)
    ISBN-0-314-20336-2 (Annotated Instructors Version)
    1. Nutrition.   2. Food.   I. Whitney, Eleanor Noss.   II. Title
OP141.S5365   1997
613.2—dc21   96-47474

To my husband, Jack Yaeger,
who never ceases to amaze me with the
depths of his goodness, with love.
Ellie

To my mother, Bernice Sienkiewicz, who heals us all;
to Harriet Harlan, for the memories we share;
to Karen Cooley and Eric Favier, mes amis;
and to wonderful Philip Webb, whom I love.
Fran

ABOUT THE AUTHORS

Eleanor Noss Whitney, Ph.D., received her B.A. in Biology from Radcliffe College in 1960 and her Ph.D. in Biology from Washington University, St. Louis, in 1970. Formerly on the faculty at the Florida State University, and a dietitian registered with the American Dietetic Association, she now devotes full time to research, writing, and consulting in nutrition, health, and environmental issues. Her earlier publications include articles in *Science, Genetics,* and other journals. Her textbooks include *Understanding Nutrition, Understanding Normal and Clinical Nutrition, Nutrition and Diet Therapy,* and *Essential Life Choices* for college students and *Making Life Choices* for high-school students. Her most intense interests presently include energy conservation, solar energy uses, alternatively fueled vehicles, and ecosystem restoration.

Frances Sienkiewicz Sizer, M.S., R.D., F.A.D.A., attended Florida State University where, in 1980, she received her B.S., and in 1982, her M.S. in nutrition. She is certified as a charter Fellow of the American Dietetic Association. She is a founding member and vice president of Nutrition and Health Associates, an information and resource center in Tallahassee, Florida, that maintains an ongoing bibliographic database that tracks research in more than 1,000 topic areas of nutrition. Her textbooks include *Life Choices: Health Concepts and Strategies; Making Life Choices; The Fitness Triad: Motivation, Training, and Nutrition;* and others. She has recently completed *Nutrition Interactive,* an instructional college-level nutrition CD-ROM. In addition to writing, she lectures at universities and at national and regional conferences.

CONTENTS IN BRIEF

CONTENTS

CHAPTER 14

CHAPTER 15

APPENDIX A

APPENDIX B

APPENDIX C

APPENDIX D

APPENDIX E

APPENDIX F

APPENDIX G

GLOSSARY GL-1

INDEX I-1

PREFACE

Six editions of *Nutrition: Concepts and Controversies* have been tested by students and professors in classrooms across the nation. In each edition, we apply what we have learned from past readers, changing the book to meet changing times. Now, as we look ahead toward a new millennium, we face an even more rapidly changing future. In this edition, we have expanded our balanced portrayal of nutrition's new frontiers, retained our accurate presentation of established nutrition knowledge, and heightened our sense of personal connection with instructors and learners alike. We still write in the informal, clear style for which we have received plaudits. For both verbal and visual learners, our style and our clear, colorful figures keep interest high and understanding at a peak. New photos and abundant figures adorn many of the pages, adding pleasure and clarity to the reading.

In the seventh edition, you will find some new practical features to connect science concepts with food choices. Sections called *Do It* invite students to apply chapter concepts to everyday encounters with nutrition. The Do Its of Chapters 1 and 10 offer ways to judge nutrition information from the media and from makers of supplements for athletes. Those of Chapters 2 through 9 guide students along approaches taken by menu planners. In one approach, demonstrated in the Do It sections of Chapters 4 through 8, the planner answers the question of how many grams, milligrams, and micrograms of nutrients a meal provides and compares the totals to a standard such as the RDA. An alternative food-based approach to menu planning, demonstrated in Chapters 2 and 9, is the food group approach. The student is asked to assess the adequacy of meals by comparing them with the Food Guide Pyramid recommendations. The final Do It of Chapter 11 ties together the previous exercises and allows students to stretch their skills by identifying meals that best meet the goals of the *Dietary Guidelines for Americans* and other recommendations.

Another powerful new feature in this edition is the *Self-Check*, a series of review questions at the end of each chapter. These sections allow students to quickly review each chapter's content, and the answers in Appendix G provide immediate feedback. These Self-Check questions were provided by Judy Kaufman who has used our text with her students at Monroe Community College for many years.

By popular demand, we have retained our *Snapshots* of vitamins and minerals, capsules of information that depict food sources and teach some salient facts about each nutrient. We have added a Snapshot to Chapter 11, emphasizing foods rich in phytochemicals, nonnutrient substances that hold promise for preventing diseases. Food sources of the energy-yielding nutrients are depicted more vividly than ever before by way of new graphics and photographs.

We hope that you will enjoy the seventh edition of our text. Chapter 1 begins with a personal challenge to nutrition students. It asks the question so many people ask of nutrition scientists: "What can I believe, when scientists keep changing their minds?" We answer with a lesson in sound scientific thinking and the context in which study results may be rightly viewed. We then introduce the nutrients and explore the concept of nutrient density. Finally, a discussion of the important role of cuisine in a person's heritage focuses on and honors this country's multicultural nature. Chapter 2 brings together the concepts of diet planning through food grouping systems and features the Daily Food Guide with its pyramid of food choices. Chapter 3 presents a thorough, but brief, introduction to the workings of the human body with major emphasis on the digestive system. Chapters 4 through 6 are devoted to the energy-yielding nutrients—carbohydrates, lipids, and proteins. Chapters 7 and 8 present the vitamins, minerals, and water, with special emphasis on the emerging importance of the antioxidant nutrients. Chapter 9 relates energy balance to body composition, obesity, and underweight and presents weight maintenance as a lifelong effort. Chapter 10 presents the relationships between fitness, physical activity, and nutrition—relationships that are of interest to the casual exerciser and athlete alike. Chapter 11 applies the essence of the first ten chapters to two broad and rapidly changing areas within nutrition: immunity and disease prevention. It also discusses the emerging importance of phytochemicals in relation to disease prevention. Chapters 12 and 13 point out the importance of nutrition throughout the life span, from gestation through old age. Chapter 14 considers the problems and advantages of food technology, with emphasis on food safety. Chapter 15 touches on the vast problems of the global food supply—world hunger, pollution, overpopulation—and shows how everyday food choices link each person with the meaningful whole.

The *Controversies* of this book's title invite you to explore beyond the safe boundaries of established nutrition knowledge. These optional readings which appear at the ends of each chapter and are printed with colored borders, delve into current scientific topics and emerging controversies. Some are new to this edition and the others have been updated. Of special current interest is Controversy 2, which compares Mediterranean foodways with those of the United States and Canada. By examining the advantages and drawbacks of each eating plan, the Controversy provides clues to which plan might hold the secret to a healthy heart. Controversy 7 sets up a lively competition between food and supplements as vitamin sources, exploring the research to date on the antioxidant vitamins. Controversy 9 tackles some pressing questions surrounding the safety and effectiveness of weight-loss diets, diet profiteers, and attitudes toward overweight people in this country. Controversy 10 presents current thinking about eating disorders. Controversy 14 evaluates new food technologies and invites the reader to look forward to and evaluate future innovations. Controversy 15 explores ways in which agriculture can ensure a high-quality food supply into the next century.

The *Food Feature* sections that appear in most chapters act as bridges between theory and practice; they are practical applications of the chapter concepts that help readers to choose foods according to nutrition principles. *Consumer Corners* present information on amino acid supplements, vitamin C and the common cold, bottled water, marketing of infant formula, and other nutrition-related marketplace issues to empower students to make informed decisions.

New or major terms in chapters are defined in the margins of the pages where they are introduced and also in the Glossary at the end of the book.

Terms in Controversy sections are grouped together and defined in tables within the sections and in the Glossary. The reader who wishes to locate any term can do so by consulting the index, which lists the page numbers of definitions in boldface type.

The appendixes have been updated. Appendix A which now presents the most complete and accurate listings ever of the nutrient contents of more than 2,200 foods. Appendix B, *Canadiana*, supplies the RNI, the Guidelines, the Food Guide, Food Labels, and the Exchange System for our Canadian readers. Appendix C demonstrates nutrition calculations, with special emphasis on finding percentage of calories from fat in a diet and percentages of the Daily Values. Appendix D provides full coverage with applications of the U.S. Exchange System. Appendix E offers an invaluable list of current addresses, telephone numbers, and Internet web sites for those interested in additional information. We have collected all chapter and controversy references in Appendix F. Older source notes have been removed but are easily available by consulting older editions of this book or by contacting the publisher.

This seventh edition has been an exciting challenge to prepare. As always, our purpose in writing it is to enhance our readers' understanding of nutrition science and motivation to apply it. We hope the information on this book's pages will reach beyond the classroom into our readers' lives. Take the information you find inside this book home with you. Use it in your life: nourish yourself, educate your loved ones, and nurture others. Stay up with the news, too. For despite all the conflicting messages, inflated claims, and even quackery that abound in news reports, true nutrition knowledge progresses with a genuine scientific spirit, and important new truths are constantly unfolding.

Acknowledgments

Our thanks to Linda Kelly DeBruyne for Chapter 10 and Controversy 10 of this edition. Thank you, Sharon Rady Rolfes for helping to perfect our table of food composition. Thanks, too, to Jan Merrit for her support of *Nutrition Interactive*, the CD-ROM that augments this text. Thanks also to Melaney Mole Jones for her upbeat energy and tireless assistance at each stage of this writing. We thank Diane Dziaken, Judy Kaufman, and Jana Kicklighter for their assistance in testing the Do It sections. Thanks to Sabrina McGriff for her help in bookkeeping and for answering the phone; thanks also to Sally Lorch for office tasks and for extra help when time ran short. Thanks, too, to our associate Lori Turner for much of the *Instructor's Manual;* thanks to Margaret Hedley, University of Guelph, who prepared the Canadian material for the manual. For the special Instructor's Edition of the text, we thank Lori Turner (lecture outlines); Judy Kaufman, Monroe Community College (margin references to overheads, videos, and videodisc); and Millicent Owens, College of the Sequoias (margin references to *Nutrition Interactive* CD-ROM). Thank you, John Woolsey and associates for bringing our figures to their full potential. To Lesly White and her associates at Photo Edit, thank you for creating the inviting photographs of food throughout the book.

Special thanks to our publisher, Peter Marshall, and to our editors Becky Tollerson, Chris Hurney, and Lisa Gunderman and to their staff, for their unflagging efforts to ensure the highest quality of all facets of this book. We appreciate the creativity and marketing expertise of Erin Ryan Titcomb and Ann Hillstrom. Thanks also to Jana Kicklighter of Georgia State University for preparing the *Student Study Guide* and the *Test Bank*. As always, we are grateful to Bob Geltz and Betty Hands and their staff at ESHA research for Appendix A and for the computerized diet analysis program that accompanies this book. Thanks, too, to Janet Ballow for our fresh new look and appealing design. To our reviewers, many heartfelt thanks for your many thoughtful ideas and suggestions:

Judy Alexander
Moorpark Community College

Sue Balinsky
College of Charleston

Ethan Bergman
Central Washington University

Mallory Boylan
Texas Tech University

Andy Bryant
Brookdale Community College

Marian Campbell
University of Manitoba

Barbara Cerio
Rochester Institute of Technology

Nancy Connor
American University

Josee Forel
University of Nebraska at Kearney

Rachel Fournet
University of Southwestern Louisiana

Joyce Gilbert
Sante Fe Community College

Linda Hahn
California State University—Los Angeles

Deloy Hendricks
Utah State University

Ann Hertzler
Virginia Polytechnic Institute and State University

Judy Kaufman
Monroe Community College

Jana Kicklighter
Georgia State University

Barbara Kilborn
Sierra Community College

Elena Kissick
California State University—Fresno

Donna Koehler
University of North Carolina—Greensboro

Billie Lane
Chattanooga State Technical Community College

Bernard Marcus
Genesee Community College

Sally McGill
Cañada College—Redwood City

Christine Medlin
Tidewater Community College

Susan Munroe
University of Tennessee—Knoxville

Amy Nickerson
St. Michael's College

Carmen Nochera
Grandvalley State University

Millicent Owens
College of the Sequoias

Jim Painter
University of Illinois

Stanley Segall
Drexel University

Anne Smith
Ohio State University

Sam Smith
University of New Hampshire

Kaye Stanek
University of Nebraska

Sara Sutton
Eastern Kentucky University

Elise West
Cornell University

Robert Wildman
University of Delaware

Joe Williford
Bowling Green State University

Fred Wolff
University of Arizona

Lisa Young
New York University

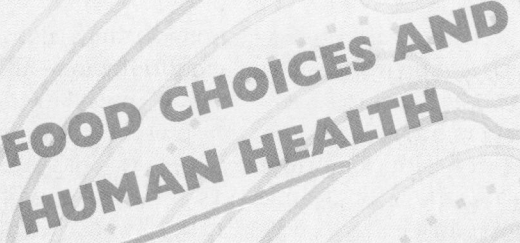

FOOD CHOICES AND HUMAN HEALTH

1

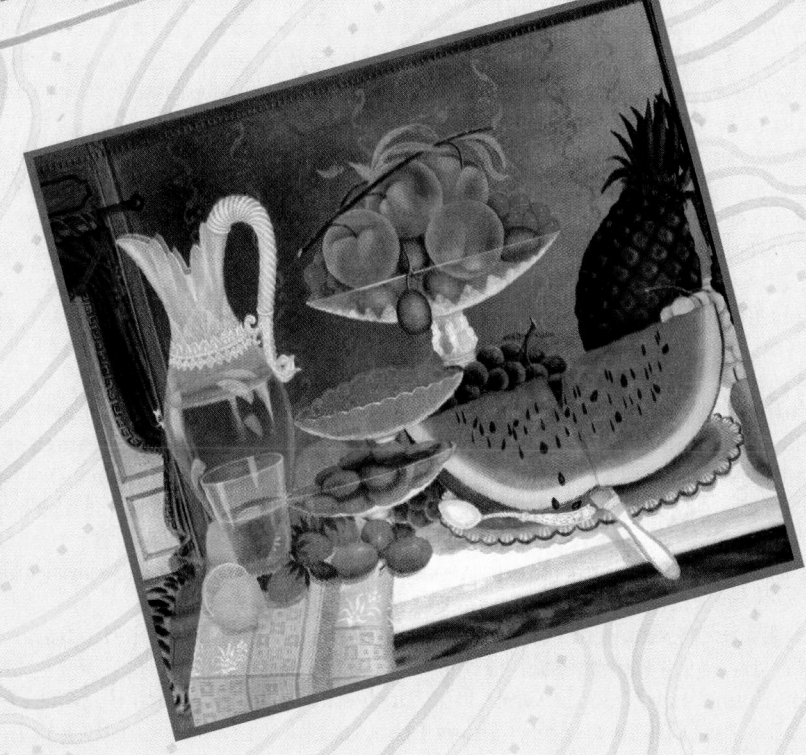

CONTENTS

Henry Church, *Still Life*, The Collection of Frances O. Stem Babinsky.

food medically, any substance that the body can take in and assimilate that will enable it to stay alive and to grow; the carrier of nourishment; socially, a more limited number of such substances defined as acceptable by each culture.

nutrition the study of the nutrients in foods and in the body; sometimes also the study of human behaviors related to food.

diet the foods (including beverages) a person usually eats and drinks.

1   If you care about your body, and if you have strong feelings about **food,** then you have much to gain from learning about **nutrition**—the study of how food nourishes the body. Nutrition is a fascinating, much talked-about subject. Each day, newspapers, radio, and television present stories of new findings on nutrition and heart health or nutrition and cancer avoidance. Daily, magazine advertisements and television commercials bombard us with multicolored pictures of tempting foods—pizza, burgers, cakes, sweet drinks, alcoholic beverages, and many more. Several times a day, you get hungry and turn from your other activities to eat a meal. And if you are like most people, you wonder, "Is this food good for me?" or you berate yourself, "I probably shouldn't be eating this."

Everyone wants to know how food affects health—naturally, because we love food and we care about our health. The study of nutrition can benefit both your physical and your mental health. When you learn which foods serve you best, you can work out ways of choosing foods, planning meals, and designing your **diet** wisely. This benefits your physical health. In addition, food facts can dispel food fears. Knowing the facts can relieve you of feeling guilty or worried that you aren't eating well. Thus, you can enhance both your diet and your enjoyment of eating, and these benefit your emotional health.

Nutrition is a science—a field of knowledge composed of organized facts. Unlike some other areas of science, such as astronomy and physics, nutrition is a relatively young science. Most nutrition research has been conducted within the past century, that is, since 1900. The first vitamin was identified in 1897, and the first protein structure was not fully described until 1945. Much remains to be learned about the effects of foods and nutrients on the body. Because nutrition science is an active, changing, growing body of knowledge, reports of scientific findings often seem to contradict one another, and those findings may be subject to several interpretations that conflict among themselves.

For this reason, people who don't understand how science operates may despair as they try to decipher current reports to learn what is really going on. They may even become distrustful: "Even the scientists themselves don't know what is true; how am I supposed to know?" Yet, other than the theories just now being investigated, many facts in nutrition are known with great certainty—enough to fill this book and many more. And where there are conflicts and contradictions, researchers are energetically attempting to resolve them. To help consumers make correct judgments regarding their food choices and diets, the first section of this chapter discusses why apparent contradictions sometimes arise in nutrition science.

This book devotes many chapters to the science of nutrition. This chapter provides a starting point by offering answers to the following questions:

1. What does food do for the body and its owner?
2. What sorts of foods should people eat today to best support their health?

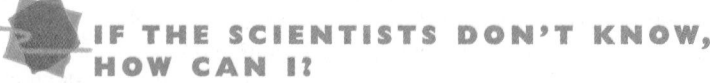

IF THE SCIENTISTS DON'T KNOW, HOW CAN I?

Everyone stampedes for oat bran, red wine, or fish oil based on today's news that these products are good for health. Then tomorrow's news reports, "it isn't true after all," and everyone drops oat bran, red wine, and fish oil and takes up the next craze. Meanwhile, they complain in frustration, "Those scientists don't know anything."

In truth, though, it is a scientist's business not to know. Scientists obtain facts by systematically asking questions—that's their job. Then they conduct experiments designed to test for various possible answers (see Figure 1-1 and Table 1-1 on the next page). When they have ruled out some possibilities and found evidence for others, they submit their findings, not to the news media, but to boards of reviewers composed of other scientists who will try to pick the findings apart. If the reviewers consider the conclusions to be well supported by the evidence, they endorse the work for publication, not in the news media, but in scientific journals where still other scientists can read it.

Once a new finding is published, it is still only preliminary. One experiment does not "prove" or "disprove" anything. The next step is for other scientists to attempt to duplicate and support the work of the first researchers or to challenge the finding by designing experiments to refute it.

Scientific journals are described in Controversy 1.

Only when a finding has stood up to rigorous, repeated testing in several kinds of experiments performed by several different researchers is it finally considered confirmed. Even then, strictly speaking, no such thing as a *fact* exists in science. Science consists of *hypotheses* that can always be challenged and revised. Some, though, like the hypothesis that the earth revolves about the sun, are so well supported by so many observations and experimental findings that they are generally accepted as facts. What we "know" in nutrition is confirmed in the same way: it results from years of replicating study findings.

The news media are hungry for new findings, though, and reporters often latch onto ideas from the scientific labs before they have been fully tested.[1] Or the reporter may misunderstand complex scientific principles, especially if the reporter lacks a strong understanding of science.[2] To tell the truth, sometimes scientists get excited about their findings, too, and leak them to the press before they have been through a rigorous review by the scientists' peers. As a result, the public often is exposed to late-breaking news stories from scientific laboratories before the findings are fully confirmed. Then, when the hypothesis being tested fails to hold up to a later challenge, consumers feel betrayed by what is simply the normal course of science at work.

It follows that if you act on science news that is hot off the press, you do so at your own risk. Applying a new nutrition finding is not like buying a new appliance: there is no warranty; it is not backed by consumer testing; and it is not a crime for the finding to be invalidated.

It also follows that people who take action based on single studies are almost always acting impulsively, not scientifically. The real scientists are trend watchers. They evaluate the methods used in each study, assess each study in light of all the evidence gleaned from other studies, and, little by little, modify their picture of what is true. As evidence accumulates, they become more and more confident about being able to make recommendations that apply to people's health and lives. Single studies are interesting, perhaps even exciting, but experienced observers learn to withhold judgment about the application of a study's findings until they have been repeated and confirmed.

Media sensationalism may even overrate the importance of true, replicated findings. This happens sometimes when a new report shows (as old reports have shown) that oat bran lowers blood cholesterol, a lipid indicative of heart disease risk. Bran is only one of several hundred factors that affect blood

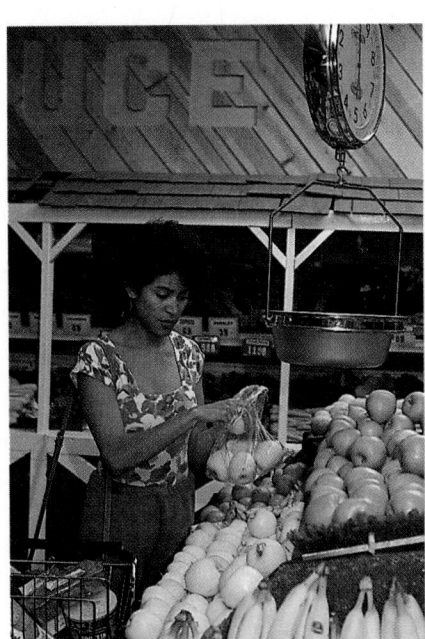

When you choose foods wisely, you can enhance your well-being.

FIGURE I-I

RESEARCH DESIGN

The source of valid nutrition information is scientific research. Nutrition is a science, an organized body of knowledge composed of facts that we believe to be true because they have been supported, time and again, in experiments designed to rule out all other possibilities. Each fact has been established by many different kinds of experiments. For example, we know that eyesight depends partly on vitamin A because animals deprived of that vitamin and only that vitamin begin to go blind; when it is restored soon enough to their diet, they regain their sight. The same fact holds true in observations of human beings.

The type of study chosen for research depends upon what sort of information the researchers require. Studies of individuals (**case studies**) yield observations that may lead to possible avenues of research. A study of a man who ate gumdrops and became a famous dancer might suggest that an experiment to be done to see if gumdrops contain dance-enhancing power.

Studies of whole populations in different areas of the world (**epidemiological studies**) provide another sort of information. Such a study can reveal a **correlation.** For example, an epidemiological study might find no worldwide correlation of gumdrop-eating with fancy footwork but, unexpectedly, might reveal a correlation with tooth decay.

Studies in which researchers actively intervene to alter people's eating habits (**intervention studies**) go a step further. In such a study, one set of subjects (the **experimental group**) receive a treatment, and another set (the **control group**) go untreated or receive a **placebo** or sham treatment. If the two groups experience different effects, then

Case Study

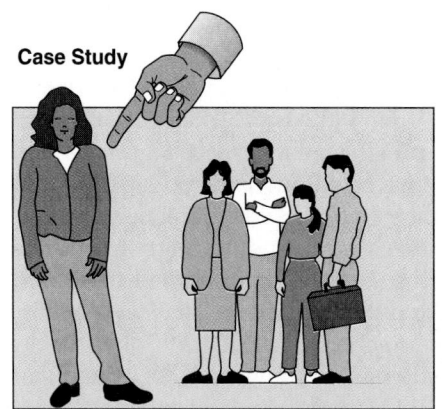

"This person eats too little of nutrient X and has illness Y."

Epidemiological Study

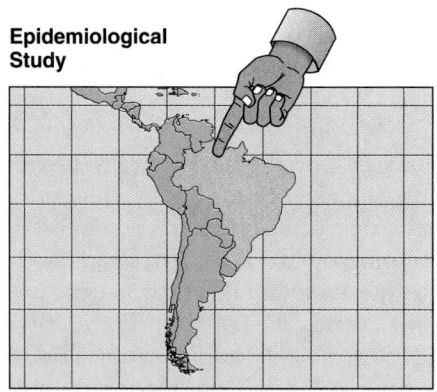

"This country's food supply contains more nutrient X and these people suffer less illness Y."

Intervention Study

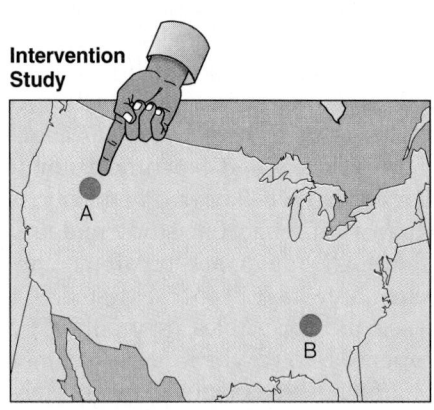

"Let's add foods containing nutrient X to city A's food supply and compare illness Y rates of city A with those of city B."

Laboratory Study

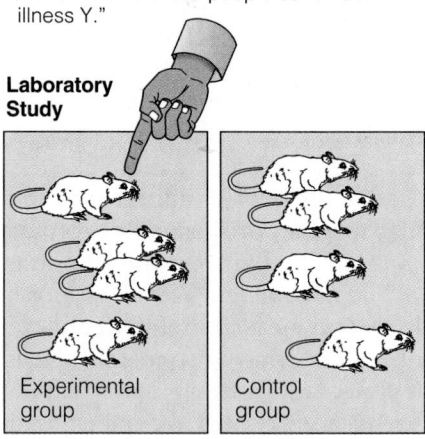

Experimental group

Control group

"Now let's prove that a nutrient X deficiency causes illness Y by inducing a deficiency in these rats."

the treatment's effect can be pinpointed. For example, an intervention study might show that withholding gumdrops, together with other candies and confections, reduced the incidence of tooth decay in an experimental population compared to that in a control population.

Finally, **laboratory studies** can pinpoint the mechanisms by which nutrition acts. What is it about gumdrops that contributes to tooth decay: their size, shape, temperature, color, ingredients? Feeding various

forms of gumdrops to rats might yield the information that sugar, in a gummy carrier, promotes tooth decay. In the laboratory, using animals or plants or cells, scientists can inoculate with diseases, induce deficiencies, and experiment with variations on treatments to obtain in-depth knowledge of the process under study. Intervention studies and laboratory experiments are among the most powerful tools in nutrition research because they show the effects of treatments.

TABLE 1-1
Research Design Terms

- **case studies** studies of individuals, usually in clinical settings where researchers can observe treatments and their apparent effects. To prove that a treatment has produced an effect requires simultaneous observation of an untreated similar subject (a *case control*).
- **control group** a group of individuals who are similar in all possible respects to the group being treated in an experiment but who receive a sham treatment instead of the real one. Also called *control subjects*. See also *experimental group* and *intervention studies*.
- **correlation** the simultaneous change of two factors, such as the increase of weight with increasing height (a *direct* or *positive* correlation) or the decrease of cancer incidence with increasing fiber intake (an *inverse* or *negative* correlation). A correlation between two factors suggests that one may cause the other, but does not rule out the possibility that both may be caused by a third factor. If the latter case turns out to be true, then the correlation is coincidental.
- **epidemiological studies** studies of populations; often used in nutrition to search for correlations between dietary habits and disease incidence; a first step in seeking nutrition-related causes of diseases.
- **experimental group** the people or animals participating in an experiment who receive the treatment under investigation. Also called *experimental subjects*. See also *control group* and *intervention studies*.
- **intervention studies** studies of populations in which observation is accompanied by experimental manipulation of some population members—for example, a study in which half of the subjects (the *experimental subjects*) follow diet advice to reduce fat intakes while the other half (the *control subjects*) do not, and both groups' heart health is monitored.
- **laboratory studies** studies that are performed under tightly controlled conditions and are designed to pinpoint causes and effects. Such studies often use animals as subjects.
- **placebo** a sham treatment often used in scientific studies; an inert harmless medication. The *placebo effect* is the healing effect that the act of treatment, rather than the treatment itself, often has.

cholesterol. A news report on oat bran may fail to mention that cutting fat intake is still the major blood cholesterol-lowering step to take. Science is constantly building on an already existing foundation of knowledge, but journalists and television reporters who do not understand science may pick isolated news items and blow them up out of proportion to the whole.

Also, new findings need definition. Oat bran is truly a cholesterol reducer; but how much bran does it take to produce the desired effects? Do little oat bran pills or powders meet the need? Do oat bran cookies? How many? Does everyone respond the same way to them? How much of a dietary indiscretion can a person commit and still rectify it with oat bran cookies? One reviewer dealing with a report on this very topic observed, "To get the equivalent of the oat fiber in one bowl of oatmeal, it would [be] necessary to eat 90 cookies."[3] An oat bran muffin eaten after a high-fat, fast-food lunch cannot undo all the damage that the meal did.

Today, oat bran's cholesterol-lowering effect is considered to be established.[4] The whole process of discovery, challenge, and vindication took almost ten years of research; some take many years longer. In science, a single finding almost never makes a crucial difference to our knowledge as a whole, but like each individual frame in a movie, it contributes a little to the big picture. It takes many such frames to tell the whole story.

✓ **KEY POINT**   **Scientists uncover nutrition facts by experimenting. Single studies must be replicated before their findings can be considered valid. New nutrition news is not always to be believed; old news has stood up to the test of time.**

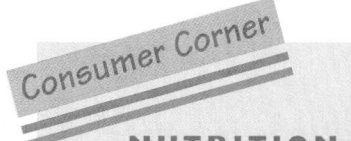

NUTRITION IN THE NEWS

A news reader, who had sworn off butter years ago for his heart's sake, bemoaned this headline: *Margarine Fat as Bad as Butter for Heart Health.* "Do you mean to say that I could have been eating butter all these years? That's it. I quit. No more diet changes for me." His response is understandable—diet changes, after all, take effort to make and commitment to sustain. Those who do make changes may feel betrayed when, years later, science appears to have turned its advice upside down. This reader might have avoided information burnout had he known some facts about the way science is reported in the news. He isn't alone in lacking knowledge. Most people are confused and frustrated by today's news.

It bears repeating that the findings of a single study never prove or disprove anything. Study results may constitute strong supporting evidence for one view or another, but they rarely merit the sort of finality implied by journalistic phrases such as "Now we know . . ." or "The answer has been found." Misinformed readers who look for simple answers to complex nutrition problems often take such phrases literally.

To read headline stories with an educated eye, keep these points in mind:

■ Valid reports also describe previous research. Some reporters regularly follow developments in a research area and thus acquire the background knowledge they need to report meaningfully in that area; others simply "drop in" for a story.

■ The report should describe the research methods used to obtain the data. For example, it matters whether the study participants numbered eight or eight thousand, or whether the researchers personally observed participants' behaviors or relied on self-reports collected over the telephone.

■ The subjects of the study may have been single cells, animals, or human beings, and the report should clearly make this distinction. If the study subjects were human beings, the more you have in common with them (age and gender, for example), the more applicable the findings may be for you.

Finally, ask yourself if the study makes common sense. Even if it turns out that the fat of margarine is damaging to the heart, do you eat enough margarine to worry about its effects? Before making a decision, learn more about the effects of fats on the arteries in Chapters 5 and 11. Then weigh new evidence against what you already know about fat and about yourself.

When a headline touts a shocking new "answer" to a nutrition question, read the story with a critical eye. It may indeed be a carefully researched report, but often it is a sensational story intended to catch the attention of newspaper and magazine buyers, not to offer useful nutrition information.

energy the capacity to do work. The energy in food is chemical energy; it can be converted to mechanical, electrical, heat, or other forms of energy in the body. Food energy is measured in calories, defined on page 8.

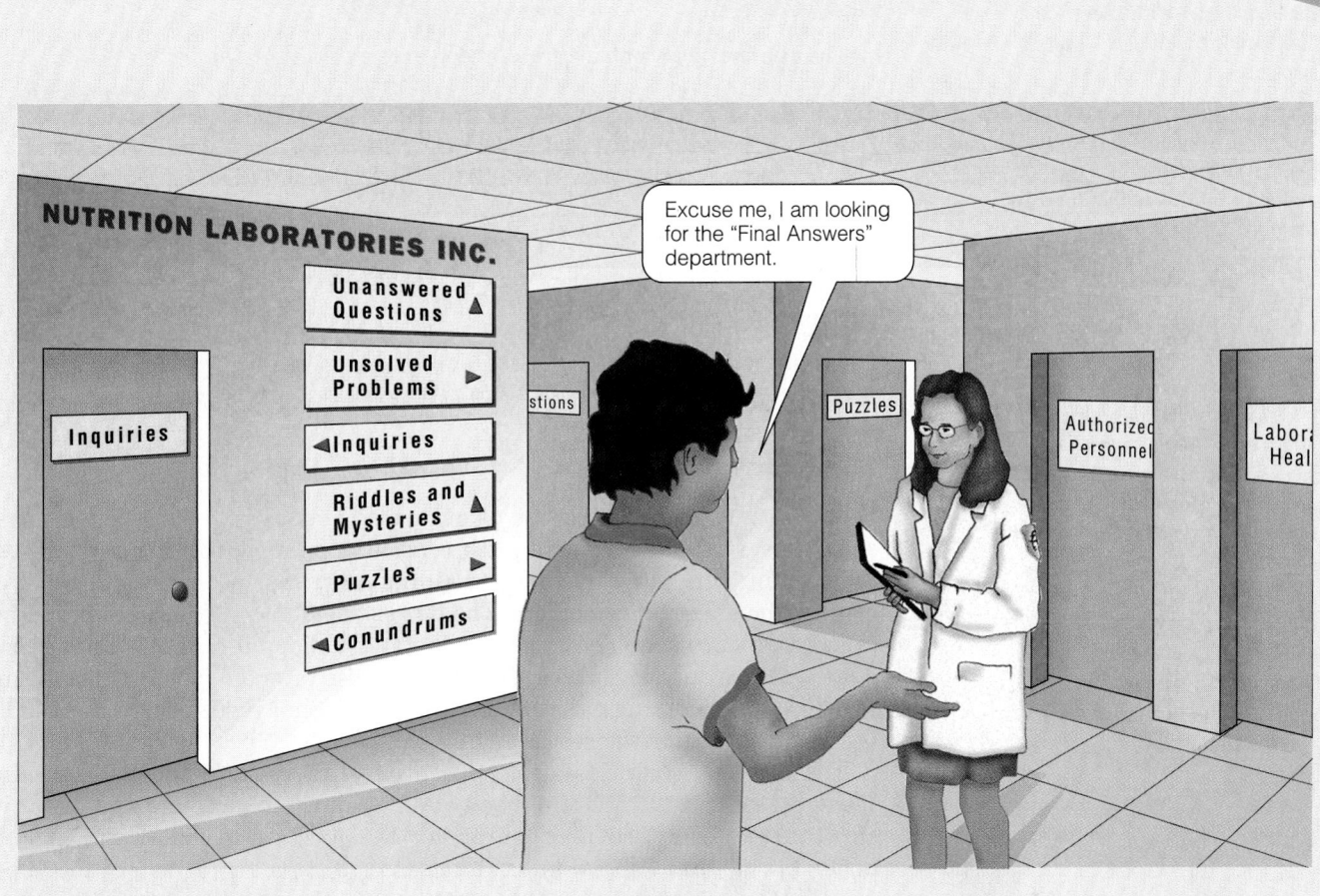

People looking for simple answers in nutrition science are often disappointed.

THE HUMAN BODY AND ITS FOOD

As your body lives each day, it moves and works, and to move or work, it must use **energy.** The energy that fuels the body's work comes indirectly from the sun by way of plants. Plants capture and store the sun's energy in their tissues as they grow. When you eat plant-derived foods such as fruits, grains, or vegetables, you obtain and use the solar energy they have stored. Plant-eating animals obtain their energy in the same way, so when you eat animal tissues, you are eating compounds containing energy that came originally from the sun.

The body also requires six kinds of **nutrients**—families of molecules indispensable to its functioning—and foods deliver these. Table 1-2 (on the next page) lists the six classes of nutrients. Four of these six are **organic;** that is, the nutrients are derived from living things that have captured solar energy, either directly or indirectly, and converted the energy into compounds containing the element carbon. The human body and foods are made of the same materials, arranged in different ways (Figure 1-2 on the next page).

nutrients components of food that are indispensable to the body's functioning. They provide energy, serve as building material, help maintain or repair body parts, and support growth. The nutrients include water, carbohydrate, fat, protein, vitamins, and minerals.

organic carbon containing. Four of the six classes of nutrients are organic: carbohydrate, fat, protein, and vitamins. Strictly speaking, organic compounds include only those made by living things and do not include carbon dioxide and a few carbon salts.

energy-yielding nutrients the nutrients the body can use for energy. They may also supply building blocks for body structures.

essential nutrients the nutrients the body cannot make for itself (or cannot make fast enough) from other raw materials; nutrients that must be obtained from food to prevent deficiencies.

calories units of energy. Strictly speaking, the unit used to measure the energy in food is a kilocalorie (*kcalorie*, or *Calorie*): it is the amount of heat energy necessary to raise the temperature of a kilogram (a liter) of water 1 degree Celsius. This book follows the common practice of using the lowercase term *calorie* (abbreviated *cal*) to mean the same thing.

FIGURE I-2

MATERIALS OF FOOD AND THE HUMAN BODY

Foods and the human body are made of the same materials.

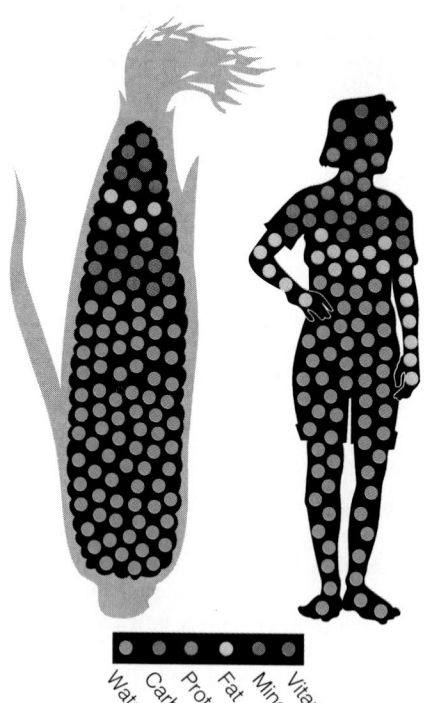

Water Carbohydrate Protein Fat Minerals Vitamins

TABLE I-2

Elements in the Six Classes of Nutrients

The nutrients that contain carbon are organic.

	Carbon	Oxygen	Hydrogen	Nitrogen	Minerals
Water		X	X		
Carbohydrate	X	X	X		
Fat	X	X	X		
Protein	X	X	X	X	b
Vitamins	X	X	X	Xa	b
Minerals					X

[a]All of the B vitamins contain nitrogen; *amine* means nitrogen.
[b]Protein and some vitamins contain the mineral sulfur; vitamin B_{12} contains the mineral cobalt.

The Nutrients in Foods

Foremost among the six classes of nutrients in foods is *water,* which is constantly lost from the body and must constantly be replaced. Among the four organic nutrients, three are **energy-yielding nutrients,** meaning that the body can use the energy they contain. The *carbohydrates* and *fats* (fats are properly called *lipids*) are especially important energy-yielding nutrients. As for *protein,* it does double duty: it can yield energy, but it also provides materials that form structures and working parts of body tissues. Alcohol yields energy, too, but it is a toxin, not a nutrient; see Table 1-3 note.

The fifth and sixth classes of nutrients are the *vitamins* and the *minerals.* These provide no energy to the body. A few minerals serve as parts of body structures (calcium and phosphorus, for example, are major constituents of bone), but all vitamins and minerals act as regulators. As regulators, the vitamins and minerals assist in all body processes: digesting food; moving muscles; disposing of wastes; growing new tissues; healing wounds; obtaining energy from carbohydrate, fat, and protein; and every other process necessary to maintain life. Later, a chapter is devoted to each of these six classes of nutrients in the order just named, except water, which is treated with the minerals.

When you eat food, then, you are not just engaging in a pleasurable activity; you are providing your body with energy and nutrients. Furthermore, some of the nutrients are **essential nutrients,** meaning that if you do not receive them from food, you will develop deficiencies; the body cannot make these nutrients for itself. Essential nutrients are found in all six classes of nutrients. Water is essential; so is a form of carbohydrate; so are some lipids, some parts of protein, all of the vitamins, and the minerals important in human nutrition, too.

To support understanding of many of the discussions that follow, two definitions and a set of numbers are needed. Food scientists measure food energy in **calories,** units of heat. Food quantities are measured in **grams,** units of weight. The most energy-rich of the nutrients is fat, which contains 9 calories in one gram. Carbohydrate and protein each contain only 4 calories in a gram (see Table 1-3).

Scientists have worked out ways to measure the energy and nutrient contents of foods. They have also calculated the amounts of energy and nutrients various types of people need—people of both sexes, of different ages, and of different walks of life. Thus, after studying human nutrient requirements (the subject of Chapter 2 of this book), you can state with some accuracy just what your own body needs—this much water, that much carbohydrate and fat, so much protein, and so forth. Might it be possible, then, to simply take pills or **supplements** in place of food? No, because, as it turns out, food offers more than just the six basic nutrients.

✔ KEY POINT   **Food supplies energy and nutrients. The most vital nutrient is water. The energy-yielding nutrients are carbohydrates, fats (lipids), and protein. The helper nutrients are vitamins and minerals. Food energy is measured in calories; food quantity is measured in grams.**

Food: More Than Just Nutrients

Nutrition science has achieved the ability to state what nutrients human beings need to *survive*—at least for a time. Scientists are becoming skilled at making **elemental diets**—diets that have a precise chemical composition and are life-saving for people in the hospital who cannot eat ordinary food. These formulas, administered to severely ill people for days and weeks at a time, support not only continued life but also recovery from nutrient deficiencies and infections and the healing of wounds.

These diets are not sufficient to enable people to thrive, however. Elemental diet formulas support life but not optimal growth and health; and they often lead to medical complications. Although these problems are rare and can be detected and corrected, they show that the composition of these diets is not yet perfect for all people in all settings.[5] Furthermore, such formula products are not needed by healthy people who eat a regular diet, even though many advertisers would have us believe that we need to buy them and drink them to ensure dietary adequacy.

Even if a person's basic nutrient needs are perfectly understood and met, concoctions of nutrients still lack something that foods provide. The story of a girl who could not eat illustrates this point. She had a severe intestinal disorder: her digestive tract was almost completely nonfunctional, so she had to be fed nutrient mixtures through a vein. Deficiencies developed and were recognized and remedied, but still something was missing—she wanted to eat food. Her health-care providers therefore occasionally allowed her to eat whatever she wanted, even though everything she ate had to be collected into a bag through an opening in her abdominal wall after only a few minutes in her intestine. Clearly, real food did something important for her emotional health:

> Her psychological outlook was completely changed. She was happy. The tastes, sounds, sights, and smells of the food gave her great gratification. But, most especially, it was interesting to note that the condition of her skin and hair improved, and the pink on her cheeks and the look of 'wellness' returned.

Whether this effect of real food was physical or psychological remains unknown. According to the physician caring for the girl, "It was just something . . . we were not able to give through a needle." This physician has abundant knowledge and years of experience and is not likely to ascribe mysterious powers to food without justification.

grams units of weight. A gram (g) is the weight of a cubic centimeter (cc) or milliliter (ml) of water under defined conditions of temperature and pressure. About 28 grams equal an ounce.

supplements pills, liquids, or powders that contain purified nutrients.

elemental diets diets composed of purified ingredients of known chemical composition; intended to supply all essential nutrients to people who cannot eat foods.

TABLE 1-3

Calorie Values of Energy Nutrients

Energy Nutrient	Energy
Carbohydrates	4 cal/g
Fat (lipid)	9 cal/g
Protein	4 cal/g

NOTE: Alcohol contributes 7 cal/g that the human body can use for energy. Alcohol is not classed as a nutrient, however, because it cannot be used to promote growth, maintenance, or repair. It is a toxin. When alcohol contributes a substantial portion of the energy in a person's diet, it damages body organs.

When you eat foods, you are receiving more than just nutrients.

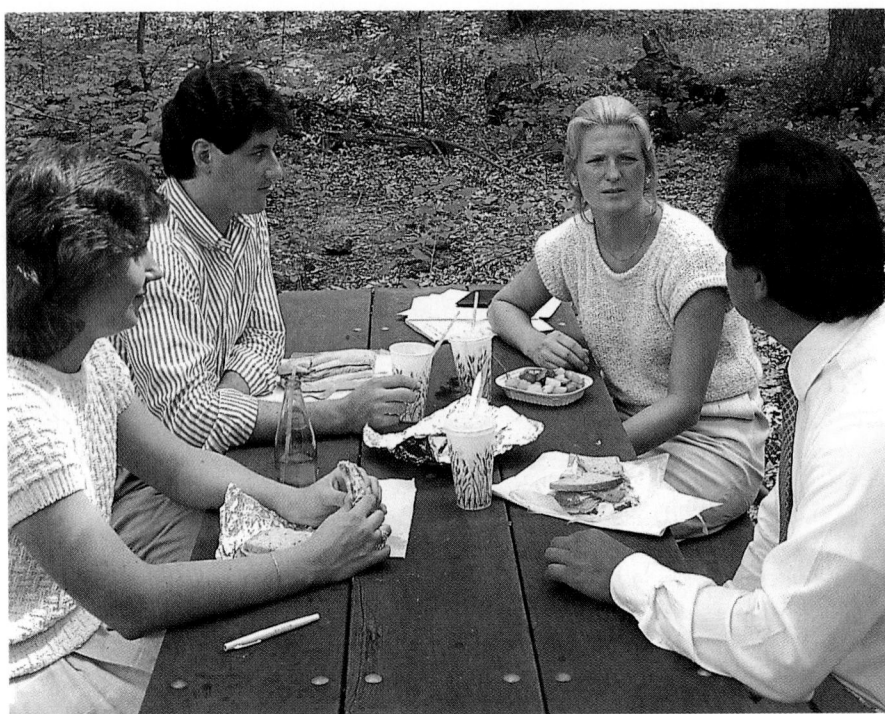

satiety (sat-EYE-uh-tee) the feeling of fullness or satisfaction that food conveys.

Science demands explanations, though: what is this mysterious "something" food offers that cannot be provided through a needle? Part of the answer may lie in the reaction of the digestive tract to food. The stomach and intestine are dynamic living organs, and they change constantly in reaction to the foods they receive. When a person is fed through a vein, the digestive organs, like unused muscles, weaken and grow smaller. Experiments have shown that when the intestine receives food, it releases hormones, chemical messengers that regulate the body's maintenance; when not fed, it fails to receive stimulation and so deteriorates. In light of this knowledge, medical wisdom now dictates that when a hospital client has to be fed through a vein, the duration should be as short as possible, and real food, taken into the intestine, should be reintroduced as early as possible.[6]

The hormones that the intestine releases in response to food also affect the brain. The messages they deliver seem to have something to do with **satiety**—the sense of satisfaction that makes a person feel, "There, that was good. Now I'm full." Both physical and emotional comfort accompany satiety: after a good meal, you can relax, enjoy entertainment, rest, or sleep. One writer says, "One cannot think well, love well, sleep well, if one has not dined well."[7]

Food does still more than maintain the intestine and convey messages of comfort to the brain. Foods are chemically complex. Even an ordinary potato contains hundreds of different compounds. People are complex, too, and the relationship between people and food is ancient. In view of all this, the fact that food gives us more than just nutrients is not surprising. If it were otherwise, that would be surprising.

✔ **KEY POINT**   In addition to nutrients, food conveys emotional satisfaction and, possibly, hormonal stimuli that contribute to health.

Nonnutrients in Foods

In addition to their many nutrients, foods also contain many other compounds that act on the body in some way. One name for these compounds is **nonnutrients.**

Among the nonnutrients of great interest today are the **phytochemicals** (*phyto* means *plant*). These include the compound that gives hot peppers their burning taste, the compound that gives garlic its pungent flavor, the pigments that give spinach and tomatoes their dark green and dark red colors, the products from yeast cells that make bread rise, and thousands upon thousands of others. Some foods contain nonnutrients that have drug effects—one in cranberries, for example, may flush some bacteria from the urinary tract and so prevent infection.[8] Some substances are toxic: one in cabbage, for example, can damage the thyroid gland when consumed in excess. That doesn't mean that cabbage is a harmful food, of course; it also contains nonnutrients that have an anticancer effect.

Many medical drugs also come from plants. The drug effects of plants, including foods, have been known to human beings for more than 20,000 years—since the Stone Age when people first began to collect plants for their medical properties. For all that time, and no doubt for thousands of years before that, people were developing a relationship with plants that involved much more than merely depending on them for nutrients. Humans learned to turn to food for comfort, for relief of pain, for pleasure, and even for the cure of some ailments.

Today, food is less valued for its medicinal effects, but it retains many other meanings for people. Cultural and social traditions are attached to the preparing, serving, eating, and sharing of food.

✓ **KEY POINT**   **Foods contain compounds other than nutrients that give them their tastes, aromas, colors, and other characteristics.**

Cultural and Social Meanings Attached to Food

Besides conveying comfort, satiety, nutrients, and nonnutrients, foods represent our cultures, our philosophies, and our beliefs. People from every country enjoy special **foodways** that represent their own histories. As a result, the sharing of food can be symbolic: people offering foods that represent their heritages are expressing a willingness to share cherished values with others. People accepting those foods are symbolically accepting not only the person doing the offering but the person's culture. This is why meetings of heads of state worldwide most often include a meal and why couples entering into cross-cultural marriages invite each other to share traditional holiday meals.

The same is true within a nation of mixed cultures such as the United States. Years ago, sociologists believed the United States was a "melting pot," creating a single, "American" culture. In reality, though, our nation resembles a mosaic more than a melting pot because people of similar heritages tend to coalesce into distinct cultural communities. This arrangement provides a wealth of unique cultural experiences for those who choose to seek them. One of the most enjoyable ways to sample other cultures is to try some of the **ethnic foods** they have to offer—that is, to sample their **cuisine.**[9] Luckily, most people living in the United States can easily do this. A menu in an "American-style" restaurant might list spaghetti (Italian), nachos (Mexican), hot dogs

nonnutrients a term used in this book to mean compounds other than the six nutrients that are present in foods.

phytochemicals nonnutrient compounds in plant-derived foods having biological activity in the body.

foodways the sum of a culture's habits, customs, beliefs, and preferences concerning food.

ethnic foods foods associated with particular cultural subgroups within a population.

cuisine a style of cooking.

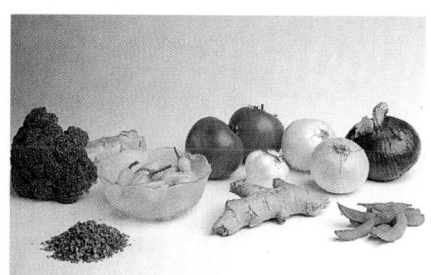

Some foods offer beneficial nonnutrients called phytochemicals.

Sharing ethnic food is a way of sharing culture.

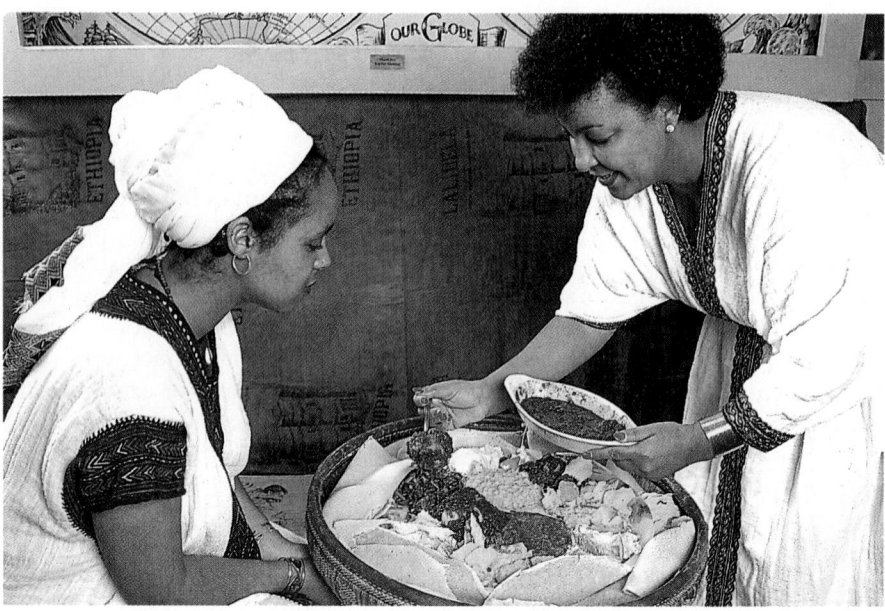

omnivores people who eat foods of both plant and animal origin, including animal flesh.

vegetarians people who exclude from their diets animal flesh and possibly animal products such as milk, cheese, and eggs. See Table 1-4, Glossary of Vegetarian Terms.

More about the effects of population, agriculture, and food choices on the earth's resources in Chapter 15 and Controversy 15.

with sauerkraut (German), croissants (French), stewed okra (African), baked squash (Native American), and egg rolls (Chinese). These traditional everyday foods, now adapted to locally available ingredients, have all become an integral part of the "American diet."

Cultural traditions regarding food are not inflexible; they keep evolving as people move about, learn new things, and teach each other. Today, some people are ceasing to be **omnivores** and are becoming **vegetarians,** as they discover the health and other advantages associated with low-meat and no-meat diets.[10]

Vegetarianism is not associated with any particular culture, but many different groups choose it for many different reasons. Some believe that we should not kill animals to eat their meat. Some believe that we should not even partake of animal products such as milk, cheese, and eggs. Others also shun honey and items made of leather, wool, or silk. Many are upset when livestock animals are treated inhumanely in feedlots and slaughterhouses. Today, on learning that the human population is straining the earth's resources of land and water and that raising grains for direct consumption by people requires less land and water than does raising grains to feed animals, some believe we should eat less meat for environmental reasons.

People who eat meat also do so for a variety of reasons. Some find that a hamburger makes a convenient lunch while providing a concentrated source of energy and nutrients. Others enjoy the taste of roasted chicken or beef stew. Others wouldn't know what to eat without meat; they are accustomed to seeing it on the plate. Romantic notions of cattle drives and barbecues on the Western frontier lead some people to associate consumption of meat, and especially beef, with masculinity. In another land, a host may honor special guests in the traditional way—by killing a lamb for dinner. To some indigenous peoples, killing a food animal is a sacred act that requires prayers for the animal's spirit. Indeed, modern-day hunters in this country may hold that allowing animals to roam freely in nature and killing them only when they are needed for food is more humane than raising them industrially and slaughtering them impersonally. A small glossary of terms related to vegetarianism appears in Table 1-4. Controversy 6 delves into the nutrition implications of vegetarian traditions.

All of these considerations—physical, psychological, cultural, social, and philosophical—make up the framework within which people choose the foods they eat. Still other consideratioons bear more immediately on a person's day-to-day food choices. Among factors people cite to explain daily food choices are:

- *Availability.* There are no others to choose from.
- *Convenience.* They are quick and easy to prepare.
- *Economy.* They are within your means.
- *Emotional comfort.* Foods can make you feel better for a while.
- *Ethnic heritage.* They are the foods of your ethnic group.
- *Habit.* They are familiar; you always eat them.
- *Personal preference.* You like them.
- *Positive associations.* They are eaten by people you admire, or they indicate status, or they remind you of fun.
- *Region of the country.* They are foods favored in your area.
- *Social pressure.* They are offered; you feel you can't refuse them.
- *Values or beliefs.* They fit your religious tradition, square with your political views, or honor the environmental ethic.
- *Nutritional value.* You think they are good for you.

Only the last of these reasons for choosing foods assigns a high priority to nutritional health. Similarly, the choice of where, as well as of what, to eat is often based more on social needs than on nutrition judgments. College students often choose to eat at fast-food and other restaurants to socialize, to get out, to save time, and to date; they are not always conscious of the need to obtain healthful food.[11]

In conclusion, then, food does many things for people. One of them, though—and the one that is most crucial to physical health—is that it nourishes the body. That function of food is the focus of this book.

✔ **KEY POINT**   **Cultural traditions and social values revolve around food. Some values are expressed through foodways.**

Food as Nourishment

If you live for 65 years or longer, you will have consumed more than 70,000 meals, and your remarkable body will have disposed of 50 tons of food. The foods you choose have cumulative effects on your body. At 65 years of age, you will see and feel those effects, if you know what to look for.

Your body renews its structures continuously, and each day it builds a little muscle, bone, skin, and blood, replacing old tissues with new. It may also add a little fat, if you consume excess food energy, or subtract a little, should you consume less than you require. In this way some of the food you eat today becomes part of "you" tomorrow. The best food for you, then, is the kind that

TABLE 1-4

Glossary of Vegetarian Terms

- **lacto-vegetarians** people who use milk and milk products but no meats in their diets.
- **lacto-ovo vegetarians** people who use milk, milk products, and eggs, but no meats in their diets.
- **vegans (VAY-guns, VEJ-uns)** people who include no animal-derived products in their diets. These people are also called *strict vegetarians.*
- **semivegetarians** people who eat only small amounts of meats, or who exclude just certain meats, such as red meats.

malnutrition any condition caused by excess or deficient food energy or nutrient intake or by an imbalance of nutrients. Nutrient or energy deficiencies are classed as forms of undernutrition; nutrient or energy excesses are classed as forms of overnutrition.

chronic disease long-duration degenerative diseases characterized by deterioration of the body organs; examples include heart disease, cancer, and diabetes.

supports the growth and maintenance of strong muscles, sound bones, healthy skin, and sufficient blood to cleanse and nourish all parts of your body. This means you need food that provides not only energy but also sufficient nutrients in all of the classes named earlier: water, carbohydrates, fats, protein, vitamins, and minerals. If the foods you eat provide too little or too much of any of these, your health will suffer a little. If the foods you eat provide too little or too much of one or more nutrients every day for years, then, by the time you are old, you may well suffer severe disease effects.

The point is that a well-chosen array of foods supplies enough energy and enough of each nutrient to prevent **malnutrition.** Malnutrition includes deficiencies of nutrients, imbalances, and excesses, which can all take a toll on health over time.

✔ KEY POINT   **The nutrients in food support growth, maintenance, and repair of the body. Deficiencies, excesses, and imbalances of nutrients bring on the diseases of malnutrition.**

Nutrition and Disease Prevention

Your choice of diet profoundly influences your long-term health prospects. Only two common lifestyle habits are more influential: smoking and other tobacco use, and excessive drinking of alcohol.[12] Many older people suffer from debilitating conditions that could have been largely prevented had they known the nutrition principles that we know today and applied those principles throughout their lives.

The poor health conveyed by a poor diet consists not only of the various forms of malnutrition just described, but also of other diseases, especially the **chronic diseases:** heart disease, diabetes, some kinds of cancer, dental disease, adult bone loss, and others. We should hasten to say that while diet powerfully influences these diseases, they cannot be prevented just by a good diet; they are to some extent determined by people's genetic constitutions, activities, and lifestyles.[13] Within the range set by your inheritance, however, the likelihood that you will develop these diseases is strongly influenced by your food choices.

Some people overestimate and some underestimate the influence of diet in preventing diseases and poor health. It is difficult to get diet's exact role in perspective—difficult not only for individual people, but also for research scientists who are spending their working lives trying to figure out exactly how diet relates to health and various diseases. Three different views of the relationship may help to show the connections.

First, remember the role of genetics. Different diseases are differently influenced by genetics and nutrition, as shown in Figure 1-3. A disease such as sickle-cell anemia, for example, is purely hereditary. Nothing a person eats affects the person's chances of contracting this anemia, although nutrition therapy may help ease its course. Sickle-cell anemia is shown at the left in the figure as a nutrition-unrelated, genetic disease. In contrast, a condition such as "low birthweight," listed at the right in the figure, is often a nutrition-related condition. An infant's low birthweight is usually not genetic, but is caused by the mother's poor nutrition during pregnancy; it can lead to severe illness and death of the infant. Diseases and conditions of poor health appear all along the spectrum from purely genetic to purely nutritional; the more nutrition-related

FIGURE I-3

NUTRITION AND DISEASE

Not all diseases are equally influenced by diet. Some are purely genetic, like sickle-cell anemia. Some may be inherited (or the tendency to develop them may be inherited) but may be influenced by diet, like some forms of diabetes. Some are purely dietary, like the vitamin and mineral deficiency diseases.

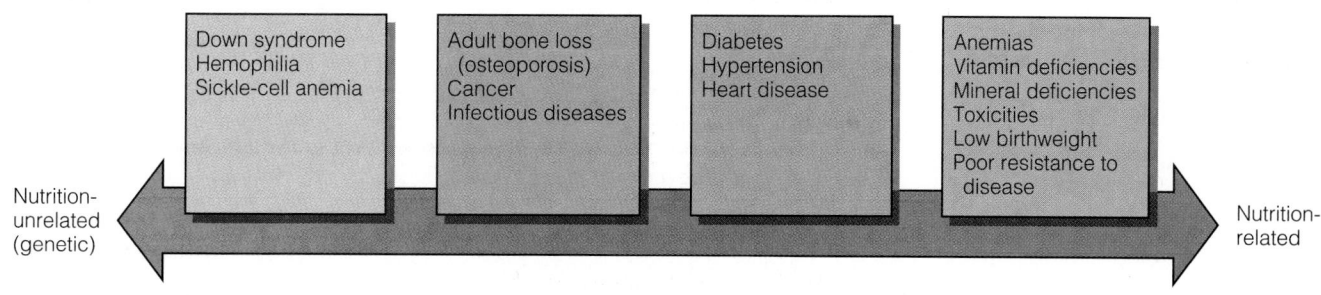

Down syndrome
Hemophilia
Sickle-cell anemia

Adult bone loss
  (osteoporosis)
Cancer
Infectious diseases

Diabetes
Hypertension
Heart disease

Anemias
Vitamin deficiencies
Mineral deficiencies
Toxicities
Low birthweight
Poor resistance to
  disease

Nutrition-
unrelated
(genetic)

Nutrition-
related

a disease or health condition is, the more successfully sound nutrition can pre-vent it.

Second, remember that some diseases, such as heart disease and cancer, are not one disease but many. Two people may both have heart disease, but not the same form. People differ genetically from each other in thousands of ways. One person's heart disease may be nutrition-related, another's may not be. No simple statement can be made about the extent to which diet can help a given person avoid or slow the course of a disease.

Third, remember that other lifestyle choices people make, besides their choices of what foods to eat, also affect their health. Tobacco and alcohol use were already mentioned, and other substance abuse can be equally destructive of health. Other major health determinants include physical activity, sleep, stress, and home and job conditions, including environmental quality.

Within all of these contexts, healthful nutrition can help prevent some dis-eases. Table 1-5 on page 16 shows some of the relationships, and later chapters return to examine these relationships in detail.

More about sickle-cell anemia in Chapter 6; low-birthweight infants are a topic of Chapter 12.

✔ KEY POINT   **Choice of diet influences long-term health, within the range set by genetic inheritance. Nutrition has no influence on some dis-eases but is closely linked to others.**

Nutrition Goals for the Nation

On September 5, 1990, the U.S. Department of Health and Human Services (U.S. DHHS) released *Healthy People 2000*, a set of health objectives for the nation.[14] The objectives numbered 297 in all and covered 22 different priority areas, of which nutrition was one. The objectives listed under "Nutrition" pro-vide a quick scan of the health goals that the department thought were within the province of nutrition science (see Table 1-6).

The first four U.S. DHHS objectives indicate that nutrition can influence four health conditions for better or worse. The next eight objectives identify the factors in the diet best known to influence the risks of contracting these conditions. The last nine objectives are intended to improve delivery of nutrition services. These lists provide a summary of what the nation's top health agency thinks is most important in the nutrition picture.

TABLE 1-5

Nutrition Measures to Prevent Diseases

Adequate Intake of Essential Nutrients, Especially *Protein*, and *Energy* from Food Helps Prevent
In Pregnancy
    Low birthweight
    Poor resistance to disease
    Some forms of birth defects
    Some forms of mental/physical retardation
In Infancy and Childhood
    Growth deficits
    Poor resistance to disease
In Adulthood and Old Age
    Poor resistance to infectious diseases
    Susceptibility to some forms of cancer
Moderation in Intake of *Energy* from Food Helps Prevent
    Obesity and related diseases, such as diabetes and hypertension
Moderation in *Fat* Intake Helps Prevent
    Susceptibility to obesity, some cancers, and atherosclerosis
Adequate *Fiber* Intake Helps Prevent
    Digestive malfunctions such as constipation and diverticulosis and possibly
        colon or other cancers
    Possibly heart disease
Moderation in *Sugar* Intake Helps Prevent
    Dental caries
Moderation in *Alcohol* Intake Helps Prevent
    Liver disease
    Malnutrition
Adequate Intake of *Any Essential Nutrient* Prevents
    Deficiency diseases such as cretinism, scurvy, and folate-deficiency anemia
Moderation in Intake of *Essential Nutrients* Prevents
    Toxicity states
Adequate *Calcium* Intake Helps Prevent
    Adult bone loss
    Possibly colon cancer and hypertension
Adequate *Iron* Intake Helps Prevent
    Iron-deficiency anemia
Adequate *Fluoride* Intake Helps Prevent
    Dental caries
Moderation in *Sodium* Intake Helps Prevent
    Hypertension and related diseases of the heart and kidney
Adequate *Vitamin* Intake Helps Prevent
    Susceptibility to certain cancers and possibly heart disease
    Certain birth defects

TABLE I-6

Nutrition-Related Health Objectives for the Nation, Year 2000

Disease-Related Objectives

1. Reduce *heart disease* deaths.
2. Reverse the rise in *cancer* deaths.
3. Reduce the prevalence of *overweight*.
4. Reduce *growth retardation* among low-income children.

Nutrient and Food Objectives

5. Reduce *dietary fat* intake.[a]
6. Increase intakes of complex *carbohydrate* and *fiber*-containing foods.[b]
7. Increase the proportion of *overweight* people taking effective steps to control their weight.
8. Increase *calcium* intakes among teenagers, pregnant women, women who are breastfeeding their infants, and adults in general.
9. Reduce *salt* intakes and purchases of foods high in salt.
10. Remedy *iron* deficiencies in children and women.
11. Encourage *breastfeeding* of infants immediately after birth and the continuation of breastfeeding for at least six months after birth.
12. Teach parents *infant-feeding practices* that will minimize the chances of tooth decay.[c]

Nutrition Information and Service Objectives

13. Promote people's learning of how best to use *food labels* to correctly select nutritious foods.
14. Make food labels more informative and complete.
15. Make more low-fat, low-saturated fat foods available.
16. Encourage more restaurants and institutions to serve low-fat, low-calorie foods.
17. Improve the nutrition quality of school lunches and breakfasts and child-care foodservice meals.
18. Make sure as many elderly people as possible receive home food services.
19. Offer nutrition education in more schools from preschool through 12th grade.
20. Encourage workplaces to provide nutrition education and/or weight-management programs for their employees.
21. Support health-care providers in offering nutrition assessment, nutrition counseling, and referrals to qualified nutrition experts as part of their services.

[a]The exact objective is to reduce fat intake to an average of 30 percent of calories or less, and saturated fat intake to less than 10 percent of calories. How to do this is described in Chapter 5.

[b]The objective is spelled out: increase these intakes in the diets of adults to five or more daily servings of vegetables (including legumes) and fruits and to six or more daily servings of grain products.

[c]The objective emphasizes *nursing-bottle syndrome,* discussed in Chapter 12.

SOURCE: *Healthy People 2000: National Health Promotion and Disease Prevention Objectives* (Washington, D.C.: U.S. Department of Health and Human Services, 1990).

In 1995, five years after the U.S. DHHS objectives were published, progress toward achieving these goals was mixed.[15] Heart disease deaths had fallen slightly, and grocery shelves overflowed with low-fat foods and foods bearing meaningful labels. On the negative side, though, the number of overweight people had jumped significantly.

Nutrition monitoring of the U.S. population is ongoing. To make it easier than it has been in the past, the agencies involved agreed in 1990 to cooperate, rather than to compete. According to a ten-year plan embodied in the National Nutrition Monitoring Act of 1990, the principal government agencies monitoring the nation's nutrition use the same standards, units, and research designs so that they can compare and compile their results meaningfully. They also

Agencies active in nutrition policy and monitoring:

✓ U.S. DDHS.
✓ USDA.
✓ CDC.

Ongoing national nutrition research projects:

✓ National Food Consumption Surveys (NFCS).
✓ Health and Nutrition Examination Surveys (HANES).

share results, using computer links, so that each agency can easily access what the others have done.

Among the agency names you may hear in connection with these efforts are the U.S. DHHS already mentioned, the U.S. Department of Agriculture (USDA), and the Centers for Disease Control and Prevention (CDC). You are also likely to hear of two research projects. The Health and Nutrition Examination Surveys (HANES) involve:

■ Asking people what they have eaten.
■ Recording measures of their health status.

The National Food Consumption Surveys (NFCS) involve:

■ Recording what people have actually eaten for two days.
■ Comparing the foods they have chosen with recommended food selections.

All of these government efforts reflect ambitious goals for our health and food choices. Now, how should we go about choosing foods to achieve these goals?

✓ **KEY POINT** **The U.S. Department of Health and Human Services has published a set of health objectives for the nation. The goals are to reduce the incidence of heart disease, cancer, overweight, and growth retardation; to improve nutritional health; and to improve delivery of nutrition services.**

THE CHALLENGE OF CHOOSING FOODS

The foods you choose should fit your tastes, personality, family and cultural traditions, lifestyle, and budget. At their best, well-planned meals convey pleasure, too, and they should also be nutritious, or at least the diet you build from them should be. Foods today come in astounding numbers and varieties. Consumers can lose track of what they contain and how they can best be put together into health-promoting diets. A few guidelines can help a lot.

The content of fat in food is often expressed as "percent of calories," and "30 percent of calories from fat" is a key limit to keep in mind. A food whose fat content is higher than 30 percent contributes too much fat to the diet, unless it is eaten with low-fat foods to bring the average down. The goal is to eat a *diet* that provides 30 percent or less of calories from fat. But people standing at a food counter or in line in a cafeteria do not choose a "diet"—they choose "macaroni and cheese," "baked fish," or "carrots." *Diet* is an academic concept built of the real-life food choices people make, one by one. The way to achieve a *diet* with less than 30 percent of calories from fat, then, is to consider how individual foods contribute to the whole. Chapter 5 explains more about controlling the fat in the diet.

The Variety of Foods to Choose From

If someone had listed the variety of foods available several hundred years ago, the list might have been relatively short. It would have consisted of basic foods—foods that have been around for a long time such as vegetables, fruits, meats, and grains. These foods have variously been called unprocessed, nat-

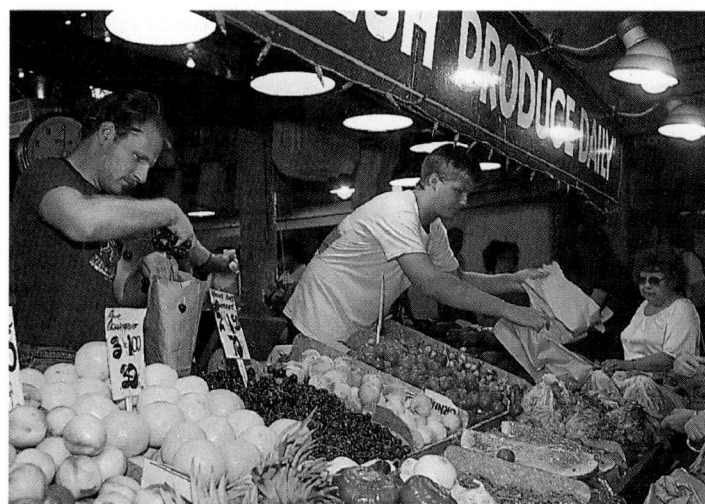

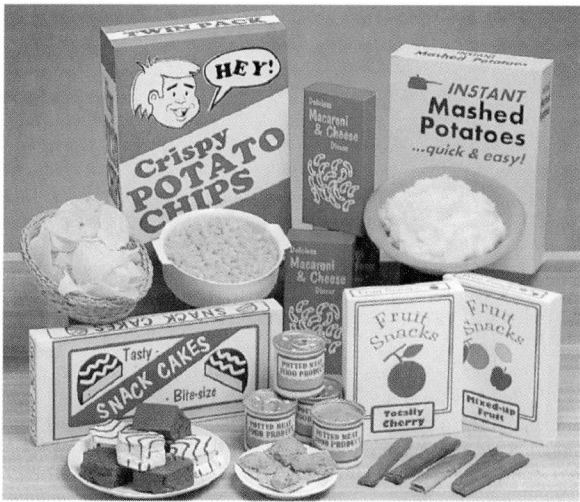

Foods once looked like this . . .

. . . but now foods often look like this.

ural, whole, or farm foods. An easy way to obtain a nutritious diet is to consume a variety of selections from among these foods each day, but data from a
recent HANES Survey show that on a given day as many as 45 percent of our
people consume no fruits or fruit juices and that, while people generally consume a serving or two of vegetables, the vegetable they most often choose is
potatoes, and usually prepared as french fries.[16]

Ironically, the variety of foods available to us today may make it more difficult, rather than easier, to plan nutritious diets. The food industry offers thousands of foods, many of which are mixtures of the basic ones, and some of
which are even constructed mostly from artificial ingredients.

Table 1-7 on the next page presents a glossary of terms related to foods. A
reading of the terms will reveal that all types of food—including fast foods and
processed foods—offer various constituents to the eater. To what extent foods
are nutritious depends on the nutrients and calories they contain.[17] In short, to
select well among foods, as among people, you need to know more than their
names; you need to know the foods' inner qualities.

Even more importantly, you need to know how to combine foods into nutritious diets. Foods are not nutritious by themselves; each is of value only in so
far as it contributes to a nutritious diet.[18] A key to wise diet planning is to make
sure that the foods you eat daily, your staple foods, are especially nutritious.

✔ KEY POINT   **Foods come in a bewildering variety in the marketplace,
but the foods that form the basis of a nutritious diet are ordinary milk and
milk products; meats, fish, and poultry; vegetables and dried peas and
beans; and fruits and grains.**

The Construction of Nutritious Diets from Foods

A nutritious diet has five characteristics. One is **adequacy:** the foods provide
enough of each essential nutrient, fiber, and energy. Another is **balance:** the
choices do not overemphasize one nutrient or food type at the expense of

adequacy the dietary characteristic of
providing all of the essential nutrients,
fiber, and energy in amounts sufficient
to maintain health and body weight.

balance the dietary characteristic of
providing foods of a number of types in
proportion to each other, such that foods
rich in some nutrients do not crowd out
of the diet foods that are rich in other
nutrients. Also called *proportionality*.

TABLE I-7

Glossary of Food Types

The purpose of this little glossary is to show that good-sounding food names don't necessarily signify that foods are nutritious. Read the comment at the end of each definition.

- **basic foods** milk and milk products; meats and similar foods such as fish and poultry; vegetables, including dried beans and peas; fruits; and grains. These foods are generally considered to form the basis of a nutritious diet. Also called *whole foods*.
- **enriched foods** and **fortified foods** foods to which nutrients have been added. If the starting material is a whole, basic food such as milk or whole grain, the result may be highly nutritious. If the starting material is a concentrated form of sugar or fat, the result may be less nutritious.
- **fast foods** restaurant foods that are available within minutes after customers order them—traditionally, hamburgers, french fries, and milkshakes; more recently, salads and other vegetable dishes as well. These foods may or may not meet people's nutrient needs well, depending on the selections made and on the energy allowances and nutrient needs of the eaters.
- **natural foods** a term that has no legal definition.
- **partitioned foods** foods composed of parts of whole foods, such as butter (from milk), sugar (from beets or cane), or corn oil (from corn). Partitioned foods are usually empty of nutrients and are not nutritious.
- **processed foods** foods subjected to any process, such as milling, alteration of texture, addition of additives, cooking, or others. Depending on the starting material and the process, a processed food may or may not be nutritious.
- **staple foods** foods used frequently or daily, for example, rice (in the Far East) or potatoes (in Ireland). If well chosen, these foods are nutritious; certainly, they should be.
- **organic foods** understood to mean foods grown without synthetic pesticides or fertilizers; in chemistry, however, all foods are made mostly of organic (carbon-containing) compounds.

calorie control control of energy intake, a feature of a sound diet plan.

moderation the dietary characteristic of providing constituents within set limits, not to excess.

variety the dietary characteristic of consuming a wide selection of foods—the opposite of monotony.

another. The third is **calorie control:** the foods provide the amount of energy you need to maintain appropriate weight—not more, not less. The fourth is **moderation:** the foods do not provide excess fat, salt, sugar, or other unwanted constituents. The fifth is **variety:** the foods chosen differ from one day to the next.

Any nutrient could be used to demonstrate the importance of dietary *adequacy*. Iron provides a familiar example. It is an essential nutrient; you lose some every day, so you have to keep replacing it; and you can get it into your body only by eating foods that contain it.* If you eat too few of the iron-containing foods, you can develop iron-deficiency anemia: with anemia you can feel weak, tired, cold, sad, and unenthusiastic; you may have frequent headaches; and you can do very little muscular work without disabling fatigue. If you add iron-rich foods to your diet, you soon feel more energetic.

---

*A person can also take supplements containing iron, but as later discussions demonstrate, this is not as effective as eating iron-rich foods.

Some foods are rich in iron; others are notoriously poor. Meat, fish, poultry, and legumes are in the iron-rich category, and an easy way to obtain the needed iron is to include these foods in your diet regularly.

To appreciate the importance of dietary *balance*, consider a second essential nutrient, calcium. Most foods that are rich in iron are poor in calcium. Calcium's best food sources are milk and milk products, which happen to be extraordinarily poor iron sources. A diet lacking calcium causes poor bone development during the growing years and increases a person's susceptibility to disabling bone loss in adult life. Children and adults are advised to consume enough milk, milk products, or other calcium-rich foods each day to meet their calcium needs—but not so much as to crowd iron-rich foods out of the diet.

Clearly, to obtain enough of both iron and calcium, which seldom appear together in the same foods, people have to balance their food choices. Balancing the whole diet to provide enough but not too much of every one of the 40-odd nutrients the body needs for health is a juggling act that requires considerable skill. As you will see in Chapter 2, food group plans can help you achieve dietary adequacy and balance because they recommend specific amounts of foods of each type.

Energy intakes should not exceed energy needs. Nicknamed *calorie control*, this diet characteristic ensures that energy intakes from food balance energy expenditures in activity. The eater of such a diet achieves control of body fat content and weight. The many strategies that promote this goal appear in Chapter 9.

Intakes of certain food constituents such as fat, cholesterol, sugar, and salt should be limited for health's sake (more on health effects in later chapters). A major guideline already mentioned is to keep fat intake below 30 percent of total calories. Some people take this to mean that they must never indulge in a delicious beefsteak or hot-fudge sundae, but they are misinformed, since *moderation*, not total abstinence, is the key. A steady diet of steak and ice cream might be harmful, but once a week as part of an otherwise moderate diet plan, these foods may have little impact; as a once-a-month treat, these foods would have practically no effect at all. Moderation also means that limits are necessary, even for desirable food constituents. For example, while a certain amount of fiber in foods contributes to the health of the digestive system, too much fiber leads to nutrient losses.

As for *variety*, it is generally agreed that people should not eat the same foods day after day, for two reasons. One reason is that some less-known nutrients and some nonnutrient food components could be important to health; some foods may be better sources of these than others. Another reason is that a monotonous diet may deliver large amounts of toxins or contaminants. Each such undesirable item in a food is diluted by all the other foods eaten with it and is even further diluted if several days are skipped before it is eaten again. Last, variety adds interest—trying new foods can be a source of pleasure.

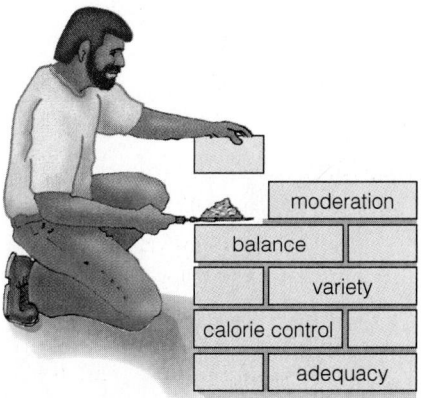

All of these factors help to build a nutritious diet.

According to the experts, adults in the United States are not very successful at meeting these objectives. In particular, people seem to consume diets that are either adequate or moderate, but not both. They behave as though they had to choose between two alternatives—getting all their nutrients but overconsuming fat calories in the process, or keeping their fat in line but running short on nutrients.[19] Only 2 percent of several thousand adults who were surveyed

nutrient density a measure of nutrients provided per calorie of food.

managed to do both. That finding defines the challenge for the health-conscious eater: try to achieve adequacy and moderation at the same time. Because this challenge is the key to good nutrition, this chapter's Food Feature is devoted to the skill required to meet it. The Food Feature offers a tool to help make it easy—the concept of **nutrient density.**

✔ KEY POINT **A well-planned diet is adequate in nutrients, is balanced with regard to food types, offers food energy that matches energy expended in activity, is moderate in unwanted constituents, and offers variety. Foods of high nutrient density form the foundation of such a diet.**

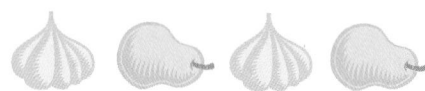

FOOD FEATURE

GETTING THE MOST NUTRIENTS FOR YOUR CALORIES

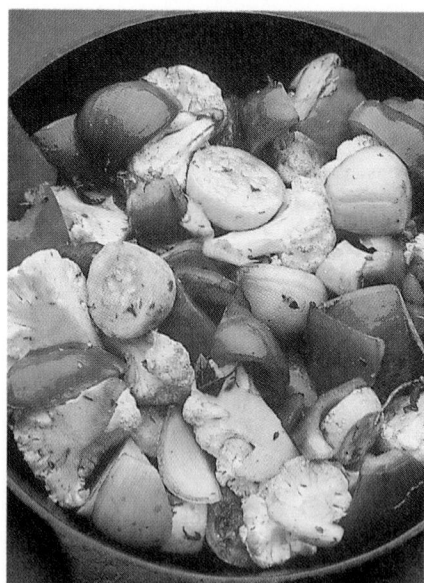

Would it take more time to prepare this dish than to prepare a batch of cookies? No, less time and less cleanup, too.

The planner who is trying to control calories while balancing the diet and making it adequate is bound to find certain foods especially useful. These are foods that are rich in nutrients relative to their energy contents, that is, foods with high nutrient density. Consider calcium sources, for example. Ice cream and nonfat milk both supply calcium, but the milk is "denser" in calcium per calorie. A cup of ice cream contributes more than 200 calories, a cup of nonfat milk only 90—and with a little more calcium. Or consider iron. A 3-ounce serving of high-fat beef pot roast offers about the same amount of iron as a 3-ounce serving of water-packed tuna, but the beef contains over 300 calories, the tuna about 100. Most people cannot, for their health's sake, afford to choose foods without regard to their energy contents. Those who do very often fill up their calorie allowances while leaving nutrient needs unmet.

For the person who plans and prepares the meals for a family, consciousness of nutrient density is especially important. In fact, the family food-preparer is well advised to *center* the meal on foods of high nutrient density. The foods that present the most nutrients per calorie are the vegetables, especially the non-starchy vegetables such as broccoli, carrots, mushrooms, peppers, and tomatoes. These take time to prepare, but time invested this way pays off in nutritional health. Twenty minutes spent peeling and slicing vegetables for a salad is a better investment in nutrition than 20 minutes spent fixing a fancy, high-fat, high-sugar dessert.

Investing meal preparation time in nutritious foods is especially important when time is limited. In today's households, although both men and women spend some 71 hours a week sleeping and taking care of personal needs, women still do most of the cooking and food shopping. Since more women are employed today than earlier, they can spend only a very little time on food preparation—most spend less than 30 minutes preparing the evening meal, and 20 percent spend less than 15 minutes.[20] Busy chefs should seek out convenience foods, such as bags of frozen vegetables, that are nutrient dense. Other selections, such as most pot pies, are less so because they contain too little of the vegetables and too much fat.

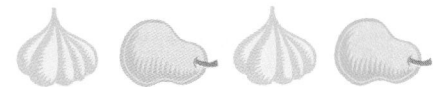

Nutrient density is such a useful concept in diet planning that experts recommend it be used on food labels. That is, food labels should express their nutrient contents "per calorie" in the food.[21] While labels have not yet evolved to this stage, this book encourages you to think in those terms. Watch for the tables and figures in later chapters that show the best buys among foods, not in nutrients per dollar, but in nutrients per calorie. Figure 1-4 offers a preview of the way this viewpoint can help you distinguish between more and less nutritious foods.

FIGURE 1-4

HOW THE EXPERTS JUDGE WHICH FOODS ARE MOST NUTRITIOUS

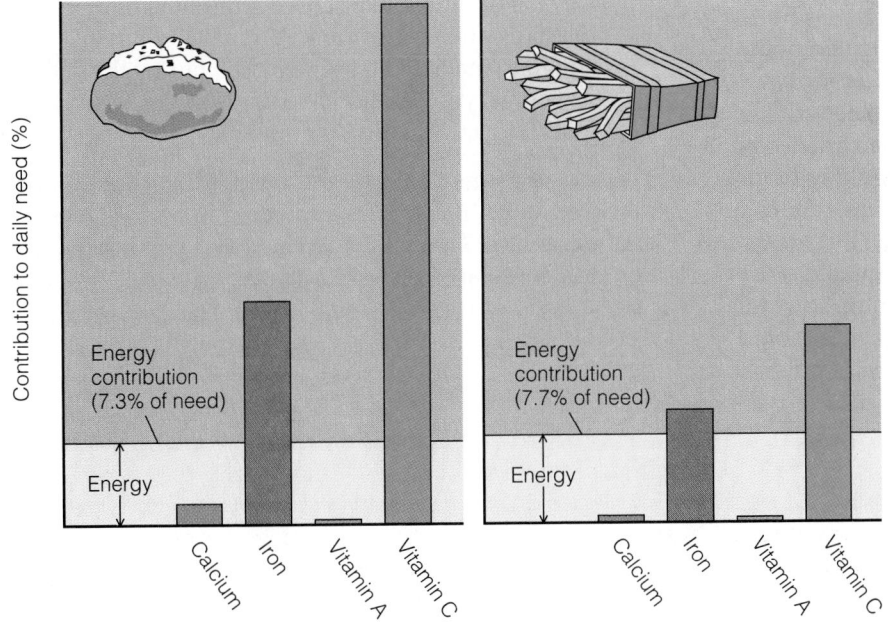

All of this discussion leads to the principle that is central to achieving nutritional health. It is not the individual foods you choose, but the way you combine them into meals and the ways you arrange meals to follow one another over days and weeks that determine how well you are nourishing yourself. Nutrition is a science, not an art, but it can be used artfully to create a pleasing, nourishing diet. The remainder of this book is dedicated to helping you make informed choices and combine them artfully to meet all the body's needs.

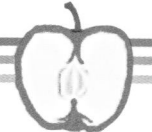

Do It!

ANALYZE NUTRITION NEWS

This chapter has pointed out the importance of reading nutrition news with an educated eye. Here is a chance to practice your skills. Read your local newspaper or any publication that carries nutrition news. On a copy of Form 1-1, answer these questions:

1. What sort of language does the writer use? Do the words imply sensationalism or conclusive findings? Phrases such as "startling revelation" or "now we know" or "the study proved" are clues to whether the report is a sensational one. Does the author take a tentative approach, using words such as *may, might,* or *could?* What do these words imply?

2. Is the report given in the context of previous nutrition findings? Does it imply that the current finding wipes out all that has gone before it? Can you detect a broad understanding of nutrition on the writer's part? From what clues? For example, an article about folate deficiency and heart disease should mention that saturated fat probably plays the major nutrition role in heart disease development.

3. Does the article mention whether the quoted research is published in a medical or nutrition journal? The following Controversy section has more information about which types of journals publish valid scientific findings and which do not.

4. How were the results obtained? Can you tell from the report whether this was a case study, an epidemiological study, an intervention study, or a laboratory study? How does that information affect your understanding of what the results have contributed to nutrition science?

5. Does the finding apply to you? Should you change your eating patterns because of it? In what ways did the subjects resemble or differ from you? Were there enough subjects to make the study seem valid? (In a serious evaluation, a statistical analysis would be used to answer this question.)

6. Does the finding make sense to you in light of what you know about nutrition? You may not know enough to make this judgment yet, but by the end of this course, you should have developed a "feel" for identifying information that fits with reality.

This sort of assessment can guide you through the numerous nutrition articles appearing in newspapers and magazines. That way, you can avoid making nutrition decisions based on passing fads.

FORM 1-1

Critiquing Nutrition News

The news report I am critiquing comes from _____ (publication), dated_____ (attach the report to this form).

1. I evaluate the language used in the publication as follows: _____

   _____

   _____

   _____

2. I believe the author's understanding of previously reported findings to be: _____

   _____

   _____

   _____

3. I judge the credibility of the item to be: _____

   _____

   _____

   _____

4. The methods used to obtain these results were: _____

   _____

   _____

   _____

5. The results of the study apply to the following populations: _____

   _____

   _____

   _____

6. To a reader without extensive nutritional background, the results of a study may be misleading. This report might mislead by:

   _____

   _____

   _____

   _____

✔ SELF-CHECK

Answers to these Self-Check questions are in Appendix G.

1. Studies of whole populations that reveal correlations between dietary habits and disease incidence are referred to as:
   a. case studies
   -b. intervention studies
   c. laboratory studies
   (d.) epidemiological studies

2. Energy-yielding nutrients include all of the following *except:*
   (a.) vitamins
   b. carbohydrates
   c. fat
   d. protein

3. Organic nutrients include all of the following *except:*
   a. minerals
   b. fat
   c. carbohydrates
   d. protein

4. One of the characteristics of a nutritious diet is that it provides no constituent in excess. This principle of diet planning is called:
   a. adequacy
   b. balance
   c. moderation
   d. variety

5. A slice of apple pie supplies 350 calories with 3 grams of fiber; an apple provides 80 calories and the same 3 grams of fiber. This is an example of:
   a. calorie control
   b. nutrient density
   c. variety
   d. essential nutrients

6. For breakfast, a vegan might eat a scrambled egg but omit the bacon.   T   F

7. Heart disease and cancer are due to genetic causes only, and diet has no effect on whether or not they occur.   T   F

8. Both carbohydrates and protein provide 4 calories per gram.   T   F

9. Once a new finding about nutrition is published, you can feel confident about changing your diet accordingly.   T   F

10. A registered dietitian (RD) has the educational background necessary to deliver reliable nutrition advice. (Read about this in the upcoming Controversy.)   T   F

NOTES

Notes are in Appendix F.

Who Speaks on Nutrition?

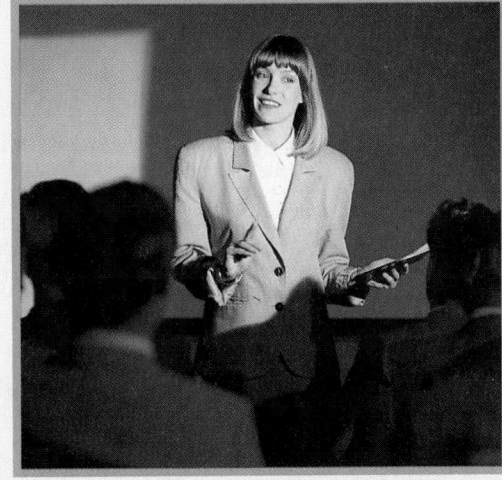

Today more than ever before, people want to know what nutrition news they can believe and safely use. They want to know how best to take care of themselves. Some people seek miracles too: supplements for weight loss without effort, nutrients to forestall aging or prevent baldness or increase sexual potency. People's heightened interest in nutrition translates into a deluge of dollars spent on services and products peddled by both legitimate and fraudulent businesses.[1] Consumers who obtain legitimate care can improve their health. Those enticed into scams, however, may lose their health, their savings, or both.[2] Unfortunately, nutrition and other **fraud** (**quackery,** defined in Table C1-1) rings cash registers to the tune of $14 billion annually. Ironically, quacks spread useless or even dangerous advice, sham products, and unproven procedures that not only rob people of the very health they are seeking, but also delay their use of legitimate strategies that could truly improve health.[3]

How can people distinguish valid nutrition information from misinformation? One excellent approach is to notice who is purveying the information: quacks or qualified sources. At the extremes, science and quackery may be easy to tell apart, but between the extremes lies an abundance of less easily recognized nutrition information and misinformation. An instructor at a gym, a physician, a health-store clerk, an author of a book (and seller of juice machines) all recommend nutrition regimens. Can you believe these people? A famous movie star speaks out to advise the U.S. Congress about pesticides in foods. What qualifies this person to give this advice? Would following the advice be helpful or harmful? In short, how can you tell whom to believe about nutrition?

IDENTIFYING QUACKS

Identifing nutrition quacks would not be difficult if they still rode into town in wooden wagons hawking snake oil to "cure what ails you" for 50 cents a bottle. But those days are gone. Today's quacks manipulate consumers in less obvious ways. Fraudulent claims sound logical, but they lack the research support found in nutrition science. In fact, you can learn to recognize fraud by the unscientific characteristics shown in Figure C1-1.

The makers of fraudulent claims are usually not credentialed professionals. Usually, their qualifications are nothing more than words on paper. Occasionally, though, a person with all the earmarks of the real thing turns out to be just plain dishonest.

The scope of the problem of nutrition misinformation almost defies description. Fraud in weight loss alone often claims the attention of Congress, whose members struggle to control it. At a subcommittee meeting on the problem of deception and fraud, the chairman said this about nutrition fraud:

> This subcommittee has found the medical field is riddled with hucksters who ply their dubious wares and their miracle cures, while Government regulators sit snoozing on the sidelines.[4]

In short, quackery respects neither science nor honesty in its pursuit of money.

TABLE C1-1
Misinformation Terms

- **anecdotal evidence**   information based on interesting and entertaining, but not scientific, personal accounts of events.
- **fraud** or **quackery**   the promotion, for financial gain, of devices, treatments, services, plans, or products (including diets and supplements) that alter or claim to alter a human condition without proof of safety or effectiveness. (The word *quackery* comes from the term *quack-salver,* meaning a person who quacks loudly about a miracle product—a lotion or a salve.)

FIGURE CI-1

EARMARKS OF NUTRITION QUACKERY

The more of these claims you hear about nutrition information, the less likely it is to be valid.

Too good to be true
The claim presents enticingly simple answers to complex problems. It says what most people want to hear. It sounds magical.

Suspicions about food supply
The person or institution pushing the product or service urges distrust of the current methods of medicine or suspicion of the regular food supply, with "alternatives" for sale (providing profit to the seller) under the guise that people should have freedom of choice.

Testimonials
The evidence presented to support the claim is in the form of praise by people who have been "healed," "made younger," and the like by the product or treatment.

Fake credentials
The person or institution making the claim is titled "doctor," "university," or the like, but has simply created or bought the title and is not legitimate.

Unpublished studies
Scientific studies are cited, but are nowhere published and so cannot be critically examined.

Persecution claims
The person or institution pushing the product or service claims to be persecuted by the medical establishment or tries to convince you that physicians "want to keep you ill so that you will continue to pay for office visits."

Authority not cited
The studies cited sound valid, but are not referenced, so that it is impossible to check and see if they were conducted scientifically.

Motive: personal gain
The person or institution making the claim stands to make a profit if it is believed.

Advertisement
The claim is being made by an advertiser who is paid to make claims for the product or procedure. (Look for the word "Advertisement," probably in tiny print somewhere on the page.)

Unreliable publication
The studies cited are published, but in a newsletter, magazine, or journal that publishes misinformation.

Logic without proof
The claim seems to be based on sound reasoning but hasn't been scientifically tested and shown to hold up.

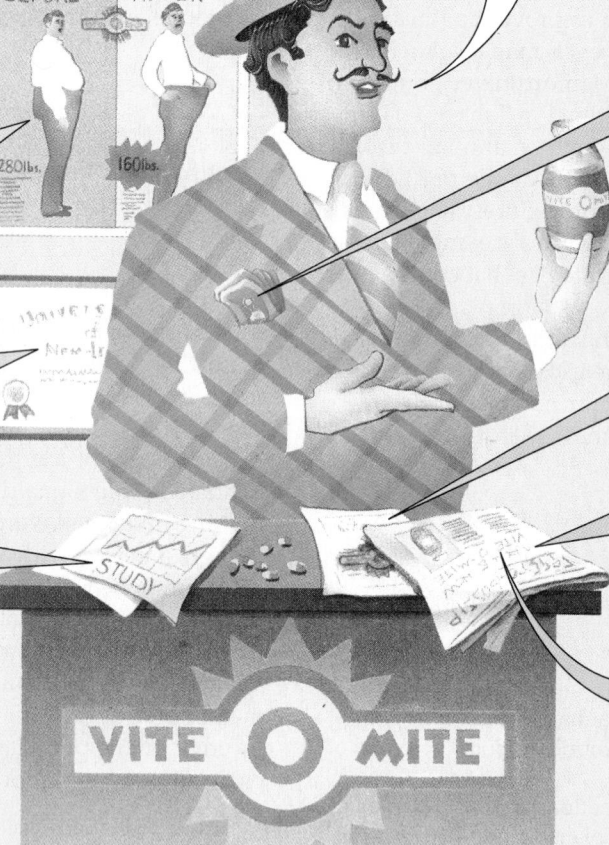

IDENTIFYING VALID NUTRITION INFORMATION

As Chapter 1 explained, nutrition is a science; that is, it derives information from scientific research. Scientists must systematically conduct research studies and cautiously interpret the findings before they can provide practical nutrition information. The following are characteristics of scientific research:

- Scientists test their ideas by conducting properly designed scientific experiments. They report their methods and procedures in detail so that other scientists can verify the findings through replication.
- Scientists recognize the inadequacy of **anecdotal evidence** or testimonials.
- Scientists who use animals in their research do not apply their findings directly to human beings.
- Scientists may use specific segments of the population in their research. When they do, they are careful not to generalize the findings to all people.
- Scientists report their findings in respected scientific journals. Their work must survive a screening review by their peers before it is accepted for publication.

With each report from scientists, the field of nutrition changes a little—each finding contributes another piece to the whole body of knowledge. Table C1-2 lists some sources of credible nutrition information.

WHO ARE THE TRUE NUTRITION EXPERTS?

Most people turn to their physicians for dietary advice. Physicians are expected to know all about health-related matters. But are physicians the best sources of accurate and current information on nutrition? Only about half of all medical schools in the United States require students to take even one nutrition course.[5] Students attending these classes receive an average of 20 hours of nutrition instruction—an amount most graduates consider inadequate.[6] While many experts call for a greatly expanded role for nutrition in the medical curriculum, they acknowledge that the curriculum carries a heavy burden already. Many see it as a challenge to integrate adequate, meaningful nutrition information into already existing courses.

In 1990, Congress passed a law mandating that:

students enrolled in United States medical schools and physicians practicing in the United States [must] have access to adequate training in the field of nutrition and its relationship to human health.[7]

Plans are now in the works to make nutrition education a standard course in medical schools. Enlarging on this idea, the American Dietetic Association (ADA) asserts that nutrition education should be part of the curricula for all sorts of health-care professionals: physician's assistants, dental hygienists, physical and occupational therapists, social workers, and all others who provide services directly to clients.[8] This way more people would have access to reliable nutrition information.

Even though most physicians are not schooled adequately in nutrition, some are superbly qualified to speak on nutrition. All physicians appreciate the connections between health and nutrition because of their course work in biochemistry and physiology. Those who have specialized in the area called clinical nutrition in medical schools that offer that specialty are

TABLE C1-2
Credible Sources of Nutrition Information

Professional health organizations, government health agencies, volunteer health agencies, and consumer groups provide consumers with reliable health and nutrition information. Credible sources of nutrition information include:

- Professional health organizations, especially the American Dietetic Association's National Center for Nutrition and Dietetics (NCND); also the Society for Nutrition Education and the American Medical Association.
- Government health agencies such as the Federal Trade Commission (FTC), the U.S. Department of Health and Human Services (U.S. DHHS), the Food and Drug Administration (FDA), and the U.S. Department of Agriculture (USDA).
- Volunteer health agencies such as the American Cancer Society, the American Diabetes Association, and the American Heart Association.
- Reputable consumer groups such as the Better Business Bureau, the Consumers Union, the American Council on Science and Health, and the National Council on Science and Health, and the National Council Against Health Fraud.

Appendix E provides addresses for these and other organizations.

SOURCE: Data from J. M. Ashley and W. T. Jarvis, Position of the American Dietetic Association: Food and nutrition misinformation, *Journal of the American Dietetic Association* 95 (1995): 705–707.

especially well qualified. Membership in the American Society for Clinical Nutrition, whose journal is cited many times throughout this text, is another sign of nutrition knowledge. Still, few physicians have the knowledge, time, or experience to develop diet plans and provide detailed diet instruction for clients. Often physicians wisely refer their clients to nutrition specialists for diet advice. Table C1-3 lists the best specialists to choose.

Fortunately, the credential that indicates a qualified nutrition expert is easy to spot—you can confidently call on a **registered dietitian (RD).** Additionally, some states require that **nutritionists,** as well as **dietitians,** receive a **license to practice.** Meeting these established criteria certifies that an expert is the genuine article.

Dietitians are easy to find in most communities because they perform a multitude of duties in a variety of settings. They work in foodservice operations, pharmaceutical companies, the food industry, home health agencies, long-term care institutions, private clinics, public health departments, cooperative extension offices,* research centers, education settings, some fitness centers, and hospitals.

Dietitians can assume a number of different responsibilities depending on their work settings and positions.[9] Dietitians in hospitals have many subspecialties. Administrative dietitians manage the foodservice system; clinical dietitians provide client care (see Table C1-4); and nutrition support team dietitians coordinate nutrition care with the efforts of other health-care professionals. In the food industry, dietitians conduct research, develop products, and market services. Dietitians who specialize in public health nutrition work in government-funded agencies to provide nutrition services to populations. Among their many roles, **public health nutritionists** help plan, coordinate, and evaluate programs; act as consultants to other agencies; manage finances; and much more.[10] Those nutrition graduates with advanced degrees or course work in public health are well placed for employment in this vast field.

DETECTING FAKE CREDENTIALS

In contrast to RDs, thousands of people possess fake nutrition degrees and claim to be nutrition counselors, nutritionists, or "dietists." These and other such titles

may sound meaningful, but most of these people lack the established credentials of the ADA-sanctioned

TABLE C1-3
Terms Associated with Nutrition Advice

- **American Dietetic Association (ADA)**   the professional organization of dietitians in the United States. The Canadian equivalent is the Dietitians of Canada (DC),[a] which operates similarly.
- **dietitian**   a person trained in nutrition, food science, and diet planning. See also *registered dietitian*.
- **license to practice**   permission under state or federal law, granted on meeting specified criteria, to use a certain title (such as *dietitian*) and to offer certain services. Licensed dietitians may use the initials LD after their names.
- **medical nutrition therapy**   nutrition services used in the treatment of injury, illness, or other conditions; includes assessment of nutrition status and dietary intake, and corrective applications of diet, counseling, and other nutrition services.
- **nutritionist**   someone who engages in the study of nutrition. Some nutritionists are RDs, whereas others are self-described experts whose training is questionable and who are not qualified to give advice. In states with responsible legislation, the term applies only to people who have masters of science (MS) or doctor of philosophy (PhD) degrees from properly accredited institutions.
- **public health nutritionist**   a dietitian who specializes in public health nutrition.
- **registered dietitian (RD)**   a dietitian who has graduated from a university or college after completing a program of dietetics. The program must be approved or accredited by the American Dietetic Association (or Dietitians of Canada). The dietitian must serve in an approved internship, coordinated program, or preprofessional practice program to practice the necessary skills; pass the five parts of the association's *registration* examination; and maintain competency through continuing education.[b] Many states also require licensing for practicing dietitians.
- **registration**   listing with a professional organization that requires specific course work, experience, and passing of an examination.

[a]A new organization comprised of the former Canadian Dietetic Association (CDA) and 10 provincial dietetic associations.

[b]The five content areas included on the registration examination for dietitians are nutrition services, foodservice systems, management, education and communication, and evaluation and standards. L. C. Webb and J. O. Maillet, The development of test specifications for the registration examinations, *Journal of the American Dietetic Association* 90 (1990): 1134–1135.

---

*Cooperative Extension agencies are associated with land grant colleges and universities and may be found in the phone book's county government listings.

dietitian. If you look closely, you can see signs that their expertise is fake.

Take, for example, a nutrition expert's educational background. The minimal standards of education for a dietitian specify a bachelor of science (BS) degree in food science and human nutrition (or related fields) from an **accredited** college or university (Table C1-5 defines this and related terms). Such a degree generally requires four to five years of study. In contrast, a fake nutrition expert may display a degree from a six-month correspondence course; such a degree is simply not the same.* In some cases, schools posing as legitimate **correspondence schools** offer even less—they are actually **diploma mills,** fraudulent businesses that sell certificates of competency to anyone who pays the fees, from under a thousand dollars for a bachelor's degree to several thousands for a doctorate. Buyers ordering multiple degrees are even given discounts. To obtain these "degrees," a candidate need not read any books or pass any examinations.

Lack of proper accreditation is the identifying sign of a fake educational institution. To guard educational quality, an accrediting agency recognized by the U.S. Department of Education (DOE) certifies that certain schools meet the criteria defining a complete and accurate schooling, but in the case of nutrition, quack accrediting agencies cloud the picture. Fake nutrition degrees are available from schools "accredited" by more than 30 phony accrediting agencies.†

To dramatize the ease with which anyone can obtain a fake nutrition degree, one writer enrolled for $82 in a nutrition diploma mill that billed itself as a correspondence school. She made every attempt to fail. She intentionally answered all the examination questions incorrectly. Even so, she received a "nutritionist" certificate at the end of the course, together with a letter from the "school" explaining that they were sure she must have just misread the test.

In a similar stunt, Ms. Sassafras Herbert was named a "professional member" of a nutrition association. For

*To find out whether a correspondence school is accredited, write the National Home Study Council, Accrediting Commission, 1601 Eighteenth Street NW, Washington, DC 20009, or call (202) 234-5100.
†The American Council on Education published a directory of accredited institutions, professionally accredited programs, and candidates for accreditation in *Accredited Institutions of Postsecondary Education Programs Candidates* (available from many libraries). For additional information, write the Council on Postsecondary Accreditation, One Dupont Circle, Suite 305, Washington, DC 20036, or call (202) 452-1433.

TABLE C1-4
Responsibilities of a Clinical Dietitian

The first six items on this list play essential roles in **medical nutrition therapy** as part of a medical treatment plan.

- Assesses clients' nutrition status.
- Determines clients' nutrient requirements.
- Monitors clients' nutrient intakes.
- Develops, implements, and evaluates clients' nutrition care plans.
- Counsels clients to cope with unique diet plans.
- Teaches clients and their families about nutrition and diet plans.
- Provides training for other dietitians, nurses, interns, and dietetics students.
- Serves as liaison between clients and the foodservice department.
- Communicates with physicians, nurses, pharmacists, and other health-care professionals about clients' progress, needs, and treatments.
- Participates in professional activities to enhance knowledge and skill.

her efforts, Sassafras has received a wallet card and is listed in a sort of fake *Who's Who* in nutrition that is distributed at health fairs and trade shows nationwide. Sassafras is a poodle. Her master, Victor Herbert, MD, paid $50 to prove that she could be awarded these honors merely by sending in her name. Mr. Charlie Herbert also is a professional member of such an organization; Charlie is a cat.

State laws don't necessarily help consumers distinguish experts from fakes; some states allow anyone to use the titles *dietitian* or *nutritionist*. But some states are beginning to respond to the need by allowing only RDs or people with certain graduate degrees to call

TABLE C1-5
Terms Describing Institutions of Higher Learning, Legitimate and Fraudulent

- **accredited**   approved; in the case of medical centers or universities, certified by an agency recognized by the U.S. Department of Education.
- **correspondence school**   a school that offers courses and degrees by mail. Some correspondence schools are accredited; others are *diploma mills*.
- **diploma mill**   an organization that awards meaningless degrees without requiring its students to meet educational standards.

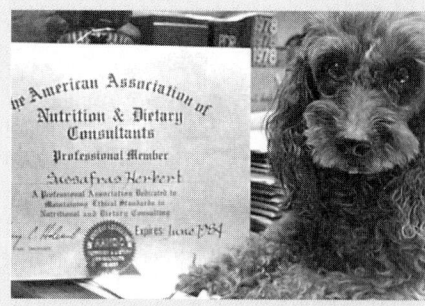 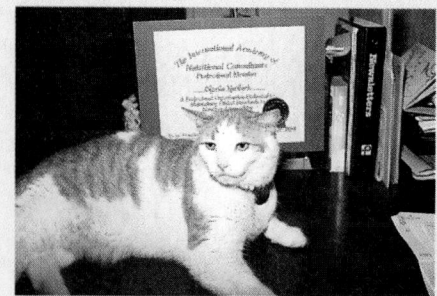

Sassafras and Charlie display their professional credentials.

themselves dietitians and many have licensing requirements.[11] Licensing provides a way to identify people who have met minimal standards of education and experience.

By knowing who is qualified to speak on nutrition, consumers are one step ahead of the nutrition quacks. Does the instructor at the spa have a degree in nutrition from an accredited university? No? Better check the instructor's advice with someone who does. Is the author of the magazine article an RD? If not, you cannot know whether to believe what you've read. Have you seen the health-store clerk's license to practice as a dietitian? If not, seek a qualified source—an RD or a person with an advanced degree in nutrition.

In summary, to check a provider's qualifications, first look for the degrees and credentials listed by the person's name (such as MD, RD, MS, PhD, or LD). Then find out what you can about the reputations of the institutions that awarded the degrees. Then call and ask your state's health-licensing agency if dietitians are licensed in your state. If they are, find out whether the person giving you dietary advice has a license—and if not, find someone better qualified. Your health is your most precious asset.

NOTES

Notes are in Appendix F.

NUTRITION STANDARDS AND GUIDELINES

2

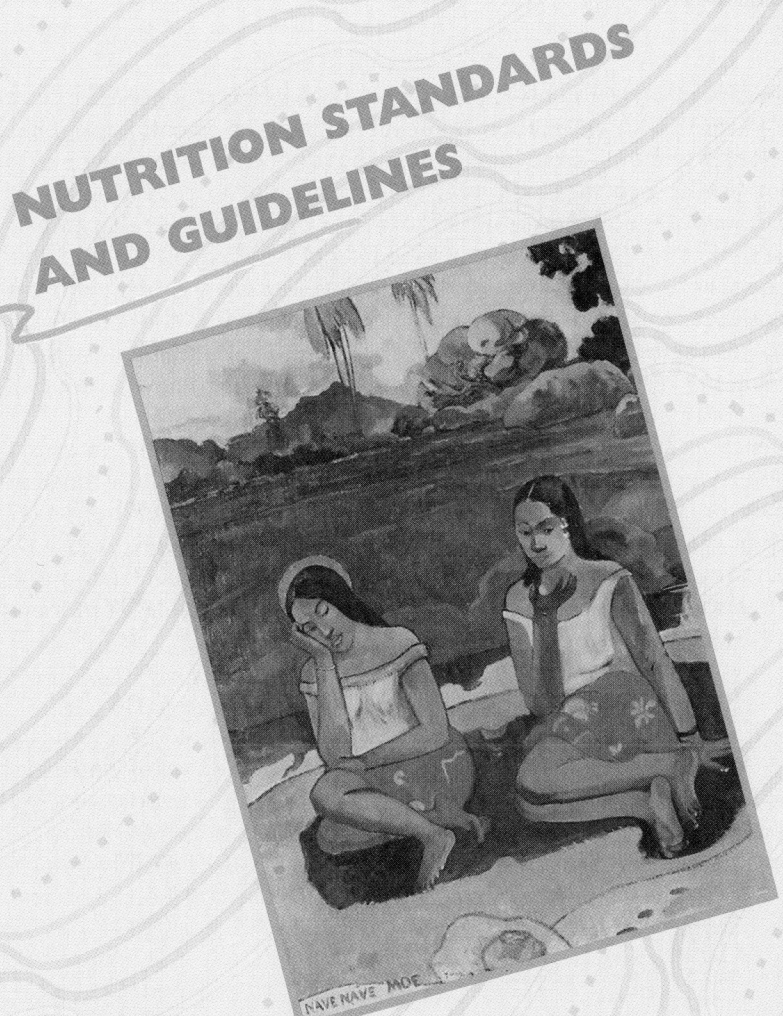

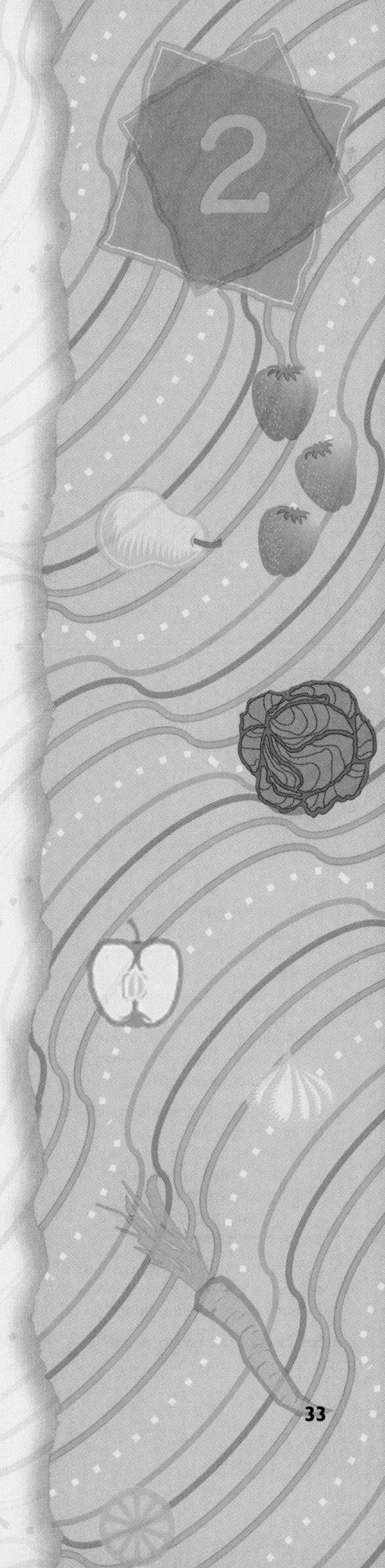

CONTENTS

Paul Gauguin 1848–1903, French, *Spring of Miracles*, Hermitage Museum, St. Petersburg, Russia, © SuperStock.

Recommended Dietary Allowances (RDA) daily consumption levels of energy and selected nutrients judged by the Food and Nutrition Board to meet the known nutrient needs of practically all healthy people.

Eating well is easy, in principle. All you have to do is choose a selection of foods that supplies appropriate amounts of the essential nutrients, fiber, and energy without excess intakes of fat, sugar, and salt. A few people do this automatically, but most do not.[1] Many people are overweight, or undernourished, or suffer from nutrient excesses or deficiencies that impair their health—that is, they are malnurished. You may not think that this statement applies to you, but you may already have less-than-optimal nutrient intakes without knowing it. Accumulated over years, the effects of malnutrition can seriously impair the quality of your life. Putting it positively, you can enjoy the best of vim, vigor, and vitality if you learn now to nourish yourself optimally.

To master the task of meeting your nutrition needs, you may find it useful to learn the answers to several questions. How much energy and how much of each nutrient do you need? Which types of foods supply which nutrients? How much of each type of food do you have to eat to get enough? And how can you eat all these foods without gaining weight and without getting too much fat or sugar? This chapter begins by identifying some ideals for nutrient intakes and ends by showing how to achieve them.

NUTRIENT RECOMMENDATIONS

The **Recommended Dietary Allowances (RDA)** are a set of yardsticks used in the United States as a standard for measuring healthy people's energy and nutrient intakes. The Canadian equivalents, the Recommended Nutrient Intakes for Canadians (RNI), are presented in Appendix B. The Daily Values, listed on page C of the inside front cover, are standards used on food labels and are described later.

RDA

RDA are set for:
- ✔ Energy.
- ✔ Protein.
- ✔ Vitamins:
  A, C, D, E, K, thiamin, riboflavin, niacin, B_6, B_{12}, folate.
- ✔ Minerals:
  Calcium, phosphorus, magnesium, iron, zinc, iodine, selenium.

Estimated safe and adequate intakes are given in ranges for:
- ✔ Vitamins:
  Biotin, pantothenic acid.
- ✔ Minerals (trace elements):
  Copper, maganese, fluoride, chromium, molybdenum.

Estimated minimum requirements of healthy persons are given for:
- ✔ Sodium, potassium, chloride.

See inside front cover for the RDA charts.

A committee of qualified nutrition experts appointed by the government publishes *recommendations* concerning appropriate nutrient intakes for the general population of this country.* These are the Recommended Dietary Allowances (RDA), and they are used and referred to so often that they are presented on pages A through C of the inside front cover of this book. As you can see, the main RDA table includes recommendations for protein, 11 vitamins, and 7 minerals, while the additional tables include 2 more vitamins and 8 more minerals as well as energy (calories). Periodically, the committee on the RDA meets to reexamine and to revise these recommendations on the basis of new research regarding people's nutrient needs. It then publishes an updated set of RDA.[2]

The RDA have been much misunderstood. One young woman, on first learning of their existence, was outraged: "You mean Uncle Sam tells me that I must eat exactly 46 grams of protein every day?" This is not the committee's intention, and the RDA are recommendations, not commandments. The following facts will help put the RDA in perspective:

■ The ongoing creation of the RDA is funded by the government, but the committee that determines the RDA is composed of scientists representing a variety of specialties.

---

*This is a committee of the Food and Nutrition Board (FNB) of the National Academy of Sciences/National Research Council (NAS/NRC).

- The RDA are based on reviews of available scientific research to the greatest extent possible and are revised periodically to keep them up to date.
- Except for sodium, potassium, and chloride, the RDA are not minimum requirements, nor are they optimal intakes. They are safe and adequate intakes that include a generous margin of safety.
- The RDA are recommended daily intakes. They are set high enough to ensure that body nutrient stores are kept full to meet needs during periods of inadequate intakes lasting a day or two for some nutrients and up to a month or two for others.
- The RDA are most appropriately used to plan diets for population groups such as schoolchildren or military personnel, but people like to use them to estimate the adequacy of their own individual intakes. The RDA can be used this way if compared with intakes over a significant period of time.
- The RDA are estimates of the needs of healthy persons only. Medical problems alter nutrient needs.

Separate recommendations are made for different sets of people: men, women, pregnant women, children, and other groups. The recommendations also vary by age. Children aged 4 to 6 years, for example, have their own RDA. Each individual can look up the recommendations for his or her own age and sex group.

No RDA is set for carbohydrate or fat. The assumption is that you will use a certain portion of your daily energy allowance meeting your protein RDA and then will distribute the remaining calories between carbohydrate and fat to meet your energy RDA. Later, this chapter will show how to balance energy sources to best support health. The next three sections describe the processes the committee goes through in selecting the RDA values, first for nutrients, then for energy.

✓ KEY POINT   **The RDA used in the United States and the RNI used in Canada represent suggested daily intakes of energy and selected nutrients for healthy people in the population.**

RDA for Nutrients

If you use the RDA to estimate the adequacy of your own diet, you need to be aware that individuals' nutrient needs vary and that the allowances are designed primarily for use with whole populations. A theoretical discussion will illustrate these points.

Suppose we were the committee members, and we had the task of setting an RDA for nutrient X (any essential nutrient). Ideally, our first step would be to try to find out how much of that nutrient various healthy individuals need. We would review studies of deficiency states, of nutrient stores and their depletion, and of the factors influencing them. We would try to select the most valid data for use in our work. Among the experiments we might review or conduct would be a **balance study.** We would take measures of the body's intake and excretion (in the case of nutrients that aren't changed before they are excreted) to find out how much of an intake is required to balance excretion. For each individual subject, we could determine a **requirement** to achieve balance for nutrient X. With an intake below the requirement, a person would slip into negative balance or experience declining stores that could, over time, lead to deficiency of the nutrient.

balance study a laboratory study in which a person is fed a controlled diet and the intake and excretion of a nutrient are measured. Balance studies are valid only for nutrients like calcium (chemical elements) that do not change while they are in the body.

requirement the amount of a nutrient that will just prevent the development of specific deficiency signs; distinguished from the RDA, which is a generous allowance with a margin of safety.

FIGURE 2-1

INDIVIDUALITY OF NUTRIENT REQUIREMENTS
Each square represents a person. A, B, and C are Mr A, Mr B, and Mr C. Each has a different requirement.

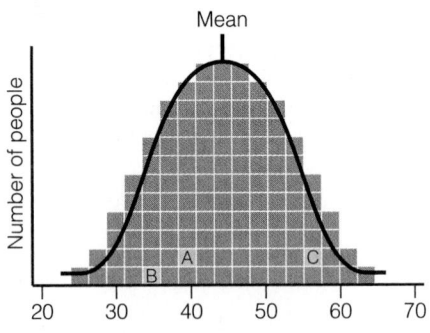

With sufficient study, we would find that different individuals, even of the same age and gender, have different requirements. Mr A might need 40 units of the nutrient each day to maintain balance; Mr B might need 35; Mr C, 57. If we looked at enough individuals, we might find that their requirements were distributed as shown in Figure 2-1—with most requirements near the midpoint (here, 45), and only a few at the extremes.

To set the RDA, we would then have to decide what intake to recommend for everybody. Should we set it at the mean (shown in Figure 2-1 at 45 units)? This is the average requirement for nutrient X; it is probably the closest to everyone's need, assuming the distribution shown in Figure 2-1. (Actually, the data for most nutrients other than protein indicate a distribution that is much less symmetrical.) But if people took us literally and consumed exactly this amount of nutrient X each day, half the population would begin to develop internal deficiencies and possibly even observable symptoms of deficiency diseases. Mr C (at 57) would be one of those people.

Perhaps we should set the RDA for nutrient X at or above the extreme, say, at 70 units a day, so that everyone would be covered. (Actually, we didn't study everyone, so some individual we didn't happen to test might have a still higher requirement.) This might be a good idea in theory, but what about a person like Mr B, who requires only 35 units a day? The recommendation would be twice his requirement, and to follow it, he might spend money needlessly on foods containing nutrient X to the exclusion of foods containing other nutrients he needs.

The choice we would finally make, with some reservations, would be to set the RDA high enough so that the bulk of the population would be covered but not so high as to be excessive. In this example, a reasonable choice might be 63 units a day. Moving the RDA further toward the extreme would pick up a few additional people but would inflate the recommendation for most people, including Mr A and Mr B.

The committee makes judgments of this kind when setting the RDA for nutrients. The RDA for nutrients are set well above the mean or average requirement that the committee has determined from available information. In theory, then, relatively few healthy people have individual requirements that are not covered by the RDA.

For these reasons the RDA are not intended to be taken personally by any individual; that is, they do not tell you exactly what your own personal requirement is. The committee members make several assumptions that may not apply to you at all. For example, they assume that you are eating a diet that includes adequate energy, protein, and all the other nutrients. They also assume that you receive your nutrients in the form of foods, not supplements, because food components affect nutrient absorption. This description may fit you exactly; then again, it may not.

✓ **KEY POINT** **The RDA are a set of yardsticks for measuring the adequacy of nutrient intakes of groups of people. They are based on valid scientific data and are designed to cover the needs of virtually all healthy people.**

"R" Is for "Recommended"

With few exceptions, the RDA are not minimum requirements. R stands for "recommended," not for "required." The RDA are allowances, and they are generous. Even so, they do not necessarily cover each individual for every nutrient. On average, one should probably try to get 100 percent or more of the RDA for every nutrient to ensure an adequate intake over time.

Beyond a certain point, though, it is unwise to consume large amounts of any nutrient. It is naive to think of the RDA simply as minimum nutrient intakes. A more accurate view is to see nutrient needs as falling within a range, with danger zones both below and above the range. Figure 2-2 illustrates this point. The RDA for the trace minerals (inside front cover), which are stated in terms of "safe (not too high) and adequate (not too low)" ranges of intakes, reflect this consideration especially clearly.

The RDA committee decided to estimate minimum requirements for sodium, potassium, and chloride. For sodium and its partner, chloride, calling the high end of the intake scale "safe" could be dangerous because people differ in their sensitivities to salt. A level that may be harmless in one person could easily worsen high blood pressure in another. A range for potassium proved difficult to justify, so the committee also provided a minimum for potassium. For each of these three minerals, the committee estimated the amount needed for growth and replacement of normal daily losses and then set the minimum requirement at that level.

The RDA and other such recommendations are for the maintenance, not the restoration, of health. Under the stress of serious illness or malnutrition, a person may require a much higher intake of certain nutrients or may not be able to handle even the RDA amount. Therapeutic diets adjust the RDA upward to account for increased needs from medical conditions, such as recovery from surgery, burns, fractures, illnesses, or addictions.

Those who use the RDA are anxiously awaiting a new edition. Although the RDA are intended for use with groups, many individuals take the recommendations personally. The experts planning the revision acknowledge the widespread personal application of the RDA, and they are planning a special book for consumers to help them use the RDA effectively.[3] The book will stress the importance of meeting nutrient needs with foods, not supplements, because food provides not just nutrients but important nonnutrients as well. The committee is also considering the theory that some supplementation may be of benefit to some people for prevention of chronic diseases, but they stress that too much of a nutrient can be as detrimental as too little.[4] The next RDA edition promises to be more flexible and applicable than ever before.

✔ KEY POINT   **Nutrient needs fall within a safety zone, with danger points above and below. Some RDA values are stated in terms of "safe and adequate."**

RDA for Energy

In setting allowances for food energy intakes, the committee took a different approach than for the nutrients. The committee had set generous allowances for protein, vitamins, and minerals, believing that a little bit extra, for a nutrient, would fill body stores enough to last through brief periods of deficient intakes. However, extra energy, even a little bit extra, on a daily basis would be harmful because it would lead to obesity. The committee therefore centered the energy RDA around the mean requirements for each age and sex group. The committee defined an acceptable energy intake range extending 20 percent

FIGURE 2-2

THE NAIVE VIEW VERSUS THE ACCURATE VIEW OF OPTIMAL NUTRIENT INTAKES
Consuming too much of a nutrient endangers health, just as consuming too little does. The RDA fall within a range of safe intake levels.

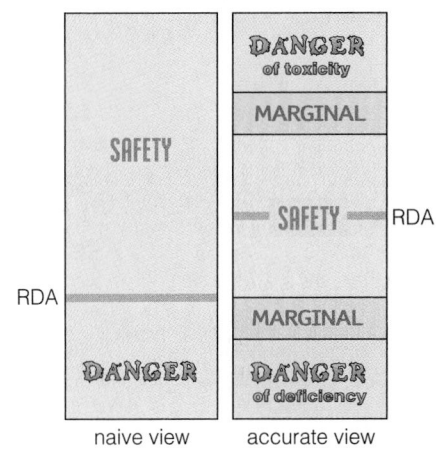

naive view   accurate view

FIGURE 2-3

THE DIFFERENCES BETWEEN THE NUTRIENT RDA AND THE ENERGY RDA
The nutrient RDA are set so that they will meet the requirements of nearly all people (boxes represent people). The energy RDA are set at the average, or mean, so that half the population's requirements will fall below and half above them.

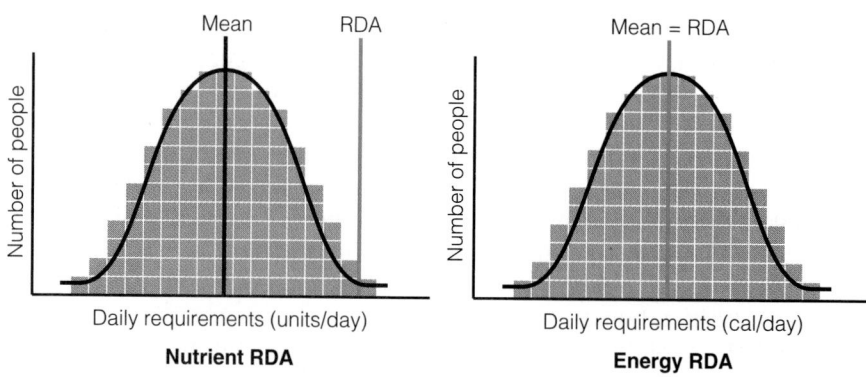

Nutrient RDA   Energy RDA

---

average a mathematical point found by adding a series of values and then dividing by the number of those values; also called the mean.

reference woman and man actual median figures for heights and weights of people of each age-sex group in the U.S. population.

above the mean, to accommodate growth, large body size, or physical activity (these require more energy), and 20 percent below this amount for most aging people or those of small body size (these require less energy). Figure 2-3 illustrates the differences between the nutrient RDA and the energy RDA set by the committee.

The energy RDA listed on the inside front cover are thus recommendations for **average** persons within groups of particular age, sex, height, weight, and activity levels according to data from extensive surveys of the U.S. population. For example, the **reference woman** aged 19 to 24 years stands 5 feet 5 inches tall and weighs 128 pounds. The **reference man** of the same age stands 5 feet 10 inches tall and weighs 160 pounds. Very few people exactly fit the average for their groups, but as Figure 2-3 showed, most people's energy needs fall close to the RDA. The best way to ensure that your food energy intake actually fits your own particular requirement is to monitor your weight compared to your food energy intake over a period of time. Chapter 9 revisits the energy RDA and shows how to control your energy intake to meet your needs.

As mentioned previously, no RDA is set for carbohydrate or fat. The committee expects that you will use the energy RDA as a guide when deciding how much carbohydrate and fat to include in your diet.

✔ KEY POINT   **The energy RDA is set at the mean of people's needs to discourage overconsumption of food energy.**

Other Nutrient Standards

Various nations and international groups have published sets of standards similar to the RDA. The RNI for Canadians are shown in Appendix B; they differ from the RDA in some respects, partly because of different interpretations of the data from which they were derived and partly because people's food intakes and daily lives in Canada differ somewhat from those in the United States.

Countries other than the United States and Canada use other standards. Many countries use recommendations developed by two international groups: the World Health Organization (WHO) and the Food and Agriculture Organization (FAO). The WHO/FAO recommendations are considered sufficient for the maintenance of health in nearly all healthy people worldwide.

The Canadiana Appendix, letter B, presents the RNI.

Appendix E, Nutrition Resources, provides addresses for WHO, FAO, and other agencies.

✓ KEY POINT **Many nations and groups issue recommendations for nutrient and energy intakes appropriate for specific groups of people.**

DIETARY GUIDELINES

So far you know that the RDA provide a standard for people's nutrient and energy intakes. Why, then, are "guidelines" needed as well? One reason is that while the RDA do much to ensure nutrient adequacy, they do little for moderation. The RDA were developed to ensure adequate nutrient intakes, and so they make specific recommendations for protein, vitamin, and mineral intakes. They also make some general statements about energy intakes, but they do little to protect people from excess intakes of fat, sugar, salt, and other food constituents believed to be related to chronic diseases. Guidelines go a step further in recommending physical activity to improve or maintain body weight. Also, the RDA refer to nutrients, not foods. People need guidance in selecting the foods they consume each day.

To ensure dietary moderation where needed, the governments of many of the developed countries have published separate sets of recommendations. These include one from the United States, two from Canada, and one intended for all the people of the world. These sets of standards are, respectively, the *Dietary Guidelines for Americans* (Table 2-1), the *Nutrition Recommendations for Canadians* (Table 2-2), Canada's Guidelines for Healthy Eating (Table 2-3), and the *World Health Organization's (WHO) Population Nutrient Goals* (Table 2-4). Only the WHO Goals set both upper and lower limits for nutrients, and they have been proposed as an international set of guidelines. Many other sets of recommendations have been published, and all offer similar advice on which nutrients to emphasize and which to control for health's sake.

Notice that these guidelines do not require that you give up your favorite foods or eat strange, unappealing foods. Many studies show that almost anyone's diet, with minor adjustments, can fit most of these recommendations.[5] The secret seems to be to modify the diet in four ways. First, learn to watch portion sizes, especially of fat-rich foods such as meat and dairy products. Second, strictly limit a few foods, especially pure fats and sugar, such as margarine and sugary soft drinks. Third, make substitutions, such as nonfat for high-fat dairy products. Finally, eat more of some foods, such as grains, fruits,

---

TABLE 2-1

Dietary Guidelines for Americans, 1995

- Eat a variety of foods.
- Balance the food you eat with physical activity—maintain or improve your weight.
- Choose a diet with plenty of grain products, vegetables, and fruits.
- Choose a diet low in fat, saturated fat, and cholesterol.
- Choose a diet moderate in sugars.
- Choose a diet moderate in salt and sodium.
- If you drink alcoholic beverages, do so in moderation.

SOURCE: *Nutrition and Your Health: Dietary Guidelines for Americans,* United States Department of Agriculture, Home and Garden Bulletin Number 232 (Washington, D.C.: Government Printing Office).

and vegetables. These four tactics, together with physical activity to balance energy intake, can change a potentially harmful diet into a nutrient-dense one that supports nutrition and health superbly.

The changes just described sound simple, but do not be deceived. Even nutrition experts struggle to design diets of appealing, nutrient-dense foods that meet both the RDA and the *Dietary Guidelines*.[6] The achievement of such a diet is a worthy goal, however, and details to help accomplish it are provided throughout this book. You will see these recommendations again wherever diet changes and the health of the body are discussed.

If the experts who develop such documents were to ask us, we would add one more recommendation to their lists: choose foods that you enjoy. While choosing foods that meet nutrient needs is of prime importance, seeking out delicious foods that meet our needs for pleasure and fun is especially important. The joys of eating are physically beneficial to the body because they trigger health-promoting changes in the nervous, hormonal, and immune systems.

Dietary recommendations encourage the health of individuals and are also best for the earth itself. Chapter and Controversy 15 explore the relationships among people, their food choices, and the planet's well-being.

TABLE 2-2

Nutrition Recommendations for Canadians

- The Canadian diet should provide energy consistent with the maintenance of *body weight* within the recommended range.
- The Canadian diet should include *essential nutrients* in amounts recommended.
- The Canadian diet should include no more than 30% of energy as *fat* (33 grams/1,000 calories or 39 grams/5,000 kilojoules) and no more than 10% as saturated fat (11 grams/1,000 calories or 13 grams/5,000 kilojoules).
- The Canadian diet should provide 55% of energy as *carbohydrate* (138 grams/1,000 calories or 165 grams/5,000 kilojoules) from a variety of sources.
- The *sodium* content of the Canadian diet should be reduced.
- The Canadian diet should include no more than 5% of total energy as *alcohol*, or two drinks daily, whichever is less.
- The Canadian diet should contain no more *caffeine* than the equivalent of four regular cups of coffee per day.
- Community water supplies containing less than 1 milligram per liter should be *fluoridated* to that level.

NOTE: Italics added to highlight areas of concern.

SOURCE: Health and Welfare Canada, *Nutrition Recommendations: The Report of the Scientific Review Committee* (Ottawa: Canadian Government Publishing Centre, 1990).

TABLE 2-3

Canada's Guidelines for Healthy Eating

- Enjoy a variety of foods.
- Emphasize cereals, breads, other grain products, vegetables, and fruits.
- Choose lower-fat dairy products, leaner meats, and foods prepared with little or no fat.
- Achieve and maintain a healthy body weight by enjoying regular physical activity and healthy eating.
- Limit salt, alcohol, and caffeine.

SOURCE: These guidelines derive from *Action Towards Healthy Eating: The Report of the Communications/Implementation Committee and Nutrition Recommendations . . . . A Call for Action: Summary Report of the Scientific Review Committee and the Communications/Implementation Committee*, which are available from Branch Publications Unit, Health Services and Promotion Branch, Department of Health and Welfare, 5th Floor, Jeanne Manice Building, Ottawa, Ontario K1A 1B4.

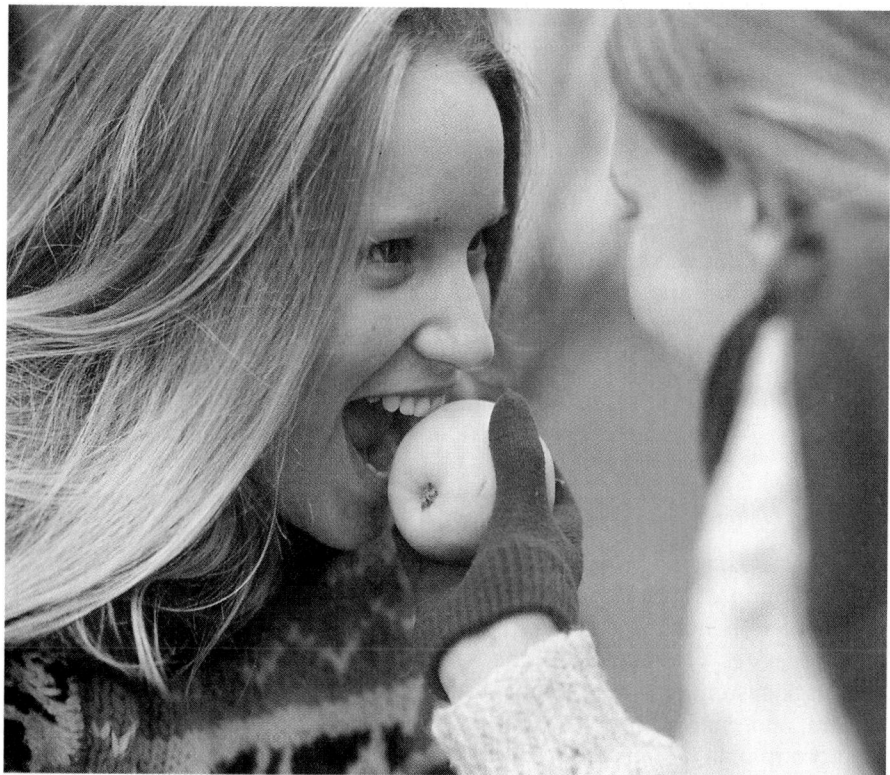

Choose foods that you enjoy.

TABLE 2-4

The WHO Population Nutrient Goals

	LIMITS FOR POPULATION AVERAGE INTAKES	
	Lower Limit	Upper Limit
Total fat	15% of energy	30% of energy[a]
Saturated fatty acids	0% of energy	10% of energy
Polyunsaturated fatty acids	3% of energy	7% of energy
Dietary cholesterol	0 mg/day	300 mg/day
Total Carbohydrate	55% of energy	75% of energy
Complex carbohydrate[b]	50% of energy	75% of energy
Dietary fiber[c]	27 g/day	40 g/day
Sugars[d]	0% of energy	10% of energy
Protein	10% of energy	15% of energy
Salt	0 g/day	6 g/day[c]

NOTE: The lower limit defines the minimum intake needed to prevent deficiency diseases, while the upper limit expresses the maximum intake compatible with the prevention of chronic diseases. This set of guidelines is proposed by WHO for acceptance as a set of international standards.

[a]An interim goal for nations with high fat intakes; further benefits would be expected by reducing fat intake toward 15% of total energy.

[b]A daily minimum intake of about 2 cups vegetables and fruits, including about a half-cup of legumes, nuts, and seeds.

[c]From mixed food sources.

[d]Added refined sugars, not the sugars found naturally in fruits, vegetables, and milk.

SOURCE: Reproduced, by permission, from *Diet, Nutrition and the Prevention of Chronic Diseases. Report of a WHO Study Group.* Geneva, World Health Organization, 1990, p. 108 (WHO Technical Report Series, No. 797).

food group plans diet planning tools that sort foods into groups based on origin and nutrient content and then specify that people should eat certain minimum numbers of servings of foods from each group.

exchange system a diet planning tool that organizes foods with respect to their nutrient contents and calorie amounts. Foods on any single exchange list can be used interchangeably. See the U.S. Exchange System, Appendix D, for details.

The five groups are:
- ✓ Bread, cereal, rice, and pasta.
- ✓ Vegetables.
- ✓ Fruit.
- ✓ Meat, poultry, fish, dry beans, eggs, and nuts.
- ✓ Milk, yogurt, and cheese.

The fats, oils, and sweets are extra and are not counted among the groups.

TABLE 2-5

Canada's Food Guide to Healthy Eating[a]

Food Group	Servings/Day
Grain products	5–12
Vegetables and fruits	5–10
Milk products	
Children aged 4–9 years:	2–3
Youth aged 10–16 years:	3–4
Adults:	2–4
Pregnant and breastfeeding women:	3–4
Meat and alternatives	2–3

[a]Canada's *Food Guide* and other Canadian guidelines are presented in full in the Canadiana Appendix B.

They ensure that people will eat and thus obtain the nutrients needed for healthy body systems, along with healthy skin, glossy hair, and the natural good looks that accompany health. People tend to repeat what brings them pleasure, and so they are most likely to stay with foods they like. Remember to enjoy your foods.

✓ KEY POINT   **The *Dietary Guidelines for Americans, Nutrition Recommendations for Canadians*, and other recommendations address the problems of overnutrition and undernutrition. To implement the recommendations requires controlling portions, limiting fat intakes, substituting nutrient-dense for fat-rich foods, and amplifying servings of low-fat grains, fruits, and vegetables.**

DIET PLANNING WITH THE DAILY FOOD GUIDE AND THE FOOD GUIDE PYRAMID

Diet planning connects nutrition theory with the food on the table. To help people plan menus, **food group plans** describe food groups and dictate numbers and sizes of servings to choose each day. Another planning tool, the **exchange system,** can help people estimate the amounts of carbohydrate, fat, protein, and energy (calories) that each type of food provides. The Canadian food group plan, *Food Guide to Healthy Eating,* is presented in full in Appendix B, and a brief description appears in Table 2-5 in the margin.

The Daily Food Guide

In past decades, schoolchildren learned about the Four Food Group Plan, which taught generations of people to recognize key nutrients provided by certain related groups of foods. Today the Daily Food Guide (see Figure 2-4, pages 44 and 45) is based on five groups instead of four, but many of the original concepts still apply. The Food Guide Pyramid is a visual representation of the new plan.

The foods in each group are well-known contributors of certain key nutrients, but you can count on them to supply many other nutrients as well. If you design your diet around this plan, it is assumed that you will obtain adequate amounts not only of the nutrients named in the figure but also of the other two dozen or so essential nutrients because they are distributed among the same groups of foods. This is true in theory. In practice, however, diet planners must be sure to choose mostly nutrient-dense foods in each group because some processes strip foods of some nutrients and add calories from fat. Figure 2-4 identifies a few foods in each group as having high, moderate, or low nutrient density to give you an idea of which are which. With this caution, the Daily Food Guide can provide a reasonable road map for diet planning.

✓ KEY POINT   **The Daily Food Guide and other food group plans sort foods into groups based on their nutrients and origins. Then they suggest patterns of intake by group that will cover nutrient needs.**

Using the Daily Food Guide and the Food Guide Pyramid

As mentioned, the pyramid-shaped diagram at the bottom of Figure 2-4 is a graphic depiction of the Daily Food Guide. The illustration was designed to depict variety, moderation, and also proportions: the size of each section reflects the number of daily servings recommended. The pyramid shape, with its broad base of grains at the bottom, conveys the idea that you should eat more grain foods than anything else: grains form the foundation of a healthful diet. Next in volume are the fruits and vegetables. Meats and milks are dense in nutrients such as protein and are important sources of vitamins and minerals, but the number of servings must be limited because these foods can also be high in fat and calories.

Fats, oils, and sweets occupy only a tiny triangle at the top of the Food Guide Pyramid, an indication that they should be used sparingly. These foods do not comprise a food group, since servings of them are optional, that is, not required to promote health. Alcoholic beverages provide no nutrients and are excluded from the Food Guide Pyramid altogether. They are high in calories, however, and must be counted in a day's tally, so a glass of wine appears in Figure 2-4 as a reminder. Spices, coffee, tea, and diet soft drinks, also excluded from the pyramid, provide few, if any, nutrients, but can add flavor and pleasure to meals as well as some potentially beneficial nonnutrients, such as those of tea.

The beauty of the Food Guide Pyramid lies in its simplicity. Also, although it may appear rigid, it can actually be very flexible once its intent is understood. For example, the user can substitute cheese for milk because both supply the key nutrients for the milk, yogurt, and cheese group. The user can choose legumes (beans) and nuts as alternatives to meats. One can adapt the plan to mixed dishes such as casseroles as well as to national and cultural cuisines as Figure 2-5 on page 46 shows.

As mentioned the Food Guide Pyramid tends to deemphasize meats and animal products such as milk, cheese, and eggs and to emphasize grains, fruits, and vegetables. This scheme can assist vegetarians in their food choices, while encouraging others to choose foods from plants most often. The food group that includes the meats also includes *meat alternates*—foods such as legumes, nuts, and tofu. As for the food group that includes milk and milk products, people who choose not to use dairy foods can substitute soy "milk"—a product made from soybeans that fills the same nutrient needs, provided that it is fortified with calcium and vitamin B$_{12}$. In short, people who choose to eat no meats or products taken from animals can still use the Food Guide Pyramid to make their diets adequate.

Vegetarians will find more tips for choosing the right foods to supply the nutrients they need in the chapters to come.

☑ KEY POINT **The Daily Food Guide and its visual image, the Food Guide Pyramid, convey the basics of planning a diet adequate in nutrients.**

Drawbacks to the Food Guide Pyramid

The Food Guide Pyramid does have drawbacks, however. It does not limit food choices to foods low in calories. People who select the minimum number of servings from among the most nutrient-dense foods in each group and who strictly limit their use of fats, sweets, and alcoholic beverages can keep their

FIGURE 2-4

THE DAILY FOOD GUIDE AND THE FOOD GUIDE PYRAMID

> **KEY: Nutrient Density**
> ■ Foods generally highest in nutrient density (preferable first choice).
> ■ Foods moderate in nutrient density (reasonable second choice).
> ■ Foods lowest in nutrient density (limit selections).

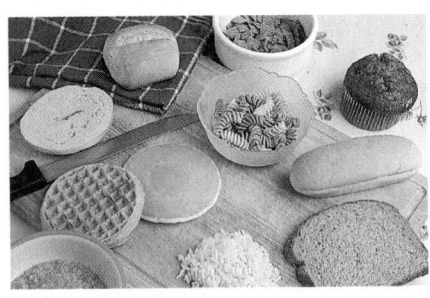

BREAD, CEREAL, RICE, AND PASTA GROUP

These foods contribute complex carbohydrates and fiber, plus riboflavin, thiamin, niacin, iron, protein, magnesium, and other nutrients.
6 to 11 servings per day.
Serving = 1 slice bread: ½ c cooked cereal, rice, or pasta: 1 oz ready-to-eat cereal; ½ bun, bagel, or English muffin; 1 small roll, biscuit, or muffin; 3 to 4 small or 2 large crackers.

■ Whole grains (wheat, oats, barley, millet, rye, bulgur), enriched breads, rolls, tortillas, cereals, bagels, rice, pastas (macaroni, spaghetti), air-popped corn.
■ Pancakes, muffins, cornbread, crackers, low-fat cookies, biscuits, presweetened cereals, granola.
■ Croissants, fried rice, doughnuts, pastries, sweet rolls.

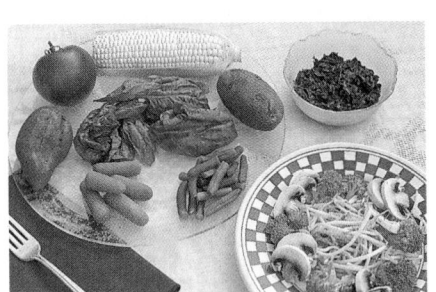

VEGETABLE GROUP

These foods contribute fiber, vitamin A, vitamin C, folate, potassium, and magnesium.
3 to 5 servings per day (use dark green, leafy vegetables and legumes several times a week).
Serving = ½ c cooked or raw vegetables; 1 c leafy raw vegetables; ½ c cooked legumes;[a] ¾ c vegetable juice.

■ Bean sprouts, broccoli, brussels sprouts, cabbage, carrots, cauliflower, cucumbers, green beans, green peas, leafy greens (spinach, mustard, and collard greens), legumes, lettuce, mushrooms, summer and winter squash, tomatoes.
■ Corn, potatoes, sweet potatoes, yams.
■ French fries, olives, tempura vegetables.

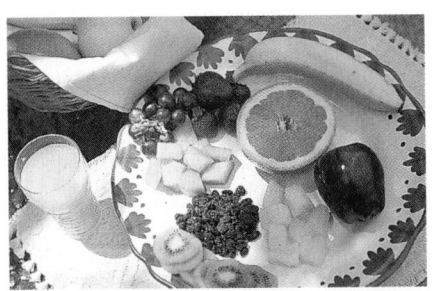

FRUIT GROUP

These foods contribute fiber, vitamin A, vitamin C, and potassium.
2 to 4 servings per day.
Serving = typical portion (such as 1 medium apple, banana, or orange, ½ grapefruit, 1 melon wedge; ¾ c juice; ½ c berries; ½ c diced, cooked, or canned fruit; ¼ c dried fruit.

■ Apricots, cantaloupe, grapefruit, oranges, orange juice, peaches, strawberries, applies, bananas, pears.
■ Canned or frozen fruit.
■ Avocados, dried fruit.

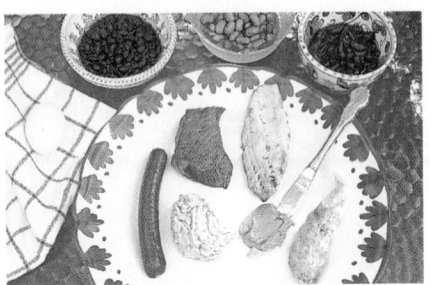

MEAT, POULTRY, FISH, DRY BEANS, EGGS, AND NUTS

These foods contribute protein, phosphorus, vitamin B_6, vitamin B_{12}, zinc, magnesium, iron, niacin, and thiamin.
2 to 3 servings per day.
Serving = 2 to 3 oz lean, cooked meat, poultry, or fish (total 5 to 7 oz per day); count 1 egg, ½ c cooked legumes,[a] or 2 tbs peanut butter as 1 oz meat (or about ⅓ serving).

■ Poultry, fish, lean meat (beef, lamb, pork, veal), legumes, egg whites.
■ Fat-trimmed beef, lamb, pork; refried beans; egg yolks, tofu, tempeh.
■ Hot dogs, luncheon meats, peanut butter, nuts (including coconut), sausage, bacon, fried fish or poultry, duck.

MILK, YOGURT, AND CHEESE

These foods contribute calcium, riboflavin, protein, vitamin B_{12}, and, when fortified, vitamin D and vitamin A.

2 servings per day.

3 servings per day for teenagers and young adults, pregnant/lactating women, women past menopause.

4 servings per day for pregnant-lactating teenagers.

Serving = 1 c milk or yogurt; 2 oz process cheese food; 1½ oz cheese.

- Nonfat and 1% low-fat milk (and nonfat products such as buttermilk, cottage cheese, cheese, yogurt); fortified soy milk.
- 2% low-fat milk (and low-fat products such as yogurt, cheese, cottage cheese); sherbet; ice milk.
- Whole milk (and whole-milk products such as cheese, yogurt, cottage cheese); custard; milk shakes; pudding; ice cream.

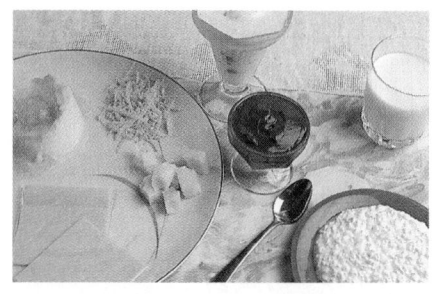

FATS, OILS, AND SWEETS

These foods contribute sugar, fat, alcohol, and food energy (calories). Their consumption should be limited because these foods provide few nutrients. Alcoholic beverages are not classed as foods on the pyramid; they contribute few nutrients, but they do contribute calories, and so are mentioned here.

- Foods high in fat include butter, margarine, salad dressings, oils, mayonnaise, cream, sour cream, cream cheese, gravy, and sauces.
- Foods high in sugar include candy fruit rolls, other candies, soft drinks, fruit drinks, jelly, syrup, gelatin, desserts, sugar, and honey.
- Alcoholic beverages include wine, beer, and liquor.

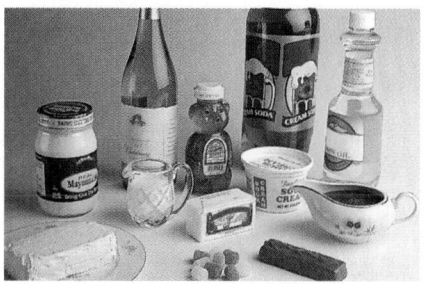

---

aThe Daily Food Guide lists legumes (dried beans, lentils, and peas) both under vegetables, for their starch, fiber, and vitamins, and under meats, for their protein and minerals.
NOTE: Serve children at least the lower number of servings from each group, but in smaller amounts (for example, ¼ to ⅓ cup rice). Children should receive the equivalent of 2 cups of milk each day; but in smaller quantities per serving (for example, 4 half-cup portions). Pregnant women may require additional servings of fruits, vegetables, meats, and breads to meet their higher needs for energy, vitamins, and minerals.

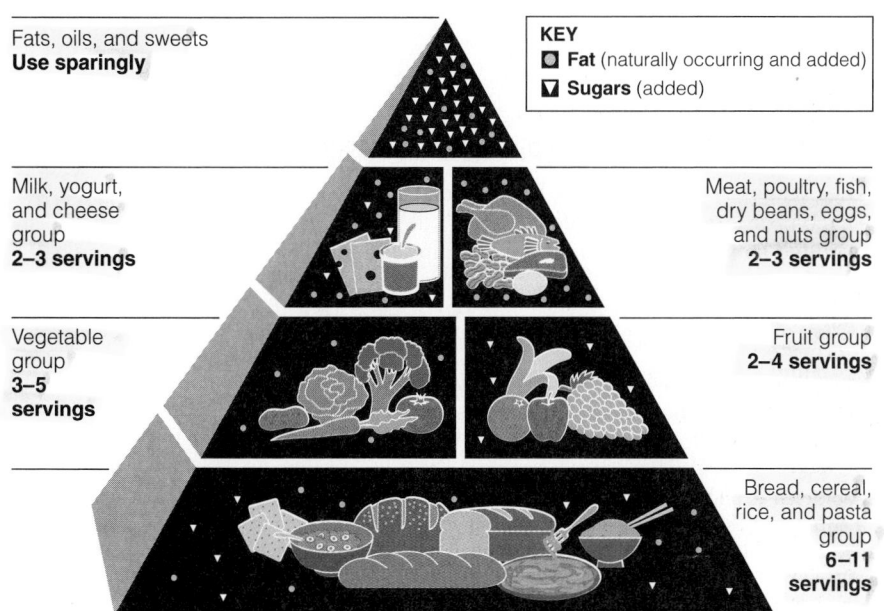

Fats, oils, and sweets
Use sparingly

KEY
- **Fat** (naturally occurring and added)
- **Sugars** (added)

Milk, yogurt, and cheese group
2–3 servings

Meat, poultry, fish, dry beans, eggs, and nuts group
2–3 servings

Vegetable group
3–5 servings

Fruit group
2–4 servings

Bread, cereal, rice, and pasta group
6–11 servings

FOOD GUIDE PYRAMID: A GUIDE TO DAILY FOOD CHOICES
The breadth of the base shows that grains (breads, cereals, rice, and pasta) deserve the most emphasis in the diet. The tip is smallest: use fats, oils, and sweets sparingly.

FIGURE 2-5

ADDING VARIETY WITH ETHNIC AND REGIONAL FOODS

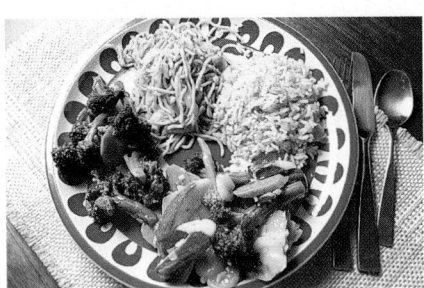

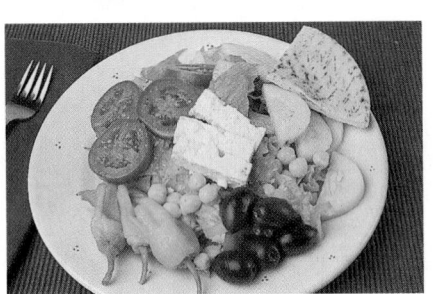

KEY: Nutrient Density

■ Foods generally highest in nutrient density (preferable first choice).

■ Foods moderate in nutrient density (reasonable second choice).

■ Foods lowest in nutrient density (limit selections).

CHINESE[a]

Bread, Cereal, Rice, and Pasta Group

■ Millet; rice; rice noodles.
■ Fried rice.

Vegetable Group

■ Bamboo shoots; bean sprouts; cabbages; scallions; seaweed; snow peas; soybeans; water chestnuts.
■ Fried vegetables.

Fruit Group

■ Plums, oranges, pears, and other fresh fruit.

Meat, Poultry, Fish, Dry Beans, Eggs, and Nuts Group

■ Broiled or stir-fried fish and seafood; egg whites.
■ Broiled or stir-fried beef or pork; egg yolks; tofu.
■ Deep-fried meats and seafood; egg foo young; pine nuts and cashews.

Fats, Oils, and Sweets

■ Lard or oil for deep-frying.

Seasonings and Sauces[b]

■ Bean sauce; garlic; ginger root; hoisin sauce;[c] oyster sauce;[c] plum sauce;[c] rice wine; scallions; soy sauce.[c]
■ Sesame oil; other oils.

GREEK

Bread, Cereal, Rice, and Pasta Group

■ Greek breads.

Vegetable Group

■ Eggplant; lentils and beans; onions; peppers; tomatoes.
■ Olives.

Fruit Group

■ Dates; figs; grapes; lemons; raisins.

Milk, Yogurt, and Cheese Group

■ Low-fat yogurt.
■ Feta cheese; goat cheese.

Meat, Poultry, Fish, Dry Beans, Eggs, and Nuts Group

■ Egg whites; fish and seafood; lentils and beans.
■ Egg yolks; lamb; poultry; beef.
■ Ground lamb; ground beef; gyros; walnuts; almonds.

Fats, Oils, and Sweets

■ Olive oil; baklava (honey-soaked nut pastry); honey; cakes.

Seasonings and Sauces

■ Garlic; herbs; lemons; egg and lemon sauce.
■ Olive oil.

---

[a]Traditional cuisines of China and of West African influence exclude fluid milk as a beverage for adults and use few or no milk products in cooking. Calcium and certain other nutrients of milk are supplied by other foods, such as small fish eaten with the bones or large servings of leafy green vegetables.
[b]Most Chinese sauces are fat-free.
[c]May be high in sodium.

MEXICAN

Bread, Cereal, Rice, and Pasta Group

- Cereal; corn or flour tortillas; macaroni; rice.
- Graham crackers.
- Fried tortilla shells; tortilla chips.

Vegetable Group

- Cabbage; cactus; iceberg lettuce; legumes; squash; tomatoes.
- Corn; potatoes.
- Olives.

Fruit Group

- Bananas; guava; oranges; papaya; pineapple.
- Avocados.

Milk, Yogurt, and Cheese Group

- Evaporated low-fat milk; powdered nonfat milk.
- Cheddar or jack cheese; custard.

Meat, Poultry, Fish, Dry Beans, Eggs, and Nuts Group

- Fish; lean beef, poultry, lamb, and pork; many bean varieties.
- Egg yolks; refried beans.
- Bacon; fried fish, pork, or poultry; nuts; sausages.

Fats, Oils, and Sweets

- Butter; candy; cream cheese; lard; margarine; pastries; soft drinks; vegetable oil; sour cream.

Seasonings and Sauces[d]

- Herbs; hot peppers; garlic; pico de gallo; salsas; spices.
- Guacamole; lard.

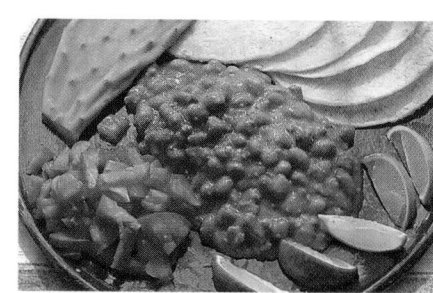

DEEP SOUTH (WEST AFRICAN INFLUENCE)[a]

Bread, Cereal, Rice, and Pasta Group

- Rice.
- Biscuits; cornbread; pastries.

Vegetable Group

- Beans; black-eyed peas; collards (other leafy greens); okra; tomatoes.
- Corn; sweet potatoes; hominy.
- Fried green tomatoes; fried okra.

Fruit Group

- Apples; berries; melons; peaches; pears.
- Fried pies; fruit pastries.

Meat, Poultry, Fish, Dry Beans, Eggs, and Nuts Group

- Beans and peas; grilled or smoked poultry and fish.
- Braised or roasted meats (beef, poultry).
- Bacon; boiled peanuts;[e] fried chicken or pork; ham hocks; peanut butter; salted pork; sausage; spareribs.

Fats, Oils, and Sweets

- Butter; lard; shortening; gravy.

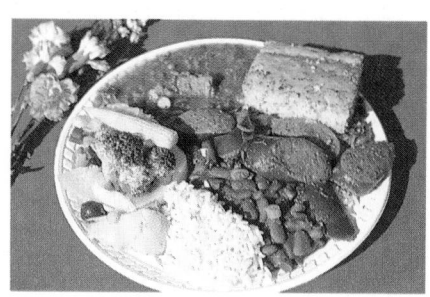

---

[d]Many Mexican sauces are fat-free.
[e]The peanut, a native of South America, was carried to West Africa by Portuguese explorers.

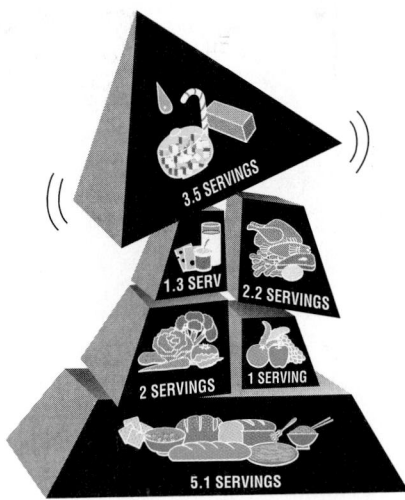

Here's how the typical U.S. diet stacks up.

SOURCE: National Livestock and Meat Board, courtesy of the National Cattlemen's Beef Association.

Details of Canada's *Food Guide to Healthy Eating* are found in the Canadiana Appendix, letter B.

energy intakes low, but people who use the higher-calorie foods in each group and who eat large servings, even without extra fats, sweets, or alcohol added in, can easily obtain too many calories.

In the cheese-for-milk substitution mentioned earlier, sufficient cheddar cheese to meet a day's calcium requirement would also provide almost 700 calories, over 70 percent of them from fat. A day's calcium from nonfat milk comes with fewer than 350 calories and with hardly any fat. Less obvious but significant over time are energy differences between sliced bread and biscuits, fish and hot dogs, or even green beans and sweet potatoes—all proper substitutions according to the Food Guide Pyramid. High-calorie choices may be just what some people, such as athletes, need to meet their high energy requirements, but for others such choices can dramatically boost energy intakes and, over time, add too much to body fat stores.

The Food Guide Pyramid attempts to caution consumers about fats and added sugars in food groups by sprinkling symbols for those two constituents across the pictures of the groups most likely to contain them. This scheme may be difficult to put into practical use, however. The bread group, for example, is sprinkled with the symbols for both fat and added sugar because baked goods can be high in those constituents. No attempt is made, however, to point out individual high-fat or high-sugar foods within the groups. As the drawing in the margin shows, most people in the United States consume far more fat and sugar than dietary wisdom would allow—and fall short in the areas of nutritious foods. They need more guidance in selecting foods.

Another criticism of the Food Guide Pyramid is that a person may choose the right number of servings from each group, yet make consistently nutrient-poor choices, and so fail to meet the day's needs for some nutrients. A diet can easily lack vitamin E or certain essential fatty acids, for example, because these nutrients are easily destroyed in processing or refined out of foods.[7]

✓ KEY POINT **Among the drawbacks of the Food Guide Pyramid is its failure to show how to use nutrient-dense foods to form the bulk of food selections from each food group.**

Planning a Diet with the Food Guide Pyramid

The Food Guide Pyramid assists you in planning a day's meals with all the needed servings from each class of nutritious foods. By using it wisely, and by learning about the energy-yielding nutrients in foods, you can achieve the goals of a nutritious diet mentioned in Chapter 1: *a*dequacy, *b*alance, *c*alorie control, *m*oderation, and *v*ariety.

To achieve adequacy, adults using the Food Guide Pyramid must choose at least six servings from the bread, cereal, rice, and pasta group; three from the vegetable group; two from the fruit group; two from the meat, poultry, fish, dry beans, eggs, and nuts group; and two from the milk, yogurt, and cheese group. Many people use shorthand to remember the pattern; six, three, two, two, and two. These are the minimum numbers of servings. The plan's makers suggest that to meet additional energy needs, a person should choose more servings of foods from these very same groups.

Note that for each food group the table presents a range of numbers of servings. Find yourself among the descriptions of people at the top of Table 2-6,

Remember: six, three, two, two, and two.

TABLE 2-6

How Many Servings?

	Sedentary Women, Some Older Adults	Children, Teenage Girls, Active Women, Sedentary Men	Teenaged Boys, Active Men
Calories[a]	About 1,600	About 2,000	About 2,800
Breads, cereals, rice, and pastas group	6	9	11
Vegetable group	3	4	5
Fruit group	2	3	4
Milk, yogurt, and cheese group[b]	2–3	2–3	2–3
Meat, poultry, fish, dry beans, eggs, and nuts group	2 (5 oz total)	2 (6 oz total)	3 (7 oz total)
Total fat (g)	53	73	93
Added sugar (tsp)	6	12	18

[a]Assumes mostly low-fat and low-calorie food choices.

[b]Women who are pregnant or lactating, teenagers, and young adults to age 24 need three servings.

SOURCE: U.S. Department of Agriculture, *Home and Garden Bulletin* 252 (1992): 9.

then look at the column of numbers below for the approximate number of servings to take from each food group to meet your calorie goal.

Clearly, a sedentary person can meet the plan's requirements and still eat only about 1,600 calories (see Table 2-7). If you are only moderately active, you can probably eat an additional 600 to 1,200 calories without gaining weight. The more active you are, the higher the energy allowance you "earn." A wise choice is to invest many of these additional calories in additional nutrient-dense vegetables, legumes, fruits, and whole-grain foods and only a few in luxury items such as sweet desserts, butter, margarine, oil, or alcohol. If you make additions from the latter group, make them by conscious choice rather than through the unintentional use of high-calorie foods. With judicious selections, the diet can supply all the necessary nutrients and provide some luxury items as well.

For a person wishing to use the Food Guide Pyramid meaningfully, it still remains to clarify what is meant by the word *serving,* for it can mean different things to different people.[8] Owners of restaurants, whose patrons want their money's worth, often deliver impressive colossal-sized servings to ensure repeat business; a server on a cafeteria line may be instructed to deliver "about a spoonful" of the foods offered; makers of frozen entrées fill up partitioned trays with whatever amounts of foods fit within the sections; fast-food burgers range from a one-ounce miniburger to a half-pound double deluxe; and so on. The trend in the United States has been toward consuming larger portions of just about everything (see Figure 2-6). At the same time body weights have been creeping upwards demonstrating an increasing need to control portions.

Remember the goals of a good diet: ABCMV.

In contrast, serving sizes in the Food Guide Pyramid are specific and precise and can be relied upon to deliver certain amounts of key nutrients in foods. Among volumetric measures, one "cup" refers to an 8-ounce measuring cup (not a teacup or drinking glass), filled to level (not heaped up, nor shaken or pressed down). Tablespoons and teaspoons refer to measuring spoons (not flatware) filled to level (not rounded). Ounces signify weight, not volume. Two ounces of meat, for example, refers to ⅛ pound of cooked meat. One ounce (weight) of granola cereal measures ¼ cup (volume), but take care: one ounce of crispy rice cereal measures a full cup. The Table of Food Composition, Appendix A lists both weights and volumes to ease conversions.

Wise diners also read labels of packaged foods to help them determine the foods' nutrient contents and to decide how the foods may fit into their total eating plan. This chapter's Consumer Corner explains how to gain insight from the information on food labels.

✔ KEY POINT **The Food Guide Pyramid can ease diet planning. The pyramid provides the framework that ensures adequacy and balance, but it's up to the diner to achieve calorie control and moderation.**

TABLE 2-7

Sample Diet Planned with the Food Guide Pyramid

Breakfast: Cornflakes with milk and sugar; toast; coffee; orange juice.
Lunch: Small cheeseburger; macaroni salad; banana; diet cola.
Supper: Chili with beans, beef, and rice; spinach salad with dressing; corn on the cob with margarine; water.

Pattern from the Pyramid	Example	Energy Cost (cal)[a]
Breads, cereals, rice, and pastas group—6 servings	½ c white rice	134
	½ c macaroni salad	106
	1 oz cornflakes	110
	2 slices	181
	1 bun	91
Meat, poultry, fish, dry beans, eggs, and nuts group—2 servings (2 to 3 oz each)	½ c chili beans	85
	3 oz extra lean ground beef	225
Fruit group—2 servings	1 banana	105
	¾ c orange juice	84
Vegetable group—3 servings	½ c tomato sauce	37
	1 c spinach leaves	12
	1 medium corn on cob	83
Milk, yogurt, and cheese group—2 servings	1 c nonfat milk	86
	2 oz processed cheese	213
Added fat	2 pats reduced fat margarine	38
	1 tbs low-calorie salad dressing	22
Added sugar—1 tsp	12 oz diet cola	0
	1 tsp sugar	16
		Total: 1,628

[a]Values from the Table of Food Composition, Appendix A.

FIGURE 2-6

U.S. TREND TOWARD *COLOSSAL CUISINE*

Food	Food Guide Pyramid	Typical 1977	Super 1996
cola	—	10 oz bottle, 120 cal	40–60 oz fountain, 580 cal
bagel	½ bagel, 90 cal	2–3 oz, 230 cal	5–7 oz, 550 cal
french fries	10, 160 cal	about 30, 475 cal	about 50, 790 cal
hamburger	2–3 oz meat, 240 cal	3–4 oz meat, 330 cal	6–8 oz meat, 650 cal
steak	2–3 oz, 170 cal	8–12 oz, 690 cal	16–22 oz, 1,260 cal
pasta	½ cup, 100 cal	1 cup, 200 cal	2–3 cups, 600 cal
baked potato	3–4 oz, 110 cal	5–7 oz, 180 cal	one pound, 420 cal
candy bar	—	1½ oz, 220 cal	3–4 oz, 580 cal
popcorn	—	1½ cups, 80 cal	8–16 cup tub, 880 cal

NOTE: Calories are rounded values for the largest portions in a given range.

SOURCE: Data for most entries from L. R. Young and M. Nestle, Portion sizes in dietary assessment: Issues and implications, *Nutrition Reviews* 53 (1995): 149–158.

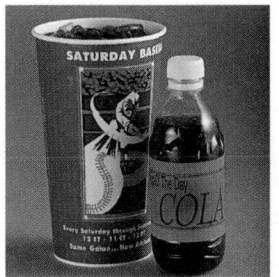
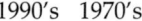

1990's 1970's

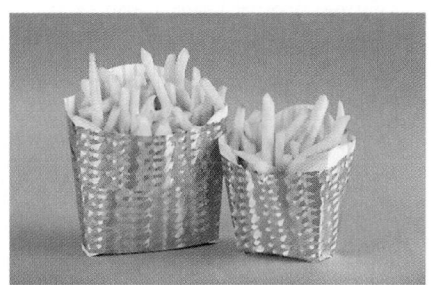

1990's   1970's

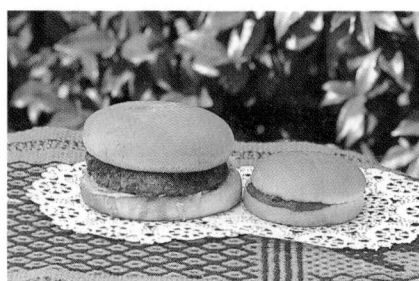

1990's   1970's

A Note about Exchange Lists

Exchange lists are lists of food portions that specify the carbohydrate, fat, and protein contents of each portion and also provide an estimate of the calories. Exchange systems are popular among careful diet planners, especially those who wish to control calories (weight watchers) and those who must control carbohydrate intakes (people with diabetes) or their intakes of fat and saturated fat (almost everyone).

You can use the exchange lists to ensure that your diet is up to standards set not only for adequacy but also for moderation and calorie control—the special advantages of exchange systems. The exchange system also highlights a fact that the Food Guide Pyramid overlooks: most foods provide more than just one energy nutrient. Meat, for example, is famous for protein, but many meats deliver more calories from fat than from protein. Pasta and bread contain significant protein with their carbohydrates. Milk products contain carbohydrates and protein, but their fat values vary; and so on. To explore this powerful aid to diet planning, spend some time studying the U.S. Food Exchange System in Appendix D, or the Canadian Exchange System, Appendix B.

✔ KEY POINT **Exchange lists facilitate calorie control by providing an understanding of how much carbohydrate, fat, and protein are in each food group.**

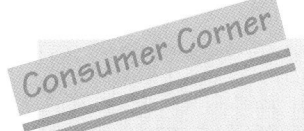

Consumer Corner

CHECKING OUT FOOD LABELS

A package of potato chips must tell you on its label that it contains potato, fat, and salt; and it must also reveal its nutrient composition. In contrast, a potato is a potato, and it bears no label to tell you what nutrients it contains. So how can you know what useful roles fresh foods play in your diet? In regard to the potato, you may be able to read about it on a sign or handout near the potato bin at the grocery store. Grocers often voluntarily post placards in fresh-food departments to provide consumers with nutrition information for the 20 most popular types of fruits, vegetables, and seafoods.

As for most packaged foods, you can use them artfully in diet planning if you can interpret their labels. The Nutrition Education and Labeling Act of 1990 brought sweeping changes in the requirements for label information. According to the law, every food label must state the following:

■ The common or usual name of the product.
■ The name and address of the manufacturer, packer, or distributor.
■ The net contents in terms of weight, measure, or count.

Then, the label must list the following in ordinary language:

■ The ingredients, in descending order of predominance by weight.

Most food labels must conform with all these requirements.[9]

Ingredient List

Knowing how to read an ingredient list puts you many steps ahead of the naive buyer. Whatever is listed first is the ingredient that predominates

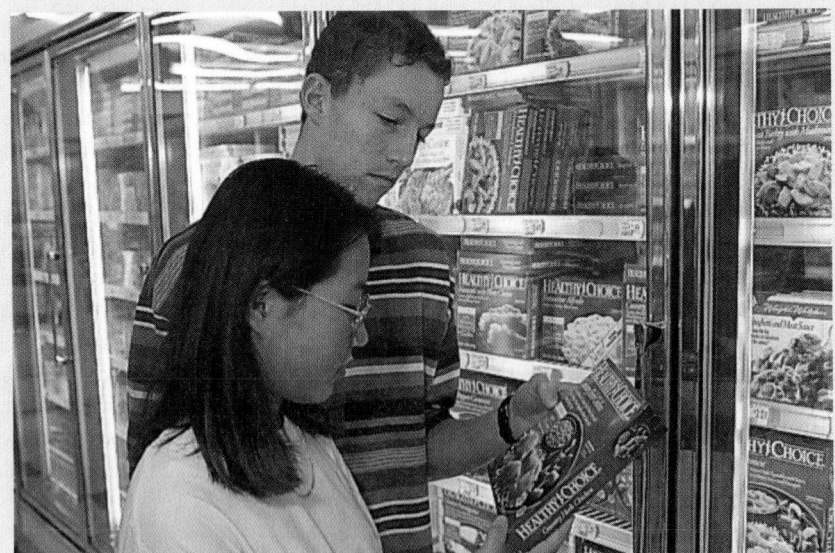

Modern-day entertainment: Reading food labels.

by weight. Consider the ingredient list on an orange drink powder whose first three ingredients are "sugar, citric acid, orange flavor." You can tell that sugar is the chief ingredient. Now look at a canned juice whose ingredient list begins with "water, orange juice concentrate, pineapple juice concentrate." This product is clearly made of reconstituted juice. Water is first on the label because it is the main constituent of juice. Sugar is nowhere to be found among the ingredients because sugar has not been added to the product. Sugar does occur naturally in juice, though, so the label *does* specify sugar grams; details are in Chapter 4.

Now look at a cereal whose entire list contains just one item: "100 percent shredded wheat." No question, this is a whole-grain food with nothing added. Finally, consider a cereal whose first three ingredients are "puffed milled corn, sweeteners (sugars: corn syrup, sucrose, honey, dextrose), salt." If you can recognize that sugar, corn syrup, honey, and dextrose are all different versions of sugar (and you will, after Chapter 4), you'll know that this product may contain close to half its weight as sugar.

Daily Values

The **Daily Values** were designed solely for listing nutrients on U.S. food labels. They are based partly on the RDA and partly on a set of standards designed especially for food labels. Students who learn about the RDA ask why experts deemed it necessary to develop a whole new set of standards for food labels. Why not just use the RDA? One answer is that the RDA values vary from group to group, whereas on a label, one set of values must apply to everyone. Another answer is that a label must specify daily amounts of nutrients not covered by the RDA, such as fat. The Daily Values do two things, then: they set *adequacy* standards for some nutrients that are desirable in the diet, such as the vitamins and fiber, and they also set *moderation* standards for other nutrients that must be limited, such as fat, cholesterol, and sodium according to the *Dietary Guidelines*. The amount of each of these nutrients in the food is expressed as a percentage of the Daily Value. To obtain enough of the hard-to-get nutrients while limiting those nutrients that can pose problems, a reasonable goal is to consume a diet that provides about 100 percent of all the nutrients listed on labels.

The calculations that determine the "% Daily Value" figures on a label are based on a 2,000-calorie diet. Of course, people's actual calorie intakes vary widely, with some people needing fewer than 2,000 calories, and some needing many more. Still, knowing a food's general nutrient profile can give an indication of how well the food fits any person's nutrient needs.

The Daily Values are intended to be easy to interpret. They are the basis upon which foods may claim to be "low" in cholesterol or a "good

(*continued on next page*)

source" of vitamin A. A rule of thumb states that any food containing less than 5 percent of the Daily Value for a nutrient provides just a small amount of the nutrient.[10] The Daily Values are listed on the inside front cover, page C, and on labels they appear in the "Nutrition Facts" panel, described next.

Nutrition Facts

When you read a "Nutrition Facts" panel, be aware that only the top portion of the panel conveys information specific to food inside the package. The bottom portion of the label lists the Daily Values for a 2,000-calorie diet as a handy reference for label-readers. The top portion of the panel provides the following nutrient information pertaining to the food in the package:

- Standard serving size expressed in both common household and metric measures to allow comparison of foods within a food category.
- Number of servings or portions per box, can, package, or other unit.
- Total food energy (calories) per serving.
- Food energy (calories) from fat per serving.
- Fat (grams) per serving with a breakdown showing saturated fat (grams) and cholesterol (milligrams).
- Sodium (milligrams) per serving.
- Carbohydrate (grams) per serving.
- Fiber and sugars (grams) per serving.
- Protein (grams) per serving.

In addition, for each of the nutrients just named plus vitamins A and C and the minerals calcium and iron, amounts in a serving of the food must be stated as percentages of the Daily Values for a person requiring 2,000 calories per day.

The side panel of the box of cereal in Figure 2-7 provides all this information. The chicken label shows a condensed format, and the candy package provides only a phone number, as is allowed for the tiniest labels.

Health Messages On Labels

At one time, a food manufacturer who hoped to promote a food as offering special benefits for health labeled it a "health food." Today that term is banned from use because it implies that to gain health, the consumer need only choose and eat that food. Some claims about health are allowed, however, as long as they meet a strict set of guidelines set forth by the Food and Drug Administration (FDA).

Claims linking nutrients and food constituents to disease states are allowable in the United States under FDA guidelines. The margin list describes them, and the terms in bold are defined in Table 2-8. Health claims are permitted on food labels because they are well supported by the available scientific evidence.

Labels may bear health claims regarding:

✔ Calcium as related to osteoporosis. Foods making this claim must be **high** in calcium.

✔ Sodium as related to hypertension (high blood pressure). Food must be **low sodium.**

✔ Dietary fat and cancer. Food must be **low fat.**

✔ Dietary saturated fat and cholesterol as related to coronary heart disease. Food must be **low saturated fat, low cholesterol,** and **low fat.**

✔ Fiber-containing grain products, fruits, and vegetables and cancer. The food must be **low fat,** and without added fiber, it must be a **good source** of dietary fiber.

✔ Fruits, vegetables, and grain products that contain fiber, particularly soluble fiber, and risk of coronary heart disease. Foods must be **low saturated fat, low fat,** and **low cholesterol.** They must also contain at least 0.6 gram of soluble fiber (explained in Chapter 4) per serving.

✔ Fruits and vegetables and cancer. Food must be **low fat,** and without added nutrients, it must be a **good source** of fiber, vitamin A, or vitamin C.[11]

✔ The vitamin folate and birth defects of the brain and spinal cord (neural tube defects). Foods must be a **good source** of folate.

✔ Sugar alcohols do not promote tooth decay. Frequent between-meal snacks, high in sugars and starch, promote tooth decay.

FIGURE 2-7

INTRODUCING A FOOD LABEL

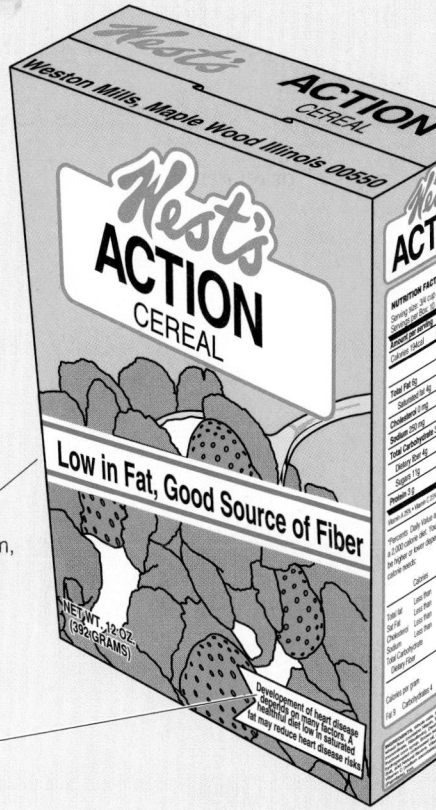

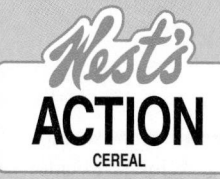

What's on a Label

The package must always state the product name, the name and address of the manufacturer, and the weight or measure.

The label may state information about sodium, calories, fat, or other constituents.

Approved health claims may be made, but only in terms of total diet.

Low in Fat, Good Source of Fiber

NET WT. 12 OZ. (392 GRAMS)

Calorie/gram reminder

Ingredients in descending order of predominance

A container with fewer than 40 square inches of surface area can present fewer facts in this format.

Nutrition Facts

Serving size ³/₄ cup (55g)
Servings per Box 10

Amount per serving	
Calories 167	Calories from Fat 27

	% Daily Value*
Total Fat 3g	5%
Saturated Fat 1g	5%
Cholesterol 0mg	0%
Sodium 250mg	10%
Total Carbohydrate 32g	11%
Dietary fiber 4g	16%
Sugars 11g	
Protein 3g	

Vitamin A 25%	•	Vitamin C 25%
Calcium 2%	•	Iron 25%

*Percent Daily Values are based on a 2,000 calorie diet. Your daily values may be higher or lower depending on your calorie needs.

	Calories	2,000	2,500
Total Fat	Less than	65g	80g
Sat Fat	Less than	20g	25g
Cholesterol	Less than	300mg	300mg
Sodium	Less than	2,400mg	2,400mg
Total Carbohydrate		300g	375g
Dietary Fiber		25g	30g

Calories per gram
Fat 9 • Carbohydrate 4 • Protein 4

INGREDIENTS. Whole oats, Milled corn, Enriched wheat flour (contains Niacin, Reduced iron, Thiamin mononitrate, Riboflavin), Dextrose, Maltose, High-fructose corn syrup, Brown sugar, Partially hydrogenated cottonseed oil, Coconut oil, Walnuts, Salt, and Natural flavors. Vitamins and minerals: Vitamin C (sodium ascorbate), Vitamin A (Palmitate), Iron.

Serving size and calorie information

Percentages of Daily Values for nutrients

Reference values

This compares some values for nutrients in a serving of the food to the needs of a person requiring 2,000 or 2,500 calories per day.

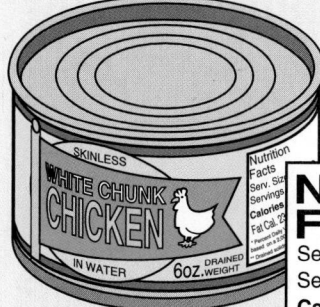

Nutrition Facts

Serv. Size ¹/₃ cup (85g)**
Servings 2
Calories 111
   Fat Cal. 23

*Percent Daily Values (DV) are based on a 2,000 calorie diet.
** Drained solids only

Amount/serving		%DV*	Amount/serving		%DV*
Total Fat	3g	5%	**Total Carb.**	0g	0%
Sat. Fat	1g	5%	Dietary Fiber	0g	0%
Cholest.	60mg	20%	Sugars	0g	
Sodium	200mg	8%	**Protein**	21g	

Vitamin A 0% • Vitamin C 0% • Calcium 0% • Iron 2%

Packages with fewer than 12 square inches of surface area need not carry nutrition information, but they must provide an address or telephone number for obtaining more information.

Serving sizes in household and metric measures

1 tsp	=	5 ml
1 tbs	=	15 ml
1 cup	=	240 ml
1 fl oz	=	30 ml
1 oz	=	28 g

Key

tsp	=	teaspoon
tbs	=	tablespoon
fl oz	=	fluid ounce
oz	=	ounce
ml	=	milliliter
g	=	gram

(continued on next page)

TABLE 2-8

Terms Used on Food Labels

Energy Terms

- **low calorie** 40 calories or less per serving.
- **reduced calorie** at least 25% lower in calories than a "regular," or reference, food.
- **calorie free** fewer than 5 calories per serving.

Fat Terms (Meat and Poultry Products)

- **extra lean**
  - less than 5 g of fat *and*
  - less than 2 g of saturated fat *and*
  - less than 95 mg of cholesterol per serving.
- **lean**[a]
  - less than 10 g of fat *and*
  - less than 4 g of saturated fat *and*
  - less than 95 mg cholesterol per serving.

Fat and Cholesterol Terms (All Products)

- **cholesterol free**
  - less than 2 mg cholesterol *and*
  - 2 g or less saturated fat per serving.
- **fat free** less than 0.5 g of fat per serving.
- **low cholesterol**
  - 20 mg or less of cholesterol *and*
  - 2 g or less saturated fat per serving.
- **low fat** 3 g or less fat per serving.
- **low saturated fat** 1 g or less saturated fat per serving.
- **percent fat free** may be used only if the product meets the definition of *low fat* or *fat free*. Requires disclosure of g fat per 100 g food.
- **reduced or less cholesterol**
  - at least 25% less cholesterol than a reference food *and*
  - 2 g or less saturated fat per serving.
- **reduced saturated fat**
  - 25% or less of saturated fat *and*
  - reduced by more than 1 gram saturated fat per serving compared with a reference food.

Regarding health claims, a food label may say only that a substance "may" or "might" reduce disease risks. This tentative wording reflects that science is still accumulating evidence concerning the rules of diet in diseases. Also, claims must state that the development of a disease rests on many factors. A permissible health claim might look like this:

Development of heart disease depends on many factors. A healthful diet low in saturated fat and cholesterol may lower blood cholesterol levels and may reduce the risk of heart disease.

TABLE 2-8

Terms Used on Food Labels continued

- **saturated fat free**
  - less than 0.5 g of saturated fat *and*
  - less than 0.5 g of *trans*-fatty acids.

Fiber Terms

- **high fiber** 5 g or more per serving. (Foods making high-fiber claims must fit the definition of low fat, or the level of total fat must appear next to the high-fiber claim.)
- **good source of fiber** 2.5 g to 4.9 g per serving.
- **more or added fiber** at least 2.5 g more per serving than a reference food.

Other Terms

- **free, without, no, zero** none or a trivial amount. *Calorie free* means containing fewer than 5 calories per serving; *sugar free* or *fat free* means containing less than half a gram per serving.
- **fresh** raw, unprocessed, or minimally processed with no added preservatives.
- **good source** 10 to 19% of the Daily Value per serving.
- **healthy** low in fat, saturated fat, cholesterol, and sodium and containing at least 10% of the Daily Value for vitamin A, vitamin C, iron, calcium, protein, or fiber.
- **high** 20% or more of the Daily Value for a given nutrient per serving; synonyms include "rich in" or "excellent source."
- **less, fewer, reduced** containing at least 25% less of a nutrient or calories than a reference food. This may occur naturally or as a result of altering the food. For example, pretzels, which are usually low in fat, can claim to provide less fat than potato chips, a comparable food.
- **light** this descriptor has three meanings on labels:
  1. a serving provides one-third fewer calories or half the fat of the regular product.
  2. a serving of a low-calorie, low-fat food provides half the sodium normally present.
  3. the product is light in color and texture, so long as the label makes this intent clear, as in "light brown sugar."
- **more, extra** at least 10% more of the Daily Value than in a reference food. The nutrient may be added or may occur naturally.

Sodium Terms

- **low sodium** 140 mg or less sodium per serving.
- **sodium free** less than 5 mg per serving.
- **very low sodium** 35 mg or less sodium per serving.

[a]The word *lean* as part of the brand name (as in "Lean Supreme") indicates that the product contains fewer than 10 grams of fat per serving.

When you choose a food that makes a health claim, or even one with the word **healthy** as part of its name, you can rely on it to live up to its claim.* Such a food cannot contain any nutrient or food constituent in an

---

*Restaurants making "heart healthy" claims for menu items are also required to provide nutrient information for consumers.

(*continued on next page*)

amount known to increase disease risk. Specifically, a serving of the product may contain no more than 20 percent of the Daily Value for the following:

■ Total fat.
■ Saturated fat.
■ Cholesterol.
■ Sodium.

This means that whole milk, even though it is a rich source of calcium, may not make a claim about osteoporosis because it contains too much saturated fat to qualify. Low-fat and nonfat milks, however, do qualify to bear the calcium and osteoporosis claim.

Health claims on labels are so carefully controlled that consumers can rely on them instead of worrying about grams, percentages, and other mathematical speed bumps that would slow them down in grocery store aisles. Much of the math previously required of nutrition-conscious shoppers has now been performed by food manufacturers, and the results are printed on the labels. Between the honest and accurate numbers and the carefully defined words, shoppers who take the time to read food labels can learn a lot about the foods they are buying.

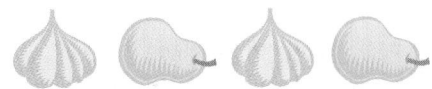

FOOD FEATURE

GETTING A FEEL FOR THE NUTRIENTS IN FOODS

Figure 2-8 illustrates a playful contrast between two days' meals. One set, labeled "Monday's Meals," shows the result of following the recommendations of this chapter. The other set of choices, "Tuesday's Meals," were chosen more for convenience and familiarity than out of concern with nutrition. The two sets of meals were made similar in energy (calories) so that other differences would stand out.

Now, how can a person compare these sets of meals with regard to the nutrients they provide? One way is to look up each food in a table of food composition, write down the food's nutrient values, and compare each one to a standard such as the Daily Values, as we've done in Figure 2-8. The computer is a time saver—it performs nutrient calculations with lightning speed. This convenience may make working with paper, pencils, and erasers seem a bit old-fashioned, but computers are rarely available on line for diners in cafeterias or fast-food counters where real-life decisions must be made. Those who can "see" the nutrients in their foods can make informed choices before eating meals, while others must wait until they visit their computers to find out how well they did in choosing. By the time you reach Chapter 11 of this text, you will be ready to test your skill at "seeing" the nutrients in foods in that chapter's Do It section. This chapter's Do It provides an alternative method for judging the adequacy of diets that employs the Food Guide Pyramid as its standard.

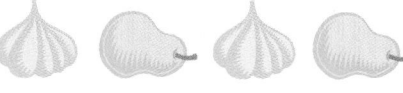

FIGURE 2-8

TWO DAYS' MEALS COMPARED WITH FIVE DAILY VALUES

MONDAY'S MEALS

Monday's meals reflect nutrient-dense choices from the Food Guide Pyramid.

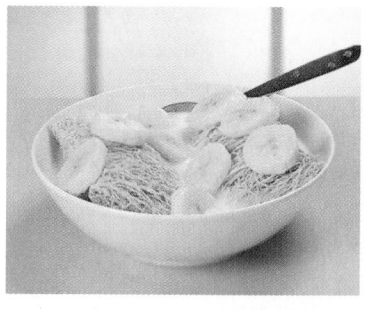

Foods	Energy (cal)	Fiber (g)	Total Fat (g)	Saturated Fat (g)	Vitamin C (mg)
Before heading off to class, a student eats breakfast:					
2 shredded wheat biscuits	166	5	—	—	—
1 c 1% low-fat milk	102	—	3	2	2
½ banana (sliced)	52	1	—	—	5
Then goes home for a quick lunch:					
1 turkey sandwich on whole-wheat bread with mayonnaise and mustard	294	4	12	2	—
1 c vegetable juice	46	2	—	—	67
While studying in the afternoon, the student eats a snack:					
4 whole-wheat crackers	80	2	3	—	—
1 oz low fat cheddar cheese	49	—	2	1	—
1 apple	82	3	—	—	8
That night, the student makes dinner:					
A salad:					
1 c raw spinach leaves, shredded carrots, and sliced mushrooms	29	3	—	—	19
⅓ c garbanzo beans	135	4	2	—	1
5 lg olives and 1 tbs ranch salad dressing	80	1	8	1	—
A main course:					
1 c spaghetti with meat sauce	332	8	12	3	22
½ c green beans	18	2	—	—	6
2 tsp butter	68	—	8	5	—
And for dessert:					
Strawberry shortcake made with: 1¼ c strawberries 1 piece spongecake 2 tbs whipped cream	293	3	8	4	102
Later that evening, the student enjoys a bedtime snack:					
3 graham crackers	89	—	2	—	—
1 c 1% low-fat milk	102	—	3	2	2
Totals:	2,017	38	63	20	234
Daily Values:[a]	2,000	25	65	20	60
Percentage of Daily Values:	101%	152%	97%	100%	390%

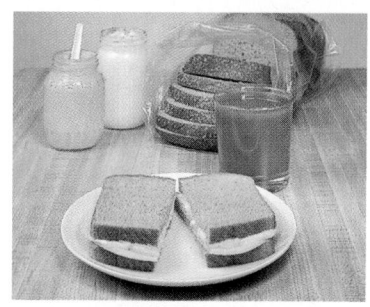

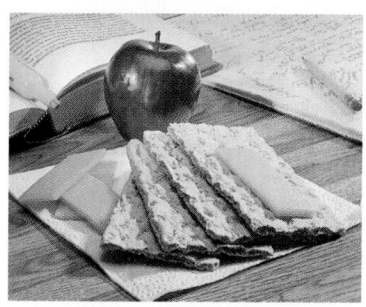

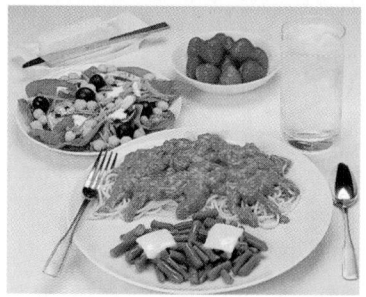

Percentage of Calories from Fat: 30%

[a]Daily Values based on a 2,000 calorie diet.

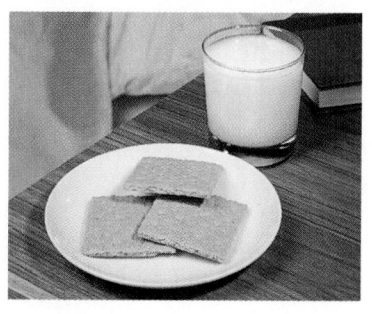

(continued on next page)

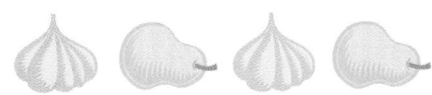

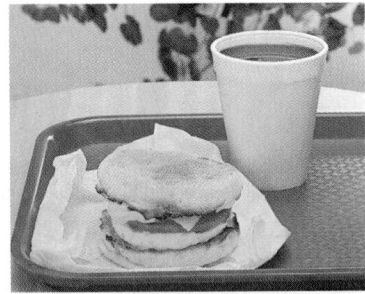

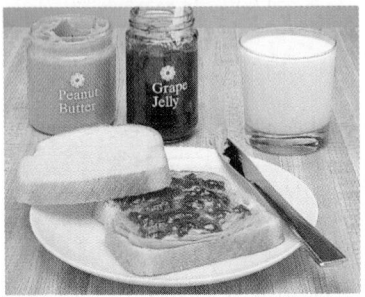

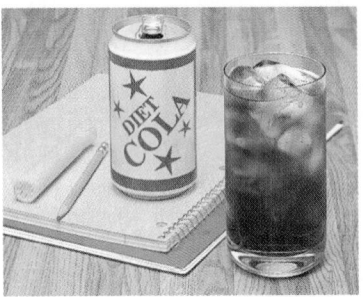

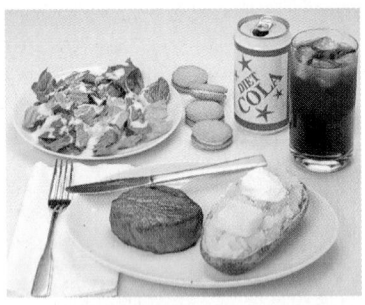

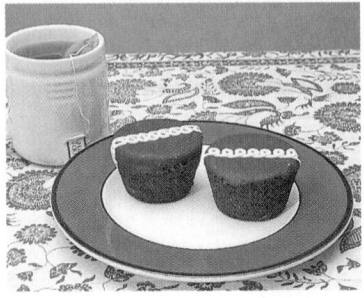

FIGURE 2-8

TWO DAYS' MEALS COMPARED WITH FIVE DAILY VALUES (CONTINUED)

TUESDAY'S MEALS
Tuesday's meals are lower on the nutrient density scale.

Foods	Energy (cal)	Fiber (g)	Total Fat (g)	Saturated Fat (g)	Vitamin C (mg)
Today, the student starts the day with a fast-food breakfast:					
1 c coffee	5	—	—	—	—
1 English muffin with egg, cheese, and bacon	383	2	20	9	1
Between classes, the student returns home for a quick lunch:					
1 peanut butter and jelly sandwich on white bread	350	3	14	3	—
1 c whole milk	150	—	8	5	2
While studying, the student has:					
12 oz diet cola	—	—	—	—	—
Bag of chips (14 chips)	228	2	15	5	13
That night for dinner, the student eats:					
A salad: 1 c lettuce					
1 tbs blue cheese dressing	84	1	8	1	3
A main course:					
6 oz steak	343	—	14	5	—
½ baked potato (large)	110	2	—	—	13
1 tbs butter	102	—	12	7	—
1 tbs sour cream	31	—	3	2	—
12 oz diet cola	—	—	—	—	—
And for dessert:					
4 sandwich-type cookies	189	1	8	2	—
Later on, a bedtime snack:					
2 creme-filled snack cakes	214	—	8	2	—
1 c herbal tea	—	—	—	—	—
Totals:	2,189	11	110	41	32
Daily Values:[a]	2,000	25	65	20	60
Percentage of Daily Values:	109%	44%	169%	205%	53%
Percentage of Calories from Fat: 45%					

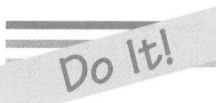 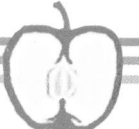

SCORE YOUR DIET WITH THE FOOD GUIDE PYRAMID

This activity examines your diet for adherence to the Food Guide Pyramid and for variety. How can you tell if your diet meets the ideals of the Food Guide Pyramid? Part of the story is told by the number of servings the diet provides from each food group. More is revealed by the variety of foods *within* each group. The rest of the tale unfolds as you learn, in the chapters to come, about the carbohydrates, lipids, protein, vitamins, and minerals in foods.

In this activity, your diet will receive six scores (Form 2-2). When added together, these six scores yield a single number. The first five scores measure how well your diet meets the ideals of the Food Guide Pyramid. The sixth score is awarded for variety among your food choices.

In this exercise, 60, not 100, is the highest score attainable. This is to serve as a reminder that the Food Guide Pyramid gives just a partial accounting of a diet's attributes.* The *Dietary Guidelines* concerning moderation in fat, salt, sugar, and alcohol are important, too. Try to keep them in mind as you review your food choices.

Your study begins with the next section. Make several copies of Form 2-1, one to use now and others in case you want to repeat this activity later.

PREPARING YOUR FOOD RECORD

Step 1. Record all of the foods you ate and all of the beverages you drank in one typical 24-hour period. Write them on the left-hand side of Form 2-1.

Step 2. As closely as possible, record the numbers of servings or fractions of servings you obtained from each food group (see Figure 2-4 for serving sizes, pages 44–45). List the numbers on the right-hand side of the form and total each column. To do this accurately, as you eat the food, you must make careful note of its amount. Estimate the amount to the nearest ounce, quarter-cup, tablespoon,

---

*This exercise represents six of the ten test categories of the *Healthy Eating Index (HEI)*, a diet assessment tool developed by the United States Department of Agriculture's (USDA's) Center for Nutrition Policy and Promotion in 1995. The full HEI also tests the diet for adherence to the *Dietary Guidelines for Americans*. For a copy of the entire HEI, contact the USDA (see the Nutrition Resources Appendix).

or other common measure. The Aids to Calculation section at the end of the book can help with conversion factors. Foods that belong in the tip of the Pyramid, the Fats, Oils, and Sweets are ignored in this exercise.

In guessing at serving sizes, use these rules of thumb:

- A 3-ounce serving of meat is about the size of the palm of a woman's hand or A deck of cards.
- A standard piece of fruit or potato is the size of a regular (60 watt) lightbulb.
- A 1½-ounce piece of cheese is the size of a nine-volt battery.
- A standard slice of lunch meat or American-type cheese weighs 1 ounce.
- A pat (1 tsp) of a quarter-pound stick of butter or margarine is about as thick as 280 pages of this book (pressed together).

You may have to break down mixed dishes into their ingredients to decide how many servings a food represents. For example, one cup of tuna noodle casserole may provide:

- an ounce of tuna (½ serving of meat, poultry, fish, dry beans, eggs, and nuts)
- a half-cup of noodles (1 serving of breads, cereals, rice, and pasta)
- a quarter-cup of a combination of peas, carrots, and onions (½ serving of vegetables).

Errors of up to 20 or 30 percent are expected and tolerated.

Step 3. On Form 2-1 write the suggested total number of servings from each food group for someone whose energy need is similar to yours. Table 2-6 on page 49 lists energy needs for some groups of people.

SCORING AGAINST THE FOOD GUIDE PYRAMID

Step 4. Compare your own totals on Form 2-1 with the suggested total number of servings for each food group and score yourself. Then transfer your scores to the pyramid of Form 2-2.

(continued on page 64)

FORM 2-1

Food Record

FOOD/AMOUNT	NUMBER OF SERVINGS FROM EACH FOOD GROUP				
	Breads, Cereals, Rice and Pasta	Vegetables	Fruit	Milk, Yogurt and Cheese	Poultry, Fish, Dry Beans, Eggs and Nuts
Breakfast: _____ _____ _____ _____					
Snack: _____ _____ _____					
Lunch: _____ _____ _____ _____					
Supper: _____ _____ _____ _____					
Snack: _____ _____ _____ _____					
Your totals:					
Suggested totals (From Table 2-6, p. 49)					
Your *Score* (Transfer to Form 2-2)					

FORM 2-2
Do It Scoreboard

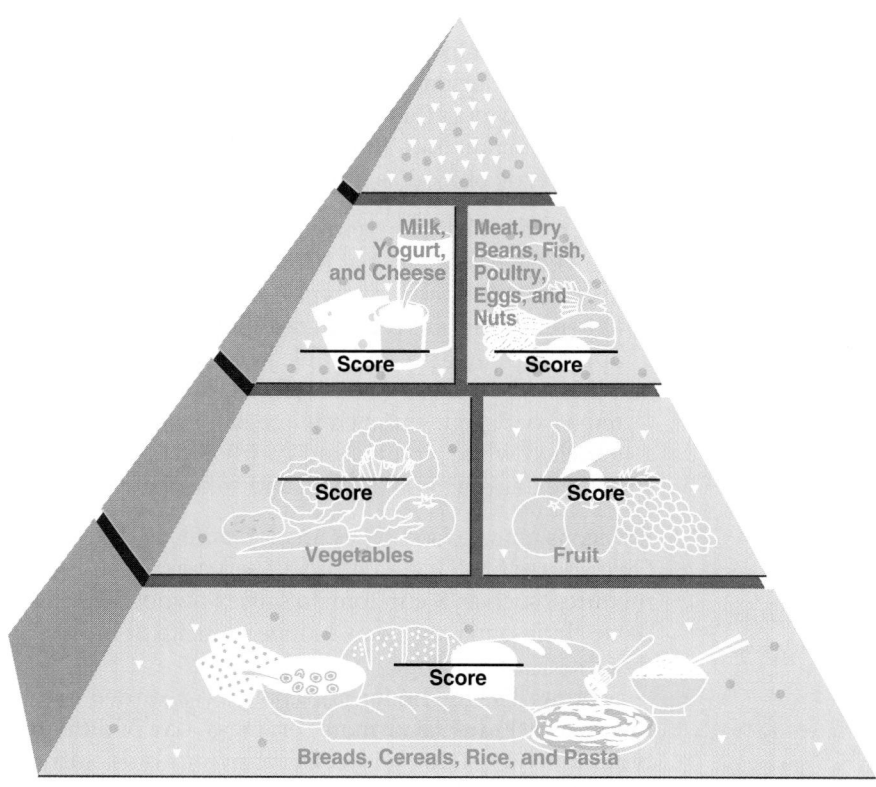

TABLE 2-10

Scoring Variety (see text instructions)

If You Ate This Many Servings of Different Types of Foods:	You Receive This Score:
9.5 or more	10
9.0	9
8.5	8
8.0	7
7.5	6
7.0	5
6.5	4
6.0	3
5.5	2
5.0	1
4.5 or fewer	0

A. Transfer your scores from Form 2-1 to the boxes of the Pyramid above. Add the 5 scores to obtain a single number as your Pyramid total.

Pyramid total: _____

B. Determine your score for variety by the method described in the text. Add your variety score and your pyramid total to obtain your total score:

Variety score: _____

+ Pyramid total: _____

Final score: _____

(continued on next page)

Score as follows:

- 10 points for each food group in which you ate all or more of the recommended number of servings.
- 0 points for no servings from a group.
- For values between these extremes, find your score by dividing the number of servings you ate by the recommended number and multiplying by 10. To help clarify the process we use a student's diet as our example:

Joe is an active young adult who needs 2,800 calories.

	Joe Needed This Many Servings	Joe Consumed
Breads, cereals, rice, or pasta:	11	6
Vegetables:	5	5
Fruit:	4	0
Milk, yogurt, or cheese:	2	3
Meat, poultry, fish, dry beans, eggs, and nuts:	3	5

After analyzing his diet on Form 2-1, Joe finds that he consumed 6 bread, cereal, rice, or pasta foods. Thus he ate 6 of 11 recommended servings of breads, cereals, rice, or pasta.

$$(6 \div 11) \times 10 = 5.5 \text{ points}$$

He consumed 5 vegetable servings, right on target, so he gets 10 points for these. He ate no fruit, so here he scores a zero.

For the milk group he ate more than the recommended 2 servings, but he gets no extra points. He receives the maximum 10 points. The same is true for the meat group: a maximum of 10. After adding the points earned for each of the five food groups, Joe finds that his total points were 35.5 out of a possible 50.

Add up your scores and write the total on the Pyramid total line of Form 2-2, part A.

SCORING VARIETY

The final scoring component, variety, is subjective. It asks you to use your own judgment in your assessment.

Step 5. Look over your food intake record and jot down the approximate number of different types of foods listed. Note that the food types referred to are not the *groups* of foods specified in the Food Guide Pyramid. Here food types mean any of the individual foods that make up those groups. For example, a person choosing milk and cheese in a day counts them as two types of foods because milk and cheese differ significantly from each other. A person choosing milk and pudding, on the other hand, counts them both as the same food because pudding is made from fluid milk and so is counted as the same type of food as milk. Other examples:

- Beef and lamb differ from each other enough to count as two types of food, but hamburger and beef steak are counted as the same type.
- Different fruits are counted as different foods, but apples, applesauce, and apple juice are all of one type.
- Whole-wheat bread and enriched white bread are different foods, but enriched white hamburger rolls, enriched white biscuits, and enriched white bread are counted as one type of food, and so on.

Divisions among food types are not perfectly described. Give yourself half a credit for half-servings of foods in mixtures, such as ¼ cup tomato sauce (a whole serving is ½ cup) in lasagna, or ¼ cup chopped tomato or onion that dresses a hot dog.

Scoring: The top honor of 10 points is awarded to the diet that includes 9.5 or more servings a day of different types of foods. A day with fewer than four types earns a zero. Use the table on Form 2-2 to obtain a score; enter your score on Form 2-2, part B.

THE FINAL SCORE

Step 6. Total your score by adding all six scores (five Pyramid scores plus variety) on the Do It Scoreboard (Form 2-2). You may interpret the score as follows: A score of 60 means that the diet is excellent with regard to both numbers of servings in each group and variety in each group.

Score	Diet characteristics
60	excellent variety and choices
50-59	fairly adequate and varied diet
less than 50	diet needs study and improvement

ANALYSIS

Answer these questions:

1. How well did your diet's overall score compare with the perfect score of 60 points?
2. Did you consume the recommended minimum numbers of servings for each of the five groups of the Food Guide Pyramid?
3. Which groups of foods, if any, are underrepresented in your diet? Reasons for failing to consume all of the servings from all of the Food Groups include allergies and intolerances, but people often simply choose their diets impulsively with inadequate planning for nutrition. If you did not consume the minimum number of servings from each group, list some reasons why.
4. Did your diet provide an adequate variety of foods, or were your choices monotonous? How can you expand your field of choices?

Keep your extra copies of Form 2-1 to help you track changes in your score over time. If you perform this analysis every week or so throughout the course, you will have a fairly accurate representation of your food habits and the adequacy and variety of your diet. You may also see changes in your eating habits as you learn more about the effects of nutrition on health.

SELF-CHECK

Answers to these Self-Check questions are in Appendix G.

1. The Recommended Dietary Allowances (RDA) used in the United States include recommendations concerning intakes of all of the following *except:*
   a. carbohydrate
   b. protein
   c. fiber
   d. a and c

2. The Recommended Dietary Allowances (RDA) list safe and adequate intakes for which of the following?
   a. sodium
   b. potassium
   c. chloride
   d. all of the above

3. According to the Food Guide Pyramid, which foods should form the foundation of a healthy diet?
   a. vegetables
   b. breads, cereals, rice, and pasta
   c. fruits
   d. milk, yogurt, and cheese

4. Which of the following adjustments in one's diet would agree with the *Dietary Guidelines for Americans, 1995?*
   a. eating baked potatoes rather than french fries
   b. drinking skim milk rather than 2% milk
   c. eating fruits rather than cakes and pies
   d. all of the above

5. According to the World Health Organization's (WHO) Population Nutrient Goals, the upper limit of total fat in one's diet should be:
   a. 5 percent
   b. 10 percent
   c. 20 percent
   d. 30 percent

6. The energy RDA are centered around the average requirements for each age and sex group. (T) F

7. The Recommended Dietary Allowances (RDA) are for all people, regardless of their medical history. T (F)

8. People who choose not to eat animals or their products need to find an alternative food guide to use instead of the Food Guide Pyramid when planning their diets. T (F)

9. By law, food labels must state as a percentage of the Daily Values the amounts of vitamin C, vitamin A, niacin, and thiamin present in a food. T (F)

10. In order for a food to be labeled "low fat," it must contain 3 grams or less fat per serving. (T) F

11. Overall, the diets of the Mediterranean are high in animal protein and low in carbohydrates and fiber. (Read about this in the upcoming Controversy.) T (F)

NOTES

Notes are in Appendix F.

The Mediterranean Diet:
Does It Hold the Secret for a Healthy Heart?

Much has been said lately in favor of eating the Mediterranean way. This is because people who eat traditional Mediterranean diets die much less frequently from heart disease and certain cancers than do people who eat diets typical of northern Europe and North America.[1] Would people in the United States be healthier if they abandoned traditional American foods and adopted Mediterranean ones? Does this diet of ample grains, vegetables, fruits, olive oil, and cheese, accompanied by

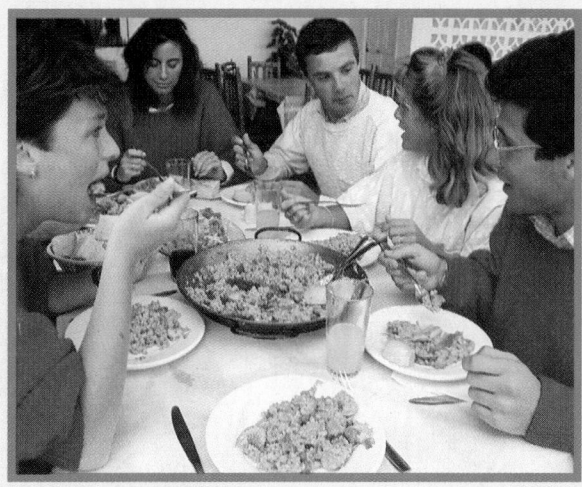

Should we be eating the Mediterranean way?

wine, hold special benefits? Some experts think so. This Controversy explores this idea from the scientific point of view.

Anyone beginning to explore these ideas runs into some paradoxes. For example, the diet of one Mediterranean country, Greece, provides up to 42 percent of its calories as fat, mostly from olive oil and olives.[2] Many Greeks carry more body fat than is considered prudent in the United States.[3] According to U.S. guidelines, then, the Greek population would be urged to eat less fat and to lose weight to protect their hearts. Yet Greeks living in Greece enjoy one of the longest life expectancies worldwide and die from cardiovascular disease far less often than do Westerners.[4]

Should Americans eat like Greeks? The suggestion has been made that perhaps a diet similar to the Greeks' might achieve heart disease rates here as low as those in Greece. Such a diet might also be easier to follow than the very-low-fat diet traditionally prescribed for heart health in the United States.[5]

Greece is not alone in having heart disease risks lower than those of the United States; many nations of the Mediterranean region do, and nobody knows why. A suggestion has been made that genetics might bestow resistance to heart disease upon Mediterranean people. However, this idea has been all but abandoned because the risks seem to follow regional diets, not individual people. Mediterranean immigrants to the West who adopt a Western diet suffer heart disease and cancer at the same rates as native-born U.S. citizens.

Further, as "American-style" foods advance across the Mediterranean region, disease rates shift toward those more typical of Western nations.[6] These pieces of evidence support the idea that diet, not genetics, is the primary variable that confers disease risk or protection. Indeed, the World Health Organization is campaigning to try to persuade countries with historically low disease rates to continue or renew use of their traditional diets rather than adopting the heavily marketed foods from the West.

DEFINING THE MEDITERRANEAN DIET

Scientists who try to define a single "Mediterranean" diet run into a problem.[7] The vast Mediterranean region includes the diets of Spain, Portugal, France, Syria, Israel, and others, all different from one another. As an example, Greeks eat abundant olive oil, but southern Italians keep total fat intakes low.[8] Because low death rates from heart disease characterize all these nations, advisers to the countries are reluctant to suggest "improvements" for their diets.[9]

Some researchers have turned to the foodways of the ancient Greeks, Spaniards, and Romans to help establish a characteristic Mediterranean eating pattern.[10] These classic diets were founded on grain foods such as crusty breads, honey-sweetened cakes, rice, seeds including lentils and beans, fish, other seafood, goat cheese, olives and olive oil, vegetables, fruits (especially grapes and figs), and wine mixed half-and-half with water. Today, traditional diets of those countries follow much the same patterns.[11] Meats are for special occasions only; the favored cooking fat is oil pressed from olives; butter is shunned. Overall, then, the diets of the Mediterranean are:

- Low in saturated fat.
- High in monounsaturated fats (such as olive oil).
- Low in animal protein.
- High in carbohydrates and fiber.

FIGURE C2-I

TWO PYRAMID PLANS

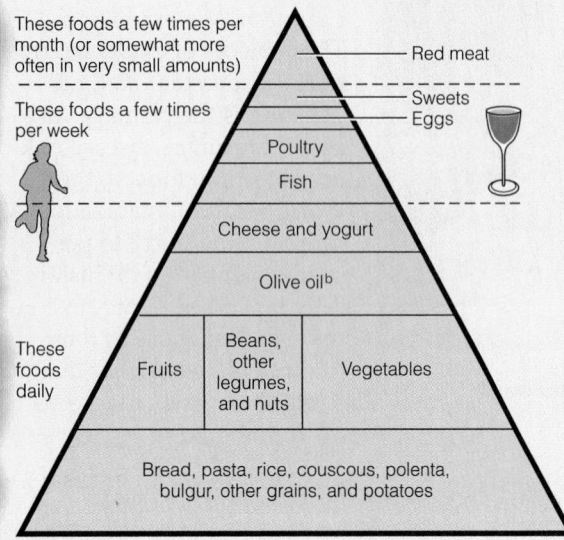

MEDITERRANEAN DIET PYRAMID^a

These foods a few times per month (or somewhat more often in very small amounts)

These foods a few times per week

These foods daily

Red meat
Sweets
Eggs
Poultry
Fish
Cheese and yogurt
Olive oil^b
Fruits
Beans, other legumes, and nuts
Vegetables
Bread, pasta, rice, couscous, polenta, bulgur, other grains, and potatoes

^aThe authors of this pyramid also recommend regular physical exercise and moderate consumption of wine.
^bOther oils rich in monounsaturated fats, such as canola or peanut oil, can be substituted for olive oil. People who are watching their weight should limit their oil consumption.

Source: 1994 Oldways Preservation & Exchange Trust, by permission.

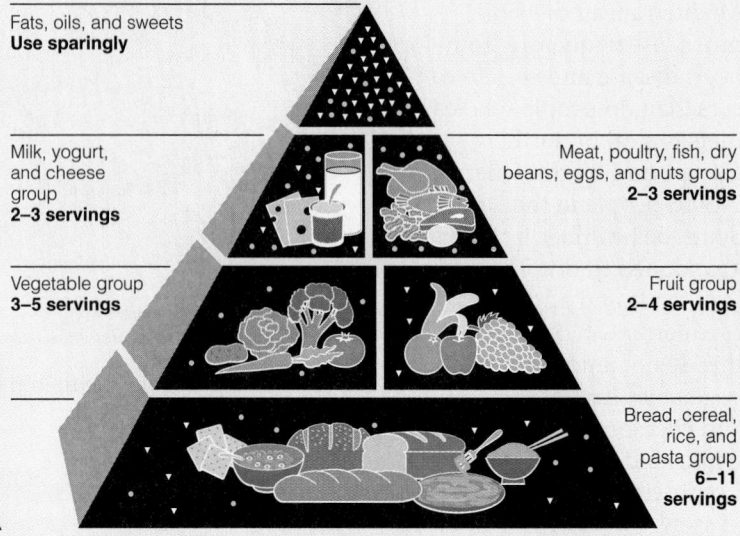

USDA's FOOD GUIDE PYRAMID

Fats, oils, and sweets
Use sparingly

Milk, yogurt, and cheese group
2–3 servings

Meat, poultry, fish, dry beans, eggs, and nuts group
2–3 servings

Vegetable group
3–5 servings

Fruit group
2–4 servings

Bread, cereal, rice, and pasta group
6–11 servings

Source: U.S. Department of Agriculture/U.S. Department of Health and Human Services

KEY TO SYMBOLS
▢ **Fat** (naturally occurring and added)   ▼ **Sugars** (added)
These symbols show that fat and added sugars come mostly from fats, oils, and sweets, but can be part of or added to foods from the other food groups as well.

Based on these observations, a group of researchers have proposed a Mediterranean Pyramid, similar to the U.S. Food Guide Pyramid. Figure C2-1 shows the pyramids side by side, and the rest of this Controversy compares them. Later chapters revisit many of the issues discussed here because they are among the top concerns of nutrition scientists today.

THE BOTTOM BASE—CARBOHYDRATES AND FIBER

Right away, some similarities between the pyramids of Figure C2-1 are apparent. Both have wide bottom bases of breads, cereals, pasta, rice, and other grains, signifying that the two diets are built on the same foundation. This wise choice supplies abundant carbohydrate-rich foods to the eater, foods that in their unrefined state provide needed energy, vitamins, minerals, and fiber with almost no fat. Such foods meet the body's needs

for these nutrients without elevating the person's risk of disease. In fact, diets high in fiber are thought to reduce risks of heart disease and cancer substantially. So far, both plans agree.

VEGETABLES AND FRUITS

In both pyramid diets, vegetables and fruits appear next in predominance but with one important difference: the Mediterranean plan requires servings of legumes (dried beans) or nuts every day. In Spain, a plateful of raw or cooked vegetables commonly precedes a main meal; melon or figs serve as dessert. So much is said in later chapters about the virtues of vegetables and fruits in the diet, let it suffice to say that the case for their role in disease prevention is virtually ironclad. Vegetables provide fiber, phytochemicals, antioxidants, and other nutrients (see Controversy 7), all of which correlate with reduced incidence of chronic diseases. Further, with few exceptions, these foods are extraordinarily low in fat. Without a doubt, vegetables and fruits are allies to those who seek a healthful diet.

THE CLASSIFICATION OF LEGUMES

As noted, a difference between the U.S. and Mediterranean Pyramids is their handling of legumes (dried beans and peas). Legumes are difficult to classify in any food grouping plan because they have desirable qualities in common with so many other foods. For example, the U.S. Pyramid classes legumes with meats because, like meats, legumes are high in protein. Legume protein is not quite identical to that of meat, however; while legumes can approach the *quantity* of protein in meat, the *quality* of their protein varies (Chapter 6 delves into this issue). A serving or two of either meat or legumes in a balanced diet amply meets the body's need for protein.

Legumes also supply iron and other minerals typically associated with meats. The similarities end there, however. Meats are notoriously high in fat, much of it the heart-clogging saturated kind, and they provide no fiber or carbohydrate. Legumes, on the other hand, supply abundant fiber and carbohydrate with little or no fat, a combination that the heart prefers. In some ways, certain legumes even resemble dairy products: they combine ample calcium and protein in one food.

In light of legumes' high fiber and mineral contents, the Mediterranean system lists legumes separately from meats and on a plane with the vegetables. Mediterranean main dishes often include some form of legumes, sometimes as part of the dish, sometimes as garnish. In Spain, cooked legumes are deep-fried in olive oil and served as snack foods, similar to potato chips in this country. While legumes are hard to categorize, the following evidence concerning their health effects leaves no doubt about their importance.

ARGUMENTS FOR REQUIRING LEGUMES

"Why should I eat a bowl of beans every day when I can afford to eat meat?" asks a student who observes that legumes and meats are interchangeable in the U.S. Pyramid. The answer invokes evidence on legumes' fiber and their health effects.

The fiber of legumes is a constituent often lacking in U.S. diets. A reviewer reported recently that "an overwhelming consensus among health organizations advises increased consumption of fruits and vegetables, dried peas and beans, and whole grains" to help people meet current dietary recommendations.[12] Dry beans have more dietary fiber per serving than almost any other unprocessed food, and they provide a balance of the types of fibers that exert various beneficial effects on health.

Fiber alone cannot explain all of the findings about legumes and health, however. What is it about beans, for example, that enhances the performance of endurance athletes? Why do people with diabetes use beans in their diets to help modulate their blood sugar levels? Research has yielded this evidence:

- Endurance athletes who eat legumes in the hours before competition may extend their glucose fuel availability during competition.[13]
- Legumes contain a form of starch believed to help control blood glucose in people with diabetes.[14]
- Legumes are rich in the type of fiber most strongly associated with low blood cholesterol and low rates of heart disease.[15]
- Replacement of meat *protein* in the diet with soybean protein may lower blood lipids, thereby lowering heart disease risk, even when dietary *fats* are held constant.[16]
- Legumes contain substances believed to inhibit the growth of certain cancers (see Chapter 11).[17]
- A meal that includes legumes satisfies hunger longer.[18]

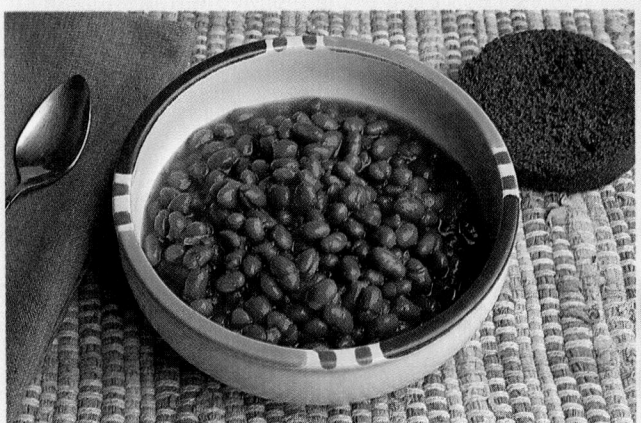

Legumes: remarkable foods.

The last of these attributes may have importance for weight control. A person who achieves a feeling of fullness sooner during a meal and stays full longer has less trouble resisting unneeded snacks.

As wonderful as legumes are, however, they are not "perfect foods" nor do they comprise an adequate diet when eaten alone. They lack the vitamins A and C of vegetables and fruits and the vitamin B_{12} of meats and dairy products. To overconsume legumes to the exclusion of other foods would be as poor a choice as never to include a bean in the diet.

ARGUMENT CONCERNING FATS AND MEATS

One of the most startling differences between the two pyramids, and the one that draws the most controversy, concerns fat. The Mediterranean plan suggests that the next most predominant daily dietary constituent after fruits and vegetables should be olive oil—a source of pure fat. In the U.S. Pyramid, olive oil joins other fats at the tip-top, flagged with a warning to use all fats sparingly.

U.S. guidelines warn us to restrict fat intakes to no more than 30 percent of daily calories. Further, the guidelines recommend reducing saturated fat to 10 percent of calories. This recommendation is based on abundant research revealing correlations between low total fat intakes, low saturated fat intakes, and low risks of heart disease (a topic of Chapter 11). It does not seem to matter which fats (other than saturated fats) contribute energy to the diet, so long as total fat and saturated fat are held in check.

As noted, the Mediterranean plan delivers much more fat than would be thought prudent under the U.S. guidelines. People following the Mediterranean plan receive some 40 percent of their calories from fat, mostly from olive oil. Advocates of this high fat intake write:

> Although additional data are sorely needed, we believe that the majority of dietary fatty acids should be monounsaturated [the olive oil–type] rather than polyunsaturated. . . . The Mediterranean alternative . . . appears to be at least as healthful, and may . . . improve the lipid profile, and will provide more variety and greater satisfaction to many.[19]

Some scientific evidence to support this view exists. For example, researchers have found that olive oil is metabolized differently in the body from the oil of soybeans.[20] As a result, olive oil may conserve a beneficial

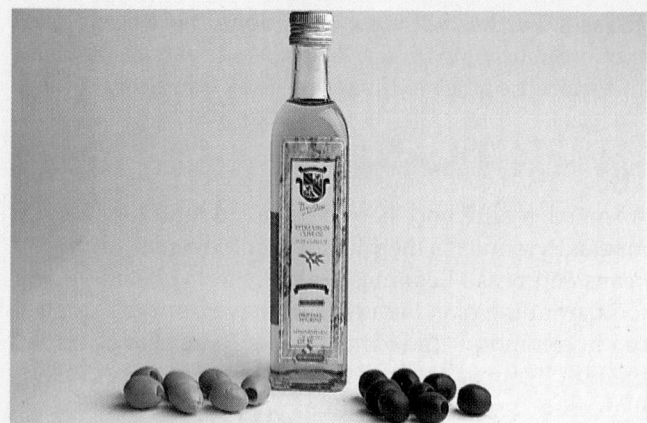

Olives and olive oil.

blood lipid (HDL) associated with low risk of heart disease, while lowering the riskier types.[21] Furthermore, olive oil stands out among unsaturated fats in being resistant to oxidation (see Chapter 5), which is a possible cause of heart disease.[22]

Not everyone agrees that research to date has made a sufficient case for a protective effect from olive oil. Not enough data exist, they say, to make recommendations for its use.[23] In addition, critics of the Mediterranean Pyramid note that foods such as avocados, nuts, and canola oil have oils similar to the oil of olives, but these foods are ignored by the plan. Also, critics point out that olive oil is fattening, providing 9 calories per gram, as do all fats. While some very active people of the Mediterranean may burn off the excess calories from their high-fat diets, many people from that region are also overweight. Obesity and its many associated ills remain major threats to health in the United States, and high-fat diets seem to promote greater body fatness than do low-fat diets. Accordingly, these critics conclude that the recommendation to consume such a high-fat diet is unwise, even if the fat itself is easy on the heart.

MEATS AND SWEETS

Returning to the differences between the two pyramids, the Mediterranean plan does not restrict total fat, but does limit *animal* fat (and this is mostly saturated fat). The U.S. Pyramid makes no such distinction. In fact, a person who uses the U.S. Pyramid as a guide may run into problems in trying to meet U.S. guidelines for fat. The pyramid allows red meats, with their associated saturated fat, at every meal if a diner so chooses. Yet the diner who eats this much meat cannot help exceeding the recommended limit on fat intake.

People following the Mediterranean plan typically consume less than 10 percent of their calories from saturated fat—a goal of both plans. People following the USDA plan find meeting this goal difficult, however. Notice that fish dominates poultry in the Mediterranean plan, and that eggs and sweets dominate red meats. Notice, too, that recommendations for consuming poultry and red meats are in terms of servings *per week or month*, not two-to-three servings *per day* as suggested by the USDA plan. The average daily consumption of meat in the United States is more than half a pound per person per day; in the Mediterranean region, it is about half a pound per person per *week*. The difference in meat intake, and therefore in saturated fat intake, is significant.

Concerning the treatment of sweets in the plans, look back at Figure C2-1 and take note of the position of sweets in the two pyramid plans. The Mediterranean plan suggests that only one food—red meats—be eaten less frequently than sweets. The USDA plan gives no specific guidance concerning intake of sweets but cautions us to "use sparingly."

EVIDENCE ABOUT YOGURT

The Mediterranean plan suggests daily cheese or yogurt but fails to mention nonfat milk, the staple milk source in the USDA plan. Mediterranean people eat yogurt or cheese each day, and they may use milk to lighten their coffee, but milk by itself is not used as a beverage by adults. Cheese contains the nutrients of milk but is typically very high in saturated fat. Yogurt is really just fermented milk. Besides all of the nutrients in milk, yogurt contains the fermenting agent, *Lactobacillus*, a type of bacteria, and the products formed during fermentation. These attributes have generated interest in yogurt's effects on the body.

Interest in yogurt often stems from a century-old study of some healthy, aged people of another culture who credited their long lives to daily meals of yogurt. This study was discredited when the discovery was made that this culture highly valued the elderly, so people often made false claims about their age. Still, researchers have studied yogurt to find out if it has special health-promoting qualities.

Early research on yogurt seemed to point to a connection between yogurt consumption and cancer prevention. Occasionally, small studies arise to suggest a correlation between tumor suppression and yogurt or *Lactobacillus* consumption. No serious conclusions are possible about implications for human cancer at this time, however.[24]

Another claim made for yogurt is that it prevents infections. One group of researchers studying vaginal yeast infections found a threefold decrease in the number of infections suffered by women who daily consumed 8 ounces of yogurt containing the live *Lactobacillus* culture.[25] Another small study is reported to have found a correlation between live-culture yogurt consumption and increased immune system activity.[26] We can only wait for further research to support or refute these ideas.

The Mediterranean preference for yogurt over milk may stem from the likelihood that adults of the region may have some problems in digesting the sugar of milk and therefore experience digestive distress when they consume milk. Yogurt contains somewhat less lactose than does fresh milk (Chapter 4 provides details). People of northern European descent, on the other hand, retain milk-digesting abilities throughout adult life. In whatever form, milk and its products provide calcium in abundance, and most adults need more calcium in their diets.

EVIDENCE ABOUT WINE

Most controversial among the suggestions of the Mediterranean Pyramid is the advice to partake moderately of wine. The major concern, of course, is that encouraging wine drinking may invite development of alcoholism or an increase in alcohol-related traffic accidents. These would be consequences too severe to risk even if wine's supposed action against heart disease was a certainty—and it is not.

Does red wine protect the French and other Mediterranean people from heart disease? While not proven, the idea probably has some validity. Studies show low rates of heart disease in populations that use moderate amounts of wine (red or white) as a beverage with meals.

Alcohol itself (one or two drinks a day) may reduce the risk of heart disease by raising beneficial blood lipids (HDL) and preventing blood clot formation.[27] These benefits are most apparent in people over age 50 and in those most likely to develop heart disease.[28] However, studies also report that heavy alcohol consumption (three or more drinks a day) *increases* the risk of death from other causes.[29] Alcohol has many negative effects on body systems, and later sections of this book describe them.

SHOULD AMERICANS EAT THE MEDITERRANEAN WAY?

Questions surrounding the Mediterranean Pyramid remain unanswered. For one, while heart disease rates may be low in Mediterranean countries, no one can explain why the incidence of stroke is almost double that of the United States. If the diet can receive the credit for heart health, should it also be blamed for increased incidence of stroke?

Also, while the link between diet and heart disease overall is strong, no one knows for sure what parts of the diet form that link. Perhaps the olive oil is a key factor, but both nutrients and phytochemicals found in vegetables, legumes, seafood, or seasonings such as garlic or herbs offer protective effects, too.[30] Active lifestyles may play a role, as may differences in tobacco use; exercise reduces heart disease risk, and smoking greatly increases it.

Critics of the Mediterranean plan have expressed concerns that it may be inadequate in calcium and iron—two problem nutrients for many people, especially women and children.[31] Because these nutrients are typically lacking in many people's diets, it seems unwise to restrict calcium selections to cheeses and yogurt and iron-rich meat consumption to a few times a month.

Should everyone abandon the U.S. Pyramid, then, and take up eating Mediterranean style? Certainly, some benefit is likely from adopting a few of its suggestions. Including legumes as part of a balanced daily diet seems like a good idea, as does *replacing* saturated fats such as butter and meat fat with unsaturated fats like olive oil. The authors of this book would not stop there, however. They would urge you to reduce fats from all sources; choose small portions of the leanest meats just occasionally, fish and poultry most often; and include fresh foods from all the groups each day. Also, exercise daily, as the Mediterraneans do. As for wine, this is a personal choice, but one to approach with extreme caution, for no other dietary choice has such destructive potential.

CONCLUSION

Recommendations will continue to evolve as nutrition science unfolds. Meanwhile, you must choose foods every day. Be assured that you can confidently build your diet according to the unchanging foundation principles of adequacy, balance, calorie control, moderation, and variety.

NOTES

Notes are in Appendix F.

THE REMARKABLE BODY

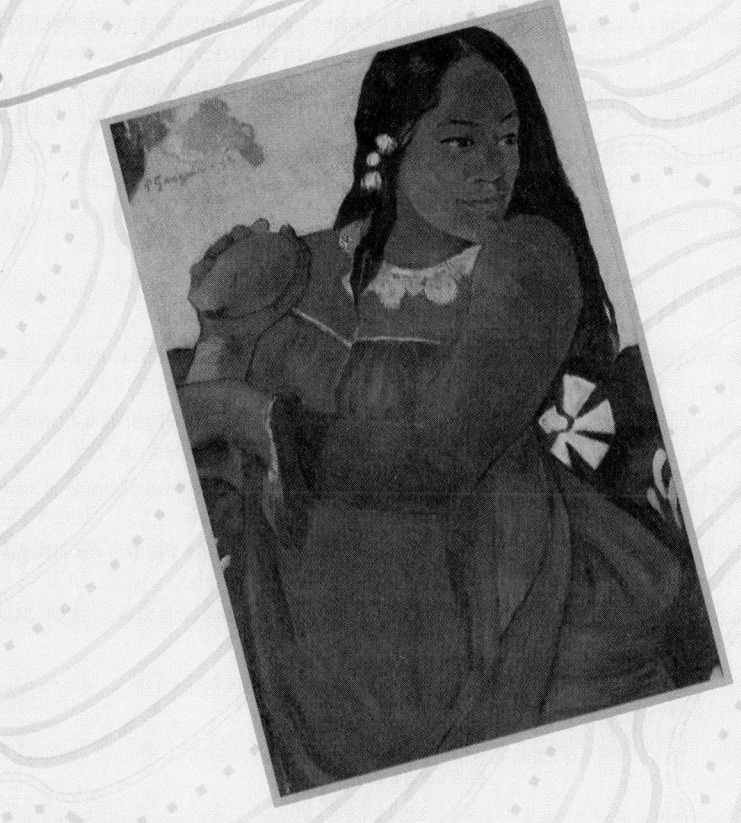

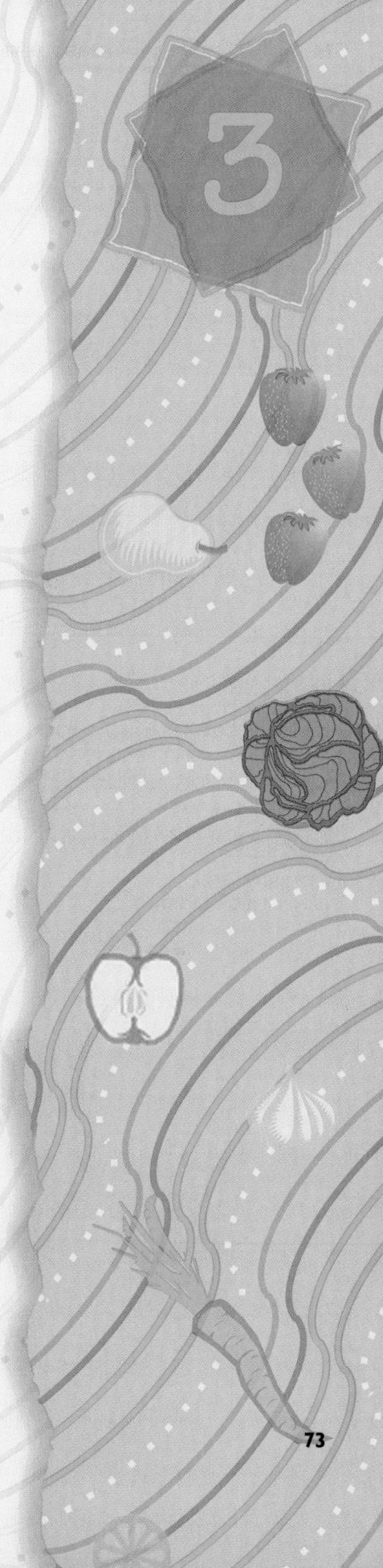

CONTENTS

Paul Gauguin, *Woman of the Mango*, 1892, The Baltimore Museum of Art; The Cone Collection, formed by Dr. Clairbel Cone and Miss Etta Cone of Baltimore, Maryland, BMA 1950, 213.

cells the smallest units in which independent life can exist. All living things are single cells or organisms made of cells.

3 At the moment of conception, you received from your mother and father the genes that determine how your body works. Many of these genes are thousands of centuries old and have not changed since the Stone Age, when your ancestors walked the earth coated with fur and carrying clubs. Your body has changed very little since then, but you are living with the food, the luxuries, the smog, the additives, and all the other pleasures and problems of the twentieth century. In this country's melting pot of cultures and traditions, you may not have learned any time-tested and proven way of patterning your food intake. There is no guarantee that your diet, haphazardly chosen, will meet the needs of your Stone Age body. Unlike your ancestors, you must learn how your body works and what it needs from food to serve it best. Hence the study of nutrition, so that you can bring your mind into the act of nourishing your body.

THE BODY'S CELLS

The human body is composed of billions of **cells,** and none of them knows anything about food. *You* may get hungry for fruit, milk, or bread, but each cell of your body needs nutrients—the vital components of foods. The ways in which the body's cells cooperate to obtain and use nutrients are the subjects of this chapter.

Each of the body's cells is a self-contained, living entity (see Figure 3-1), although each depends on the rest of the body to supply its needs. Among the cells' most basic needs are energy and the oxygen with which to burn it. Cells also need water to maintain the environment in which they live. They need

FIGURE 3-1

A TYPICAL CELL (SIMPLIFIED DIAGRAM)

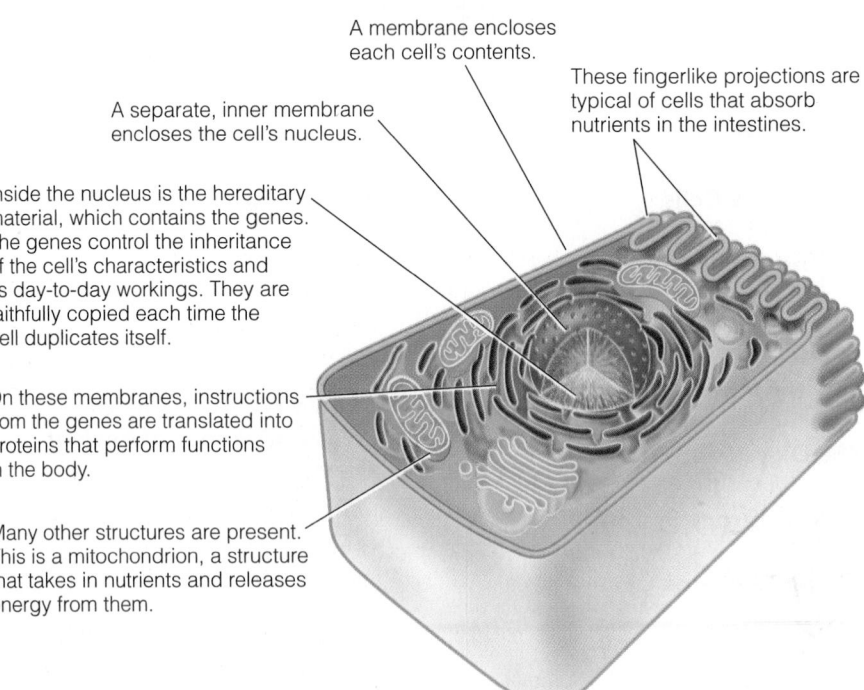

A membrane encloses each cell's contents.

These fingerlike projections are typical of cells that absorb nutrients in the intestines.

A separate, inner membrane encloses the cell's nucleus.

Inside the nucleus is the hereditary material, which contains the genes. The genes control the inheritance of the cell's characteristics and its day-to-day workings. They are faithfully copied each time the cell duplicates itself.

On these membranes, instructions from the genes are translated into proteins that perform functions in the body.

Many other structures are present. This is a mitochondrion, a structure that takes in nutrients and releases energy from them.

building blocks and control systems. They especially need the nutrients they cannot make for themselves, the essential nutrients first described in Chapter 1, which must be supplied from food. The first principle of diet planning is that the foods we choose must provide energy, water, and the essential nutrients.

In the human body, every cell works in cooperation with every other cell to support the whole. The cell's **genes** determine the nature of that work. Each gene is a blueprint that directs the production of a piece of protein machinery, most often an **enzyme,** that helps to do the cell's work. Each cell contains a complete set of genes, but different ones are active in different types of cells. For example, in some intestinal cells, the genes for making digestive enzymes are active; in some of the body's **fat cells,** the genes for making enzymes that metabolize fat are active.

Cells are organized into **tissues** that perform specialized tasks. For example, individual muscle cells are joined together to form muscle tissue, which can contract. Tissues, in turn, are grouped together to form whole **organs.** In the organ we call the heart, for example, muscle tissues, nerve tissues, connective tissues, and other types all work together to pump blood. Some body functions are performed by several related organs working together as part of a **body system.** For example, the heart, lungs, and blood vessels cooperate as parts of the cardiovascular system to deliver oxygen to all the body cells. The next few sections present the body systems with special significance to nutrition.

✔ KEY POINT   **The body's cells need energy, oxygen, water, and nutrients to remain healthy and do their work. Genes direct the making of each cell's machinery, including enzymes. Specialized cells are grouped together to form tissues and organs; organs work together in body systems.**

THE BODY FLUIDS AND THE CARDIOVASCULAR SYSTEM

Body fluids supply the tissues continuously with energy, oxygen, water, and building materials. The fluids constantly circulate to pick up fresh supplies and deliver wastes to points of disposal. Every cell continuously draws oxygen and nutrients from those fluids and releases carbon dioxide and other waste products into them.

The body's main fluids are the **blood** and **lymph.** Blood travels within the **arteries, veins,** and **capillaries,** as well as within the heart's chambers (see Figure 3-2). Lymph travels in separate vessels of its own. Other fluids circulate around the cells, such as the plasma of the blood and the fluid surrounding muscle cells (see Figure 3-3). Fluid surrounding cells **(extracellular fluid)** is derived from the blood in the capillaries; it squeezes out through the capillary walls and flows around the outsides of cells, permitting exchange of materials. Some of the fluid outside the cells returns to the blood by reentering the capillaries. The fluid remaining outside the capillaries forms lymph, which travels around the body by way of lymph vessels. The lymph eventually returns to the bloodstream near the heart where large lymph and blood vessels join. In this way, all cells are served by the cardiovascular system.

The fluid inside cells provides a medium in which all cell reactions take place. Its pressure also helps the cells hold their shape. The fluid inside cells is drawn from the fluid on the outside that bathes the cells.

genes units of a cell's inheritance, made of the chemical DNA (deoxyribonucleic acid). Each gene directs the making of a protein to do the body's work. (Proteins are described fully in Chapter 6.)

enzyme a protein that promotes a chemical reaction, described in Chapter 6.

fat cells cells that specialize in the storage of fat and that form the fat tissue.

tissues systems of cells working together to perform specialized tasks. Examples are muscles, nerves, blood, and bone.

organs discrete structural units made of tissues that perform specific jobs, such as the heart, liver, and brain.

body system a group of related organs that work together to perform a function. Examples are the circulatory system, respiratory system, and nervous system.

blood the fluid of the cardiovascular system, composed of water, red and white blood cells, other formed particles, nutrients, oxygen, and other constituents.

lymph (LIMF) the fluid that moves from the bloodstream into tissue spaces and then travels in its own vessels, which eventually drain back into the bloodstream.

arteries blood vessels that carry blood containing fresh oxygen supplies from the heart to the tissues (see Figure 3-2).

veins blood vessels that carry blood, with the carbon dioxide it has collected, from the tissues back to the heart (see Figure 3-2).

capillaries minute, weblike blood vessels that connect arteries to veins and permit transfer of materials between blood and tissues (see Figures 3-2 and 3-3).

extracellular fluid fluid residing outside the cells.

FIGURE 3-2

BLOOD FLOW IN THE CARDIOVASCULAR SYSTEM

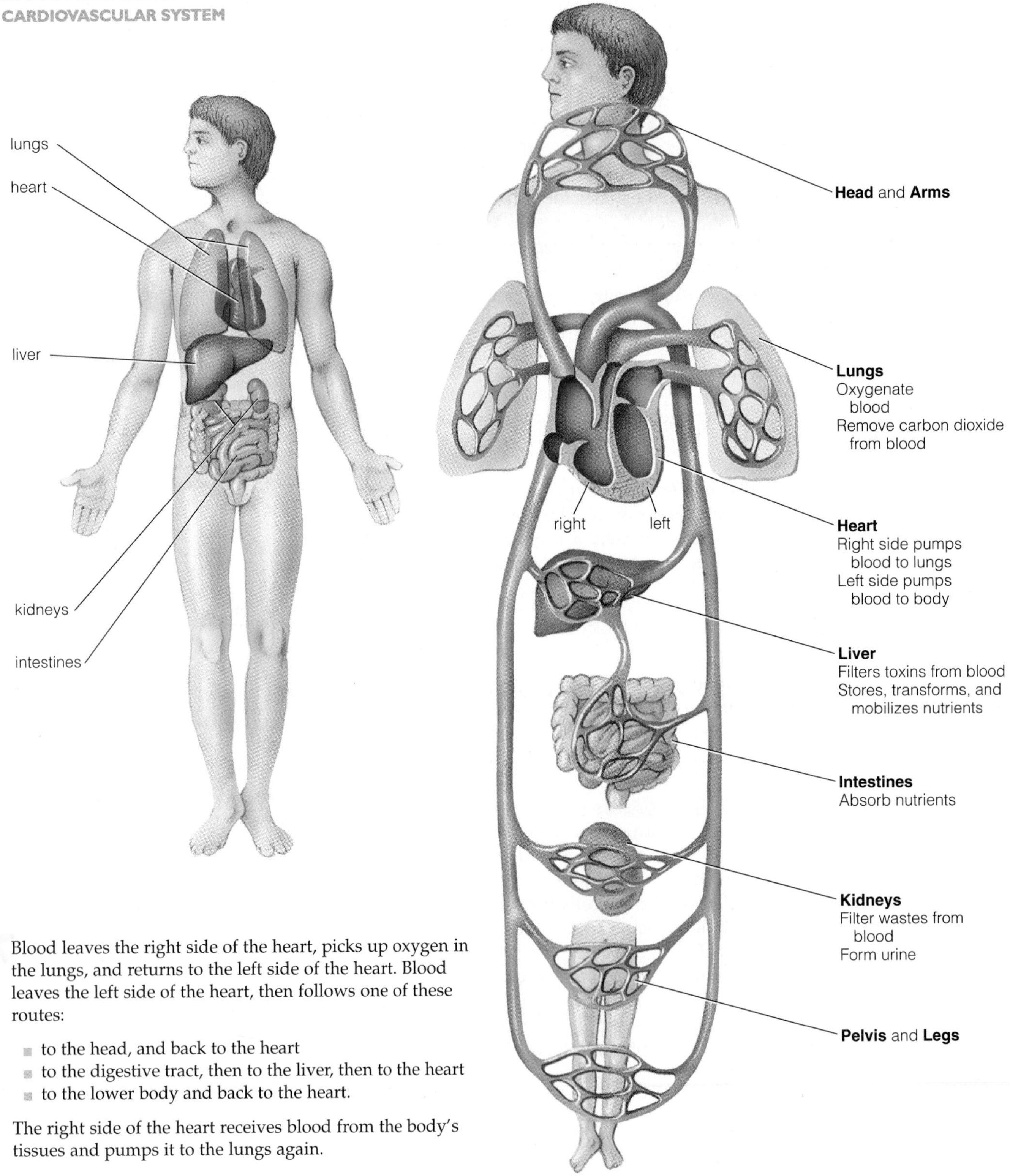

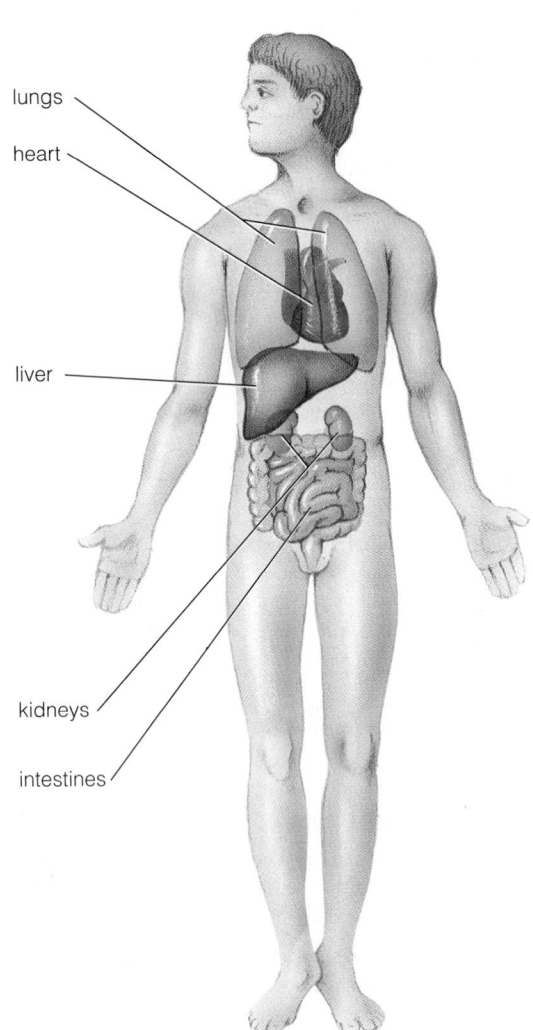

lungs

heart

liver

kidneys

intestines

Head and **Arms**

Lungs
Oxygenate
  blood
Remove carbon dioxide
  from blood

right   left

Heart
Right side pumps
  blood to lungs
Left side pumps
  blood to body

Liver
Filters toxins from blood
Stores, transforms, and
  mobilizes nutrients

Intestines
Absorb nutrients

Kidneys
Filter wastes from
  blood
Form urine

Pelvis and **Legs**

Blood leaves the right side of the heart, picks up oxygen in the lungs, and returns to the left side of the heart. Blood leaves the left side of the heart, then follows one of these routes:

- to the head, and back to the heart
- to the digestive tract, then to the liver, then to the heart
- to the lower body and back to the heart.

The right side of the heart receives blood from the body's tissues and pumps it to the lungs again.

As the blood travels through the cardiovascular system, it delivers materials cells need and picks up their wastes. The blood picks up oxygen in the **lungs** and also releases carbon dioxide there, as Figure 3-4 on the next page shows. All the blood circulates to the lungs, then returns to the heart, where it receives powerful impetus from the pumping heartbeats that push it out to all body tissues. Thus all tissues receive oxygenated blood fresh from the lungs.

As it passes through the digestive system, the blood delivers oxygen to the cells there and picks up most nutrients other than fats from the **intestine** for distribution elsewhere. Lymphatic vessels pick up most fats from the intestine and then transport them to the blood. All blood leaving the digestive system is routed directly to the **liver,** which has the special task of chemically altering the absorbed materials to make them better suited for use by other tissues. Later, in passing through the **kidneys,** the blood is cleaned of wastes. In summary, the blood is routed as follows (look again at Figure 3-2):

- Heart to tissues to heart to lungs to heart (repeat).

The portion of the blood that flows by the intestine travels from:

- Heart to intestine to liver to heart.

To ensure efficient circulation of fluid to all your cells, you need an ample fluid intake. This means drinking sufficient water to replace the water lost each

lungs the body's organs of gas exchange. Blood circulating through the lungs releases its carbon dioxide and picks up fresh oxygen to carry to the tissues.

intestine the body's long, tubular organ of digestion and the site of nutrient absorption.

liver a large, lobed organ that lies just under the ribs. It filters the blood, removes and processes nutrients, manufactures materials for export to other parts of the body, and destroys toxins or stores them to keep them out of the circulation.

kidneys a pair of organs that filter wastes from the blood, make urine, and release it to the bladder for excretion from the body.

FIGURE 3-3

HOW THE BODY FLUIDS CIRCULATE AROUND CELLS
The upper box shows a tiny portion of tissue with blood flowing through its network of capillaries (greatly enlarged). The lower-box illustrates the movement of the extracellular fluid.

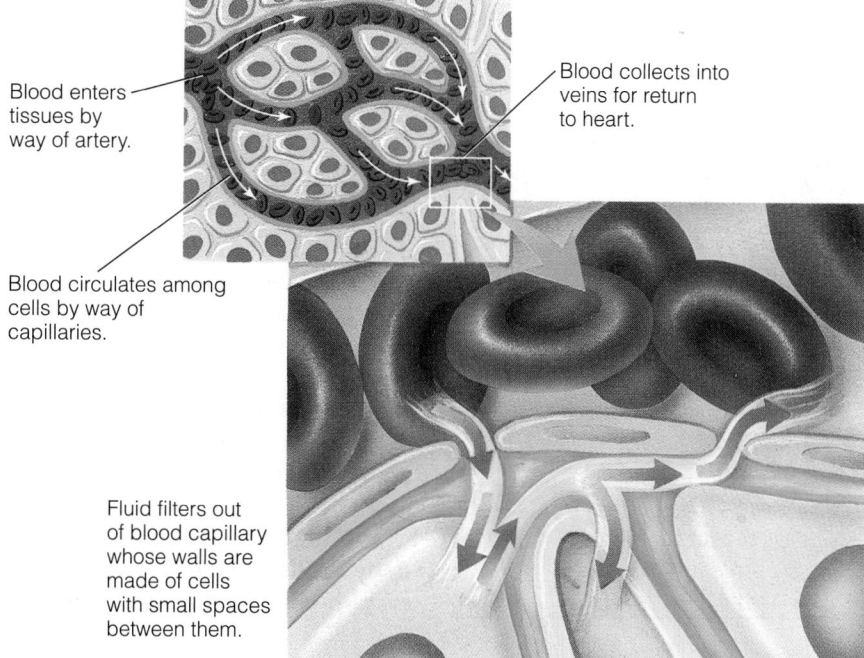

Blood enters tissues by way of artery.

Blood collects into veins for return to heart.

Blood circulates among cells by way of capillaries.

Fluid filters out of blood capillary whose walls are made of cells with small spaces between them.

Exchange of materials takes place between cell fluid and extracellular fluid.

Fluid may flow back into capillary or into lymph vessel. Lymph enters the bloodstream later through a large lymphatic vessel that empties into a large vein.

FIGURE 3-4

OXYGEN–CARBON DIOXIDE
EXCHANGE IN THE LUNGS

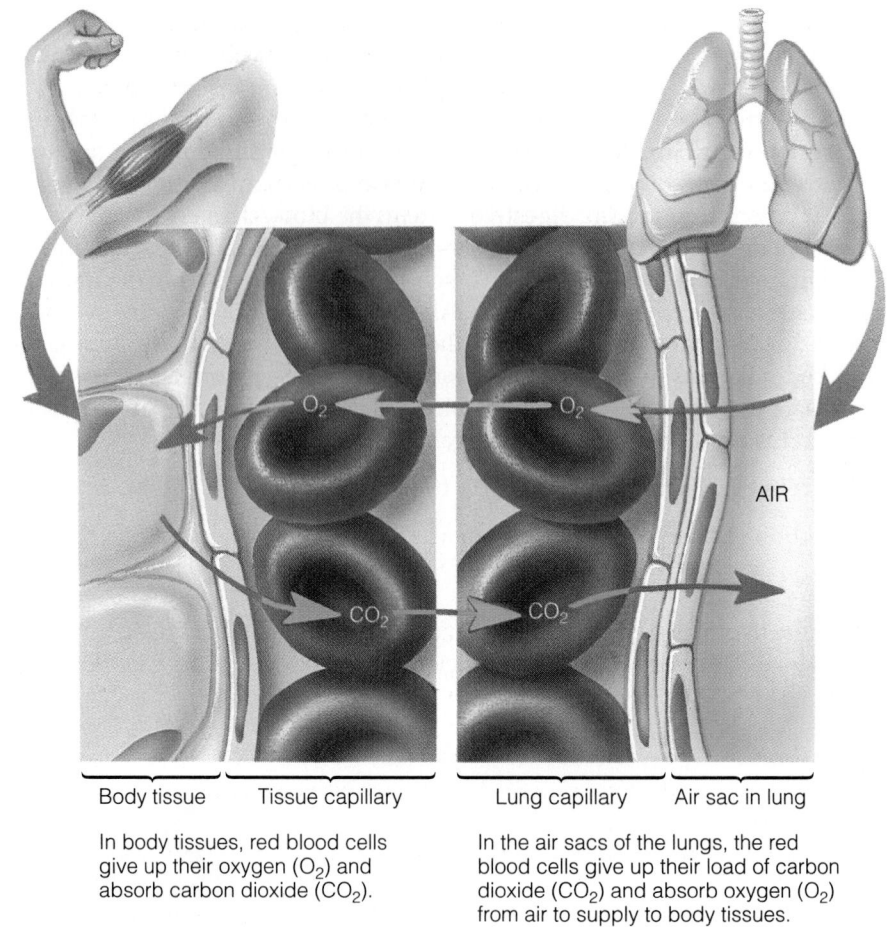

| Body tissue | Tissue capillary | Lung capillary | Air sac in lung |

In body tissues, red blood cells give up their oxygen (O_2) and absorb carbon dioxide (CO_2).

In the air sacs of the lungs, the red blood cells give up their load of carbon dioxide (CO_2) and absorb oxygen (O_2) from air to supply to body tissues.

---

hormones chemicals that are secreted by glands into the blood in response to conditions in the body that require regulation. These chemicals serve as messengers, acting on other organs to maintain constant conditions.

day. Cardiovascular fitness is essential, too, and constitutes an ongoing project that requires attention to both nutrition and physical activity. Healthy red blood cells also play a role, for they carry oxygen to all the other cells, enabling them to use fuels for energy. Since red blood cells arise, live, and die within about four months, your body replaces them constantly, a manufacturing process that requires many essential nutrients from food. Many kinds of blood disorders are caused by dietary deficiencies or imbalances of vitamins or minerals; the blood is very sensitive to malnutrition.

✓ KEY POINT **Blood and lymph deliver oxygen and nutrients to all the body's cells and carry waste materials away from them. The cardiovascular system ensures that these fluids circulate properly among all organs.**

THE HORMONAL AND NERVOUS SYSTEMS

In addition to nutrients, oxygen, and wastes the blood also carries chemical messengers, **hormones,** from one system of cells to another. Hormones communicate changing conditions that demand responses from the body organs. Hormones are secreted and released directly into the blood by organs known as glands. For example, when the **pancreas** (a gland) detects a high concentration of the blood's sugar, glucose, it releases **insulin,** a hormone. Insulin stimulates muscle and other cells to remove glucose from the blood and to store it. When the blood glucose level falls, the pancreas secretes another hormone, **glucagon,** to which the liver responds by releasing into the blood some of the glucose it stored earlier. Thus normal blood glucose levels are maintained.

Glands and hormones abound in the body. Each gland monitors a condition and produces one or more hormones to regulate it. Each hormone acts as a messenger that stimulates various organs to take appropriate actions.

Nutrition affects the hormonal system. Fasting, feeding, and exercise alter hormonal balances. People who become very thin have an altered hormonal balance that may make them unable to maintain their bones.[1] People who eat high-fat diets have hormone levels that may make them susceptible to certain cancers.

Hormones also affect nutrition. Along with the nervous system, they regulate hunger and affect appetite. They carry messages to regulate the digestive system, telling the digestive organs what kinds of foods have been eaten and how much of each digestive juice to secrete in response. Hormones also regulate the menstrual cycle in women, and they affect the appetite changes many women experience during the cycle and in pregnancy. An altered hormonal state is thought to be at least partly responsible, too, for the loss of appetite that sick people experience. Hormones also regulate the body's reaction to stress, suppressing hunger and the digestion and absorption of nutrients. When questions about a person's nutrition are asked, the state of that person's hormonal system is often part of the answer.

The body's other major communication system is, of course, the nervous system. With the brain and spinal cord as central controllers, the nervous system receives and integrates information from sensory receptors all over the

pancreas an organ with two main functions. One is an endocrine function—the making of hormones such as insulin, which it releases directly into the blood (*endo* means "into" the blood). The other is an exocrine function—the making of digestive enzymes, which it releases through a duct into the small intestine to assist in digestion (*exo* means "out" into a body cavity or onto the skin surface).

insulin a hormone from the pancreas that helps glucose enter cells from the blood (details in Chapter 4).

glucagon a hormone from the pancreas that stimulates the liver to release glucose into the bloodstream.

Details about hormones, menstruation, and the bones appear in Controversy 8 and Controversy 10.

All the body's cells live in water.

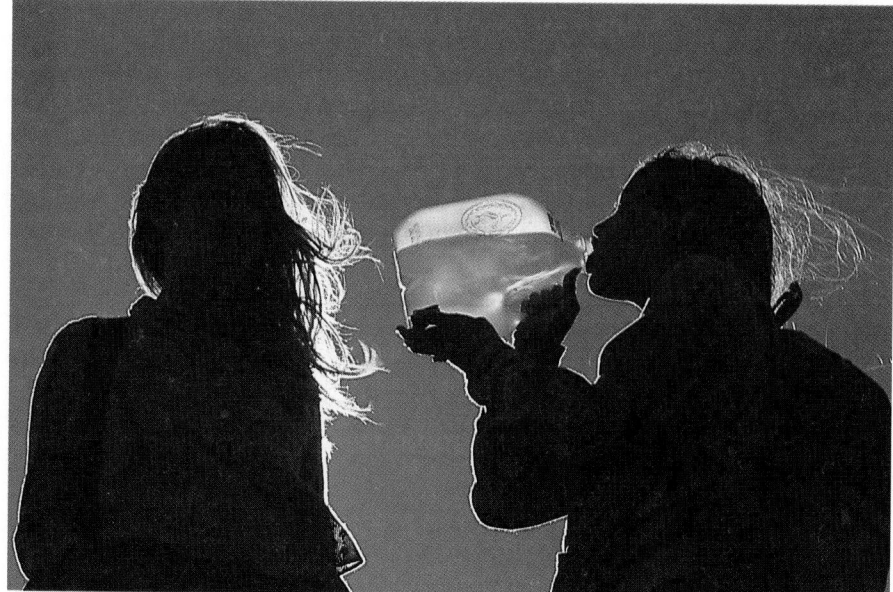

cortex the outermost layer of something. The brain's cortex is the part of the brain where conscious thought takes place.

hypothalamus (high-poh-THAL-uh-mus) a part of the brain that senses a variety of conditions in the blood, such as temperature, glucose content, salt content, and others. It signals other parts of the brain or body to adjust those conditions when necessary.

fight-or-flight reaction the body's instinctive hormone- and nerve-mediated reaction to danger. Also known as the *stress response.*

epinephrine the major hormone that elicits the stress response.

norepinephrine a compound related to epinephrine that helps to elicit the stress response.

body—sight, hearing, touch, smell, taste, and others—which communicate to the brain the state of both the outer and inner worlds, including the availability of food and the need to eat. The nervous system also sends instructions to the muscles and glands, telling them what to do.

The nervous system's role in hunger regulation is coordinated by the brain. The sensations of hunger and appetite are perceived by the brain's **cortex,** the thinking, outer layer. Much of the brain's regulatory work, however, goes on in the deep brain centers without the person's (or the cortex's) awareness. Deep inside the brain, the **hypothalamus** (see Figure 3-5) monitors many body conditions, including the availability of nutrients and water. The digestive tract sends messages to the hypothalamus by way of hormones and nerves that signal hunger, the physiological need for food. The signals also stimulate the stomach to intensify its contractions and secretions, causing hunger pangs (and gurgling sounds). When your cerebral cortex becomes conscious of hunger, you eat. The conscious mind of the cortex, however, can override such signals and allow a person to choose to delay eating despite hunger or to eat when hunger is absent.

A marvelous adaptation of the human body, the ability to respond to physical danger, involves the workings of both the hormonal and nervous systems. Known as the **fight-or-flight reaction** or the *stress response,* this adaptation is present with only minor variations in all animals, showing how universally important it is to survival. It is a magnificently well-coordinated response. When danger is detected, nerves fire and glands supply the compounds **epinephrine** and **norepinephrine.*** Every organ of the body responds. The pupils of the eyes widen so that you can see better; the muscles tense up so that you can jump, run, or struggle with maximum strength; breathing quickens and deepens to provide more oxygen. The heart races to rush the oxygen to the muscles, and the blood pressure rises to deliver efficiently the fuel the muscles need for energy. The liver pours forth glucose from its stores, while the fat cells release fat. The digestive system shuts down to permit all the body's systems to serve the muscles and nerves. With all action systems at peak efficiency, the body can respond with amazing speed and strength to whatever threatens it.

In ancient times, stress usually involved physical danger, and the response to it was violent physical exertion. In the modern world, stress is seldom physical, but the body's reaction to it is still the same. What stresses you today may be a checkbook out of control or a teacher who suddenly announces a pop quiz. Under these stresses, you are not supposed to fight or run as your Stone Age ancestor did. You smile at the "enemy" and suppress your fear. But your heart races, you feel it pounding, and hormones still flood your bloodstream with glucose and fat.

Your number-one enemy today is not a saber-toothed tiger prowling outside your cave, but a disease of modern civilization: atherosclerosis. Years of fat and other constituents accumulating in the arteries and stresses that strain the heart often lead to heart attacks, especially when chronic underexertion pairs with sudden high blood pressure. Daily exercise as part of a healthy lifestyle releases pent-up stress and strengthens the heart's defenses against atherosclerosis.

---

*Strictly speaking, norepinephrine is a neurotransmitter.

FIGURE 3-5

FIGURE 3-5

CUTAWAY SIDE VIEW OF THE BRAIN SHOWING THE HYPOTHALAMUS AND CORTEX
The hypothalamus monitors the body's conditions and sends signals to the brain's thinking portion, the cortex, which decides on actions.

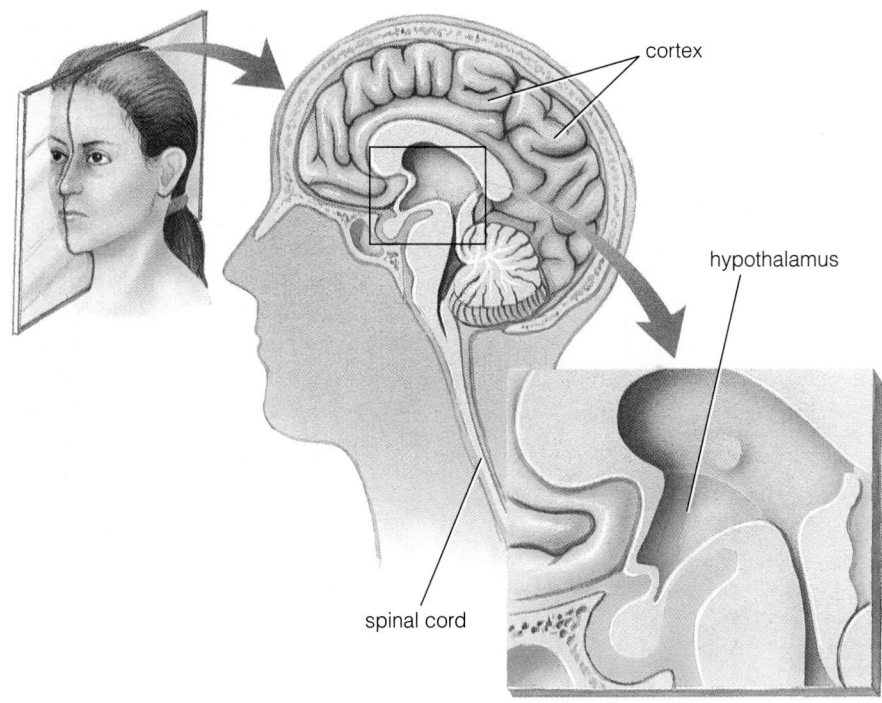

cortex

hypothalamus

spinal cord

✔ KEY POINT   **The hormonal and nervous systems regulate body processes through communication among all the organs. They respond to the need for food, govern the act of eating, regulate digestion, and call for the stress response.**

THE DIGESTIVE SYSTEM

When your body needs food, your brain and hormones alert your conscious mind to the sensation of hunger. Then, when you eat, your taste buds guide you in judging whether foods are acceptable (see Figure 3-6).

Sweet and salty tastes seem to be universally desirable, but most people have aversions to bitter and sour tastes in isolation (see Figure 3-7). The enjoyment of sweetness encourages people to consume ample energy, especially from foods containing sugars, the energy fuel for the brain. The pleasure of a salty taste prompts them to consume sufficient amounts of two very important minerals—sodium and chloride. The aversion to bitterness affects people's liking for foods in general. People born with great sensitivity to bitter tastes are apt to avoid foods with slightly bitter tastes, such as turnips or broccoli.[2]

The instinctive liking for sugar and salt can lead to drastic overeating of these substances. Sugar has become available in pure form only in the last hundred years, so it is relatively new to the human diet. While salt is much older, today both are being added liberally to foods by manufacturers to tempt us to eat their products.

Once you have eaten, your brain and hormones direct the many organs of the **digestive system** to **digest** and **absorb** the complex mixture of chewed and

digestive system the body system composed of organs that break down complex food particles into smaller, absorbable products. The *digestive tract* and *alimentary canal* are names for the tubular organs that extend from the mouth to the anus. The whole system, including the pancreas, liver, and gallbladder, is sometimes called the *gastrointestinal*, or *GI*, system.

digest to break molecules into smaller molecules, a main function of the digestive tract with respect to food.

absorb to take in, as nutrients are taken into the intestinal cells after digestion, the main function of the digestive tract with respect to nutrients.

peristalsis (perri-STALL-sis) the wave-like muscular squeezing of the esophagus, stomach, and small intestine that pushes their contents along.

stomach a muscular, elastic, pouchlike organ of the digestive tract that grinds and churns swallowed food and mixes it with acid and enzymes, forming chyme.

sphincter (SFINK-ter) a circular muscle surrounding, and able to close, a body opening.

chyme (KIME) the fluid resulting from the actions of the stomach upon a meal.

swallowed food. A diagram showing the digestive tract and its associated organs appears in Figure 3-8. The tract itself is a flexible, muscular tube extending from the mouth through the throat, esophagus, stomach, small intestine, large intestine, and rectum to the anus, for a total length of about 26 feet. In a sense the human body is itself a tube surrounding this digestive canal. When you have swallowed something, it still is not inside the body; it is only inside the inner bore of this tube. Only when a nutrient or other substance passes through the wall of the digestive tract does it actually enter the body's tissues. Many things pass into the digestive tract and out again, unabsorbed. A baby playing with beads may swallow one, but the bead will not really enter the body. It will emerge from the digestive tract within a day or two.

The digestive system's job is to digest food to its component nutrients and then to absorb those nutrients, leaving behind the substances, such as fiber, that are appropriate to excrete. To do this the system works at two levels: one, mechanical; the other, chemical.

The Mechanical Aspect of Digestion

The job of mechanical digestion begins in the mouth, where large, solid food pieces such as bites of meat are torn into shreds that can be swallowed without choking. Chewing also adds water in the form of saliva to soften rough or sharp foods, such as fried tortilla chips, to prevent them from tearing the esophagus. Saliva also moistens and coats each bite of food, making it slippery and able to pass easily down the esophagus.

Nutrients trapped inside indigestible skins, such as seeds, must be liberated by breaking these skins before they can be digested. Chewing bursts open kernels of corn, for example, which would otherwise traverse the tract and exit undigested. Once food has been mashed and moistened for comfortable swallowing, longer chewing times provide no additional advantages to digestion. In fact, for digestion's sake, a relaxed, peaceful attitude during a meal aids digestion much more than chewing for an extended time.[3]

Other organs take up the task of liquefying foods through the various mashing and squeezing actions of the stomach and intestines. The best known of these actions is **peristalsis,** a series of squeezing waves that start with the tongue's movement during a swallow and pass all the way down the esophagus (see Figure 3-9. The stomach and the intestines also push food through the tract by waves of peristalsis. Besides these actions, the **stomach** holds swallowed food for a while and mashes it into a fine paste; the stomach and intestines also add water, so that the paste becomes more fluid as it moves along.

Figure 3-10 shows the muscular stomach. Notice the circular **sphincter** muscle at the base of the esophagus.* It squeezes the opening at the entrance to the stomach to narrow it and prevent the stomach's contents from creeping back up the esophagus as the stomach contracts. The stomach stores swallowed food in a lump in its upper portion and squeezes the food little by little to its lower portion. There the food is ground and mixed thoroughly, ensuring that digestive chemicals mix with the entire thick liquid mass, now called **chyme.** Chyme bears no resemblance to the original food. The starches have been

*The circular stomach muscle is the cardiac spincter, so named for its proximity to the heart.

FIGURE 3-6

THE TASTE BUDS
Four basic kinds of taste buds are located on specific areas of the tongue. Each senses a single taste sensation: sweet, sour, bitter, or salty. Other factors that affect a food's flavor are aroma, texture, and temperature. In fact, the detection of a food's aroma is thousands of times more sensitive than detection of taste. The nose can detect just a few molecules responsible for the aroma of frying bacon, for example, even if they are diluted in several rooms full of air.

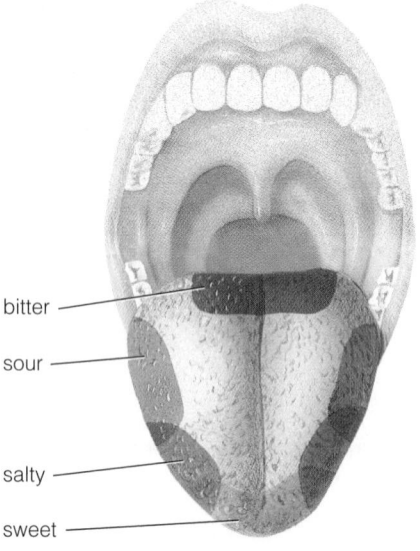

bitter

sour

salty

sweet

FIGURE 3-7

THE INNATE PREFERENCE FOR SWEET TASTE

This newborn baby is (a) resting (b) tasting distilled water, (c) tasting sugar, (d) tasting something sour, and (e) tasting something bitter.

SOURCE: Taste-induced facial expressions of neonate infants from the classic studies of J. E. Steiner, in *Taste and Development: The Genesis of Sweet Preference,* ed. J. M. Weiffenbach, HHS publication no. NIH 77–1068 (Bethesda, Md.: U.S. Department of Health and Human Services, 1977), pp. 173–189, with permission of the author.

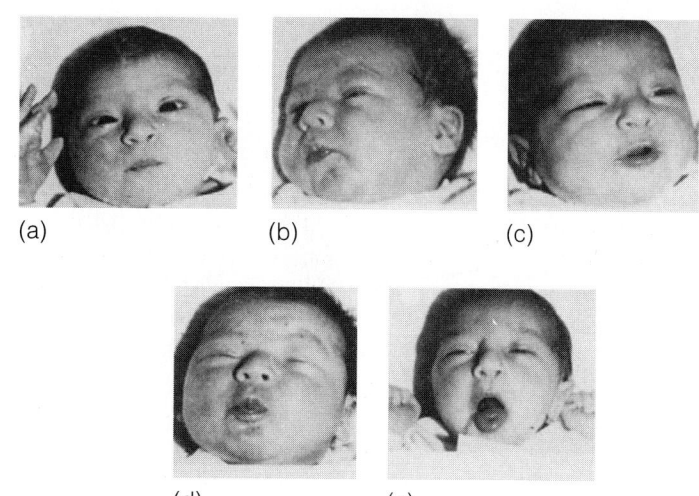

(a)   (b)   (c)

(d)   (e)

partly split, proteins have been uncoiled and clipped, and fat has separated from the mass.

The process of digestion is complicated, and the stomach acts as a holding tank, releasing only small amounts of food into the **small intestine** at one time. The muscular **pyloric valve** at the stomach's lower end (look again at Figure 3-10 controls the exit of the chyme, allowing only a little at a time to be squirted forcefully into the small intestine. Within a few hours after a meal, the stomach empties itself by means of these powerful squirts. The small intestine contracts rhythmically to move the contents along its length.

By the time the intestinal contents have arrived in the **large intestine** (also called the **colon**), digestion and absorption are nearly complete. The colon's task is mostly to reabsorb the water donated earlier by digestive organs and to absorb minerals, leaving a paste of fiber and other undigested materials, the **feces,** suitable for excretion. The fiber provides bulk against which the muscles of the colon can work. The rectum stores this fecal material to be excreted at intervals. From mouth to rectum, the transit of a meal is accomplished in as short a time as a single day or as long as three days.

Some people wonder whether the digestive tract works best at some hours in the day and whether the timing of meals can affect how a person feels. Timing of meals is important to feeling well, not because the digestive tract is unable to digest food at certain times, but because the body requires nutrients to be replenished every few hours. Digestion is virtually continuous, being limited only during sleep and exercise. For some people, eating late may interfere with normal sleep. As for exercise, it is best pursued a few hours after eating because digestion can inhibit physical work (see Chapter 10 for details).

KEY POINT **The digestive tract moves food through its various processing chambers by mechanical means. The mechanical actions include chewing, mixing by the stomach, adding fluid, and moving the tract's contents by peristalsis. After digestion and absorption, wastes are excreted.**

small intestine the 20-foot length of small-diameter intestine, below the stomach and above the large intestine, that is the major site of digestion of food and absorption of nutrients.

pyloric (pye-LORE-ick) **valve** the circular muscle of the lower stomach that regulates the flow of partly digested food into the small intestine. Also called *pyloric sphincter.*

large intestine the portion of the intestine that completes the absorption process.

colon the large intestine.

feces waste material remaining after digestion and absorption are complete; eventually discharged from the body.

FIGURE 3-8

THE DIGESTIVE SYSTEM

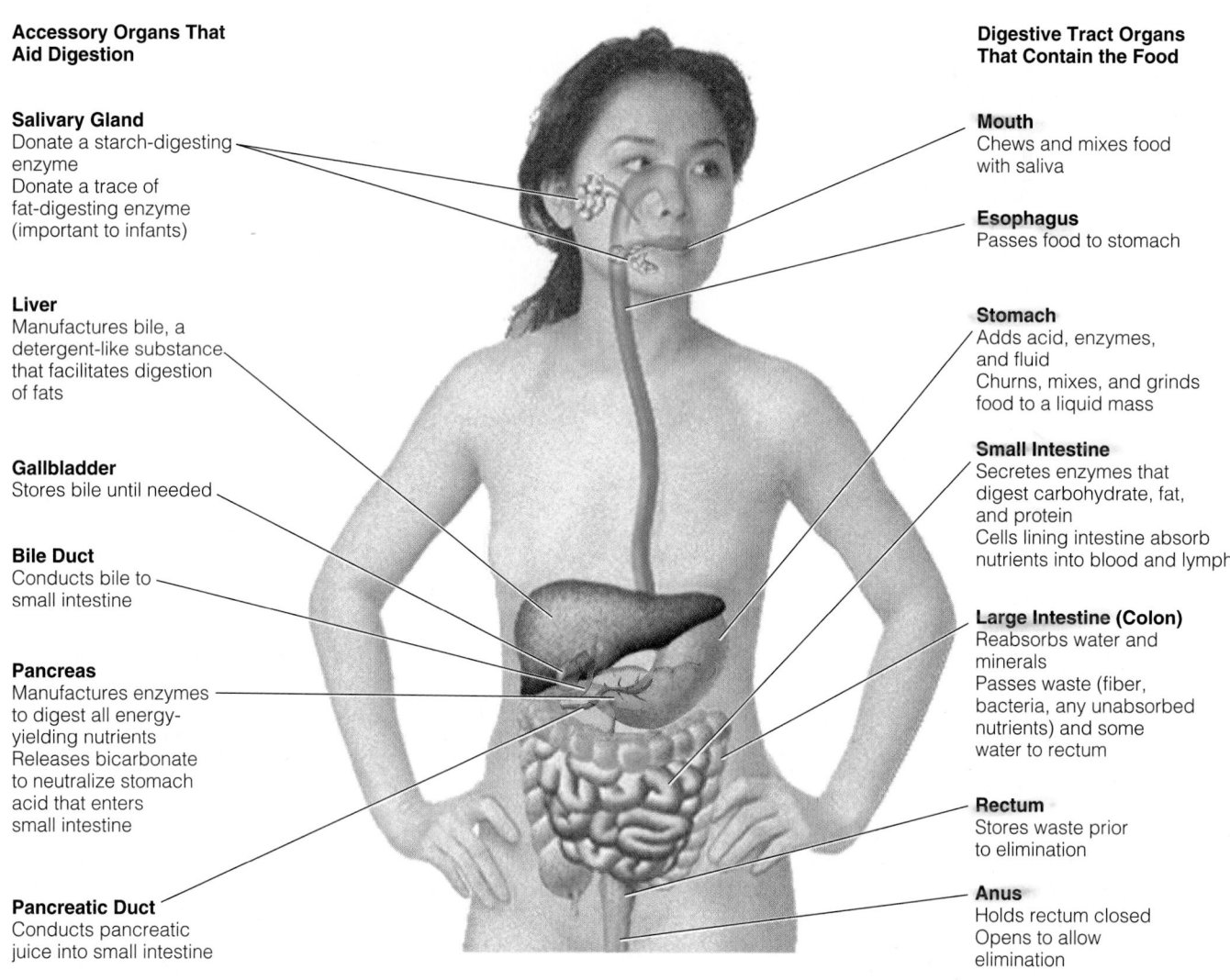

**Accessory Organs That
Aid Digestion**

Salivary Gland
Donate a starch-digesting
enzyme
Donate a trace of
fat-digesting enzyme
(important to infants)

Liver
Manufactures bile, a
detergent-like substance
that facilitates digestion
of fats

Gallbladder
Stores bile until needed

Bile Duct
Conducts bile to
small intestine

Pancreas
Manufactures enzymes
to digest all energy-
yielding nutrients
Releases bicarbonate
to neutralize stomach
acid that enters
small intestine

Pancreatic Duct
Conducts pancreatic
juice into small intestine

**Digestive Tract Organs
That Contain the Food**

Mouth
Chews and mixes food
with saliva

Esophagus
Passes food to stomach

Stomach
Adds acid, enzymes,
and fluid
Churns, mixes, and grinds
food to a liquid mass

Small Intestine
Secretes enzymes that
digest carbohydrate, fat,
and protein
Cells lining intestine absorb
nutrients into blood and lymph

Large Intestine (Colon)
Reabsorbs water and
minerals
Passes waste (fiber,
bacteria, any unabsorbed
nutrients) and some
water to rectum

Rectum
Stores waste prior
to elimination

Anus
Holds rectum closed
Opens to allow
elimination

gastric juice the digestive secretion of
the stomach.

pH a measure of acidity on a point
scale. A solution with a pH of 1 is a
strong acid; a solution with a pH of 7 is
neutral; a solution with a pH of 14 is a
strong base.

The Chemical Aspect of Digestion

Several organs of the digestive system secrete special digestive juices that perform the complex chemical processes of digestion. Digestive juices contain
enzymes that break nutrients down into their component parts. The digestive
organs are the salivary glands, the stomach, the pancreas, the liver, and the
small intestine. Their secretions are listed in Figure 3-8, above.

Digestion begins in the mouth. An enzyme in saliva starts rapidly breaking
down starch, and another enzyme initiates a little digestion of fat, especially
the digestion of milk fat, important in infants. Saliva also helps maintain the
health of the teeth in two ways: by washing away food particles that would
otherwise foster decay and by neutralizing decay-promoting acids produced
by bacteria in the mouth.

FIGURE 3-9

PERISTALTIC WAVE PASSING DOWN
THE ESOPHAGUS

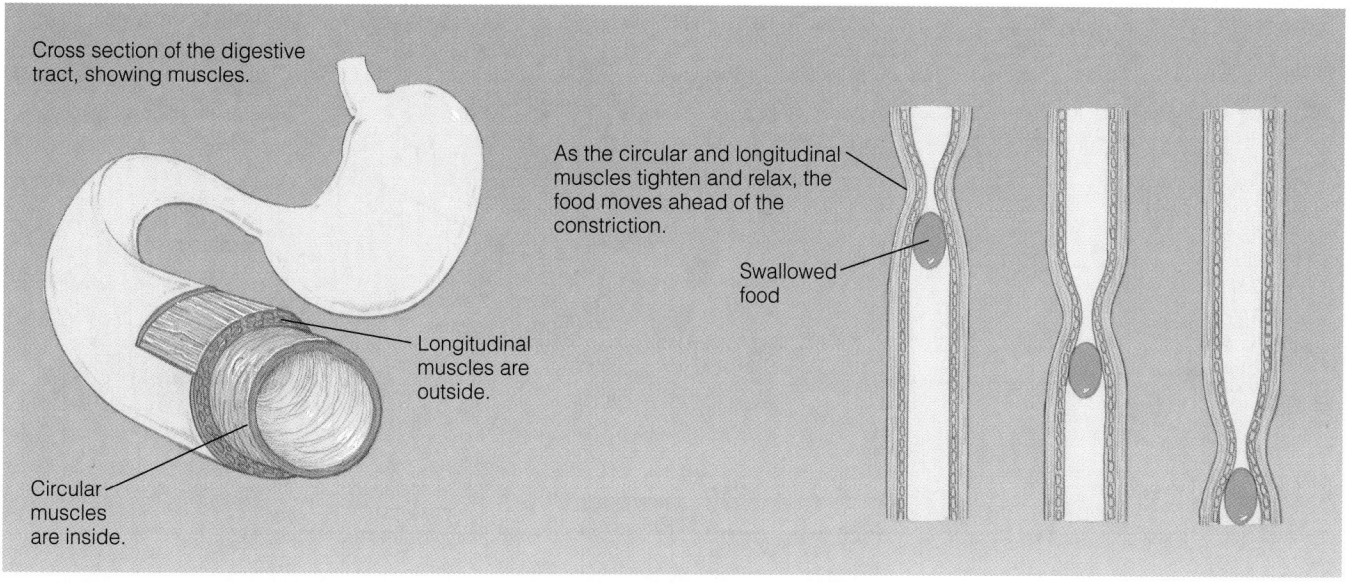

Cross section of the digestive tract, showing muscles.

As the circular and longitudinal muscles tighten and relax, the food moves ahead of the constriction.

Swallowed food

Longitudinal muscles are outside.

Circular muscles are inside.

In the stomach, protein digestion begins. Cells in the stomach release **gastric juice,** a mixture of water, enzymes, and hydrochloric acid. A strong acid is needed to activate a protein-digesting enzyme and to initiate digestion of protein. As you might guess from the presence of acid and enzymes, protein digestion is the stomach's main function. The strength of an acid solution is expressed as its **pH.** Figure 3-11 demonstrates that saliva is only weakly acidic, while the stomach's gastric juice is much more strongly acidic.

Upon learning of the powerful digestive juices and enzymes within the digestive tract, students often wonder how the tract's own cellular lining escapes being digested along with the food. Indeed, if it were not for specialized cells that secrete a thick, viscous substance known as **mucus,** the structures of the tract lining would be exposed to chemical attack. Mucus coats and protects the digestive tract lining.

In the small intestine, the digestive process gets under way in earnest. The small intestine is "the" organ of digestion and absorption, and it finishes what the mouth and stomach have started. The small intestine works with the precision of a laboratory chemist. As the thoroughly liquefied and partially digested nutrient mixture arrives there, hormonal messengers signal the gallbladder to contract and to squirt the right amount of the **emulsifier, bile,** into the intestine. Other hormones notify the pancreas to release **pancreatic juice** containing the alkaline compound **bicarbonate** in amounts precisely adjusted to neutralize the stomach acid that has reached the small intestine. All of the actions just described alter the intestinal environment to perfectly support the work of the digestive enzymes.

Meanwhile, the pancreatic and intestinal enzymes act on the chemical bonds that hold the large nutrients together, so that smaller and smaller pieces

mucus (MYOO-cus) a slippery coating of the digestive tract lining (and other body linings) that protects the cells from exposure to digestive juices (and other destructive agents). The adjective form is *mucous* (same pronunciation). The digestive tract lining is a *mucous membrane.*

emulsifier (ee-MULL-sih-fire) a compound with both water-soluble and fat-soluble portions that can attract fats and oils into water to form an emulsion.

bile a compound made by the liver, stored in the gallbladder, and released into the small intestine when needed. It emulsifies fats and oils to ready them for enzymatic digestion (described in Chapter 5).

pancreatic juice fluid secreted by the pancreas that contains enzymes to digest carbohydrate, fat, and protein as well as sodium bicarbonate, a neutralizing agent.

bicarbonate a common alkaline chemical; a secretion of the pancreas; also, the active ingredient of baking soda.

FIGURE 3-10

THE MUSCULAR STOMACH

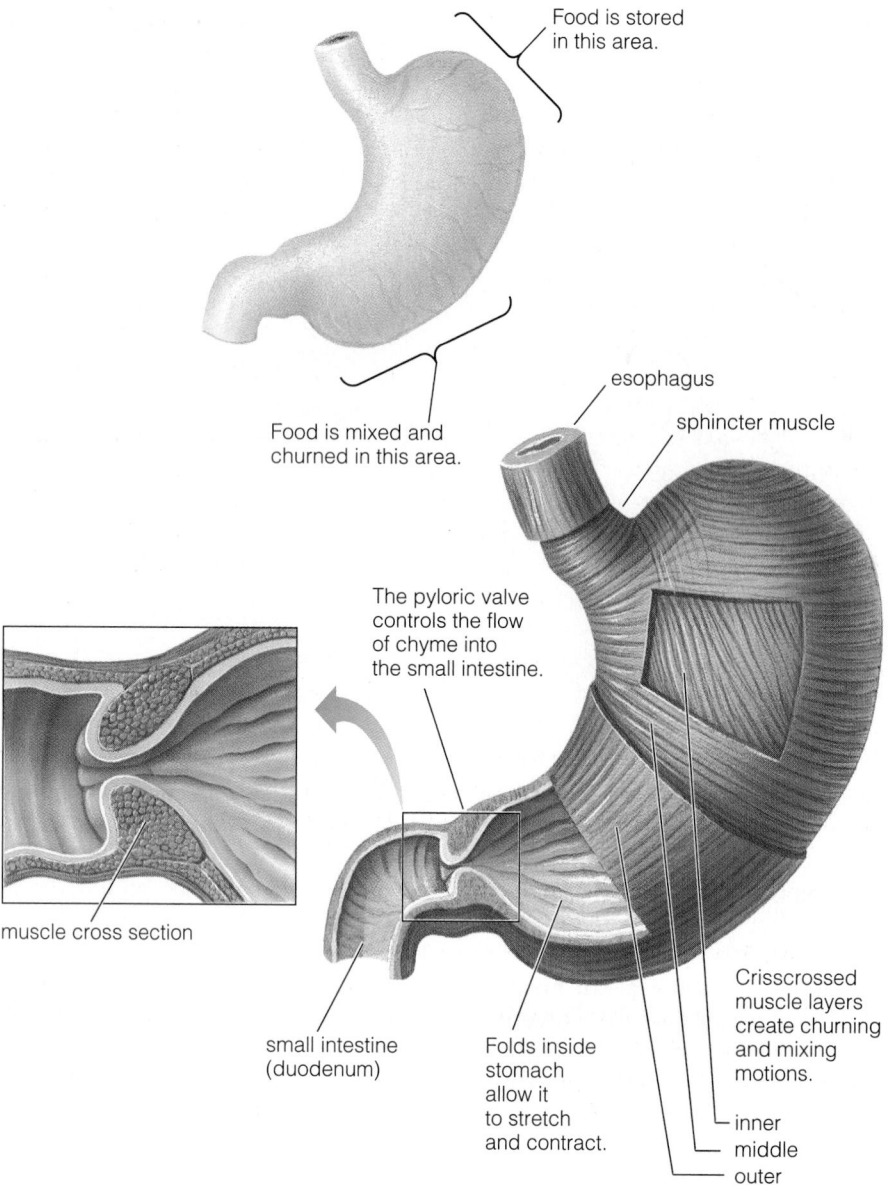

Food is stored in this area.

Food is mixed and churned in this area.

esophagus

sphincter muscle

The pyloric valve controls the flow of chyme into the small intestine.

muscle cross section

small intestine (duodenum)

Folds inside stomach allow it to stretch and contract.

Crisscrossed muscle layers create churning and mixing motions.

inner
middle
outer

are released into the intestinal fluids. The cells of the intestinal wall also hold some digestive enzymes on their surfaces, which perform last-minute breakdown reactions required before nutrients can be absorbed. Finally, the digestive process releases pieces small enough for the cells to absorb and use. Digestion and absorption of carbohydrate, fat, and protein are essentially complete by the time the intestinal contents enter the colon. Water, fiber, and some minerals, however, remain in the tract. Table 3-1 provides a summary of all the processes involved.

The digestive system can adjust to whatever mixture of foods is presented to it. People sometimes wonder if the digestive tract has trouble digesting certain foods in combination—for example, fruit and meat. Proponents of the fad of "food combining" claim that the digestive tract cannot perform certain digestive tasks at the same time, but this is a gross underestimation of the tract's capabilities. The truth is that all foods, regardless of identity, are broken down by enzymes into the basic molecules that make them up. In fact, scientists who study digestion suggest that the tract analyzes the diet's nutrient contents and delivers juice and enzymes appropriate for digesting those nutrients.[4] The pancreas is especially sensitive in this regard and has been observed to adjust its output of enzymes to digest carbohydrate, fat, or protein to an amazing degree. The pancreas of a person who suddenly consumes a meal unusually high in carbohydrate, for example, would begin increasing its output of carbohydrate-digesting enzymes within 24 hours, while reducing outputs of other types.[5] This sensitive mechanism ensures that foods of all types are used fully by the body.

The next section reviews the major processes of digestion by showing how the nutrients in a mixture of foods are handled. The foods used to illustrate the digestive process are those in a peanut butter and banana sandwich. But whether the nutrients in the digestive tract occurred originally in this meal or in a chili dog makes little difference to the digestive tract, which can promptly polish off either or both.

✔ KEY POINT **Chemical digestion begins in the mouth, where food is mixed with an enzyme in saliva that acts on carbohydrates. Digestion continues in the stomach, where stomach enzymes and acid break down protein. Digestion continues in the small intestine, where the liver and gallbladder contribute bile that emulsifies fat, and where the pancreas and small intestine donate enzymes that continue digestion so that absorption can occur.**

The Digestive Fate of a Sandwich

The process of rendering foods into nutrients and absorbing them into the body fluids is remarkably efficient. Within about 24 to 48 hours of eating, a healthy body digests and absorbs about 90 percent of the carbohydrate, fat, and protein in a meal. Here, we follow a peanut butter and banana sandwich on whole-wheat, sesame seed bread through the tract for the purpose of reviewing digestive processes in order of their occurrence in the body.

In the Mouth   In each bite, food components are crushed, mashed, and mixed with saliva by the teeth and the tongue. The sesame seeds are crushed and torn open by the teeth, which break through the indigestible fiber coating so that digestive enzymes can reach the nutrients inside the seeds. The peanut butter is the "extra crunchy" type, but the teeth grind the chunks to a paste before the bite is swallowed. The carbohydrate-digesting enzyme of saliva begins to break down the starches of the bread, banana, and peanut butter to sugars. Each swallow triggers a peristaltic wave that travels the length of the esophagus and carries one bite of food to the stomach.

In the Stomach   The stomach collects bite after swallowed bite in its upper storage area, where starch continues to be digested until the gastric juice mixes with the salivary enzymes and halts their action. Small portions of the mashed sandwich are pushed into the digesting area of the stomach where

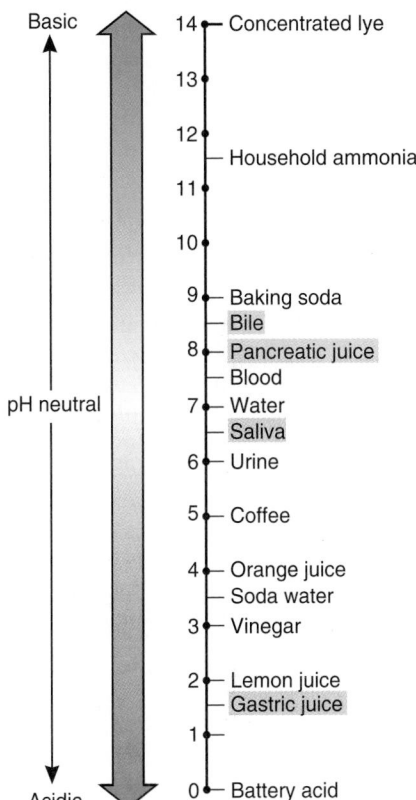

FIGURE 3-11

pH VALUES OF DIGESTIVE JUICES AND OTHER COMMON FLUIDS

A substance's acidity or alkalinity is measured in pH units. Each step down the scale indicates a tenfold increase in concentration of hydrogen particles. For example, a pH of 2 is 1,000 times stronger than a pH of 5.

Basic	14 — Concentrated lye
	13
	12
	— Household ammonia
	11
	10
	9 — Baking soda
	— Bile
	8 — Pancreatic juice
	— Blood
pH neutral	7 — Water
	— Saliva
	6 — Urine
	5 — Coffee
	4 — Orange juice
	— Soda water
	3 — Vinegar
	2 — Lemon juice
	— Gastric juice
	1
Acidic	0 — Battery acid

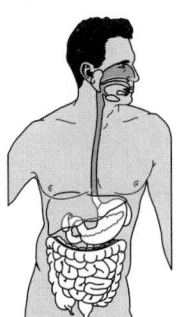

Time in mouth, less than a minute.

TABLE 3-1

Summary of Chemical Digestion

	Mouth	Stomach	Small Intestine, Pancreas, Liver, and Gallbladder	Large Intestine (Colon)
Sugar and Starch	The salivary glands secrete saliva to moisten and lubricate food; chewing crushes and mixes it with a salivary enzyme that initiates starch digestion.	Digestion of starch continues while food remains in the upper storage area of the stomach. In the lower digesting area of the stomach, hydrochloric acid and an enzyme of the stomach's juices halt starch digestion.	The pancreas produces a starch-digesting enzyme and releases it into the small intestine. Cells in the intestinal lining possess enzymes on their surfaces that break sugars and starch fragments into simple sugars, which then are absorbed.	Undigested carbohydrates reach the colon and are partly broken down by intestinal bacteria.
Fiber	The teeth crush fiber and mix it with saliva to moisten it for swallowing.	No action.	Fiber binds cholesterol and some minerals.	Most fiber excreted with feces; some fiber digested by bacteria in colon.
Fat	Fat-rich foods are mixed with saliva. The tongue produces traces of a fat-digesting enzyme that accomplishes some breakdown, especially of milk fats. The enzyme is stable at low pH and is important to digestion in nursing infants.	Fat tends to rise from the watery stomach fluid and foods and float on top of the mixture. Only a small amount of fat is digested. Fat is last to leave the stomach.	The liver secretes bile; the gallbladder stores it and releases it into the small intestine. Bile emulsifies the fat and readies it for enzyme action. The pancreas produces fat-digesting enzymes and releases them into the small intestine to split fats into their component parts (primarily fatty acids), which then are absorbed.	Some fatty materials escape absorption and are carried out of the body with other wastes.
Protein	Chewing crushes and softens protein-rich foods and mixes them with saliva.	Stomach acid works to uncoil protein strands and to activate the stomach's protein-digesting enzyme. Then the enzyme breaks the protein strands into smaller fragments.	Enzymes of the small intestine and pancreas split protein fragments into smaller fragments or free amino acids. Enzymes on the cells of the intestinal lining break some protein fragments into free amino acids, which then are absorbed. Some protein fragments are also absorbed.	The large intestine carries undigested protein residue out of the body. Normally, almost all food protein is digested and absorbed.
Water	The mouth donates watery, enzyme-containing saliva.	The stomach donates acidic, watery, enzyme-containing gastric juice.	The liver donates a watery juice containing bile. The pancreas and small intestine add watery, enzyme-containing juices; pancreatic juice is also alkaline.	The large intestine reabsorbs water and some minerals.

gastric juice mixes with the mass. Acid in gastric juice unwinds proteins; an enzyme clips into pieces the protein strands from the bread, seeds, and peanut butter. The sandwich has now become chyme. The watery carbohydrate- and protein-rich part of the chyme enters the small intestine first; a layer of fat follows closely behind.

In the Small Intestine   Some of the sweet sugars in the banana require so little digesting that they begin to cross the linings of the small intestine immediately on contact. Nearby, the liver donates bile through a duct into the small intestine. The bile blends the fat from the peanut butter and seeds with the watery enzyme-containing digestive fluids. The nearby pancreas squirts enzymes into the small intestine to break down the fat, protein, and starch in the chemical soup that just an hour ago was a sandwich. The cells of the small intestine itself produce enzymes to complete these processes. As the enzymes do their work, smaller and smaller chemical fragments are liberated from the chemical soup and are absorbed into the blood and lymph through the cells of the small intestine's wall. Vitamins and minerals are absorbed here, too. They all eventually enter the bloodstream to nourish the tissues.

In the Large Intestine (Colon)   Only fiber fragments, fluid, and some minerals are absorbed in the large intestine. The fibers from the seeds, whole-wheat bread, peanut butter, and banana are partly digested by the bacteria living in the colon, and some of the products are absorbed.[6] Most fiber is not absorbed, however, and, along with some other components, passes out of the colon, excreted as feces.

✔ **KEY POINT** **The mechanical and chemical actions of the digestive tract break foods down to nutrients, and large nutrients to their smaller building blocks, with remarkable efficiency.**

Absorption and Transportation of Nutrients

Once the digestive system has broken food down to its nutrient components, the rest of the body awaits their delivery. First, though, every molecule of nutrient must traverse one of the cells of the intestinal lining. These cells absorb nutrients from the mixture within the intestine and deposit them in the blood and lymph. The cells are selective: they recognize some of the nutrients that may be in short supply in the body. The mineral calcium is an example. The less calcium in the body, the more calcium the intestinal cells absorb. The cells are also extraordinarily efficient: they absorb enough nutrients to nourish all the body's other cells.

The cells of the intestinal tract lining are arranged in sheets that poke out into millions of finger-shaped projections **(villi).** Every cell on every villus has a brushlike covering of tiny hairs **(microvilli)** that can trap the nutrient particles. Each villus (projection) has its own capillary network and a lymph vessel so that as nutrients move across the cells, they can immediately mingle with the body fluids. Figure 3-12 provides a close look at these details.

The small intestine's lining, villi and all, is wrinkled into thousands of folds, so that its absorbing surface is enormous. If the folds, and the villi that poke out from them, were spread out flat, they would cover a third of a football

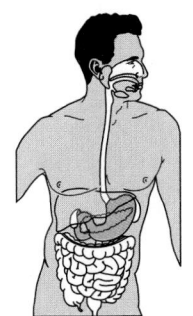

Time in stomach, about 1–2 hours.

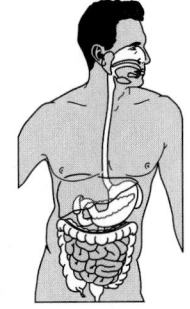

Time in small intestine, about 7–8 hours.*

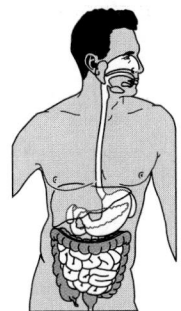

Time in colon, about 12–14 hours.*

*Based on a 24-hour transit time. Actual times vary widely.

villi (VILL-ee, VILL-eye) fingerlike projections of the sheets of cells that line the intestinal tract. The villi make the surface area much greater than it would otherwise be (singular: *villus*).

microvilli (MY-croh-VILL-ee, MY-croh-VILL-eye) tiny, hairlike projections on each cell of every villus that can trap nutrient particles and transport them into the cells (singular: *microvillus*).

FIGURE 3-12

DETAILS OF THE
SMALL INTESTINAL LINING

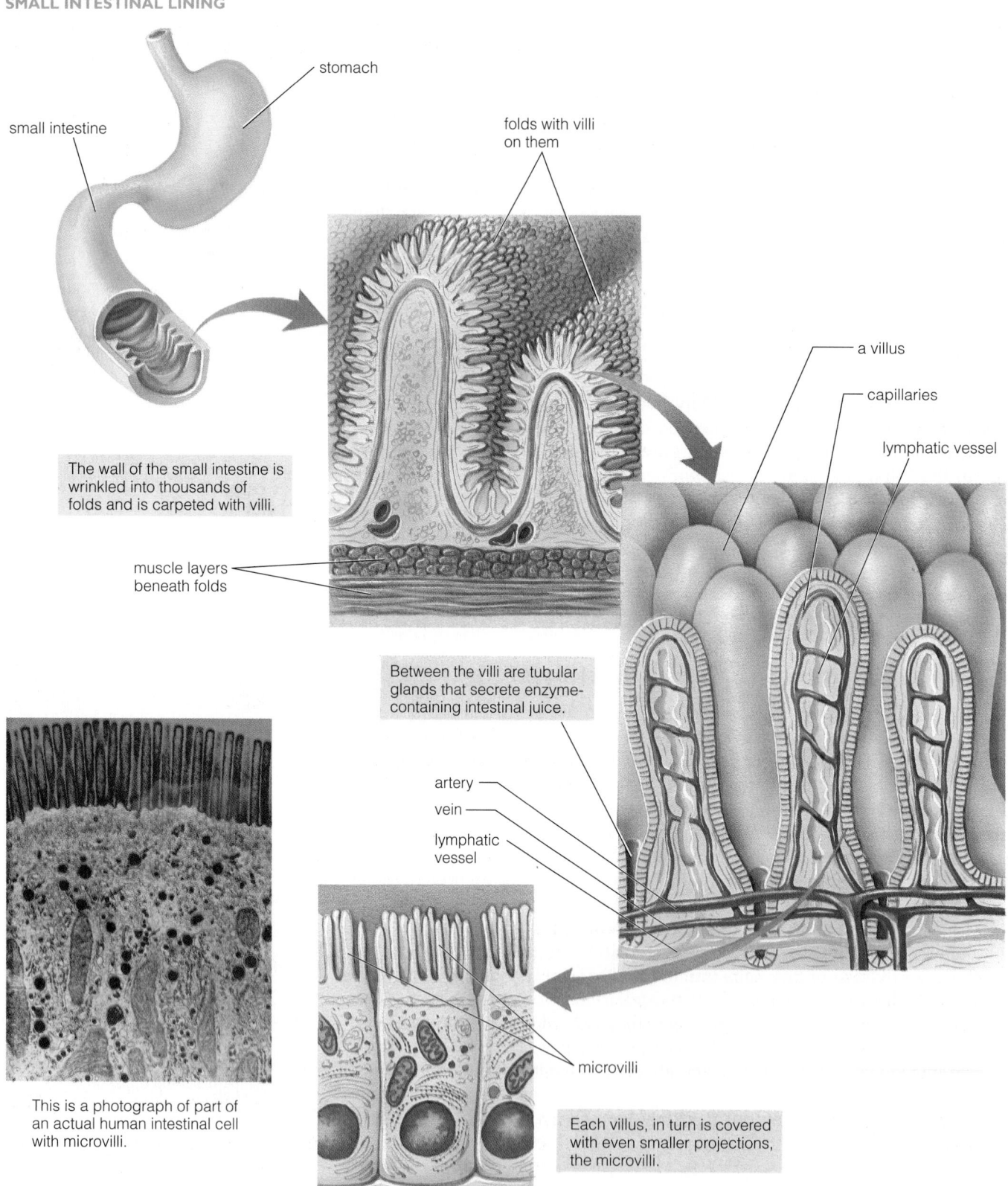

stomach

small intestine

folds with villi
on them

a villus

capillaries

lymphatic vessel

The wall of the small intestine is
wrinkled into thousands of
folds and is carpeted with villi.

muscle layers
beneath folds

Between the villi are tubular
glands that secrete enzyme-
containing intestinal juice.

artery

vein

lymphatic
vessel

microvilli

This is a photograph of part of
an actual human intestinal cell
with microvilli.

Each villus, in turn is covered
with even smaller projections,
the microvilli.

field. The billions of cells of that surface weigh only 4 to 5 pounds, yet they absorb enough nutrients to nourish the other 150 or so pounds of body tissues.

After the nutrients pass through the cells of the villi, the blood and lymph take over the job of transporting the nutrients to their ultimate consumers, the body's cells. The lymphatic vessels initially transport most of the products of fat digestion and a few vitamins, later delivering them to the bloodstream. The blood vessels carry the products of carbohydrate and protein digestion, most vitamins, and the minerals from the digestive tract to the liver. Thanks to these two transportation systems, every nutrient soon arrives at the place where it is needed.

The digestive system's millions of specialized cells are themselves sensitive to an undersupply of energy, nutrients, or dietary fiber. In cases of severe under-nutrition of energy and nutrients, the absorptive surface of the small intestine shrinks. The surface may be reduced to a tenth of its normal area, preventing it from absorbing what few nutrients a limited food supply may provide. With-out sufficient fiber to provide an undigested bulk for the tract's muscles to push against, the muscles become weak from lack of exercise. Malnutrition that impairs digestion is self-perpetuating because impaired digestion makes mal-nutrition worse. In fact, the digestive system's needs are few, but important. The body has much to say to the attentive listener, stated in a language of symptoms and feelings that you would be wise to study. The next section takes a light-hearted look at what your digestive tract might be trying to tell you.

✔ **KEY POINT** **The digestive system feeds the rest of the body and is itself sensitive to malnutrition. The folds and villi of the small intestine enlarge its surface area to facilitate nutrient absorption through uncount-able cells to the blood and lymph. These transport systems then deliver the nutrients to all the body cells.**

A Letter from Your Digestive Tract

To My Owner,

You and I are so close; I hope that I can speak frankly without offending you. I know that sometimes I *do* offend, with my gurgling noises and belching at quiet times and, oh yes, the gas. But please understand that when you chew gum, drink carbonated beverages, or eat hastily, you gulp air with each swal-low. I can't help making some noise as I move the air along my length or release it upward in a noisy belch. And if you eat or drink too fast, I can't help getting **hiccups.** Please sit and relax while you dine. You will ease my task and we'll both be happier.

Also, when someone offers you a new food, you gobble away, trusting me to do my job. I try. It would make my life easier, and yours less gassy, if you would start with small amounts of new foods, especially those high in fiber. The bacteria that break down fiber produce gas in the process. I can handle just about anything if you introduce it slowly. But please: if you do notice more gas than normal from a specific food, avoid it. If the gas becomes exces-sive, check with a physician—the problem could be something simple, or it could be serious.

When you eat or drink too much, it just burns me up. Overeating causes **heartburn** because the acidic juice from my stomach backs up into my esoph-agus. Acid poses no problem to my healthy stomach, whose walls are coated

hiccups spasms of both the vocal cords and the diaphragm, causing periodic, audible, short, inhaled coughs. Can be caused by irritation of the diaphragm, indigestion, or other causes. Hiccups usually resolve in a few minutes, but can have serious effects if prolonged. Breath-ing in to a paper bag (inhaling carbon dioxide) or dissolving a teaspoon of sugar in the mouth may stop them.

heartburn a burning sensation in the chest (in the area of the heart) area caused by backflow of stomach acid into the esophagus.

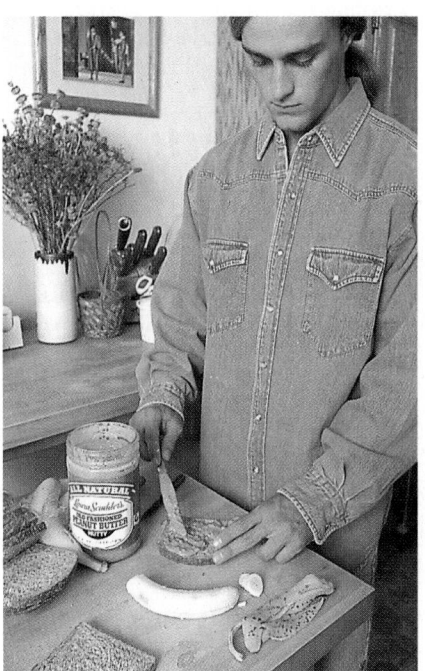

To become part of your body, food must first be digested and absorbed.

antacids medications that react directly and immediately with the acid of the stomach, neutralizing it. Antacids are most suitable for treating occasional heartburn. More about antacids appears in Controversy 8.

ulcers erosions in the topmost, and sometimes underlying, layers of cells that form linings. Ulcers of the digestive tract commonly form in the esophagus, stomach, or upper small intestine.

acid reducers and **acid controllers** drugs that reduce the acid output of the stomach. They are most suitable for treating severe, persistent forms of heartburn, but are useless for neutralizing acid already present in the stomach. Previously sold as prescription ulcer medications, the drugs are now sold freely, but the packages bear warnings of side effects; some types interfere with the stomach's ability to destroy alcohol, so more of the alcohol in a drink enters the bloodstream.

hernia a protrusion of an organ or part of an organ through the wall of the body chamber that normally contains the organ. An example is a *hiatal* (high-AY-tal) *hernia*, in which part of the stomach protrudes up through the diaphragm into the chest cavity, which contains the esophagus, heart, and lungs.

constipation infrequent, difficult bowel movements often caused by diet, inactivity, dehydration, or medication. (Also defined in Chapter 4.)

diarrhea frequent, watery bowel movements usually caused by diet, stress, or irritation of the colon. Severe, prolonged diarrhea robs the body of fluid and certain minerals, causing dehydration and imbalances that can be dangerous if left untreated.

with thick mucus to protect them. But when my too-full stomach squeezes some of its contents back up into the esophagus, the acid burns its unprotected surface. Also, those tight jeans you wear constrict my stomach, squeezing the contents upward into the esophagus. Just leaning over or lying down after a meal may allow the acid to escape up the esophagus because the muscular closure separating the two spaces is much looser than other such muscles. When heartburn is a problem, do me a favor: try to eat smaller meals; drink liquids an hour before or after, but not during, meals; wear reasonably loose clothing; and relax after eating, but sit up (don't lie down).

Sometimes your food choices irritate me. Specifically, chemical irritants in foods, such as the "hot" component of chili peppers, chemicals in coffee, fat, chocolate, and alcohol, can worsen heartburn.[7] Avoid the ones that cause trouble. Above all, do not smoke. Smoking makes my heartburn worse—and you should hear your lungs bellyache about it.

By the way, I can tell you've been taking heartburn medicines again. You must have been watching those TV commercials and letting them mislead you. You need to know that **antacids** are designed only to temporarily relieve pain from conditions such as heartburn and **ulcers,** while antibiotics and other medications help to heal ulcers. But in my case, the antacids trigger my stomach, which is normal, to produce *more* acid. That's because when my normal stomach acidity is reduced, I respond by producing more acid to restore the normal acid condition. Also, the ingredients in antacids can interfere with my ability to absorb nutrients. And don't take **acid reducers** and **acid controllers** for my sake; these reduce my acid so much that my job of digesting becomes much harder. In fact, the drugs can *cause* indigestion and diarrhea. They can also mask the symptoms of a **hernia** or an ulcer. A hernia can cause food to back up in the esophagus, and so feels like heartburn. Ulcer pain can be temporarily relieved by acid reducers and controllers. Treating only the symptoms of a hernia or an ulcer can delay its diagnosis and cure.

When you eat too quickly, I worry about choking (see Figure 3-13). Please take time to cut your food into small pieces, and chew it until it is crushed and moistened with saliva. Also, refrain from talking or laughing before swallowing, and never attempt to eat when you are breathing hard. Also, for our sake and the sake of others, learn the Heimlich maneuver as shown in Figure 3-14.

When I'm suffering, you suffer, too. When **constipation** and **diarrhea** strike, neither of us is having fun. Slow, hard, dry bowel movements can be painful, and failing to have a movement for too long brings on headaches and ill feelings. Listen carefully for my signal that it is time to defecate, and make time for it even if you are busy. The longer you ignore my signal, the more time the colon has to extract water from the feces, hardening them. Also, please choose foods that provide enough fiber (Chapter 4 lists some of these foods). Fiber attracts water, creating softer, bulkier stools that stimulate my muscles to contract, pushing the contents along. Fiber helps my muscles to stay fit, too, making elimination easier. Be sure to drink enough water, because dehydration causes the colon to absorb all the water it can get from the feces. And please work out regularly; exercise strengthens not just the muscles of your arms, legs, and torso, but those of the colon, too.

When I have the opposite problem, diarrhea, my system will rob you of water and salts. In diarrhea my intestinal contents have moved too quickly,

FIGURE 3-13

SWALLOWING AND CHOKING

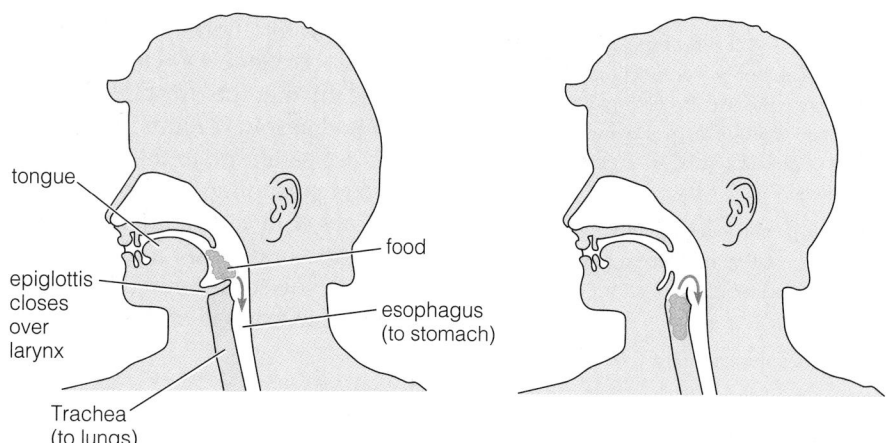

tongue

epiglottis
closes
over
larynx

Trachea
(to lungs)

food

esophagus
(to stomach)

A normal swallow. The epiglottis acts as a flap to seal the entrance to the lungs (trachea) and direct food to the stomach via the esophagus.

Choking. A choking person cannot speak or gasp because food lodged in the trachea blocks the passage of air. The red arrow points to where the food should have gone to prevent choking.

FIGURE 3-14

THE HEIMLICH MANEUVER

SOURCE: Adapted from H. J. Heimlich and M. H. Uhley, The Heimlich maneuver, *Clinical Symposia* 31 (1979): 1–32.

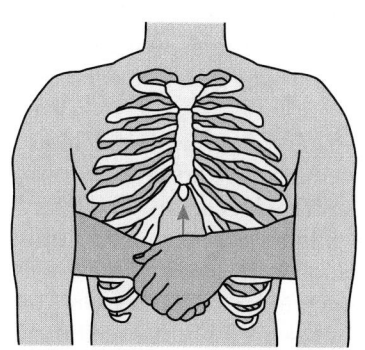

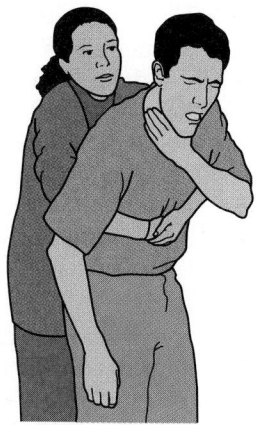

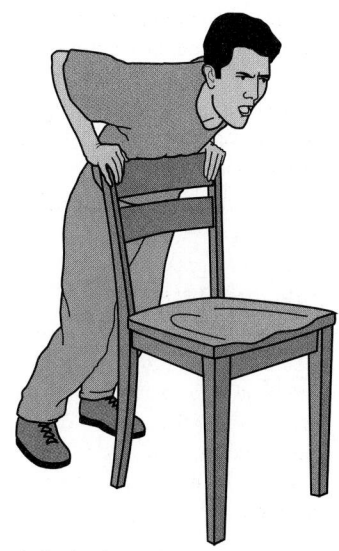

Rescuer positions fist directly against victim's abdomen as shown.

1. Rescuer stands behind victim and wraps her arms around victim's waist.

2. Rescuer makes a fist with one hand and places the thumb side of the fist against the victim's abdomen, slightly above the navel and below the rib cage.

3. Rescuer grasps fist with other hand and rapidly squeezes it inward and upward three or four times in rapid succession.

4. Rescuer repeats the process if necessary.

If the victim is alone, the victim positions himself or herself over edge of fixed horizontal object, such as a chair back, railing, or table edge, and presses abdomen into edge with quick movement.

irritable bowel syndrome intermittent disturbance of bowel function, especially diarrhea or alternating diarrhea and constipation, associated with diet, lack of physical activity, or psychological stress.

nephrons the working units in the kidneys, consisting of intermeshed blood vessels and tubules.

bladder the sac that holds urine until time for elimination.

Food poisoning and its prevention are topics of Chapter 14.

drawing water and minerals from your tissues into the contents. When this happens, please rest a while and drink fluids. To avoid diarrhea, try not to change my diet too drastically or quickly. I'm willing to work with you and learn to digest new foods, but if you suddenly change your diet, we're both in for it. I hate even to think of it, but one likely cause of diarrhea is dangerous food poisoning. If diarrhea lasts longer than just a day or two, or if it alternates with constipation, the cause could be **irritable bowel syndrome,** and you should go see a physician.

Thank you for listening. I know we'll both benefit from communicating like this, since we're in this together for the long haul.

Affectionately,

Your Digestive Tract

So much for digestion of foods, absorption of nutrients, and the workings of the digestive tract. The next section introduces the body's primary organs of waste removal, the kidneys, and describes how these marvelous organs monitor and adjust the amounts of dissolved substances in the blood.

✔ KEY POINT **The digestive tract has many ways to communicate its needs. By taking the time to listen, you will obtain a complete understanding of the mechanics of the digestive tract and its signals.**

THE EXCRETORY SYSTEM

Cells generate a number of wastes, and all of them must be eliminated. Many of the body's organs play roles in removing wastes. Carbon dioxide waste from the cells travels in the blood to the lungs, where it is exchanged for oxygen, as already mentioned. Other wastes are pulled out of the bloodstream by the liver. The liver processes these wastes and either tosses them out into the digestive tract with bile, to leave the body with the feces, or prepares them to be sent to the kidneys for disposal in the urine. Organ systems work together to dispose of the body's wastes, but the kidneys are waste- and water-removal specialists.

The kidneys straddle the cardiovascular system and filter the passing blood. Waste materials, dissolved in water, are collected by the kidneys' working units, the **nephrons.** These wastes become concentrated as urine, which travels through tubes to the urinary **bladder.** The bladder empties periodically, removing the wastes from the body. Thus the blood is purified continuously throughout the day, and dissolved materials are excreted as necessary. One dissolved mineral, sodium, helps to regulate blood pressure, and its excretion or retention by the kidneys is a vital part of the body's blood pressure–controlling mechanism. As you might expect, the kidneys' work is regulated by hormones secreted by glands that respond to conditions in the blood (such as the sodium concentration).

Because the kidneys remove toxins that could otherwise damage body tissues, whatever supports the health of the kidneys supports the health of the whole body. A strong cardiovascular system and an abundant supply of water are important to keep blood flushing swiftly through the kidneys. In addition, the kidneys need sufficient energy to do their complex sifting and sorting job, and many vitamins and minerals serve as the cogs in their machinery. Exercise and nutrition are vital to healthy kidney function.

✓ **KEY POINT**   **The kidneys adjust the blood's composition in response to the body's needs, disposing of everyday wastes and helping remove toxins. Nutrients, including water, and exercise help keep them healthy.**

STORAGE SYSTEMS

The human body is designed to eat at intervals of about four to six hours, but cells need nutrients around the clock. Providing the cells with a constant flow of the needed nutrients requires the cooperation of many body systems. These systems store and release nutrients to meet the cells' needs between meals. Among the major storage places are the liver and muscles, which store carbohydrate, and the fat cells, which store fat as well as other things.

Nutrients collected from the digestive system sooner or later all move through a vast network of capillaries that weave among the liver cells. This arrangement ensures that liver cells have access to the newly arriving nutrients for processing. Later chapters provide the details, but it is important to know now that the liver converts excess energy-containing nutrients into two forms. It makes some into **glycogen** (a carbohydrate) and some into fat. The liver stores the glycogen to meet the body's ongoing glucose needs. Liver glycogen can sustain cell activities when the intervals between meals become long. Without glucose absorbed from food, the cells (including the muscle cells) draw on liver glycogen. Should no food be available, the liver's glycogen supply dwindles; it can be effectively depleted within as few as three to six hours. Muscle cells make and store glycogen, too, but selfishly reserve it for their own use.

Whereas the liver stores glycogen, it ships out fat in packages (see Chapter 5) to be picked up by cells that need it. All body cells may withdraw the fat they need from these packages, and the fat cells pick up the remainder and store it to meet long-term energy needs. Unlike the liver, fat tissue has virtually infinite storage capacity. It can continue to supply the body's cells with fat for days, weeks, or possibly even months when no food is eaten.

These storage systems for glucose and fat ensure that the body's cells will not go without energy even if the body is hungry for food. Body stores also exist for many other nutrients, each with a characteristic capacity. For example, liver and fat cells store many vitamins, and bones provide reserves of calcium, sodium, and other minerals. Stores of nutrients are available to keep the blood levels constant and to meet cellular demands.

Some nutrients are stored in the body in much larger quantities than others are. For example, certain vitamins are stored without limit, even if they reach toxic levels within the body. Other nutrients are stored in only small amounts, regardless of the amount taken in, and these can readily be depleted. As you learn how the body handles various nutrients, pay particular attention to their storage so that you can know your tolerance limits. For example, you needn't eat fat at every meal, since fat is stored abundantly. On the other hand, you normally do need to have a source of carbohydrate at intervals throughout the day because the liver stores less than one day's supply of glycogen.

glycogen a storage form of carbohydrate energy (glucose), described more fully in Chapter 4.

✓ **KEY POINT** **The body's energy stores are of two principal kinds: fat in fat cells (in potentially large quantities) and glycogen in muscle and liver cells (in smaller quantities). Other tissues store other nutrients.**

OTHER SYSTEMS

In addition to the systems described above, the body has many more: bones, an immune system, muscles, reproductive organs, and others. All of these cooperate, enabling each cell to carry on its own life. Each system ensures, through hormonal or nerve-mediated messengers, that its needs will be met by the others, and each contributes to the welfare of the whole by doing its own specialized work. For example, the skin and body linings defend other tissues against microbial invaders, while being nourished and cleansed by tissues specializing in these tasks. Each system needs a continuous supply of many specific nutrients to maintain itself and carry out its work. Calcium is particularly important for bones, for example; iron for muscles; glucose for the brain. But all systems need all nutrients, and every system is impaired by an undersupply or oversupply of them.

While external events clamor and vie for attention, the body quietly continues its life-sustaining work. Of the billions of cells in the body, only a small percentage make up the cortex of the brain, where the conscious mind resides. When the cells of the cortex receive messages from other cells, the person "becomes conscious" of a need for decision and action. In modern life the need may be complex, as when a person feels anxious and decides to consult an adviser, or simple, as when a person feels hungry and decides, "I'd better eat."

Most of the body's work is directed automatically by the unconscious portions of the brain and nervous system, and this work is finely regulated to achieve a state of well-being. But you need to involve your cerebral cortex, your consciousness, so as to cultivate an understanding and appreciation of your body's needs. In doing so, attend to nutrition first. The rewards are liberating—ample energy to tackle life's tasks, a robust attitude, and the glowing appearance that comes from the best of health. Indulge in the foods that best meet your body's needs and support its health. Read on, and learn to let nutrition principles guide your choices.

Immunity and nutrition are discussed in Chapter 11.

✓ **KEY POINT** **To achieve optimal function, the body's systems require nutrients from outside. These have to be supplied through a human being's conscious food choices.**

✓ **SELF-CHECK**

Answers to these Self-Check questions are in Appendix G.

1. All blood leaving the digestive system is routed directly to the:
   a. heart
   b. kidney
   c. liver
   d. lungs

2. Which of the following can affect the hormonal system?
   a. fasting
   b. eating
   c. exercise
   d. all of the above

3. Chemical digestion of which nutrient begins in the mouth?
   a. starch
   b. vitamins
   c. protein
   d. all of the above

4. Which chemical substance released by the pancreas neutralizes stomach acid that has reached the small intestine?
   a. mucus
   b. enzymes
   c. bicarbonate
   d. bile

5. Which nutrient passes through the large intestine mostly unabsorbed?
   a. starch
   b. vitamins
   c. minerals
   d. fiber

6. The organs that work together to perform functions are parts of the body systems.   T   F

7. The process of digestion occurs mainly in the stomach.   T   F

8. To digest food efficiently, people should not combine certain foods, such as meat and fruit, at the same meal.   T   F

9. The gallbladder stores bile until it is needed to emulsify fat.   T   F

10. Absorption of the majority of nutrients takes place across the mucus-coated lining of the stomach.   T   F

11. Stone Age people achieved their abundant nutrient intakes using only two of the four food groups: meats and milk and milk products. (Read about this in the upcoming Controversy).   T   F

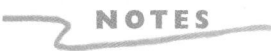
NOTES

Notes are in Appendix F.

Should We Be Eating the "Natural" Foods of Ancient Diets?

Some people are unwilling to follow the food group plans advocated by traditional nutrition teaching. They'd rather have simpler rules to follow. Our popular notion is that you can "just eat the way our ancestors did—they were healthy." This Controversy looks at that proposition and applies some scientific criticism to it.

It's true that you may be clothed in the latest fashions, and your car may be the maker's latest model, but your body is of prehistoric design—it is a caveperson body (actually, our earliest ancestors were not cave dwellers and are properly called the people of the Stone Age). You have come a long way from the Stone Age in many ways: in language skills, in the arts, in medicine, and especially in the use of machinery. But it is true that your body handles food and physical activity in virtually the same way as your ancient ancestors' bodies did. The muscles, heart, and lungs have hardly changed at all, and the brain, too, responds in the same ways to what the body sees, smells, and tastes.

The world, however, has changed vastly, especially in the last hundred years. The earth is far more crowded than it used to be. Our ancestors roamed the wilderness; today, more than half of the world's people live in cities. Extremes contrast with each other: poverty and death from malnutrition and related causes are common in the developing world; health problems caused by overabundance are common in the developed countries. The processed foods of developed countries are often much higher in fat, salt, and sugar and lower in fiber, vitamins, and minerals than the wild foods eaten by our ancestors. Too, most people's lifestyles offer much less physical activity than did the lives of their ancestors. Many people face new technological by-products in their environments, too, such as smog and water pollution. Your Stone Age body is stressed by contending with these new prob-

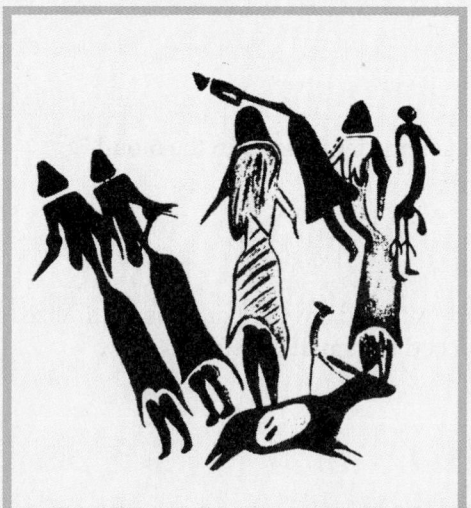

lems. Naturally, people are inclined to wonder whether we should live and eat more nearly as our ancestors did.

THE TIME AND WORLD OF OUR ANCESTORS

Before arriving at any conclusions, researchers need to know what our ancestors ate and how healthy they were. They have to begin by deciding which ancestors to study—our farmer forebears and the early agricultural people who preceded them, or the hunter-gatherer people who lived still longer ago.

People have farmed the land for 10,000 years or more, 50 times longer than the period since the beginning of the industrial era, about A.D. 1800. Ten thousand years may seem long, but try a second comparison. Imagine all of the three-million-year history of human existence on earth compressed into the last 24 hours. Then the agricultural era would have begun only 3½ minutes ago, and the industrial era would have begun 4 *seconds* ago.[1] People who grow their own food have thus occupied the earth for only a few *hundred* generations, while people who hunted for their food roamed the earth for *thousands* of generations. Figure C3-1 depicts the magnitude of the differences between the earlier people's times on earth and our own.

One group of people to study therefore is the earliest one, the hunter-gatherers before agriculture. They were the people of the Stone Age, the Paleolithic period, which lasted from 10,000 to about 500,000 years ago (*paleo* means "ancient"; *lith* means "stone," referring to the stone tools they used). Thus Stone Age people's way of life and diet persisted for close to half a million years. Enough time elapsed to permit natural selection of genes for traits that favored survival of generation after generation under the conditions of that period including the diet. Many of the genes for those traits persist in our inheritance today. Thousands of years

FIGURE C3-1

A PERSPECTIVE ON MODERN HUMAN BEINGS' TIME ON EARTH

If all human existence on earth is collapsed into 1 year's time, then agriculture began yesterday, and the current A.D. calendar began 4 hours ago. The *space* occupied in the pyramid is in proportion to the *time* spent on earth.

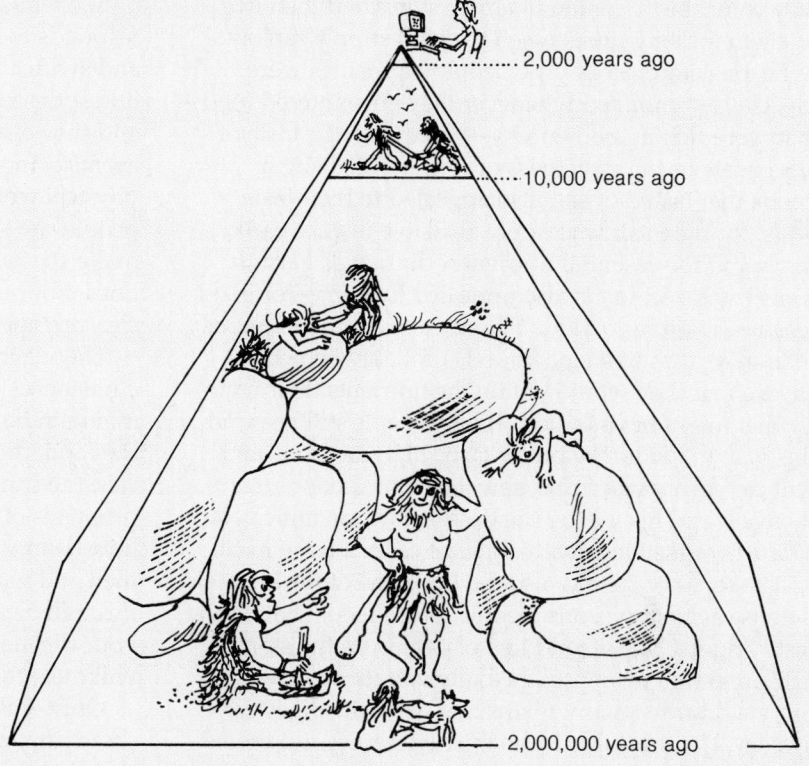

- 2,000 years ago
- 10,000 years ago
- 2,000,000 years ago

old, those genes still support physical characteristics in us that favored survival in those early times. The more we know about the Stone Age people, then, the better we can understand our bodies' needs today.

Modern-day hunting-gathering peoples are also worth studying in this regard. A few such groups remain on earth today, and from them we can learn of the effects on health of a changing diet.

THE ANCIENT BODY IN THE MODERN WORLD

Food was not available all the time for Stone Age people. Times of plenty alternated with times of famine. The human body adapted well to this state of affairs. It was omnivorous—able to digest and to use the nutrients from both plants and animals. This made wide food choices possible and reduced the likelihood of starvation in the face of a food supply that depended on place and season. The body could also store excess energy in its fat tissues when food was plentiful. Then

people could draw on that fuel supply during famine or illness.

Our bodies can do the same things today. We too can eat many kinds of food. We too efficiently store surplus energy in body fat. Today, though, these abilities confer less of an advantage. Not all the foods available to us today benefit our health, and in food-abundant societies, times of famine never come. Our overeating and storage of excess fat often produce conditions that shorten life. Excess body fatness precipitates diabetes in susceptible people, aggravates high blood pressure, renders certain cancers more likely, and worsens arthritis, among other things.

The body feels hungry at approximately four- to six-hour intervals, even though it may have sufficient fat stores to last for many days. This adaptation served Stone Age people well, for it drove them to continue stocking fuel within their bodies as often as their digestive systems could perform the task. They ate whenever food was available, even when they had sufficient body fat and nutrient stores for temporary needs. As a result, they were able to maintain ample stores and then live on them for long times when the food supply ran out.

Furthermore, Stone Age people's appetites were especially stimulated whenever they encountered foods that were rich in food energy—those with the taste of oils or fats or the sweetness of concentrated sugar. Foods that tasted of salt also appealed to their taste buds, for pure salt was rarely available in very early times and the essential nutrient sodium was hard to come by. Novel foods also appealed to them—for good reasons. For long periods their diets were monotonous; their eagerness to try new foods probably helped to ensure that they would obtain the nutrients their regular diet might have lacked. Today, people still respond this way to foods. We prefer tasty, high-fat foods and will eat even when full if new delicious foods present themselves. This is why the dessert cart can entice you to stuff yourself, even after you've eaten a large meal.

The sense of taste is also the front line of the body's defense against poisons: people refuse foods that don't taste "right." The second line of defense is the stomach's rejection response: the body vomits up or washes out via diarrhea many toxins that enter the digestive system. The third line is the liver's filtering and detoxifying systems. Toxins that get into the bloodstream are removed from it by the liver cells, which then render the toxins harmless and put them away in permanent storage or release them for excretion in the urine.

For example, protection against the harmful effects of one ancient and familiar substance—alcohol—is built into the body's genes. One of those genes, expressed in the liver, codes for an enzyme that converts alcohol into substances the body can use or excrete. So long as the liver is not overwhelmed with alcohol, the system works efficiently.

The same is not true of all poisons. Alcohol has been around since the first fruit ripened and fermented, so there have been millions of years for natural selection to mold a detoxifying system for it. On the other hand, most of the additives intentionally put into foods and the pollutants and toxins that get in by mistake are new to the body. If it can't excrete them, it may accumulate harmful quantities or convert them to odd, unfamiliar substances that can interfere with metabolism or cause cancer or birth defects. An important new area of study in nutrition is concerned with the body's handling of these substances.

In other ways, too, the body is adapted to the conditions of earlier times. Heredity has given each human being a body that can *develop* itself to run after prey,

fight enemies, or carry heavy burdens long distances; it responds to physical exertion by becoming stronger and swifter. Among the muscles that become stronger in response to exercise are the heart and lung muscles, and they also (like all muscles) become weaker without exercise. In ancient times, vigorous activity and hard physical work were part of everyone's life, but today people can sit around for months at a time. We have to make special efforts to plan exercise into our daily routines if our muscles, including our heart and lung muscles, are not to become weak.

These and other differences add up to a set of circumstances that challenge your body and mind to maintain health against many odds. You are living with the food, the labor-saving devices, the medical miracles, the contaminants, and all the other pleasures and problems of the twentieth century. However, you are housed in a body adapted to a world in which strong men and women survived on simple foods obtained through hard physical labor. There is no guarantee that your diet and exercise routine, haphazardly chosen, will meet the needs of your Stone Age body.

Only with your brain can you compensate for these disadvantages of modern life. Stone Age people used their brains to discover ways to obtain food; you must use yours, sometimes, to refuse delicious food and to battle the ancient instincts that cry out for you to eat. Stone Age people used their ingenuity to save their energy when they could; you may have to use yours to find ways to spend energy so that you can maintain appropriate weight and keep your heart and muscles fit. You have an advantage, though. Unlike your ancestors, you can learn more about how your body works and what it needs from food.

THE STONE AGE DIET

Researchers have studied what Stone Age people actually ate. Analysis of their probable diet from fossilized remains of their meals and excretions has produced a picture of what foods they ate and how much of each nutrient they received. The figures are undoubtedly not exact, but it is interesting to compare them with those of today. Early people probably consumed 3,000 calories per day and apparently were never obese. (Today we consume fewer than 2,000 calories a day, yet many of us are obese because we get so little exercise.)

Given their large energy allowances and the exclusively nutrient-dense food options from which they were forced to choose, Stone Age people probably met

FIGURE C3-2

SELECTED DIFFERENCES BETWEEN ANCIENT AND MODERN DIETS

The percentages referred to here are the percent of total daily caloric intake from fat, starch, and refined sugar. Daily fiber is shown in grams.

SOURCE: Data for hunter-gatherers and agriculturists from WHO Study Group, Diet, nutrition, and the prevention of chronic diseases. World Health Organization Technical Report Series 797 (Geneva: WHO, 1990). 43: Data for U.S. population averages from *Diet and Health: Implications for Reducing Chronic Disease Risk* (Washington, D.C.: National Academy Press, 1989), pp. 41–84 and Interagency, Board for Nutrition Monitoring, *Third Report on Nutrition Monitoring in the United States* (Washington, D.C.: Government Printing Office, 1995), pp. ES-3, 49.

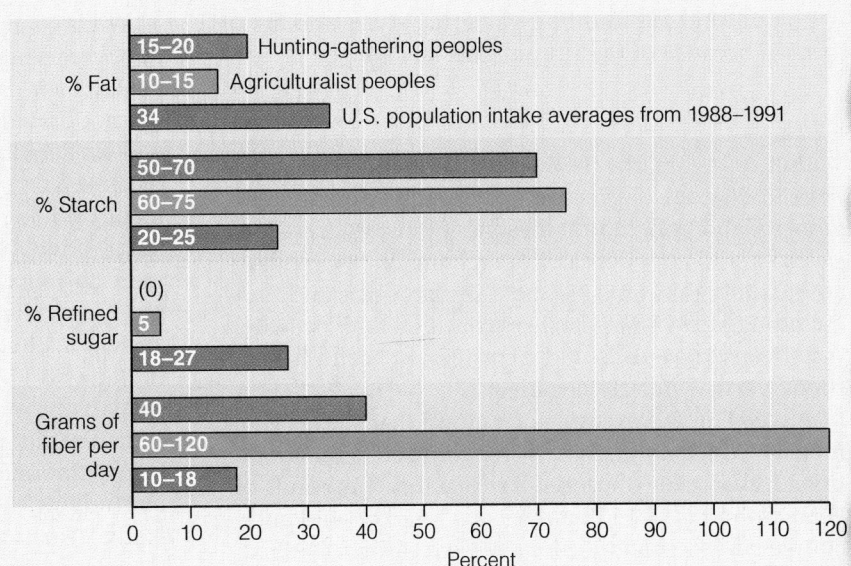

all of their nutrient needs well. For example, although they drank no milk and made no cheese, their intakes of calcium were probably close to 1,500 milligrams a day, thanks to the fruits and vegetables they consumed. Today we fall short of 800 milligrams, although recommendations state that many people (and especially young people) need more than 1,000 milligrams to preserve the integrity of their bones. Stone Age people probably consumed close to 400 milligrams of vitamin C a day, whereas we take in less than 100 milligrams. They ingested much more fiber than we do today, 45 grams or so, compared with our 20 grams or less. Counterbalancing these pluses, they also ate more dirt, and even gravel![2] Figure C3-2 provides other comparisons of the diets of agriculturist peoples, hunter-gatherers, and the U.S. population.

Stone Age people achieved their abundant nutrient intakes using only two of the four groups of foods we think of as important: meat and fruits/vegetables. Their intakes of meat, and therefore of protein, were two to five times higher than ours are today, but most of their meats were lean, whereas many of ours are high in fat. The fats in their meats included a type thought to be preventive against heart disease and cancer and known to be lacking from our meats today, the so-called omega-3 fatty acids described in Chapter 5. They apparently consumed cereal grains rarely, if at all, and they

had no dairy foods whatsoever. (Remember, they lived before the dawn of agriculture, and kept no cattle.)

Although their total energy intakes were higher than ours, the people of the Stone Age had lower intakes of two no-no's that plague modern eaters: fat and sodium. Their cholesterol intakes were similar to ours, however, because even lean meat contains cholesterol. Also, their diet seldom contained concentrated sweets such as honey, and there was no such thing as table sugar.

Were earlier people healthier, then, than we are today? Not necessarily. Many died of starvation during times of climatic extremes. Many must have suffered vitamin deficiencies and food-borne diseases.[3] Stone Age people died younger than we do, and this is one reason why the so-called degenerative diseases of old age were less common then than they are today.

Our longer lives are not the only reason for the modern prevalence of cancer and heart disease, though; our diets share the blame. Researchers have learned this from studying primitive people living today: tribes in Africa and other places whose diets and ways of life resemble those of Stone Age people. These people's lifestyles enable them to attain the age of 60 years relatively free of degenerative diseases. Others living today within a generation or two of ancient foodways are Native Americans. The traditional diets of the tribes most often studied are a blend of agricultural and hunting-gathering styles and are of interest because of their rapid rates of change.

NATIVE AMERICAN DIETS

Within 200 years, the foodways of Native Americans have undergone unprecedented changes. The hunter-gatherer and agricultural lifestyles of history have given way to a modern culture relying on fast foods, abundant high-fat meats, and dairy products and including alcohol. Researchers conclude that for Native Americans, the effects of the changes on health have been overwhelmingly negative.

A well-studied example of a group that suffers enormously from the effects of a "modernized" diet are the Pima Indian tribe of central Arizona. For thousands of years up to 1930, the Pima diet consisted of wild and cultivated desert legumes, cactus leaves and fruit, fish, venison (deer meat), small seeds, mesquite pods, acorns, and corn.[4] Then in 1930, a change began. The tribe largely replaced their traditional wild foods, which had become scarce, with modern ones such as refined wheat flour, lard, sugar, coffee, and ready-to-eat cereals that were easily obtained. The result has been tragic—the Pima now suffer the highest per capita rate of diabetes (roughly 50 percent) known among any people of the world.[5] Genetics may make diabetes especially likely to develop in Pimas who adopt modern foodways.[6] Likewise, the Sioux Indians rarely ever suffered heart disease when consuming their traditional diets, but now suffer one of the highest known rates of heart and artery disease. Navajos also now suffer high rates of diabetes and cardiovascular disease.[7] And Alaskan natives, among whom obesity and diabetes were rare before 1960, now suffer greatly from these twin threats.[8]

The Pima, Navajo, and Sioux tribes changed not only their diets, but also their highly active lifestyles. Modern-day Pima and Sioux no longer hunt game on the windswept plains, toil in the fields, or gather wood to cook over stone fireplaces as their ancestors once did. They now drive to supermarkets to purchase convenience foods to cook in microwave ovens. The Sioux also traded their occasional ceremonial pipes for daily cigarette smoking, a new habit that is especially damaging to the heart.

While changed diets and lifestyles almost certainly have contributed to the changes in Native American health, their native diets were not perfect, either.[9] They did not provide adequate amounts of some nutrients, and availability of foods depended on such unpredictable factors as weather changes and herd movements. While modern foods are usually safe and sanitary, Native Alaskans eating traditional foods suffer more botulism (a deadly food poisoning) than any other group worldwide. Modern descendants changed the ancient methods of preserving meat, fish, and blubber (fat) in slight but critical ways that encourage the growth of the bacteria that cause botulism.[10] The point is that all diets, even those that have supported human beings through many centuries, have drawbacks. Still, by studying them, scientists are learning that when Native Americans consumed their ancient diets of high-fiber, low-fat native foods, their hearts and bodies benefited.

Does this mean we should abandon the use of today's foods and eat only meat and wild fruits and vegetables? No—even if we did, we would not be eating like the Stone Age people or today's few remaining primitive tribes. Our foods are different. Our meats differ in the amounts and types of fat they contain. Our fruits and vegetables are totally different. And ancient people's environments, with their vast, cityless open spaces, no longer exist for us.

Still, even if we cannot eat the same foods they did, we can attempt to duplicate their activity and nutrient intake levels using the foods available to us. Clearly, we should emulate them in incorporating more physical activity into our days. If we exercise more, we can eat more without getting fat; if we eat more, we can obtain more nutrients; and if we obtain more nutrients, we are better protected against deficiencies.

In conclusion, no one can go back in time to live as the ancient people did. We can learn from them, though, the importance of getting more exercise and of eating wholesome foods that will support our health as well as, or even better than, theirs did.

NOTES

Notes are in Appendix F.

THE CARBOHYDRATES: SUGAR, STARCH, GLYCOGEN, AND FIBER

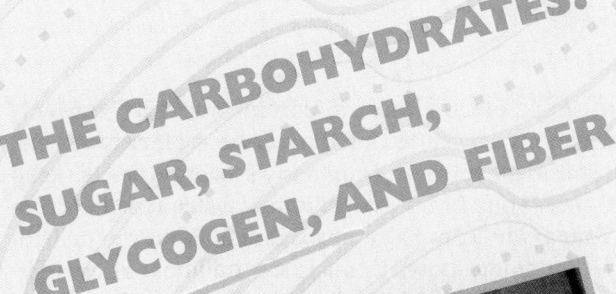

4

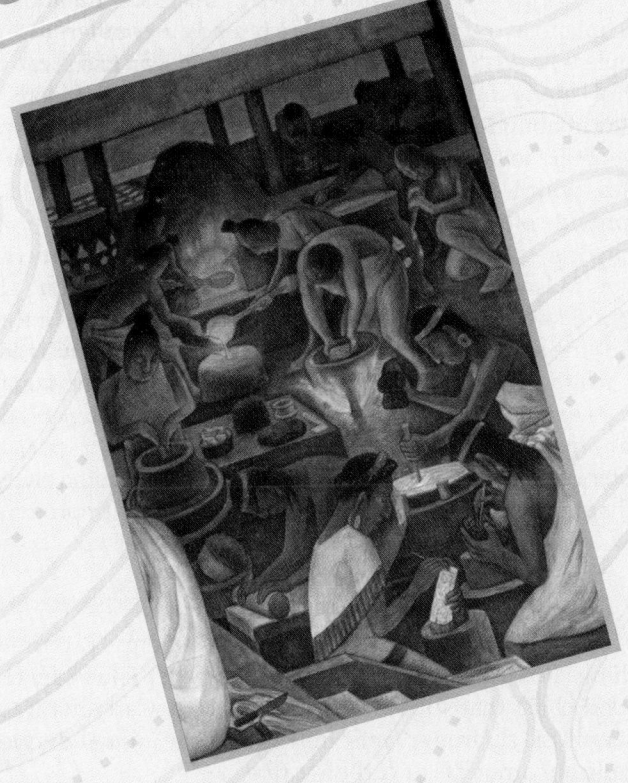

CONTENTS

Diego Rivera, Detail of *Le Civilization Zapotec;* Charles and Josette Lenars, Corbis.

carbohydrates compounds composed of single or multiple sugars. The name means "carbon and water," and a chemical shorthand for carbohydrate is CHO, signifying carbon (C), hydrogen (H), and oxygen (O).

complex carbohydrates long chains of sugar units arranged to form starch or fiber; also called *polysaccharides*.

simple carbohydrates sugars, including both single sugar units and linked pairs of sugar units. The basic sugar unit is a molecule containing six carbon atoms, together with oxygen and hydrogen atoms.

FIGURE 4-1

CARBOHYDRATE—MAINLY GLUCOSE—IS MADE BY PHOTOSYNTHESIS

The sun's energy becomes part of the glucose molecule—its calories, in a sense. In the molecule of glucose on the leaf here, dots represent the carbon atoms; bars represent the chemical bonds that contain energy.

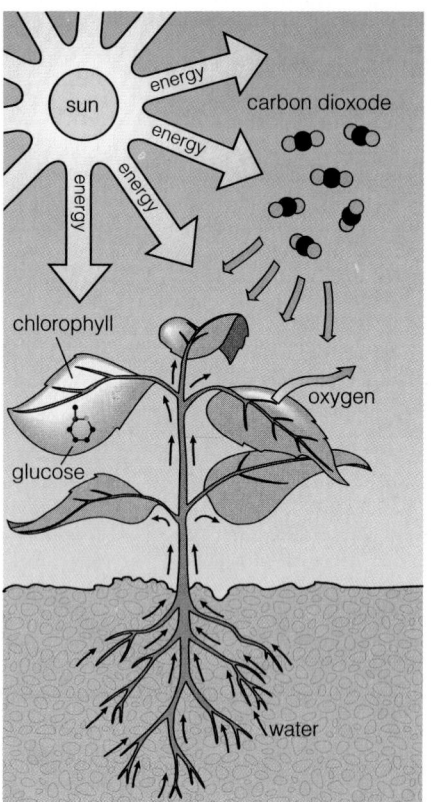

4 It is impossible to single out the most important nutrient. Nutrients work together in harmony, each affecting the functions of many others. **Carbohydrates,** however, are ideal to meet your body's energy needs, keep your digestive system fit, feed your brain and nervous system, and, within calorie limits, help keep your body lean. False propaganda about the evils of carbohydrate's supposed "fattening power" misleads millions of weight-conscious people to avoid carbohydrate-rich foods, a counterproductive tactic. In truth, people who wish to lose fat and to maintain lean tissue can do no better than to control calories and design their diets around low-fat foods that supply carbohydrates in abundance. Digestible carbohydrates, together with fats and protein, give bulk to foods and provide energy for the body. Indigestible carbohydrates, which comprise most of the fibers in foods, yield little or no energy but provide other important benefits.

All carbohydrates are not equal as far as nutrition is concerned. This chapter invites you to learn to distinguish between foods containing the **complex carbohydrates** (starch and fiber), which are put to good use in the body, and those made of the **simple carbohydrates** (sugars), which can be less valuable to people's health. The Controversy then asks whether the sugar added to foods harms health and whether the alternative sweeteners designed to replace sugar are preferable.

This chapter on the carbohydrates is the first of three on the energy-yielding nutrients. Chapter 5 deals with the fats and Chapter 6 with protein.

A CLOSE LOOK AT CARBOHYDRATES

Carbohydrates contain the sun's radiant energy, captured in a form that living things can use to drive the processes of life. Thus they form the first link in the food chain that supports all life on earth. Carbohydrate-rich foods come almost exclusively from plants; milk is the only animal-derived food that contains significant amounts of carbohydrate.

Green plants make carbohydrate through **photosynthesis** in the presence of **chlorophyll** and sunlight. In this process water (H_2O), absorbed by the plant's roots, donates hydrogen and oxygen, while carbon dioxide gas (CO_2), absorbed into its leaves, donates carbon and oxygen. Water and carbon dioxide combine to yield the most common of the **sugars,** the single sugar **glucose.** Scientists know the reaction in the minutest detail, but have never been able to reproduce it from scratch; green plants are required to make it happen (see Figure 4-1).

Light energy from the sun drives the photosynthesis reaction. The light energy becomes the chemical energy of the bonds that hold six atoms of carbon together in the sugar glucose. Glucose provides energy for the work of all cells of the stem, roots, flowers, and fruits of the plant. For example, in the roots, far from the energy-giving rays of the sun, each cell draws upon some of the glucose made in the leaves, breaks it down (to carbon dioxide and water), and uses the energy thus released to fuel its own growth and water-gathering activities.

Some energy remains in the sugars stored in plants. This is the part of photosynthesis that is important to our survival. The next few sections describe the forms that carbohydrates take, with their treasures of stored energy awaiting use in the human body.

✔ **KEY POINT** **Through photosynthesis, plants combine carbon dioxide, water, and the sun's energy to form glucose. Carbohydrates are made of**

carbon, hydrogen, and oxygen held together by energy-containing bonds: *carbo* **means "carbon";** *hydrate* **means "water."**

Sugars

Altogether, six sugar molecules are important in nutrition. These are single sugars, or **monosaccharides.** The other three are double sugars, or **disaccharides.** All of their chemical names end in *ose,* which means *sugar,* and although they all sound alike to the newcomer, they take on distinct characteristics to the nutrition enthusiast who quickly gets to know each individually.

The three monosaccharides are glucose, already described, **fructose,** and **galactose.** Fructose, or fruit sugar, the intensely sweet sugar of fruit, is made by rearranging the atoms in glucose molecules. Fructose occurs mostly in fruits, in honey, and as part of table sugar. Glucose and fructose are the most common monosaccharides in nature.

The other monosaccharide, galactose, has the same numbers and kinds of atoms, but they are arranged still differently. Galactose is one of the two single sugars bound together to form the pair that make up the sugar of milk. It does not occur free in nature, but instead is tied up in milk sugar until it is freed during digestion.

The three other sugars important in nutrition are disaccharides, linked pairs of single sugars. All three contain glucose. In **lactose,** the sugar of milk just mentioned, glucose is linked to galactose.

In malt sugar, or **maltose,** there are two glucose units. Maltose appears wherever starch is being broken down. It occurs in germinating seeds and arises during the fermentation process that yields alcohol. It also arises during the digestion of starch in the human body.

The last of the six sugars, **sucrose,** is the most familiar. It is table sugar, the product most people think of when they use the term *sugar.* In sucrose, fructose and glucose are bonded together. Table sugar is obtained by refining the juice from sugar beets or sugar cane, but sucrose also occurs naturally in many vegetables and fruits. It tastes sweet, as does fruit sugar, because it, too, contains the sweet monosaccharide fructose. Sucrose is of major importance in human nutrition, and research about its effects on the human body is a topic of Controversy 4.

When you eat a food containing single sugars, you can absorb then directly into your blood. When you eat disaccharides, though, you must digest them first. Enzymes in your intestine must split the disaccharides into separate monosaccharides so that they can enter the bloodstream. The blood then delivers all products of digestion first to the liver, which possesses enzymes to modify nutrients, making them useful to the body. Glucose is the most-used monosaccharide inside the body, so the liver quickly converts fructose or galactose to glucose or to smaller pieces that can serve as building blocks for either glucose or fat.

When people learn that the energy of many vegetables and fruit comes from sugars, they may think that eating sweet-tasting fruit is the same as eating concentrated sweets such as candy or cola beverages. Not so. Like vegetables, fruits differ from concentrated sweets in nutrient density. The sugars of fruits arrive in the body diluted in large volumes of water, packaged with fiber, and mixed with many vitamins and needed minerals. In contrast, all types of refined sugars, even honey, arrive in the body in concentrated form, practically

photosynthesis the synthesis of carbohydrates by green plants from carbon dioxide and water using the green pigment chlorophyll to capture the sun's energy (*photo* means "light"; *synthesis* means "making").

chlorophyll the green pigment of plants that captures energy from sunlight for use in photosynthesis.

sugars simple carbohydrates, that is, molecules of either single sugar units or pairs of those sugar units bonded together.

glucose (GLOO-cose) a single sugar used in both plant and animal tissues for quick energy; sometimes known as blood sugar or *dextrose.*

monosaccharides single sugar units (*mono* means "one"; *saccharide* means "sugar unit").

disaccharides pairs of single sugars linked together (*di* means "two").

fructose (FROOK-tose) a monosaccharide; sometimes known as fruit sugar (*fruct* means "fruit"; *ose* means "sugar").

galactose (ga-LACK-tose) a monosaccharide; part of the disaccharide lactose (milk sugar).

lactose a disaccharide composed of glucose and galactose; sometimes known as milk sugar (*lact* means "milk"; *ose* means "sugar").

maltose a disaccharide composed of two glucose units; sometimes known as malt sugar.

sucrose (SOO-crose) a disaccharide composed of glucose and fructose; sometimes known as table, beet, or cane sugar.

Single sugars are monosaccharides.

Pairs of sugars are disaccharides.

polysaccharides another term for complex carbohydrates; compounds of long strands of glucose units linked together (*poly* means "many").

starch a plant polysaccharide composed of glucose; highly digestible by human beings.

granules small grains. Starch granules are packages of starch molecules. Various plant species make starch granules of varying shapes.

Strands of many sugar units are polysaccharides.

devoid of nutrients. From the body's point of view, fruits are vastly different from purified sugars, except that both provide glucose in abundance.

✔ KEY POINT **Glucose is the most important monosaccharide in the human body. Most other monosaccharides and disaccharides become glucose in the body.**

Starch

Glucose occurs in foods not only in sugars but also in long strands of thousands of glucose units strung together. These are the **polysaccharides**. Starch is a polysaccharide as are glycogen and some of the fibers.

Starch is a plant's storage form of glucose. As a plant matures, it not only provides energy for its own needs but also stores energy in its seeds for the next generation to use. For example, after a corn plant reaches its full growth and has many leaves manufacturing glucose, it stores packed clusters of **starch** molecules in **granules,** and packs the granules into its seeds to provide energy for the growth of new plants next season.[1] Glucose is soluble in water and would be washed away by rains while the seed lay in the soil. Starch is an insoluble substance that will stay with the seed and nourish it until it forms shoots with leaves that can catch the sun's rays. A kernel of corn, then, is really a seed packed with this nutritive material. The starch of corn and other foods is nutritive for human beings, too, because they can digest the starch to glucose and extract the sun's energy stored in its chemical bonds. A later section describes starch digestion in greater detail.

✔ KEY POINT **Starch is the storage form of glucose in plants that is nutritive for human beings.**

Glycogen

Just as plants store glucose in long chains of starch, animal bodies store glucose in long chains of **glycogen** (sometimes called *animal starch*). Glycogen resembles starch in that it consists of glucose molecules linked together to form chains, but its chains are longer and more highly branched. A later section describes the body's handling of these packages of stored glucose. The relationships among the monosaccharides, dissacharides, and polysaccharides are summed up in Figures 4-2 and 4-3.

Carbohydrate plays a prominent role in the global carbon cycle. Carbon dioxide, water, and energy are combined in plants to form glucose; the plants may store the glucose in the polysaccharide starch. Then animals or people eat the plants and retrieve glucose from it. In the body, the liver and muscles may store the glucose as the polysaccharide glycogen, but ultimately it becomes glucose again. The glucose delivers the sun's energy to fuel the body's activities. In the process, glucose breaks down to waste products, carbon dioxide and water, which are excreted. Later, these compounds are used again by plants as raw materials to make carbohydrate. Chapter 15 comes back to humankind's relationship with the earth's food chain.

✔ KEY POINT **Glycogen is the storage form of glucose in animals, including human beings.**

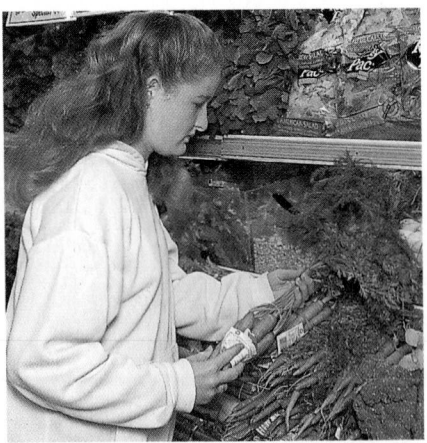

The sugars in these carrots are diluted with water and packaged with vitamins, minerals, and fiber.

FIGURE 4-2

HOW MONOSACCHARIDES JOIN TO FORM DISACCHARIDES

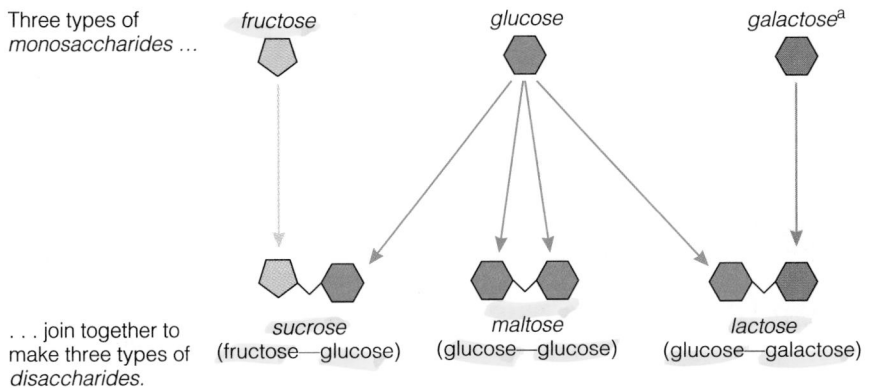

Three types of *monosaccharides* ...

fructose   *glucose*   *galactose*[a]

. . . join together to make three types of *disaccharides*.

sucrose (fructose—glucose)   *maltose* (glucose—glucose)   *lactose* (glucose—galactose)

A note on the glucose symbol:
The glucose molecule is really a ring of 5 carbons and one oxygen plus a carbon "flag."

carbons   oxygen

For convenience, in this and other illustrations, glucose is symbolized as   or

[a]Galactose does not occur in foods singly but as part of lactose.

Fiber

The **fibers** of a plant contribute the supporting structures of its leaves, stems, and seeds. Most fibers are polysaccharides—chains of sugars—just as starch is, but in fibers the sugar units are held together by bonds that human digestive enzymes cannot break. Most fibers therefore pass through the human body without providing energy for its use. The best known of these polysaccharides are *cellulose* (shown in Figure 4-3), *hemicellulose*, and *pectin*. (Other fibers are *gums, mucilages,* and *lignins*.) Cellulose and hemicellulose are found in the familiar strings of celery, the skins of corn kernels, and the membranes surrounding kernels of wheat. In the body these two provide what a grandparent might have called **roughage**—fiber that aids in digestion and elimination. Pectin, isolated from plants such as apples or citrus fruits, may be used as a food additive to thicken jelly, keep salad dressing from separating, and otherwise alter the texture and consistency of processed foods.

The term *dietary fiber* describes substances that cannot be broken down by human digestive enzymes. They are, however, somewhat vulnerable to breakdown by the enzymes of bacteria that reside in the digestive tracts of human beings. Some fibers are changed by intestinal bacteria into products that are absorbed and contribute a few calories' worth of energy or have other effects on the body. How much fiber is broken down varies greatly depending upon the nature of both the fiber and the bacteria in the tract.[2]

Some animals, such as cattle, depend heavily on their intestinal bacteria to make available the energy of glucose from the abundant fiber cellulose in their fodder. When we eat beef, we receive indirectly some of the sun's energy that was originally stored in the fiber of the plants the cattle ate. Beef, of course, contains no fiber itself; no meats or dairy products contain fiber.

Chemists classify fiber types according to how readily they dissolve in water. Some types are **insoluble fiber;** some, **soluble fiber.** Each type of fiber exerts important effects on people's health; these effects will be described later.

glycogen (GLY-co-gen) a polysaccharide composed of glucose, made and stored by liver and muscle tissues of human beings and animals as a storage form of glucose. Glycogen is not a significant food source of carbohydrate and is not counted as one of the complex carbohydrates in foods.

fibers the indigestible polysaccharides in food, comprised mostly of cellulose, hemicellulose, and pectin. Also called *nonstarch polysaccharides.*

roughage (RUFF-idge) the rough parts of food; an imprecise term that has largely been replaced by the term *fiber.*

insoluble fibers the tough, fibrous structures of fruits, vegetables, and grains; indigestible food components that do not dissolve in water.

soluble fibers indigestible food components that readily dissolve in water and often impart gummy or gel-like characteristics to foods. An example is pectin from fruit used to thicken jellies.

FIGURE 4-3

HOW GLUCOSE MOLECULES JOIN TO FORM POLYSACCHARIDES

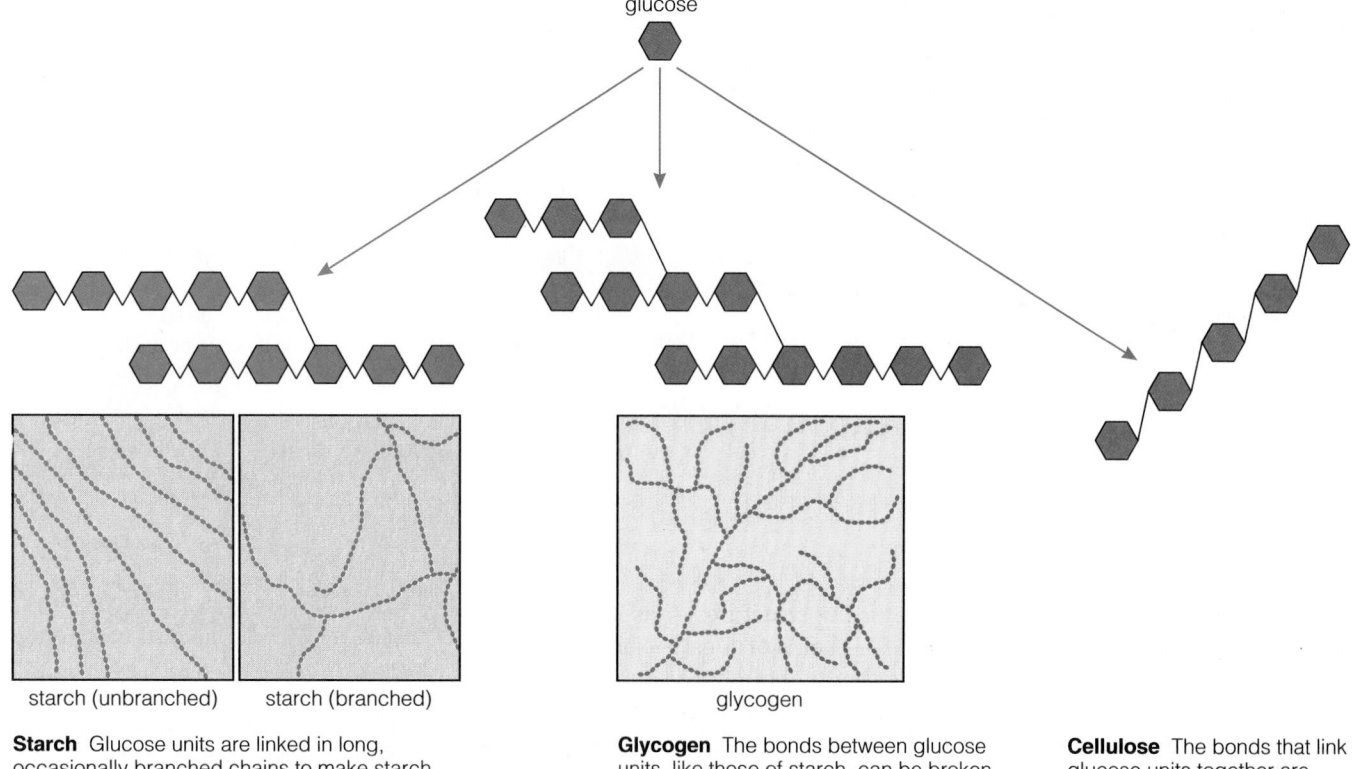

glucose

Starch Glucose units are linked in long, occasionally branched chains to make starch. Human digestive enzymes can digest these bonds, retrieving glucose. Real glucose units are so tiny that you can't see them, even with the highest-power light microscope.

starch (unbranched)   starch (branched)

Glycogen The bonds between glucose units, like those of starch, can be broken by human enzymes, but the chains are more highly branched.

glycogen

Cellulose The bonds that link glucose units together are different from the bonds in starch or glycogen. Human enzymes cannot digest them.

✓ KEY POINT   **Little fiber is digested by the enzymes in the human digestive tract. Most fiber passes through the digestive tract unchanged.**

THE NEED FOR CARBOHYDRATES

Glucose from carbohydrate is the preferred fuel for most body functions. Only two other nutrients provide energy to the body: protein and fats. Protein-rich foods are usually expensive, and when used to make fuel for the body, provide no advantage over carbohydrates. In fact, their overuse has disadvantages, as explained in Chapter 6. Fats are not normally used as fuel by the brain and central nervous system, and diets high in fats are associated with many disease states. Thus, of the possible alternatives, glucose is the preferred energy source. It is especially important as the chief fuel of nerve cells, including those of the brain, which depend almost exclusively on glucose for their energy. And starchy foods, or complex carbohydrates, are the preferred source of glucose.

The Truth about Carbohydrates

A myth about complex carbohydrates wrongly accuses them of being the "fattening" ingredients of foods. Some people are still startled to hear that we need to consume more starchy foods rather than less. Yet much evidence supports this assertion. Gram for gram, carbohydrates donate fewer calories than do dietary fats, so a diet of high-carbohydrate foods is likely to be lower in calories than a diet of high-fat foods. Also, to convert glucose to fat in the body requires chemical conversions that cost many of the glucose's original calories, making glucose even less fattening. Government agencies in many countries, recognizing the value of complex carbohydrates, urge their citizens to consume abundant foods that contain them. Table 4-1 reviews the U.S. recommendations and goals first presented in Chapters 1 and 2 as well as the World Health Organization's recommended upper and lower limits for carbohydrate intakes.

TABLE 4-1

Recommendations Concerning Intakes of Carbohydrates

1. Recommendations for Complex Carbohydrates

   Dietary Guidelines
   - Every day eat 5 to 9 servings[a] of a combination of vegetables and fruits. Also, increase intake of starches and other complex carbohydrates by eating 6 to 11 daily servings of a combination of breads, cereals, and legumes.

   Daily Values[b]
   - 300 grams of complex carbohydrate, or 60% of total calories.

   Healthy People 2000
   - Increase complex carbohydrate and fiber-containing foods in the diets of adults to 5 or more daily servings for vegetables (including legumes) and fruits and to 6 or more daily servings for grain products.

   World Health Organization
   - Lower limit: 50% of total calories from complex carbohydrates
   - Upper limit: 75% of total calories from complex carbohydrates

2. Recommendations for Refined Sugars

   Dietary Guidelines
   - Use sugars only in moderation.

   World Health Organization
   - Lower limit: 0% of total calories from refined sugars
   - Upper limit: 10% of total calories from refined sugars

3. Recommendations for Dietary Fiber

   Dietary Guidelines
   - Increase your fiber intake by eating more of a variety of foods that contain fiber naturally.

   Daily Values[b]
   - 25 grams of fiber per day, or 11.5 grams per 1,000 calories.

   World Health Organization
   - Lower limit: 27 grams of dietary fiber a day
   - Upper limit: 40 grams of dietary fiber a day

[a]Serving sizes were presented in Figure 2-4 of Chapter 2.
[b]Daily Values are for a 2,000 calorie diet.

constipation hardness and dryness of bowel movements, associated with discomfort in passing them from the body.

hemorrhoids (HEM-or-oids) swollen, hardened (varicose) veins in the rectum, usually caused by the pressure resulting from constipation.

appendicitis inflammation and/or infection of the appendix, a sac protruding from the intestine.

diverticulosis (dye-ver-tic-you-LOH-sis) outpocketing or ballooning out of areas of the intestinal wall, caused by weakening of the muscle layers that encase the intestine.

Unlike complex carbohydrates, pure sugars displace nutrient-dense foods from the diet. Purified, refined sugar (sucrose) contains no other nutrients—protein, vitamins, minerals, or fiber—and so can be termed as empty-calorie food. If you choose 400 calories of sugar in place of 400 calories of starchy food such as whole-grain bread, you lose not only the starch but also the vitamins, minerals, and fiber of the bread. You can afford to do this only if you have already met your nutrient needs for the day and still have calories to spend. This chapter's Food Feature offers more about the sugars in foods.

✓ KEY POINT **Complex carbohydrates are the preferred energy source for the body.**

The Benefits of Fiber

Foods containing starch offer additional benefits if fibers come with the starch, as they do naturally. Fibers benefit health in all these ways:

- Promote feelings of fullness because they absorb water and swell. Soluble fibers in a meal also slow the movement of food through the upper digestive tract, so you feel full longer.
- Reduce energy consumption by displacing calorie-dense concentrated fats and sweets from the diet while donating little energy. Fibers therefore can help in weight control.
- Help prevent **constipation, hemorrhoids,** and other intestinal problems by keeping the contents of the intestine moist and easy to eliminate.
- Help prevent bacterial infection of the appendix **(appendicitis)** by the same mechanism.
- Are associated with reduced incidence of colon cancer (see Chapter 11). Insoluble fibers bind or dilute cancer-causing materials and speed their transit through the colon. Lignin may have an independent effect, described later.
- Stimulate the muscles of the digestive tract so that they retain their health and tone. This prevents **diverticulosis,** in which the intestinal walls become weak and bulge out in places.
- May reduce the risks of heart and artery disease by lowering blood cholesterol (see Figure 4-4).[3] Also, some soluble fibers are digested by intestinal bacteria to yield small, fatlike products that, when absorbed, may inhibit the liver's production of cholesterol.[4] High-fiber foods also displace fatty, cholesterol-raising foods from the diet.[5]
- Improve the body's handling of glucose perhaps by slowing the digestion or absorption of carbohydrate. A high-fiber meal eaten for breakfast continues to exert regulatory effects on blood glucose after lunch.

In general, then, fibers:

- *Moderate nutrient absorption* rates by entrapping nutrient molecules and preventing their contact with absorptive surfaces.
- *Delay cholesterol and other sterol absorption,* probably by the same mechanism.
- *Stimulate bacterial fermentation* in the colon (described below).
- *Increase stool weight* by holding water within the feces.

FIGURE 4-4

ONE WAY FIBER IN FOOD MAY LOWER CHOLESTEROL IN THE BLOOD

In some ways, the liver is like the body's vacuum cleaner, sucking up cholesterol from the blood, converting the cholesterol to bile, and discharging the bile into its storage bag, the gallbladder. The gallbladder empties its bile into the intestine, where bile performs necessary digestive tasks. In the intestine, some of the bile links up with fiber and is carried out of the body in feces.

A. When the diet is rich in fiber, much of the cholesterol (as bile) is carried out of the body.

B. When the diet is low in fiber, most of the cholesterol is reabsorbed and returned to the bloodstream.

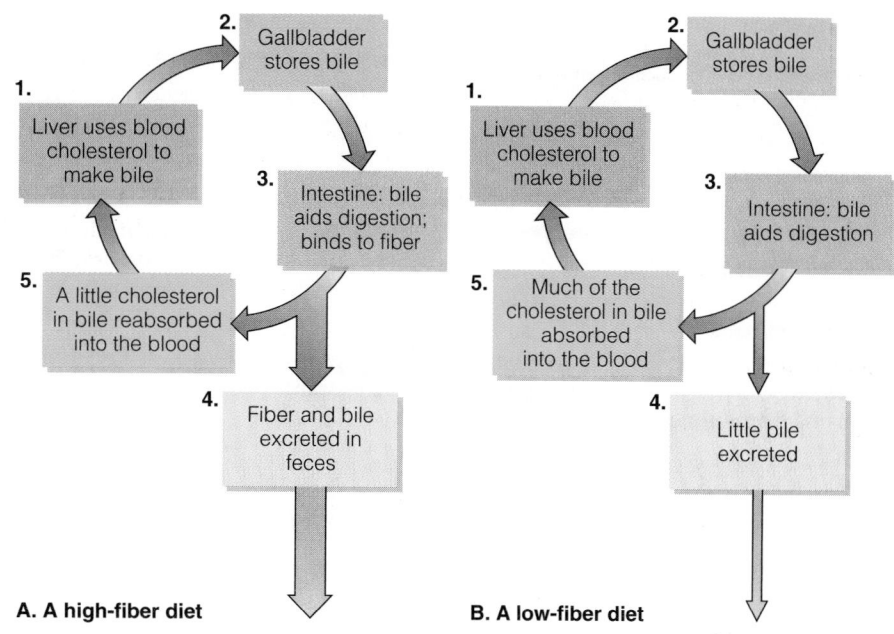

A. A high-fiber diet

1. Liver uses blood cholesterol to make bile
2. Gallbladder stores bile
3. Intestine: bile aids digestion; binds to fiber
4. Fiber and bile excreted in feces
5. A little cholesterol in bile reabsorbed into the blood

B. A low-fiber diet

1. Liver uses blood cholesterol to make bile
2. Gallbladder stores bile
3. Intestine: bile aids digestion
4. Little bile excreted
5. Much of the cholesterol in bile absorbed into the blood

These four actions underlie the many health benefits attributed to dietary fibers.[6]

People choosing high-fiber foods in hopes of receiving some of these benefits are wise to seek out a variety of fiber sources. Wheat bran, which is composed mostly of insoluble fibers, is one of the most effective stool-softening fibers; oat bran and other more soluble fibers have a greater cholesterol-lowering effect.[7] The fibers of legumes, apples, and carrots may also lower blood cholesterol.

One fiber already mentioned, lignin, has created a stir among research scientists who are investigating its role against some forms of cancer. Bacteria in the human colon transform lignin into hormonelike compounds called lignans that are absorbed into the body.[8] In animals, lignans seem to block the growth of hormone-sensitive tumors, such as those of the prostate gland, colon, and breast. Evidence in people is still scanty, but research is progressing. Table 4-2 shows the diverse effects of different fibers; it also shows that most unrefined plant foods contain a mix of fiber types. To consumers, this means that although a food may play a starring role in providing one type of fiber, to receive the whole range of fiber benefits, one must choose a variety of whole foods each day.

Like any other substances, fibers can cause harm if taken in excess. Fibers carry water out of the body and can cause dehydration. Most iron is absorbed at the beginning of the intestinal tract, and excess insoluble fibers may limit iron's absorption by speeding up the transit of foods through the upper part of the digestive system. Binders in some fibers act as **chelating agents** and link chemically with nutrient minerals (iron, zinc, calcium, and others) and then carry them out of the body. Too much bulk in the diet can limit the total

chelating (KEE-late-ing) **agents** molecules that surround other molecules and are therefore useful in either preventing or promoting movement of substances from place to place.

Chelating agents are often sold by supplement vendors to "remove poisons" from the body. Some valid medical uses such as treatment of lead poisoning exist, but most of the chelating agents sold over-the-counter are promoted based on unproven claims.

TABLE 4-2

Water Solubilities, Sources, and Health Effects of Fiber

Fiber Type	Major Food Sources	Possible Health Effects
Water Soluble		
Gums, mucilages, pectins, psyllium[a], some hemicellulose	Barley, fruits, legumes, oats, oat bran, rye, seeds, vegetables	These fibers lower blood cholesterol; slow glucose absorption; slow transit of food through upper digestive tract; hold moisture in stools, softening them; partly fermentable into fragments the body can use.
Water Insoluble		
Cellulose Lignin Some hemicellulose	Brown rice, fruits, legumes, seeds, vegetables, wheat bran, whole grains	These fibers soften stools; regulate bowel movements; speed transit of material through small intestine; increase fecal weight and speed fecal passage through colon; reduce colon cancer risk; reduce risks of diverticulosis, hemorrhoids, and appendicitis.

[a]Psyllium, a fiber laxative and a cereal additive, has both soluble and insoluble properties.

amount of food consumed and cause deficiencies of both nutrients and energy. The malnourished, the elderly, and children who consume no animal products are especially vulnerable to this chain of events.

The average fiber intake in the United States is lower than has previously been thought. On a given day, women report an intake of about 12 grams of fiber per day, while men report an intake of about 18 grams per day.[9] Most people do not consume as much fiber as they need for their health. There is no Recommended Dietary Allowance (RDA) for fiber, but the committee on RDA acknowledges the need for fiber and recommends that people meet it by eating unprocessed, fiber-containing foods and not by eating refined fiber sources such as bran.[10] As Table 4-1 showed, the World Health Organization recommends a daily intake of 27 to 40 grams of fiber.[11]

The addition of purified fibers, such as oat or wheat bran, to foods is easily taken to extreme. One report tells of a man who required emergency intestinal surgery for the removal of a blockage formed by too many oat bran muffins; the bran had rendered his digestive system unable to work.[12] This doesn't mean that people should avoid bran-containing foods, but that they should use bran, separated from its original food product, with moderation. A less extreme concern is that purified fiber might displace nutrients from the diet. Purified fibers are, in one way, like refined sugars: the nutrients that may have originally accompanied the fibers have been lost. Furthermore, a purified fiber such as cellulose may not affect the body the same way as the cellulose in whole grains. This chapter's Consumer Corner provides information about choosing wisely among grain foods, and the Do It Feature shows which foods provide fiber.

KEY POINT **Fibers aid in maintaining the health of the digestive tract and help to prevent or control certain diseases. Most people probably need 27 to 40 grams of fiber each day. Fiber needs are best met with whole foods. Purified fiber in large doses can have undesirable effects.**

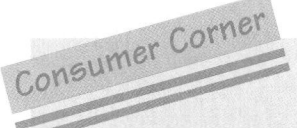

REFINED, ENRICHED, AND WHOLE-GRAIN BREAD

For many people, bread supplies much of the carbohydrate, or at least most of the starch, in a day's meals. Any food used in such abundance in the diet should be scrutinized closely, and if it doesn't measure up to high nutrition standards, it should be replaced with a food that does. For people who eat bread, the meanings of the words associated with the wheat flour that makes up the bread—**refined, enriched, fortified,** and **whole grain**—hold the key to understanding this product, in which they invest many calories per day (see Table 4-3).

The part of the wheat plant that is made into flour and then into bread and other baked goods is the seed or kernel. The wheat kernel (a whole grain) has four main parts: the **germ,** the **endosperm,** the **bran,** and the **husk,** as shown in Figure 4-5. The germ is the part that grows into a wheat plant and therefore carries with it concentrated food to support the new life. It is especially rich in vitamins and minerals. The endosperm is the soft, white, inside portion of the kernel, containing starch and proteins that help nourish the seed as it sprouts. The kernel is encased in the

(continued on next page)

TABLE 4-3

Terms That Describe Grain Foods

- **bran** the protective fibrous coating around a grain; the chief fiber donator of a grain.
- **endosperm** the bulk of the edible part of a grain, the starchy part.
- **enriched, fortified** refers to addition of nutrients to a refined food product. As defined by U.S. law, these terms mean that specified levels of thiamin, riboflavin, niacin, folate, and iron have been added to refined grains and grain products. The terms *enriched* and *fortified* can refer to addition of more nutrients than just these five; read the label.[a]
- **germ** the nutrient-rich inner part of a grain.
- **husk** the outer, inedible part of a grain.
- **refined** refers to the process by which the coarse parts of food products are removed. For example, the refining of wheat into flour involves removing three of the four parts of the kernel—the chaff, the bran, and the germ— leaving only the endosperm, composed mainly of starch and a little protein.
- **unbleached flour** a beige-colored endosperm flour with texture and nutritive qualities that approximate those of regular white flour.
- **wheat flour** any flour made from wheat, including white flour.
- **white flour** an endosperm flour that has been refined and bleached for maximum softness and whiteness.
- **whole grain** refers to a grain milled in its entirety (all but the husk), not refined.
- **whole-wheat flour** flour made from whole-wheat kernels; a whole-grain flour.

[a]Formerly, *enriched* and *fortified* carried distinct meanings with regard to the nutrient amounts added to foods, but a change in the law has made these terms virtually synonymous.

FIGURE 4-5

A WHEAT PLANT AND A SINGLE KERNEL OF WHEAT

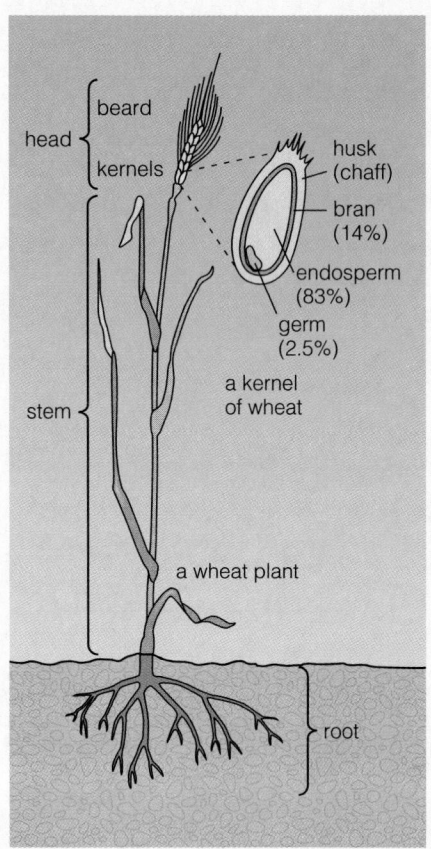

head { beard
kernels }

stem {

husk (chaff)
bran (14%)
endosperm (83%)
germ (2.5%)
a kernel of wheat

a wheat plant

root

In Western societies, bread is the staff of life.

bran, a protective coating that is similar in function to the shell of a nut; the bran is also rich in nutrients and fiber. The husk, commonly called chaff, is the dry outermost layer and is inedible but can be used in animal feed.

In earlier times people milled wheat by grinding it between two stones, blowing or sifting out the chaff, and retaining the nutrient-rich bran and germ as well as the endosperm. Then milling machinery was "improved," or so the makers thought, and it became possible to remove the dark, heavy germ and bran as well, leaving a whiter, smoother-textured flour. People came to look on this flour as more desirable than the crunchy, dark brown, "old-fashioned" flour.

In turning to white bread, bread eaters suffered a tragic loss of needed nutrients. Many people developed deficiencies of iron, thiamin, riboflavin, and niacin—nutrients that they had formerly received from whole-grain bread. Finally, the problem was recognized, and Congress passed the Enrichment Act requiring that iron, niacin, thiamin, and riboflavin be added to refined grain products before they were sold. (The Enrichment Act of 1942 is still in effect in the United States today.) This doesn't make a single slice of refined bread "rich" in these nutrients, but people who eat several or many slices of bread a day obtain significantly more of the nutrients than they would from unenriched white bread, as Figure 4-6 shows.

Today you can almost take for granted that all breads, grain products such as rice, macaroni, and spaghetti, and all types of cereals have been enriched with at least the four nutrients just mentioned. You will also soon see grain foods that have been enriched with the vitamin folate, or "folic acid" as it may be called on food labels. The Enrichment Act was amended

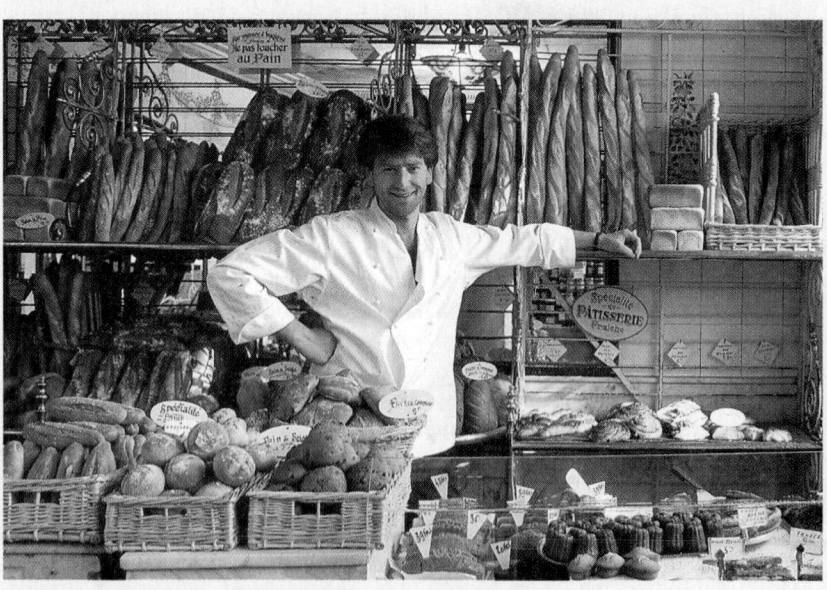

FIGURE 4-6

NUTRIENTS IN WHOLE-GRAIN,
ENRICHED WHITE, AND UNENRICHED
WHITE BREADS

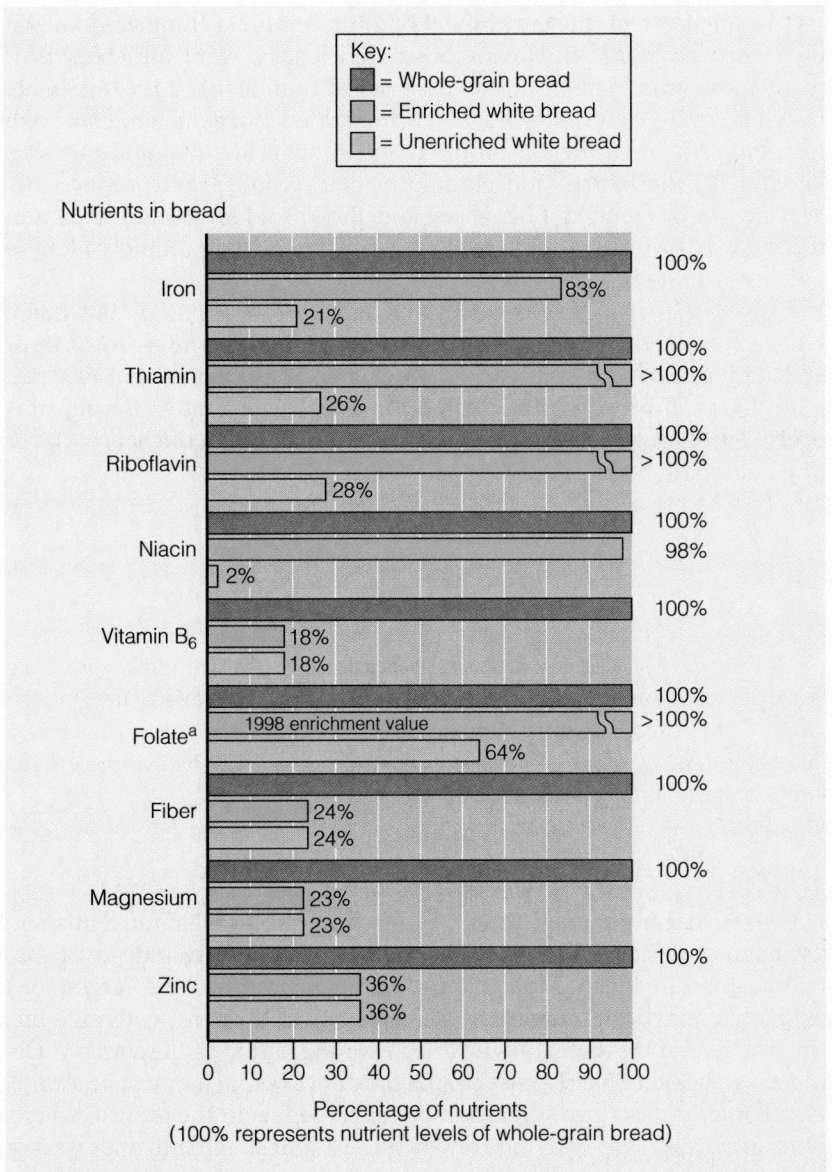

[a]By 1998, folate will be added to enriched bread and other enriched grain products in amounts that equal or exceed the whole-grain values for folate. Folic acid fortification, *Nutrition Reviews* 54 (1996): 94–95.

for the first time in 1996 to include this vitamin, with the intent of preventing serious birth defects, as Chapters 7 and 12 explain.[13] The folate values in Figure 4-6 show how the new fortification will affect the folate content of a slice of bread. Food manufacturers may add folate to foods right away, but by 1998, all refined grain foods must be enriched with folate.

To a great extent, the enrichment of grain products eliminated known deficiency problems, but many other deficiencies went undetected for many more years. The trouble with enriched flour is that it is comparable to whole grain only with respect to the added nutrients and not with respect to others. Enriched products still contain less magnesium, zinc, vitamin B_6, vitamin E, and chromium than whole-grain products do. When a grain is refined, fiber is lost, too. Bread sold for weight-reduction dieting may be fortified with pure cellulose, but adding cellulose alone is not enough; the bread still lacks other fibers.

Only *whole-grain* flour contains all nutritive portions of the grain. Notice, too, the distinctions between **wheat flour** and **whole-wheat flour** and **white flour** and **unbleached flour** among the terms that describe grain foods. If bread is a staple food in your diet—that is, if you eat it every day—you would be well advised to learn to like the hearty flavor of whole-grain bread.

Grams of Fiber in One Cup of Flour:

✔ Dark rye, 18 g.
✔ Whole-grain cornmeal, 15 g.
✔ Whole wheat, 15 g.
✔ Light rye, 14 g.
✔ Buckwheat, 8 g.
✔ Enriched white, 3 g.

FROM CARBOHYDRATES TO GLUCOSE

The body's cells cannot use foods such as bread or even whole molecules of lactose, sucrose, or starch for energy, but they need the glucose in them, and they need it continuously. An important task of the various body systems, then, is to make glucose available to the cells, not all at once when it is eaten, but at a steady rate all day.

Digestion and Absorption of Carbohydrate

To obtain glucose from newly eaten food, the digestive system must first render the starch and disaccharides from the food into monosaccharides that can be absorbed through the cells that line the small intestine. The largest of the digestible carbohydrate molecules, starch, requires the most extensive breakdown. The rate of this breakdown varies with the nature of the starch.[14] Disaccharides, on the other hand, must be split only once before they can be absorbed.

As Chapter 3 described, digestion of starch begins in the mouth, where an enzyme in saliva mixes with food and begins to split starch into maltose. While chewing a bite of bread, you may have noticed that a slightly sweet taste develops. This is because maltose is being liberated from starch by the enzyme. The salivary enzyme continues to act on the starch in the swallowed bite of bread while it remains tucked in the stomach's storage area together with other swallowed bites. Slowly, each chewed lump is pushed downward, to be thoroughly mixed with the stomach's acid and other juices. Enzyme molecules are made of protein, and as such, they eventually succumb to deactivation by the stomach's protein-digesting acid. (The only exception is the protein-digesting enzyme that works in the stomach; its structure protects it from the stomach's acid.) Starch digestion therefore ceases in the stomach, but it resumes at full speed in the small intestine, where another starch-splitting enzyme is delivered by the pancreas. This enzyme breaks starch down entirely into disaccharides and small polysaccharides.[15]

Sucrose and lactose from food, and maltose and small polysaccharides freed from starch, undergo one more split to yield free monosaccharides before they are absorbed. This split is accomplished by enzymes that are attached to the cells of the lining of the small intestine. The conversion of a bite of bread to nutrients for the body is completed when monosaccharides cross these cells and are washed away in a rush of circulating blood that carries them to the waiting liver. Figure 4-7 presents a quick review of carbohydrate digestion.

Once in the body, the absorbed carbohydrates travel to the liver, which converts fructose and galactose to glucose or products of glucose metabolism (such as fats). The circulatory system transports the glucose and fats to the cells. Liver and muscle cells may store circulating glucose as glycogen; all cells may split glucose for energy.

As mentioned, molecules of fiber are not changed by human digestive enzymes. Some dietary fibers can, however, be digested by the billions of living inhabitants of the human digestive tract, the resident bacteria. So active are these inhabitants in breaking down substances from food that one expert claims they constitute "an organ of intense metabolic activity that is involved in nutrient salvage."[16] Digestion of fibers by resident bacteria yields waste products, mainly small fat fragments that the body absorbs and can use to provide a tiny bit of energy.[17] A by-product of fiber breakdown is any of several odorous gases, which may make people want to avoid fiber-containing foods altogether. Don't give up on high-fiber foods if they cause gas. Instead, start with small amounts and gradually increase them over several weeks' time; chew foods thoroughly to break up hard-to-digest lumps that can ferment in the intestine; and try many fiber-rich foods until you find some that do not cause the problem. In some people, persistent painful gas may indicate that the digestive tract has undergone a change in its ability to digest the sugar in milk, a condition known as lactose intolerance.

✓ KEY POINT   **With respect to starch and sugars, the main task of the various body systems is to convert them into glucose to fuel the cells' work. Fibers help regulate digestion and contribute a little energy.**

Lactose Intolerance and Milk Allergy

About 80 percent of the world's people, as they age, lose the ability to produce enough of the enzyme **lactase** to digest the milk sugar lactose.[18] In children of nonwhite races, **lactose intolerance** may appear as early as age four. Thereafter, on drinking milk or eating lactose-containing products, these people experience nausea, pain, diarrhea, and excessive gas. The undigested lactose remaining in the intestine demands dilution with fluid from surrounding tissue, and ultimately from the bloodstream. Intestinal bacteria use the undigested lactose for their own energy, a process that produces gas and intestinal irritants. The tendency to develop lactose intolerance appears to be primarily

lactase the intestinal enzyme that splits the disaccharide lactose to monosaccharides during digestion.

lactose intolerance inability to digest lactose due to a lack of the enzyme lactase.

FIGURE 4-7

HOW CARBOHYDRATE IN FOOD BECOMES GLUCOSE IN THE BODY

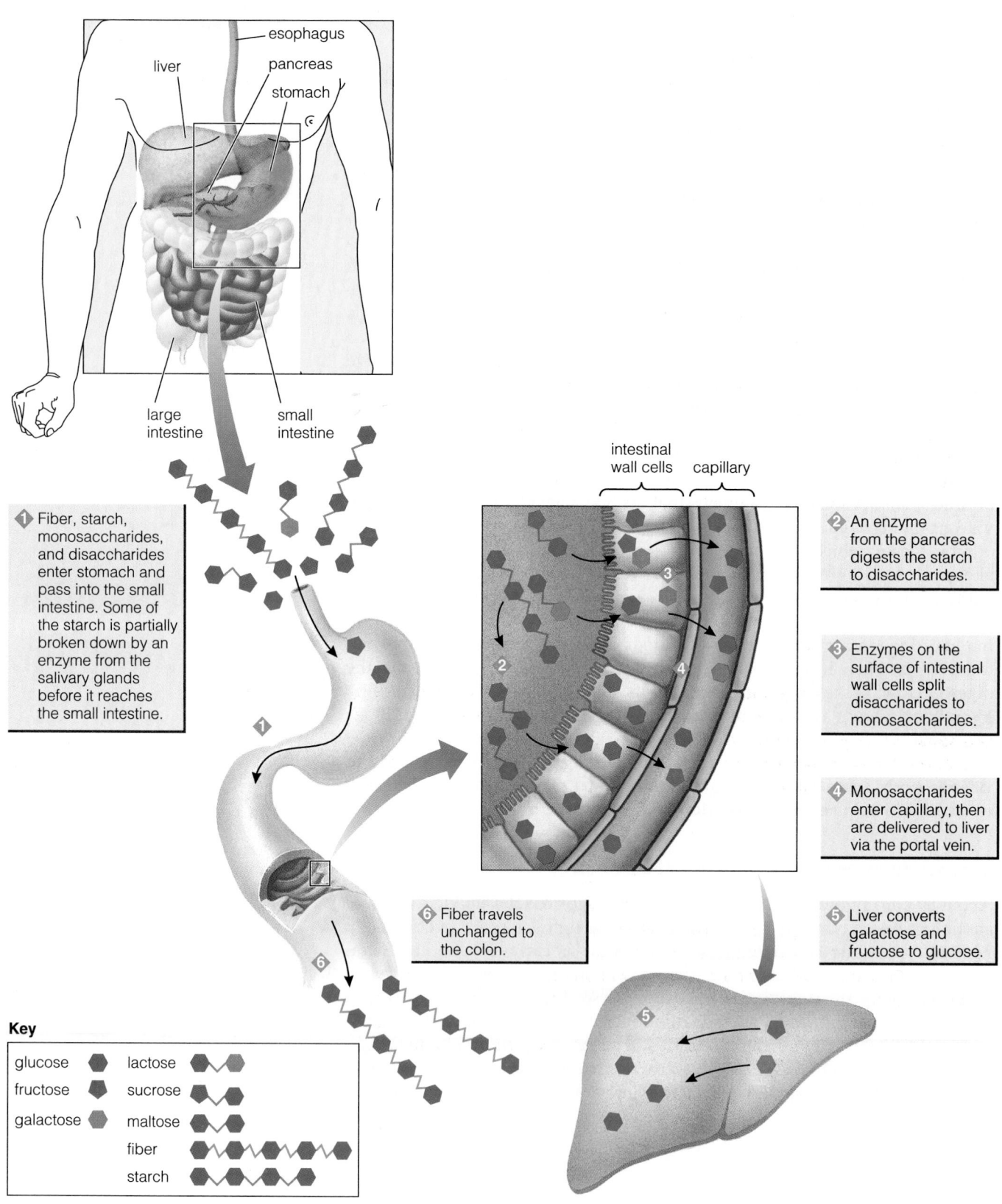

esophagus

liver

pancreas

stomach

large intestine

small intestine

intestinal wall cells

capillary

① Fiber, starch, monosaccharides, and disaccharides enter stomach and pass into the small intestine. Some of the starch is partially broken down by an enzyme from the salivary glands before it reaches the small intestine.

② An enzyme from the pancreas digests the starch to disaccharides.

③ Enzymes on the surface of intestinal wall cells split disaccharides to monosaccharides.

④ Monosaccharides enter capillary, then are delivered to liver via the portal vein.

⑥ Fiber travels unchanged to the colon.

⑤ Liver converts galactose and fructose to glucose.

Key

glucose	⬡	lactose	⬡⬡
fructose	⬡	sucrose	⬡⬡
galactose	⬡	maltose	⬡⬡
		fiber	⬡⬡⬡⬡⬡
		starch	⬡⬡⬡⬡

an inherited trait but anyone who is malnourished or sick may develop lactose intolerance for a short time, making avoidance of milk and milk products a temporary necessity. Lactose intolerance affects people to differing degrees. Some can tolerate as much as a cupful of milk; some tolerate lactose-reduced milk; others cannot tolerate lactose in any amount.[19]

Because milk is an almost indispensable source of the calcium a child needs for growth, a milk substitute must be found for any child who becomes lactose intolerant. Women who fail to consume enough calcium during youth may later develop weak bones, so it is urgent that young women, too, search for substitutes if they become unable to tolerate milk. Sometimes yogurt or aged cheese makes an acceptable substitute: the bacteria or molds that help create these products digest lactose as they convert milk to a fermented product. Yogurts that contain added milk solids are too high in lactose to be used this way; milk solids are listed among the ingredients on the label.

Alternatively, people can choose milk products that have undergone treatment with lactose-digesting enzymes, or they may treat the products themselves. Enzyme pills or drops can be purchased over-the-counter. When the pills are taken with milk-containing meals, or drops added to milk-based foods, these products help to digest lactose by replacing the missing natural enzymes. In all cases, the trick is to find ways of splitting lactose to glucose and galactose so that the body can absorb the products, rather than leaving the lactose undigested to feed the bacteria of the colon.

Sometimes sensitivity to milk is due not to lactose intolerance but to an allergic reaction to the protein in milk. Milk allergy arises as other allergies do—from sensitization of the immune system to a substance. In this case, the immune system overreacts when it encounters the protein of milk.

Children and adults with milk allergy often cannot tolerate cheese or yogurt either, and they have to find nondairy calcium sources. Good choices are calcium-fortified orange juice or soy milk, where available, or canned sardines or salmon with the bones. Controversy 8 examines the topic of milk in adult diets in relation to the adult bone disease, osteoporosis.

✔ **KEY POINT   Lactose intolerance is a common condition in which the body fails to produce sufficient amounts of the enzyme needed to digest the sugar of milk. Uncomfortable symptoms result and can lead to milk avoidance. Lactose-intolerant people and those allergic to milk need milk alternates that contain calcium.**

THE BODY'S USE OF GLUCOSE

Carbohydrates serve structural roles in the body, such as forming part of the internal organs' protective coatings of mucus, but their main role is to serve as an energy source. Glucose is not only the main original unit from which carbohydrate-rich foods are made, it is also the basic carbohydrate unit that each cell of the body uses for energy. The body handles its glucose judiciously. It maintains an internal supply for use in case of need, and it tightly controls its blood glucose concentration to ensure that glucose remains available for ongoing use.

Percentages of People with Lactose Intolerance:

✔ >80% Asian Americans.
✔ 80% Native Americans
✔ 75% African Americans
✔ 70% Mediterranean peoples.
✔ 60% Inuits (Native Alaskans).
✔ 50% Hispanics.
✔ 20% Caucasians.
✔ <10% Northern Europeans.

Food allergies are a topic of Chapter 13.

FIGURE 4-8

THE BREAKDOWN OF GLUCOSE
YIELDS ENERGY AND
CARBON DIOXIDE

The bonds between the carbon atoms in glucose are split apart by cell enzymes, liberating the energy stored there for the cell's use. The first split yields two 3-carbon fragments. The two-way arrows mean that these fragments can also be rejoined to make glucose again. Once they are broken down further into 2-carbon fragments, however, they cannot rejoin to make glucose. The carbon atoms liberated when the bonds split are combined with oxygen and released into the air, via the lungs, as carbon dioxide. Although not shown here, water is also produced at each split.

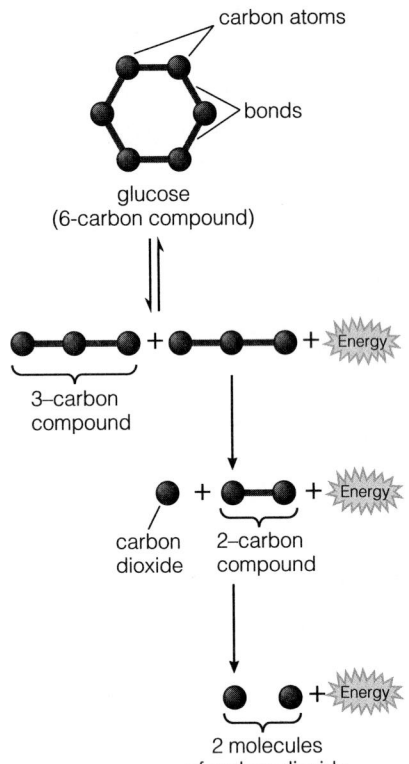

carbon atoms

bonds

glucose
(6-carbon compound)

3–carbon
compound

carbon
dioxide

2–carbon
compound

2 molecules
of carbon dioxide

Splitting Glucose for Energy

Glucose fuels the work of most of the body's cells. When a cell splits glucose for energy, it performs an intricate sequence of maneuvers that are of great interest to the biochemist—and of no interest whatever to most people who eat bread and potatoes. One fact that everybody needs to understand, though, is that there is no good substitute for carbohydrate. That is why carbohydrate was mentioned as *essential* in Chapter 1. The following details are given to make this point clear.

At a certain point, glucose is forever lost to the body, and this can have serious consequences. Inside a cell, the glucose is broken in half, releasing some energy. These halves have two pathways open to them. They can be put back together to make glucose, or they can be further broken apart into smaller fragments. If they are broken into smaller fragments, they can never again be reassembled to form glucose. The smaller fragments can yield still more energy and in the process break down completely to carbon dioxide and water; or they can be hitched together into units of body fat. Figure 4-8 shows how glucose is broken down to yield energy and carbon dioxide.

Although glucose can be converted into body fat, body fat can never be converted into glucose to feed the brain adequately. This is one reason why fasting and low-carbohydrate diets are dangerous. When there is a severe carbohydrate deficit, the body has two problems. Having no glucose, it has to turn to protein to make some (it has this ability), thus diverting protein from vitally important functions of its own such as maintaining the body's immune defenses. Protein's functions in the body are so indispensable that carbohydrate should be kept available precisely to prevent the use of protein for energy. This is called the **protein-sparing action** of carbohydrate.

Also, without sufficient carbohydrate, the body cannot use its fat in the normal way. (Carbohydrate has to combine with fat fragments before they can be used for energy.) Using fat without the help of carbohydrate causes the body to go into **ketosis,** a condition in which unusual products of fat breakdown **(ketone bodies)** accumulate in the blood, disturbing the normal acid-base balance. Ketosis during pregnancy can cause brain damage to the fetus with irreversible mental retardation after birth.

The minimum amount of carbohydrate needed to ensure complete sparing of body protein and avoidance of ketosis is around 100 grams a day in an average-sized person. This has to be digestible carbohydrate, and considerably more (three or four times more) than this minimum is recommended.[20] The servings of vegetables, fruits, and grains recommended in Table 4-1 (page 109) would deliver 125 grams at a minimum and 200 to 400 grams on average.

✓ KEY POINT   **Without glucose the body is forced to alter its uses of protein and fats. The body breaks down its own muscles and other protein tissues to make glucose and converts its fats into ketone bodies, incurring ketosis.**

Storing Glucose as Glycogen

After a meal, as blood glucose rises, the pancreas is the first organ to respond. It releases the hormone **insulin,** which signals the body's tissues to take up surplus glucose. From some of this excess glucose, muscle and liver cells build the polysaccharide glycogen. The muscles hoard two-thirds of the body's total glycogen and use it just for themselves. The liver stores the other one-third and is more generous with its glycogen, making it available as blood glucose for the brain or other organs when the supply runs low.

Glycogen is wondrously designed for its task of releasing glucose on demand. Instead of having long chains with occasional branches, as starch does, that are cleaved linearly during digestion, glycogen is many-branched, so that hundreds of ends stick out at each molecule's surface. When the blood glucose concentration drops and cells need energy, a pancreatic hormone, **glucagon,** floods the bloodstream. Thousand of enzymes within the liver cells respond by attacking a multitude of ends simultaneously to release a surge of glucose into the blood for use by all the other body cells. Another hormone, epinephrine, does the same thing as part of the body's defense mechanism in times of danger.

To a person living in the Stone Age, this internal source of quick energy was indispensable. Life was fraught with physical peril. The person who stopped and ate before running from a saber-toothed tiger did not survive to produce our ancestors. The quick-energy response in a stress situation works to our advantage today as well. For example, it accounts for the energy you suddenly have to clean up your room when you learn that a special person is coming to visit. To meet such emergencies, we are well advised to eat and to store carbohydrate every four to six waking hours.

You may rightly ask, "What kind of carbohydrate?" Candy bars and sugary beverages supply sugar energy quickly, but they are not the best choices. Balanced meals, eaten on a regular schedule, help the body to maintain its blood glucose. Meals containing starch and fiber along with some protein and a little fat slow down digestion so that glucose enters the blood gradually in an ongoing steady supply. Such meals also provide an assortment of other nutrients, not found in candy and soft drinks, that help cells to use their glucose.

✔ **KEY POINT**   **Glycogen is the body's form of stored glucose. The liver stores glycogen for use by the whole body. Muscles have their own private glycogen stock for their exclusive use. The hormone glucagon acts to liberate stored glucose from liver glycogen.**

Returning Glucose to the Blood

Should your glucose supplies ever fall too low, you would feel dizzy and weak. Should your blood glucose ever climb abnormally high, you might become confused or have difficulty breathing. Both conditions could be dangerous, but luckily the body normally guards against such occurrences.

The maintenance of a normal blood glucose concentration depends on the two safeguards already mentioned. When blood glucose starts to fall too low, it is replenished by drawing on liver glycogen stores. When it starts to rise too high, the body siphons off the excess into the liver, to be converted to glycogen or fat, and into the muscle, to be converted to glycogen.

To replenish blood glucose, the hormone glucagon triggers the breakdown of liver glycogen to free glucose. Other hormones also act in this manner, including epinephrine (the stress hormone) and some that promote the conversion of protein into glucose. The liver's glycogen stores can be depleted within half a waking day, however. As for protein, only a little can be spared.

protein-sparing action the action of carbohydrate and fat in providing energy that allows protein to be used for purposes it alone can serve.

ketosis (kee-TOE-sis) an undesirably high concentration of ketone bodies, such as acetone, in the blood or urine.

ketone (KEE-tone) **bodies** acidic, fat-related compounds that can arise from the incomplete breakdown of fat when carbohydrate is not available.

insulin a hormone secreted by the pancreas in response to a high blood glucose concentration. It assists cells in drawing glucose from the blood.

glucagon a hormone of the pancreas that stimulates the liver to release glucose into the blood when blood glucose concentration dips.

glycemic (gligh-SEEM-ic) **effect** a measure of the extent to which a food raises the blood glucose concentration and elicits an insulin response as compared with pure glucose.

When body protein is used, it is taken from blood, muscle, or organ proteins; no surplus of protein is stored specifically for emergencies. As for fat, it cannot regenerate enough glucose to make a difference.

Obviously, when blood glucose falls and stores are depleted, a meal or a snack can replenish the supply. The meal or snack you choose may flood the blood with glucose, however, requiring the body to protect itself against too *high* a blood glucose concentration.

Within limits, some foods elevate blood glucose and insulin concentrations higher than others do. The effect, called the **glycemic effect,** is worth a moment's attention. Scientists measure the glycemic effect by administering a food or a meal and then observing how fast and how high the blood glucose rises and how quickly the body responds by bringing it back to normal. Most people can quickly adjust, but people with abnormal carbohydrate metabolism may experience extreme blood glucose levels. These people do well to choose most often foods with a low glycemic effect such as dried beans, pasta, barley, bulgur (wheat), pumpernickel bread, and any food with the soluble fiber psyllium added.[21] These foods produce a slow, sustained rise in blood glucose.[22] In addition, eating small, frequent meals spreads glucose absorption across the day and prevents a large influx.

Many factors work together to determine a food's glycemic effect, and the result is not always what a person might expect. Ice cream, for example, produces less of a response than potatoes; baked potatoes produce less of a response than mashed; a sweet, juicy apple produces a low response (probably due to the apple's soluble fiber); and dried beans and legumes of all kinds are notable for keeping blood glucose remarkably steady. Importantly, a food's glycemic effect differs depending on whether it is eaten alone or as part of a mixed meal. The glycemic effects of foods in mixed meals tend to balance each other. Most people eat a variety of foods in a meal and so need not worry at all about the glycemic effect of the foods they choose.

✔ **KEY POINT** **Blood glucose regulation depends mainly on the hormones insulin and glucagon. Certain carbohydrate foods produce a greater rise and fall in blood glucose than do others. Most people have no problem regulating their blood glucose, especially when they consume regular mixed meals.**

Converting Glucose to Fat

When food is tempting, people may continue to eat beyond the amount they need. After meeting the body cells' immediate energy needs and filling glycogen stores to capacity, the body takes a third path for handling incoming carbohydrates. Say you have eaten and are now sitting on the couch, eating pretzels and drinking a cola as you watch a ball game on television. Your digestive tract is delivering molecules of glucose to your bloodstream, and your blood is carrying these molecules to your liver and other body cells. The body cells use what glucose they can for their energy needs of the moment. More glucose is linked together and stored as glycogen until the muscles and liver are full to capacity with glycogen. Still the glucose keeps coming, and the liver has no choice but to handle the excess. The liver breaks the extra glucose into small fragments and puts them together into more permanent energy-storage compounds—fats. (This would happen with excess protein or fat, too.) The fats are then released into the blood, carried to the fatty tissues of the body, and deposited there. Unlike the liver cells, which can store only about four to six hours' worth of glycogen, the fat cells can store practically unlimited quantities of fats. Moral: you had better play the game if you are going to eat the food.

Even though excess carbohydrate is converted to fat and stored, a balanced diet that is high in complex carbohydrates helps control body weight and maintain lean tissue. Researchers are beginning to understand this seeming paradox, and the results of the work are fascinating; they are presented in full in Controversy 5. The current thrust seems to be that, calorie for calorie, carbohydrate-rich foods contribute less to body fatness than do fat-rich foods.[23] Had you chosen fatty potato chips instead of low-fat pretzels for your ball game snack, your body would have stored even greater amounts of fat for the calories taken in. Thus, if you want to stay within your calorie limits, eat until full, never skip a meal, and remain lean, you should make every effort to choose foods that, together, comprise a diet with 55 percent or more of its calories from mostly complex carbohydrates and 30 percent or less from fats. The Food Feature of this chapter provides the first set of tools required for the job of designing such a diet. Once you have learned to identify the carbohydrates in foods, you must then learn where the fats come in (Chapter 5's Food Feature) and how to obtain adequate protein without overdoing it (Chapter 6).

✔ KEY POINT **The liver converts extra energy compounds into fat, a more permanent and unlimited energy-storage compound than glycogen.**

DIABETES AND HYPOGLYCEMIA

Some people have physical conditions that render their bodies unable to handle carbohydrates in the normal way. One of these, **diabetes,** is common in developed nations and can be detected by way of a timed blood test. Another, hypoglycemia, is rare as a true disease condition, but many people believe they experience its symptoms at times.

Diabetes

Diabetes can lead to or contribute to any of a number of other diseases and is itself among the top ten killers of adults and the leading cause of blindness in the United States. Several diseases have been called diabetes, but by far the most common ones are the two main forms of diabetes mellitus described here. Both types are disorders of blood glucose regulation. Both produce warning signs that can signal their presence (see Table 4-4).

In the first, less common type, **Type I diabetes** (about 20 percent of cases), the person's own immune system attacks the cells of the pancreas that normally synthesize the hormone insulin. Researchers suspect genetics, toxins, a virus, and a disordered immune system as causes. Soon the pancreas can no longer produce insulin, and after each meal, blood glucose remains elevated, even though body tissues are simultaneously starving for glucose. The person must receive insulin periodically to assist the cells in taking up the needed glucose from the blood; therefore this type of diabetes is called *insulin-dependent diabetes mellitus (IDDM).*

diabetes (dye-uh-BEET-eez) a disease (technically termed *diabetes mellitus*) characterized by inadequate or ineffective insulin, which renders a person unable to regulate blood glucose normally.

Type I diabetes the type of diabetes in which the person produces no insulin at all; also known as *juvenile-onset* or *insulin-dependent diabetes,* although some cases arise in adulthood.

TABLE 4-4

Warning Signs of Diabetes

- Excessive urination and thirst.
- Glucose in the urine.
- Weight loss with nausea, easy tiring, weakness, or irritability.
- Cravings for food, especially for sweets.
- Frequent infections of the skin, gums, vagina, or urinary tract.
- Vision disturbances; blurred vision.
- Pain in the legs, feet, or fingers.
- Slow healing of cuts and bruises.
- Itching.
- Drowsiness.
- Abnormally high glucose tolerance test results.

Type II diabetes the type of diabetes in which the fat cells resist insulin; also called *adult-onset* or *noninsulin-dependent diabetes.*

Insulin is a protein, and if it were taken orally, the digestive system would digest it. Insulin must therefore be injected, either by daily shots or by an insulin pump that delivers insulin through an implanted needle. Medical researchers are working to learn how to transplant healthy tissue into the pancreas to get it working again or to develop a vaccine or other drug that may prevent IDDM by preventing the body's attack on its own pancreas.

The second and predominant type of diabetes mellitus, **Type II diabetes** (80 percent of cases), is characterized by insulin resistance of the body's cells, including fat cells.[24] Insulin may be present, often in abnormally large amounts, and it does stimulate cells to take up glucose, but they do so more slowly than normal. Blood glucose rises too high, as in IDDM, but in this case blood insulin also rises. This type of diabetes is therefore called *noninsulin-dependent diabetes mellitus (NIDDM).* Eventually, the pancreas becomes less able to make insulin.[25] At this point, some people with NIDDM must take insulin to supplement their own supply, especially late in the course of the disease. If drugs are necessary, a preferred therapy is to take a drug that stimulates the person's own pancreas to secrete insulin. The characteristics of the two types of diabetes are summarized in Table 4-5.

NIDDM tends to occur late in life and tends to run in families. People with the disease often become obese because they overeat due to their cells' resistance to insulin—while they are waiting for their cells to be fed, so to speak. Figure 4-9 depicts one theory on how this may become a cycle—the larger the fat cells become, the more insulin resistant they become, and the more obese the person. Obesity worsens insulin resistance, which, in turn, worsens obesity. Weight loss in overweight people with diabetes often helps control the disease. Even moderate weight gain in adults has been observed to predict diabetes.[26] The incidence of this type of diabetes also increases with increasing age, for in all people, the pancreatic cells that produce insulin progressively lose their function with time.[27] In some people this age-related decline in cell function is more rapid or more severe than in others, and these people especially need to beware of excess weight gain and also to watch their alcohol intakes. Heavy use of alcohol makes development of NIDDM more likely.[28]

Chapter 12 discusses a form of diabetes seen only in pregnancy—*gestational diabetes.*

TABLE 4-5

Diabetes Types I and II Compared

	IDDM (Type I Diabetes)	NIDDM (Type II Diabetes)
Age of onset	Childhood or mid-life	Adulthood
Body cells	Responsive to insulin action	Resistant to insulin action
Body fatness	Generally low to average	Generally high
Insulin shots required	Yes	Possibly[a]
Insulin-stimulating drugs may be effective	No	Yes
Natural insulin	Pancreas makes too little or none	Panceras makes enough or too much.
Pancreatic function	Insulin-producing cells impaired or nonfunctional	Insulin-producing cells normal
Severity of symptoms	Relatively severe	Relatively mild

[a]People past age 40 who suffer from NIDDM may lose pancreatic function and become dependent on insulin.

Diabetes can be diagnosed by means of a **glucose tolerance** test, in which the body is challenged to handle a sudden, large amount of glucose. After fasting overnight, the subject is fed a sugary drink. Four or six hours later, when blood glucose should be normal, the person's blood glucose will still be elevated **(hyperglycemia),** and possibly the blood insulin will be, too.[29]

Although the symptoms of diabetes are controllable for the most part, its effects can be severe and may progress even when blood glucose is controlled by drugs.[30] Problems may include impaired circulation leading to disease of the feet and legs, often necessitating amputation; kidney disease, sometimes requiring hospital care or kidney transplant; impaired vision or blindness due to cataracts and damaged retinas; nerve damage; skin damage; and strokes and heart attacks.[31] The root cause of all these conditions is probably the same. Diabetes causes fatty blockage or destruction of capillaries that feed the body organs, and tissues die from lack of nourishment.[32] The person is advised to control not only weight but also all possible risk factors that might contribute to heart and blood vessel disease (artherosclerosis and hypertension, discussed in Chapter 11).

A diet constructed of a balanced pattern of foods is best for controlling diabetes, and also for controlling weight and supporting physical activity. Such a diet also has all the characteristics important to prevention of chronic diseases and meets most of the *Dietary Guidelines for Americans*. The diet can vary, depending on personal tastes and on how much restriction is required to control an individual's blood glucose and lipid values.[33] In general, the diet:

- Is adequate (deficiencies in trace minerals, especially chromium, may hasten diabetes onset).
- Provides the recommended amount of fiber (fiber helps regulate blood glucose concentration).
- Is moderate in concentrated sugar (the amount allowed varies with an individual's blood glucose response).[34]
- Is high in complex carbohydrates (thought to assist in blood glucose regulation).
- Is low in fat and saturated fat (helping to protect against cardiovascular disease).
- Is not too high in protein (to protect the kidneys).[35]

A person at risk for diabetes can do no better than to adopt such a diet long before any symptoms appear.

Exercise is important, too. It not only helps to maintain a desirable body weight, but it also heightens tissue sensitivity to insulin and is considered by some to help prevent or forestall NIDDM.[36] Like a juggler who keeps three circus balls constantly in motion, the person with diabetes must constantly balance three lifestyle factors—diet, exercise, and medication—to control the blood glucose level.

✔ **KEY POINT** **Diabetes is an example of the body's abnormal handling of glucose. Inadequate or ineffective insulin leaves blood glucose high and cells undersupplied with glucose energy. This causes blood vessel and tissue damage. Weight control and exercise may be most effective in preventing the predominant form of diabetes (Type II) and the illnesses that accompany it.**

glucose tolerance the ability of the body to respond to dietary carbohydrate by regulating its blood glucose concentration promptly to a normal level.

hyperglycemia (HIGH-per-gligh-SEEM-ee-uh) an abnormally high blood glucose concentration (*hyper* means "too much"; *glyce* means "glucose"; *emia* means "in the blood").

FIGURE 4-9

THE OBESITY–DIABETES CYCLE

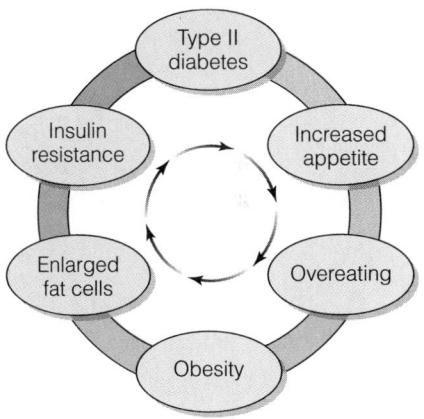

The exchange system introduced in Chapter 2 and presented in full in Appendix D was developed to help people with diabetes control calorie, carbohydrate, sugar, and fat intakes.

hypoglycemia a blood glucose concentration below normal, a symptom that may indicate any of several diseases, including impending diabetes (NIDDM).

postprandial hypoglycemia a drop in blood glucose that follows a meal and is accompanied by symptoms of the stress response. Also called *reactive hypoglycemia.*

fasting hypoglycemia hypoglycemia that occurs after 8 to 14 hours of fasting.

Hypoglycemia

The term **hypoglycemia** refers to a *symptom,* low blood glucose, and to a variety of conditions, including *disease conditions,* that cause that symptom. One such condition is **postprandial hypoglycemia,** literally, "low blood glucose after (or caused by) a meal." The symptoms are fatigue, weakness, irritability, a rapid heartbeat, anxiety, sweating, trembling, hunger, and headaches—symptoms common enough from many causes so that people easily misdiagnose themselves as having this meal-induced condition.

It takes more than guesswork to diagnose postprandial hypoglycemia, though. A diagnosis requires a test to detect low blood glucose while the symptoms are present to confirm that both occur simultaneously.[37] When they do, the diagnosis is confirmed.

A different kind of hypoglycemia exists in a person who has symptoms while well advanced into the fasting state (for example, overnight). The symptoms of **fasting hypoglycemia** are different from those of postprandial hypoglycemia: headache, mental dullness, fatigue, confusion, amnesia, and even seizures and unconsciousness.

Only a few people suffer from truly abnormal conditions that cause hypoglycemia. Many of the cases result from serious disease that endangers health and life. Conditions such as cancer, pancreatic damage, infection of the liver with accompanying damage (hepatitis), or advanced alcohol-induced liver disease can all produce hypoglycemia.[38]

In a very few other cases, symptoms occur together with a drop in blood glucose that cannot be explained by a disease state, and that can be relieved by eating.[39] In a study of people with postprandial hypoglycemia, researchers determined that a portion of hard-to-digest starch (raw cornstarch in this case) eaten with sugar effectively prevented a drop in blood glucose together with the associated symptoms.[40] The authors of the study suggest what some people have suspected for a long time—that a sugary meal promotes symptoms in those few people who have postprandial hypoglycemia, but that certain starches and other nutrients taken with the sugar can prevent the problem.

Hypoglycemia can be experimentally produced in just about everyone but only through extreme measures. To produce even mild hypoglycemia and its symptoms in normal, healthy people requires administering drugs that overwhelm the body's glucose-controlling hormones, insulin and glucagon. Without such intervention, those hormones rarely fail to keep blood glucose within normal limits. Symptoms that people ascribe to hypoglycemia hardly ever correlate to low blood glucose in blood tests.

Medical science cannot fully explain why many people with normal blood glucose test results report symptoms of hypoglycemia. Perhaps these people experience symptoms when their blood glucose drops just slightly, but still remains within the range considered normal.[41]

For people who seem to experience postprandial hypoglycemia after meals, it may help to avoid oscillating between low-carbohydrate dieting and sudden large sugar doses. Two findings suggest that these pointers may be on the mark:

1. A person with *normal* glucose regulation can develop the symptoms of hypoglycemia on taking a large dose of simple sugar after three days of following a low-carbohydrate diet.

2. A person who appears to have postprandial hypoglycemia by traditional testing may have it only after a simple-sugar load, and not after eating mixed meals.

If you are *not* prone to such symptoms, you still might bring them on if you deprived your system of carbohydrate for days and then dumped in a large dose all at once. If you do experience symptoms between meals, try to eliminate them by eating regular mixed meals rather than sugary snacks. Eat regularly timed, balanced meals to hold blood glucose steady.[42]

Part of eating right is choosing wisely among the many foods available. Two features follow that can help with choices of carbohydrate-containing foods. First, the Food Feature explains how to integrate foods into a diet that meets the body's needs for carbohydrates. The Do It section then asks you to critique your diet with regard to the fiber it contains.

✓ **KEY POINT** **Postprandial hypoglycemia is a rare medical condition in which blood glucose falls too low. It can be a warning of organ damage or disease. Many people believe they experience symptoms of hypoglycemia, but their symptoms normally do not accompany below-normal blood glucose.**

So far, this chapter has explored the body's responses to carbohydrate, processes that occur largely without your awareness. Now it asks that you take the controls by learning which foods supply the carbohydrates your body needs.

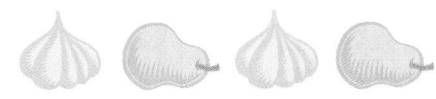

To best support health, a diet must supply enough carbohydrate-rich foods to meet the body's needs. The Daily Value suggests a goal of 300 grams of mostly complex carbohydrate each day for a person who eats a 2,000-calorie diet. This Food Feature illustrates how you can obtain the carbohydrate-rich foods you need while using the Food Guide Pyramid as a guide. Breads, cereals, vegetables, fruits, and milk are the foods noted for their contributions of valuable energy-yielding carbohydrates: starches and dilute sugars. Among those foods, many are also rich sources of fiber, and this chapter's Do It section helps to point them out.

BREAD, CEREAL, RICE, AND PASTA

A serving of most foods in this group—a slice of whole-wheat bread, half an English muffin or bagel, a 6-inch tortilla, or a half-cup of rice, pasta, or cooked cereal—provides about 15 grams of carbohydrate, mostly as starch.* People who like breads and other starchy foods are happy to learn that nutrition authorities encourage people to use them in abundance. They know that if calories are a problem, they should first cut out some added sugar or fat from

FOOD FEATURE

MEETING CARBOHYDRATE NEEDS

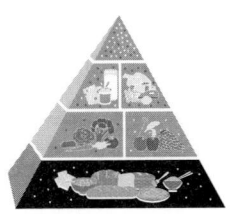

_____

*Gram values in this section are adapted from the 1995 exchange system.

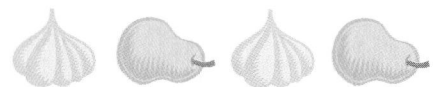

foods and limit total calories. Some foods in this group, especially baked goods such as biscuits, croissants, muffins, and snack crackers, do contain added sugar and/or fat, however.

The Exchange System section at the end of the book lists carbohydrate values for a variety of foods.

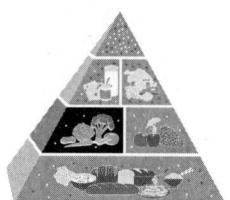

VEGETABLES

Some vegetables are major contributors of starch in the diet—just a small white or sweet potato or a half-cup of cooked dry beans, corn, peas, plantain, or winter squash provides 15 grams of carbohydrate, as much as in a slice of bread, though as a mixture of sugars and starch. A half-cup portion of carrots, okra, onions, tomatoes, cooked greens, or most other nonstarchy vegetables or a cup of salad greens provides about 5 grams as a mixture of starch and sugars.

FRUITS

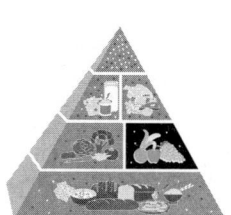

Different forms of fruit are assigned different serving sizes. A typical fruit serving—three-quarters of a cup of juice; a small banana, apple, or orange; a half-cup of most canned or fresh fruit; or a quarter-cup of dried fruit—contains an average of about 15 grams of carbohydrate, mostly as sugars, including the fruit sugar fructose. Fruits vary greatly in their water and fiber contents, and therefore their sugar concentrations vary also. With the exception of avocado, which is high in fat, fruits contain insignificant amounts of fat and protein.

MILK, CHEESE, AND YOGURT

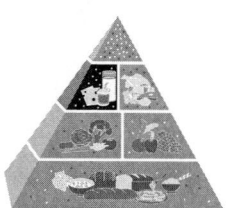

A serving (a cup) of milk or yogurt is a generous contributor of carbohydrate, donating about 12 grams. Among cheeses, cottage cheese provides about 6 grams of carbohydrate per cup, while most other types contain little if any carbohydrate. These foods also contribute high-quality protein (a point in their favor), as well as several important vitamins and minerals. All milk products vary in fat content, an important consideration in choosing among them; Chapter 5 provides the details.

Cream and butter, although dairy products, are not equivalent with milk because they contain little or no carbohydrate and insignificant amounts of the other nutrients important in milk. They are appropriately placed with the fats at the top of the pyramid.

MEAT, POULTRY, FISH, DRY BEANS, EGGS, AND NUTS

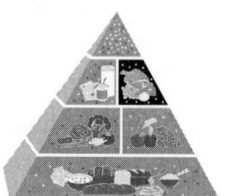

With two exceptions, foods of this group provide almost no carbohydrate to the diet. The exceptions are nuts, which provide a little starch and fiber along with their abundant fat, and dry beans, revered by diet-watchers as low-fat sources of both starch and fiber. Just a half-cup serving of beans provides 15 grams of carbohydrate, an amount equaling the richest sources in the Food

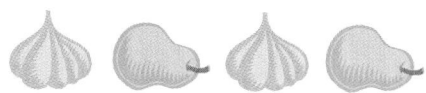

Guide Pyramid. Among providers of fiber, they are peerless, totaling 8 grams in a half cup.

FATS, OILS, AND SWEETS

Fats are devoid of carbohydrate, of course, but since sweets supply carbohydrate, it is useful to account for them in the diet. Most people enjoy sweets and frequently include them in their diets, so it is useful, too, to learn something of the nature of these foods.

In the last half-decade, scientists have been arguing about what constitutes "sugar" and how to measure it in the diet. Some experts wish to abandon the idea of measuring the sugars in foods. They accurately point out that a sugar molecule arising in an orange by way of photosynthesis is indistinguishable in laboratory tests from one added at the jam factory to sweeten orange marmalade. How can we measure the **added sugars**, they ask, when we cannot separate them from the **naturally occurring sugars** in foods? Besides, they say, the body handles all the sugars in the same ways, whatever the source.

Nutritionists argue back that chemical structures of sugars are not at issue; the addition of a concentrated energy source reduces the nutrient density of the foods and this can affect the body adversely. Manufacturers measure sugar when they add it to food products, so laboratory tests are not needed to determine the amounts in foods.

Both sides of the argument have validity, and as the spat continues, some useful distinctions between sugars are emerging. A new term, **carbohydrate sweeteners,** shifts the focus from separating sugars by their chemical structures to including sweet sugars from all sources. It is clear that the carbohydrate sweeteners from beets, corn, grapes, honey, and sugar cane are alike. All arise naturally and, through processing, are purified of most or all of the original plant material—bees process honey, while machines process the other types.[43] Nutrition authorities discourage the liberal use of added sugars, but we consume dramatically more added sugar than people did a century ago when most forms of purified sugar were unknown. Today, our intakes of added sugars exceed recommendations and nutrition authorities recommend we use them more sparingly (see Controversy 4).

THE NATURE OF SUGAR

Each teaspoonful of any sweet can be assumed to supply about 20 calories and 4 grams of carbohydrate. You may not think of candy or molasses in terms of *teaspoons*, but we've done this to emphasize that all sugary items are like white sugar, in spite of many people's belief that some are different or "better." See Table 4-6, which defines sugar terms. For a person who uses ketchup liberally, it may help to remember that a tablespoon of it contains a teaspoon of sugar. And for the soft drink user, a 12-ounce can of sugar-sweetened cola contains about 8 or more teaspoons of sugar. Figure 4-10 shows that processed foods contain surprisingly large amounts of sugar.

added sugars sugars added to a food for any purpose, such as to add sweetness or bulk or to aid in browning (baked goods).

naturally occurring sugars sugars present as original constituents of the unaltered food, and not added, such as the sugars of fruit or milk.

carbohydrate sweeteners ingredients composed of carbohydrates that contain sugars used for sweetening food products, including glucose, fructose, corn syrup, concentrated grape juice, and other sweet carbohydrates.

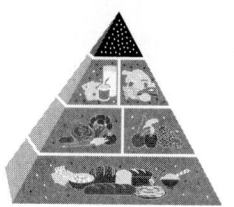

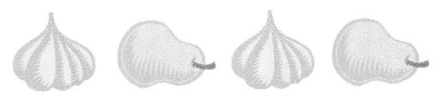

FIGURE 4-10

SUGAR IN PROCESSED FOODS

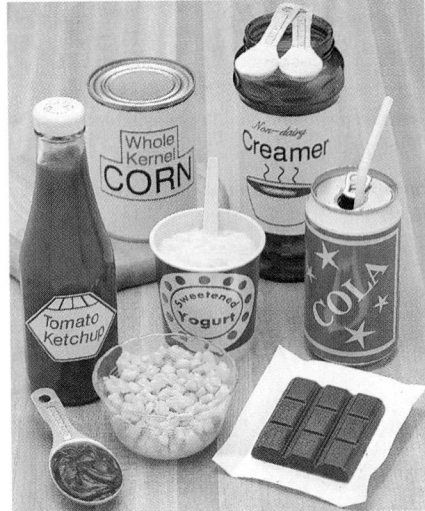

½ c canned corn = 3 tsp sugar[a]
12 oz cola = 8 tsp sugar
1 tbs ketchup = 1 tsp sugar
1 tbs creamer = 2 tsp sugar
8 oz sweetened yogurt = 7 tsp sugar
2 oz chocolate = 8 tsp sugar

[a]Values based on 1 tsp = 4 g.

Sugars on a Nutrition Facts panel of a food label reflect both added and naturally-occurring sugars in foods. Sugars listed among the ingredients are all added. Products listing sugars among the first few ingredients contain substantial amounts per serving.

What about the nutritional value of a product such as molasses or honey compared to white sugar? Molasses contains more than 3 milligrams of iron per tablespoon and so if used frequently can contribute some of this important nutrient. Molasses is less sweet than the other sweeteners, however, so it takes more molasses to provide the same sweetness as sugar. Also, the iron comes from the iron machinery in which the molasses is made and is in the form of an iron salt not easily absorbed by the body. And honey is no better for health than other sugars by virtue of being "natural." As a matter of fact, honey is chemically almost indistinguishable from sucrose. Honey contains the two

TABLE 4-6

Terms That Describe Sugar

Note: The term *sugars* here refers to all of the monosaccharides and disaccharides. On a label's ingredient list, the term *sugar* means sucrose. See Controversy 4 for terms concerning *artificial sweeteners* and *sugar alcohols*.

- **brown sugar** white sugar with molasses added, 95% pure sucrose.
- **concentrated fruit juice sweetener** a concentrated sugar syrup made from dehydrated, deflavored fruit juice, commonly grape juice; used to sweeten products that can then claim to be "all fruit."
- **confectioner's sugar** finely powdered sucrose, 99.9% pure.
- **corn sweeteners** corn syrup and sugar solutions derived from corn.
- **corn syrup** a syrup, mostly glucose, partly maltose, produced by the action of enzymes on cornstarch. *High-fructose corn syrup (HFCS)* is mostly fructose; glucose (dextrose) and maltose make up the balance.
- **dextrose** an older name for glucose.
- **fructose, galactose, glucose** the monosaccharides.
- **granulated sugar** common table sugar, crystalline sucrose, 99.9% pure.
- **honey** a concentrated solution primarily composed of glucose and fructose produced by enzymatic digestion of the sucrose in nectar by bees.
- **invert sugar** a mixture of glucose and fructose formed by the splitting of sucrose in an industrial process. Sold only in liquid form and sweeter than sucrose, invert sugar forms during certain cooking procedures and works to prevent crystallization of sucrose in soft candies and sweets.
- **lactose, maltose, sucrose** the disaccharides.
- **levulose** an older name for fructose.
- **maple sugar** a concentrated solution of sucrose derived from the sap of the sugar maple tree, mostly sucrose. This sugar was once common but is now usually replaced by sucrose and artificial maple flavoring.
- **molasses** a syrup left over from the refining of sucrose from sugar cane; a thick, brown syrup. The major nutrient in molasses is iron, a contaminant from the machinery used in processing it.
- **raw sugar** the first crop of crystals harvested during sugar processing. Raw sugar cannot be sold in the United States because it contains too much filth (dirt, insect fragments, and the like). Sugar sold as "raw sugar" domestically is not actually raw but has gone through more than half of the refining steps.
- **turbinado** (ter-bih-NOD-oh) **sugar** raw sugar from which the filth has been washed; legal to sell in the United States.
- **white sugar** pure sucrose, produced by dissolving, concentrating, and recrystallizing raw sugar.

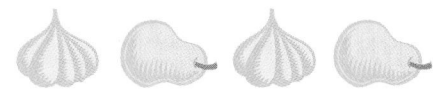

TABLE 4-7

The Empty Calories of Sugar

At first glance, honey, jelly, and brown sugar look more nutritious than plain sugar, but when compared with a person's nutrient needs, none contributes anything to speak of. The cola beverage is clearly an empty-calorie item, too.

Food	Energy (cal)	Protein (g)	Fiber (g)	Calcium (mg)	Iron (mg)	Magnesium (mg)	Potassium (mg)	Zinc (mg)	Vitamin A (re)	Thiamin (mg)	Riboflavin (mg)	Niacin (mg)	Vitamin B$_6$ (mg)	Folate (μg)	Vitamin C (mg)
Sugar (1 tbs)	45	0	0	0	0.0	0	0	0.0	0	0	0	0.0	0	0	0
Honey (1 tbs)	64	0	0	1	0.1	0	11	0.0	0	0	0	0.0	0	<1	0
Molasses (1 tbs)	55	0	0	42	1.0	50	300	0.1	0	0	0	0.2	0	0	0
Jelly (1 tbs)	49	0	0	1	0.0	1	12	0.0	0	0	0	0.0	0	0	<1
Brown sugar (1 tbs)	34	0	0	8	0.2	3	31	0.0	0	0	0	0.0	0	0	0
Cola beverage (12 fl oz)	152	0	0	11	0.1	4	4	0.1	0	0	0	0.0	0	0	0
Daily Values	2,000	56	25	1,000	18.0	400	3,500	15.0	1,000	1.5	1.7	20.0	2.0	400	60

monosaccharides glucose and fructose in approximately equal amounts. Sucrose contains the same monosaccharides but joined together in the disaccharide form. Spoon for spoon, however, sugar contains fewer calories than honey because the dry crystals of sugar take up more space than the sugars of honey dissolved in its water. No form of sugar is "more healthy" than white sugar, as Table 4-7 shows.

It would be absurd to rely on any sugar for nutrient contributions. A tablespoon of honey (64 calories) does offer 0.1 milligram of iron, but an adult would need to eat 150 tablespoons of honey a day—9,600 calories—to obtain the needed 15 milligrams of iron. The nutrients of honey just don't add up as fast as its calories. Thus if you choose molasses, brown sugar, or honey, choose them not for their nutrient contributions but for the pleasure they give. These tricks can help magnify the sweetness of foods without boosting their calories:

Sugar alcohols, discussed in the Controversy section, help protect against tooth decay.

- Serve sweet food warm (heat enhances sweet tastes).
- Add sweet spices such as cinnamon, nutmeg, allspice, or clove.
- Add a tiny pinch of salt; it will make food taste sweeter.
- Try reducing the sugar added to recipes by one-third.
- Select fresh fruits or fruit juice, or those prepared without added sugar.
- Use small amounts of sugar substitutes in place of sucrose.
- Read food labels for clues on sugar content.

Finally, enjoy whatever sugar you do eat. Sweetness is one of life's great sensations, and you need not forgo it completely. The person who cares about nutrition and loves sweets can artfully combine the two by using moderate amounts of sugar with creative imagination to enhance the flavors of nutritious foods.

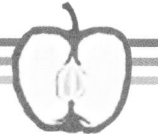

Do It!

INVESTIGATE YOUR FIBER INTAKE

This activity guides you in estimating the grams of the fiber in your diet and helps you to recognize the fiber in the foods of the Food Guide Pyramid.

PREPARING YOUR FOOD AND FIBER RECORD

Step 1. List on a copy of Form 4-1 all the foods you ate and beverages you drank in one day. Take care to record portion sizes accurately. It makes a big difference whether you ate a half or quarter of a cup of beans, berries, or any other foods. If you need guidance in doing this, reread the section called *Preparing Your Food Record* on page 61 of Chapter 2.

Step 2. List the fiber grams in each of the foods. Fiber values for many common foods are listed in Figure 4-11; look there first for convenience. The fiber values of other foods can be found in Appendix A.

Step 3. Add the numbers in the vertical columns to obtain subtotals of fiber; then add the subtotals across to obtain your grand total fiber intake for the day.

ANALYSIS

Answer the following questions:

1. Did your fiber total meet the recommended minimum 25 grams? Did it approach or exceed the maximum value of 40 grams?
2. Do you think your intake was too low, just right, or too high? Why do you think so?
3. Did your diet meet the minimum number of servings of foods from each fiber-containing group? One of the reasons the Food Guide Pyramid recommends a minimum of 3 servings of vegetables, 2 of fruit, and 6 of grains is to meet fiber needs.
4. Which fiber-containing groups fell short of the recommended intake?
5. Which specific foods provided the most fiber to the day's meals? Which provided the least? Identify trends in your food choices that would affect your fiber intakes. For example, if you consistently choose whole grains, your fiber intake benefits.

6. What alterations might you make among your vegetable, fruit, meat and alternates, or grain choices to increase the fiber in your meals?
7. Looking at the foods listed in Figure 4-11, how do juices differ from whole foods with regard to fiber? Turn to Appendix A and look up some of the energy values for whole vegetables and fruits and their juices. If a person consistently chooses juices over whole foods, how does this choice affect the diet's fiber and calorie values?
8. Among the juices listed in Figure 4-11, is any relatively rich in fiber? What type of fiber do you think juices might contain? (Hint: The main constituent of juice is water.)
9. What contributions do meats or milk products make to the day's fiber total? What advice about fiber would you give to someone who emphasizes meat and milk products at each meal? Hint: A quick way to direct someone to the fiber in foods is to guide them to the *bottom half* of the Food Guide Pyramid, which accounts for 11 of the 15 food servings recommended for a day.
10. Did your meals include fiber-rich bean dishes, such as chili, bean burritos, beans in a salad, or split pea soup? How many grams of fiber did those foods contribute to the total? Look up the fiber contents of a few legumes in Figure 4-11 or in Appendix A. Anyone interested in obtaining fiber should find ways to eat some legumes each day.

Constructed mostly of refined foods and meats and lacking in plant-derived foods, the average U.S. diet supplies just half the amount of fiber recommended and does a disservice to the health of the eater.[44] Does this mean that you should never consume low-fiber foods such as white rolls, white rice, meats, potato chips, or apple juice? No, but such foods should be included in moderation among abundant fruit, vegetables, legumes, and whole grains. Constructed from a variety of whole foods, the diet can easily meet the recommended 25 or more grams of dietary fiber daily.

FORM 4-1

Food and Fiber Record

Instructions: In the left-hand column, list the foods and amounts that you ate. Then list the grams of fiber in the food in the appropriate column to the right. For example, for a piece of wheat toast eaten at breakfast, list 2 grams of fiber in the Breads, Cereals, Rice, and Pasta column. For a glass of milk, list zero grams in the Milk, Yogurt, and Cheese column.

FOOD/AMOUNT	Breads, Cereals, Rice and Pasta	Vegetables	Fruit	Milk, Yogurt and Cheese	Poultry, Fish, Dry Beans, Eggs and Nuts
Breakfast:					
Snack:					
Lunch:					
Supper:					
Snack:					
Your subtotals:					

Suggested minimum fiber intake: 25g

Your Grand Total: _____ g

(continued on next page)

FIGURE 4-11

FINDING THE FIBER IN FOODS

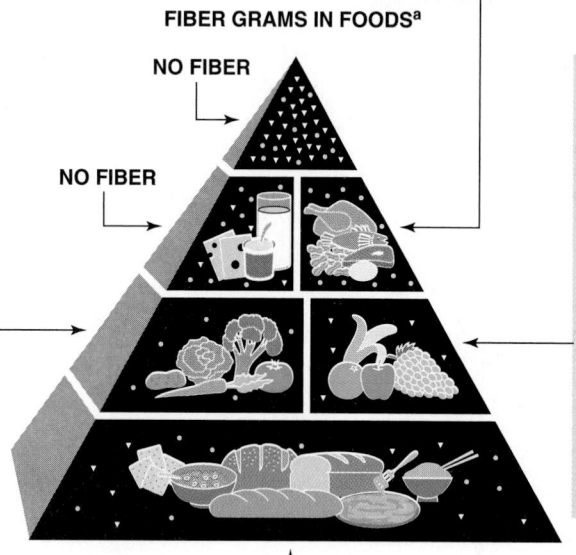

FIBER GRAMS IN FOODS[a]

Meat, Poultry, Fish, Dry Beans, Eggs, and Nuts Group

Food	Fiber g
Dried beans, 1/2 c	8
Lentils or peas, 1/2 c	5
Nuts, 1/4 c	2
Peanut butter, 2 tbs	2

Vegetable Group

Food	Fiber g
Baked potato with skin, 1	3
Brussels sprouts, 1/2 c	3
Carrot juice, 3/4 c	2
Broccoli, 1/2 c	2
Asparagus, 1/2 c	2
Corn, 1/2 c	2
Eggplant, 1/2 c	2
Green beans, 1/2 c	2
Spinach, 1/2 c	2
Baked potato, no skin, 1	2
Cauliflower, 1/2 c	2
Carrots, 1/2 c	2
Cabbage, 1/2 c	2
Onions, 1/2 c	1
Tomato, raw, 1 medium	1
Celery, 1/2 c	1
Lettuce, raw, 1 c	1
Bell peppers, 1/2 c	1
Dill pickle, 1 whole	1
Tomato juice, canned, 3/4 c	1

NO FIBER

NO FIBER

Fruit Group

Food	Fiber g
Prunes, cooked, 1/4 c	4
Pear, raw, 1 medium	4
Apple/orange, raw, 1 medium	3
Blackberries/raspberries, raw, 1/2 c	3
Apricots, raw, 3 each	2
Banana, raw, 1	2
Other berries, raw, 1/2 c	2
Peach, raw, 1 medium	2
Fruit cocktail, canned, 1/2 c	2
Raisins, dry, 1/4 c	1
Cantaloupe, raw, 1/2 c	1
Cherries, raw, 1/2 c	1
Apple juice, 3/4 c	<1
Orange juice, 3/4 c	<1

Breads, Cereals, Rice, and Pasta Group

Food	Fiber g
100% bran cereal, 1 oz	8
Barley, 1/2 c	7
Muffin, bran, 1	4
Wheat flakes, 1 oz	3
Shredded wheat, 1 large biscuit	2
Oatmeal, 1/2 c	2
Puffed wheat, 1 1/2 c	2
Whole-wheat bread, 1 slice	2
Light rye bread, 1 slice	2
Pumpernickel bread, 1 slice	2
Popcorn, 2 c	2
Brown rice, 1/2 c	2
Cheerios, 1 oz	2
Corn flakes, 1 oz	1
Pasta,[b] 1/2 c	1
Muffin, blueberry, 1	1
White rice, 1/2 c	<1
White bread, 1 slice	<1

[a]All values are for ready-to-eat or cooked foods, unless otherwise noted. Fruit values include edible skins. All values are rounded values.
[b]Pasta includes spaghetti noodles, lasagna noodles, and other noodles.

✔ SELF-CHECK

Answers to these Self-Check questions are in Appendix G.

1. The dietary monosaccharides include:
   a. sucrose, fructose, and glucose
   b. glucose, fructose, and galactose
   c. lactose, maltose, and glucose
   d. glycogen, starch, and fiber

2. The primary form of stored glucose in plants is:
   a. galactose
   b. glycogen
   c. cellulose
   d. starch

3. The polysaccharide that helps form the supporting structures of plants is:
   a. cellulose
   b. maltose
   c. glycogen
   d. sucrose

4. Digestible carbohydrates are absorbed as _____ through the small intestinal wall and are delivered to the liver where they are all converted to _____.
   a. disaccharides; sucrose
   b. glucose; glycogen
   c. monosaccharides; glucose
   d. galactose; cellulose

5. When blood glucose concentrations rise, the pancreas secretes _____, and when blood glucose levels fall, the pancreas secretes _____.
   a. glycogen; insulin
   b. insulin; glucagon
   c. glucagon; glycogen
   d. insulin; fructose

6. When the body uses fat for fuel without the help of carbohydrate, this results in the production of:
   a. ketones
   b. glucose
   c. starch
   d. galactose

7. In the body, the liver and muscles may store glucose as the polysaccharide glycogen.   T   F

8. The body converts excesses of glucose into glycogen or fat.   T   F

9. Type II diabetes is characterized by insulin resistance of the body's cells.   T   F

10. Type I diabetes is most often controlled by successful weight-loss and maintenance.   T   F

11. Around the world, most people are lactose intolerant.   T   F

12. By law, enriched white bread must equal whole-grain bread in nutrient content.   T   F

13. The fiber-rich portion of the wheat kernel is the bran layer.   T   F

14. The prevention of constipation and a lowered risk of colon cancer are achieved by eating a diet high in fructose.   T   F

15. Using artificial sweeteners has been proven to help people lose weight. (Read about this in the upcoming Controversy.)   T   F

NOTES

Notes are in Appendix F.

Sugar and Alternative Sweeteners: Are They "Bad" for You?

For every person in the United States today, 174 pounds of sugar disappear from the marketplace annually. In 1860, that amount was less than 20 pounds per year. *Disappearance* means that the sugar (all carbohydrate sweeteners) was available for use, but not that it was used. Much sugar is purchased but not eaten: the sugar of fruit packed in syrup, in the brine of sweet pickles, in jam that spoils and is thrown away, and sugar added pet and livestock feed. In 1995, U.S. consumers used up about 3 percent more added sugar than in the year before, a part of an upward trend of several years' duration.[1]

Another way of looking at sugar use is to estimate the amount of sugar a typical consumer actually eats in a year.[2] Currently, each man, woman, and child is estimated to consume an average of about 50 pounds per year, or about one pound per week.

In the past few years, U.S. sugar consumption has increased.[3] At the same time, overall calorie intakes have gone up dramatically, which may reflect people's consumption of more reduced-fat foods. Many new low-fat foods contain much more sugar than their full-fat counterparts, and the same number of calories, too.

Another recent trend is a steady rise in the consumption of artificial sweeteners. It seems that instead of substituting artificial sweeteners for sugar, people chose to consume both.

Do sugars harm people's health? And if they do, are sugar substitutes a better choice? This Controversy addresses these questions and, in the process, demonstrates how nutrition researchers pursue their answers, step by step, via scientific inquiry.

EVIDENCE CONCERNING SUGAR

Sugar is accused by some of causing nutrition problems. It is said to (1) promote and maintain obesity, (2) cause and aggravate diabetes, (3) increase the risk of heart disease, (4) disrupt behavior in children and adults, and (5)

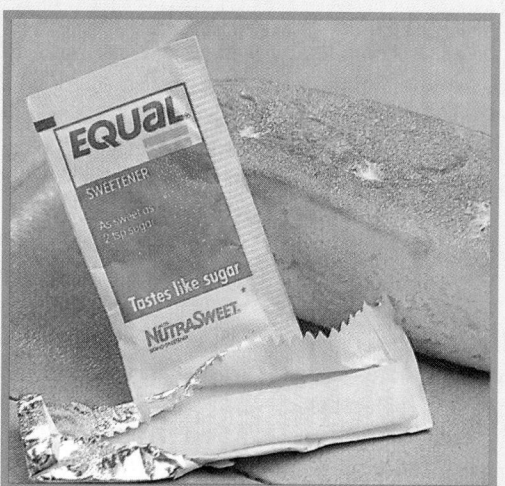

cause dental decay and gum disease. Is it guilty or innocent of these charges?

Obesity Does sugar cause obesity? The evidence suggests that this is unlikely. For example, rats fed a sucrose-rich diet did not become fatter, but their fat distribution changed. The diet high in sucrose seemed to cause deposits of more belly fat than did a diet of regular rat chow. This change might be significant if it held true for people because central obesity is associated with human heart disease. So far, evidence for the effect is lacking.

More direct evidence on obesity in people comes from population studies. In many countries incidence of obesity increases as sugar consumption rises. But this evidence does not all point to sugar as the sole cause. Wherever sugar intake increases, fat and total calorie intakes also rise. Simultaneously, physical activity declines. On the other hand, obesity also occurs where sugar intakes are low, and obese people in many instances eat less sugar than thin people do.[4] Fat is more calorie dense than sugar and often occurs together with sugar in sweet treats and snacks. Studies of populations by themselves cannot separate the effects of eating sugar from those of eating too much fat or of exercising too little.

Concentrated sweets do make it easy for people to consume large amounts of calories quickly, however, and that is why most diet plans recommend avoiding them. Some people believe that eating even small amounts of sugar triggers binges; for them, conscientious sugar avoidance is an important part of weight-loss dieting. For others the inclusion of small amounts of sugar in a weight-loss plan makes the plan easier to follow. In short, the effects of sugar on a person's eating style and body weight depend on the user.

Diabetes Does sugar cause or contribute to Type II diabetes? Recall from the chapter that in diabetes, insulin secretion or tissue responsiveness to it becomes abnormal. This, of course, affects the body's ability to manage sugar. At one time people thought that eating sugar caused diabetes by "overstraining the pancreas," but now we know that this is not the case. Body fatness is more closely related to diabetes than diet is. High rates of diabetes have not been reported in any society where obesity is rare. Still, it can be asked whether people with the genetic tendency to develop this type of diabetes should avoid eating sugar. The evidence on this point is conflicting and interesting.

In populations around the world, a profound increase, by as much as tenfold, in the incidence of diabetes has occurred simultaneously with an increase in sugar consumption. This has been true for the Japanese, Israelis, Africans, Native Americans, Eskimos, Polynesians, and Micronesians. Yet in other populations, no relationship has been found between sugar intake and diabetes. Wherever starch, rather than sugar, is the major carbohydrate in the diet, diabetes is rare. But this does not prove that sugar causes diabetes or that starch prevents it. The apparent protective effect of starch might be due, for example, to the chromium or fiber that comes with it. Sugar is not thought to raise blood glucose levels any more than do starches.[5] The fairest conclusion that can be drawn is that obesity is a major causal factor but that sugar may share in the guilt as a contributor to the obesity that accompanies Type II diabetes.

Once a person has diabetes, is it all right to use moderate amounts of sugar? Most authorities agree that, as part of the carbohydrate in a controlled diet, an amount of sucrose equaling 5 to 10 percent of total calories consumed is acceptable.[6] *Other* body responses must also be considered, however, among them raised blood lipids, which suggest a high risk of heart disease (discussed next).

Heart Disease   Does eating sugar increase the risk of heart disease? Again, a research study using rats provides some clues. When researchers fed rats a diet with sucrose as the only carbohydrate source, the rats sustained microscopic damage to their arteries, and their blood tested high for both triglycerides and cholesterol.[7] Rats fed starch instead of sugar did not develop the damage or the elevated blood lipids. Keep in mind that the rats consumed sucrose as their only source of carbohydrate; even people with a highly unusual craving for sweets wouldn't choose to live on such a diet. Among human beings, most studies show a similar result—that is, in response to diets high in sucrose and fructose, blood lipids associated with heart

disease rise, and those believed to be protective fall.[8] The diets evoking this response are almost twice the nation's average intake of added sugars, though; current intake levels are thought to be below the amount that may adversely affect blood lipids.[9] Still, the American Heart Association's *Dietary Guidelines* suggest choosing a diet moderate in sugar because high-sugar diets are often high in calories and low in fiber and nutrients.[10]

Saturated fat is clearly the major *dietary* culprit in the heart disease susceptibility of most people, but there is a *hereditary* culprit, too, and some people may have inherited the tendency to develop raised blood lipid levels in response to carbohydrate and alcohol. If their heart disease risk is assessed as high, they are told to restrict their intakes of carbohydrate and alcohol.

Experiments implicating sugar in heart and artery disease have used diets so high in sugar that the results may not reflect the effects of people's real sugar intakes. No one has shown conclusively, throughout many years of research, that moderate amounts of sugar (10 percent of total calories) affect the disease process in healthy human beings.

Behavior   What about sugar and behavior? In the 1970s and 1980s, claims appeared that eating sugary foods caused children to become unruly and adolescents and adults to exhibit antisocial and even criminal behavior. Sugar was labeled a toxin and an addictive drug. The brain is dependent on blood glucose for its energy, and some proponents of the sugar-behavior idea believe that eating sucrose causes wide fluctuations in blood glucose levels, leading to frequent hypoglycemia and irrational and violent behavior. A criminal defense was even won on the argument that the defendant was not responsible for his actions because he was in the habit of eating high-sugar "junk food," notably Twinkies, and had thereby become hypoglycemic.

A decade of research following those years yielded only mixed or negative results. While most experts agree that the "sugar-behavior" theory has been put to rest, many teachers, parents, grandparents, and others still believe that the children they know react behaviorally to sugar.

In the 1990s, research has once again become active on the idea that sugar may somehow influence behavior. There are many ways in which it might do so: by altering the levels of chemicals in the brain that affect mood, by inducing nutrient deficiencies, and others. One group of researchers studying children propose that behavior changes may be brought about by the series of hormones the body releases after consuming sugar.[11] It is known that blood glucose is regulated not by diet but by hormones, and one of those is the stress hormone, norepinephrine.

The researchers fed a syrupy beverage to 9 adults and 14 children and then tested their blood norepinephrine levels three hours later, after insulin had had time to store the sugar. The blood *sugar* levels of both groups had dropped only slightly, but the blood *norepinephrine* was elevated. In the children it had shot up to double the level seen in the adults. The children also complained of symptoms such as weakness and nervousness during the test period. While it is tempting to declare as proven the idea that sugar elevates blood norepinephrine levels in children and that this leads to behavior changes, many more studies are needed before the theory can be confirmed as fact.

Another way sugar has been theorized to affect behavior is by providing energy. In a study of 13 children hospitalized for psychiatric disorders, researchers gave the children either plain orange juice or orange juice sweetened with sucrose or fructose. The children given the sugar-added drinks became more active and exhibited more inappropriate behavior than the children who had received the plain drinks. The researchers concluded that the added calories from sugar permitted the children to exert more energy (the so-called Halloween effect); they did not suggest that sugar, specifically, had a negative effect on behavior.

Another group of researchers set out to discover whether children diagnosed as hyperactive became more aggressive or less attentive after eating sugar.[12] These researchers tested sugar and two noncaloric sweeteners. When 17 children with hyperactivity and 9 children without the disorder were given a high-sugar breakfast, neither group behaved more aggressively. The children with hyperactivity, however, became more distractible (paid less attention) than usual after the sugary breakfast. This effect was not seen after a breakfast sweetened with aspartame or saccharin. Perhaps some children with hyperactivity are especially sensitive to sugar's effects.

Several well-controlled studies have shown that sugar calms normal children, a finding consistent with convincing biochemical evidence. One such study showed no differences in activity, social interactions, learning performance, or mood in children given artificial sweeteners, but found that sugar made the children less active.[13] In other studies, sugar has calmed juvenile delinquents with pronounced behavioral problems.[14]

Overwhelmingly, studies have failed to demonstrate any consistent effects of sucrose on behavior in either normal or hyperactive children.[15] In conclusion, occasional behavioral reactions to sugar may be possible, but until research proves otherwise, the idea that sugar alone directly affects behavior adversely in most healthy children or adults remains all but ruled out.

DENTAL CARIES

Does sugar cause **dental caries?** Caries are a serious public health problem. They afflict nearly everyone in the country, half by the time they are two years old. (A very lucky few *never* get caries because they have inherited resistance to them.) One of the most successful measures taken to reduce the incidence of dental decay is fluoridation of community water. But sugar has something to do with dental caries, too.

Caries develop as acids produced by bacterial growth in the mouth eat into tooth enamel. Bacteria establish colonies known as **plaque** whenever they can get a foothold on tooth surfaces. Once established, they multiply and affix themselves more and more firmly unless they are brushed, flossed, or scraped away. Eventually, the acid of plaque creates pits that deepen into cavities. Below the gum line, plaque works its way down until the acid erodes the roots of teeth and jawbone in which they are embedded, loosening the teeth and leading to infections of the gums. Gum disease severe enough to threaten tooth loss afflicts the majority of our population by their later years. Flossing every 24 hours greatly reduces this risk. Table C4-1 defines some terms related to caries.

Bacteria thrive on carbohydrate. Carbohydrate as sugar has been named as the main causative factor in forming cavities.[16] However, starch also supports bacterial growth if the bacteria are allowed sufficient time to work on it. Of prime importance is the length of time the food stays in the mouth, and this depends on the food's composition, how sticky it is, how often you eat

TABLE C4-1
Dental Terms

- **dental caries** decay of the teeth (*caries* means "rottenness").
- **plaque** (PLACK) a mass of microorganisms and their deposits on the crowns and roots of the teeth, a forerunner of dental caries and gum disease. (The term *plaque* is used in another connection—arterial plaque in atherosclerosis. See Chapter 11.)

it, and especially on whether you brush your teeth afterward.[17]

Bacteria produce acid for 20 to 30 minutes after exposure to sugar. Thus, if you were to eat three pieces of candy, one right after the other, your teeth would be exposed to approximately 30 minutes of acid demineralization. Should you eat the candy pieces at half-hour intervals, though, the acid exposure time would be 90 minutes. Likewise, slowly sipping a sugary soft drink may be more harmful than drinking quickly and emptying the mouth of sugar.

Some forms of candy, such as milk chocolate and caramels, may be less harmful than once believed because the sugar dissolves completely and is washed away in saliva. Particles from breads, granola bars, sugary cereals, oatmeal cookies, raisins, salted crackers, and chips, on the other hand, may be worse than once thought, because they get stuck in the teeth and do not dissolve. These particles may remain in contact with tooth surfaces for hours, providing a feast for bacteria and greatly increasing the likelihood of caries.[18] A table in Chapter 13 lists foods of both high and low caries potential. The punchline seems to be: Brush your teeth after eating.

Total sugar intakes still play a major role in caries incidence, though, and populations with diets of more than 10 percent of calories from sugar are demonstrated to have an unacceptably high incidence of dental caries.[19] Worldwide, many governing agencies urge their citizens to consume no more than 10 percent of calories from sugar because of sugar's link with dental caries. It is clear that sugar is an energy source for the bacteria that cause tooth decay and that when exposure is sufficient in susceptible people, sugar is guilty as charged.[20]

PERSONAL STRATEGY FOR USING SUGAR

Controversy about sugar is health effects has all but resolved in the minds of scientists.[21] Meanwhile, consumers wonder whether they should avoid sugar or reduce their intakes. The *Dietary Guidelines* suggest only that people "use moderation" concerning sugar, not that they avoid it altogether. The World Health Organization's recommendations are more specific and recommend that sugar should not contribute more than 10 percent of a person's total calorie intake.[22] A person who eats 2,000 calories of energy a day, then, is allowed 200 calories from sugar. Those 200 calories of sugar, 10 teaspoons or so, sound like quite a lot. But

when you add up all the sugar teaspoons present in common foods, 200 calories' worth may start to seem restrictive. The U.S. average sugar intake is 18 percent of calories.

One way that people may attempt to limit their sugar intakes is by using artificial sweeteners or sugar substitutes. These do provide sweetness without sucrose, but people are curious about their safety.

People who wish to avoid sugar may choose from two sets of alternative sweeteners. One set is the sugar alcohols, which are energy-yielding sweeteners sometimes referred to as nutritive sweeteners. The other is the artificial sweeteners, which provide virtually no energy and are thus sometimes referred to as nonnutritive sweeteners.

EVIDENCE CONCERNING SUGAR ALCOHOLS

The sugar alcohols are familiar to people who use special dietary products. Many new low-calorie food products appearing on grocery shelves depend on sugar alcohols for their bulking and sweetening powers.[23] Among the sugar alcohols are **mannitol, sorbitol, xylitol,** and **maltitol.** All the sugar alcohols can be metabolized by human beings, and generally speaking, they provide about as much energy as sucrose (3–4 calories per gram).

A proven benefit of sugar alcohols is that ordinary mouth bacteria metabolize them less rapidly than other carbohydrates. As a result, sugar alcohols do not contribute as much to dental caries.

Mannitol is the least satisfactory of the sugar alcohols just named. It is less sweet than sucrose, so large amounts have to be used to obtain the same sweetness (see Table C4-2). It lingers unabsorbed in the intestine for a long time, available to intestinal bacteria for their energy. As they consume the mannitol, the bacteria multiply, attract water, produce irritating waste, and cause diarrhea.

More practical than mannitol, sorbitol sweetens sugar-free gums and candies, but it, too, has drawbacks. At least two teaspoons as much sorbitol (with twice the calories) must be used to deliver the sweetness of one teaspoon of sucrose. Also, like mannitol, it can cause diarrhea when consumed in large quantities.

Xylitol is popular, especially in chewing gums, thanks to reports that it helps to prevent dental caries. It not only doesn't support caries-producing bacteria, it may actually inhibit their production of acid and prevent them from adhering to the teeth.[24] Xylitol occurs naturally in many fruits and also arises in the body during normal metabolic processes. Most people can tolerate the small amounts present in food. In large amounts, xylitol slows down the emptying of the stomach but also stimulates release of a hormone (motilin) that speeds up intestinal activity and so causes diarrhea.[25]

Maltitol is used in some carbonated beverages and canned fruits, as well as in sweets that are said not to cause tooth decay. Maltitol may donate somewhat fewer calories, gram for gram, than sucrose to the body because it is poorly absorbed and because some of it may be lost in diarrhea. Maltitol is expensive to make, however, and costs limit its use.

The person who wishes to reduce energy intake should be aware that the sugar alcohols *do* provide energy. The body handles them differently from sugar, but they are not calorie-free.

EVIDENCE CONCERNING ARTIFICIAL SWEETENERS

Like the sugar alcohols, artificial sweeteners make foods taste sweet without promoting dental decay. Unlike sugar alcohols, they have the added attraction of being calorie-free. Also unlike sugar alcohols, the human taste buds perceive the artificial sweeteners as supersweet. But are they safe? All substances are toxic if high enough doses are consumed. Artificial sweeteners, their components, and metabolic by-products are not exceptions. The questions to ask are whether artificial sweeteners are harmful to human beings at levels normally used, and how much is too much. The Food and Drug Administration (FDA) has proposed answers by setting **acceptable daily intake (ADI)** levels for some of the artificial sweeteners used in the United States. Table C4-3 defines some sugar substitute terms. The big three synthetic sweeteners are **saccharin, acesulfame-K,** and **aspartame.**

Saccharin   Saccharin has had a rocky history of acceptance, although it is now consumed by millions of Americans primarily in prepared foods and beverages, secondarily as a tabletop sweetener. Questions about its safety surfaced in the late 1970s, when experiments suggested that it caused bladder tumors in rats. As a result, the FDA proposed banning it. The public outcry in favor of retaining it was so loud, however, that Congress placed a moratorium on any action, and the ban proposal was eventually withdrawn. At this writing, products containing saccharin still must carry the warning label familiar to all consumers of diet products: "Use of this product may be hazardous to your health. This product contains saccharin, which has been determined to cause cancer in laboratory animals."

Does saccharin cause cancer? The evidence that it does so in animals is as follows. Rats that had been fed diets containing saccharin from the time of weaning to adulthood were mated. The offspring of those rats were then fed saccharin throughout their lives and were found to have a higher incidence of bladder tumors than comparable animals not fed saccharin. In Canada, on the basis of these findings, all uses of saccharin were banned except use as a tabletop sweetener to be sold in pharmacies with a warning label.

In human beings, a large-scale population study involving 9,000 people seemed to show a slightly elevated risk of cancers in women who drank two or more saccharin-sweetened diet sodas a day and in men and women who both smoked heavily and used artificial

TABLE C4-2
Sweetness of Sugar Substitutes

Sugar Substitute	Relative Sweetness[a]
Sugars	
Sucrose	1.0
Fructose	1.7
Sugar Alcohols	
Sorbitol	0.5
Mannitol	0.7
Maltitol	0.9
Xylitol	1.0
Noncaloric Sweeteners	
Acesulfame-K	200.0
Cyclamate	45.0
Aspartame	200.0
Saccharin	300.0
Sucralose	600.0
Alitame	2,000.0

[a] The relative sweetness depends on the temperature, acidity, and other flavors of the foods in which the substance occurs. The sweetness of pure sucrose is the standard with which the approximate sweetness of sugar substitutes is compared.

SOURCES: Data from W. L. Dills, Sugar alcohols as bulk sweeteners, *Annual Review of Nutrition* (1989): 161–186, S. A. Schlicker and C. Regan, Innovations in calorie-reduced foods: A review of fat and sugar replacement technologies. *Topics in Clinical Nutrition,* November 1990, pp. 50–60; V. M. Sardesai and T. H. Waldsham, Natural and synthetic intense sweeteners, *Journal of Nutritional Biochemistry* 2 (1991): 236–244.

TABLE C4-3

Sugar Substitute Terms

- **acceptable daily intake (ADI)** the estimated amount of sweetener that can be consumed daily over a person's lifetime without any adverse effects.
- **acesulfame** (AY-sul-fame) **potassium,** also called **acesulfame-K** a zero-calorie sweetener approved by the FDA and Health Canada.
- **alitame** a noncaloric sweetener formed from the amino acids L-aspartic acid and L-alanine. In the United States, the FDA is considering its approval.
- **aspartame** a compound of phenylalanine and aspartic acid that tastes like the sugar sucrose but is much sweeter. It is used in both the United States and Canada.
- **cyclamate** a zero-calorie sweetener under consideration for use in the United States and used with restrictions in Canada.
- **maltitol, mannitol, sorbitol, xylitol** sugar alcohols that can be derived from fruits or commercially produced from dextrose; absorbed more slowly and metabolized differently than other sugars in the human body and not readily used by ordinary mouth bacteria.
- **saccharin** a zero-calorie sweetener used freely in the United States but restricted in Canada.
- **sucralose** a noncaloric sweetener derived from a chlorinated form of sugar that travels through the digestive tract unabsorbed. Canada has approved the sweetener; in the United States, the FDA is considering its approval.

sweeteners. Other studies involving more than 5,000 people showed no excess risk of bladder cancers.[26]

A solid clue has emerged from the laboratory based on some physiological differences between the urinary systems of rats and human beings.[27] Rats excrete far less water in their urine than people do. As a result, rats can make highly concentrated solutions of substances in just small amounts of water in their urine. Dissolved substances in such high concentrations are likely to crystallize. In safety tests, saccharin overdoses caused crystals to form in the rats' bladders, and the crystals probably caused the tumors. Human beings cannot concentrate urinary substances to such a degree, so they would never form saccharin crystals, even if they consumed larger-than-normal doses of saccharin. They would, however, lose large amounts of water as the kidneys struggled to free the blood of the overload.

It goes without saying that overloading on huge saccharin doses is probably not safe, but consuming moderate amounts almost certainly does not cause bladder cancer in human beings. Although no ADI has been set for saccharin, the amount of saccharin that can be commercially added to foods or drinks is limited to about 30 milligrams per serving. The FDA also suggests that adults not exceed total daily saccharin intakes of 1,000 milligrams and that children not exceed 500 milligrams.[28]

Acesulfame-K   For 15 years of testing and use, the artificial sweetener 'acesulfame potassium' (or acesulfame-K) has been used without reported health problems. An ADI of 15 milligrams per kilogram of body weight was set for acesulfame-K on its approval. Marketed under the trade names Sunette and Sweet One, this sweetener is about as sweet as aspartame and is used in chewing gum, beverages, instant coffee and tea, gelatins, and puddings, as well as for table use. Acesulfame-K holds up well during cooking.

Acesulfame-K is 200 times as sweet as sucrose but leaves a slight aftertaste. Blending it with other sweeteners solves the problem. Acesulfame-K is not recognized by the body's metabolic equipment and therefore is excreted unchanged by the kidneys.

Aspartame   Aspartame is one of the most thoroughly studied substances ever to be approved for use in foods.[29] Within only a few years after aspartame received the FDA's approval, manufacturers began using it under the name *Nutrasweet* to sweeten dozens of products including diet drinks, candies, chewing gum, presweetened cereal, gelatins, baked goods and mixes, and pudding. Aspartame provides 4 calories per gram, as does protein, but because so little is needed, it is virtually calorie-free. Under the brand name *Equal*, aspartame is also available as a powder to use at home in place of sugar. In powdered form it is mixed with lactose, so a 1-gram packet contains 4 calories.

Aspartame's amazing popularity is mostly due to its flavor, which is almost identical to that of sugar. Another lure drawing people to aspartame is the hope that it may be completely harmless, unlike some other sweeteners, whose laboratory records seem tarnished. Furthermore, aspartame is touted as safe for children, so families wishing to limit their children's sugar intakes are offering them Nutrasweet products instead.

Aspartame is a simple chemical compound: two protein fragments (the amino acids phenylalanine and aspartic acid) joined together. In the digestive tract, the two fragments are split apart, absorbed, and metabolized just as they would be if they had come from protein in food. The flavors of the components give no clue to the combined effect; one of them tastes bitter, and the other is tasteless. But aspartame is 200 times sweeter than sucrose.

An inherited metabolic disease known as phenyl-ketonuria (PKU) poses problems with respect to aspartame. People with PKU have the hereditary inability to dispose of phenylalanine eaten in excess of the need for building proteins. Unusual products made from phenylalanine build up and damage the tissues. PKU causes irreversible, progressive brain damage if left untreated in early life. Newborns in the United States are tested for PKU; if they have it, the treatment is to limit dietary intake of phenylalanine.

For a compelling reason, children with PKU should not get their phenylalanine from aspartame. Phenylalanine occurs in such protein-rich and nutrient-rich foods as milk and meat, and the PKU child is allowed only a limited amount of these foods. The child has difficulty obtaining the many essential nutrients, such as calcium, iron, and the B vitamins, found along with phenylalanine in these foods. To suggest that such a child squander any of the limited phenylalanine allowance on the purified phenylalanine of aspartame, with none of the associated nutrients to support normal growth, would be to invite nutritional disaster. People with PKU need to know which products contain aspartame and how to avoid them. Product labels offer special warnings for people with PKU.

Other concerns about aspartame's safety have had to do with compounds that arise briefly during its metabolism. These compounds (methyl alcohol, formaldehyde, and diketopiperazine, or DKP) are not toxic at the levels generated, and concerns about them have been laid to rest.

An important safety concern is what effects, if any, aspartame might have on the brain. While no experimental evidence has shown a connection, some 5,500 individual complaints have been received by the Centers for Disease Control (CDC), many of which claim that aspartame gives people headaches.[30]

Every day, millions of people use aspartame. Every day, millions of people have headaches. Anyone who claims, on this basis, that aspartame causes headaches is using personal experience to jump to conclusions. In the case of sweeteners and headaches, only casual reports of a link, no true connections, have been shown. Some of the headache sufferers might indeed be reacting to the artificial sweetener, but they might also be reacting to another substance such as caffeine or to factors in their lives unrelated to foods.

Other complaints, about 250 in all, have linked aspartame intakes to seizures. People who experienced seizures reported to the FDA that they believed their seizures were related to ingesting aspartame. When the reports were scrutinized scientifically, though, the seizures were found to be unrelated to aspartame intake. The authors who analyzed the evidence suggested that the topic warranted no further research.[31]

On approving aspartame for U.S. consumers, the FDA assumed that no one would consume more than the ADI of 50 milligrams per kilogram of body weight in a day. In Canada, the acceptable level is set at 40 milligrams per kilogram.[32] These seem to be reasonable numbers. Most adults in the United States and other countries consume less than 10 milligrams per kilogram, significantly less than the ADI level. Still, the ADI amount is not impossible to exceed. For a 132-pound person, it adds up to 80 packets of Equal. About 15 soft drinks sweetened only with aspartame provide this maximum amount. A child who drinks a quart of Kool-Aid on a hot day and who also has pudding, chewing gum, cereal, and other products sweetened with aspartame can pack in more than the daily ADI limit. Infants or toddlers under two years old should probably not be fed artificially sweetened foods and drinks.

Other Artificial Sweeteners   Two other artificial sweeteners are awaiting FDA approval—**cyclamate** and **sucralose,** already approved in Canada, and **alitame.** Sucralose is a chlorinated form of sugar that travels through the digestive tract unabsorbed and therefore is noncaloric. Cyclamate was once approved but then banned in the United States when it was suspected, but never proved, to cause cancer in rats. In Canada, cyclamate is restricted to use as a tabletop sweetener on the advice of a physician and as a sweetening additive in medicines. Alitame resembles aspartame in being composed of two amino acids, but unlike aspartame it remains stable when heated.

Do Artificial Sweeteners Help with Weight Control?   Many people eat and drink products sweetened with artificial sweeteners in the belief that the products help control weight. Do they work? Ironically, studies of rats report that intense sweeteners, such as saccharin, stimulate appetite and lead to weight *gain* instead of loss.[33] Many studies on *people,* however, find either no change or a decline in feelings of hunger. Researchers conclude that most people's food intakes do not change much when they use artificial sweeteners.[34]

In studying the effects of artificial sweeteners on food intake and body weight, different researchers ask different questions and take different approaches in searching for the answers. It matters, for example, whether the people used in the study were of a healthy weight or obese and whether they were on weight-loss diets or not. Motivations for using sweeteners differ, too, and this influences a person's actions. For example, a person might drink a low-calorie beverage now so as to be able to eat a high-calorie food later. This person's energy intake might stay the same or increase. On the other hand, a person trying to control food energy intake might use the artificial sweetener and then choose low-calorie foods consistently. This person might achieve a lower-than-normal energy intake in this way.

Researchers must also distinguish between the effects of the experience of tasting something sweet and the physiological effects of a particular substance on the body. If a person experiences hunger or feels full shortly after eating an artificially sweetened snack, is that because tasting something sweet stimulates or depresses the appetite? Or is it because the artificial sweetener itself somehow affects the appetite through nervous, hormonal, or other means? Furthermore, if appetite is stimulated, does that actually lead to increased food intake?

One recent study was designed to answer questions concerning appetite and artificial sweeteners. Researchers fed normal-weight people one of four breakfasts and then measured their food intakes at later meals throughout the day.[35] Two of the breakfasts provided 700 calories: one contained sucrose, and the other aspartame with enough starch to equalize the calories. The other two breakfasts provided 300 calories: one was plain, and the other contained aspartame. Subjects who ate either lower-calorie breakfast, regardless of sweetness, were hungrier later. Those who ate either higher-calorie breakfast stayed fuller longer. Sweet taste and the presence of aspartame seemed to have no effect on hunger or subsequent food energy intakes. At the end of the day, both groups who had eaten the 700-calorie breakfasts had higher total energy intakes, because although they were less hungry at lunch, they still consumed ample food energy at lunch and supper.

Overall it seems that artificial sweeteners alone do not stimulate or depress appetite.[36] If the sweeteners have the effect of lowering calorie intakes, however, this may leave people hungry, so that they compensate at later meals. Whether a person overcompensates or partially or fully compensates for the reduction in energy intake depends on several factors, including the person's characteristics. Using artificial sweeteners will not automatically lower energy intake; to control energy intake successfully, a person will need to make informed diet and activity decisions throughout the day (as Chapter 9 explains).

Another sweetener, however, has shown a clear, strong ability to cut the appetite and to reduce food intake. That sweetener is sugar.[37] The common belief that sugar "spoils the appetite" has proved true.

PERSONAL STRATEGIES FOR USING ARTIFICIAL SWEETENERS

Current evidence indicates that moderate intakes of artificial sweeteners pose no health risks.[38] For those who choose to include artificial sweeteners in their diets, moderation is the key. When used in the context of a nutritious diet, artificial sweeteners are generally safe for consumption by healthy people.[39] While they are clearly not magic bullets in fighting overweight, they probably do not hinder weight-loss efforts, either, and they are safer for the teeth than carbohydrate sweeteners.

NOTES

Notes are in Appendix F.

THE LIPIDS: FATS, OILS, PHOSPHOLIPIDS, AND STEROLS

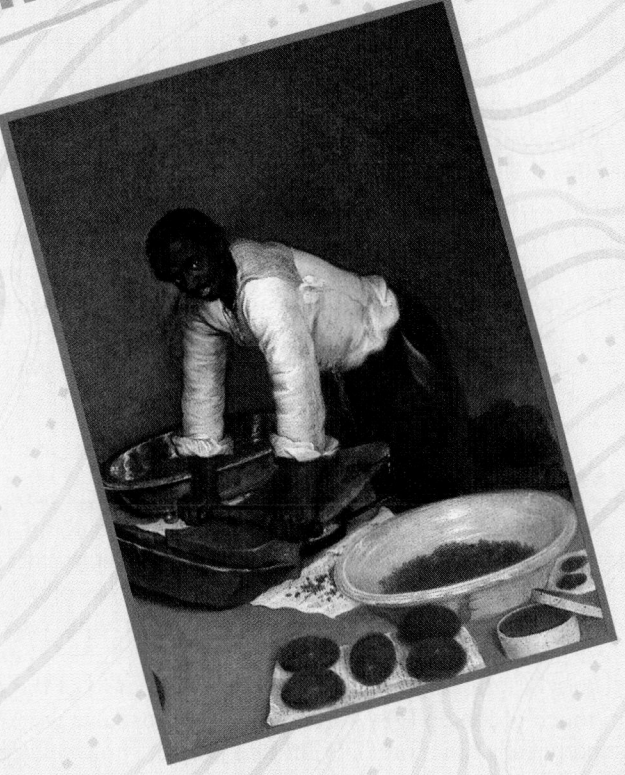

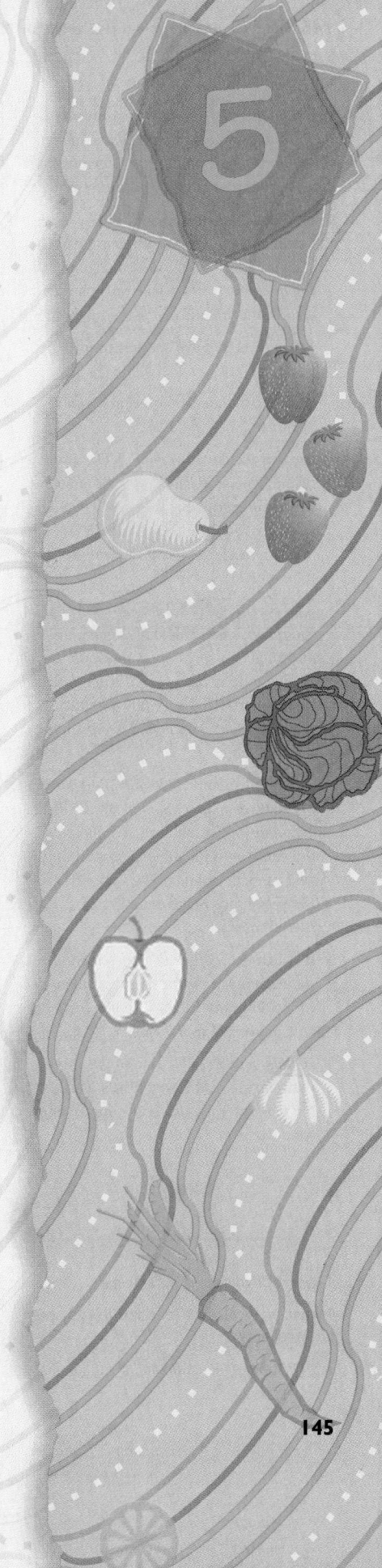

CONTENTS

Anonymous (Spanish, eighteenth century?), *A Man Scraping Chocolate*, c. 1680–1780, North Carolina Museum of Art, Raleigh, gift of Mr. and Mrs. Benjamin Cone.

lipid (LIP-id) a family of compounds soluble in organic solvents but not in water. Lipids include triglycerides (fats and oils), phospholipids, and sterols.

cholesterol (koh-LESS-ter-all) a member of the group of lipids known as sterols; a soft waxy substance made in the body for a variety of purposes and also found in animal-derived foods.

fats lipids that are solid at room temperature (70°F or 25°C).

oils lipids that are liquid at room temperature (70°F or 25°C).

cardiovascular disease (CVD) disease of the heart and blood vessels, also called *coronary heart disease (CHD)*. The two most common forms of CVD are atherosclerosis and hypertension (Chapter 11).

triglycerides (try-GLISS-er-ides) one of the three main classes of dietary lipids and the chief form of fat in foods. A triglyceride is made up of three units known as fatty acids and one unit called glycerol. (Fatty acids and glycerol are defined later.)

phospholipids (FOSS-foh-LIP-ids) one of the three main classes of dietary lipids. These lipids are similar to triglycerides, but each has a phosphorus-containing acid in place of one of the fatty acids. Phospholipids are present in all cell membranes.

lecithin (LESS-ih-thin) a phospholipid manufactured by the liver and also found in many foods; a major constituent of cell membranes.

sterols (STEER-alls) one of the three main classes of dietary lipids. Sterols have a structure similar to that of cholesterol.

1 g carbohydrate = 4 calories.

1 g fat = 9 calories (but see this chapter's Controversy).

1 g protein = 4 calories.

5 Your bill from a medical laboratory reads, "Blood **lipid** profile—$125." A health-care provider reports, "Your blood **cholesterol** is high." Your physician advises, "You must cut down on the **fats** and **oils** in your diet to lower your **cardiovascular disease (CVD)** risk." Blood lipids, cholesterol, fats, and oils—all contribute to health and detract from it.

INTRODUCTION TO THE LIPIDS

The lipids in foods and in the human body fall into three classes. About 95 percent are **triglycerides.** Other classes of the lipid family are the **phospholipids** (of which **lecithin** is one) and the **sterols** (cholesterol is the best known of these).

No doubt you have been expecting to hear that these fat-related compounds have the potential to harm your health. It may come as a surprise to hear that lipids are also valuable. In fact, lipids are absolutely necessary, and some lipids must be present in your foods if you are to maintain good health. Luckily, traces of fats and oils are present in almost all foods, so you needn't make an effort to eat any extra.

Usefulness of Fats

When people speak of fat, they are usually talking about triglycerides. The term *fat* is more familiar, though, and we will use it here. Fat is the body's chief storage form for the energy from food eaten in excess of need. The storage of fat is a valuable survival mechanism for people who must live a feast-or-famine existence: stored during times of plenty, it enables them to remain alive during times of famine. In addition, fats provide most of the energy needed to perform much of the body's work, especially muscular work.

Most body cells can store only limited fat, but some cells are specialized for storing fat. These, the fat cells, seem able to expand almost indefinitely. The more fat they store, the larger they grow. An obese person's fat cells may be many times the size of a thin person's. A fat cell is shown in Figure 5-1.

You may be wondering why the carbohydrate glucose is not the body's major form of stored energy. As mentioned in Chapter 4, glucose is stored in the form of glycogen. One characteristic of glycogen is that it holds a great deal of water, and as a result, it is quite bulky and heavy. The body cannot store enough glycogen to provide energy for very long. Fats, however, pack tightly together without water and can store much more energy in a small space.[1] The body fat found on a normal-weight, healthy person contains sufficient energy to fuel a marathon run to the finish or to give a sick person who cannot eat the energy to battle disease.

By the same token, foods rich in fat are valuable in many situations. A gram of fat or oil delivers more than twice as many calories as a gram of carbohydrate. A hunter or hiker needs to consume a large amount of food energy to travel long distances or to survive in intensely cold weather. As Figure 5-2 shows, such a person can carry more energy in fat-rich foods than in carbohydrate-rich foods. On the other hand, high-fat foods may deliver many unneeded calories in only a few bites to the person who is not expending much energy in physical work.

People like high-fat foods. Fat carries with it many dissolved compounds that give foods enticing aromas and flavors, such as the aroma of frying bacon

FIGURE 5-1

A FAT CELL
Within the fat cell, lipid is stored in a droplet. This droplet can greatly enlarge, and the fat cell membrane will grow to accommodate its swollen contents. More about fat cells and obesity in Chapter 9.

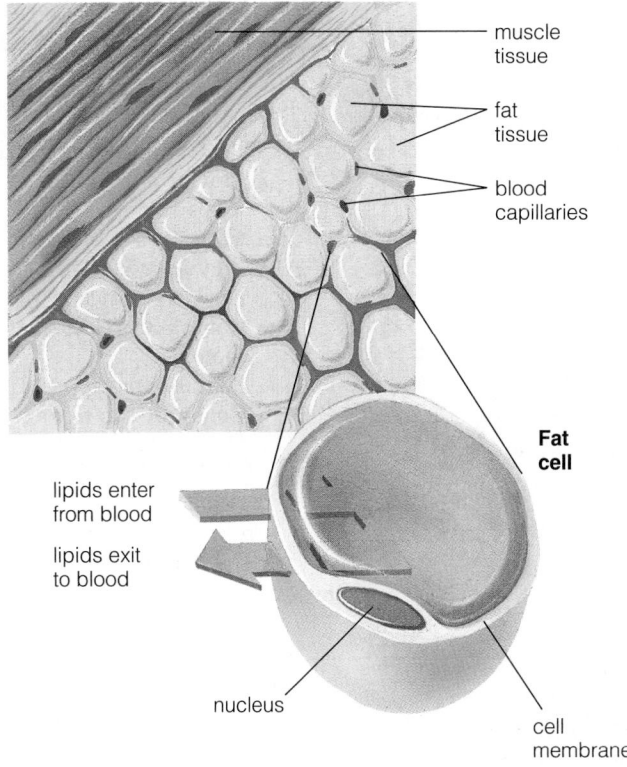

muscle tissue

fat tissue

blood capillaries

Fat cell

lipids enter from blood

lipids exit to blood

nucleus

cell membrane

or french fries. In fact, when a person refuses food, foods flavored with some fat may tempt that person to eat again. Fats also help make foods such as meats and baked goods tender.

Scientists once thought that because fat in food slows digestion, fat was especially powerful at bringing a lasting feeling of fullness to the eater. Recently, however, research has revealed that **satiety** results from many interrelated factors. Fat in food may act at the end of a meal, by sending a signal that enough food has been eaten. Carbohydrate and protein in food seem to provide a more lasting feeling of fullness.[2] Chapter 9 comes back to the topic of appetite and its control.

In the body, fat serves many purposes. Pads of fat surrounding the vital organs serve as shock absorbers. Thanks to the fat pads cushioning your internal organs, you can ride a horse or a motorcycle for many hours with no serious internal injuries. The fat blanket under the skin also insulates the body from extremes of temperature, thus assisting with internal climate control.

Some essential nutrients are soluble in fat and therefore are found mainly in foods that contain fat. These nutrients are the fat-soluble vitamins: A, D, E, and K. Other essential nutrients, the **essential fatty acids,** constitute parts of the fats themselves. A later section shows that the essential fatty acids serve as raw materials from which the body makes molecules it needs. Lipids are also important to all the body's cells as part of their surrounding envelopes, the cell membranes. Table 5-1 sums up the usefulness of fats, both in foods and in the body.

satiety (sat-EYE-uh-tee) the feeling of fullness or satisfaction that people feel after meals.

essential fatty acids fatty acids that the body needs but cannot make in amounts sufficient to meet physiological needs.

FIGURE 5-2

TWO LUNCHES

Both lunches contain the same number of calories, but the fat-rich lunch takes up less space and weighs less.

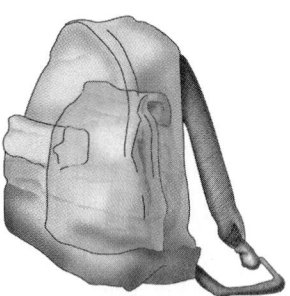

carbohydrate-rich lunch
1 low-fat muffin
1 banana
2 oz carrot sticks
8 oz fruit yogurt

calories   = 550
weight (g) = 500

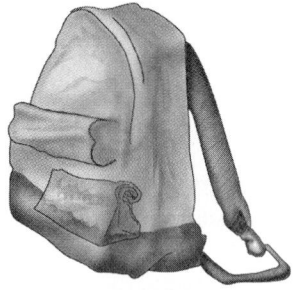

fat-rich lunch
6 butter-style crackers
1½ oz American cheese
2 oz trail mix with candy

calories   = 550
weight (g) = 115

---

fatty acids organic acids composed of carbon chains of various lengths. Each fatty acid has an acid end and hydrogens attached to all of the carbon atoms of the chain.

glycerol (GLISS-er-all) an organic compound, three carbons long, of interest here because it serves as the backbone for triglycerides.

TABLE 5-1

The Usefulness of Fats

Fats in Food	Fats in the Body
■ Provide essential fatty acids. ■ Provide a concentrated energy source in foods. ■ Carry fat-soluble vitamins. ■ Provide raw material for making needed products. ■ Contribute to taste and smell of foods. ■ Stimulate the appetite. ■ Contributes to feelings of fullness. ■ Help make foods tender.	■ Are the body's chief form of stored energy. ■ Provide most of the energy to fuel muscular work. ■ Serve as an emergency fuel supply in times of illness and diminished food intake. ■ Fat pads inside body cavity protect internal organs from shock. ■ Fat layer under skin insulates against temperature extremes. ■ Form the major material of cell membranes. ■ Are converted to other compounds as needed.

✔ **KEY POINT** **Lipids not only serve as energy reserves but also contribute to feelings of fullness at a meal, enhance food's aroma and flavor, cushion the vital organs, protect the body from temperature extremes, carry the fat-soluble nutrients, serve as raw materials, and provide the major material of which cell membranes are made.**

A CLOSE LOOK AT FATS

As mentioned, the term *fat* refers to triglycerides, the major form of lipid found in foods. Triglycerides, in turn, are made of fatty acids and glycerol.

Triglycerides: Fatty Acids and Glycerol

Very few **fatty acids** are found free in the body or in foods. Usually, the fatty acids are incorporated into large, complex compounds: triglycerides. The name almost explains itself: three fatty acids (*tri*) are attached to a molecule of **glycerol**. Figure 5-3 shows how glycerol and three fatty acids combine to make a triglyceride molecule. Tissues all over the body can easily assemble triglycerides or disassemble them as needed. Many triglycerides eaten in foods are transported to the fat depots—muscles, breasts, the insulating fat layer under the skin, and others—where they are stored.

Fatty acids may differ from one another in two ways: in chain length and in degree of saturation (explained next). Depending on which fatty acids are incorporated into a triglyceride, the resulting fat will be soft or hard. Triglycerides that contain the shorter-chain fatty acids or the more unsaturated ones are softer and melt more readily. Each species of animal (including people) makes its own characteristic kinds of triglycerides, a function governed by genetics. Fats in the diet, though, can affect the types of triglycerides made. For

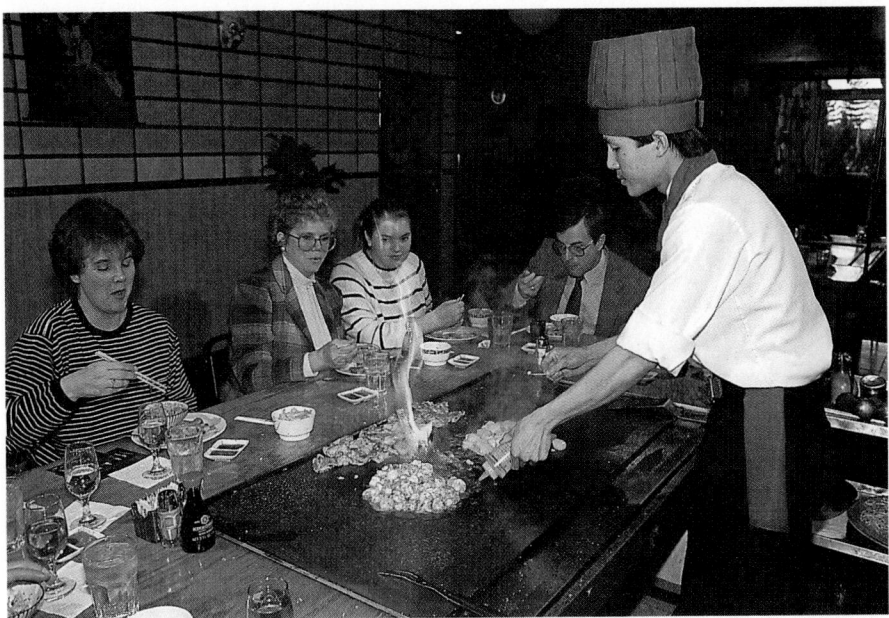

Small amounts of fat offer eaters both pleasure and needed nutrients.

example, animals raised for food can be fed diets containing softer or harder triglycerides to give the animals softer or harder fat, whichever consumers demand.

✔ KEY POINT   **The body combines three fatty acids with one glycerol to make a triglyceride, its storage form of fat. Fatty acids in food influence the composition of fats in the body.**

FIGURE 5-3

TRIGLYCERIDE FORMATION
Glycerol, a small, water-soluble carbohydrate derivative, plus three fatty acids, equals a triglyceride.

glycerol

3 fatty acids of differing lengths

A triglyceride formed from 1 glycerol + 3 fatty acids

FIGURE 5-4

THREE FATTY ACIDS

The more carbon atoms in a fatty acid, the longer it is. The more hydrogen atoms attached to those carbons, the more saturated the fatty acid is.

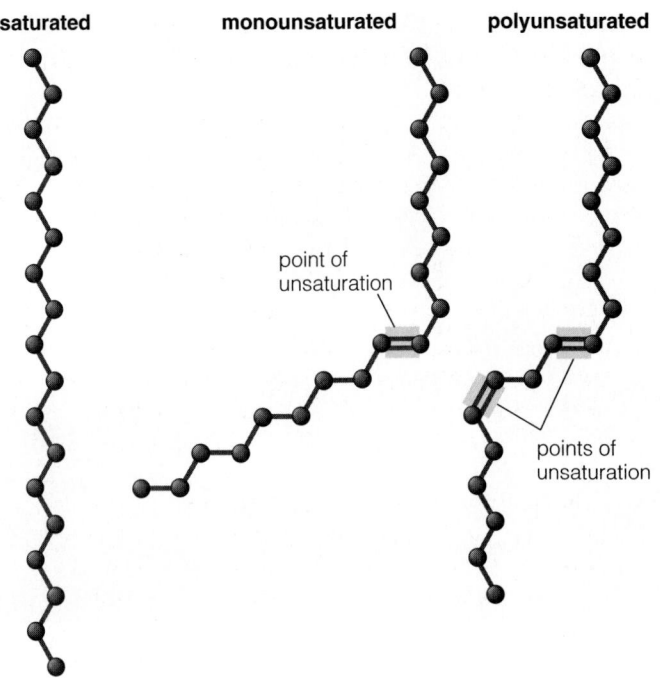

saturated   monounsaturated   polyunsaturated

point of unsaturation

points of unsaturation

saturated fatty acid a fatty acid carrying the maximum possible number of hydrogen atoms (having no points of unsaturation). A saturated fat is a triglyceride that contains three saturated fatty acids.

point of unsaturation a site in a molecule where the bonding is such that additional hydrogen atoms can easily be attached.

unsaturated fatty acids a fatty acid that lacks some hydrogen atoms and has one or more points of unsaturation. An unsaturated fat is a triglyceride that contains one or more unsaturated fatty acids.

monounsaturated fatty acid a fatty acid containing one point of unsaturation.

polyunsaturated fatty acid (PUFA) a fatty acid with two or more points of unsaturation.

saturated fats triglycerides in which all the fatty acids are saturated.

Saturated versus Unsaturated Fatty Acids

Saturation refers to the number of hydrogens a fatty acid chain is holding. If every available bond from the carbons is holding a hydrogen, the chain forms a **saturated fatty acid**; it is filled to capacity with hydrogen. The zigzag structure on the left in Figure 5-4 represents a saturated fatty acid.

Sometimes, especially in the fatty acids of plants and fish, there is a place in the chain where hydrogens are missing, an "empty spot," or **point of unsaturation.** A fatty acid carbon chain that possesses one or more points of unsaturation is an **unsaturated fatty acid.** If there is one point of unsaturation, then the fatty acid is a **monounsaturated fatty acid** (see the second structure in Figure 5-4). If there are two or more points of unsaturation, then it is a **polyunsaturated fatty acid** (examples are given later in the chapter; and see the third structure in Figure 5-4). You sometimes see polyunsaturated fatty acids abbreviated as **PUFA.**

The degree of saturation of fatty acids in a fat affects the temperature at which the fat melts. Generally, the more unsaturated the fatty acids of a fat, the more liquid the fat is at room temperature. In contrast, the more saturated a fat, the firmer it is. Thus of three fats—lard (which comes from pork), chicken fat, and safflower oil—lard is the most saturated and the hardest; chicken fat is less saturated and somewhat soft; and safflower oil, which is the most unsaturated, is a liquid at room temperature. Thus, if a health-care provider recommends limiting **saturated fats** and using **monounsaturated fats** or **polyunsaturated fats** instead, you can generally judge by the hardness of the fats which ones to choose. To determine whether an oil you use contains saturated fats, place the oil in a clear container in the refrigerator and watch for cloudiness. The least saturated oils remain clearest.

Generally speaking, vegetable and fish oils are rich in polyunsaturates. Some vegetable oils, especially olive oil, are also rich in monounsaturates, and animal fats are generally the most saturated. But you have to know your oils. To obtain polyunsaturated oils, it is not enough to choose foods with labels claiming plant oils over those containing animal fats. Some nondairy whipped dessert toppings use coconut oil, one of the so-called tropical oils, in place of cream (butterfat). Coconut oil does come from a plant, but it disobeys the rule that plant oils are more liquid than animal fats; coconut oil is actually more saturated than cream and seems to add to heart disease risk. Palm oil, used frequently in food processing, is also highly saturated and seems to affect blood lipids in ways not yet fully understood, but it has not been proved to add to heart disease risk.[3]

A benefit to health is seen when monounsaturated fat is used in place of saturated fat in the diet.[4] As the Controversy section of Chapter 2 made clear, olive oil does not harm the health of the heart. When it replaces other fats in the diet, olive oil may even benefit heart health, if the low rates of heart disease among the people of Mediterranean regions serve as an indicator. Lately, canola oil, another rich source of monounsaturated fatty acids, has appeared on U.S. grocery shelves. Figure 5-5 compares fats and oils in terms of their percentages of saturated, monounsaturated, and polyunsaturated fatty acids.

monounsaturated fats triglycerides in which one or more of the fatty acids has one point of unsaturation (is monounsaturated).

polyunsaturated fats triglycerides in which one or more of the fatty acids has two or more points of unsaturation (is polyunsaturated).

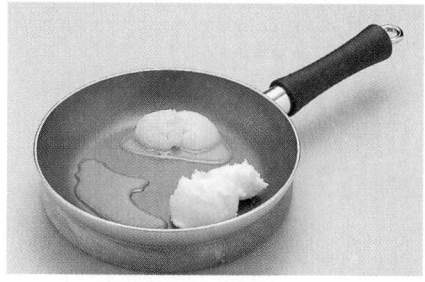

The more unsaturated a fat, the more liquid it is at room temperature. The more saturated a fat, the higher the temperature at which it melts.

FIGURE 5-5

FATTY ACID COMPOSITION OF COMMON FOOD FATS

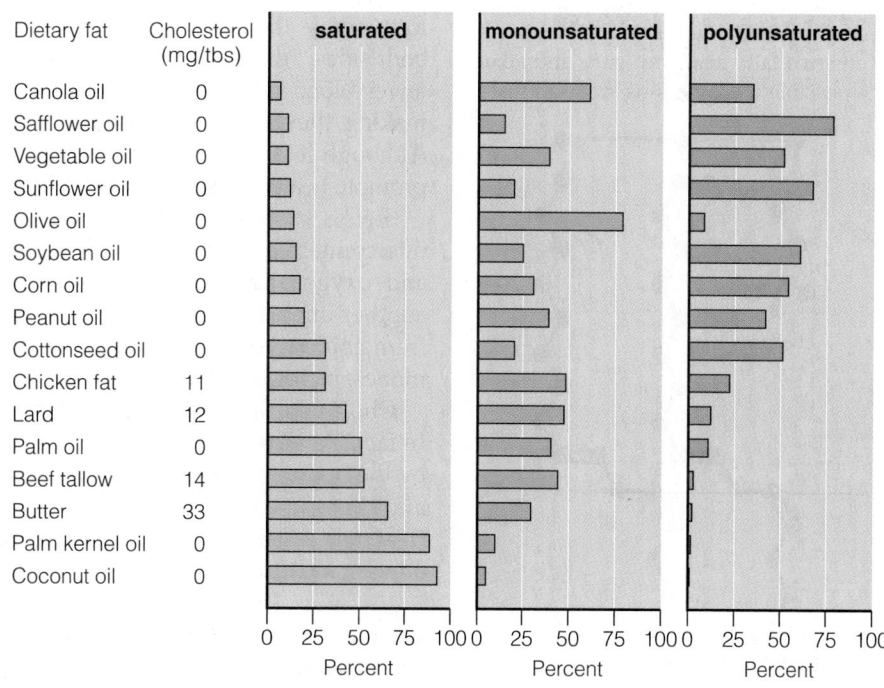

emulsifier a substance that mixes with both fat and water and permanently disperses fat in water, forming an emulsion.

emulsification the process of mixing lipid with water, by adding an emulsifier.

bile an emulsifier made by the liver from cholesterol and stored in the gallbladder. Bile does not digest fat as enzymes do but emulsifies it so that enzymes in the watery fluids may contact it and split the fatty acids from their glycerol for absorption.

FIGURE 5-6

A MOLECULE OF LECITHIN
A molecule of lecithin is like a triglyceride but contains only two (polyunsaturated) fatty acids. The third position is occupied by choline (a compound containing phosphorus and related to the B vitamins). The identity of the two fatty acids can vary, and all of the possible combinations are lecithins.

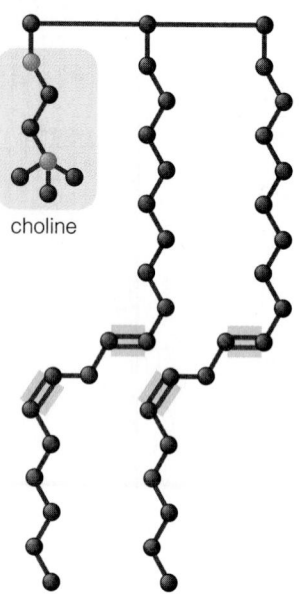

choline

✔️ KEY POINT   **Fatty acids are energy-rich carbon chains that can be saturated (filled with hydrogens) or monounsaturated (with one point of unsaturation) or polyunsaturated (with more than one point of unsaturation). The degree of saturation of the fatty acids in a fat determines the fat's softness or hardness.**

Other Members of the Lipid Family

The foregoing sections have dealt with just one of the three classes of lipids—the triglycerides and their component fatty acids. These lipids represent 95 percent of all the lipids in the diet and in the body. The word *fat*, used properly, refers to the triglycerides.

The other two classes—phospholipids and sterols—merit a moment's attention, though, because they play important roles in the body. A phospholipid, like a triglyceride, consists of a molecule of glycerol with fatty acids attached, but it contains two, rather than three, fatty acids. In place of the third is a molecule containing phosphorus, which makes the phospholipid soluble in water, while its fatty acids make it soluble in fat. This versatility permits any phospholipid to play a role in keeping fats dispersed in water; it can serve as an **emulsifier.**

Food processors often blend fat with watery ingredients by way of **emulsification.** Some salad dressings separate to form two layers—vinegar on the bottom, oil on the top. Other dressings, such as mayonnaise, are also made from vinegar and oil but never separate. The difference lies in a special ingredient of mayonnaise, the emulsifier lecithin in egg yolks. Lecithin, a phospholipid, blends the vinegar and oil in a permanent emulsion.

Lecithins and other phospholipids also play key roles in the structure of cell membranes. Because phospholipids are emulsifiers, they have both water-loving and fat-loving characteristics, which enable them to help fats travel back and forth across the lipid-containing membranes of cells into the watery fluids on both sides. Almost magical health-promoting properties, such as the ability to lower blood cholesterol, are sometimes attributed to lecithin, but the people making the claims are those who stand to gain from selling supplements. Although it is an important lipid to the body, lecithin has no special ability to promote health. A molecule of lecithin is shown in Figure 5-6.

Sterols such as cholesterol are large, complicated molecules consisting of interconnected *rings* of carbon atoms with side chains of carbon, hydrogen, and oxygen attached. Cholesterol serves as the raw material for making another important emulsifier, **bile.** Other sterols are vitamin D, which is made from cholesterol, and several important hormones, the so-called steroid hormones, including the sex hormones.

Cholesterol is an important sterol in the structure of brain and nerve cells. In fact, cholesterol is a part of every cell. Like lecithin, cholesterol can be made by the body, so it is not an essential nutrient. Though widespread in the body and necessary to its function, cholesterol is also the major part of the plaques that narrow the arteries in atherosclerosis, the underlying cause of heart attacks and strokes.

✔️ KEY POINT   **Phospholipids, including lecithin, play key roles in cell membranes; sterols play roles as part of bile, vitamin D, the sex hormones, and other important compounds.**

LIPIDS IN THE BODY

In handling lipids, the body must solve the problem of how to thoroughly mix them with its own watery fluids. The digestive system solves this problem through the use of bile, which emulsifies the fat in food in the watery digestive fluids. Thus, to digest fats, the digestive system first mixes them with its bile-containing digestive juices; once the fats are emulsified, the fat-digesting enzymes can break them down. After fats have been digested, they face another watery barrier, the watery layer of mucus that coats the absorptive lining of the digestive tract. Fats must traverse this layer to enter the cells of the digestive tract lining. Then the cells face another challenge: to package lipids so that they can travel in the watery fluids on the circulatory system. The next two sections describe the body's superb adaptations to meet all these needs for lipid digestion and transport.

Digestion of Fats

When you partake of animal products such as meat, fish, poultry, or eggs, you are eating fat and protein. When you eat oil-containing plant foods, such as nuts, coconut, or olives, you are eating fat and carbohydrate along with some protein. Of the fats and oils in foods, 95 percent are triglycerides that have been made in living animal or plant tissues, mostly from carbohydrate, the same way the human body makes them.

Food fat can end up in fat stores in the body, but first it has to be digested, absorbed, and transported to its cell destinations. A bite of food in the mouth first encounters the enzymes of saliva. One enzyme, produced by the tongue, acts on long-chain fatty acids, especially those of milk. The enzyme plays a major role in milk fat digestion in infants, but is thought to be of little importance to fat digestion in adults.[5] Once the food has been chewed and swallowed, it travels to the stomach, where the fat separates from other components and floats as a layer on the top. Since fat does not mix with the stomach fluids, little fat digestion takes place.

By the time fat enters the small intestine, the gallbladder, which stores the liver's output of bile, has contracted and squirted its bile into the intestine. Bile mixes fat particles with watery fluid by emulsifying them (see Figure 5-7), suspending them in the fluid until the fat-digesting enzymes contributed by the pancreas can split them for absorption. A bile molecule, made from cholesterol, works because one of its ends attracts and holds fat, while the other end is attracted to and held by water.

People sometimes wonder how a person without a gallbladder can digest food. The gallbladder is just a storage organ. Without it, the liver still produces bile, but delivers it continuously into the small intestine. People who have had their gallbladders removed must reduce their fat intakes because they can no longer store bile and release it at mealtimes. As a result, their systems can handle only a little fat at a time.

Once the intestine's contents are emulsified, fat-splitting enzymes act on triglycerides to split fatty acids from their glycerol backbones. Free fatty acids, glycerol, and **monoglycerides** cling together in balls surrounded by bile and are shuttled across the watery layer of mucus to the waiting absorptive cells of the intestinal villi.[6] The bile may be absorbed and reused by the body, or it may exit with the feces as shown in Figure 4-4 of the previous chapter.

monoglycerides (mon-oh-GLISS-er-ides) a product of the digestion of lipids; glycerol molecules with one fatty acid attached (*mono* means "one"; *glyceride* means "a compound of glycerol").

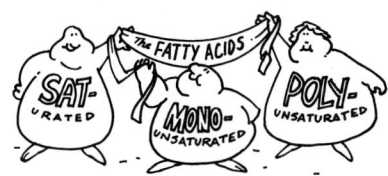

A trio of fatty acids—saturated, monounsaturated, and polyunsaturated.

Chapter 3 first described the action of bile and gave details of the digestive system.

FIGURE 5-7

THE ACTION OF BILE
IN FAT DIGESTION

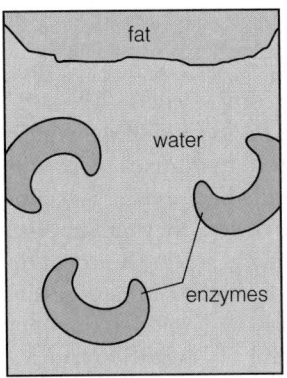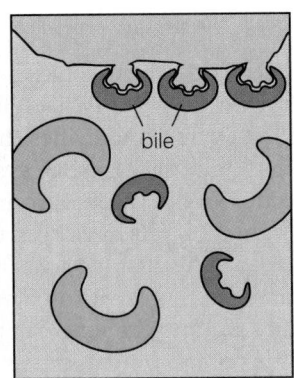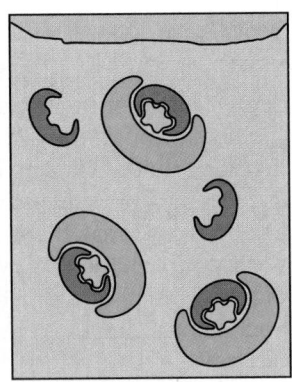

Fat and water tend to separate. Enzymes are in the water and can't get at the fat.

Bile (an emulsifier) arrives. Bile has an affinity for both fat and water and can therefore bring the fat into the water.

After emulsification, the fat is mixed in the water solution, so fat-digesting enzymes have access to it.

Detergents are emulsifiers and work the same way, which is why they are effective in removing grease spots from clothes. Molecule by molecule, the grease is dissolved out of the spot and suspended in the water, where it can be rinsed away.

chylomicrons (KYE-low-MY-krons) clusters formed when lipids from a meal are combined with carrier proteins in the intestinal lining. Chylomicrons transport food fats through the watery body fluids to the liver and other tissues.

lipoproteins (LIP-oh-PRO-teens) clusters of lipids associated with protein, which serve as transport vehicles for lipids in blood and lymph. Major lipoprotein classes are the chylomicrons, the LDL, and the HDL.

The small products of lipid digestion, glycerol and shorter-chain fatty acids, can pass directly through the cells of the digestive tract lining into the bloodstream. From there they can travel without help to the tissues that need them.

The larger products of lipid digestion, monoglycerides and long-chain fatty acids, need some help to get to their destinations via the bloodstream. Once inside the intestinal cells, they are re-formed into triglycerides and incorporated into **chylomicrons,** clusters of proteins and the digested lipids. Chylomicrons are a class of **lipoproteins,** described later.

The digestive tract absorbs triglycerides from a meal with up to 98 percent efficiency. In other words, little fat is excreted by a healthy system.[7] The process of fat digestion takes time, though, so the more fat taken in at a meal, the slower the digestive system action becomes. The efficient series of events just described is depicted in Figure 5-8.

✔ KEY POINT In the stomach, fats separate from other food components. In the small intestine, bile emulsifies the fats, enzymes digest them, and the intestinal cells absorb them. Small lipids can travel alone in the blood after absorption, but large lipids must be incorporated into chylomicrons for transport.

Lipid Transport in the Body Fluids

Within the body, many fats travel from place to place as passengers in lipoproteins. For example, the monoglycerides and long-chain fatty acids liberated from digested food fat are too large to be released directly into the bloodstream. Without some mechanism to keep them dispersed, these lipids would separate out and float in globules, disrupting the blood's normal functions. Therefore, before releasing the lipids, the intestinal cells allow them to cluster together, rejoin them as triglycerides, and combine them with protein to form the chylomicrons mentioned earlier. The protein and phospholipid in the clusters act as emulsifiers: they attract both water and fat. Their association with both substances enables them to transport lipids in the watery body fluids. The tissues of the body can extract whatever fat they need from these clusters. The remnants that are left are picked up by the liver, which dismantles them and reuses their parts.

The chylomicrons are the special class of lipoproteins that the body uses to carry fats from the intestine to the liver. Other lipoproteins are the **low-density lipoproteins (LDL),** which carry fats made in the liver to the body cells, and the **high-density lipoproteins (HDL),** which carry fats from body cells to the liver.* The carrier proteins for both are made in the liver, and both carry large quantities of cholesterol; the HDL also carry many phospholipids. Figure 5-9 depicts a lipoprotein.

Lipoproteins are very much on the minds of health-care providers who measure people's blood lipid profiles. They are interested not only in the types of fats in the blood (triglycerides and cholesterol) but also in the lipoproteins that carry them. The distinction between LDL and HDL is of great importance

LDL (low-density lipoproteins) lipoproteins, containing a large proportion of cholesterol, that transport lipids from the liver to other tissues such as muscle and fat.

HDL (high-density lipoproteins) lipoproteins, containing a large proportion of protein, that return cholesterol from storage places to the liver for dismantling and disposal.

---

*Another class of lipoproteins is the very-low-density lipoproteins (VLDL), an early version of the LDL. VLDL become LDL as they lose triglycerides and gain cholesterol.

FIGURE 5-8

THE PROCESS OF LIPID DIGESTION AND ABSORPTION

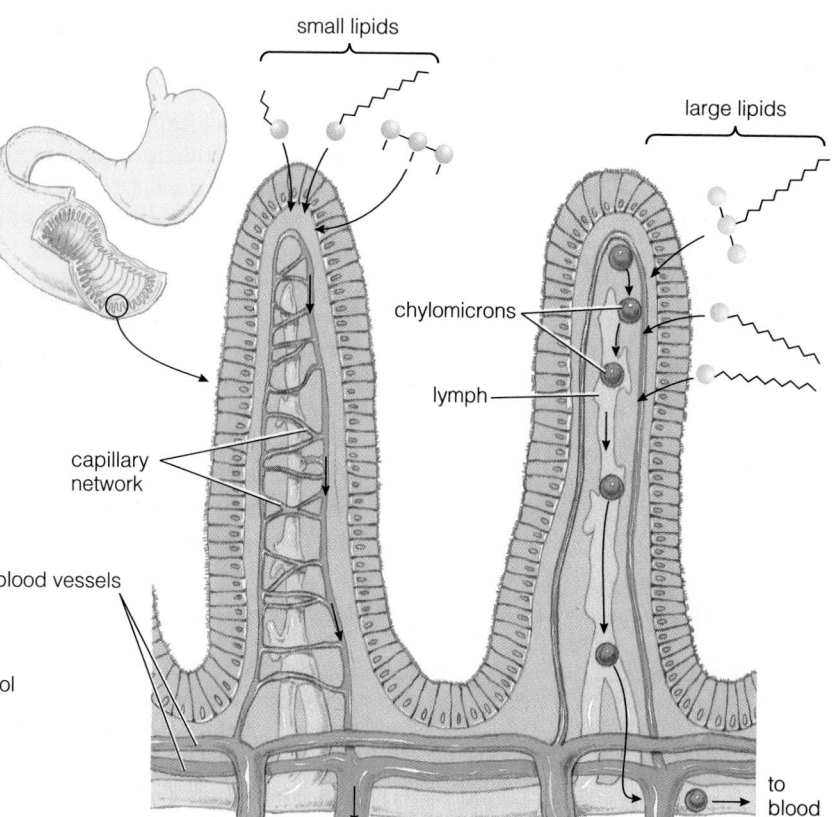

Inside the digestive tract:

Digestive enzymes accomplish most fat digestion in the small intestine where bile emulsifies fat, making it available for enzyme action. The enzymes cleave triglycerides into free fatty acids, glycerol, and monoglycerides.

At the intestinal lining:

The parts are absorbed by intestinal villi. Large lipid fragments, such as monoglycerides and long-chain fatty acids are converted back into triglycerides and combined with protein, forming chylomicrons that travel in the lymph vessels. Small lipid particles such as glycerol and short-chain fatty acids are small enough to enter directly into the bloodstream without further processing.

In this diagram, molecules of fatty acids are shown as large objects, but, in reality, molecules of fatty acids are too small to see even with a powerful microscope, while villi are visible to the naked eye.

small lipids

large lipids

chylomicrons

lymph

capillary network

blood vessels

to blood

to liver

FIGURE 5-9

A LIPOPROTEIN
An LDL has a high ratio of lipid to protein (about 80 percent lipid to 20 percent protein); an HDL has more protein relative to its lipid content (about equal parts lipid and protein).

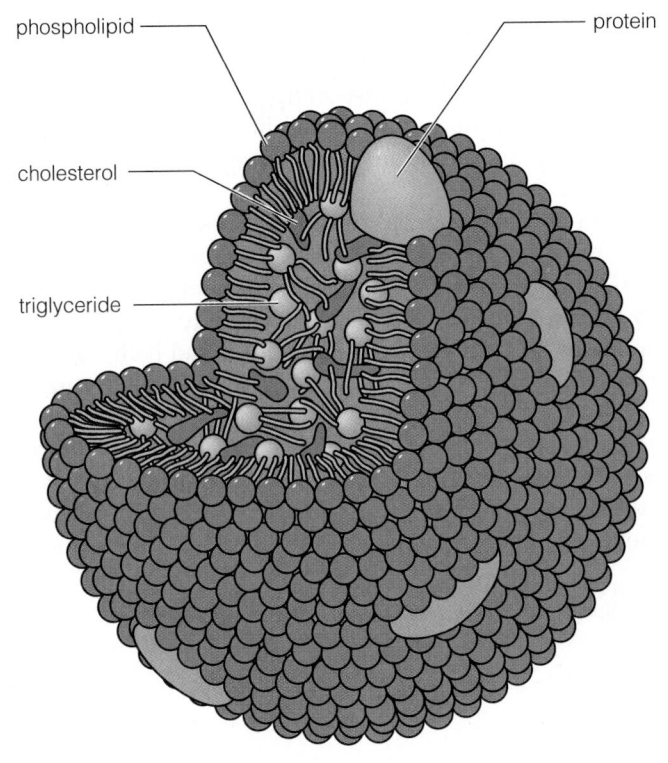

because it has implications for the health of the heart and blood vessels. The more lipid in the lipoprotein molecule, the lower the density; the more protein, the higher the density. Both LDL and HDL carry lipids around in the blood, but LDL are larger, lighter, and more lipid filled; HDL are smaller, denser, and packaged with more protein. LDL deliver triglycerides and cholesterol from the liver to the tissues; HDL scavenge excess cholesterol and phospholipids from the tissues and return them to the liver for disposal. Elevated LDL concentrations in the blood are a sign of high risk of heart attack, whereas elevated HDL concentrations are associated with a low risk.[8] A later section clarifies this relationship.

✓ KEY POINT   **Blood and other body fluids are watery, so fats need special transport vehicles, to carry them around the body, in these fluids. The chief lipoproteins are chylomicrons, LDL, and HDL.**

Use of Stored Fat for Energy

Excess fat carried in LDL is stored by the body's fat cells for later use. An earlier section described the body's remarkable ability to store excess energy as body fat. When a person's body starts to run out of fuel available from food, it begins to retrieve its stored fat to use for energy and also its glycogen, as the last chapter showed. Fat cells respond to the call for energy by dismantling stored fat molecules and releasing their components into the blood. Upon receiving these components, the energy-hungry cells break them down further into small fragments. Finally, each fat fragment is combined with a fragment

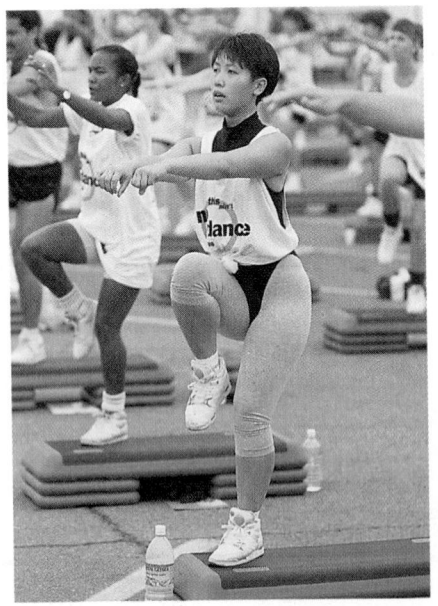

Body fat supplies much of the fuel these muscles need to do their work.

derived from glucose, and the energy-releasing reaction continues, liberating energy, carbon dioxide, and water.

Thus, whenever body fat is broken down to provide energy, carbohydrate must be available as well. Without carbohydrate, ketosis will occur, as described in the last chapter, and products of incomplete fat breakdown (ketones) will appear in the blood and urine. Because this process and its consequences are so important in weight control, Chapter 9 describes them in greater detail.

The body can also store excess glucose as fat, but this conversion is not energy efficient. Figure 5-10 illustrates a simplified series of steps from carbohydrate to fat. As it shows, before excess glucose can be stored as fat, it must first be broken into tiny fragments and then reassembled into fatty acids, steps that require energy to perform. Fat, on the other hand, goes through fewer chemical steps before storage. Thus, given the same number of calories from excess dietary fat or carbohydrate, the body stores more calories from the fat than from the carbohydrate. In short, you may get fatter on fat calories than on the same number of carbohydrate calories. The Controversy that follows this chapter revisits this changing research area and tells what, if any, significance it holds for meal planners who wish to control the amounts of energy they store as body fat.

✔ KEY POINT **When low on fuel, the body draws on its stored fat for energy. Glucose is necessary for the complete breakdown of fat; without carbohydrate, ketosis occurs.**

Harmful Potential of Fats

High dietary fat intakes are associated with serious diseases. A person who chooses a diet too high in certain fats may be inviting the risk of heart and artery disease, or CVD.[9] Heart disease is this nation's number-one killer of adults. The person who eats a high-fat diet also incurs a greater-than-average risk of developing some forms of cancer, another leading killer disease.[10] Much research has focused on the links between diet and disease, and later a whole chapter is devoted to these connections (Chapter 11). A few points about fats and heart health are presented here because they underlie dietary recommendations concerning fats (see Table 5-2).

Of great importance in regard to fat and disease is a medical test, the blood lipid profile, which reveals the amounts of various lipids, especially triglycerides and cholesterol, in the blood. It also identifies the protein carriers with

To estimate the approximate number of fat grams allowed in a day to limit fat calories to 30% of total, use this rule of thumb:

General equation:

Total energy need (in calories)

Drop last digit = x

$\dfrac{x}{3}$ = g fat/day

Example: 2,300-calorie energy need

$\dfrac{230\!\!\!/0}{3}$ = 77 g fat/day

SOURCE: K. McNutt, Fat traps, tips, and tricks, *Nutrition Today*, May/June 1992, pp. 47–49.

As of the early 1990s, less than a fifth of children, adolescents, and adult males and a quarter of adult females consumed diets with less than 30% calories from fat.

SOURCE: Federation of American Societies for Experimental Biology, *Third Report on Nutrition Monitoring in the United States* (Washington, D.C.: Government Printing Office, 1995), p. ES–3.

FIGURE 5-10

GLUCOSE TO FAT

Glucose can be used for energy, or it can be changed into fat and stored.

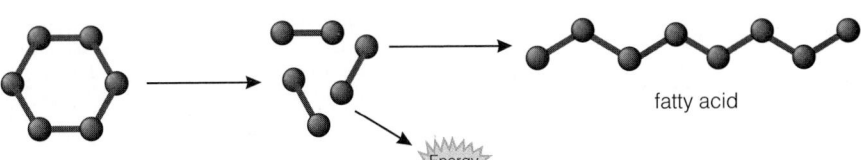

fatty acid

Glucose is broken down into fragments.

The fragments can provide immediate energy for the tissues.

Energy

Or, if the tissues need no more energy, the fragments can be reassembled, not back to glucose but into fatty acid chains.

TABLE 5-2

Recommendations Concerning Intakes of Fats

1. Total Fat[a]

   Dietary Guidelines
   - Choose a diet low in fat.

   Daily Values[b]
   - 65 grams fat per day.

   Healthy People 2000
   - Reduce dietary fat intake to an average of 30% of energy or less (people age 2 years and older).

   World Health Organization[e]
   - Lower limit for total fat intake: 15% of total calories from fat.[c]
   - Upper limit for total fat intake: 30% of total calories from fat.[d]

2. Saturated Fat

   Dietary Guidelines
   - Choose a diet low in saturated fat.

   Daily Values[b]
   - 20 grams of saturated fat per day.

   Healthy People 2000
   - Reduce saturated fat intake to an average of less than 10% of energy (people age 2 years and older).

   World Health Organization
   - Lower limit for saturated fat intake: 0% of total calories from saturated fat.
   - Upper limit for saturated fat intake: 10% of total calories from saturated fat.

3. Polyunsaturated Fatty Acids

   World Health Organization
   - Lower limit for polyunsaturated fat intake: 3% of total calories from polyunsaturated fatty acids.
   - Upper limit for polyunsaturated fat intake: 7% of total calories from polyunsaturated fatty acids.

4. Cholesterol

   Dietary Guidelines
   - Choose a diet low in cholesterol.

   Daily Values[b]
   - 300 milligrams cholesterol per day.

   World Health Organization
   - Lower limit for cholesterol intake: 0 milligrams cholesterol per day.
   - Upper limit for cholesterol intake: 300 milligrams cholesterol per day.

[a]Includes monounsaturated fatty acids.
[b]The Daily Values are for a 2,000-calorie diet.
[c]Except for women of reproductive age, who should consume at least 20% of energy from fat.
[d]Sedentary individuals. Active individuals may consume up to 35% of total energy from fat if saturated fat does not exceed 10% of calories and the diet is otherwise adequate.
[e]WHO and FAO Joint Consultation, Fats and oils in human nutrition, *Nutrition Reviews* 53 (1995): 202–205.

which these lipids are traveling. The results of this test tell much about a person's risk of CVD.

Most important in regard to CVD is blood cholesterol.* A person's blood cholesterol concentration is considered to be a predictor of that person's likelihood of suffering a fatal heart attack or stroke, and the higher the cholesterol, the earlier the episode is expected to be. Blood cholesterol is one of the three major risk factors for CVD (the other two are smoking and high blood pressure, or hypertension). The importance of blood cholesterol cannot be overemphasized.

Now, what does *food* cholesterol have to do with *blood* cholesterol? The answer is that saturated food *fats* (triglycerides) raise blood cholesterol more than food *cholesterol* does. People often fail to understand this point. When told that cholesterol doesn't matter as much as fat, people often jump to the wrong conclusion—that blood cholesterol doesn't matter. It does matter. High *blood* cholesterol is an indicator of risk for CVD. The main dietary factor associated with elevated blood cholesterol is a high *saturated fat* intake. In comparison, dietary cholesterol alone makes only a minor contribution.[11]

Heredity modifies everyone's ability to handle food cholesterol somewhat, but a few individuals have inherited a total inability to clear from their blood the cholesterol they have eaten and absorbed. This condition is rare but well known because studying it led to the discovery of how cholesterol is transported in the body. People with a genetic tendency toward high blood cholesterol must strictly limit fats and refrain from eating cholesterol in foods; perhaps this is where the general public's fear of food cholesterol has come from. The majority of people can eat eggs, liver, and other cholesterol-containing foods in moderation without fear of incurring high blood cholesterol.

An effective dietary tactic against high blood cholesterol is to trim the fat, and especially the saturated fat, from foods. The photos of Figure 5-11 show that food trimmed of fat is also trimmed of much of its energy. A pork chop trimmed of its border of fat loses almost 100 calories. A plain baked potato has half the calories of one with butter and sour cream. Choosing nonfat milk over whole milk provides a large saving of fat, saturated fat, and calories; and so forth. The single most effective step you can take to reduce a food's potential for elevating blood cholesterol is to eat it without the fat.

> ✓ KEY POINT   **An important distinction: it is not the intake of cholesterol in foods but fat intake, and especially saturated fat intake, that is the major dietary factor that raises blood cholesterol. Elevated blood cholesterol is a risk factor for cardiovascular disease.**

The 1996 American Heart Association Dietary Guidelines for Healthy American Adults are found in Table 11-12 of Chapter 11.

Significance of LDL and HDL

To repeat, cholesterol in foods contributes somewhat to cholesterol in the blood, and excesses of food cholesterol should be avoided. Dietary cholesterol is not as influential in raising blood cholesterol, however, as is total dietary fat, and especially saturated fat, which the body uses to make cholesterol. Now the link to

---

Blood, plasma, and *serum* cholesterol all refer to about the same thing; this book uses the term *blood* cholesterol. Plasma is blood with the cells removed; in serum the clotting factors are also removed. The concentration of cholesterol is not much altered by these treatments.

FIGURE 5-11

FOOD FAT AND CALORIES

Fat hides calories in food. When you trim fat, you trim calories.

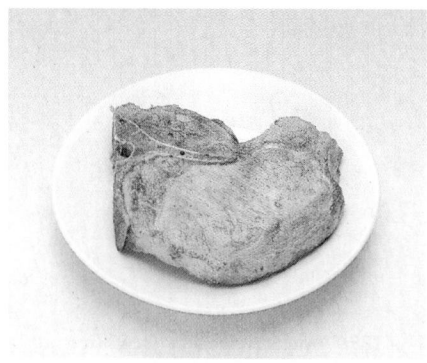

Pork chop with ½ inch of fat (353 calories; 225 calories from fat).

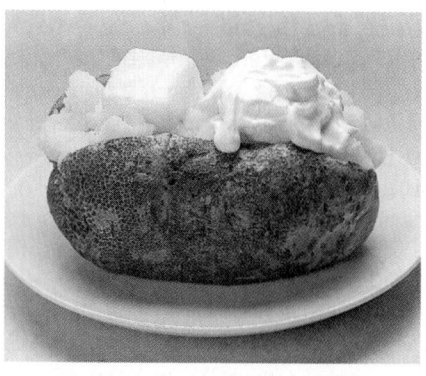

Potato with 1 tablespoon butter and 1 tablespoon sour cream (350 calories; 126 calories from fat).

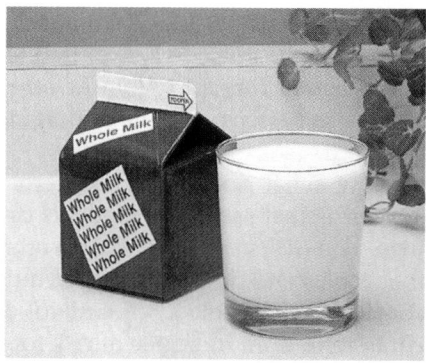

Whole milk, 1 cup (150 calories; 72 calories from fat).

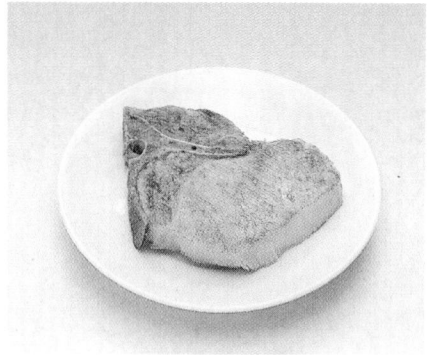

Pork chop with fat trimmed off (265 calories; 117 calories from fat).

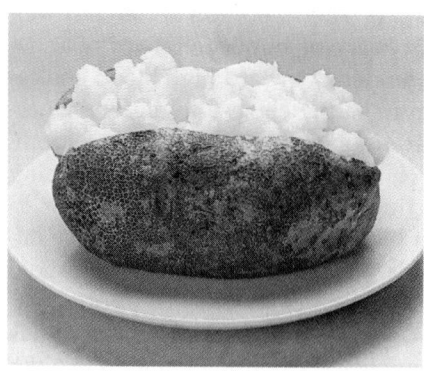

Plain potato (220 calories; fewer than 9 calories from fat).

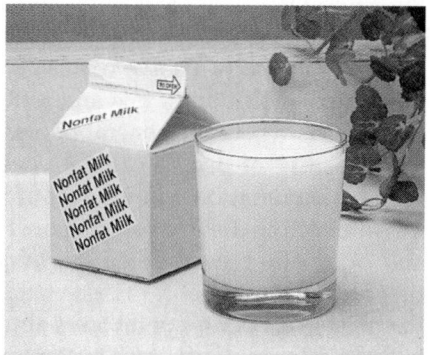

Nonfat milk, 1 cup (90 calories; fewer than 9 calories from fat).

Antioxidant nutrients are topics of Chapter 7 and its Controversy.

Here's a trick:

Remember **HDL** is **H**ealthy;

LDL is **L**ess healthy.

Desirable blood lipid values (mg/dL):

✓ Total cholesterol <200.
✓ LDL <130.
✓ HDL >35.
✓ Triglycerides <200.

the LDL can be explained. When a person's high blood cholesterol signifies a risk of heart disease, it is because the cholesterol, which is carried in LDL, is traveling to body tissues to be deposited here. If a person has high blood cholesterol in HDL, that is cause not for concern but for celebration. The vehicle matters.

Elevated LDL forecast heart and artery disease; elevated HDL signify a low disease risk. The rule of thumb is that a minimum of 35 milligrams HDL per deciliter of blood or plasma is associated with a low risk of heart attack. This measurement of HDL amount seems to be especially predictive when compared with the total cholesterol count.[12] Another rule of thumb states that total blood cholesterol should be no more than about four times higher than HDL cholesterol for an acceptable level of risk.

Fortunately, the changes in diet that reduce blood cholesterol concentration mostly do so by reducing LDL. HDL concentration remains unaffected for the most part. The most influential dietary factor thought to raise blood cholesterol is a high saturated fat intake.[13] A person who attempts to lower blood cholesterol by reducing only the total fat in the diet may have little success.[14] Better to reduce total fat *and* replace cholesterol-raising saturated fat with monounsaturated or polyunsaturated fat. No beneficial change in blood lipids is seen when monounsaturated or polyunsaturated fat is *added* to a diet rich in saturated fat. That is, an eater of a bacon double cheeseburger cannot expect health protection from adding olive oil dressing to a side salad.

An important detail about LDL concerns its susceptibility to damage by **oxidation.**[15] Oxidation of the lipid part of LDL is thought to play a role in the injury of the arteries of the heart. **Antioxidant** nutrients, such as vitamin C and vitamin E, slow LDL oxidation. Other antioxidants, the phytochemicals, may also be helpful in this regard.

Some health authorities say all adults should take steps to reduce their blood cholesterol; others say that only those medically identified as at risk for heart disease should do so. In any case, it seems desirable for most people's health's sake to limit saturated fat intake. A diet that is low in saturated fat and rich in vegetables offers many advantages for health by supplying abundant nutrients and antioxidants along with beneficial fiber.

What about cholesterol intake? People respond differently. Dietary cholesterol has only a minimal effect on the blood cholesterol of about two-thirds of people. The other third must limit intakes to keep blood cholesterol from rising too high. Eggs, shellfish, liver, and other cholesterol-containing foods are nutritious, however. Cholesterol is unlike salt and sugar in this respect: it cannot be omitted from the diet without omitting nutritious foods.

People can also take steps to raise HDL levels through exercise, weight loss in the overweight, and, for smokers, quitting smoking. Another benefit to heart health is probably unrelated to blood cholesterol, but involves consumption of the essential fatty acids mentioned earlier. These relationships deserve some discussion.

> ✓ **KEY POINT** **Dietary measures to lower LDL in the blood involve reducing saturated fat and substituting monounsaturated and polyunsaturated fats for saturated fat. A few people must also reduce cholesterol intake. Cholesterol-containing foods are nutritious and are best used in moderation.**

Essential Polyunsaturated Fatty Acids

The human body can use carbohydrate, fat, or protein to synthesize nearly all the fatty acids it needs. Two are well-known exceptions: **linoleic acid** and **linolenic acid.** These two polyunsaturated fatty acids, which the body needs for its basic functions, cannot be made from other substances in the body or from each other. They must be supplied by the diet and are therefore essential nutrients. These essential fatty acids are found in small amounts in the oils of plants and cold-water fish and are readily stored in the adult body. Both serve as raw materials from which the body makes hormonelike substances that regulate a wide range of body functions: blood pressure, blood clot formation, blood lipids, the immune response, the inflammation response to injury and

oxidation interaction of a compound with oxygen; in this case, a damaging effect by reactive oxygen.

antioxidant (anti-OX-ih-dant) a compound that protects other compounds from oxygen by itself reacting with oxygen (*anti* means "against"; *oxy* means "oxygen").

linoleic (lin-oh-LAY-ic) **acid** and **linolenic** (lin-oh-LEN-ic) **acid** polyunsaturated fatty acids that are essential nutrients for human beings.

To read about a possible relationship between polyunsaturated fatty acids and cancer, see Chapter 11.

omega-6 fatty acid a polyunsaturated fatty acid with its endmost double bond six carbons from the end of the carbon chain; long recognized as important in nutrition. Linoleic acid is an example.

omega-3 fatty acid a polyunsaturated fatty acid with its endmost double bond three carbons from the end of its carbon chain; relatively newly recognized as important in nutrition. Linolenic acid is an example.

EPA, DHA eicosapentaenoic acid, docosahexaenoic acid; omega-3 fatty acids made from linolenic acid in the tissues of fish.

These fish provide at least 1 gram of omega-3 fatty acids, including EPA and DHA, in 100 grams of fish (about 3.5 ounces):*

- ✔ Anchovy, European.
- ✔ Bluefish.
- ✔ Capelin conch.
- ✔ Herring, Atlantic, Pacific.
- ✔ Mackerel, Atlantic, chub, Japanese horse, or king.
- ✔ Mullet.
- ✔ Sablefish.
- ✔ Salmon, all varieties.†
- ✔ Saury.
- ✔ Scad, Muroaji.
- ✔ Sprat.
- ✔ Sturgeon, Atlantic or common.
- ✔ Trout, lake.
- ✔ Tuna, white albacore or bluefin (not light tuna).
- ✔ Whitefish, lake.

*The oil content of a species varies with the season and location.

†Canned varieties may be high in sodium.

infection, and many others.[16]* Essential fatty acids also serve as structural parts of cell membranes.

A deficiency of an essential fatty acid in the diet leads to observable changes in cells, some more subtle than others. When the diet is deficient in *all* of the polyunsaturated fatty acids, symptoms of reproductive failure, skin abnormalities, and kidney and liver disorders appear. In children, growth is retarded. Luckily, these deficiency disorders are seldom seen except when intentionally induced in research. They sometimes do arise, however, on rare occasions when inadequate diets are provided by mistake. One such mistake is to feed hospital clients a formula lacking essential fatty acids through a vein for long periods. Another is to feed infants exclusively on a formula that lacks polyunsaturated fatty acids. Normal food, and especially a balanced diet that includes grains, seeds, nuts, leafy vegetables, and fish, supplies all the needed forms of fatty acids in abundance and prevents deficiencies.

Linoleic acid is the primary member of a group of fatty acids named the **omega-6 fatty acid** family after their chemical structure. The body can convert linoleic acid to the other members of its omega-6 family, and these play active parts in body functioning. One plays a critical role in the cell membranes that define and protect each cell of the body. Any diet that contains vegetable oils, seeds, nuts, and whole-grain products supplies enough linoleic acid to meet the body's needs. Almost everyone eats enough.

Linolenic acid is the primary member of the **omega-3 fatty acid** family. This family has come to be appreciated for its role in health. These fatty acids comprise a large part of the brain's thinking part, the cerebral cortex, and of the eye's main center of vision, the retina. Additionally, omega-3 fatty acids are converted to hormone-like products that play roles that affect the heart. Someone thought to ask why the native people of Greenland and Alaska, who eat a diet very high in fat, have such a low death rate from heart disease.[17] The trail led to the abundance of fish and other marine life that they eat, then to the oils in those fish, and finally to two omega-3 fatty acids, **EPA** and **DHA,** in the oils. These fatty acids can be made in the body from linolenic acid to some extent or can be derived from some foods, especially fatty fish.

No Recommended Dietary Allowances (RDA) for omega-6 and omega-3 fatty acids now exist, but scientists may agree to include them in the future. Meanwhile the advice of the experts is this: eat meals of fish two or three times a week, as well as small amounts of vegetable oils, to obtain the right balance between omega-3 and omega-6 intakes. The ratio of intakes of omega-3 to omega-6 fatty acids should be about 1 to 4.[18] This ratio may even turn out to be the key to human requirements; more omega-3 acids may not necessarily be better.[19] Even one fatty fish meal per week has been associated with a reduced risk of heart attack and people who eat more than a fish meal a week suffer from strokes only half as often as those who eat no fish.[20] Purchasing and taking fish oil supplements is not recommended, as this chapter's Consumer Corner points out.

✔ **KEY POINT** **Two polyunsaturated fatty acids, linoleic acid (an omega-6 acid) and linolenic acid (an omega-3 acid), are essential nutrients used to**

*The hormonelike derivatives referred to here are short-lived *eicosanoid* (eye-COSS-a-noid) compounds, such as prostaglandins and thromboxanes.

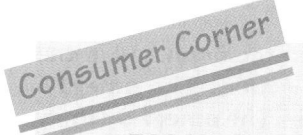

FISH OIL SUPPLEMENTS

Readers of books and magazines may see claims about fish oil: it cures arthritis, prevents cancer, reverses heart disease, or boosts the immune system. While all these claims are linked to some research, proof that fish oil can do these things for individuals or populations is lacking. Most research about fish oil and cancer consists of studies using rats as subjects, and so cannot be directly applied to human beings. The research on heart disease is more convincing than that on cancer, but it does not indicate that people can reverse the effects of smoking or being overweight simply by taking capsules of fish oil.

The Food and Drug Administration (FDA) disallows labeling claims that fish oil supplements can prevent or cure diseases because these effects are unproved.[21] The bulk of evidence supports the idea that food choices make a difference, however. Replacing two or three meals of meat each week with fish can support heart health, especially when the person takes other steps, such as increasing physical activity.[22] Eating no fish seems clearly detrimental to heart health.[23]

The idea that fish oil is beneficial and safe in any amount is erroneous. Overdoses from supplements can alter blood lipids and blood clotting and may worsen Type II diabetes.[24] Some question also remains concerning the very population that led to this line of research—Greenlanders have a high incidence of fatal strokes.

No one knows whether strokes may be related to high intakes of fish oils.[25] Omega-3 fatty acids are preferentially taken up by the brain, however. They are also among the most vulnerable of the lipids to damage by oxidation. Research subjects taking fish oil capsules experienced an increase in oxidative cell damage of 122 percent.[26] Vitamin E in high doses prevented the increase, but scientists are still working to discover how much vitamin E is needed to protect cells.[27]

Overdoses may also impair immune function.[28] Even low-dose supplements produce an undesirable elevation of LDL cholesterol. Large (7 ounces) daily servings of fatty fish have also been observed to elevate LDL cholesterol.[29] Another drawback is that fish oil supplements are made from fish skins and livers, which may have accumulated toxic concentrations of pesticides, heavy metals, and other ocean contaminants that may, in turn, be concentrated in the pills. Moreover, even without contamination, fish oil naturally contains high levels of the two most potentially toxic vitamins, A and D. Lastly, supplements of fish oil are expensive.

So little is known about the long-term effects of fish oil supplements that taking them is chancy. Besides, eating fish brings other benefits; they are leaner than most other animal protein choices, and they are richer in minerals (with the exception of iron). Go to the source for fish oil—eat fish.

More about vitamin E and other antioxidant vitamins in Controversy 7.

Chapter 14 comes back to the topic of seafood safety.

hydrogenation (high-droh-gen-AY-shun) the process of adding hydrogen to unsaturated fatty acids to make fat more solid and resistant to the chemical change of oxidation.

make hormonelike substances that are prominent in the brain and in the retina of the eye, and that perform many other functions. The omega-6 family includes linoleic acid; seed oils are rich sources. The omega-3 family includes linolenic acid, EPA, and DHA. Fish oils are rich sources of EPA and DHA.

THE EFFECTS OF PROCESSING ON FATS

Vegetable oils comprise most of the added fat in the U.S. diet because fast-food chains use them for frying, food manufacturers add them to processed foods, and consumers tend to choose margarine over butter. Food manufacturers often process vegetable oils in ways that greatly change their effects on the body.

Consumers of vegetable oils may feel safe in choosing them because they are generally less saturated than animal fats. If consumers choose a liquid oil, they may be justified in feeling secure. If the choice is a processed food, however, their security may be questionable, especially if the word *hydrogenated* appears on the label's ingredient list.

Hydrogenation of Fats

When manufacturers process foods, they often alter the fatty acids in the fat (triglycerides) the foods contain through a process called **hydrogenation.** Hydrogenation of fats makes them stay fresher longer and also changes their physical properties.

Points of unsaturation in fatty acids are like weak spots that are vulnerable to attack by oxygen. Oxidative damage is not confined to fats within body tissues but occurs anywhere oxygen mixes with fats. When the unsaturated points in the oils of food are oxidized, the oils become rancid. This is why cooking oils should be stored in tightly covered containers that exclude air. If stored for long periods, they need refrigeration to retard oxidation.

One way to prevent spoilage of unsaturated fats and also to make them harder is to change their fatty acids chemically by hydrogenation, as shown in Figure 5-12. When food producers want to use a polyunsaturated oil such as corn oil to make a spreadable margarine, for example, they hydrogenate it by forcing hydrogen into the oil. Some of the unsaturated fatty acids become more saturated as they accept the hydrogen, and the oil becomes harder. The product that results is more saturated and more spreadable than the original oil. It is also more resistant to damage from oxidation.

Once hydrogenated, oils lose their unsaturated character and the health benefits that go with it. An alternative to hydrogenation is to add a chemical preservative that will compete for oxygen and thus protect the oil. The additives are antioxidants, and they work just as vitamin E does, by reacting with oxygen before it can do damage. Examples are the well-known additives BHA and BHT* listed on snack food labels. Another alternative, already mentioned, is to keep the product refrigerated.

If you, the consumer, are looking for polyunsaturated oils to include in your diet, hydrogenated oils such as those in shortening or stick margarine will not

---

*BHA and BHT are butylated hydroxyanisole and butylated hydroxytoluene.

FIGURE 5-12

**HOW HYDROGENATION MAKES FATS
MORE SATURATED**

Points of unsaturation are places on fatty acid chains where hydrogen is missing. The bonds that would normally be occupied by hydrogen in a saturated fatty acid are shared, reluctantly, as a double bond between two carbons that both carry a slightly negative charge.

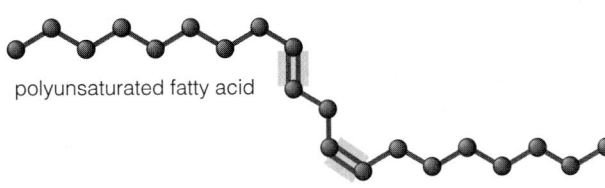

polyunsaturated fatty acid

When positively charged hydrogen is made available to one of those bonds, it readily accepts the hydrogen molecules and, in the process, becomes saturated. It no longer has a point of unsaturation.

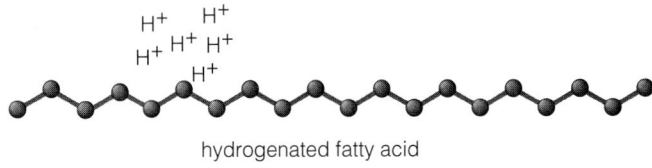

hydrogenated fatty acid

meet your need. Hydrogenated oils are easy to handle and store well. They also have a high **smoking point,** so they are suitable for purposes such as frying. Hydrogenated oils are more saturated than the oils from which they are made, however. In contrast, margarines that list liquid oil as the first ingredient are usually the most polyunsaturated, especially those made from highly unsaturated oils, such as safflower or canola. Margarines that are sold in tubs or squeeze bottles or labeled "soft" are sometimes less saturated than the stick varieties.

smoking point the temperature at which fat gives off an acrid blue gas.

trans-fatty acids fatty acids with unusual shapes that can arise when polyunsaturated oils are hydrogenated.

✔ KEY POINT   **Vegetable oils become more saturated when they are hydrogenated. Hydrogenated fats resist rancidity better, are firmer textured, and have a higher smoking point than unsaturated oils.**

*Trans-*Fatty Acids

Another concern about hydrogenation of fat centers around a change in chemical structure that occurs when polyunsaturated oils are hardened by hydrogenation processing. Some of the unsaturated fatty acids, instead of becoming saturated, end up changing their shapes (Figure 5-13). This creates unusual products that are not made by the body and that occur naturally mainly in dairy foods and beef and only to a limited extent.[30] These changed fatty acids, or ***trans-*fatty acids,** have implications for the body's health. In terms of the health of the heart and arteries, they carry a risk falling between those of saturated and unsaturated fats.[31] The risk arises because *trans-*fatty acids elevate serum LDL cholesterol and possibly lower beneficial HDL.[32] Also, a high total fat consumption is also associated with cancer susceptibility, and *trans-*fatty acids contribute to the total fat intake. No strong evidence suggests that *trans-*fatty acids by *themselves* play any specific role in promoting or causing cancer, however.[33]

When news of *trans-*fatty acids' effects on heart health first emerged, some people hastily switched from using margarine back to butter, believing oversimplified reports that margarine provided no heart health advantage over butter. It is true that most margarines and virtually all shortenings are made largely from hydrogenated fats and therefore are saturated and contain substantial *trans-*fatty acids—up to 40 percent. Some margarines, however, especially the soft or liquid varieties, are made from unhydrogenated oils. These

FIGURE 5-13

A *TRANS-*FATTY ACID

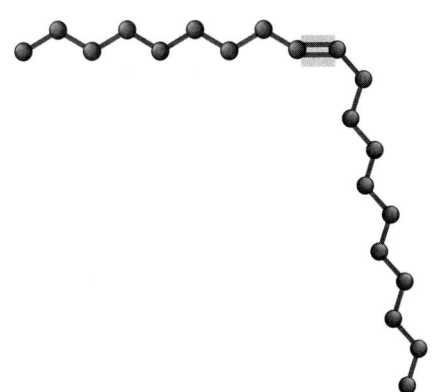

fat replacers substances added to a food that replace some or all of the fat in the food.

artificial fats zero-energy fat replacers that are chemically synthesized to mimic the sensory and cooking qualities of naturally occurring fats, but are totally or partially resistant to digestion. Also called *fat analogues*.

have long proved to be less likely to elevate serum cholesterol than the saturated fats of butter.

In regard to serum cholesterol, margarine may be just a small contributor. Foods other than margarine contribute far more *trans*-fatty acids to the diet—and more total fat, too.[34] Fast foods, chips, baked goods, and other commercially prepared foods are high in fats containing up to 50 percent *trans*-fatty acids. Overall, consumers are eating more fats containing *trans*-fatty acids than ever before and they are eating them in the form of processed foods.[35]

Food labels can be misleading in this regard. On the "Nutrition Facts" panels, *trans*-fatty acids are counted with the polyunsaturated fats from which they arose, and not with the saturated fats whose health effects they mimic. Further, fast-food chains advertise foods fried in "vegetable oil" when that oil is a hydrogenated type containing abundant *trans*-fatty acids. Some experts are calling for a separate statement of *trans*-fatty acids on food labels and for more honesty in advertising.[36]

✓ KEY POINT   **The process of hydrogenation creates *trans*-fatty acids. *Trans*-fatty acids act as saturated fats in the body.**

FAT REPLACERS

Today, shoppers choose from thousands of fat-reduced products. Many bakery goods, cheeses, frozen desserts, and other products made with **fat replacers** now offer less than half a gram of fat in a serving. While some of these products contain **artificial fats,** others use conventional ingredients in unconventional ways to achieve calorie reduction. Among the latter, manufacturers can:

- Add water or whip air into foods.
- Add nonfat milk to creamy foods.
- Use lean meats and soy protein to replace high-fat meats.
- Bake foods instead of frying them.

Other common food ingredients such as fibers, sugars, or proteins can also take the place of some food fats. Products made this way still provide calories, but far fewer calories from fat.

Many manufactured fat replacers are chemical derivatives of carbohydrate, protein, or fat. Carbohydrate-based fat replacers include dextrins, modified food starches, and gums. Maltodextrin, from corn, is flavored to resemble the taste of butter and melts like it when sprinkled as a powder on hot, moist foods such as baked potatoes. Oatrim, derived from oat fiber, has the added advantage of providing satiety—it makes the eater feel fuller. A related product, Z-trim, is a modified form of insoluble fiber that feels like fat in the mouth and can be used in some forms of cooking, but not frying. Gels used to make fat-free margarines mimic the texture of real margarine and can meet some baking needs. However, a cook who tries using a gel-based product for frying an egg or other food ends up with a panful of burned, sticky gum.

To gain the FDA's consent for the use of a new fat replacer in the food supply, U.S. manufacturers must prove that their fat replacer contributes little food energy, is nontoxic, is not stored in body tissues, and does not rob the body of needed nutrients. Two fat replacers of interest are Simplesse and the recently approved olestra.

Simplesse

The only protein-based fat replacement to receive FDA approval to date is **Simplesse,** developed for use in ice cream desserts and dairy products. Simplesse is digested and absorbed in the body, but it contributes just 4 *protein* calories per gram—a dramatic reduction from fat's 9 calories per gram. Further, just 1 gram of Simplesse replaces 3 to 4 grams of fat, greatly enhancing the calorie savings.[37] Watch out, though: some manufacturers add so much extra sugar to their fat-free ice cream that it contains almost as many calories as regular ice cream.

To make Simplesse, the manufacturer processes the proteins of milk or egg white into mistlike particles that roll over the tongue, making Simplesse feel and taste like fat. Its protein nature makes Simplesse useless for frying or baking, but it melts on hot foods, so we may soon see a Simplesse spread for toast.

Because Simplesse is changed physically, not chemically, the body handles it like protein from any other source. Also, since the proteins remain intact, people with allergies to egg or milk may have to avoid Simplesse.

✔ **KEY POINT**   **Simplesse, a protein-based fat replacer, replaces fat in ice cream desserts at a great savings in fat calories. People with milk or egg allergy may have to avoid Simplesse.**

Olestra, a Sucrose Polyester

The most recently approved artificial fat is **olestra,** brand name Olean, one member of a synthetic chemical family known as **sucrose polyester.** Olestra's chemical structure bears some similarity to that of regular fat, but olestra passes through the digestive tract unabsorbed.

A sucrose polyester consists of a core molecule of sucrose to which up to eight fatty acid molecules are bonded. In comparison, ordinary triglycerides consist of a core of glycerol to which three fatty acids are bonded. The enzymes that break down triglycerides in the digestive tract do not recognize the shape of the olestra molecule, and so cannot split the fatty acids from their sucrose.

From some points of view, olestra is the most successful of the artificial fats, for its properties are identical to those of fats and oils when used in frying, cooking, and baking. It can be heated to frying temperatures without breaking down; it performs all of the functions of fat in cakes, pie crusts, and other baked goods; and most remarkably—aside from a slight aftertaste—it tastes like fat. Nevertheless, the wonders of olestra must be weighed against evidence concerning its safety.

The company that invented olestra has been studying its safety for more than two decades. The results of the studies revealed that olestra causes digestive distress, nutrient losses, and losses of phytochemicals. The company has addressed each of these problems to the satisfaction of an FDA commission panel, who approved olestra for use in snack foods in 1996. Some nutrition experts disagree with the panel, however, and have come out strongly against olestra's approval. These issues deserve a moment's attention.

Olestra's side effects are rooted in two aspects of its nature. For one thing, because olestra replaces a major food constituent, fat, the substance is consumed in large amounts, measured in many grams per serving. Nonfat potato chips, for example, derive about a third of their weight from olestra. Also, by

Simplesse a protein-based fat replacer useful in cold foods or frozen confections.

olestra a noncaloric artificial fat made from sucrose and fatty acids; formerly called *sucrose polyester.*

sucrose polyester any of a family of compounds in which fatty acids are bonded with sugars or sugar alcohols. Olestra is an example.

design, olestra is indigestible. All of the oily olestra eaten in a food passes through the digestive tract and is excreted from the body.

Digestive Problems   The presence of olestra in the large intestine causes diarrhea, gas, cramping, and an urgent need for defecation in some people. Further, the oil can creep through the feces and leak uncontrollably from the anus, producing smelly dark yellow stains on underwear. No one yet knows who is most likely to encounter these effects, but some of these symptoms almost always occur when olestra is consumed in large quantities. The FDA commission that approved olestra decided that the digestive problems of olestra were unpleasant, but did not constitute a safety problem.

Nutrient Losses   Whenever olestra is present in the digestive tract, it dissolves fat-soluble substances in the foods being digested. For example, some vitamins dissolve in fat, and all of these (vitamins A, D, E, and K) become unavailable for absorption when olestra is present in a meal. Thus, when olestra-containing chips are eaten with other foods, the vitamins those foods contain are entrapped, and the eater is robbed of those vitamins. To compensate for this effect, olestra will be fortified with vitamin E and other vitamins. The FDA ruled that fortification removes the threat of harm from malnutrition that olestra could otherwise cause.

Other Losses   A related problem, and one to which olestra's opponents object vigorously, is the loss of many important phytochemicals from foods. Phytochemicals and their effects are described in Controversy 7. As an example, members of the carotene family, consumed over a lifetime, have been linked with prevention of a degenerative eye condition that affects many people as they age. One recent study showed that just 3 grams of olestra a day strongly reduced (by about 40 percent) the blood concentrations of lycopene, a phytochemical believed to defend the health of the eyes.[38] No studies exist to predict the effects, if any, of lifelong olestra exposure or the effects of olestra on growing children, and children often favor the foods in which olestra is allowed.

✓ **KEY POINT**   **Olestra is a lipid-based, zero-calorie, artificial fat approved for use in snack foods. Its use can cause side effects that are unpleasant, but have not been proved harmful; olestra's long-term effects are unknown.**

Fat Replacers and Weight Control

People hope, of course, that fat replacers will help fight both obesity and heart disease by lowering fat intakes. The question remains whether eating fat replacers will actually do these things. If the U.S. experience with artificial sweeteners, described in Controversy 4, is any guide, consumers are likely to eat fat-replacer products *in addition* to other high-fat foods they prefer, negating the potential benefits of the fat replacers. Preliminary studies seem to indicate that while fat replacers can cut overall fat intakes, people eating fat replacers make up for lost calories by eating more total food. The chances for weight loss, therefore, are slim.

The FDA requires olestra-containing foods to bear this warning:

"This Product Contains Olestra. Olestra may cause abdominal cramping and loose stools. Olestra inhibits the absorption of some vitamins and other nutrients. Vitamins A, D, E, and K have been added."

Used wisely, fat replacers may help some consumers achieve some of their dietary goals.[39] The next section shows where the fat resides in foods and the Food Feature gives practical advice about cutting fat in time-tested ways.

✔ KEY POINT   **More research is needed to determine whether fat reducers are effective agents for achieving weight loss or reduction of heart disease risk.**

FAT IN THE DIET

The remainder of this chapter shows you how to choose the right kinds of fat, and the right amounts, to provide optimal health and pleasure in eating. As you read, notice which foods offer naturally occurring fats and those to which fats are often added so that you can recognize both fat sources in the diet. Another useful distinction is between unsaturated fat items and saturated fat items. Your choices among them can make a difference in the unseen condition of your arteries. Labels of processed foods in the United States must now state the grams of total fat and of saturated fat.

In the Food Guide Pyramid, two groups always contain fat (the fats and the meats and nuts), and two sometimes contain fat (the milk and milk products and the breads). Most unprocessed vegetables and fruits are fat-free, but two exceptions are rich in monounsaturated fat—avocados and olives. In their natural states, grains are like fruits and vegetables in that they contain little or no fat. Keep in mind that fats may be visible on foods, such as the fat trimmed from a steak, or they may be invisible, such as the fats in the marbling of meat, the fat ground into lunch meats, or the fats in avocados, biscuits, cheese, coconuts, other nuts, olives, or fried foods.* Before reading on, look at the sandwich depicted in the margin. As you learn about the fats in foods, think of ways to reduce the fat in the sandwich. One reduced-fat version appears later, on page 177.

Added Fats

A dollop of dessert topping, a spread of butter on bread, oil or shortening in a recipe, dressing on a salad—all of these are examples of *added* fats. As a student of dietetics once pointed out: it's not so much the food itself, but the preparation that adds fat to the diet. Indeed, all sorts of fats can be added to foods during commercial or home preparation or at the table. The following amounts of these fats contain about 5 grams of pure fat, providing 45 calories and negligible protein and carbohydrate:

- 1 teaspoon oil or shortening.
- 1½ teaspoon mayonnaise, butter, or margarine.
- 1 tablespoon regular salad dressing, cream cheese, or heavy cream.
- 1½ tablespoon sour cream.

These foods provide the majority of added fats to the diet. They are the hidden fats of fried foods or baked goods, sauces and mixed dishes, and dips and spreads.

---

*Coconut is a nut, not a vegetable, although its oil is listed among vegetable oils.

A FAT QUIZ

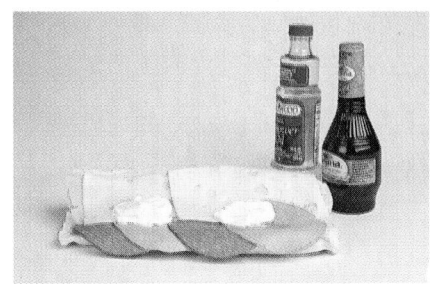

Here's a typical hoagie sandwich with 4 slices of cold cuts and 4 slices of cheese. It offers 60 grams fat, 28 of them saturated fat, and 630 calories. As you read this section, create a sandwich of your own, but with less fat and fewer calories.

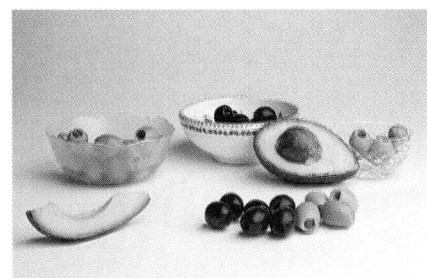

Ten small olives or a sixth of an avocado each provide about 5 grams of mostly monounsaturated fat.

✔ KEY POINT   **Fats added to foods during preparation or at the table are a major source of fat in the diet.**

Meat, Poultry, Fish, Dry Beans, Eggs, and Nuts Group

Meats conceal much of the fat—mostly saturated fat—that people unwittingly consume. Many people, when choosing a serving of meat, don't realize that they are electing to eat a large amount of fat. To help people "see" the fat in meats, the exchange lists at the back of the book present the meats in four categories according to their fat contents: very lean, lean, medium-fat, and high-fat meats. Meats in all four categories contain about equal amounts of protein, but because their fat contents differ, their calorie amounts vary significantly. Figure 5-13 shows fat and calorie data for some ground meats.

According to the Food Guide Pyramid, a serving of meat amounts to just 2 or 3 ounces—a size considered very small compared with average consumption standards. A small, fast-food hamburger, for example, weighs about 3 ounces. A steak served in a restaurant averages 12 to 16 ounces, more than a whole day's meat allowance. Of course, your judgment of what is normal differs from other people's, and you may have to weigh a serving or two of meat to see how much you are eating.

People think of meat as protein food, but calculation of its nutrient content shows a surprising fact. A big (4-ounce), fast-food hamburger sandwich contains 23 grams of protein and 20 grams of fat. Because protein offers 4 calories per gram and fat offers 9, the sandwich provides 92 calories from protein and 180 calories from fat. The calorie total, counting carbohydrates from the bun and condiments, is over 400 calories, with over 50 percent of them from fat. Hot dogs, fried chicken sandwiches, and fried fish sandwiches are also high-fat choices. Because so much of the energy in a meat eater's diet is hidden from view, people can easily overeat on high-fat food, making weight control difficult.

Animal breeders have been striving to produce beef and pork that are lower in fat. This is a help to those shoppers who choose lean cuts: they get less fat in the same quantity of meat. When choosing beef or pork, look for lean cuts named *loin* or *round* from which the fat can be trimmed. Eat small portions, too.

Chicken and turkey meat is also naturally lean, but processing and frying add fats, especially in "patties," "nuggets," "fingers," or "wings." Chicken wings are mostly skin, and a chicken stores most of its fat just under its skin. The tastiest wing snacks have also been fried in cooking fat (often a saturated type), smothered with a buttery, spicy sauce, and then dipped in blue cheese dressing, making wings an extraordinarily high-fat snack. A person who snacks on wings should plan on eating low-fat foods at other meals to balance them out.

Many people are confused, with good reason, by meat labels that state "percent fat-free" values on the front panels. Take a package of chicken hot dogs for example. The front label might proclaim "94% fat-free." A nutrition-minded consumer might feel encouraged by the label, thinking that the hot dogs supply only 6 percent of their *calories* from fat. In reality, this thinking is wrong. The value on the front label refers to *weight*, not to calories. On reading the Nutrition Facts panel and calculating the percentage of calories from fat, the person would be surprised to learn that the hot dogs actually supply 30 percent of their *calories* from fat.

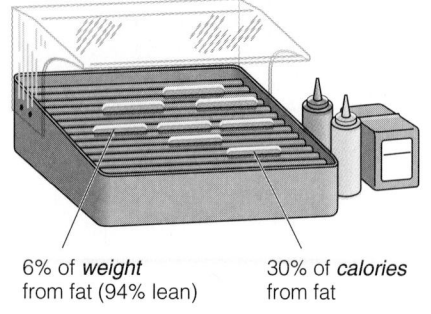

6% of *weight* from fat (94% lean)   30% of *calories* from fat

Same hot dog; two points of view.

FIGURE 5-14

FAT IN GROUND MEATS

Note that only the ground round, at 7 percent fat by weight, qualifies to bear the "lean" label. To be called "lean," products must contain fewer than 10 grams fat, 4 grams saturated fat, and 95 milligrams cholesterol per 100 grams of food. The numbers that qualify products to be called "extra lean" are, respectively, 5, 2, and 95. The red labels on these packages list rules for safe meat handling, explained in Chapter 14.

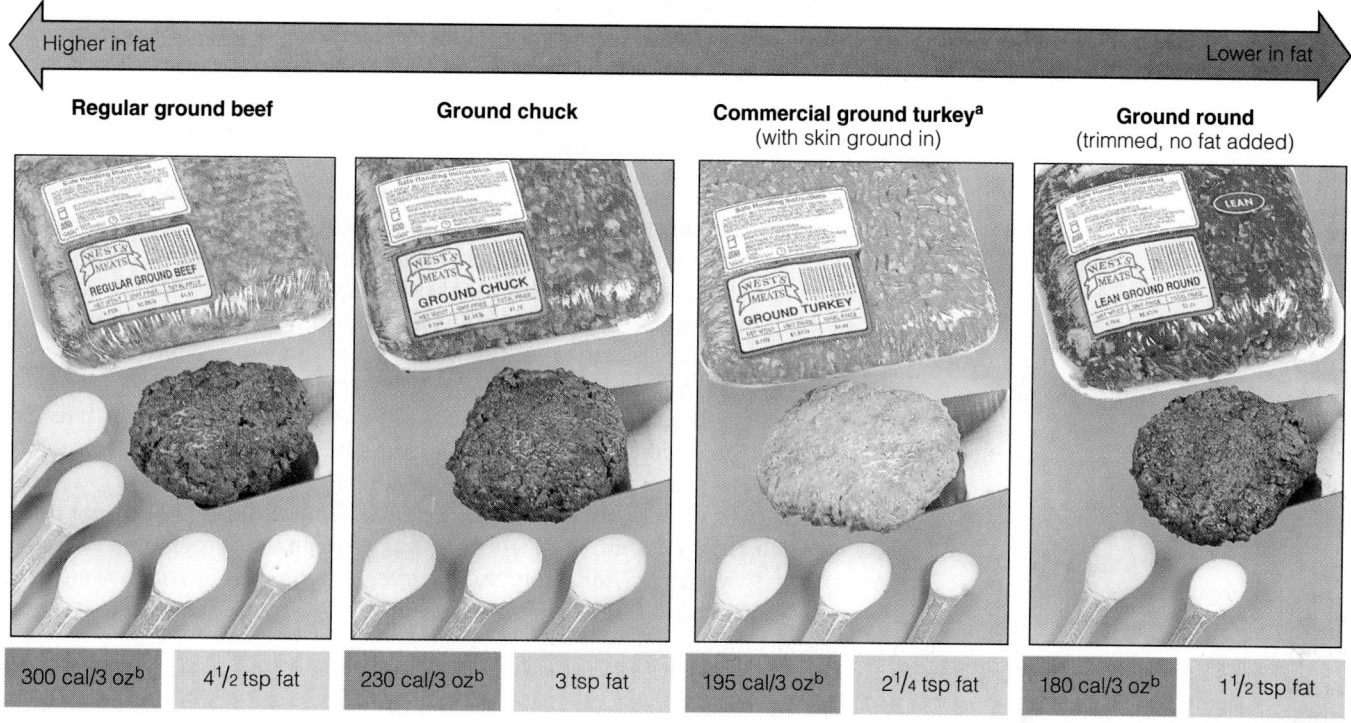

Regular ground beef	Ground chuck	Commercial ground turkey[a] (with skin ground in)	Ground round (trimmed, no fat added)
300 cal/3 oz[b]	230 cal/3 oz[b]	195 cal/3 oz[b]	180 cal/3 oz[b]
4 1/2 tsp fat	3 tsp fat	2 1/4 tsp fat	1 1/2 tsp fat

[a]Values for 3 ounces of cooked turkey breast ground without skin are 108 calories and 1/2 teaspoon fat (25% calories from fat). This type is not typically offered in many areas, but can be specially ordered from the butcher.

[b]The 3-ounce cooked serving used here may seem small to some but it is the largest allowable meat serving according to the Daily Food Guide. Larger servings will, of course, provide more fat and calories than the values listed here.

The consumer might be tempted to report an error in labeling to the hot dog manufacturer, but the label is not in error. The USDA allows some food packages to state the percentage of fat by weight; this number is virtually meaningless to those concerned with nutrition, however. The lean (fat-free) weight of the product includes water weight, and water throws off the fat calculation by contributing to the lean fraction of the product's weight without contributing to its calories. In other words, water "bulks up" the lean part of a product, making the fat portion seem smaller by comparison. About 63% of the hot dog's weight is from water; protein contributes just over 14 percent of the non-water weight; pure fat weighs in at 6 percent; carbohydrate, minerals, and other minor constituents make up the difference.

In the same way, watch out for ground turkey or chicken products. Many of these have the skin ground in to add moistness when cooked, and they can be much higher in fat than even lean beef, as Figure 5-14 has already shown. The labels of meat products may state "lower in fat," but ask yourself, "lower than what?" The box of terms that appeared on pages 56 and 57 in Chapter 2 provided some definitions concerning the fat contents of meats.

✔ **KEY POINT** **Meats hide a large proportion of the fat in many people's diets. Most people consume meat in larger servings than those recommended. Labels on processed meats often express fat as a percentage of product weight, which is not the same as percentage of calories from fat.**

Milk, Yogurt, and Cheese Group

Some milk products contain fat. In homogenizing whole milk, milk processors blend in the cream, which otherwise would float and could be removed by skimming. A cup of whole milk, then, contains the protein and carbohydrate of skim milk, but in addition contains about 60 extra calories from fat. A cup of low-fat (2 percent) milk is halfway between whole and nonfat, with 30 calories of fat. The fat occupies only a teaspoon or two of the volume but nearly doubles the calories in the milk.

Milk labels work the same way as those of meat. Would you guess that "2% milk" provides 37 percent of its calories from fat? It does, because so much of milk's weight is comprised of water. Water contributes almost 90 percent of the fat-free weight of any form of milk, protein about 3 percent, carbohydrate (lactose) about 5 percent, with the rest from minerals (largely calcium and phosphorus), vitamins, and other substances. A small change in the weight of fat in a food like milk makes a large difference in the percentage of calories from fat, as the margin shows.

Milks vary in fat:

✔ Whole milk = 3.3% fat by weight, 48% of calories from fat.

✔ 2% low-fat milk = 2% fat by weight, 37% of calories from fat.

✔ 1% low-fat milk = 1% fat by weight, 26% of calories from fat.

✔ Nonfat milk = 0% fat by weight, 0% of calories from fat.*

*Nonfat milk contains a trace of fat, but an amount too small to count.

FIGURE 5-15

LIPIDS IN MILK, YOGURT, AND CHEESE

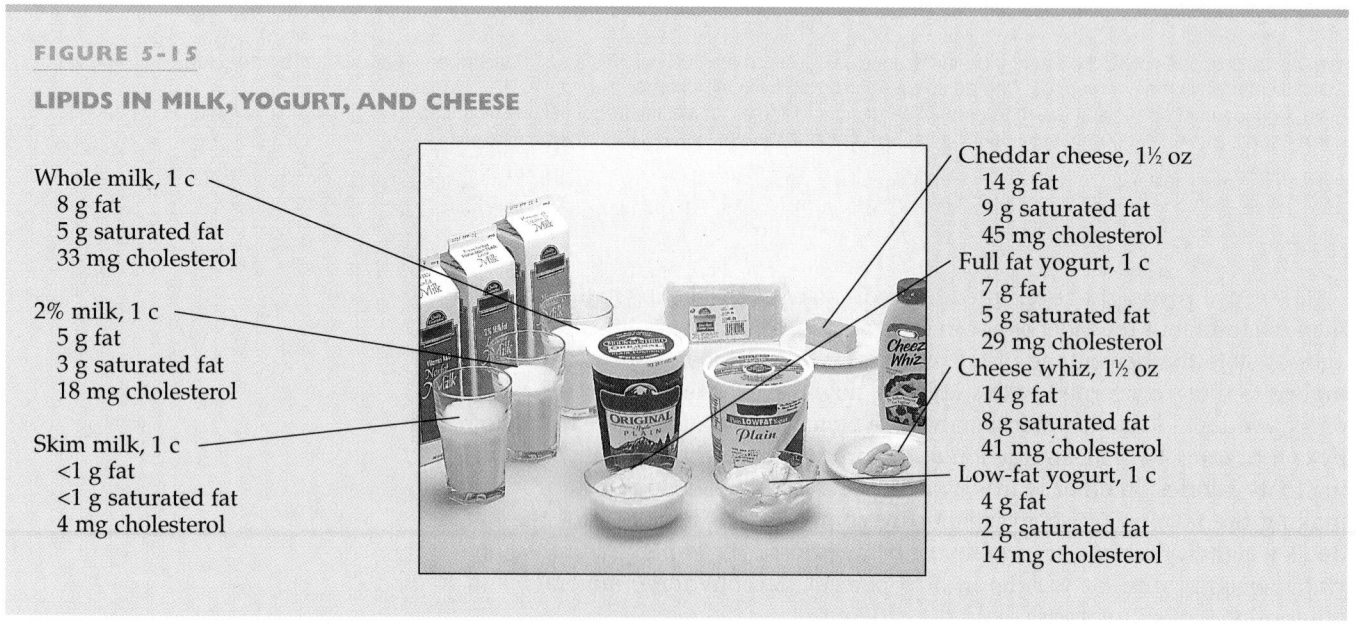

Whole milk, 1 c
  8 g fat
  5 g saturated fat
  33 mg cholesterol

2% milk, 1 c
  5 g fat
  3 g saturated fat
  18 mg cholesterol

Skim milk, 1 c
  <1 g fat
  <1 g saturated fat
  4 mg cholesterol

Cheddar cheese, 1½ oz
  14 g fat
  9 g saturated fat
  45 mg cholesterol

Full fat yogurt, 1 c
  7 g fat
  5 g saturated fat
  29 mg cholesterol

Cheese whiz, 1½ oz
  14 g fat
  8 g saturated fat
  41 mg cholesterol

Low-fat yogurt, 1 c
  4 g fat
  2 g saturated fat
  14 mg cholesterol

FIGURE 5-16

LIPIDS IN BREAD, CEREAL, RICE, AND PASTA

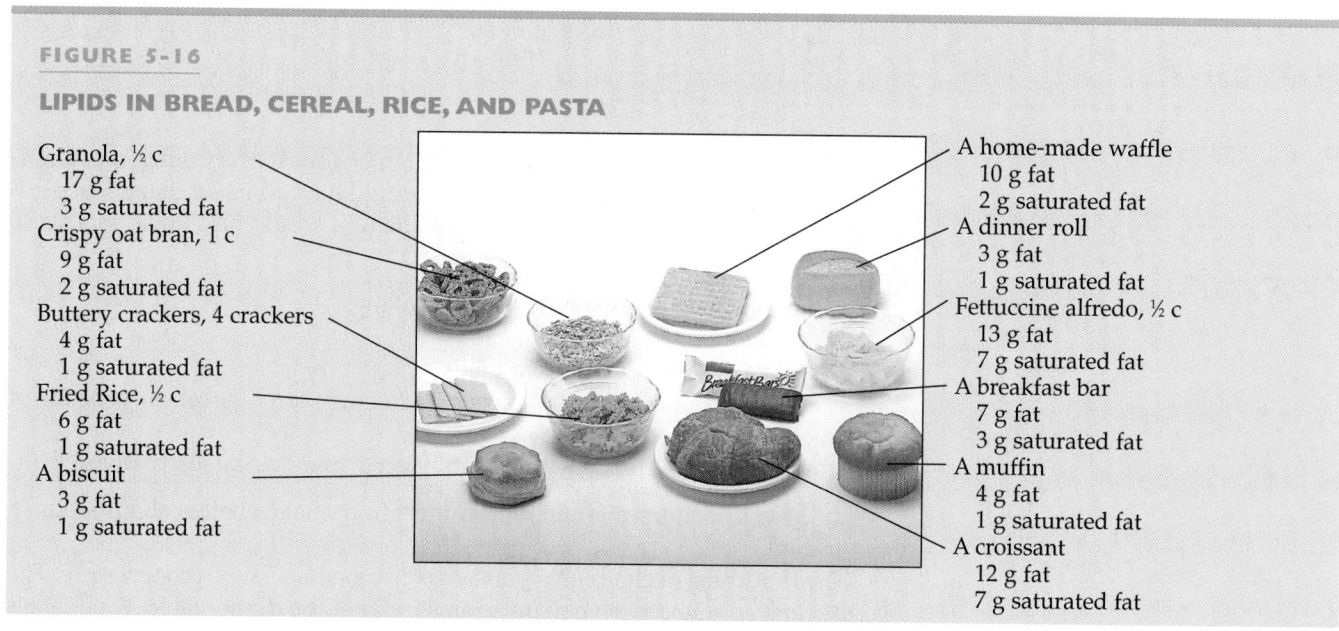

Granola, ½ c
   17 g fat
   3 g saturated fat
Crispy oat bran, 1 c
   9 g fat
   2 g saturated fat
Buttery crackers, 4 crackers
   4 g fat
   1 g saturated fat
Fried Rice, ½ c
   6 g fat
   1 g saturated fat
A biscuit
   3 g fat
   1 g saturated fat

A home-made waffle
   10 g fat
   2 g saturated fat
A dinner roll
   3 g fat
   1 g saturated fat
Fettuccine alfredo, ½ c
   13 g fat
   7 g saturated fat
A breakfast bar
   7 g fat
   3 g saturated fat
A muffin
   4 g fat
   1 g saturated fat
A croissant
   12 g fat
   7 g saturated fat

Milk and yogurt appear in the milk group, but cream and butter do not. Milk and yogurt are rich in calcium and protein, but cream and butter are not. Cream and butter are fats, as are whipped cream, sour cream, and cream cheese. That is why the food group that includes milk is carefully called the "milk, yogurt, and cheese group," and not the "dairy group." Figure 5-15 shows where the lipids are found in various kinds of milk, yogurt, and cheese.

✔ KEY POINT   **The choice between whole and nonfat milk products can make a large difference to the fat content of a diet.**

Bread, Cereal, Rice, and Pasta Group

Breads and cereals in their natural state are very low in fat, but they also may contain fat added during processing or cooking. The fat in these foods can be particularly hard to detect, and so diners must remember which foods stand out as being high in fat. Notable are granola and certain other ready-to-eat cereals, croissants, biscuits, cornbread, dinner rolls, fried rice, pasta with creamy or oily sauces, quick breads, snack and party crackers, muffins, pancakes, and home made waffles. Packaged breakfast bars often resemble candy bars in their fat and sugar contents. Figure 5-16 shows the lipid contents of many grain products.

✔ KEY POINT   **Fat in breads and cereals can be well hidden. Consumers must learn which foods of this group contain fats.**

Now that you know where the fats in foods are found, how can you reduce or eliminate them from your diet? The Food Feature that follows provides some pointers.

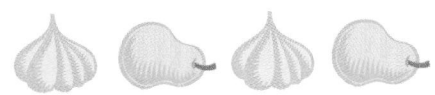

To meet the most important recommendation of almost every nutrition authority—to reduce dietary fats—most people would have to make changes according to the following five principles. The changes would also lower intakes of saturated fat.

1. Eliminate fat as a seasoning and in cooking.
2. Cut down on intake of red meat.
3. Remove the fat from high-fat foods.
4. Replace high-fat foods with specially manufactured lower-fat versions of those foods.
5. Replace high-fat foods with naturally occurring low-fat alternatives.[40]

With these principles in mind, you can begin to make choices about foods in your diet.

The first arena of choice that you as a consumer face is the grocery store. The right choices here can save many grams of fat at the dinner table. Food labels can reveal much about a processed food's fat content. Once you figure out whether or not a food is high in fat, the choice of whether to consume it depends on how you intend to use it in your diet: as a staple item, or as an occasional treat.

Once at home, one of the most effective steps for reducing fats is to limit fats used as seasonings.[41] This means serving cooked vegetables without butter, bacon, or margarine; omitting high-fat gravies and sauces; and leaving off other last-minute fat additions. Butter and regular margarine contain the same number of calories (45 per teaspoon); diet margarine contains fewer calories because water, air, or fillers have been added. Imitation butter flavoring contains no fat and few calories.

For snacks, use an air popper for popcorn, and then add butter flavoring to the popcorn, if you like it. Keep that flavoring on hand together with other low-fat cooking substitutes such as diet margarine, low-fat salad dressings, nonfat sauce mixes or recipes, and nonstick spray for frying. To replace high-fat ingredients in recipes, check Table 5-3 for hints. These replacements will not change the finished product too much, except for dramatically lowering its contents of fat and saturated fat.

If you must add fats, be sure that they are detectable in the food and that you enjoy them. For example, if you use strongly flavored fat, a little goes a long way. Sesame oil, peanut butter, and the fats of strong cheeses are equal in calories to others, but they are so strongly flavored that you can use much less. Try small amounts of grated sapsago, romano, or other hard cheeses to replace larger amounts of less flavorful cheeses.

If you use oils, trade off among types to obtain the benefits different oils offer. Peanut and safflower oils are especially rich in vitamin E. Olive and canola oil present the heart health benefits associated with monounsaturates, mentioned earlier. Canola oil also contains omega-3 fatty acids. High temperatures, such as those used in frying, destroy omega-3 acids.

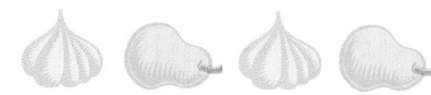

TABLE 5-3

Substitutes for High-Fat Ingredients

Use	Instead of
Nonfat milk products	Whole-milk products
Evaporated nonfat ("skim") milk (canned)	Cream
Yogurt[a] or fat-free sour cream replacer	Sour cream
Reduced-calorie margarine; butter replacers	Butter
Wine, lemon juice, or broth	Butter
Fruit butters	Butter
Part-skim or fat-free ricotta; low-fat or fat-free cottage cheese	Whole-milk ricotta
Part-skim, low-fat, or fat-free cheeses	Regular cheeses
1 tbs cornstarch (for thickening sauces)	1 egg yolk
Low-fat or fat-free mayonnaise	Regular mayonnaise
Low-fat or fat-free salad dressing (for salads and marinades)	Regular salad dressing
Water-packed canned fish and meats	Oil-packed fish and meats
Lean ground meat and grain mixture	Ground beef
Low-fat frozen yogurt or sherbet	Ice cream
Herbs, lemons, spices, fruits, liquid smoke flavoring, or oil-free dressings	Butter, bacon fat

[a]If the recipe is to be boiled, the yogurt or cottage cheese must be stabilized with a small amount of cornstarch or flour.

Here are some other tips to update old, high-fat recipes:

- Grill, roast, broil, boil, bake, stir-fry, microwave, or poach foods. Don't fry in fat.
- Add a little water or nonfat yogurt to thick, bottled salad dressings and then apply them sparingly. They'll go farther this way, and you'll use less oil.
- Cut recipe amounts of meat in half; use only lean meats. Fill in the lost bulk with shredded vegetables, legumes, pasta, grains, or other low-fat items.
- Trim all visible fat and skin from meat and poultry.
- Refrigerate meat pan drippings and broth, and lift off the fat when it solidifies. Then add the defatted broth to a recipe.
- Make prepared mixes, such as rice or potato mixtures, without the fats called for on the label. The taste is practically unchanged.

All of these suggestions work well when a person carefully plans, selects, purchases, and prepares each meal with the loving attention it deserves. But in the real world, people sometimes fall behind schedule and don't have time to cook, so they eat fast food. Figure 5-17 shows that while some fast-food choices can be remarkably high in fat and calories, other choices can be reasonable.

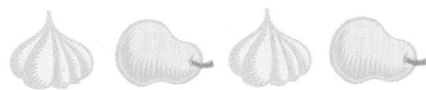

FIGURE 5-17

FAST-FOOD CHOICES

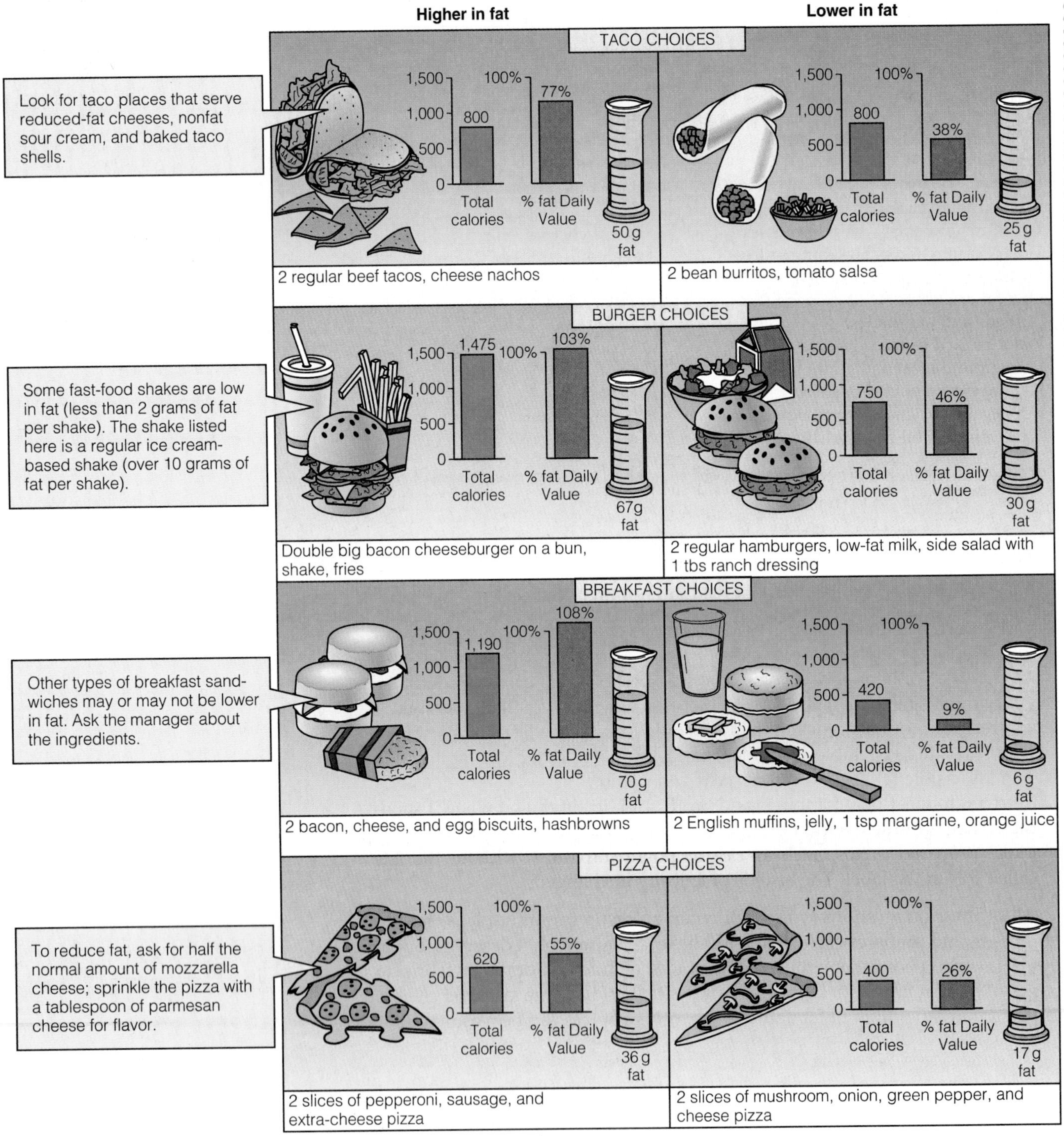

Higher in fat   **Lower in fat**

TACO CHOICES

Look for taco places that serve reduced-fat cheeses, nonfat sour cream, and baked taco shells.

800 Total calories | 77% % fat Daily Value | 50 g fat

800 Total calories | 38% % fat Daily Value | 25 g fat

2 regular beef tacos, cheese nachos | 2 bean burritos, tomato salsa

BURGER CHOICES

Some fast-food shakes are low in fat (less than 2 grams of fat per shake). The shake listed here is a regular ice cream-based shake (over 10 grams of fat per shake).

1,475 Total calories | 103% % fat Daily Value | 67 g fat

750 Total calories | 46% % fat Daily Value | 30 g fat

Double big bacon cheeseburger on a bun, shake, fries | 2 regular hamburgers, low-fat milk, side salad with 1 tbs ranch dressing

BREAKFAST CHOICES

Other types of breakfast sandwiches may or may not be lower in fat. Ask the manager about the ingredients.

1,190 Total calories | 108% % fat Daily Value | 70 g fat

420 Total calories | 9% % fat Daily Value | 6 g fat

2 bacon, cheese, and egg biscuits, hashbrowns | 2 English muffins, jelly, 1 tsp margarine, orange juice

PIZZA CHOICES

To reduce fat, ask for half the normal amount of mozzarella cheese; sprinkle the pizza with a tablespoon of parmesan cheese for flavor.

620 Total calories | 55% % fat Daily Value | 36 g fat

400 Total calories | 26% % fat Daily Value | 17 g fat

2 slices of pepperoni, sausage, and extra-cheese pizza | 2 slices of mushroom, onion, green pepper, and cheese pizza

Note: Fat Daily Value based on a 2,000 calorie diet.

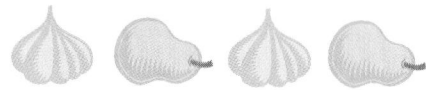

Keep these facts about fast food in mind:

- Salads are a good choice. Avoid mixed salad bar items, such as macaroni salad. Use only about a quarter of the dressing provided or use low-fat dressing.
- If you are really hungry, order a small hamburger on the side. Hold the mayonnaise: use mustard or ketchup instead. A small bowl of chili or a plain baked potato can also satisfy a bigger appetite.
- Fried fish or chicken sandwiches are at least as high in fat as hamburgers. Broiled sandwiches are far less fatty if you order them made without spreads, dressings, cheese, bacon, or mayonnaise.

Because fast foods are short on variety, let them be part of a lifestyle in which they complement the other parts. Eat differently, often, elsewhere.

By this time you may be wondering if you can realistically make all the changes recommended for your diet and keep high-fat foods completely under control. Be assured that most of the needed changes can easily become habits after a few repetitions. You need not give up all high-fat foods; you need only learn to exercise moderation. The famous French chef Julia Child makes this point about moderation:

An imaginary shelf labeled INDULGENCES is a good idea. It contains the best butter, jumbo-size eggs, heavy cream, marbled steaks, sausages and pâtés, hollandaise and butter sauces, French butter-cream fillings, gooey chocolate cakes, and all those lovely items that demand disciplined rationing. Thus, with these items high up and almost out of reach, we are ever conscious that they are not everyday foods. They are for special occasions, and when that occasion comes we can enjoy every mouthful.

JULIA CHILD, *THE WAY TO COOK*, 1989.

You decide what the treats should be and then choose them judiciously, just for pure pleasure. Meanwhile, make sure that your everyday, ordinary choices are those whole, nutrient-dense foods suggested throughout this book. Use the fat-reducing principles presented here to achieve a diet with an ideal percentage of fat and room left over for favorite foods. That way you'll meet all your body's needs for nutrients and never feel deprived.

Did you design a sandwich that is lower in fat than the original? The photo in the margin presents our ideas—half the cheese, mustard replaces mayonnaise, turkey instead of cold cuts, and lots of vegetables for flavor. To confirm that your sandwich is indeed lower in fats and calories, look up the ingredients in the Table of Food Composition, Appendix A.

QUIZ ANSWER

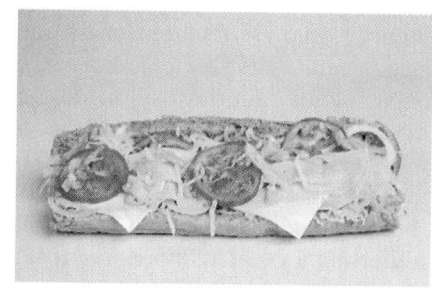

Our choice: 1 ounce cheese and all the vegetables the roll can hold.
25 grams fat.
7 grams saturated fat.
380 calories.
What's your choice?

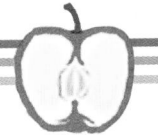

Do It!

READ ABOUT FATS ON FOOD LABELS

Figure 5-18 presents three labels from packages of lasagna and asks you to compare the fat in one serving of each with your day's allowances for fat and saturated fat. Food labels make this comparison easy for people whose energy needs are about 2,000 calories a day. For those people the Daily Values for fat and saturated fat are listed right on the food labels. Other people must perform a few calculations to arrive at meaningful numbers for themselves. This activity asks that you do three things:

■ Calculate your own personal Daily Values for *total fat* and *saturated fat.*

■ Calculate the percentage of your personal Daily Value for *total fat* contributed by each of the lasagnas.

■ Calculate the percentage of your personal Daily Value for *saturated fat* contributed by each of the lasagnas.

Then it asks you some questions.

In calculating your Daily Values for fats, you will use three numbers. First is your RDA for energy (from the inside front cover). Second is the recommendation to consume no more than 30 percent of calories from fat, or 10 percent of calories from saturated fat. The third number arises from the calorie value of fats: 9 calories for every 1 gram of fat.

FIND YOUR PERSONAL DAILY VALUES FOR TOTAL FAT AND SATURATED FAT

Step 1. Calculate your personal Daily Value for total fat. On Form 5-1, section 1, part A, copy your energy RDA from the inside front cover, page C. Transfer your energy RDA to part B and calculate 30 percent of it as shown. In part C, copy the answer of Part B and divide by 9 calories per gram to determine the number of grams of fat as shown. The answer is your personal Daily Value for total fat. Copy it into part D for later use.

Step 2. Calculate your personal Daily Value for saturated fat. On Form 5-1, section 2, part A, write in your personal energy RDA (from part A of section 1.) Transfer your energy RDA to part B and calculate 10 percent of it

as shown. Transfer this number from part B to part C and divide by 9 calories per gram to find grams of saturated fat. The answer is your personal Daily Value for saturated fat. Copy it into part D for later use.

It's wise to memorize your Daily Value for fat and saturated fat and make food choices each day that do not exceed them. These are two of the most valuable numbers you can learn.

COMPARE THE FAT IN A SERVING OF EACH OF THREE LASAGNAS WITH YOUR DAILY VALUES

Step 3. Using Form 5-2, part A, copy the grams of total fat and saturated fat per serving of lasagna from the three package labels of Figure 5-18. Then copy to part B your personal Daily Values for both total fat and saturated fat from Form 5-1. Enter these values on part C of Form 5-2 and calculate the percentage of your Daily Value for total fat presented by each lasagna. Repeat the process for saturated fat in part D.

ANALYSIS

Now use the information you have generated to respond to the following questions:

1. How many grams of fat can you consume in a day and not exceed 30 percent of calories from fat?

2. How many grams of saturated fat can you consume in a day and not exceed 10 percent of calories from saturated fat?

3. Which lasagna is highest in fat per serving? What percentage of your personal Daily Value for fat would this lasagna contribute to your day's intake?

4. What percentages of your personal Daily Value for fat do the other two lasagnas contribute?

(continued on next page)

FIGURE 5-18

COMPARISON OF THREE DIFFERENT LASAGNAS

A

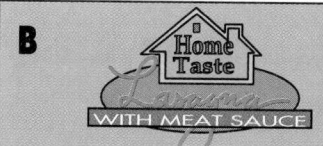

LASAGNA WITH CHEESE & VEGETABLES

Nutrition Facts

Serving size 10^1/$_2$ oz (298g)
Servings per Package 1

Amount per serving

Calories 472	Calories from Fat 252

	% Daily Value*
Total Fat 28g	43%
Saturated Fat 16g	80%
Cholesterol 125mg	42%
Sodium 820mg	34%
Total Carbohydrate 35g	12%
Dietary fiber 4g	16%
Sugars 9g	
Protein 20g	

Vitamin A 25%	•	Vitamin C <2%
Calcium 50%	•	Iron 10%

*Percent Daily Values are based on a 2,000 calorie diet. Your daily values may be higher or lower depending on your calorie needs.

	Calories	2,000	2,500
Total Fat	Less than	65g	80g
Sat Fat	Less than	20g	25g
Cholesterol	Less than	300mg	300mg
Sodium	Less than	2,400mg	2,400mg
Total Carbohydrate		300g	375g
Dietary Fiber		25g	30g

Calories per gram
Fat 9 • Carbohydrate 4 • Protein 4

INGREDIENTS, Skim Milk, Ricotta Cheese (Whole milk,Cream, Skim Milk, Vinegar and Salt), Cooked Macaroni, Spinach, Parmesan Cheese, Carrots, Onions, Butter, Soybean Oil, Modified Cornstarch, Bread Crumbs (Enriched Bleached Wheat Flour, Sugar, Corn Syrup, Partially Hydrogenated Soybean Oil, Salt, Yeast, Calcium Propionate, Spice Extractives and BHT),Corn Syrup, Long Grain Rice Meal, Potato Flakes, Malt, Yeast, Vegetable Shortening (Partially Hydrogenated Soybean Oil), Salt, Calcium Propionate, Nonfat Dry Milk Solids, Salt, Romano Cheese (made From Cow's Milk), Mushrooms, Sugar, Salt, Mono- and Diglycerides, Xanthan gum, Spices, Garlic Salt.

B

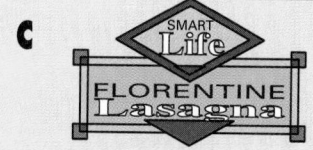

Home Taste Lasagna WITH MEAT SAUCE

Nutrition Facts

Serving size 10^1/$_2$ oz (298g)
Servings per Package 1

Amount per serving

Calories 361	Calories from Fat 117

	% Daily Value*
Total Fat 13g	20%
Saturated Fat 8g	40%
Cholesterol 87mg	29%
Sodium 860mg	36%
Total Carbohydrate 37g	12%
Dietary fiber 0g	
Sugars 8g	
Protein 26g	

Vitamin A 15%	•	Vitamin C 10%
Calcium 25 %	•	Iron 10%

*Percent Daily Values are based on a 2,000 calorie diet. Your daily values may be higher or lower depending on your calorie needs.

	Calories	2,000	2,500
Total Fat	Less than	65g	80g
Sat Fat	Less than	20g	25g
Cholesterol	Less than	300mg	300mg
Sodium	Less than	2,400mg	2,400mg
Total Carbohydrate		300g	375g
Dietary Fiber		25g	30g

Calories per gram
Fat 9 • Carbohydrate 4 • Protein 4

INGREDIENTS, Tomatoes, Cooked Macaroni Product, Dry Curd Cottage Cheese, Beef, Low-Moisture Part-Skim Mozzarella Cheese, Dehydrated Onions, Modified Cornstarch, Salt, Parmesan Cheese, Enriched Wheat Flour, Sugar, Spices, Tomato Flavor (Salt, Tomato Paste and Flavorings), Dehydrated Garlic.

C

SMART Life FLORENTINE Lasagna

Nutrition Facts

Serving size 11 oz (312g)
Servings per Package 1

Amount per serving

Calories 217	Calories from Fat 9

	% Daily Value*
Total Fat 1g	2%
Saturated Fat 0g	0%
Cholesterol 10mg	3%
Sodium 500mg	21%
Total Carbohydrate 34g	11%
Dietary fiber 5g	20%
Sugars 10g	
Protein 18g	

Vitamin A 25%	•	Vitamin C 25%
Calcium 40 %	•	Iron 10%

*Percent daily values are based on a 2,000 calorie diet. Your daily values may be higher or lower depending on your calorie needs.

	Calories	2,000	2,500
Total Fat	Less than	65g	80g
Sat Fat	Less than	20g	25g
Cholesterol	Less than	300mg	300mg
Sodium	Less than	2,400mg	2,400mg
Total Carbohydrate		300g	375g
Dietary Fiber		25g	30g

Calories per gram
Fat 9 • Carbohydrate 4 • Protein 4

INGREDIENTS, Tomato Puree, Cooked Enriched Macaroni Product (Durum Semolina,[Niacin, Ferrous Sulfate, Thiamin Mononitrate, Riboflavin], Water, Egg White Solids, Disodium Phosphate, Powdered Cellulose, Soy Protein Isolate, Soy Protein, Vital Wheat Gluten, Guar Gum), Ricotta Cheese (Pasteurized Whey, Pasteurized Milk, Vinegar, Xanthum Gum) Tomatoes, Zucchini, Cheese (Pasteurized Skim-Milk, Water, Natural Flavors, Enzyme, Calcium Chloride, Salt and Vitamin A & D), Carrots, Spinach, Onions, Water, Mushrooms, Concentrated Dealcoholized Burgundy Wine, Sugar, Modified Food Starch, Salt, Spices, Microcrystalline Cellulose, Methylcellulose, Maltodextrin, Hydrolyzed Corn Protein, Xanthum Gum, Guar Gum, Autolyzed Yeast, Calcium Chloride, Citric Acid, Garlic Extractives, Dextrin.

FORM 5-1

Calculate Your Daily Value for Fat and Saturated Fat

Section 1–Total Fat

A. Copy your energy RDA in calories from inside front cover, page C:

_____ calories.
(energy RDA)

B. Calculate the number of calories you can consume as fat in a day:

_____ cal × .3 = _____
(energy RDA)   (fat calories)

C. How many grams is this?

_____ cal ÷ 9 cal per gram= _____ grams fat
(fat calories,
from B)

D. Your personal Daily Value for total fat = _____ g
(from C)

Section 2–Saturated Fat

A. Copy your energy RDA from A in section 1: _____ calories
(energy RDA)

B. Calculate the number of calories you can consume as saturated fat each day:

_____ cal × .1 = _____
(energy RDA)   (saturated fat calories)

C. How many grams is this?

_____ cal ÷ 9 cal per gram = _____ grams saturated fat
(saturated fat
calories from B)

D. Your personal Daily Value for saturated fat = _____ g
(from C)

5. If you ate a serving of the highest-fat lasagna, how could you avoid exceeding the recommended fat intake for the day?

6. If you substituted a serving of the lowest-fat lasagna for the highest-fat choice, what effects would this have on your *other* food choices and to your calorie and nutrient intakes that day?

7. How does the saturated fat in each of the three lasagnas compare with your personal Daily Value for saturated fat?

CONSIDER THE INGREDIENTS

Read the ingredients list for each lasagna. Keep in mind that manufacturers list ingredients in descending order of their predominence in the food. Ingredients listed first are present in the largest quantities; those listed last are present in the smallest quantities. Now respond to the following questions (on page 181).

FORM 5-2

Compare Your Personal Daily Values with Fats in Three Lasagnas

A. Grams total fat per serving:

_____ _____ _____
(lasagna A) (lasagna B) (lasagna C)

Grams saturated fat per serving:

_____ _____ _____
(lasagna A) (lasagna B) (lasagna C)

B. Your personal Daily Value for total fat (from Form 5-1, section 1, part D) _____ g

Your Daily Value for saturated fat (from Form 5-1, section 2, part D) _____ g

C. What percentage of your Daily Value for total fat does a serving of each lasagna present?

Lasagna A _____ g ÷ _____ g × 100 = _____ % of personal Daily Value for total fat
(total fat)   (total fat Daily Value)

Lasagna B _____ g ÷ _____ g × 100 = _____ % of personal Daily Value for total fat
(total fat)   (total fat Daily Value)

Lasagna C _____ g ÷ _____ g × 100 = _____ % of personal Daily Value for total fat
(total fat)   (total fat Daily Value)

D. What percentage of your Daily Value for saturated fat does a serving of each lasagna present?

Lasagna A _____ g ÷ _____ g × 100 = _____ % of personal Daily Value for saturated fat
(saturated fat)   (saturated fat Daily Value)

Lasagna B _____ g ÷ _____ g × 100 = _____ % of personal Daily Value for saturated fat
(saturated fat)   (saturated fat Daily Value)

Lasagna C _____ g ÷ _____ g × 100 = _____ % of personal Daily Value for saturated fat
(saturated fat)   (saturated fat Daily Value)

8. Which ingredients contributed most to the total fat, saturated fat, and cholesterol in the highest-fat lasagna?

9. In the lowest-fat lasagna, which ingredients replaced or substituted for high-fat ingredients present in the other lasagnas? How did this help to lower the total fat content?

10. Do you agree or disagree with the following statement: "No food is good or bad based on its fat content alone." Justify your stance on this issue.

Take time to read labels, especially with regard to the fat contents of the foods you choose often. What you find there will often surprise you and may benefit your health.

✓   SELF-CHECK

Answers to these Self-Check questions are in Appendix G.

1. Which of the following is *not* one of the ways fats are useful in foods?
   a. Fats contribute to the taste and smell of foods.
   b. Fats carry fat-soluble vitamins.
   c. Fats provide a low-calorie source of energy compared to carbohydrates.
   d. Fats provide essential fatty acids.

2. Generally speaking, vegetable and fish oils are rich in:
   a. polyunsaturated fat
   b. saturated fat
   c. cholesterol
   d. *trans*-fatty acids

3. A benefit to health is seen when _____ fat is used in place of _____ fat in the diet.
   a. saturated/monounsaturated
   b. saturated/polyunsaturated
   c. monounsaturated/saturated
   d. polyunsaturated/cholesterol-type

4. Chylomicrons, a class of lipoproteins, are produced in the:
   a. gallbladder
   b. small intestinal cells
   c. large intestinal cells
   d. liver

5. Which foods from the breads, cereals, rice, and pasta group generally contain fat?
   a. biscuits
   b. muffins
   c. pasta
   d. (a) and (b)

6. Low-density lipoprotein delivers triglycerides and cholesterol from the liver to the body's tissues.   T   F

7. Given the same number of calories from excess dietary fat or carbohydrate, the body stores more calories from the fat than from the carbohydrate.   T   F

8. Consuming large amounts of *trans*-fatty acids lowers LDL cholesterol and thus lowers the risk of heart disease and heart attack.   T   F

9. When olestra is present in the digestive tract, it enhances the absorption of vitamin E.   T   F

10. The best way to diet for weight control is to keep the fat low and eat ample carbohydrates, but only up to the limit of calories needed. (Read about this in the upcoming Controversy.)   T   F

⌇ NOTES

Notes are in Appendix F.

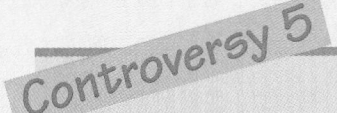
First Calories, Then Carbohydrates, Then Fat, Now What?

For years, nutritionists have taught that the body receives 9 calories from each gram of fat eaten and 4 calories from each gram of protein or carbohydrate. These are the amounts of energy found when a laboratory scientist burns the nutrients and measures the heat they give off. Logic says that the body should derive the same amounts of energy from these nutrients as the heat the scientist measures. After all, a calorie is a calorie, regardless of how it is released, right? The bodies of real people, however, do not produce such tidy numbers of calories from the nutrients.

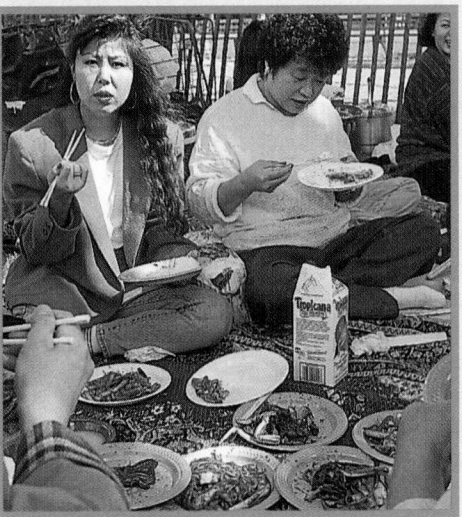

Scientists know, too, that each pound of body fat tissue represents 3,500 calories of stored energy. Logically, a person who eats 3,500 extra calories from any nutrient source should gain a pound, and a person who cuts 3,500 calories from any source should lose a pound. Yet some people seem to gain more body fat from an extra 3,500 fat calories than from an extra 3,500 carbohydrate calories. People also seem to lose body fat more efficiently when they limit their intakes of calories specifically from fat than when they limit protein or carbohydrate. In short, it may make a great difference to your body fatness whether you choose extra butter or extra potatoes.

Researchers have been investigating the possibility that fat in the diet influences body fatness more than an equal number of calories of carbohydrate.[1] This Controversy explores their findings.

DO HIGH-FAT DIETS CAUSE OBESITY?

As often happens in science, researchers were testing an unrelated theory when they stumbled onto some suggestive clues. Their study was designed to determine whether, given a fat-rich diet, rats would compensate for the extra calories by eating less food. The study proceeded as expected.[2] Rats fed a high-fat diet (42 percent of the calories from fat) voluntarily ate a smaller quantity of food than rats given a lower-fat control diet; as a result, both groups of rats consumed the same number of calories. The rats seemed to have internal

calorie counters that enabled them to eat just enough food to match the energy they expended. This was the expected result.

Then came a surprise. Even though both groups had eaten the same number of calories, one group gained more fat: the rats fed the fat-rich diet became severely obese. Their bodies became more than 50 percent body fat, whereas the control rats' bodies remained at 30 percent body fat. Thus, the researchers reported, high-fat diets could induce obesity even if food energy intakes were moderate—in rats, anyway.

This landmark study opened an enormous field of research on human beings. Scientists now want to see whether people respond to the composition of their diets the same way the rats did. Do people control their calorie intakes with "internal calorie counters?" Do people eating small amounts of high-fat foods gain more body fat than people eating large amounts of low-fat foods—if their calorie intakes are the same?

Research to answer such questions is harder to perform with human beings as subjects than with rats. Scientists can control perfectly what foods, and how much, rats eat over a lifetime, but with human beings, they can usually only observe and estimate. Also, researchers cannot easily use genetically identical human beings, and a few people carry genes for obesity that add to body fatness whatever the diet composition.[3] Given these handicaps, conclusions must be tentative, but most studies seem to show that fat in the diet does add more fat to the human body than does an equal number of calories of carbohydrate.

One group of scientists observed 155 obese men who, on average, were eating a diet that was typical for Americans at the time—about 15 percent of total calories from protein, 38 percent from carbohydrate, 41 percent from fat, and 6 percent from alcohol. Despite their obesity, their average food-energy intakes (2,570 calories per day) fell short of recommendations (2,900 calories per day).[4] The researchers found no correlation between the men's total body fat and their total food-energy intakes, but they did find a correlation with the men's fat intakes. The more fat and the less carbohydrate a man ate, the fatter his body was; conversely, the more carbohydrate and the less fat a man ate, the leaner his body was.

Another study showed the same relationship to hold true for women: those who are fed higher-fat diets develop higher body-fat contents than their total energy intakes alone would predict.[5] The effect seems especially strong in women who are genetically prone to obesity.[6] Such findings have been reported over and over, and the consensus seems to be that people tend to store body fat most efficiently from diets high in fat.[7]

Researchers curious about whether people with high fat intakes are overfat looked at the degree of British people's obesity and their intakes of high-fat or low-fat diets. People who regularly consumed high-fat diets were *19 times* more likely to be obese than those who ate low-fat diets.[8] The conclusion was that a low-fat diet, habitually consumed, offered protection against obesity development.

Findings like these have led some researchers to believe that the composition of the diet is every bit as important in the body's fat storage as total energy intake or exercise.[9] One researcher puts it this way, "The single most important thing you can do [to lose weight] is to get the fat out of the diet."[10]

The correlation between fat intake and body fat is not perfect, however, for in the British study just described, not everyone who ate a high-fat diet was obese. A few lean people habitually ate diets high in fat, leading to the suspicion that perhaps some mechanism of protection exists for a few lean people who can eat as they please and remain thin.

More questions now beg for answers. What is it about fat that makes most people fat?

1. Does the high energy value of fat combined with its irresistible taste make some people overeat?
2. Does the body control its intakes of calories by suppressing its appetite when it has consumed enough fat calories to meet its needs?
3. Do metabolic differences between the body's handling of fat and carbohydrate make fat the more fattening of the two?

The next sections explore some current work in these areas.

ARE FAT'S CALORIES THE CULPRIT?

Results from one experiment implicate fat's high calorie level in promoting body fatness. Men ate freely from three different diet plans: a low-fat diet (about 20 percent of calories from fat), a medium-fat diet (about 40 percent), and a high-fat diet (about 60 percent).[11] The foods in each diet plan were similar in taste and appearance; they differed only in the percentages of calories contributed by fat. Unlike rats, the men failed to adjust perfectly. The more fat in the food, the more calories the men consumed. The men ate the same total bulk of food whether or not the diet was high in fat. The researchers confirmed these results with a follow-up study.[12]

One reason the men may have failed to compensate is that fat occupies so little bulk. For example, only two teaspoons of fat in an 8-ounce glass of milk nearly double the calories in the milk (a cup of nonfat milk has 90 calories; a cup of whole milk, 150). Therefore, to keep calories constant while using whole milk in place of nonfat milk, one would have to reduce one's milk portion by almost half. The men did not cut down at all on total bulk of high-fat foods, and so consumed many more total calories. Other experiments designed the same way have confirmed that people do tend to overconsume calories when given high-fat diets.[13]

GIVEN MORE FAT, DO PEOPLE EAT MORE OR FEWER CALORIES?

So far, then, rats tend to eat just the right amount of food energy to maintain their normal body weights, regardless of the composition of the chow, whereas people given high-fat diets tend to overconsume calories. One group of researchers asked whether people might compensate for this after a short time lag. The researchers found that, to about the same degree, adding either fat or carbohydrate to a meal does cause people to eat less food later on.

In another experiment, the same researchers secretly manipulated the energy content of breakfasts by adding either fat or carbohydrate to yogurt.[14] They allowed the subjects free access to food at lunch later on and measured the subjects' total calorie intakes for the two meals. On average, the subjects reduced their energy intakes at lunch if they had consumed extra energy at breakfast, regardless of whether the extra energy came from carbohydrate or fat.

The ability to compensate seems to vary widely among individuals. Some compensate perfectly; others do not. Notably, lean men seem to compensate with precision, adjusting their food intakes to hold calories constant; obese people and those concerned about their weights compensate the least precisely, especially with regard to fat. The researchers suggest that perhaps some obese people are insensitive to feelings of fullness normally attributed to fat and therefore overconsume calories whenever they choose foods high in fat.[15]

It seems amazing that some people effortlessly control their energy intakes almost to the calorie. How this regulation might take place in the body is not known, but it is a subject of lively debate among nutrition researchers who are pursuing the answers.[16]

DO PEOPLE TEND TO STORE FAT AND BURN OFF CARBOHYDRATE?

Researchers have also begun to focus on the biochemical reasons why people who eat high-fat diets gain body fatness. Does the body handle excess energy differently from fat than from carbohydrate? Researchers fed men mixed meals of varying energy nutrient composition. During one experimental period, the men overate on carbohydrate; during another period, they overate on fat. Researchers monitored the study and found that the men's bodies used more of the carbohydrate for energy and stored more of the fat as body fat.[17] Why?

Evidence is accumulating to indicate that the body may regulate carbohydrate, fat, and protein separately, and that overall body energy regulation relates to all three.[18] The details of how this might occur are only now under study, but it already seems true that of the three energy-yielding nutrients, fat is most efficiently stored, even with moderate food-energy intakes.

The picture that emerges is this. Immediately after a meal, when food fat has enriched the blood with lipids, fat-storage cells avidly take them up and store them. Fat storage is a highly efficient process, requiring little energy. Once stored in adipose tissue, fat becomes less readily available to body tissues as an energy source than fuels still traveling in the bloodstream.

The body's handling of carbohydrate from food starts out the same as for fat. Glucose from food is readily taken up by tissues that store it by converting it to glycogen. Glycogen-storage space is extremely limited, however, unlike fat deposits, which can expand to hold virtually unlimited quantities of fat. Once the glycogen stores are full, excess glucose cannot remain in the blood; any glucose beyond the amount needed to fill glycogen stores must be disposed of by the body.

The body has two options for dealing with excess energy from glucose: it may use the glucose up immediately for fuel, or it may convert the glucose to fat by way of a long, energy-demanding series of reactions performed by the liver. Finally, the fat generated in this way can be shipped to the fat cells for storage. Normally, however, it seems that, when presented with excesses of both fat and carbohydrate from a meal, the body opts for the most energy-efficient processes; it tends to store fat as fat and use glucose for energy.

HOW DOES THE BODY HANDLE FAT AND CARBOHYDRATE?

Research shows that the more carbohydrate people are fed, the faster they convert it into energy. The body's cells can even metabolize some carbohydrate in ways that produce heat but perform no work. When fed excess fat, however, people exhibit no such increase in fuel use.

This effect was seen clearly in the study described earlier when researchers overfed men on diets high in either fat or carbohydrate and measured their energy expenditures.[19] Carbohydrate overfeeding produced progressive increases in carbohydrate use and total energy expenditure. As a result, the men stored just 75 to 85 percent of the excess carbohydrate energy that they took in. Alternatively, fat overfeeding did not increase the men's energy expenditures. When the men overate fat, they stored 90 to 95 percent of the excess energy.

Another study of obese women yielded similar results. The women's metabolism increased when they ate excess carbohydrate, but not when they ate excess fat.[20] These findings support the theory that the body's metabolism does store excess fat, but to some extent, burns off excess carbohydrate.

The Thermic Effect of Food   Researchers can account for these findings by their understanding of how the body produces heat from different nutrients. The heat energy produced from food is called the thermic effect of food (TEF, described in Chapter 9).[21] Only the energy that remains after the TEF is spent is available to the body to use immediately or to store as fat.

On average, a person spends about 10 percent of a meal's total energy on TEF, but this varies considerably, depending on the composition of the meal. As the percentage of dietary carbohydrate increases, the number of calories given off as body heat after a meal increases. In contrast, as the fat in the diet increases, heat production declines. Thus, while the amount of energy available from foods (as measured in calories) may seem to

OVERWEIGHT AND FAT INTAKES IN U.S. ADULTS

People in the United States have grown fatter, and the percentage of calories from fat in their diets has diminished. The data indicate that, on average, people have increased their total energy intakes during the same time.

SOURCE: Adapted from J. B. Allred, Too much of a good thing? *Journal of the American Dietetic Association* 95 (1995): 417–418.

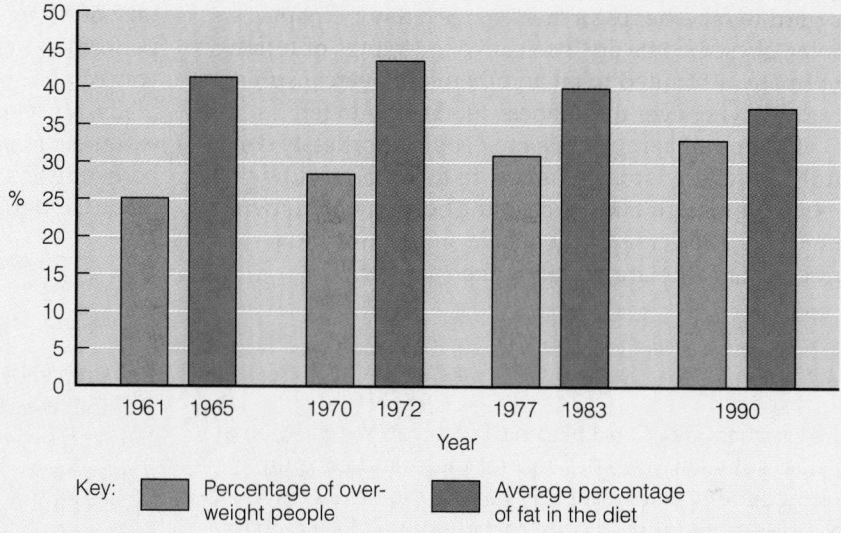

Key:
Percentage of over-weight people
Average percentage of fat in the diet

be the same in diets of different composition, the efficiency with which the body uses or stores that energy may vary considerably, depending on the diet's composition.

The Conversion of Carbohydrate to Fat It has long been known that when the body makes new fat molecules, it makes them in the liver. Also known is that the liver possesses enzymes to convert carbohydrate to fat. However, the questions remain: Does the liver routinely perform this conversion in response to excess carbohydrate in a meal? Does carbohydrate in the diet become fat in the body?

To observe the liver as it made new fat molecules after a meal, researchers injected male volunteers with a harmless tracer* that would be incorporated into the new fat molecules they made.[22] The men were then each given an amount of carbohydrate that exceeded the body's immediate energy need. If they converted excess carbohydrate to fat during the experiment, the tracer should promptly appear in their blood lipids. Very little of the tracer did appear in the subjects' blood lipids, however. This finding along with other evidence led the researchers to a conclusion that even they found startling: that under normal eating conditions, the human body rarely converts glucose to fat, even though it possesses the equipment to do so.[23]

---

*The substance was [13C] acetate.

Other thinkers disagree with this conclusion, however, based on the study's design.[24] They point out that in experiments on animals, researchers must feed carbohydrate for weeks before animal livers begin substantial conversion of carbohydrate to fat. Still needed are studies in which human subjects are overfed on high-carbohydrate meals for several weeks to allow their livers to adapt to such a diet. Then tests would reveal whether, after adaptation, they produce substantial amounts of fat from carbohydrate.

IF DIETERS LIMIT FAT INTAKE, CAN THEY EAT UNLIMITED CARBOHYDRATE?

If the body doesn't convert much carbohydrate to fat, does this mean that people can indulge freely in carbohydrate and not get fat? Most people who are not trained in nutrition seem to believe that it does. Since 1970, Americans have reduced their fat intakes somewhat, but at the same time they have consumed many more carbohydrate calories.[25] During the same period, they have become dramatically fatter (see Figure C5-1). They seem to have gone overboard eating "low-fat" foods while ignoring the carbohydrate calories those foods contribute to the diet.

But wait: this seems to show that *carbohydrate*, not fat, has caused the average adult's recent weight gain. Surely that can't mean that the piles of evidence for the fattening power of fat are not valid. Actually, no contradiction is implied by Figure C5-1. People did eat a smaller *percentage* of fat in 1990 than in 1970, but because it was a percentage of more total calories, the total *grams* of fat they ate each day stayed about the same. They increased their total food energy intakes, especially from carbohydrate, and gained weight proportionately.

This real-life "experiment," conducted spontaneously by the whole U.S. population, showed that overconsuming calories from a mixed diet causes weight gain, whatever the diet's composition. This probably reflects the trend toward consuming larger portions of food at each meal, as first mentioned in Chapter 2. The weight gain may also reflect an extraordinarily sedentary lifestyle, and sadly, this is typical for the people of this nation.[26]

While academically interesting, these insights into the body's regulation of energy metabolism do not change the old truth. As always, in the real world, too many calories and too little exercise lead to overweight. Fat may be more fattening than carbohydrate, but it seems that people who overeat either one must pay the price by gaining weight.

Clearly, from all of the experiments reported here, a diet's total fat content remains an important predictor of how much fat the body will store, but total calories can also cause weight gain. This is bad news for the wishful thinkers of yesteryear who fantasized that if they limited their fat intakes, they could eat all the carbohydrate they wanted and not get fat. Not so: the accurate view is that people must control both their fat *and* calorie intakes. The best way to diet for weight control is to keep the fat low and eat ample carbohydrates, but only up to the limit of calories allowed. This is the recommendation of every legitimate nutrition authority. It is the healthiest way to minimize disease risks, to meet the body's nutrient needs, and to control body fatness.

A full discussion of why people gain and lose weight is presented later in this book. This Controversy has focused narrowly on the body's efficiency in handling carbohydrate and fat from the diet. Besides diet composition, other factors such as genetics, age, physical activity, smoking, and alcohol intake also influence the body's metabolic efficiency. The next chapter concentrates on the last of the three energy-yielding nutrients, protein.

NOTES

Notes are in Appendix F.

THE PROTEINS AND AMINO ACIDS

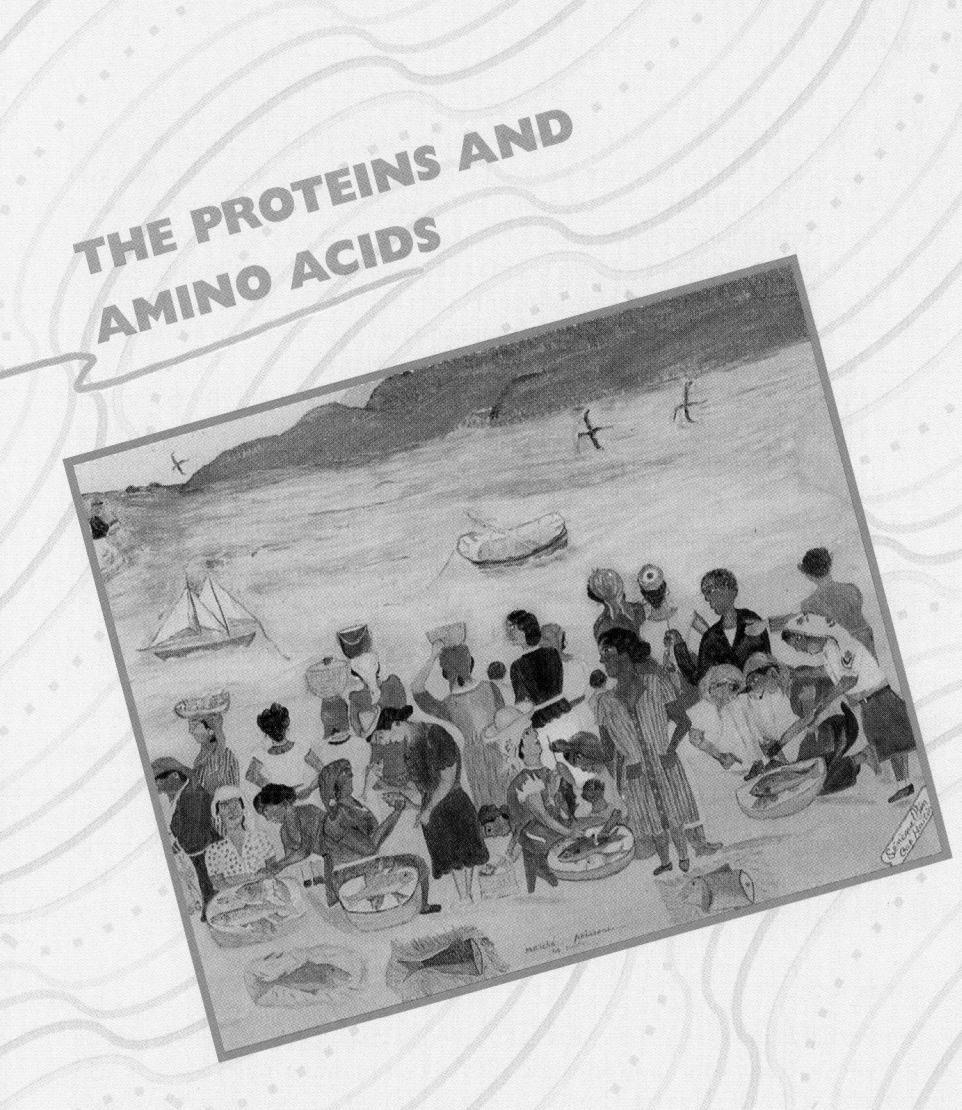

CONTENTS

Sénèque Obin 1893–1977, *Marché Poissons before 1957 (Fish Market)*, Collection of Siri von Reis, New York,
New York.

proteins compounds composed of carbon, hydrogen, oxygen, and nitrogen and arranged as strands of amino acids. Some amino acids also contain the element sulfur.

amino (a-MEEN-o) **acids** building blocks of protein. Each has an amine group at one end, an acid group at the other, and a distinctive side chain.

amine (a-MEEN) **group** the nitrogen-containing portion of an amino acid.

side chain the unique chemical structure attached to the backbone of each amino acid that differentiates one amino acid from another.

essential amino acids amino acids that either cannot be synthesized at all by the body or cannot be synthesized in amounts sufficient to meet physiological need. Also called *indispensable amino acids.*

peptide bond a bond that connects one amino acid with another, forming a link in a protein chain.

6 The **proteins** are amazing, versatile, and vital cellular working molecules. Without them, life would not exist. First named 150 years ago after the Greek word *proteios* ("of prime importance"), proteins have revealed countless secrets of the ways life processes take place, and they account for many nutrition concerns. Why are certain chemical substances essential nutrients and not others? How do we grow? How do our bodies replace the materials they lose? How does blood clot? What gives us immunity? Understanding the nature of the proteins gives us many of the answers to these questions.

Some proteins are working proteins; others form structures. Working proteins include the body's enzymes, antibodies, transport vehicles, hormones, cellular "pumps," and oxygen carriers. Structural proteins include tendons and ligaments, scars, the cores of bones and teeth, the filaments of hair, the materials of nails, and more. All protein molecules have much in common.

THE STRUCTURE OF PROTEINS

The structure of proteins enables them to perform many vital functions. One key difference from carbohydrates and fats, which contain only carbon, hydrogen, and oxygen atoms, is that proteins contain nitrogen atoms. These nitrogen atoms give the name *amino* (nitrogen containing) to the **amino acids,** the building blocks of protein. Another key difference is that in contrast to the carbohydrates, whose repeating units, glucose molecules, are identical, the amino acids in a strand of protein are different from one another. A strand of amino acids that makes up a protein may contain 20 *different* kinds of amino acids.

Amino Acids

All amino acids have a simple chemical backbone consisting of a single carbon atom with both an **amine group** (the nitrogen-containing part) and an acid group attached to it. This backbone is the same for all amino acids. The differ-

Hair, skin, eyesight, and the health of the whole body depend on protein from food.

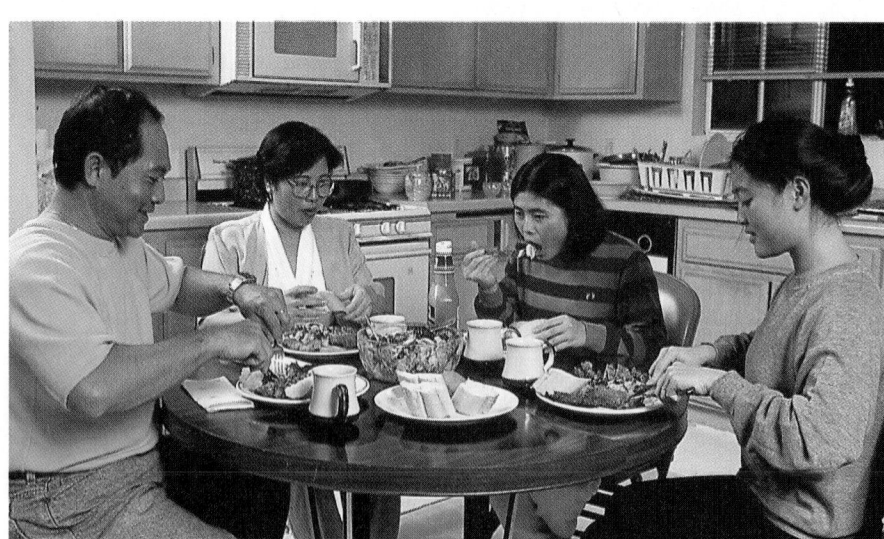

ences among amino acids depend on a distinctive structure, the chemical **side chain,** that is also attached to the center carbon of the backbone (see Figure 6-1). It is the side chain that gives identity and chemical nature to each amino acid. About 20 amino acids with 20 different side chains make up most of the proteins of living tissue. Other rare amino acids appear in a few proteins.

The side chains make the amino acids differ in size, shape, and electrical charge. Some are negative, some are positive, and some have no charge (they are neutral). The first part of Figure 6-2 is a diagram of three amino acids, each with a different side chain attached to its backbone. The rest of the figure shows how amino acids link to form protein strands. Long strands of amino acids form large protein molecules, and the side chains of the amino acids ultimately help to determine the molecules' shapes and behaviors.

The body can make about half of the 20 amino acids for itself, given the needed parts: fragments derived from carbohydrate or fat to form the backbones and nitrogen from other sources to form the amine groups. The healthy adult body makes some other amino acids too slowly to meet its needs, however, or cannot make them at all. These are the **essential amino acids.** Without these essential nutrients, the body cannot make the proteins it needs to do its work. The indispensability of the essential amino acids makes it necessary to eat often the foods that provide them.

The body not only makes some amino acids, but also breaks protein molecules apart and reuses their amino acids. Both food proteins, after digestion, and body proteins, when they have finished their cellular work, are dismantled to liberate their component amino acids. Pools of such amino acids provide the cells with raw materials from which they can build the protein molecules they need. Cells can also use the amino acids for energy and discard the nitrogen atoms as wastes. By reusing amino acids to build proteins, however, the body recycles and conserves a valuable commodity while easing its nitrogen disposal burden.[1]

This recycling system also provides a sort of emergency fund of amino acids that tissues can draw on in times of fuel or protein deprivation. At such times, tissues break down their own proteins, sacrificing working molecules before the ends of their normal lifetimes, to supply energy and protein to body tissues. The body employs a priority system in selecting the tissue proteins to dismantle—it uses the most dispensable ones first.

✔ **KEY POINT**   **Proteins are unique among the energy nutrients because they possess nitrogen-containing amine groups and are composed of 20 different amino acid units. Some amino acids are essential, and some are essential only in special circumstances.**

Proteins: Strands of Amino Acids

In the first step of making a protein, each amino acid is hooked to the next (this was shown in Figure 6-2). A bond, called a **peptide bond,** is formed between the amino end of one amino acid and the acid end of the next. The side chains bristle out from the backbone of the structure, and these give the protein molecule its unique character.

The strand of protein does not remain a straight chain. Figure 6-2 showed only the first step in making proteins, the linking of from several dozen to as

FIGURE 6-1

AN AMINO ACID
The "backbone" is the same for all amino acids. The side chain differs from one amino acid to the next. The nitrogen is in the amine group.

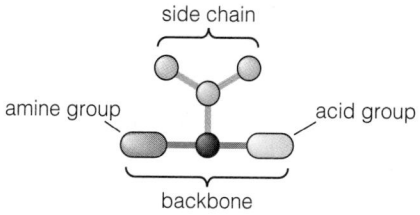

FIGURE 6-2

DIFFERENT AMINO ACIDS JOIN TOGETHER
This is the basic process by which proteins are assembled.

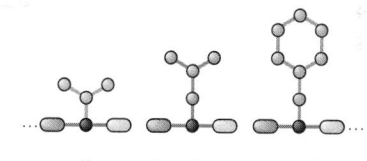

valine   leucine   tyrosine

Single amino acids with different side chains…

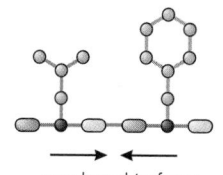

can bond to form…

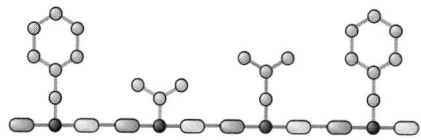

a strand of amino acids, part of a protein.

FIGURE 6-3

THE COILING AND FOLDING OF A PROTEIN MOLECULE

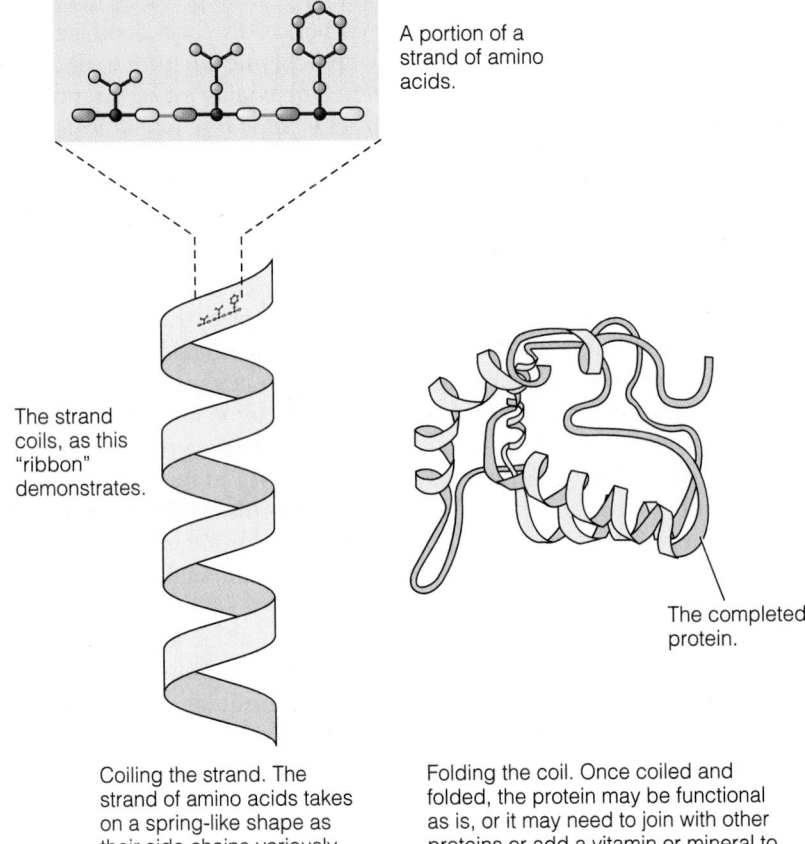

A portion of a strand of amino acids.

The strand coils, as this "ribbon" demonstrates.

The completed protein.

Coiling the strand. The strand of amino acids takes on a spring-like shape as their side chains variously attract and repel each other.

Folding the coil. Once coiled and folded, the protein may be functional as is, or it may need to join with other proteins or add a vitamin or mineral to become active.

The essential amino acids:

✔ Histidine.
✔ Isoleucine.
✔ Leucine.
✔ Lysine.
✔ Methionine.
✔ Phenylalanine.
✔ Threonine.
✔ Tryptophan.
✔ Valine.

Other amino acids important in nutrition:

✔ Alanine.
✔ Arginine.
✔ Asparagine.
✔ Aspartic acid.
✔ Cysteine.
✔ Glutamic acid.
✔ Glutamine.
✔ Glycine.
✔ Proline.
✔ Serine.
✔ Tyrosine.

many as 300 amino acid units with peptide bonds. The amino acids at different places along the strand are attracted to each other, and this attraction causes some segments of the strand to coil, somewhat like a metal spring. Also, each spot along the coiled strand is attracted to, or repelled from, other spots along its length. This causes the entire coil to fold this way and that, forming a globular structure, as shown in Figure 6-3, or a fibrous structure (not shown).

The amino acids whose side chains are electrically charged are attracted to water. In the body's watery fluids, they therefore orient themselves on the outside of the protein structure. The amino acids whose side chains are neutral are repelled by water and are attracted to one another; these tuck themselves into the center, away from the body fluids. All these interactions among the amino acids and the surrounding fluids result in the unique architecture of each protein.

One final detail may be needed for the protein to become functional. Several strands may cluster together into a functioning unit; or a metal ion (mineral) or a vitamin may join to the unit and activate it.

The dramatically different shapes of proteins enable them to perform different tasks in the body. Those of globular shape, such as some proteins of blood, are water soluble. Some are hollow balls, which can carry and store materials in their interiors. In some proteins, several coils of amino acids wind around each other and form ropelike fibers that can give strength and elasticity to body parts. Some, such as those that form tendons, are more than ten times as long as they are wide, forming stiff, rodlike structures that are somewhat insoluble in water and very strong. Still others act like glue. Among the most fascinating proteins are the **enzymes,** which act on other substances to change them chemically. The variety of proteins is endless. A model of a single large globular protein molecule, the **hemoglobin** that carries oxygen in the red blood cells, is shown in Figure 6-4.

The great variety of proteins in the world is possible because an infinite number of sequences of amino acids is possible. If you consider the size of the dictionary, in which all of the words are constructed from just 26 letters, you can visualize the variety of proteins that can be designed from 20 or so amino acids. The letters in a word must alternate between consonant and vowel sounds, but the amino acids in a protein need follow no such rules. Nor is there any restriction on the length of the chain of amino acids. Thus the number of possible proteins is much greater than the number of possible English words. A single human cell may contain as many as 10,000 different proteins, each one present in thousands of copies.

The sequences of amino acids that make up a protein molecule are specified by heredity. For each protein there is only one proper amino acid sequence. If a wrong amino acid is inserted, the result may be disastrous to health.

Sickle-cell disease, in which hemoglobin, the oxygen-carrying protein of the red blood cells, is abnormal, is an example of an inherited mistake in the amino acid sequence. Normal hemoglobin contains two kinds of chains. One of the chains in sickle-cell hemoglobin is an exact copy of that in normal hemoglobin. But in the other chain, the sixth amino acid, which should be glutamine, is replaced by valine. The protein is so altered that it is unable to carry and to release oxygen. The red blood cells collapse into crescent shapes instead of remaining disk shaped, as they normally do (see Figure 6-5 on the next page). If too many abnormal, crescent-shaped cells appear in the blood, the result is illness and death. One can detect the disease by observing the altered red blood cells under a microscope.

Each person is different from any other human being. What makes you unique are minute differences in your body proteins. These differences are determined by the amino acid sequences of your proteins, which are written into the genetic code you inherited from your parents and they from theirs. At conception each person receives a unique combination of genes. The genes, passed down to a cell from its parent cell, direct the making of all the body's proteins, as shown in Figure 6-6. Notice that it is the sequences of the amino acids in the finished protein that genes determine.

enzymes (EN-zimes) protein catalysts. A catalyst is a compound that facilitates a chemical reaction without itself being altered in the process.

hemoglobin the globular protein of red blood cells, the protein whose iron atoms carry oxygen around the body. (More about hemoglobin in Chapter 8.)

FIGURE 6-4

THE PROTEIN HEMOGLOBIN
The coiled and looped red structures are the globular proteins: the flat, jagged-edged objects are heme structures; the red center balls are iron atoms. This model represents a molecule of hemoglobin magnified 27 million times.

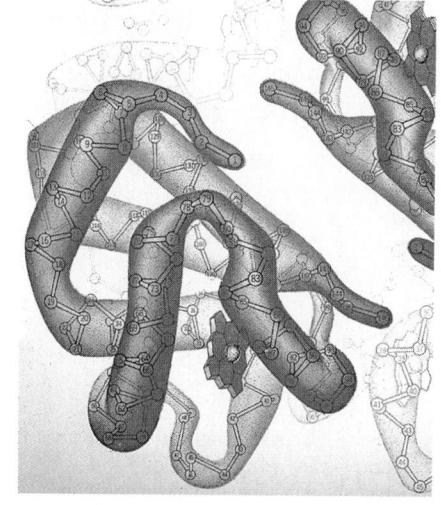

✔ KEY POINT   **Amino acids link into long strands that coil and fold to make a wide variety of different proteins. Each type of protein has a distinctive sequence of amino acids and so has great specificity.**

denaturation the change in shape of a protein brought about by heat, acids, bases, alcohol, salts of heavy metals, or other agents.

FIGURE 6-5

NORMAL RED BLOOD CELLS AND SICKLE CELLS

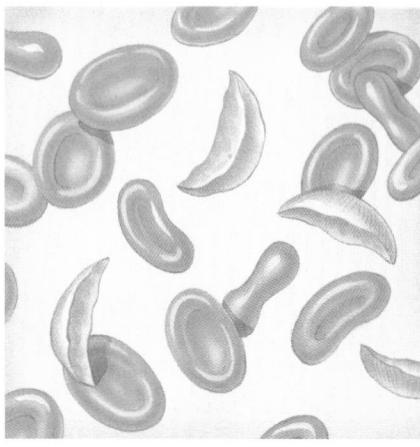

Denaturation of Proteins

Proteins can undergo **denaturation** (distortion of shape) by heat, alcohol, acids, bases, or the salts of heavy metals. The denaturation of a protein is the first step in its destruction; thus these agents are dangerous because they damage the body's proteins. In digestion, however, denaturation is useful to the body. During the digestion of a food protein, the stomach acid opens up the protein's structure, permitting digestive enzymes to make contact with the peptide bonds and cleave them. Denaturation also occurs during the cooking of foods. Cooking an egg denatures the proteins of the egg and makes it firm. Perhaps more importantly, cooking denatures two proteins in raw eggs: one that binds the B vitamin biotin and the mineral iron and another that slows protein digestion. Thus cooking eggs liberates biotin and iron and aids digestion.

Many well-known poisons are salts of heavy metals like mercury and silver; these denature proteins wherever they touch them. The common first-aid remedy for swallowing a heavy-metal poison is to drink milk. The poison then acts on the protein of the milk rather than on the protein tissues of the mouth, esophagus, and stomach. Later, vomiting is induced to expel the poison that has combined with the milk.

✔ **KEY POINT**   **Proteins can be denatured by heat, acids, bases, alcohol, or the salts of heavy metals. Denaturation may destroy body proteins.**

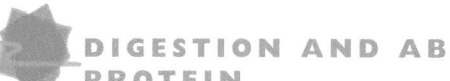

DIGESTION AND ABSORPTION OF PROTEIN

Each protein is designed for a special purpose in a particular tissue of a specific kind of animal or plant. When a person eats food proteins, whether from cereals, vegetables, beef, fish, or cheese, the body must alter them by breaking them down into amino acids before rearranging them into proteins with its own unique amino acid sequences.

Other than being crushed and moistened with saliva in the mouth, nothing happens to protein until it reaches the very strong acid of the stomach. There the acid helps to uncoil the protein's tangled strands so that molecules of the stomach's protein-digesting enzyme can attack the peptide bonds. You might expect that the stomach enzyme itself, being a protein, would be denatured by the stomach's acid. Unlike most enzymes, though, the stomach enzyme functions best in an acid environment. Its job is to break apart other protein strands into smaller pieces. The stomach lining, which is also made partly of protein, is protected against attack by acid and enzymes by a coat of mucus, secreted by its cells.

Digestion

Chapter 3 discussed the use of medicines to control the stomach's acidity and also defined pH as a measure of acidity. See page 88.

The whole process of digestion is an ingenious solution to a complex problem. Proteins (enzymes), activated by acid, digest proteins from food, denatured by acid. The coating of mucus secreted by the stomach wall protects its proteins from being affected by either acid or enzymes. The acid in the stomach is so strong (pH 1.5) that no food is acid enough to make it stronger; the pH of pure vinegar is about 3. Thus it is obvious that the stomach is supposed to be acid to do its job.

FIGURE 6-6

PROTEIN SYNTHESIS

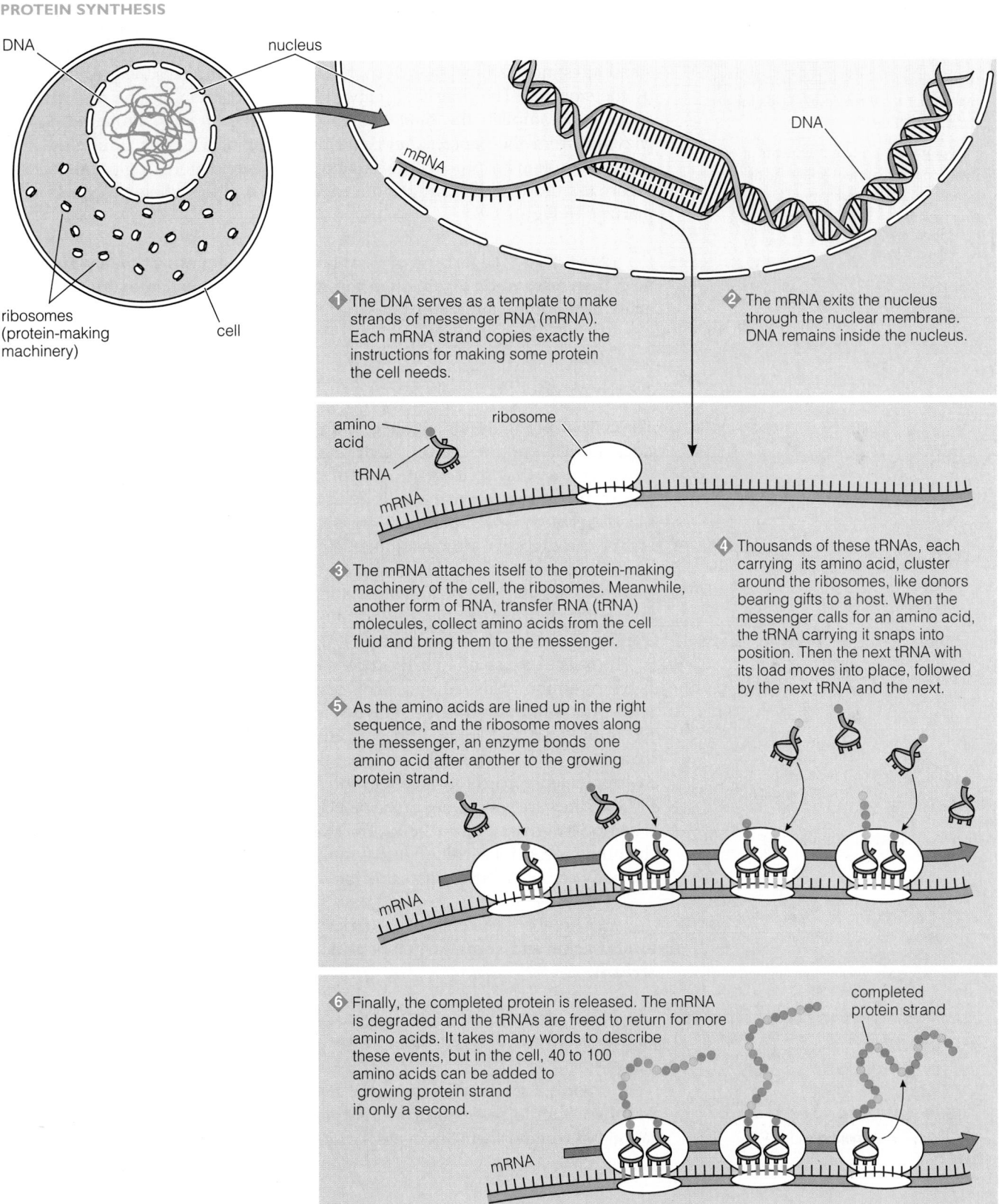

DNA

nucleus

ribosomes
(protein-making
machinery)

cell

DNA

mRNA

1 The DNA serves as a template to make strands of messenger RNA (mRNA). Each mRNA strand copies exactly the instructions for making some protein the cell needs.

2 The mRNA exits the nucleus through the nuclear membrane. DNA remains inside the nucleus.

amino
acid

ribosome

tRNA

mRNA

3 The mRNA attaches itself to the protein-making machinery of the cell, the ribosomes. Meanwhile, another form of RNA, transfer RNA (tRNA) molecules, collect amino acids from the cell fluid and bring them to the messenger.

4 Thousands of these tRNAs, each carrying its amino acid, cluster around the ribosomes, like donors bearing gifts to a host. When the messenger calls for an amino acid, the tRNA carrying it snaps into position. Then the next tRNA with its load moves into place, followed by the next tRNA and the next.

5 As the amino acids are lined up in the right sequence, and the ribosome moves along the messenger, an enzyme bonds one amino acid after another to the growing protein strand.

mRNA

6 Finally, the completed protein is released. The mRNA is degraded and the tRNAs are freed to return for more amino acids. It takes many words to describe these events, but in the cell, 40 to 100 amino acids can be added to growing protein strand in only a second.

completed
protein strand

mRNA

dipeptides (dye-PEP-tides): protein fragments that are two amino acids long. A peptide is a strand of amino acids (*di* means "two").

tripeptides (try-PEP-tides) protein fragments that are three amino acids long (*tri* means "three").

polypeptides protein fragments of many (more than ten) amino acids bonded together. (A chain of between four and ten is called an *oligopeptide*.)

By the time most proteins slip from the stomach into the small intestine, they are already broken into smaller pieces. Some are single amino acids, some are strands of two or three amino acids **(dipeptides** and **tripeptides).** The majority are longer chains **(polypeptides),** and a few are whole proteins. In the small intestine, alkaline juice from the pancreas neutralizes the acid delivered by the stomach. The pH rises to about 7 (neutral), enabling the next enzyme team to accomplish the final breakdown of the strands. Protein-digesting enzymes from the pancreas and intestine continue working until almost all pieces of protein are broken into small fragments and more single amino acids. Figure 6-7 shows a dipeptide and a tripeptide, and the whole process is summarized in Figure 6-8.

✓ KEY POINT   **Digestion of protein involves denaturation by stomach acid, then enzymatic digestion in the stomach and small intestine to amino acids, dipeptides, and tripeptides.**

Absorption

The cells all along the small intestine absorb single amino acids. As for dipeptides and tripeptides, the cells that line the small intestine have enzymes on their surfaces that split most of them into single amino acids, and the cells absorb them, too. Then the cells release all the single amino acids into the bloodstream. A few dipeptides, tripeptides, and even larger molecules can escape the digestive process altogether and cross the digestive tract wall to enter the bloodstream. It is thought that these larger particles may act as hormones to regulate body functions and provide the body with information about the environment. The larger molecules may also play a role in food allergy via the immune response.

The cells of the small intestine possess different sites for absorbing different types of amino acids. Amino acids of the same type compete for the same absorption sites. This means that when a person ingests a large dose of any single amino acid, that amino acid may limit absorption of others of its type. The Consumer Corner, presented later, cautions against taking single amino acids as supplements, partly for this reason.

Once they are circulating in the bloodstream, amino acids are available to be taken up by any cell of the body. The body cells then make proteins, either for their own use or for secretion into lymph or blood for other uses. Alternatively, the body cells can use amino acids for energy.

✓ KEY POINT   **The cells of the small intestine complete digestion, absorb amino acids and some larger peptides, and release them into the bloodstream.**

FIGURE 6-7

A DIPEPTIDE AND TRIPEPTIDE

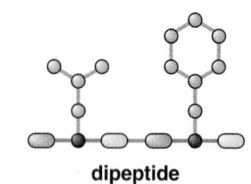

dipeptide

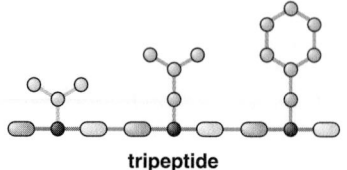

tripeptide

THE ROLES OF PROTEINS IN THE BODY

Only a sampling of the many roles proteins play can be described here, but these should serve to illustrate their versatility, uniqueness, and importance. No wonder their discoverers called them the primary material of life.

FIGURE 6-8

HOW PROTEIN IN FOOD BECOMES
AMINO ACIDS IN THE BODY

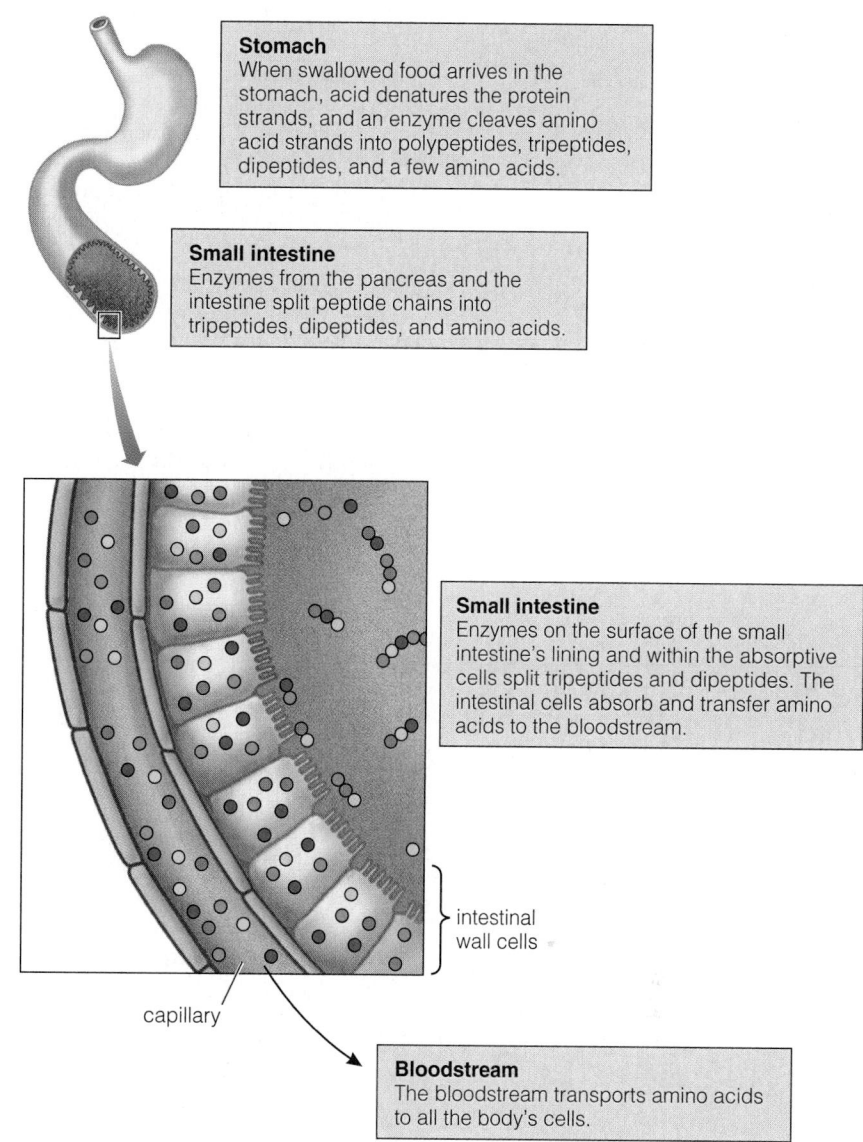

Stomach
When swallowed food arrives in the stomach, acid denatures the protein strands, and an enzyme cleaves amino acid strands into polypeptides, tripeptides, dipeptides, and a few amino acids.

Small intestine
Enzymes from the pancreas and the intestine split peptide chains into tripeptides, dipeptides, and amino acids.

Small intestine
Enzymes on the surface of the small intestine's lining and within the absorptive cells split tripeptides and dipeptides. The intestinal cells absorb and transfer amino acids to the bloodstream.

intestinal wall cells

capillary

Bloodstream
The bloodstream transports amino acids to all the body's cells.

Supporting Growth and Maintenance

Amino acids must be continuously available to build the proteins of new tissue. The new tissue may be in an embryo: in a growing child; in new blood needed to replace blood lost in burns, hemorrhage, or surgery; in the scar tissue that heals wounds; or in new hair and nails.

Less obvious is the protein that helps to replace worn-out cells in everyone's body all the time. Each of the millions of red blood cells lives for only three or four months. Then each must be replaced by a new cell produced by the bone marrow. The millions of cells that line the intestinal tract live for only three days; they are constantly being shed and need to be replaced. The cells of the skin die and rub off, and new ones grow from underneath. Nearly all cells arise, live,

FIGURE 6-9

ENZYME ACTION

Enzymes are catalysts: they speed up reactions that would happen anyway, but much more slowly. This enzyme works by positioning two compounds. A and B, so that the reaction between them will be especially likely to take place.

Compounds A and B are attracted to the enzyme's active site and park there for a moment in the exact position that makes the reaction between them most likely to occur. They react by bonding together and leave the enzyme as the new compound, AB.

A single enzyme can facilitate several hundred such synthetic reactions in a second. Other enzymes break apart compounds into two or more products or rearrange the atoms in one compound to make another one.

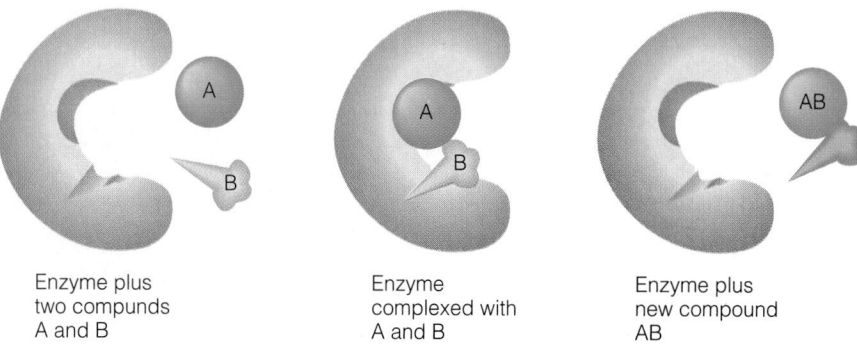

Enzyme plus two compunds A and B

Enzyme complexed with A and B

Enzyme plus new compound AB

hormones as defined in Chapter 3, chemical messengers secreted by a number of body organs in response to conditions that require regulation. Each hormone affects a specific organ or tissue and elicits a specific response.

and die this way, and while they are living, they constantly make and break down their proteins. Amino acids from food support all the new growth and maintenance of cells and the making of the working parts within them.

✓ KEY POINT **The body needs amino acids to grow new cells and to replace worn-out ones.**

Building Enzymes, Hormones, and Other Compounds

Enzymes are among the most important of the proteins formed in living cells. Thousands of enzymes reside inside a single cell, each one a catalyst that facilitates a specific chemical reaction. Figure 6-9 shows how a hypothetical enzyme works.

The body's many **hormones** are messenger molecules, and some are made from amino acids. (Recall from Chapter 5 that some hormones are made from fats.) Various body glands release hormones in response to changes in the internal environment. The hormones then elicit the responses necessary to restore normal conditions. Among hormones made of amino acids is the thyroid hormone, which regulates the metabolic rate of the body. An opposing pair of hormones, insulin and glucagon, maintain blood glucose levels, as described in Chapter 4. Many other hormones are at work in the body regulating equally critical body functions. For interest, Figure 6-10 shows how many amino acids are linked in sequence to form human insulin. It also shows how certain side groups attract one another to complete the insulin molecule and make it functional.

Not only do amino acids serve as building blocks for proteins, they also perform tasks as amino acids. For example, the amino acid tyrosine forms parts of the chemical messengers epinephrine and norepinephrine, which relay nervous system messages throughout the body. The body also uses tyrosine to make the brown pigment melanin responsible for skin, hair, and eye color. It also becomes the hormone thyroxine, which helps to regulate the body's metabolic rate. The amino acid tryptophan serves as starting material for the neurotransmitter serotonin and the vitamin niacin.

✔ KEY POINT   **The body makes enzymes, hormones, and chemical messengers of the nervous system from its amino acids.**

Building Antibodies

Of all the great variety of proteins in living organisms, the **antibodies** demonstrate best that proteins are specific to one organism. Antibodies recognize every protein that belongs in "their" body and leave it alone, but they attack foreign particles (usually proteins) that invade the body. The foreign protein may be part of a bacterium, a virus, or a toxin, or it may be present in a food that causes allergy. The body, upon recognizing that it has been invaded, manufactures antibodies specially designed to inactivate the foreign protein.

Each antibody is designed specifically to destroy just one invader. An antibody active against one strain of influenza would be of no help to a person ill with another strain. Once the body has learned to make a particular antibody, it remembers. The next time the body encounters that same invader, it destroys the invader even more rapidly. In other words, the body develops **immun**ity to the invader. This molecular memory underlies the principle of immunizations, injections of drugs made from destroyed and inactivated microbes or their products that activate the body's immune defenses. Some immunities are lifelong; others, such as that to tetanus, must be "boosted" at intervals.

✔ KEY POINT   **Antibodies are formed from amino acids to defend against foreign proteins and other foreign substances within the body.**

Maintaining Fluid and Electrolyte Balance

Proteins help to maintain the **fluid and electrolyte balance** by regulating the quantity of fluids in the compartments of the body. To remain alive, cells must contain a constant amount of fluid. Too much might cause them to rupture; too little would make them unable to function. Although water can diffuse freely into and out of cells, proteins cannot; and proteins attract water. By maintaining stores of internal proteins and also of some minerals, cells retain the fluid they need. Conversely, the cells secrete proteins (and minerals) into the spaces between them to keep the fluid volume constant in those spaces. Thus proper balance is maintained. Should this system begin to fail, too much fluid would collect outside the cells, causing **edema.**

Not only is the quantity of the body fluids vital to life, but so also is their composition. Transport proteins in the membranes of cells correct this composition continuously by transferring substances into and out of cells. For example, sodium is concentrated outside the cells, and potassium is concentrated

antibodies (AN-tee-bod-ees) large proteins of the blood, produced by the immune system in response to invasion of the body by foreign substances (antigens). Antibodies combine with and inactivate the antigens.

immunity specific disease resistance, derived from the immune system's memory of prior exposure to specific disease agents and its ability to mount a swift defense against them.

fluid and electrolyte balance the distribution of fluid and dissolved particles among body compartments (see also Chapter 8).

edema (eh-DEEM-uh) swelling of body tissue caused by leakage of fluid from the blood vessels, seen in (among other conditions) protein deficiency.

FIGURE 6-10

AMINO ACID SEQUENCE OF HUMAN INSULIN

This picture shows a refinement of protein structure not mentioned in the text. The amino acid cysteine (cys) has a sulfur-containing side group in it. The sulfur groups on two cysteine molecules can bond together, creating a bridge between two protein strands or two parts of the same strand. Insulin contains three such bridges.

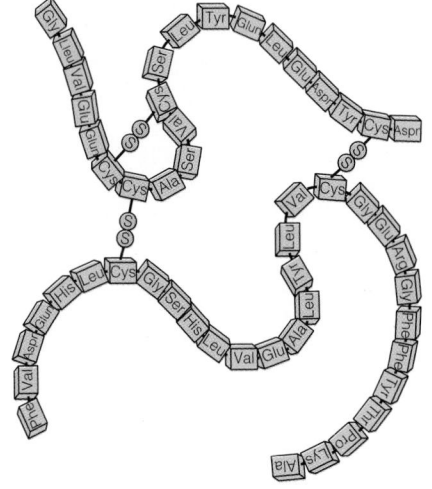

acids compounds that release hydrogens in a watery solution.

bases compounds that accept hydrogens from solutions.

acid-base balance equilibrium between acid and base concentrations in the body fluids.

buffers compounds that help keep a solution's acidity or alkalinity constant.

acidosis (acid-DOH-sis) blood acidity above normal, indicating excess acid (*osis* means "too much in the blood").

alkalosis (al-kah-LOH-sis) blood alkalinity above normal (*alka* means "base"; *osis* means "too much in the blood").

The control of water's location by particles is discussed further in Chapter 8.

inside (see Figure 6-11). A disturbance of this balance can impair the action of the heart, lungs, and brain, triggering a major medical emergency. Cell proteins work daily to avert such a disaster by holding fluids and electrolytes in their proper chambers.

✔ KEY POINT **Proteins help to regulate the body's electrolytes and fluids.**

Maintaining Acid-Base Balance

Normal processes of the body continually produce **acids** and their opposite, **bases,** which must be carried by the blood to the organs of excretion. The blood must do this without allowing its own **acid-base balance** to be affected. This feat is another trick of the blood proteins, which act as **buffers** to maintain the blood's normal pH. They pick up hydrogens (acid) when there are too many and release them again when there are too few. The secret is that negatively charged side chains of amino acids can accommodate additional hydrogens, which are positively charged, when necessary.

Blood pH is one of the most rigidly controlled conditions in the body. If it changes too much, the dangerous condition **acidosis** or the opposite, basic condition **alkalosis** can cause coma or death. The hazard of these conditions is due to their effect on proteins. When the proteins' buffering capacity is filled—that is, when they have taken on board all the acid hydrogens they can accommodate—additional acid pulls them out of shape, denaturing them and disrupting many body processes. Table 6-1 sums up the functions of protein discussed in this section and adds several others.

✔ KEY POINT **Proteins buffer the blood against excess acidity or alkalinity.**

TABLE 6-1

Summary of Functions of Proteins

- **growth and maintenance** Proteins serve as building materials for growth and repair of body tissues.
- **enzymes** Proteins facilitate needed chemical reactions.
- **hormones** Proteins regulate body processes. Some hormones are proteins or are made from amino acids.
- **antibodies** Proteins form the immune system molecules that fight diseases.
- **fluid and electrolyte balance** Proteins help to maintain the fluid and mineral composition of various body fluids.
- **acid-base balance** Proteins help maintain the acid-base balance of various body fluids by acting as buffers.
- **energy** Proteins provide some fuel for the body's energy needs.
- **transportation** Proteins help transport needed substances, such as lipids, minerals, and oxygen, around the body.
- **blood clotting** Proteins provide the netting on which blood clots are built.
- **structural components** Proteins form integral parts of most body structures such as skin, tendons, ligaments, membranes, muscles, organs, and bones.

FIGURE 6-11

PROTEINS TRANSPORT SUBSTANCES INTO AND OUT OF CELLS

A transport protein within a cell membrane acts as a sort of revolving door—it picks up substances on one side of the membrane and flips them to the other side without leaving the membrane itself. The substances being transported here are sodium and potassium. The significance of sodium in fluid and electrolyte balance is discussed in Chapter 8.

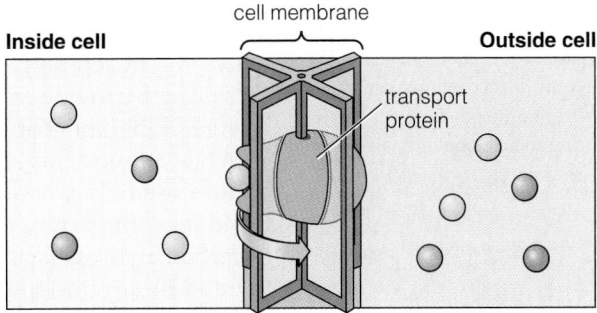

Protein flips

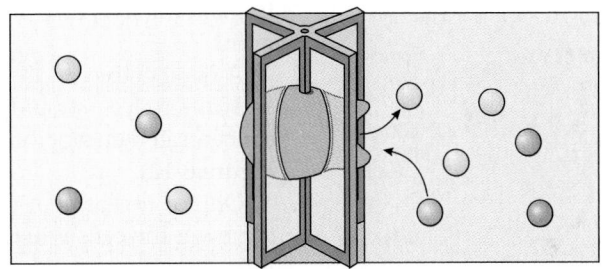

Molecules trade places

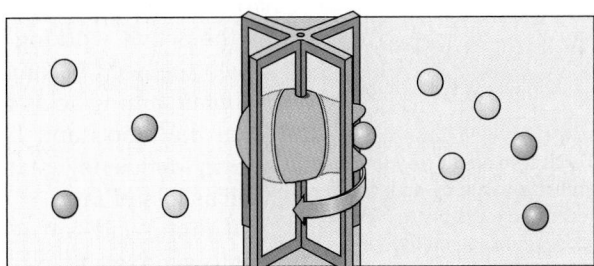

Protein flips

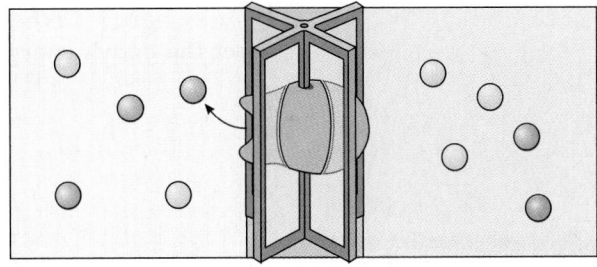

urea (yoo-REE-uh) the principal nitrogen-excretion product of metabolism, generated mostly by removal of amine groups from unneeded amino acids or from amino acids being sacrificed to a need for energy.

Providing Energy

Only protein can perform all the functions just described, but protein will be sacrificed to provide energy if need be. The body must have energy to live from moment to moment and obtaining that energy is a top-priority matter.

When amino acids are degraded for energy, their amine groups are stripped off and used elsewhere or are incorporated by the liver into **urea** and sent to the kidney for excretion in the urine. The fragments that remain are composed of carbon, hydrogen, and oxygen, as are carbohydrate and fat, and can be used to build those substances or can be metabolized like them.

Not only can amino acids supply energy, but many of them can be converted to glucose, as fatty acids can never be. Thus, if need be, protein can help to maintain a steady blood glucose level and so serve the glucose need of the brain.

A perspective on the three energy-yielding nutrients with their similarities and differences should now be clear. Carbohydrate offers energy; fat offers concentrated energy; and protein, if needed, can offer energy plus nitrogen (see Figure 6-12).

Only if the protein-sparing energy from carbohydrate and fat is sufficient to power the cells will the amino acids be used for the work only they can perform—making proteins. The body does not make a specialized energy-storage compound from protein as it does from carbohydrate and fat. Glucose is stored as glycogen and fat as triglycerides, but body protein is available only as the active working molecular and structural components of the tissues. When the need becomes urgent, the body must dismantle its tissue proteins to obtain amino acids for energy.[2] Each protein is taken in its own time: first, from the blood and liver; then, from the muscles and other organs. Thus energy deficiency (starvation) always incurs wasting of lean body tissue as well as loss of fat.

If amino acids are oversupplied, the body cannot store them. It has no choice but to remove and excrete their amine groups and then to convert the residues to glycogen or fat for energy storage.

Athletes and exercisers take note: you cannot build extra muscle tissue by eating extra protein because excess protein is burned as fuel, converted to glucose, or stored as fat. Chapter 10 gives more details about protein needs of exercisers.

✔ **KEY POINT**   **When insufficient carbohydrate and fat are consumed to meet the body's energy need, food protein and body protein are sacrificed**

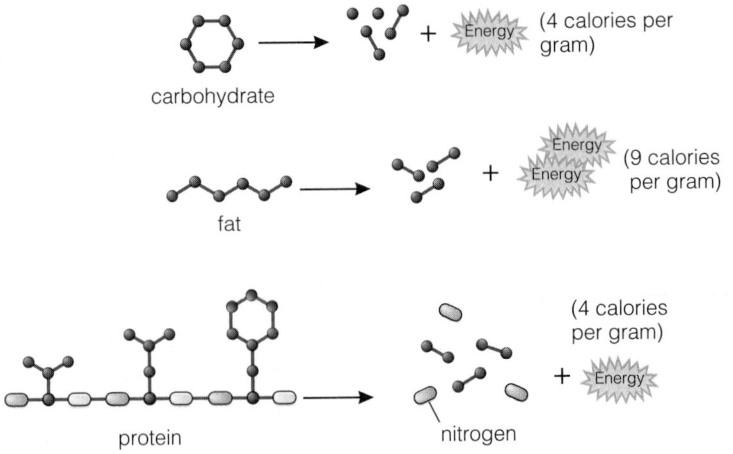

FIGURE 6-12

THREE DIFFERENT ENERGY SOURCES
Carbohydrate offers energy; fat offers concentrated energy; and protein, if necessary, can offer energy plus nitrogen. The compounds at the left yield the 2-carbon fragments shown at the right. These fragments oxidize quickly in the presence of oxygen to yield carbon dioxide, water, and energy.

carbohydrate   + Energy   (4 calories per gram)

fat   + Energy Energy   (9 calories per gram)

protein   nitrogen   + Energy   (4 calories per gram)

to supply energy. The nitrogen part is removed from each amino acid, and the resulting fragment is oxidized for energy.

The Fate of an Amino Acid

To review the body's handling of amino acids, let us follow the fate of an amino acid that was originally part of a protein-containing food. When the amino acid arrives in a cell, it may be used in several different ways, depending on the needs of the cell at the time.

The amino acid may be used as is and become part of a growing protein. It may be altered somewhat to make another needed compound. Alternatively, the cell may dismantle the amino acid and use its amine group to build a different amino acid. The remainder may be used for fuel or, if not needed, converted to glucose or fat.

Almost the same fate awaits the amino acid in a cell that is starved for energy but has no glucose or fatty acids. This amino acid may be needed to build a vital protein, but without energy, the cell would die. Therefore the amino acid is stripped of its amine group (the nitrogen part), and the remainder of its structure is used for energy. The amine group is excreted from the cell and, finally, from the body in the urine.

Another case in which amino acids are used for energy is when the body has a surplus of amino acids and energy-yielding nutrients. In this case the body does not waste this resource. It takes the amino acid apart, excretes the amine group, converts the rest to fat, and then stores the fat in the fat cells.

In summary, then, amino acids in the cell can be

- used to build proteins,
- converted to other small nitrogen-containing compounds such as the vitamin niacin, or
- converted to some other amino acids.

Stripped of their nitrogen, amino acids can be

- converted to glucose,
- burned as fuel, or
- stored as fat.

When not used to build protein or make other nitrogen-containing compounds, amino acids are "wasted" in a sense. This wasting occurs under any of four conditions: (1) when there is not enough energy from other sources; (2) when there is too much protein, so that not all is needed; (3) when there is too much of any single amino acid, such as from a supplement; or (4) when the quality of the diet's protein is too low, with too few essential amino acids, as described in the next section.

To prevent the wasting of dietary protein and permit the synthesis of needed body protein, three conditions must be met. First, the dietary protein must be adequate in quantity. Second, it must supply all essential amino acids in the proper amounts. Third, enough energy-yielding carbohydrate and fat must be present to permit the dietary protein to be used as such.

Amino acids are wasted when:
- Energy is lacking.
- Protein is overabundant.
- An amino acid is oversupplied in supplement form.
- The quality of the diet's protein is too low (too few essential amino acids).

✔ **KEY POINT**   **Amino acids can be metabolized to protein, nitrogen plus energy, glucose, or fat. They will be metabolized to protein only if sufficient energy is present from other sources. The diet should supply all essential amino acids and a full measure of protein according to guidelines.**

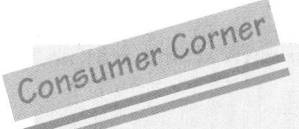

PROTEIN AND AMINO ACID SUPPLEMENTS

Why do people take protein or amino acid supplements? Athletes take them to build muscle. Dieters take them to spare their bodies' protein while losing weight. People also take individual amino acids, mixtures of two or more amino acids, or products that combine amino acids with other nutrients. Some consumers believe the products will cure herpes, induce restful sleep, or relieve pain or depression. Do protein and amino acid supplements really do any of these things? Almost never. Are they safe? No.

Enthusiastic popular reports about two amino acids have led to widespread public use. One is lysine, popularly recommended to prevent or relieve the infections that cause herpes sores on the mouth or genital organs. The other is tryptophan, popularly recommended to relieve pain, depression, and insomnia. Lysine does not relieve or cure herpes infections, and if long-term use helps prevent outbreaks, it does so only in some individuals and with unknown associated risks. Tryptophan has some interesting effects with respect to pain and sleep in responsive individuals, as Controversy 13 explains later.

Some people who elected to take tryptophan developed a blood disorder (EMS, short for *eosinophilia-myalgia syndrome*). EMS is characterized by severe muscle and joint pain, limb swelling, an elevated white blood cell count, extremely high fever, and, in at least 15 cases, death. Whether tryptophan, contaminants, or a combination of the two caused the disease remains unknown.[3] The FDA recalled tryptophan supplements and formulas to which it was added.[4] If you own a bottle of tryptophan or a formula containing it, throw it out. It is safer to derive your amino acids from protein-rich foods taken with a little carbohydrate to facilitate their use. A glass of milk or a turkey sandwich is a good choice.

Processing can render some protein supplements less digestible than protein-rich food, and they cost more than food, too. When used as a replacement for such food, protein supplements are often downright dangerous. The "liquid protein" diet, advocated some years ago for weight loss, caused the deaths of many users. Even the physician-supervised "protein-sparing" fast, also based on liquid protein, has caused abnormal heart rhythms.

More about the effects of fasting in Chapter 9.

Amino acid supplements are also unnecessary. The body is designed to handle whole proteins best. It breaks them into manageable pieces (dipeptides and tripeptides), then splits these a few at a time, simultaneously absorbing them into the blood. This slow bit-by-bit absorption is ideal, because groups of chemically similar amino acids compete for the carriers that absorb them into the blood. An excess of one amino acid can tie up a carrier and temporarily prevent the absorption of another similar amino acid. When carriers are tied up dealing with an overdose of one or a few amino acids, some other needed amino acids may pass through the body unabsorbed. The result is a deficiency. The human body evolved without encountering highly concentrated amino acids in the unbalanced arrays found in supplements and therefore lacks equipment with which to handle them.[5]

Recently, the Food and Drug Administration (FDA) asked a panel of scientists from a well-known scientific research group to review the safety of amino acid supplements.[6] When the scientists began to search the literature for well-controlled studies on the supplements, they found next to none. The panel did find evidence of adverse health effects from amino acids, however, and they therefore concluded that, without appropriate scientific research, no level of intake of these supplements could be considered safe. They also warned that any use of amino acids as dietary supplements is inappropriate for two reasons. First, some (serine and proline) present a high risk of toxicity. Second, no amino acid supplement performs any nutrient function in the human body.

The panel also singled out some groups of people whose growth or altered metabolism makes them especially likely to suffer harm from amino acid supplements:

- All women of childbearing age.
- Pregnant or lactating women.
- Infants, children, and adolescents.
- Elderly people.
- People with inborn errors of metabolism that affect their bodies' handling of amino acids.
- Smokers.
- People on low-protein diets.
- People with chronic or acute mental or physical illnesses who take amino acids without medical supervision.

Also, because they may take frequent, massive amino acid doses, weight lifters and bodybuilders may suffer harm from the supplements while believing false promises of benefits. Anyone considering taking amino acid supplements should check with a physician first.

Many of the chapters of this book present evidence on purified nutrients added to foods or taken singly. The Consumer Corner in Chapter 4 showed that the enrichment of a nutritionally inferior food (refined bread) with a few added nutrients left is still deficient in many others. The Chapter 5 Consumer Corner showed that fish oil supplements cause side effects. The same is true of amino acids. Even with all that we know about science, it is hard to improve on nature.

Muscle work builds muscle; protein supplements do not, and athletes do not need them. Chapter 10 describes how muscles are built and the diet that best supports them.

legumes (leg-GOOMS, LEG-yooms) plants of the bean and pea family having roots with nodules that contain special bacteria. These bacteria can trap nitrogen from the air in the soil and make it into compounds that become part of the seed. The seeds are rich in high-quality protein compared with those of most other plant foods.

amino acid pools amino acids dissolved in cellular fluid that provide cells with ready raw materials from which to build new proteins or other molecules.

limiting amino acid a term given to an essential amino acid present in dietary protein in an insufficient amount, so that it limits the body's ability to build protein.

Some concern exists about the formation of carcinogens in foods when fat or protein is exposed to open flame—see Chapter 11.

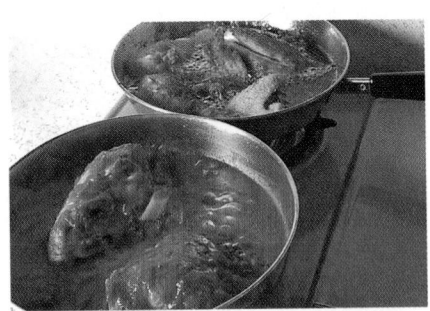

Cooking with moist heat improves protein digestibility, whereas frying makes protein harder to digest.

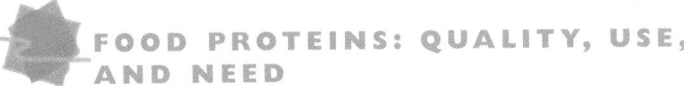

FOOD PROTEINS: QUALITY, USE, AND NEED

The body responds to different proteins in different ways, depending on many factors: the body's state of health, the food source of the protein, its digestibility, the other nutrients taken with it, and its amino acid assortment. To know whether, say, 30 grams of a particular protein is enough to meet a person's daily needs, it is necessary to account for the effects of these other factors on the body's use of the protein.

Regarding a person's state of health, malnutrition or infection may greatly increase the need for protein while making it hard to eat even normal amounts of food. In malnutrition, digestive enzyme secretion slows as the tract's lining degenerates, impairing protein digestion and absorption. When infection is present, extra protein is needed for enhanced immune functions.

Protein Digestibility

Digestibility affects protein quality profoundly, and it varies from food to food. The protein of oats, for example, is less digestible than that of eggs. Generally, amino acids from animal proteins are most easily digested and absorbed (over 90 percent). Those from **legumes** follow (about 80 percent). Those from grains and other plant foods vary (from 60 to 90 percent). Cooking with moist heat generally improves protein digestibility, whereas dry heat methods can impair it.[7]

As for taking the other nutrients with protein, the need for carbohydrate and fat has already been emphasized. To be used efficiently, protein must also be accompanied by the full array of vitamins and minerals.

✓ KEY POINT   **The body's use of a protein depends in part on the user's health and on the protein's digestibility. To be used efficiently, protein should be accompanied by all the other nutrients.**

Protein Quality

The quality of a food protein depends largely on its amino acid content. The cells, in making their own proteins, need a full array of amino acids from food, from their own **amino acid pools,** or from both. If a nonessential amino acid (that is, one the cell can make) is unavailable from food, the cell will synthesize it and continue attaching amino acids to protein strands being manufactured. If an essential amino acid (one the cell cannot make) is missing from food, the cells begin to adjust their activities almost immediately.[8] Within a single day of restricted essential amino acid intake, cells begin to conserve by restricting the breakdown of their working proteins and by reducing their use of amino acids for fuel.

These measures help cells to channel the available **limiting amino acid** to its wisest use: making new proteins. Even so, the normally fast rate of protein synthesis slows to a crawl, and cells must make do with the proteins on hand. When the limiting amino acid once again becomes available in abundance, the cells resume normal protein-related activities. If the shortage becomes chronic, however, cells begin to break down their protein-making machinery. This means that even when protein intakes become adequate, protein synthesis lags behind until cells can rebuild the needed machinery. Meanwhile, cells function less and less effectively as their proteins wear out and are only partially replaced.

Thus a diet that is short in any of the essential amino acids limits protein synthesis. An earlier analogy likened amino acids to letters of the alphabet. To be meaningful, words must contain all the right letters. For example, a print shop that had no letter "n" in the shop could not make personalized stationary for Jana Johnson. No matter how many J's, a's, o's, h's, and s's in the printer's possession, they cannot replace the missing n's. Likewise in building a protein molecule, no amino acid can fill the spot of any other. If, in building a protein, a cell cannot find a certain amino acid that is called for, then synthesis stops, and the partial protein is released.

Partially completed proteins are not held for completion at a later time when the diet may improve. Rather, they are dismantled, and the component amino acids are returned to the circulation to be made available to other cells. If they are not soon inserted into protein, their amine groups are removed and excreted, and the residues are used for other purposes. The need that prompted the call for that particular protein will not be met. Since the other amino acids are wasted, the amine groups are excreted and the body cannot resynthesize the amino acids later.

It follows that all the essential amino acids must be consumed in proportion to the body's needs, or else the body's pools of essential amino acids will dwindle to the point at which body organs are compromised. This presents no problem to people who regularly eat **complete proteins,** such as those of meat, fish, poultry, cheese, eggs, milk, and, new to this list, many soybean products.[9] The proteins of these foods contain ample amounts of all the essential amino acids. An equally sound choice is to eat two **incomplete protein** foods from plants, each of which supplies the amino acids missing in the other. In this strategy, called **mutual supplementation,** the two protein-rich foods are combined to yield **complementary proteins** (see Table 6-2); that is, proteins containing all the essential amino acids in amounts sufficient to support health. This concept is illustrated in Figure 6-13. The two proteins need not even be eaten together, so long as the day's meals supply them both, and the diet provides enough energy and total protein from a variety of sources.[10]

Concern about the quality of individual food proteins is of only theoretical interest in settings where food is abundant. Most people in the United States and Canada eat a variety of nutritious foods to meet their energy needs—not just, say, cookies, potato chips, or alcoholic beverages. They would find it next to impossible *not* to meet their protein requirements, even if they were to eat no meat, fish, poultry, eggs, cheese, or soy products. However, while *protein* is usually sufficient in North American diets, the next two chapters point out *other* nutrients to which people must attend.

Protein quality can make the difference between health and disease when food energy intake is limited (where malnutrition is widespread) or when the selection of foods available is severely limited (where a single food such as potatoes or rice provides 90 percent of the calories). Even then, protein intake may be adequate, but it may not be. To be sure, in these cases, the primary food source of protein must be checked, since its quality is crucial.

complete proteins proteins containing all the essential amino acids in the right balance to meet human needs.

incomplete proteins proteins lacking, or low in, one or more of the essential amino acids.

mutual supplementation the strategy of combining two incomplete protein sources so that the amino acids in each food make up for those lacking in the other food. Such protein combinations are sometimes called *complementary proteins.*

complementary proteins two or more proteins whose amino acid assortments complement each other in such a way that the essential amino acids missing from each are supplied by the other.

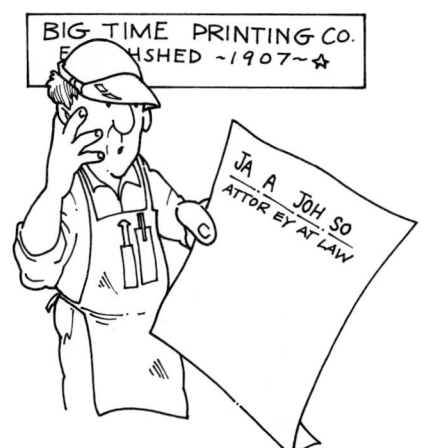

Just as each letter of the alphabet is important in forming whole words, each amino acid must be available to build finished proteins.

FIGURE 6-13

MUTUAL SUPPLEMENTATION

Proteins A and B are incomplete proteins, that is, they each lack one or more essential amino acids. Luckily for the eater, proteins A and B are complementary proteins.

After digestion and absorption, the two complementary proteins provide all of the essential amino acids from which the body can build the proteins it needs.

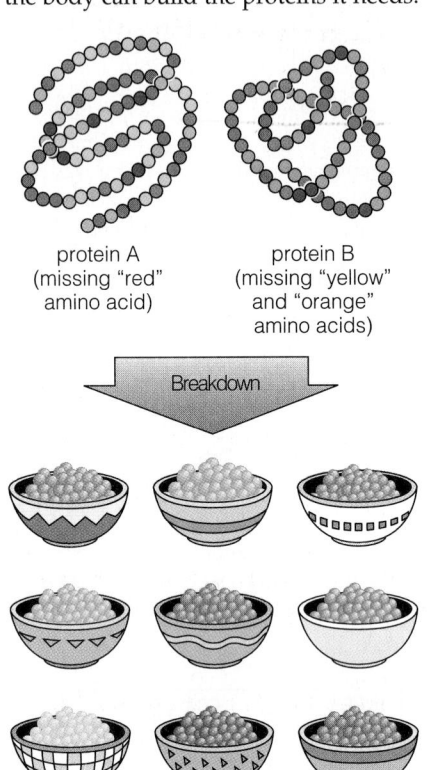

protein A
(missing "red"
amino acid)

protein B
(missing "yellow"
and "orange"
amino acids)

Breakdown

protein digestibility–corrected amino acid score (PDCAAS) a measuring tool used to determine protein quality. PDCAAS reflects a protein's digestibility as well as the proportions of amino acids that it provides.

protein efficiency ratio (PER) a measure of protein quality assessed by determining how well a given protein supports weight gain in growing rats. The PER is used to judge the quality of protein in infant formulas and baby foods.

✓ **KEY POINT**   **A protein's amino acid assortment greatly influences its usefulness to the body. Proteins lacking needed amino acids can be used only if those amino acids are present from other sources.**

Measuring Protein Quality

Researchers have developed many different methods of evaluating the quality of food protein. The most important one for consumers is the **protein digestibility–corrected amino acid score,** or **PDCAAS.** The protein values that U.S. consumers read on food labels are based on PDCAAS. Another measure of protein quality, the **protein efficiency ratio (PER),** is also used for measuring the protein quality of infant and baby foods.

The PDCAAS correction for digestibility is important. Simple measures of the total protein in foods are not useful by themselves, since even animal hair or hooves would receive a top score by those measures alone. Some PDCAAS scores are listed in Table 6-3 in the margin. A person trying to choose between peanut butter and chili in the grocery store may have no use for the PDCAAS scoring method, but scientists who must establish adequacy of protein sources for human health worldwide rely on it heavily.[11] Of more relevance to the average well-fed North American, however, is the protein RDA, discussed next.

✓ **KEY POINT**   **The quality of a protein is measured by its amino acids, its digestibility, or by how well the protein supports growth.**

TABLE 6-2

Complementary Protein Combinations

Combine foods from two or more of these columns to obtain complete protein.			
Grains	**Legumes**	**Seeds and Nuts**	**Vegetables**
Barley	Dried beans	Cashews	Broccoli
Bulgur	Dried lentils	Nut butters	Leafy greens
Cornmeal	Dried peas	Other nuts	Other
Oats	Peanuts	Sesame seeds	vegetables
Pasta	Soy products	Sunflower seeds	
Rice		Walnuts	
Whole-grain breads			

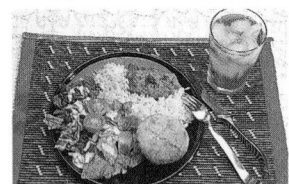
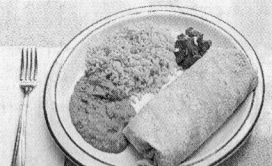
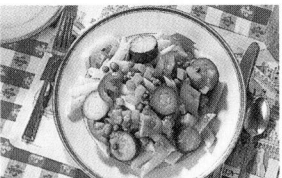
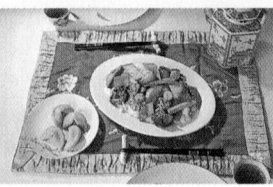
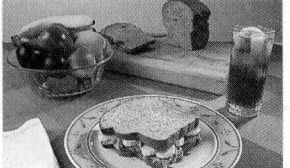

The Protein RDA

The RDA for protein is designed to cover the need to replace protein-containing tissue that people lose and wear out every day. Therefore it depends on body size: larger people have a higher protein RDA. The protein RDA is also adjusted to cover additional needs for building new tissue and so is higher for growing children and pregnant and lactating women. The Canadian recommendation for protein is similar and is based on similar assumptions. Table 6-4 reviews the recommendations concerning dietary protein, first presented in Chapter 2. These ensure that the body is well supplied with the protein it needs.

Underlying the protein RDA are **nitrogen balance** studies, which measure nitrogen lost by excretion compared with nitrogen eaten in food. In healthy adults, nitrogen-in (consumed) must equal nitrogen-out (excreted). The laboratory scientist measures the body's daily nitrogen losses in urine, feces, sweat, and skin under controlled conditions and can then estimate the amount of protein needed to replace these losses.*

Under normal circumstances healthy adults are in nitrogen equilibrium, or zero balance; that is, they have the same amount of total protein in their bodies at all times. When nitrogen-in exceeds nitrogen-out, people are said to be in positive nitrogen balance; this means that somewhere in their bodies more proteins are being built than are being broken down and lost. When nitrogen-in is less than nitrogen-out, people are said to be in negative nitrogen balance; they are losing protein. Figure 6-14 illustrates these different states.

Growing children add new blood, bone, and muscle cells to their bodies every day. These cells contain protein, so children must have more protein, and

---

*The average protein is 16 percent nitrogen by weight; that is, each 100 grams of protein contain 16 grams of nitrogen. As a rule of thumb, the scientist multiplies the nitrogen's weight by 6.25 to estimate the protein's weight.

TABLE 6-3

PDCAAS of Selected Foods

Food	PDCAAS[a]
Egg white	100
Ground beef	100
Chicken hot dogs	100
Milk protein (casein)	100
Nonfat milk powder	100
Beef salami	100
Tuna	100
Soybean protein	94
Whole wheat–pea flour	82[b]
Chick peas (garbanzos)	69
Kidney beans	68
Peas	67
Sausage, pork	63
Pinto beans	61
Rolled oats	57
Black beans	53
Lentils	52
Peanut meal	52
Whole wheat	40
Wheat protein (gluten)	25

[a]Proteins whose digestion and amino acid balance are perfect for meeting human needs are given a score of 100; others are scored against this standard.
[b]An example of mutual supplementation. Combining whole wheat and pea flours yields a protein with a higher PDCAAS than that of either product alone.

nitrogen balance the amount of nitrogen consumed compared with the amount excreted in a given time period.

TABLE 6-4

Recommendations Concerning Intakes of Protein for Adults[a]

Recommended Dietary Allowance (RDA)
- 0.8 gram protein per kilogram body weight per day.

Dietary Guidelines
- Every day eat 2 to 3 servings to total 4 to 9 ounces daily of cooked dry beans and peas, lean beef or other lean meats, poultry without the skin, fish and shellfish, and occasionally eggs and organ meats.
- Every day choose 2 to 3 servings of lowfat or nonfat milk, yogurt, or cheese.
- Eat a variety of foods to provide small amounts of protein from other sources.

Daily Values[b]
- 50 grams protein per day.

World Health Organization
- Lower limit: 10% of total calories from protein.
- Upper limit: 15% of total calories from protein.

[a]Protein recommendations for infants, children, and pregnant and lactating women are higher.
[b]The Daily Value is for a 2,000-calorie diet.

FIGURE 6-14

NITROGEN BALANCE

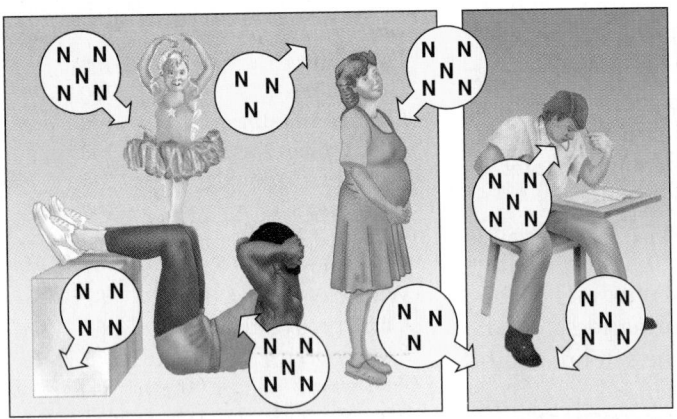

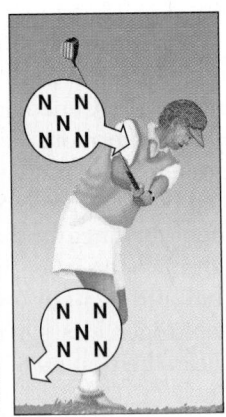
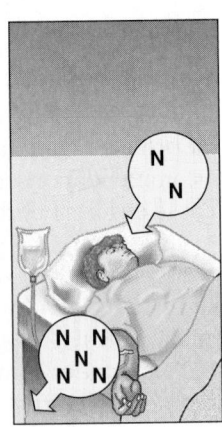

Positive Nitrogen Balance
These people, a growing child, a person building muscle, and a pregnant woman, are all retaining more nitrogen than they are excreting.

Nitrogen Equilibrium
These people, a healthy college student and a young retiree, are in nitrogen equilibrium.

Negative Nitrogen Balance
These people, an astronaut and a surgery patient, are losing more nitrogen than they are taking in.

therefore more nitrogen, in their bodies at the end of each day than they had at the beginning. A growing child is therefore in positive nitrogen balance. Similarly, when a woman is pregnant, she is, in essence, growing a new person; she too must be in positive nitrogen balance until after the birth when she once again reaches equilibrium.

Negative nitrogen balance occurs when muscle or other protein tissue is broken down and lost.[12] Consider the situation of an ill person, for example. Illness or injury triggers the release of powerful messengers that signal the body to break down nonessential proteins, such as those of the skin.* This action floods the blood with amino acids needed for building antibodies to fight the illness and for energy to fuel the body's defenses. The result is negative nitrogen balance. Astronauts, too, experience negative nitrogen balance. Nutritionists responsible for the welfare of astronauts must plan for the negative nitrogen balance that occurs after many days without gravity in space.[13] Without the exercise of supporting their bodies' weight against gravity, the astronauts' muscles waste and weaken. To minimize the inevitable loss of muscle tissue, they must do special exercises in space.

For healthy adults, the RDA for protein has been set at 0.8 grams for each kilogram (or 2.2 pounds) of body weight. Athletes need slightly more, but the increased need is well covered by a regular diet (more in Chapter 10). For infants and children who are growing, the protein RDA, like all nutrient RDA, is higher per unit of body weight.

In making its recommendations for protein intakes, the members of the committee on RDA took into consideration that the protein in a normal diet would be mixed, that is, a combination of animal and plant protein. They also

More on exercise in bone-loss prevention in Controversy 8 and Chapter 10.

———————
*The messengers are cytokines.

recognized that not all proteins are used with 100 percent efficiency and that individuals use protein with different efficiencies. Accordingly, the committee made the RDA quite generous. Many normal people can consume less than the RDA for protein and still meet their bodies' needs. What this means in terms of food selections is presented in this chapter's Food Feature.

✔ **KEY POINT**   **Nitrogen balance compares nitrogen excreted from the body with nitrogen ingested in food. The amount of protein needed daily depends on size and stage of growth. The RDA for adults is 0.8 gram of protein per kilogram of body weight.**

PROTEIN DEFICIENCY AND EXCESS

With all the attention that has been paid in recent years to the health effects of starch, sugars, fibers, fats, oils, and cholesterol, protein has been slighted. Protein deficiencies are well known because, together with energy deficiencies, they are the world's leading form of malnutrition. But the health effects of too much protein are far less well known. Both deficiency and excess are of concern.

Protein-Energy Malnutrition

Protein deficiency and energy deficiency go hand in hand. This combination—**protein-energy malnutrition (PEM)**—is the most widespread form of malnutrition in the world today, costing an estimated 13 to 18 million lives, most of them young, each year. Many more millions face imminent starvation and suffer the effects of severe malnutrition and **hunger.** PEM is prevalent in Africa, Central America, South America, the Near East, and the Far East, but developed countries including the United States are not immune to it.

PEM strikes early in childhood, but it endangers many adults as well. Inadequate food intake leads to poor growth in children and to weight loss and wasting in adults. Stunted growth due to PEM is easy to overlook because a small child can look perfectly normal. The small stature of children in impoverished nations was once thought to be a normal adaptation to the limited availability of food; now it is known to be an avoidable failure of growth due to a lack of food during the growing years.[14]

PEM seems to take two different forms. In one, the person is shriveled and lean all over; in the other, a swollen belly and skin rash are present. These forms of PEM have two different disease names: **marasmus** and **kwashiorkor,** respectively.[15*] Marasmus was thought to be caused by energy deficiency and kwashiorkor by protein deficiency. In reality, though, marasmus reflects a chronic inadequate food intake and therefore inadequate energy, vitamins, and minerals as well as too little protein. Kwashiorkor may result from severe acute malnutrition, with too little protein to support body functions.[16]

Marasmus   Marasmus occurs most commonly in children from 6 to 18 months of age in overpopulated city slums. Children in impoverished nations subsist on a weak cereal drink with scant energy and protein of low quality;

---

*A term gaining acceptance for use in place of kwashiorkor is hypoalbuminemic-type PEM.

protein-energy malnutrition (PEM) also called **protein-calorie malnutrition (PCM)** the world's most widespread malnutrition problem, including both marasmus and kwashiorkor and states in which they overlap.

hunger the physiological craving for food; the progressive discomfort, illness, and pain resulting from the lack of food. (See also Chapters 9 and 15.)

marasmus (ma-RAZ-mus) the calorie-deficiency disease; starvation.

kwashiorkor (kwash-ee-OR-core, kwashee-or-CORE) a disease related to protein malnutrition, with a set of recognizable symptoms, such as edema.

Protein RDA (adult) = 0.8 g/kg

To figure your protein RDA:
1. Find your body weight.
2. Convert pounds to kilograms (pounds divided by 2.2 lb/kg equal kilograms).
3. Multiply by 0.8 g/kg to get your RDA in grams per day.

For example:
1. Weight = 110 lb
2. 110 lb ÷ 2.2 lb/kg = 50 kg
3. 50 kg × 0.8 g/kg = 40 g

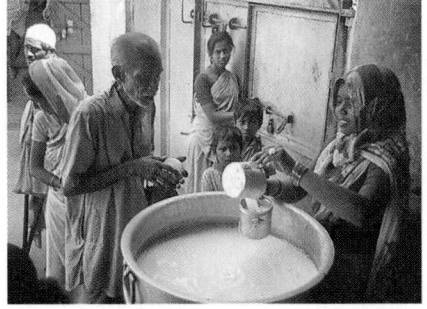

Scant supplies of donated food save some from starvation, but many others go hungry.

dysentery (DISS-en-terry) an infection of the digestive tract that causes diarrhea.

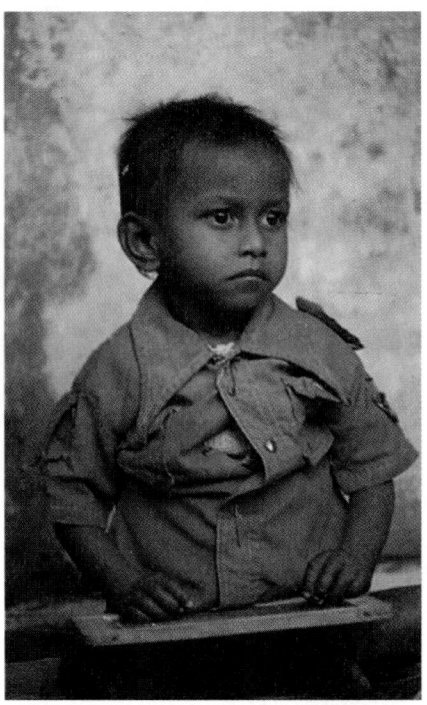

Protein malnutrition impairs learning.

The term *electrolyte balance* refers to the proper concentrations of salts within the body fluids (see Chapter 8 for details).

such food can barely sustain life, much less support growth. A starving child often looks like a wizened little old person—just skin and bones.

Without adequate nutrition, muscles, including the heart muscles, waste and weaken. Brain development is stunted and learning is impaired. Metabolism is so slow that body temperature is subnormal. There is little or no fat under the skin to insulate against cold. Hospital workers find that children with marasmus need to be wrapped up and kept warm. They also need love because they have often been deprived of parental attention as well as food.

The starving child faces this threat to life by engaging in as little activity as possible—not even crying for food. The body collects all its forces to meet the crisis and so cuts down on any expenditure of protein not needed for the heart, lungs, and brain to function. Growth ceases; the child is no larger at age four than at age two. The skin loses its elasticity and moisture, so it tends to crack; when sores develop, they fail to heal.[17] Digestive enzymes are in short supply, the digestive tract lining deteriorates, and absorption fails. The child can't assimilate what little food is eaten.

Blood proteins, including hemoglobin, are no longer produced, so the child becomes anemic and weak. The protein and energy needed for immune functions are lacking, which explains the high prevalence of infections in malnourished children. Antibodies to fight off invading bacteria are degraded to provide amino acids for other uses, leaving the child an easy target for infection.[18] Then **dysentery,** an infection of the digestive tract, causes diarrhea, further depleting the body of nutrients, especially minerals. Measles, which might make a healthy child sick for a week or two, kills a child with PEM within two or three days. In fact, infections that occur with malnutrition are responsible for two-thirds of the deaths of young children in developing countries.[19]

Ultimately, marasmus progresses to the point of no return, when the body's machinery for protein synthesis, itself made of protein, has been degraded. At this point, attempts to correct the situation by giving food or protein fail to prevent death. If caught before this time, however, the starvation of a child may be reversed by careful nutrition therapy. The fluid balances are most critical. Diarrhea will have depleted the body's potassium and upset other electrolyte balances. The combination of electrolyte imbalances, anemia, fever, and infections often leads to heart failure and sudden death. Careful correction of fluid and electrolyte balances usually raises the blood pressure and strengthens the heartbeat within a few days. Later, nonfat milk, providing protein and carbohydrate, can safely be given; fat is introduced still later, when body protein is sufficient to provide carriers.

Kwashiorkor Kwashiorkor is the Ghanaian name for "the evil spirit that infects the first child when the second child is born." In countries where kwashiorkor is prevalent, each baby is weaned from breast milk as soon as the next one comes along. The older baby no longer receives breast milk, which contains high-quality protein designed perfectly to support growth, but is given a watery cereal with scant protein of low quality. Small wonder the just-weaned child sickens when the new baby arrives.

Some kwashiorkor symptoms very much resemble those of marasmus (see Table 6-5), but often without severe wasting of body fat. Proteins and hormones that previously maintained fluid balance are now diminished, so that fluid leaks out of the blood and accumulates in the belly and legs, causing

TABLE 6-5

Features of Marasmus and Kwashiorkor in Children

Separating PEM into two classifications oversimplifies the condition, but at the extremes, marasmus and kwashiorkor exhibit marked differences. Marasmus-kwashiorkor mix presents symptoms common to both marasmus and kwashiorkor. In all cases, children are likely to develop diarrhea, infections, and multiple nutrient deficiencies.

Marasmus	Kwashiorkor
Infancy (less than 2 yr)	Older infants and young children (1 to 3 yr)
Severe deprivation, or impaired absorption, of protein, energy, vitamins, and minerals	Inadequate protein intake or, more commonly, infections
Develops slowly; chronic PEM	Rapid onset; acute PEM
Severe weight loss	Some weight loss
Severe muscle wasting, with fat loss	Some muscle wasting, with retention of some body fat
Growth: <60% weight-for-age	Growth: 60 to 80% weight-for-age
No detectable edema	Edema
No fatty liver	Enlarged, fatty liver
Anxiety, apathy	Apathy, misery, irritability, sadness
Good appetite possible	Loss of appetite
Hair is sparse, thin, and dry; easily pulled out	Hair is dry and brittle; easily pulled out; changes color; becomes straight
Skin is dry and thin and wrinkles easily	Skin develops lesions

edema, a distinguishing feature of kwashiorkor. The kwashiorkor victim's belly often bulges with a fatty liver, caused by lack of the protein carriers that transport fat out of the liver.[20] The fatty liver loses some of its ability to clear poisons from the body, prolonging their toxic effects. Without sufficient tyrosine to make melanin, the child's hair loses its color; inadequate protein synthesis leaves the skin patchy and scaly; sores fail to heal.

Melanin, a brown pigment of hair, skin, and eyes, was mentioned earlier as a product made from tyrosine.

PEM at Home PEM is common among some groups in the United States and Canada: the poor living on U.S. Indian reservations, in inner cities, and in rural areas; many elderly people; hungry and homeless children; and those suffering from the eating disorder anorexia nervosa.[21] People who are hospitalized for long periods are also at risk for PEM, as are those addicted to drugs and alcohol.

Today, millions of people who work to support their children earn so little that they cannot afford nutritious food—one child in eight under the age of 12 goes hungry. This situation presents a challenge to nutritionists.[22] Hunger, especially in children, threatens everyone's future. Hungry children do not learn as well as fed children, nor are they competitive. They are ill more often, they have higher absentee rates from school, and when they attend, they cannot concentrate for long. The forces driving poverty and hunger will require many great minds working together to find solutions. Chapter 15 comes back to the topics of hunger, food, and poverty.

✔ **KEY POINT** Protein-deficiency symptoms are always observed when either protein or energy is deficient. Extreme food-energy deficiency is marasmus; extreme protein deficiency is kwashiorkor. The two diseases overlap most of the time and together are called PEM.

Protein Excess

While many of the world's people struggle to obtain enough food and enough protein to keep themselves alive, people in developed countries must consciously limit their protein intakes to avoid excesses. Overconsumption of protein offers no benefits and may pose health risks. For one thing, as mentioned before, protein-rich foods are often high-fat foods that contribute to obesity with its accompanying health risks. Furthermore, foods providing animal protein can be high in saturated fat, a known contributor to atherosclerosis and heart disease. Independently of the effects of saturated fat, however, animal protein itself may raise blood cholesterol, thus contributing to atherosclerosis and heart disease. The protein of soybeans, on the other hand, seems to lower blood cholesterol.[23]

Animals fed experimentally on high-protein diets may develop enlarged kidneys or livers. In human beings, high-protein diets eaten over a lifetime are known to worsen existing kidney problems.[24] A preliminary study also suggests that the people who consume the most protein may face a doubled risk of developing kidney cancer.[25] This study opens the door to additional research that will strengthen or refute the finding.

High protein intakes may also accelerate adult bone loss. Calcium excretion rises as protein intake increases, especially protein from animal-derived, though not plant-derived, foods.[26] Whether excess protein depletes bone minerals depends largely upon the ratio of dietary calcium to protein.[27] An ideal ratio has not been established, but a woman whose intake just meets, but does not exceed, the RDA for both nutrients has a calcium-to-protein ratio of 16 milligrams calcium to 1 gram protein. For most women in the United States, however, average calcium intakes are lower and protein intakes are higher, yielding a 9-to-1 relationship, which may produce calcium losses that compromise bone health.[28] Regular physical activity and adequate calcium intake may help to protect against such losses.[29]

The committee on RDA has suggested an upper limit for protein intake of no more than twice the RDA amount, and the World Health Organization (WHO) suggests an even more stringent upper limit of 15 percent of total calories. In a world where protein deficiency is such a threat to so many, it is ironic that some people in developed countries should be overconsuming protein.

✓ KEY POINT   **Health risks follow the overconsumption of protein-rich foods.**

Protein RDA for women aged
19 to 24 = 46 g
Average protein intake = 65 g

Protein RDA for men aged 19 to 24 = 58 g
Average protein intake = 105 g

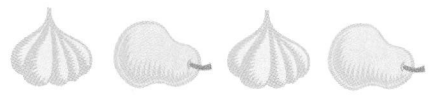

It is clear by now that people in developed nations usually eat more than ample protein. The protein RDA is generous: it more than adequately covers the estimated needs of most people, even those with unusually high requirements.

Foods in the meat, poultry, fish, dry beans, eggs, and nuts group and in the milk, yogurt, and cheese groups contribute an abundance of high-quality protein. Two others, the vegetables and bread, cereals, rice, and pasta groups, contribute smaller amounts of protein, but they can add up to significant quantities. What about the fruit group? Don't rely on fruit for protein—fruit contains only small amounts. Figure 6-15 shows the wide variety of foods that contribute most of the protein to the diet.

Protein is critical in nutrition, but too many protein-rich foods can displace other important foods from the diet. Foods richest in protein carry with them a characteristic array of vitamins and minerals, including vitamin B_{12} and iron, but they are notoriously lacking in others—vitamin C and folate, for example. In addition, many protein-rich foods such as meat are high in calories, and to overconsume them is to invite obesity.

With so many foods contributing to the protein of a day's meals, one can have confidence that one's protein intake is ample. With this knowledge, one can plan meatless or reduced-meat meals with pleasure. Of the many interesting, protein-rich meat alternates available, one has already been mentioned: the legumes.

FOOD FEATURE

GETTING ENOUGH, BUT NOT TOO MUCH, PROTEIN

FIGURE 6-15

PROTEIN IN FOODS[a]

Cooked cereal, rice, noodles, pasta, ½ c
   3 g protein

Legumes, cooked, ½ c
   7 g protein

Egg, 1 large
   6 g protein

Cheese, 1½ oz
   11 g protein

[a]Average values.

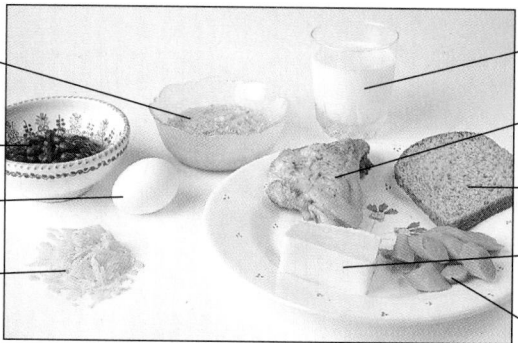

Milk or yogurt, 1 c
   8 g protein

Poultry, beef, pork or lamb, 3 oz
   26 g protein

Bread, 1 slice
   2 g protein

Tofu, 3 oz
   7 g protein

Cooked vegetables, ½ c
   2 g protein

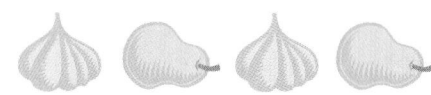

textured vegetable protein processed soybean protein used in products formulated to look and taste like meat, fish, or poultry.

tofu (TOE-foo) a curd made from soybeans, rich in protein, often rich in calcium, and variable in fat content; used in many Asian and vegetarian dishes in place of meat.

FIGURE 6-16

A LEGUME

The legumes include such plants as the kidney bean, soybean, garden pea, lentil, black-eyed pea, and lima bean. Bacteria in the root nodules can "fix" nitrogen from the air, contributing it to the beans. Ultimately, thanks to these bacteria, the plant accumulates more nitrogen than it can get from the soil and also leaves more nitrogen in the soil than it takes out. So efficient at trapping nitrogen are the legumes that farmers often grow them in rotation with other crops to fertilize fields. Legumes are shown among the meat alternatives in Figure 2-4 of Chapter 2.

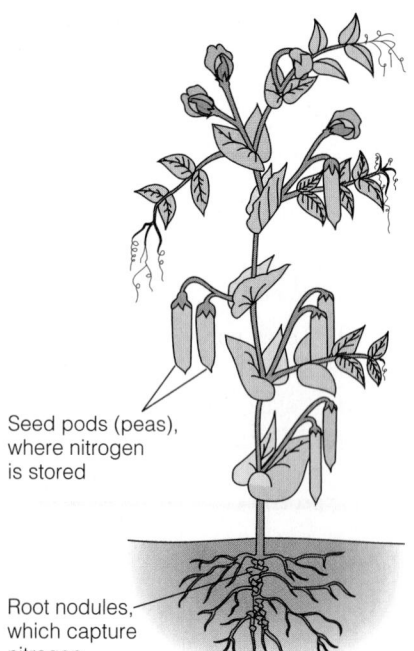

Seed pods (peas), where nitrogen is stored

Root nodules, which capture nitrogen

The protein of some legumes is of a quality almost comparable to that of meat. In fact, for practical purposes, the quality of soy protein can be considered equivalent to that of meat.[30] Figure 6-16 shows a legume plant's special root system that enables it to make abundant protein. Legumes are also excellent sources of fiber, many B vitamins, iron, calcium, and other minerals. A cup of cooked legumes contains 31 percent of the protein and 42 percent of the iron recommended daily for an adult male. Like meats, though, legumes do not offer every nutrient, and they do not make a complete meal by themselves. They contain no vitamin A, vitamin C, or vitamin B_{12}, and their balance of amino acids can be much improved by using grains and other vegetables with them.

Soybeans are versatile legumes, and people make many products from them. One problem, however, is that the heavy use of soy products in place of meat inhibits iron absorption. The effect can be alleviated by using small amounts of meat and/or foods rich in vitamin C in the same meal with soy products. Vegetarians sometimes use convenience foods made from **textured vegetable protein** (soy protein) formulated to look and taste like hamburgers or breakfast sausages. Many of these are intended to match the known nutrient contents of animal-protein foods, but often they fall short.* A wise vegetarian would use such foods sparingly, and learn to use combinations of whole foods to supply the needed nutrients.

Another form in which the nutrients of soybeans are available is as bean curd, or **tofu,** a staple used in many Asian dishes. Thanks to the use of calcium salts when some tofu is made, it can be high in calcium. Check the nutrition facts on the label.

The Food Features presented so far show that the recommendations for the three energy-yielding nutrients go hand in hand. If you reduce fat and increase carbohydrate, protein totals automatically come into line with the requirements. To help you accept that protein is abundant in most foods, the Do It section that follows asks you to complete a day's meals and watch the protein grams add up.

---

*In Canada, regulations govern the nutrient contents of such products.

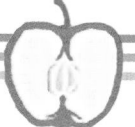

Do It!

ADD UP THE PROTEIN IN A DAY'S MEALS

Consider the sources of protein in a day's meals. Look at the meals in Figure 6-17. Breakfast and lunch are given, but supper is yet to be planned. A simple breakfast of cereal, milk, and juice provides 14 grams of protein. Lunch is a bit heartier with a ham and cheese sandwich contributing most of its 18 protein grams. Now comes a puzzle—which supper to choose? After picking a supper from among the choices, check Figure 6-18 to find out how much protein each supper contains. Then compare the protein in the meals with your protein RDA (see the calculation in the margin of page 211, or use the RDA value from the inside front cover).

FIGURE 6-17

A PROTEIN PUZZLE

The protein values listed in this exercise are from the *Food Processor Plus*, a computerized diet analysis software program developed by ESHA Research, 1996.

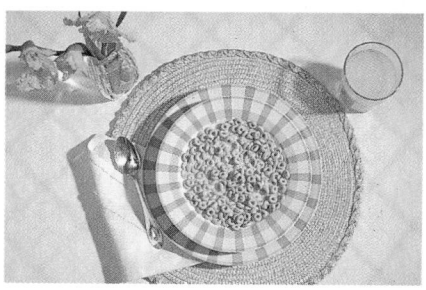

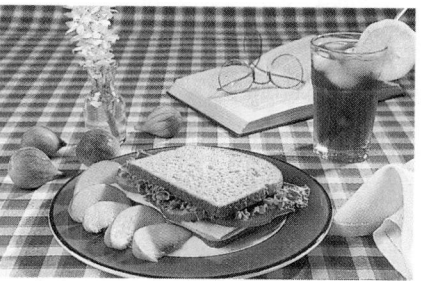

Breakfast
1 c orange juice
 2 g protein
Cheerios cereal, 1 oz
 4 g protein
1 c low-fat milk
 8 g protein
Breakfast total = 14 g protein

Lunch
iced tea
 0 g protein
ham and cheese sandwich (1 slice lunchmeat; 1 slice cheese; ¾ c lettuce and tomato; 2 slices whole-wheat bread)
 17 g protein
peaches ½ c
 1 g protein
Lunch total = 18 g protein

So far, this day's meals have contributed 32 grams of protein. On this basis, what would you choose for supper? Turn the page to see how much protein each supper adds to the day's intake.

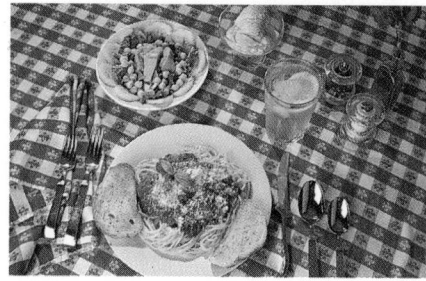

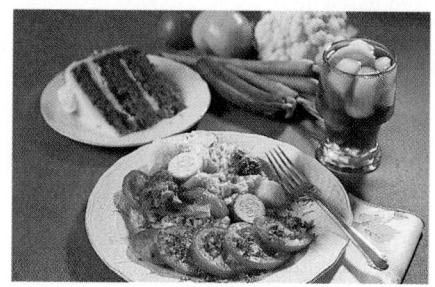

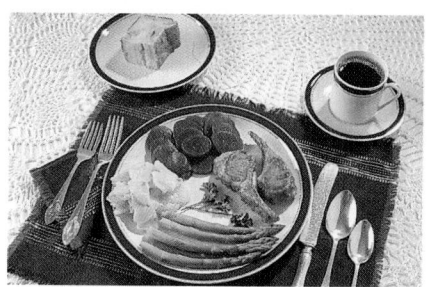

Supper A = ? protein

Supper B = ? protein

Supper C = ? protein

Two of the supper options are meatless (the spaghetti supper and the vegetable-rice supper), and one contains meat. To quickly assess the protein in such meals, remember that the fruits provide only a little protein, but that meats, milk, and cheeses are the richest sources, followed by legumes, grains, breads, and vegetables.

Settle on a supper choice and consider these questions:

1. Did the supper you chose add up to a protein total that meets, but does not exceed, your protein RDA? Which other suppers also qualify?

2. If your answer to question 1 was no, which foods might you substitute to achieve your goal without shorting yourself on nutrients? Hint: To keep from vastly overconsuming protein, you may need to restrict something, and an obvious "something" to restrict is some of the meat.

3. Make some educated guesses concerning the other two energy-yielding nutrients, fat and carbohydrate. Which foods contribute abundant fat and saturated fat to this day's meals? Which contribute carbohydrates and fiber?

4. Note that breakfast, while it contains no meat, provides almost as much protein as the ham and cheese sandwich at lunch. Which foods in this breakfast provide protein? Is the protein of each of these foods complete or incomplete? Is the total breakfast protein complete or incomplete? Why?

5. Which plant food shown in Figure 6-18 is the richest in protein? Which is next richest? Hint: If you have eliminated or are considering eliminating meat from your diet, read the Controversy that follows—it points out the pros and cons of both vegetarian and meat-containing diets.

6. If you were to design a day's meals around the lamb supper, yet did not want to consume too much protein, how would you change breakfast and lunch? What foods would you substitute for some of the protein-rich foods listed in Figure 6-17? Another hint: If you are considering doing away with the milk or cheese, remember that you must then provide other sources of calcium (you may reconsider this decision when you discover in Chapter 8 that few foods other than milk supply an abundance of calcium).

FIGURE 6-18

PROTEIN PUZZLE ANSWERS

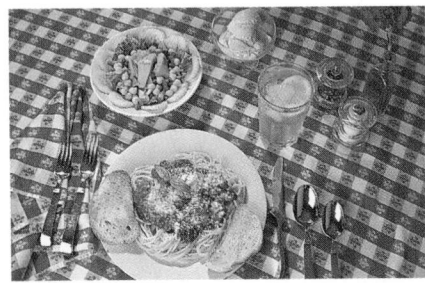

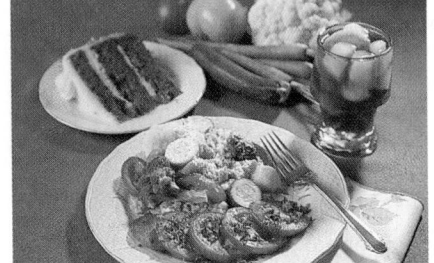

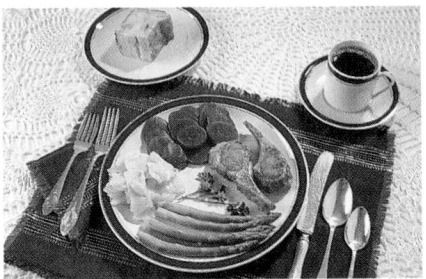

Choice A.
iced water/lemon
  0 g protein
garlic bread, 2 pieces
  6 g protein
large salad with ¼ c each garbanzo beans, artichoke and cucumber
  6 g protein
spaghetti, 1 c; parmesan cheese, 1 tbs
  13 g protein
sherbet, 1 c
  2 g protein
Totals:
Supper A total =
  27 g protein
Entire day's protein = 59 g

Choice B.
iced tea/lemon
  0 g protein
tomato slices, ½ c
  1 g protein
grated cheese, 1 tbs
  3 g protein
mixed vegetables, 1 c
  4 g protein
brown rice, 1 c
  6 g protein
carrot cake, 1 pce
  4 g protein
Totals:
Supper B total = 18 g protein
Entire day's protein = 50 g

Choice C.
coffee, black, 1 c
  0 g protein
bread pudding, ½ c
  7 g protein
asparagus, ½ c
  2 g protein
potatoes au gratin, ½ c
  6 g protein
lamb chops, 2-oz
  35 g protein
sliced beets, ½ c
  1 g protein
Totals:
Supper C total = 51 g
Entire day's protein = 83 g

SELF-CHECK

Answers to these Self-Check questions are in Appendix G.

1. The basic building blocks for protein are:
   a. glucose units
   b. amino acids
   c. side chains
   d. saturated bonds

2. Protein digestion begins in the:
   a. mouth
   b. stomach
   c. small intestine
   d. large intestine

3. Which of the following can form enzymes?
   a. carbohydrates
   b. lipids
   c. proteins
   d. (b) and (c)

4. For healthy adults, the RDA for protein has been set at:
   a. 0.8 gram per kilogram of body weight
   b. 2.2 pounds per kilogram of body weight
   c. 12 to 15 percent of total calories
   d. 100 grams per day

5. Which of the following conditions occur(s) less frequently in people who consume vegetarian diets? (Read about this in the upcoming Controversy.)
   a. obesity
   b. high blood pressure
   c. diverticular disease
   d. all of the above

6. Under certain circumstances, protein can be converted to glucose and so serve the energy needs of the brain.   T   F

7. Too little protein in the diet can have severe consequences, but excess protein has no adverse effects.   T   F

8. Although protein-energy malnutrition (PEM) is prevalent in developing nations, it is not seen in the United States.   T   F

9. Partially completed proteins are not held for completion at a later time when the diet may improve.   T   F

10. An example of a person in negative nitrogen balance is an astronaut.   T   F

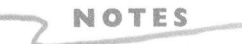

NOTES

Notes are in Appendix F.

Vegetarians versus Meat Eaters: Whose Diet Is Best?

One young professional person rejects all animal products, shuns grains, and seeks out vegetables, fruits, and herbs. Another young professional relishes meat at every meal and usually orders "a steak and potato: hold the rabbit food." These two have a lot more in common than either would probably believe. Both are extremists in their choices of foods. Both may be jeopardizing their health by their rigid, unbalanced eating styles. But both vegetarian diets and meat-containing diets have elements in their favor, provided that they are not taken to

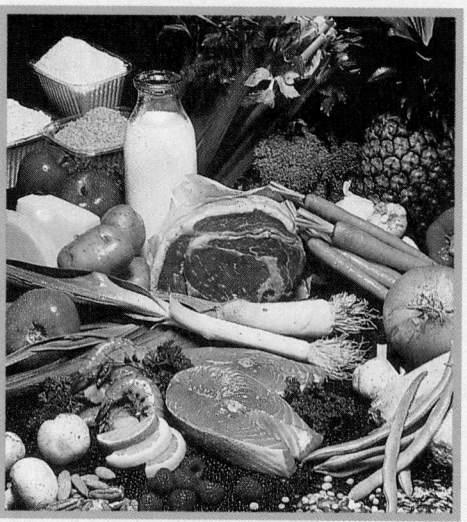

extremes. This Controversy looks first at the positive health aspects of vegetarian diets, then at the positive aspects of meat eaters' diets. It concludes by showing how both types of eaters can maximize the benefits and minimize the risks of their diets.

POSITIVE HEALTH ASPECTS OF VEGETARIAN DIETS

In 1995, for the first time, the *Dietary Guidelines for Americans* acknowledged that some vegetarian diets are consistent with excellent health.[1] This statement came in response to strong research links between vegetarian diets and reduced incidence of chronic diseases. Such research results are not easily obtained. It would be easy if vegetarians differed from others only in not consuming meat, but they also have *increased* intakes of fruits and vegetables, the primary contributors of phytochemicals believed to reduce disease risks, and more fiber, also associated with reduced disease risks.[2] Also, though there are exceptions, vegetarians typically use no tobacco, use alcohol in moderation if at all, and are physically active. Researchers must account for the effects of these lifestyle differences on disease development before they can see how health correlates with diet. Even then, *correlations* are not causes. Without more evidence, conclusions must be tentative.

Still, with all these qualifications, research findings are intriguing. They seem to indicate that a vegetarian diet may offer some protection against six conditions: obesity, diabetes, high blood pressure, heart disease,

digestive disorders, and some forms of cancer. It matters, however, what form the vegetarian diet takes. Vegetarians differ, as Table C6-1 demonstrates. What is known about the relationships between vegetarianism and disease follows.[3]

Obesity and Diabetes

Vegetarians tend to be leaner than nonvegetarians. Perhaps they consciously control their calorie intakes and make an effort to exercise regularly. Perhaps their diet, which tends to be high in fiber-rich bulky foods, is automatically lower in calories than the average diet based on meat.

The fattening power of fat, described in Controversy 5, may also be a factor: vegetarians tend to have low intakes of fat, which is easily stored in the body, and high intakes of carbohydrate, which is harder to store. One study found vegetarians have higher rates of metabolism than nonvegetarians.[4] This finding is consistent with the idea that carbohydrate calories are used most readily for fuel in a mixed diet, while fat calories are most readily stored. In any case, a healthy body weight combined with high intakes of complex carbohydrates and fiber reduces the risks of diabetes and several other obesity-related diseases. A limited body of research implies a connection between meat-containing diets and increased incidences of diabetes, even without obesity.[5]

Blood Pressure Vegetarians often are found to have lower blood pressure than nonvegetarians. Various combinations of lifestyle factors and diet seem to influence blood pressure. Among lifestyle factors, smoking and alcohol intake raise blood pressure, and exercise lowers it. Diet alone may be significant, however. A recent review of the literature in this area concluded that "there is now convincing evidence for a blood-pressure-lowering effect of . . . the type [of diet] eaten by some vegetarians."[6] The authors qualify this by saying that the effect is associated with diets low in fat and saturated fat and high in fiber, fruits, and

TABLE C6-1

Terms Used to Describe Vegetarians

- **fruitarian** includes only raw or dried fruits, seeds, and nuts.
- **lacto-ovo vegetarian** includes dairy products, eggs, vegetables, grains, legumes, fruits, and nuts; excludes flesh and seafood.
- **lacto-vegetarian** includes dairy products, vegetables, grains, legumes, fruits, and nuts; excludes flesh, seafood, and eggs.
- **macrobiotic diet follower** observes a vegan diet that progressively eliminates more and more foods. Ultimately, only brown rice and small amounts of water or herbal tea are consumed; taken to extremes, macrobiotic diets have resulted in malnutrition and even death.
- **ovo-vegetarian** includes eggs, vegetables, grains, legumes, fruits, and nuts; excludes flesh, seafood, and milk products.
- **partial vegetarian** includes seafood, poultry, eggs, dairy products, vegetables, grains, legumes, fruits, and nuts; excludes or strictly limits red meats.
- **pesco-vegetarian** same as partial vegetarian, but eliminates poultry.
- **vegan** includes only food from plant sources: vegetables, grains, legumes, fruits, seeds and nuts; also called *strict vegetarian*.

SOURCE: Adapted from E. Antonian, Are vegetarian diets healthful? *Priorities*, March 1995, p. 37.

vegetables; they also say that meat itself need not be totally excluded. It would be oversimplifying to say that including or excluding any one food or nutrient lowers blood pressure. Apparently, many factors act together.

Heart Disease Fewer vegetarians than meat eaters suffer from diseases of the heart and arteries, even when the people being compared are all nonsmokers. The dietary factor most directly related to coronary artery disease is saturated fat intake, but other factors may also play a role.[7] Research is currently concentrating on the sources of protein in the diet and on the antioxidant nutrients and phytochemicals found in plants.

When vegetarians are fed meat, which contains saturated fat, their lipid profiles change for the worse; when meat eaters are fed a low-fat vegetarian diet, their lipid profiles improve. One study compared two low-fat diets, one vegetarian and another containing lean meats. Both diets lowered blood cholesterol, but the vegetarian diet's effects were greater.[8] People can achieve lower blood cholesterol and still eat meat: researchers found lowered blood cholesterol in subjects

Phytochemicals and antioxidants are discussed in Controversy 7.

who ate meat but also kept intakes of saturated fat to a minimum.[9] Even so, vegetarian diets lower blood cholesterol most dramatically.[10]

Protein itself may affect blood cholesterol. Experimental diets containing purified proteins from animal sources (milk, fish, and egg) raise blood cholesterol higher than do similar diets containing purified soybean protein, at least in some animals. When rabbits were fed diets containing 50 percent of calories from purified animal protein along with high cholesterol, the animals suffered rapid advancement of atherosclerosis.[11] Rabbits are naturally vegetarians, though, so this may not be a fair test of what happens in human beings. Another problem in the study concerns the use of soybean protein as a control. Soybean protein itself seems to have a cholesterol-lowering effect.[12]

People eat foods, not purified proteins, so the question of whether animal or vegetable proteins by themselves raise or lower blood cholesterol is academic. The purified proteins that experimentally raise blood cholesterol are milk protein (casein) and the protein of fish. If the whole foods are used instead of the isolated proteins, the contrast between animal and vegetable proteins is not seen. Milk *lowers* blood cholesterol just as soy does, and meals of fish provide benefits to heart health, as Chapter 5 made clear.

Vegetarians eat vegetables, and vegetables contain some constituents thought to be protective against

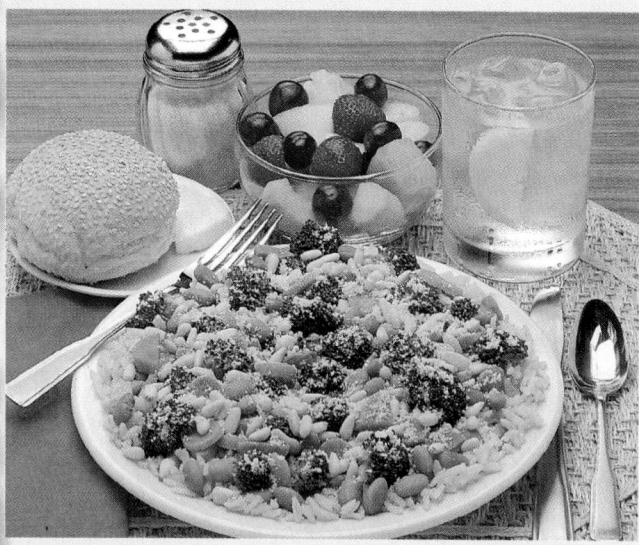

A balanced meal need not include meat to be nutritious.

heart disease. The antioxidant nutrients and phyto-chemicals are believed to oppose a crucial step in the formation of arterial plaques (see Controversy 7). Against heart disease, then, a vegetarian diet may offer these advantages:

- promotes leaner body composition and lower blood pressure.
- provides less saturated fat.
- provides more vegetable protein, fiber, antioxidant nutrients, and phytochemicals.

Digestive Disorders   Constipation and diverticular disease are less common in people who consume high-fiber vegetarian or semivegetarian diets than in people who consume typical meat-based diets. Chapter 4 presented possible ways fiber might influence the health of the digestive tract.

Cancer   Seventh-Day Adventists, an often-studied vegetarian group, enjoy a significantly lower cancer rate than the rest of the population, even when cancers linked to smoking and alcohol are taken out of the picture.[13] Their low cancer mortality may possibly be due to their low meat intakes, to their high intakes of fruits, vegetables, and cereal grains, to both, or to other lifestyle factors.

Some scientific findings support the idea that vegetarian diets may reduce the risks of colon cancer.[14] People with colon cancer seem to eat more meat, less fiber, and more saturated fat than others without colon cancer. Something about high-fat, high-protein, low-fiber

diets creates an environment in the human colon that may promote the development of cancer. Additionally, such a diet has been associated with a form of cancer of the lymphatic system.[15]

In general, then, many vegetarians have lower risks of developing obesity, high blood pressure, heart disease, digestive disorders, and cancer than do meat eaters. Two million people in the United States follow vegetarian diets. If they plan their diets correctly, they obtain all the nutrients they need to support good health.

POSITIVE HEALTH ASPECTS OF THE MEAT EATER'S DIET

The meat-loving character introduced at the start of this Controversy was exaggerated to make a point. Those who really eat like that place themselves in immediate peril of malnutrition. In reality, few people shun all vegetables. To be healthy, people must either eat foods from all five food groups presented in Chapter 2, or if they omit foods from one group, they must make careful substitutions to compensate. No substitutes can take the place of fruits and vegetables (not even antioxidant supplements, as the next chapter points out). This section considers a balanced diet of which meat is a part.

Growth   Meats, eggs, and other foods from animal sources support growth well. Without them, children's growth often lags behind the growth of peers. Populations existing on monotonous grain diets, either for reasons of meat taboos or of economic necessity, are often found to be malnourished, as revealed by their short stature, low resistance to diseases, short life span, and high infant mortality.

Even in populations with more varied diets, the children who eat the most animal-derived products have been observed to grow the best.[16] Even when the protein amounts are equal, children whose protein intakes are from plant sources may not grow as well as those eating animal products.[17] Protein may not be the only nutrient affecting growth, however; families who can afford to buy animal products are also likely to consume a larger variety of fruits and vegetables. These foods provide the vitamins and minerals also needed for growth.[18]

Foods of plant origin generally offer much less energy for their bulk than do foods of animal origin. A child's small stomach can hold only so much food, and a vegetarian child may feel full before having eaten enough food to supply nutrients and energy sufficient to support growth. For obesity-prone adults, a bulky diet can be advantageous, but a child fed without meat, milk, or eggs may face stunted growth that lasts a lifetime.

Are animal and dairy products superior to plants as protein-rich foods? It is true that animal and dairy foods contain complete, more digestible proteins. It seems to be true that children of milk- and meat-eating populations are generally larger, fatter, and more resistant to infections than are those of grain-eating populations. They are also protected from the vitamin D–deficiency disease rickets, which is especially likely to strike vegans in cold climates who are rarely exposed to the sun.[19]

It is also true, however, that meat itself may not be necessary for children to achieve healthy growth. Many children grow normally when milk and eggs accompany a vegetarian diet and when knowledgeable adults plan and deliver the diet with care. An example is again found among the Seventh-Day Adventists—the growth of children of that lacto-ovo vegetarian community is practically identical to the growth of children who eat meat.[20]

Support During Critical Times   Meat eaters can generally rely on their diets during critical times of life. In contrast, a vegan woman who doesn't meet her nutrient needs may enter pregnancy too thin; have inadequate stores of iron, zinc, and vitamin B_{12}; and fail to gain enough weight during pregnancy to support the normal growth and development of her fetus. Eaters of meats, eggs, and dairy products are much less likely to face these problems.

Unlike vegans, eaters of meats and dairy products can be sure of receiving enough vitamin B_{12}, vitamin D,

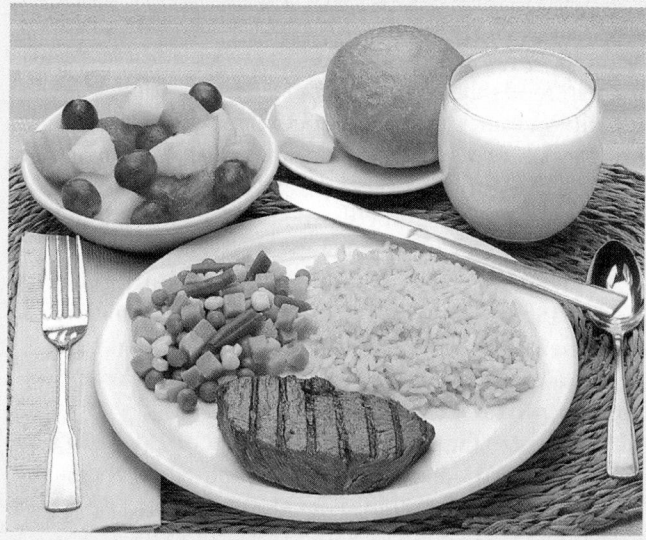

Two meat servings of the size depicted here present the maximum daily meat intake suggested by the Daily Food Guide as health promoting.

calcium, iron, and zinc, as well as protein, without supplements or fortified foods. Well-nourished vegetarian women, on the other hand, may habitually consume more folate and other nutrients associated with vegetables and fruits. The importance of adequate folate, especially for women in the childbearing years, will become evident in the next chapter.

CONCLUSIONS

Both the vegetarian's and the meat eater's diets have the potential to benefit health. Many of the benefits attributed to the vegetarian diet may be due to its low fat content, but a meat eater who keeps fat intakes low gains the same advantages. Diets including the recommended 2- to 3-ounce portions of such lean meats as skinless turkey breast and fish, as well as providing the needed low-fat grains, fruits, and vegetables, probably support health as well as vegetarian diets. The vegetarian diet's other chief advantage, that it is high in fiber, can also be true of the judicious meat eater's diet.

Have you noticed the lack of concern about protein for adult vegetarians? Protein is not the problem it was once thought to be for adults eating a varied diet. Even in vegans, protein deficiency is rare in those who consume adequate calories of various nutritious foods.[21]

With planning, both the meat eater's and the vegetarian's diets can contribute to their good health. Conversely, both diets can be high in saturated fat and so pose a threat to the health of the heart. A vegetarian who dines on cheddar cheese, butter sauces, sour cream, and deep-fried vegetables invites the same health hazards as the overeater of high-fat meats. And both diets, if not properly balanced, can lack nutrients.

For both eaters, then, planning is the key to obtaining adequate nutrients. Those who eliminate meats can follow a plan such as the Daily Food Guide for Vegetarians presented in Table C6-2.

To obtain calcium, U.S. consumers who use no milk can purchase calcium-fortified soy milk or calcium-fortified orange juice. Alternatively, large servings of calcium-rich green vegetables such as broccoli or kale make a sizable calcium donation to the diet. In addition, the nutrients iron, zinc, vitamin D, and vitamin B_{12} require special attention from strict vegetarians. Meat provides much of the iron and zinc in the meat-eater's diet, and vitamin D and vitamin B_{12} are found reliably only in animal-derived foods. Vegetarians can obtain iron and zinc from plant foods such as legumes, dark green, leafy vegetables, fortified cereals, and whole-grain breads and cereals. An interesting note is that well-fed vegetarians are not found to be deficient in iron

TABLE C6-2

Daily Food Guide for Vegetarians

Food Group	Suggested Daily Servings	Serving Sizes
Bread, cereal, rice, and pasta	6 or more	1 slice bread ½ bun, bagel, or English muffin ½ c cooked cereal, rice, or pasta 1 oz dry cereal
Vegetables Legumes and other meat substitutes	4 or more 2 to 3	½ c cooked or 1 c raw ½ c cooked beans 4 oz tofu or tempeh 8 oz soy milk 2 tbs nuts or seeds (these tend to be high in fat, so use sparingly if you are following a low-fat diet)
Fruit	3 or more	1 piece fresh fruit ¾ c fruit juice ½ c canned or cooked fruit
Milk, yogurt, cheese	Optional—up to 3 servings daily	1 c low-fat or skim milk 1 c low-fat or nonfat yogurt 1½ oz low-fat cheese
Eggs	Optional—limit to 3 to 4 yolks per week	1 egg or 2 egg whites
Fats, sweets, and alcohol	Use sparingly	Oil, margarine, and mayonnaise Cakes, cookies, pies, pastries, and candies Beef, wine, and distilled spirits

SOURCE: *Eating Well—the Vegetarian Way* (Chicago: American Dietetic Association, 1992).

or zinc any more often than are meat eaters. A strict vegetarian diet cannot meet vitamin D needs without a supplemental source or adequate exposure to sunlight (the next chapter provides details).[22] Substitutions take planning, but yield results.

Eggs, for those who eat them, can meet vitamin B_{12} needs; vegans must rely on vitamin B_{12}-fortified cereals and other sources or on supplements.[23] Fermented plant products such as tempeh, made from soybeans, may contain some vitamin B_{12} contributed by the bacteria that did the fermenting, but unfortunately, much of the vitamin B_{12} found in these products may be in an inactive form.

This comparison has shown that there is nothing mysterious about either the meat eater's or the vegetarian's diet. Both can be analyzed scientifically. In particular, vegetarianism is not a religion like Buddhism or Hinduism; it is merely an eating plan that selects plant foods to deliver needed nutrients. Some people make much of the distinctions between types of vegetarians, and the distinctions are useful academically, but they do not represent uncrossable lines. Many combinations of these categories exist. Some people use meat as a condiment or seasoning for vegetable or grain dishes. Some people eat meat only once a week and use plant protein foods the rest of the time. Many people rely mostly on milk products to meet their protein needs, but eat fish occasionally, and so forth. To force people into the categories of "vegetarians" and "meat eaters" leaves out all these in-between styles of eating that have much to recommend them.

To the person just beginning to study nutrition, consider adopting the attitude that the choice to make is not whether to be a meat eater or a vegetarian, but where along the spectrum to locate yourself. Your preferences, whatever they are, should be honored, and the only caveat is that you make your diet adequate, balanced, and varied and use moderation when choosing foods high in saturated fat or calories.

NOTES

Notes are in Appendix F.

THE VITAMINS

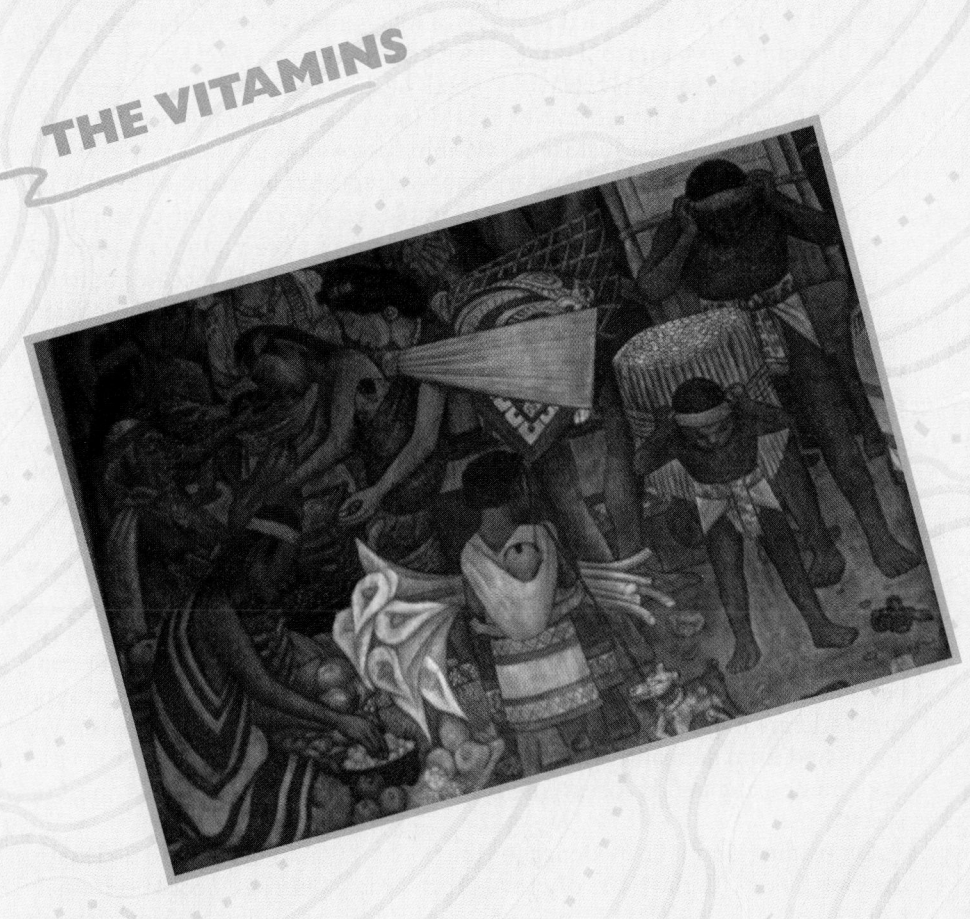

Diego Rivera, Detail of *Le Grand Tenochtitlan*; Charles and Josette Lenars, Corbis.

vitamins organic compounds that are vital to life and indispensable to body function, but are needed only in minute amounts; noncaloric essential nutrients.

7 At the turn of this century, the romance and thrill of discovery of the first **vitamins** captured the world's heart. People loved the vitamins. Catapulted from the shrouded mystery of folk cures into the technological era that brought us vitamin pills, they seemed a perfect answer to people who were looking for an easy way to good health. Only today are scientists beginning to uncover how complex are the interactions of vitamins in the body.

From a review of the history of vitamin discoveries, it is easy to see why people were so impressed. The story line was repeated over and over with the discovery of each new vitamin. For example, whole groups of people were unable to walk (or were going blind or bleeding profusely) until an alert scientist stumbled onto the substance missing from their diets. According to the plot, the scientist usually confirmed the discovery by feeding vitamin-deficient feed to laboratory animals. The animals responded by becoming unable to walk (or going blind or bleeding profusely). Then, miraculously, they recovered when the one missing ingredient was restored to their diet. Miraculous cures of people followed as they, too, received the vitamins they lacked.

It took a sophisticated knowledge of chemistry and biology to isolate the vitamins and to learn their chemical structures. More scientific advances brought an understanding of the biological roles that vitamins play in maintaining health and preventing deficiency diseases. Now, our knowledge of the vitamins has entered a new era of hope and discovery.[1]

Today, people's excitement is growing as research hints that two of the major scourges of humankind, cardiovascular disease (CVD) and cancer, may be somehow linked with low intakes of vitamins. Research laboratories around the world are issuing new theories postulating new relationships between vitamins and human health and disease. Can it be that vitamins will protect us from life-threatening diseases? There is much still to learn before this question is settled.

On reading dramatic evidence for the power of vitamins to cure deficiency diseases, and with the hope of preventing chronic diseases, people can easily come to believe that vitamin pills will cure almost any ailment. Many people take supplements of vitamin C in the belief that they will cure a cold or the flu, a topic addressed in this chapter's Consumer Corner. This chapter's Controversy section focuses on emerging knowledge about antioxidant nutrients and biologically active nonnutrients, the phytochemicals first defined in Chapter 1. Meanwhile, the media still bombard us with a never-ending stream of overly simple claims for "miracle vitamins," and the supplement business is a multi-*billion* dollar industry.

For now, we can still say this with certainty: the only disease a vitamin will *cure* is the one caused by a deficiency of that vitamin. As for disease prevention, the evidence is still emerging.

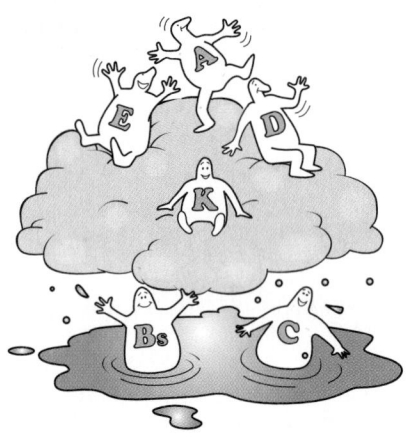

Vitamins fall into two classes—fat soluble and water soluble.

The only disease a vitamin can cure is the one caused by a deficiency of that vitamin.

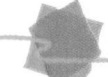

DEFINITION AND CLASSIFICATION OF VITAMINS

A child once defined a vitamin as "what, if you don't eat, you get sick." Although the grammar left something to be desired, the definition was accurate. Less imaginatively, a vitamin is defined as an essential, noncaloric, organic nutrient needed in tiny amounts in the diet. The role of many vitamins is to help make possible the processes by which other nutrients are digested, absorbed, and metabolized or built into body structures. Although small in size and quantity, the vitamins accomplish mighty tasks, some of which are still being discovered.

As they were discovered, the vitamins were named, and many were also given letters and numbers. This led to the confusion that still exists today. This chapter uses the names shown in Table 7-1; alternative names are given in Tables 7-5 and 7-6 at the end of the chapter.

Some of the vitamins occur in foods in a form known as **precursors,** or **provitamins.** Once inside the body, these are transformed chemically to one or more active vitamin forms. Thus, in measuring the amount of a vitamin found in food, it is often most accurate to count not only the amount of the true vitamin but also the vitamin activity potentially available from its precursors. Tables 7-5 and 7-6 show which vitamins have precursors.

The vitamins fall naturally into two classes: fat soluble and water soluble. Solubility imparts to vitamins many of their characteristic behaviors and determines how they are absorbed into and transported around the bloodstream, whether they can be stored in the body, and how easily they are lost from the body. In general, like other fats, fat-soluble vitamins are absorbed into the lymph. They travel in the blood associated with protein carriers. Fat-soluble vitamins can be stored with other lipids in fatty tissues, and because they are stored, some of them can build up to toxic concentrations. The water-soluble vitamins, on the other hand, are generally absorbed directly into the bloodstream, where they travel freely. They are not stored in tissues to any great extent; rather, excesses are excreted in the urine. Thus the risks of immediate toxicities are not as great as for fat-soluble vitamins, except in cases of extremely high doses. This chapter addresses first the fat-soluble vitamins and then the water-soluble ones. Some of the most important facts will be discussed separately for each vitamin, and the tables at the end of the chapter sum up the basic facts about all of them.

✔ KEY POINT **Vitamins are essential, noncaloric nutrients, needed in tiny amounts in the diet, that help to drive cell processes. The fat-soluble vitamins are vitamins A, D, E, and K; the water-soluble vitamins are the B vitamins and vitamin C.**

THE FAT-SOLUBLE VITAMINS

The fat-soluble vitamins—A, D, E, and K—generally occur together in the fats and oils of foods. Like the lipids, these vitamins require bile for absorption. Once absorbed, they are stored in the liver and fatty tissues until the body needs them. For this reason the body can easily survive weeks of consuming foods that lack them, as long as the diet as a whole provides *average* amounts that approximate the Recommended Dietary Allowances (RDA).[2] The capacity to be stored also sets the stage for toxic buildup, should an excess be taken in, especially in the form of supplements. Excesses of vitamins A, D, and K can reach toxic levels especially easily.

Deficiencies of the fat-soluble vitamins are likely when the diet is consistently low in them or when they are inadvertently lost from the digestive tract dissolved in undigested fat. We know that any disease that produces fat malabsorption (such as liver disease that prevents bile production) can bring about deficiencies of the fat-soluble vitamins. Deficiencies are also likely when people eat diets that are extraordinarily low in fat; such diets interfere with the

precursors, provitamins compounds that can be converted into active vitamins.

TABLE 7-1

Vitamin Names

Fat-soluble vitamins
   Vitamin A
   Vitamin D
   Vitamin E
   Vitamin K
Water-soluble vitamins
   B vitamins
      Thiamin (B$_1$)
      Riboflavin (B$_2$)
      Niacin (B$_3$)
      Folate
      Vitamin B$_{12}$
      Vitamin B$_6$
      Biotin
      Pantothenic acid
   Vitamin C

Vitamin names established by the International Union of Nutritional Sciences Committee on Nomenclature.

The RDA tables are on the inside front cover.

Characteristics fat-soluble vitamins share:
✔ Dissolve in lipid.
✔ Require bile for absorption.
✔ Are stored in tissues.
✔ May be toxic in excess.

Colorful foods often are rich in vitamins.

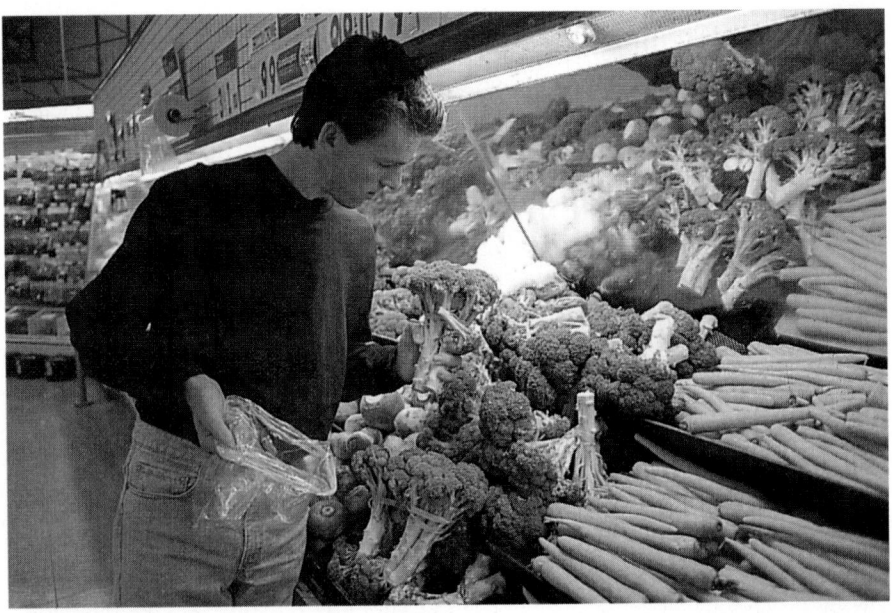

beta-carotene an orange pigment with antioxidant activity; a vitamin A precursor made by plants and stored in human fat tissue.

retinol one of the active forms of vitamin A made from beta-carotene in animal and human bodies; an antioxidant nutrient. Other active forms are *retinal* and *retinoic acid*.

retina (RET-in-uh) the layer of light-sensitive nerve cells lining the back of the inside of the eye.

cornea (KOR-nee-uh) the hard, transparent membrane covering the outside of the eye.

An acne medication and a wrinkle cream contain retinoic acid—see Chapter 13.

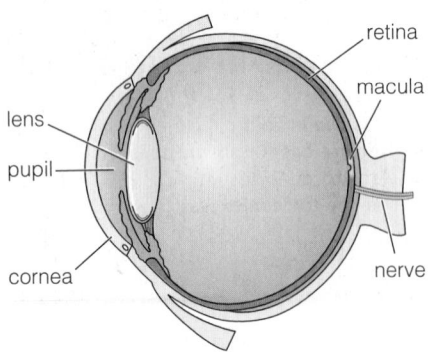

An eye (sectioned).

absorption of these vitamins. A worry about the indigestible artificial fat olestra is that fat-soluble vitamins readily dissolve in it and are carried out of the body unabsorbed. Time will tell whether heavy users of olestra will suffer vitamin deficiencies.[3] Likewise, a person who uses mineral oil (which the body can't absorb) as a laxative risks losing the fat-soluble vitamins by excretion.

The roles that the fat-soluble vitamins play in the body are diverse. Vitamin A is, among many other things, a visual pigment. Vitamins A and D may act somewhat like hormones, directing cells to convert one substance to another, to store this, or to release that. Vitamin E flows all over the body, preventing oxidative destruction of tissues. Vitamin K is necessary for blood to clot. Each is worth a book in itself.

Vitamin A

Vitamin A has the distinction of being the first fat-soluble vitamin to be recognized. Today, after more than 75 years of research, vitamin A and its plant-derived precursor, **beta-carotene,** are still the focus of much research.

Vitamin A is certainly one of the most versatile vitamins, with roles in such diverse functions as vision, immune defenses, maintenance of body linings and skin, bone and body growth, normal cell development, and reproduction.[4] In short, vitamin A is needed everywhere. Three forms of vitamin A are active in the body; one of the active forms, **retinol,** is stored in the liver. The liver makes retinol available to the bloodstream and thereby to the body cells. The cells convert retinol to its other two active forms, retinal and retinoic acid, as needed.

Roles of Vitamin A—It's a Jack of All Trades Perhaps the most familiar function of vitamin A is in eyesight. Vitamin A plays two indispensable roles in the eye: in the events of light perception at the **retina** and in the maintenance of a healthy, crystal-clear outer window, the **cornea** (see the margin drawing).

When light falls on the eye, it passes through the clear cornea and strikes the cells of the retina, bleaching many molecules of the pigment **rhodopsin** that lie within them. Vitamin A is a part of the rhodopsin molecule. The vitamin is broken off when bleaching occurs, initiating the signal that conveys the sensation of sight to the optic center in the brain. The vitamin then reunites with the pigment, but a little vitamin A is destroyed each time this reaction takes place, and fresh vitamin A arriving in the blood regenerates the supply. If the supply is low, a lag occurs before the eye can see again after a flash of bright light at night (see Figure 7-1). This lag in the recovery of night vision, termed **night blindness,** may indicate a vitamin A deficiency. A bright flash of light can temporarily blind even normal, well-nourished eyes, but if you experience a long recovery period before vision returns, your health-care provider may want you to check your vitamin A intake.

A deficiency of vitamin A that has progressed well beyond the night blindness stage may be reflected in an accumulation of a protein, **keratin,** that clouds the eye's outer vitamin A–dependent part, the cornea. The condition is known as **keratinization,** and it can progress to **xerosis** (drying) and then to thickening and permanent blindness, **xerophthalmia.** Tragically, vitamin A–deprived children become blind from this often preventable condition. If the deficiency

rhodopsin the light-sensitive pigment of the cells in the retina; it contains vitamin A (*rhod* refers to the rod-shaped cells; *opsin* means "visual protein").

night blindness slow recovery of vision after exposure to flashes of bright light at night; an early symptom of vitamin A deficiency.

keratin (KERR-uh-tin) the normal protein of hair and nails.

keratinization accumulation of keratin in a tissue; a sign of vitamin A deficiency.

xerosis drying of the cornea; a symptom of vitamin A deficiency.

xerophthalmia (ZEER-ahf-THALL-meuh) hardening of the cornea of the eye in advanced vitamin A deficiency that can lead to blindness (*xero* means "dry"; *ophthalm* means "eye").

FIGURE 7-1

NIGHT BLINDNESS
This is one of the earliest signs of vitamin A deficiency.

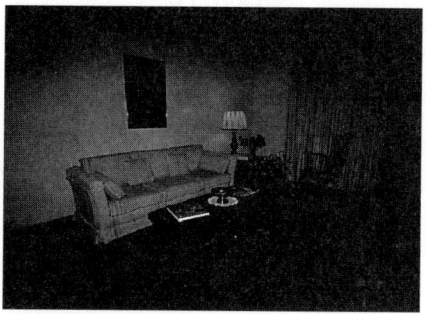

In dim light, you can make out the details in this room.

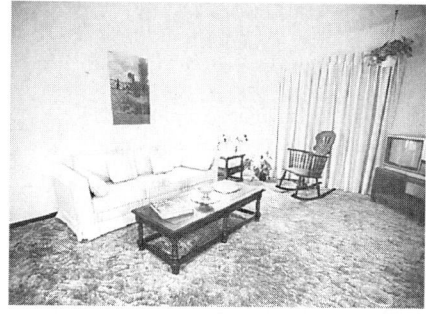

A flash of bright light momentarily blinds you as the pigment in the retina is bleached.

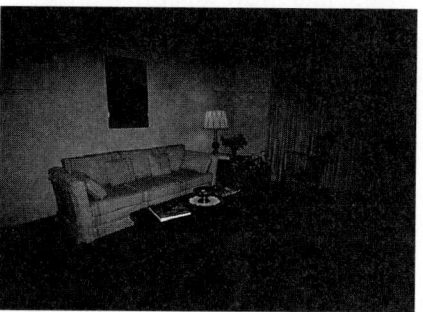

You quickly recover and can see the details again in a few seconds.

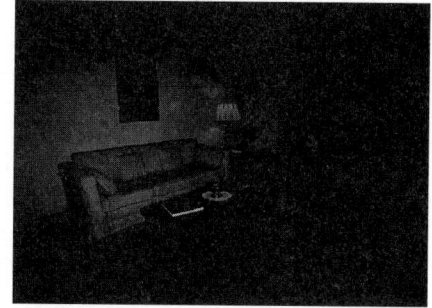

With inadequate vitamin A, you do not recover but remain blind for many seconds; this is night blindness.

FIGURE 7-2

THE SKIN IN VITAMIN A DEFICIENCY
The hard lumps reflect accumulations of keratin in the epithelial cells.

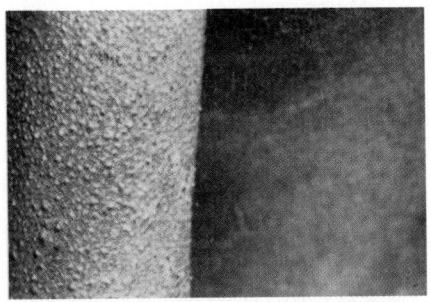

Retin A, a vitamin A acid cream for acne, is discussed in Chapter 13.

---

epithelial (ep-ih-THEE-lee-ull) **tissue** the layers of the body that serve as selective barriers to environmental factors. Examples are the cornea, the skin, the respiratory lining, and the lining of the digestive tract.

RE (retinol equivalent) a measure of vitamin A activity; the amount of retinol that the body will derive from a food containing vitamin A (preformed retinol) or its precursor carotene.

IU (international unit) a measure of fat-soluble vitamin activity. For methods to convert IU to RE, see Aids to Calculations, Appendix C.

---

is discovered early, it can be reversed by capsules containing 60,000 RE of vitamin A taken twice each year.[5] Better still, a child fed fruits and vegetables regularly is virtually assured protection from ever incurring the problem.[6]

Vitamin A is needed by all **epithelial tissue** (external skin and internal linings), not just by the cornea.[7] The skin and all of the protective linings of the lungs, intestines, vagina, urinary tract, and bladder serve as barriers to infection by bacteria and to damage from other sources. If vitamin A is deficient, some of the cells in these areas are displaced by cells that secrete keratin, the same protein that provides toughness in hair and fingernails. Keratin makes the surfaces dry, hard, cracked, and vulnerable to infection (see Figure 7-2). The cells then fail to function and eventually die. The dead cells accumulate on the surface and become hosts to bacterial infection. In the cornea, as described, keratinization leads to xerophthalmia; in the lungs, the displacement of mucus-producing cells makes respiratory infections likely; in the vagina, the same process leads to vaginal infections.

The body's other defenses against infection also depend on vitamin A.[8] When the defenses are weak, especially in vitamin A–deficient children, an illness such as measles can become severe. A downward cycle of malnutrition and infection can set in. The child's body must devote its scanty store of vitamin A to the immune system's fight against measles viruses.[9] The infection causes vitamin A to be spilled into the urine.[10] Without adequate vitamin A, the infection worsens. More vitamin A is needed for the fight, but it is unavailable, and the infection gains ground. Even if the child survives the measles infection, blindness is likely. The corneas, already damaged by the chronic vitamin A shortage, degenerate rapidly as their meager supply of vitamin A is diverted to the immune system. Vitamin A deficiency–induced blindness often follows bouts of infection.[11] In Asia alone vitamin A deficiency causes permanent blindness in a quarter of a million children each year.[12]

Vitamin A also assists in bone growth. Normal children's bones grow longer, and the children grow taller by remodeling each old bone into a new, bigger version. This requires dismantling the old bone structures and replacing them with new, larger bone parts. Growth cannot take place just by adding on to the small bone; vitamin A is needed in the critical dismantling steps. By helping reshape the jawbone as it grows, vitamin A permits normal tooth spacing. Crooked teeth and poor dental health can result from deficiencies in prenatal or early postnatal life. In children, failure to grow is one of the first signs of poor vitamin A status; when vitamin A is restored in such children, they gain weight and grow taller.

Vitamin A Deficiency around the World Although relatively rare in developed countries, vitamin A deficiency has been a vast problem worldwide, placing a heavy burden on society. More than 3 million of the world's children suffer from signs of severe vitamin A deficiency—not only blindness but stunted growth with poor appetite. A staggering 275 million more children suffer from milder deficiency, sufficient to impair immunity and promote infections.[13] In just one country, Indonesia, vitamin A deficiency is responsible for the deaths of 150,000 preschool children each year. In other countries, the toll is many times greater. In some countries, supplementing such children with vitamin A has reduced their rates of death by as much as half.[14] The World Health Organization (WHO) and UNICEF (United Nations International Children's Emergency Fund) are tracking the progress toward their goal of eliminating vitamin A deficiency and improving child survival throughout the developing world.

Vitamin A Toxicity As Figure 7-3 shows, toxicity presents a danger equal to that of deficiency for people who take excess vitamin A in supplements.[15] Toxicity's many symptoms include hair loss, joint pain, stunted growth, bone and muscle soreness, cessation of menstruation, nausea, diarrhea, rashes, damage to the liver, and enlargement of the spleen. Pregnant women should take note—chronic use of vitamin A supplements equaling three to four times the RDA have been observed to cause birth defects.[16] Even one massive vitamin A dose (100 times the RDA) will do so. Children are also likely to be hurt from vitamin A excesses because they need less and are more sensitive to overdoses than adults are. Serious toxicity is seen in infants and young children whose overzealous parents have given them more than ten times the recommended amount for weeks at a time. Children who mistake chewable vitamin pills for candy may also overdose. Early symptoms of overdoses in children are loss of appetite, growth failure, and itching of the skin.

Healthy people can eat vitamin A–rich foods in large amounts without risking toxicity, with the possible exception of liver. One report describes children falling ill after eating liver daily for years, but this is a medical rarity. Inuit people and Arctic explorers know that polar bear livers contain large enough amounts of the vitamin to be a dangerous food source because the bears eat fish whole including the livers.

Sources of Vitamin A As far as vitamin A supplements go, the National Research Council (NRC) and other nutrition agencies recommend that people avoid taking supplements in excess of the RDA.[17] A table later on in the chapter lists a safe dose of vitamin A that will not be toxic even over a long period of time. But the best way to ensure a safe vitamin A intake is to steer clear of supplements and instead to eat foods to obtain it. Snapshot 7-1 shows a sampling of the richest food sources of both preformed vitamin A and beta-carotene. This chapter's Food Feature discusses the best ways to obtain sufficient amounts of all of the vitamins.

The definitive fast-food meal, the hamburger, fries, and cola popular since its birth in the 1950s, lacks vitamin A. Some fast-food restaurants, however, now offer salads with cheese, carrots, and other vitamin A–rich foods as alternatives to plain burgers. These selections greatly improve the nutritional quality of a fast-food meal.

The amount of vitamin A a person needs is proportional to the person's body weight. Although the RDA for vitamin A is given as a daily amount, the vitamin need not be consumed every day. An average intake that meets the daily RDA over several months is sufficient. According to the RDA, a man needs a daily average of about 1,000 **RE (retinol equivalents);** a woman needs about 800 RE and more during lactation; children need less.

Vitamin A recommendations are expressed in RE, but some food tables still express vitamin A contents using a different unit, the **IU (international unit).** Note that this book's Table of Food Composition (Appendix A) uses RE for your convenience, but be careful to notice whether other food tables or supplement labels use RE or IU. See the Aids to Calculations section for help in converting the units. People working with the amounts of vitamin A in foods

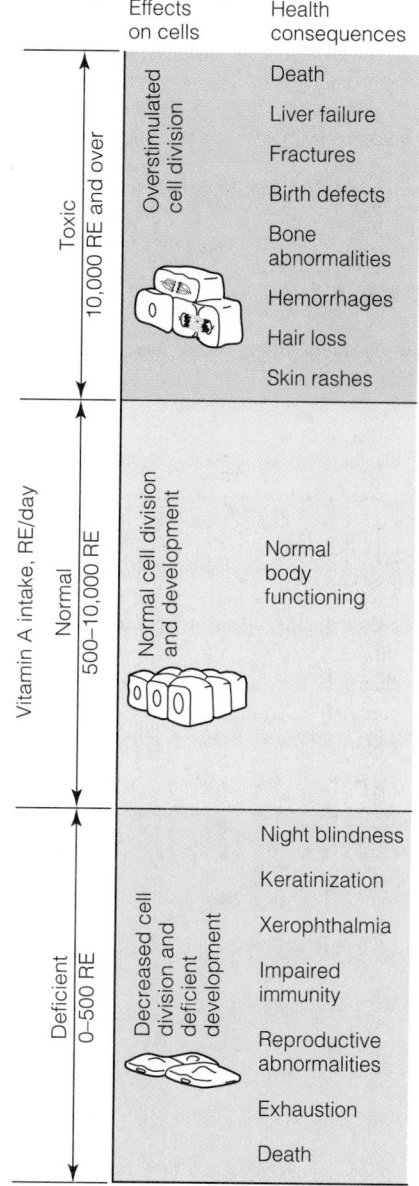

FIGURE 7-3

VITAMIN A DEFICIENCY AND TOXICITY Danger lies both above and below a normal range of intakes of vitamin A.

The effects of excessive vitamin A intakes during pregnancy are discussed in Chapter 12.

SNAPSHOT 7-1

VITAMIN A AND BETA-CAROTENE

RDA for men: 1,000 RE/day
RDA for women: 800 RE/day

Sweet potato 1,936 RE[b] per ½ c mashed

Carrots 1,914 RE[b] per ½ c cooked

Fortified milk 150 RE[a] per 1 c

Beef liver 9,124 RE[a] per 3 oz fried

Spinach 739 RE[b] per ½ c cooked

Apricots 277 RE[b] per 3 fresh apricots

[a]This food item contains preformed vitamin A.
[b] This food item contains beta-carotene.

macular degeneration a common, progressive loss of function of that part of the retina that is most crucial to focused vision (the macula is shown on p. 228). This degeneration often leads to blindness.

have to remember to make sure that the amounts are all expressed in the same units before making comparisons.

✓ **KEY POINT** **Vitamin A is essential to vision, integrity of epithelial tissue, growth of bone, reproduction, and more. Vitamin A deficiency causes blindness, sickness, and death and is a major problem worldwide. Liver and milk are rich sources of active vitamin A. Overdoses are possible and cause many serious symptoms.**

Beta-Carotene

In plants, vitamin A exists only in its precursor forms. Beta-carotene, the most abundant of these precursors, has the highest vitamin A activity. For many years scientists believed beta-carotene to be of interest solely as a vitamin A precursor, but now they also recognize beta-carotene and its other carotene relatives for their antioxidant actions in the body.

Studies of populations suggest that people whose diets are low in foods that contain beta-carotene have a high incidence of certain types of cancer.[18] Likewise, a common form of blindness in the aged, **macular degeneration,** is linked with a lifelong diet that excludes foods rich in beta-carotene. Interestingly, research has all but ruled out a protective effect of supplements of beta-carotene against these diseases.[19] Evidence is growing, however, to support the link between eating beta-carotene–rich *foods* regularly and low rates of diseases. The Controversy following this chapter offers more explanation of why this might be so.

Retinol in excess is toxic, but beta-carotene is not; it is not converted to retinol efficiently enough to cause toxicity symptoms. Beta-carotene has, however, been known to turn people bright yellow if they eat too much. Beta-carotene builds up in the fat just beneath the skin and imparts a yellow cast.

More about carotenes and disease prevention in this chapter's Controversy.

When beta-carotene is converted to retinol in the body, losses occur. This is why nutrition scientists do not express the amounts of beta-carotene in foods, but instead use the RE, which expresses the amount of retinol the body actually derives from a plant food after conversion. The body can make one unit of retinol from about three of beta-carotene.

Many foods from plants contain beta-carotene. Some are such a bright orange color that they decorate the plate. Carrots, sweet potatoes, pumpkins, cantaloupe, and apricots are all rich sources. Another colorful group, *dark green vegetables*, such as spinach, other greens, and broccoli, owe their color to chlorophyll and beta-carotene. The orange and green pigments together give a deep dark green color to the vegetables.

Other colorful vegetables, such as iceberg lettuce, beets, and sweet corn, can fool you into thinking they contain beta-carotene, but these foods derive their colors from other pigments and are poor sources of beta-carotene. As for "white" plant foods such as grains and potatoes, they have none. Some confusion exists concerning the term *yam*. A white-fleshed Mexican root vegetable called "yam" is devoid of beta-carotene, while the orange-fleshed sweet potato termed *yam* in this country is one of the richest beta-carotene sources known. Recommendations state that a person should eat *deep* orange or *dark* green vegetables and fruits regularly.

✔ **KEY POINT**   **The vitamin A precursor in plants, beta-carotene, is an effective antioxidant in the body. Brightly colored plant foods are richest in beta-carotene.**

Vitamin D

Vitamin D is different from all the other nutrients in the body in that the body can synthesize it with the help of sunlight. Therefore, in a sense, vitamin D is not an essential nutrient. Given enough sun each day, you need consume no vitamin D at all in the foods you eat. Folk wisdom has always held that sunshine promotes health. People of past generations cared for those with tuberculosis by taking them outside into the sunshine long before scientists worked out the details of vitamin D synthesis. Now vitamin D is appreciated for its role in assisting the tissues of immunity in fighting all kinds of infections. (Of course, too much sun is dangerous—it may trigger the start of skin cancer.)

Roles of Vitamin D   The best-known role of vitamin D is as a member of a large and interacting team of nutrients and hormones that continuously maintain blood calcium levels and thereby bone integrity, especially important during growth. Vitamin D ensures that sufficient calcium and phosphorus are available in the blood to support the growing bone structure.

Calcium is also indispensable to the proper functioning of all tissues of the body; cells of muscles, nerves, glands, and others all draw calcium from the blood as they need it. The skeleton serves as a vast warehouse of stored calcium that can be tapped when the blood supply begins to run low. To raise the level of blood calcium, the body can draw from only two other places: the digestive tract, where food brings calcium in, and the kidneys, which can recycle calcium into the body from blood filtrate destined to become urine. When calcium is needed, vitamin D acts at all three locations to raise the blood calcium level.

Chapter 8 and Controversy 8 present more about bone minerals and their regulation and about osteoporosis, the bone-weakening disease.

rickets the vitamin D–deficiency disease in children; characterized by abnormal growth of bone and manifested in bowed legs or knock-knees, outward-bowed chest, and knobs on the ribs.

osteomalacia (OS-tee-o-mal-AY-shuh) the vitamin D–deficiency disease in adults (*osteo* means "bone"; *mal* means "bad"). Symptoms include bending of the spine and bowing of the legs.

Vitamin D acts like a hormone, a compound manufactured by one organ of the body that acts on other organs or tissues. In addition to its actions in the bones, intestines, and kidneys, vitamin D is known to play roles in the brain, pancreas, skin, reproductive organs, and some cancer cells, but these are not yet fully understood.[20] Like vitamin A, vitamin D stimulates maturation of cells, including cells of the immune system.[21]

Too Little Vitamin D—A Danger to Bones   The most obvious sign of vitamin D deficiency is abnormality of the bones. The disease **rickets,** caused in children by vitamin D deficiency, has been recognized for several centuries, and even in the 1700s it was known to be curable by cod-liver oil, which is rich in the vitamin. More than a hundred years later, a Polish physician linked sunlight exposure to prevention and cure of rickets. At the turn of this century, enough was finally known about rickets to reproduce it in laboratory animals. Today the bowed legs, knock-knees, and protruding (pigeon) chests of children with rickets are no longer common sights. Tragically, some children still suffer the ravages of rickets largely because of inadequate food due to poverty combined with a lack of sunlight.[22]

Adult rickets, or **osteomalacia,** occurs most often in women with low calcium intakes and little exposure to the sun (therefore little opportunity to make vitamin D) who have repeated pregnancies and then breastfeed their babies. Under these conditions, calcium is withdrawn from the bones but is not picked up efficiently from the intestine or recycled by the kidneys. The bones lose their minerals and protein understructure, becoming porous, soft, and easy to break. The bones of the legs and spine may soften to such an extent that a young woman who is tall and straight at the age of 20 years may, after several pregnancies, become bowlegged and bent by age 30.

Too Much Vitamin D—A Danger to Soft Tissues   Vitamin D is the most potentially toxic of all vitamins. Ingestion of as little as four to five times the recommended daily intake can cause toxicity symptoms including diarrhea, headache, and nausea. If overdoses continue, the vitamin raises the blood mineral level to dangerous extremes, forcing calcium to be deposited in soft tissues such as the heart and kidneys. If calcium deposits form in the arteries of the heart, the consequence of overdosing is death.

The likeliest victims of vitamin D poisoning are infants whose well-intended but misguided parents think that if some is good, more is better. People who take supplements containing vitamin D may also easily overdose, not realizing that their tissues are building up stockpiles of the vitamin. Intakes of only five times the RDA have been associated with signs of vitamin D toxicity in young children and adults.[23] Recently, some people fell ill with vitamin D toxicity, and two died, after drinking milk from a dairy that had mistakenly overfortified the milk with up to 500 times the standard requirement of vitamin D.[24] While such occurrences are rare, the incident renewed awareness of the potential for harm from vitamin D and the need for close monitoring of those who fortify the nation's foods with vitamins.

Sources of Vitamin D   Most of the world's population relies on natural exposure to sunlight to maintain adequate vitamin D nutrition. When the sun

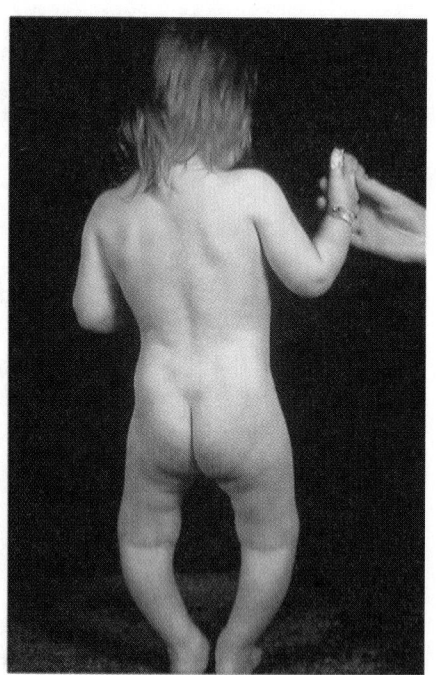

This child has the vitamin D–deficiency disease rickets.

shines on a cholesterol compound in human skin, the compound is transformed into a vitamin D precursor and is absorbed directly into the blood. Slowly, over the next day and a half or so, the liver and kidneys finish converting the precursor to the active form of vitamin D. Diseases that affect either the liver or the kidneys may impair the conversion of the inactive precursor to the active vitamin and therefore produce symptoms of vitamin D deficiency.

Unlike concentrated supplements, the sun presents no risk of vitamin D toxicity; the sun itself begins breaking down excess vitamin made in the skin. Sunbathers run *other* risks, of course, such as premature wrinkling of the skin and the increased risk of skin cancer, mentioned earlier. Sunscreens with sun protection factors (SPF) of 8 and above can reduce these risks, but unfortunately they also prevent vitamin D synthesis.[25] A strategy to solve this dilemma is to wait until enough time has elapsed to make some vitamin D, then apply sunscreen. In reality, production of vitamin D doesn't demand idle hours of sunbathing. Just being outdoors, even in lightweight clothing, is sufficient. Dark-skinned people require long exposure to direct sun (up to three hours, depending on the climate) for several days' worth of vitamin D, while light-skinned people need much less time (10 or 15 minutes). Tanning booths may or may not promote vitamin D synthesis, but the Food and Drug Administration (FDA) has declared them risky because their unfiltered rays may promote skin cancer and damage the blood vessels and eyes. Daily doses of vitamin D are not necessary because the body stores enough vitamin D in its fat tissue to last through the dark winter months.

The ultraviolet rays of the sun that promote vitamin D synthesis cannot penetrate clouds, smoke, smog, heavy clothing, window glass, or even window screens. In the United States and Canada, almost all cases of rickets show up in dark-skinned people who live in smoggy northern cities or who lack exposure to sunlight. Worldwide, rickets is still a major health problem, especially in societies where people traditionally clothe themselves in concealing garments. People who are housebound or institutionalized or who work at night may incur (over years) a vitamin D deficiency that leads to a deficiency of calcium severe enough to damage their bones.

As Snapshot 7-2 shows, the few significant food sources of vitamin D are butter, cream, egg yolks, liver, fatty fish such as salmon, and fortified margarine. In the United States and Canada, milk, whether fluid, dried, or evaporated, is fortified with vitamin D, so that a daily quart (or liter) will supply the amount of the vitamin recommended for a young adult. That way the young adult who drinks the recommended 2 cups a day receives half the RDA; the other half comes from sun exposure and other food sources. Children who drink 2 cups or more of milk will have a head start toward meeting their vitamin D needs for growth. Strict vegetarians, and especially their children, may have low vitamin D intakes because only two fortified plant sources exist: margarine and, in the United States, certain fortified cereals.

The RDA for vitamin D is 5 micrograms per day for adults older than 24 years. The RDA is higher during pregnancy, lactation, childhood, and adolescence. It remains high in early adult life, while bones continue to gain density. Adults who can tolerate milk can get both vitamin D and calcium from it; those who are sensitive to milk need alternative calcium sources and should make a point of spending time outdoors.

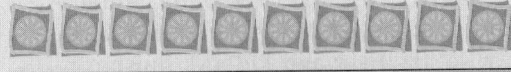

SNAPSHOT 7-2

VITAMIN D

RDA for adults (19–24 yr):
10 µg/day
RDA for adults (25–50 yr):
5 µg/day

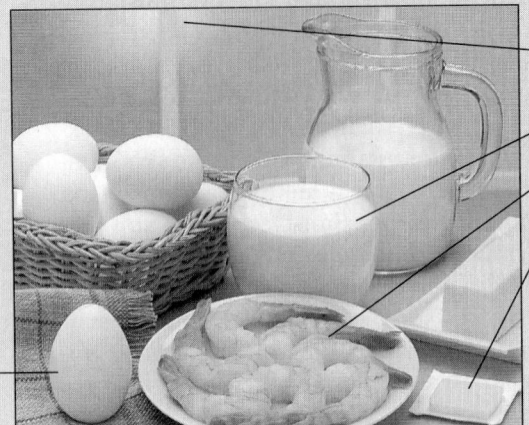

Sunlight promotes vitamin D
synthesis in the skin.ᵃ

Fortified milk 2.5 µg per 1 c

Shrimp 3 µg per 3 oz boiled

Fortified margarine 0.5 µg per
teaspoon

Eggs 0.7 µg per egg

ᵃ Avoid prolonged exposure to the sun.

---

tocopherol (tuh-KOFF-er-all) a kind of
alcohol. The active form of vitamin E is
alpha-tocopherol.

✔ **KEY POINT** **Vitamin D raises blood minerals, notably calcium and phosphorus, permitting bone formation and maintenance. A deficiency in childhood can cause rickets or, in later life, osteomalacia. Vitamin D is the most toxic of all the vitamins, and excesses are dangerous or deadly. People exposed to the sun make vitamin D from a cholesterol-like compound in their skin; fortified milk is an important food source.**

Vitamin E

More than 70 years ago, researchers discovered a compound in vegetable oils necessary for reproduction in rats. This compound was named **tocopherol** from *tokos*, a Greek word meaning "offspring." A few years later, the compound was named vitamin E. Eventually, four different tocopherol compounds were discovered, and each was designated by one of the first four letters of the Greek alphabet: alpha, beta, gamma, and delta.

See the Controversy section for details about antioxidants, vitamins, and diseases.

The Extraordinary Bodyguard   Vitamin E, because it can be oxidized, serves as one of the body's main defenders against oxidative damage.[26] By being oxidized itself, vitamin E protects the polyunsaturated fats and other vulnerable components of the cells and their membranes from destruction. Vitamin E protects all the cells' lipids and related compounds, such as vitamin A, from oxidation.

Vitamin E exerts an especially important antioxidant effect in the lungs, where the cells are exposed to high oxygen concentrations that can destroy their membranes. As the red blood cells carry oxygen from the lungs to other tissues, vitamin E protects their cell membranes, too. Vitamin E may also help defend against heart disease; this chapter's Controversy section provides details. Normal nerve development also depends on vitamin E. Vitamin E also protects the white blood cells that defend the body against disease. Vitamin E may also play other roles in normal immunity, and supplements of the vitamin were found to improve the immune response in healthy older adults.[27]

Vitamin E Deficiency   A deficiency of vitamin E produces a wide variety of symptoms in laboratory animals. Most of these symptoms have not been reproduced in human beings, however, despite many attempts. Three reasons have been given for this. First, the vitamin is so widespread in food that it is almost impossible to create a vitamin E–deficient diet. Second, the body stores so much vitamin E in its fatty tissues that a person could not keep on eating a vitamin E–free diet for long enough to deplete these stores and produce a deficiency. Third, the cells recycle their working supply of vitamin E, using the same molecules over and over, warding off deficiency.[28]

The classic vitamin E–deficiency symptom in human beings occurs in premature babies. Some of these babies are born before the transfer of the vitamin from the mother to the infant that takes place in the last weeks of pregnancy. Without sufficient vitamin E, the infant's red blood cells rupture **(erythrocyte hemolysis),** and the infant becomes anemic. Common symptoms of vitamin E deficiency in adults include loss of muscle coordination and reflexes and impaired vision and speech. Vitamin E treatment corrects these symptoms.

In adults, vitamin E deficiency is usually associated with diseases, notably those that cause malabsorption of fat. These include disease or injury of the liver (which makes bile, necessary for digestion of fat), the gallbladder (which delivers bile into the intestine), and the pancreas (which makes fat-digesting enzymes), as well as a number of hereditary diseases involving digestion and use of nutrients.

It may be, however, that rare vitamin E deficiencies are seen in people without diseases. Deficiencies are most likely in those who for years eat diets extremely low in fat; or use fat substitutes, such as diet margarines and salad dressings, as their only sources of fat; or consume diets composed largely of highly processed or "convenience" foods, since vitamin E is destroyed by extensive heating in the processing of these foods.

Although vitamin E deficiency is rare, extravagant claims are being made that vitamin E cures all sorts of things because its deficiency affects animals' muscles and reproductive systems. Vitamin E deficiency does not affect the organs of human beings as it affects animals, however. Research has clearly discredited claims that vitamin E improves athletic endurance and skill, enhances sexual performance, or cures sexual dysfunction in males.

Vitamin E Requirements, Toxicity, and Sources   The RDA for vitamin E is based on body size: it is 8 milligrams a day for women, 10 for men. Note that the RDA gives values for vitamin E in units known as alpha TE (alpha-tocopherol equivalents). One of these units, 1 alpha TE, equals 1 milligram of active vitamin E. The need for vitamin E rises as people consume more polyunsaturated oil because the oil requires antioxidant protection by the vitamin. Luckily, most raw oils also contain vitamin E so people who eat the oil also receive the vitamin. Heat processing, such as frying, destroys vitamin E, as does oxidation, so most processed, fast, deep-fried, and convenience foods retain little intact vitamin E.

Cases of vitamin E toxicity are rare, and high doses taken over a short period seem to have no adverse effects.[29] The medical literature contains isolated reports of adverse effects on laboratory animals and occasionally of nausea, intestinal distress, and other vague complaints in human beings. Large doses may augment the effects of anticoagulant medication used to oppose

erythrocyte (eh-REETH-ro-sight) **hemolysis** (he-MOLL-ih-sis) rupture of the red blood cells, caused by vitamin E deficiency (*erythro* means "red"; *cyte* means "cell"; *hemo* means "blood"; *lysis* means "breaking").

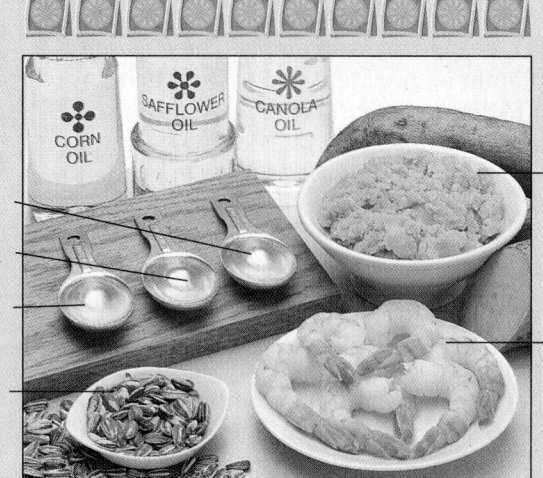

Sweet potato 0.5 mg per ½ c mashed

Shrimp 1.5 mg per 3 oz boiled

For perspectives on possible risks and benefits of vitamin E supplements, see the Controversy.

unwanted blood clotting; people taking such drugs risk uncontrollable bleeding when they also take large doses of vitamin E. For most individuals, however, daily doses below 300 milligrams may be harmless. We say "may be" because preliminary research has linked long-term use of even low-dose vitamin E supplements with brain hemorrhages, a form of stroke.

Vitamin E is widespread in foods. About 20 percent of the vitamin E people consume comes from vegetable oils and products made from them, such as margarine, salad dressings, and shortenings (see Snapshot 7-3). Another 20 percent comes from fruits and vegetables. Fortified cereals* and other grain products contribute about 15 percent of the vitamin E in the diet, and meats, poultry, fish, eggs, nuts, and seeds contribute smaller percentages.[30] Wheat germ oil and soybean oil are rich in vitamin E while animal fats, such as milk fat or the fat of meats, have almost none.

✔ **KEY POINT** **Vitamin E acts as an antioxidant in cell membranes and is especially important for the integrity of cells that are constantly exposed to high oxygen concentrations, namely, the lungs and blood cells, both red and white. Vitamin E deficiency is rare in human beings, but it does occur in newborn premature infants. The vitamin is widely distributed in plant foods; it is destroyed by high heat; toxicity is rare.**

Vitamin K

Have you ever thought about how remarkable it is that blood can clot? The liquid turns solid in a life-saving series of reactions. If blood cannot clot, then wounds will bleed for a dangerously long time; this is why people's blood is drawn to measure clotting time before they go into surgery. Vitamin K, needed for the synthesis of proteins that help clot the blood, is sometimes administered before operations to reduce bleeding in surgery. Vitamin K may be of value at

K stands for the Danish word *koagulation* (clotting).

*Cereals fortified with vitamin E are not available in Canada.

SNAPSHOT 7-4

VITAMIN K[a]

RDA for men:
(19–24 yr) 70 µg/day
(25–50 yr) 80 µg/day
RDA for women:
(19–24 yr) 60 µg/day
(25–50 yr) 65 µg/day

_____

[a] Techniques to analyze vitamin K in foods are changing rapidly. Values based on the newest analytical techniques are not yet available.

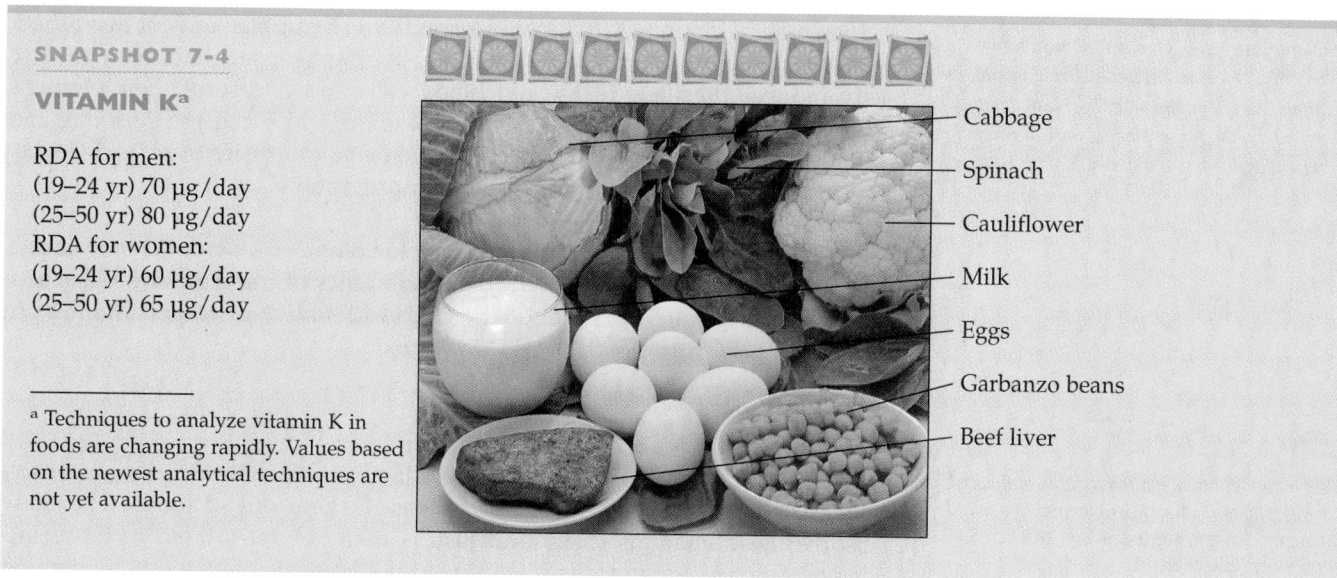

- Cabbage
- Spinach
- Cauliflower
- Milk
- Eggs
- Garbanzo beans
- Beef liver

this time, but only if a vitamin K deficiency exists. Vitamin K does not improve clotting in those with other bleeding disorders, such as the genetic disease hemophilia.

In some heart problems there is a need to _prevent_ the formation of clots within the circulatory system. This is popularly referred to as "thinning" the blood. One of the best-known medicines for this purpose is dicumarol, which interferes with the action of vitamin K in promoting clotting. Vitamin K therapy is necessary for people taking dicumarol if uncontrolled bleeding occurs.

Vitamin K is also necessary for the synthesis of a key protein in bone formation.[31] Together with the more famous bone vitamin, vitamin D, vitamin K ensures that the bones produce this protein normally so that bones can properly bind the minerals they need.

Like vitamin D, vitamin K can be obtained from a nonfood source—in this case, the intestinal bacteria. Billions of bacteria normally reside in the intestines, and some of them synthesize vitamin K. The extent to which the body uses the vitamin K synthesized by these bacteria is not known, but it is thought that people may obtain about half of their daily needs from this source.

An RDA for vitamin K was published for the first time in 1989 (see the RDA tables on the inside front cover). As Snapshot 7-4 shows, vitamin K's richest plant food sources are dark green, leafy vegetables, which provide from 50 to 800 micrograms per 3-ounce serving, and members of the cabbage family. There is also one rich animal food source, liver.[32] Milk, meats, eggs, cereals, and fruits provide smaller but still significant amounts. Food tables do not include vitamin K contents of foods because they are not well enough known.

It seems unlikely that many U.S. adults experience vitamin K deficiency, even if they seldom eat vitamin K–rich foods.[33] Exceptions are newborn infants whose intestinal tracts are not yet inhabited by bacteria and people who have taken antibiotics that have killed their intestinal bacteria. Supplements of the vitamin are needed in these cases.

coenzyme (co-EN-zime) a small molecule that works with an enzyme to promote the enzyme's activity. Many coenzymes have B vitamins as part of their structure (*co* means "with").

The water-soluble vitamins require special consideration in food preparation to avoid losing or destroying them. See the Food Feature of Chapter 14.

Characteristics water-soluble vitamins share:

✔ Dissolve in water.
✔ Are easily absorbed and excreted.
✔ Are not stored extensively in tissues.
✔ Seldom reach toxic levels.

For others, vitamin K toxicity can result when supplements of a synthetic version of vitamin K are given, especially to infants or pregnant women. Toxicity induces breakage of the red blood cells and release of their pigment, which colors the skin yellow.* Vitamin K toxicity also causes brain damage. Because the vitamin K contained in supplements can easily reach toxic levels, it is available as a single vitamin only by prescription.

✔ **KEY POINT** **Vitamin K is necessary for blood to clot; deficiency causes uncontrolled bleeding. The bacterial inhabitants of the digestive tract produce vitamin K, and most people derive about half their requirement from them and half from food. Excesses are toxic.**

THE WATER-SOLUBLE VITAMINS

All of the other vitamins, the B vitamins and vitamin C, are water soluble. Cooking and washing water can leach them out of foods. The body absorbs these vitamins easily and just as easily excretes them in the urine. Under ordinary circumstances, you need not be concerned about consuming modest excesses. Some of the water-soluble vitamins can remain in the lean tissues for periods of a month or more, but these tissues are actively exchanging materials with the body fluids at all times. At any time, the vitamins may be picked up by the extracellular fluids, carried away by the blood, and excreted in the urine. Generally, the RDA committee suggests that you make sure your three-day intake average meets the RDA by choosing foods that are rich in water-soluble vitamins.[34]

Foods never deliver toxic doses of the water-soluble vitamins, but the large doses concentrated in some vitamin supplements can reach toxic levels. Normally, though, the most likely hazard to the supplement taker is to the wallet. As one person aptly noted, "If you take high-dose supplements of the water-soluble vitamins, you may have the most expensive urine in town."

The B Vitamins and Their Relatives

The B vitamins act as part of coenzymes. A **coenzyme** is a small molecule that combines with an enzyme to make it active. (Recall that enzymes are large proteins that do the body's building, dismantling, and other work; see page 198.) Sometimes the vitamin part of the enzyme is the active site, where the chemical reaction takes place. The substance to be worked on is attracted to the active site and snaps into place; the reaction proceeds instantaneously. The shape of each enzyme predestines it to accomplish just one kind of job. Without its coenzyme, however, the enzyme is as useless as a car without wheels. Figure 7-4 shows how a coenzyme enables an enzyme to do its job.

Each B vitamin has its own special character, and the amount of detail known about each one is overwhelming. To simplify things, this introduction describes some of the ways in which the B vitamins work together as a group

---

*A toxic dose of a vitamin K compound such as menadione causes the liver to release the blood cell pigment (bilirubin) into the blood (instead of excreting it into the bile) and leads to jaundice. When bilirubin invades the brain of an infant, the condition is often fatal.

and emphasizes the consequences of deficiencies. The sections that follow present more details about the vitamins as individuals.

✔ **KEY POINT** **As part of coenzymes, the B vitamins help enzymes do their jobs.**

B Vitamin Roles in Metabolism

Figure 7-5 shows some body organs and tissues in which the B vitamins help the body metabolize carbohydrates, lipids, and amino acids. It is not presented to teach details; that is best left to courses in biochemistry. The purpose of the figure is to give an impression of where the B vitamins work together with enzymes in the metabolism of energy nutrients and in the making of new cells.

Many people mistakenly believe that B vitamins give the body energy. They do not, at least not directly. The energy-yielding nutrients, carbohydrate, fat, and protein, give the body fuel for energy; the B vitamins help the body use that fuel. More specifically, the B vitamins thiamin, riboflavin, niacin, pantothenic acid, and biotin participate in the release of energy from carbohydrate, fat, and protein. Vitamin B_6 helps the body use amino acids to make protein; the body then puts the protein to work in many ways—to build new tissues, to make hormones, to fight infections, or to serve as energy fuel, to name a few.

Folate and vitamin B_{12} help cells to multiply; this is especially important to cells with short life spans that must replace themselves rapidly. Such cells include both the red blood cells (which live an average of six weeks) and the cells that line the digestive tract (which replace themselves every three days). These cells deliver energy to all the others. In short, each and every B vitamin is involved, directly or indirectly, in energy metabolism.

The B vitamin amounts that people need are determined differently for each vitamin. For three of the B vitamins, thiamin, riboflavin, and niacin, recommendations are proportional to energy intake. For vitamin B_6, the recommendation is proportional to protein intake.

✔ **KEY POINT** **The B vitamins facilitate the work of every cell. Some help generate energy; others help make protein and new cells. B vitamins work everywhere in the body tissues to metabolize carbohydrate, fats, and protein.**

B Vitamin Deficiencies and Toxicities

As long as B vitamins are present, their presence is not felt. Only when they are missing does their absence manifest itself in a lack of energy and a multitude of other symptoms, as you can imagine after looking at Figure 7-5. The reactions by which B vitamins facilitate energy release take place in every cell, and no cell can do its work without energy. Thus, in a B vitamin deficiency, every cell is affected. Among the symptoms of B vitamin deficiencies are nausea, severe exhaustion, irritability, depression, forgetfulness, loss of appetite and weight, pain in muscles, impairment of the immune response, loss of control of the limbs, abnormal heart action, severe skin problems, teary or bloodshot eyes, and many more. Because cell renewal depends on energy and protein, and because these depend on the B vitamins, the digestive tract and the blood are

FIGURE 7-4

COENZYME ACTION

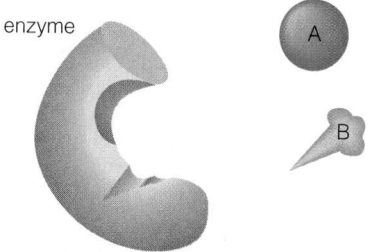

enzyme

Without the coenzyme, compounds A and B don't respond to the enzyme.

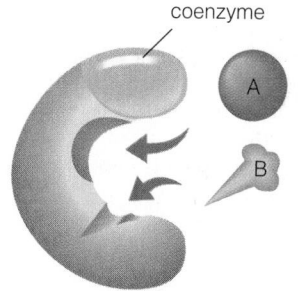

coenzyme

With the coenzyme in place, compounds A and B are attracted to the active site on the enzyme, and they react.

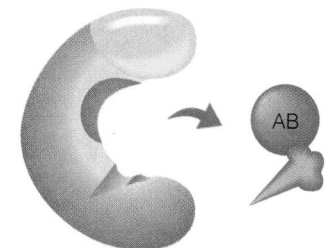

The reaction is completed with the formation of a new product. In this case the product is AB.

FIGURE 7-5

SOME ROLES OF THE B VITAMINS IN METABOLISM: EXAMPLES

This figure does not attempt to teach intricate biochemical pathways or names of B vitamin–containing enzymes. Its sole purpose is to show a few of the many tissue functions that depend on B vitamin–containing enzymes. The B vitamins work in every cell, and this figure displays less than a thousandth of what they actually do.

Every B vitamin is part of one or more coenzymes that make possible the body's chemical work. For example, the niacin, thiamin, and riboflavin coenzymes are important in the energy pathways. The folate and vitamin B_{12} coenzymes are necessary for making RNA and DNA and thus new cells. The vitamin B_6 coenzyme is necessary for processing amino acids and, therefore, protein. Many other relationships are also critical to metabolism.

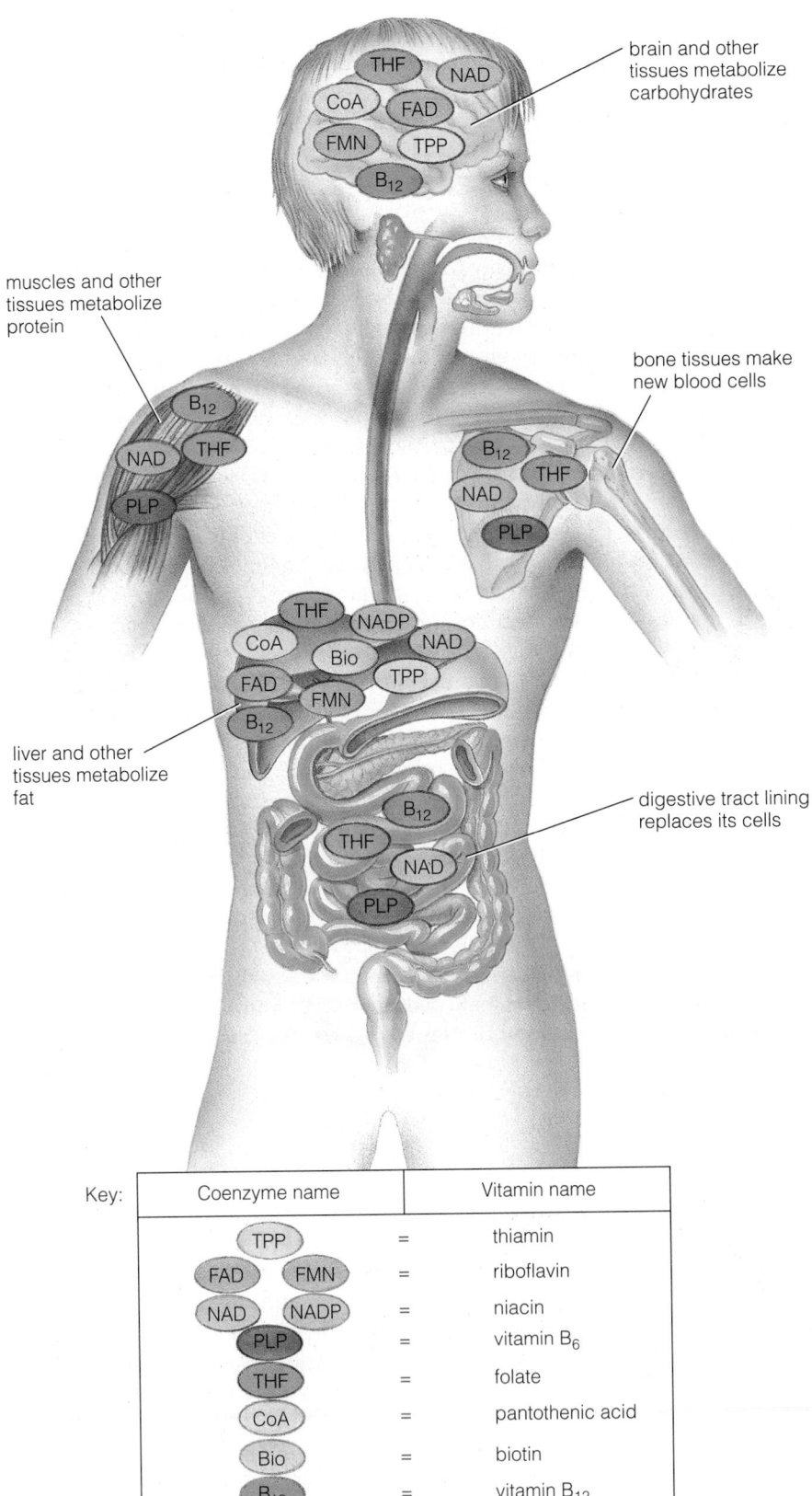

brain and other tissues metabolize carbohydrates

muscles and other tissues metabolize protein

bone tissues make new blood cells

liver and other tissues metabolize fat

digestive tract lining replaces its cells

Key:	Coenzyme name		Vitamin name
	TPP	=	thiamin
	FAD FMN	=	riboflavin
	NAD NADP	=	niacin
	PLP	=	vitamin B_6
	THF	=	folate
	CoA	=	pantothenic acid
	Bio	=	biotin
	B_{12}	=	vitamin B_{12}

invariably damaged. In children, full recovery may be impossible. In the case of a thiamin deficiency during growth, permanent brain damage can result.

In academic discussions of the vitamins, different sets of deficiency symptoms are given for each one. Actually, such clear-cut sets of symptoms are found only in laboratory animals that have been fed contrived diets that lack just one ingredient. In real life, a deficiency of any one B vitamin seldom shows up by itself because people don't eat nutrients singly; they eat foods that contain mixtures of nutrients. One deficiency of a B vitamin may appear responsible for a cluster of deficiencies, but subtler deficiencies may accompany it, unseen. If treatment involves giving wholesome food rather than single supplements, the subtler deficiencies will be corrected along with the major one. The symptoms of B vitamin deficiencies and toxicities are listed in Table 7-6 at the end of the chapter. The next few sections treat each B vitamin separately.

Thiamin and Riboflavin   All cells use **thiamin,** which plays a critical role in their energy metabolism. Thiamin also occupies a special site on nerve cell membranes. Consequently, nerve processes and their responding tissues, the muscles, depend heavily on thiamin.

The thiamin-deficiency disease **beriberi** was first observed in the Far East, where rice provided 80 to 90 percent of the total calories most people consumed and was therefore their principal source of thiamin. When the custom of polishing rice (removing its brown coat, which contained the thiamin) became widespread, beriberi swept through the population like an epidemic. Scientists wasted years of time and effort hunting for a microbial cause of beriberi before they realized that the cause was not something present in the environment but something absent from it.

Just before the year 1900, an observant physician working in a prison in the Far East discovered that beriberi could be cured with proper diet. The physician noticed that the chickens at the prison developed a stiffness and weakness similar to that of the prisoners who had beriberi. The chickens were being fed the rice left on prisoners' plates. When the rice bran, which had been discarded in the kitchen, was given to the chickens, their paralysis was cured. As might be expected, the physician met resistance when he tried to feed the rice bran, the "garbage," to the prisoners, but it worked—dramatically. Later, extracts of rice bran were used to prevent infantile beriberi; still later, thiamin was synthesized.

Thiamin occurs in small amounts in many nutritious foods. Pork, ham, leafy green vegetables, whole-grain cereals, and legumes are especially rich in thiamin (see Snapshot 7-5). People who keep empty-calorie foods to a minimum and include ten or more servings of nutritious foods each day will easily meet their thiamin needs.

People addicted to alcohol, though, may develop thiamin deficiency. Alcohol contributes energy, but carries almost no nutrients with it and often displaces food. In addition, alcohol impairs absorption of thiamin from the digestive tract and hastens its excretion in the urine, tripling the risk of deficiency.

Like thiamin, **riboflavin** plays a role in the energy metabolism of all cells. When thiamin is deficient, riboflavin may be lacking, too, but its deficiency symptoms may go undetected because those of thiamin deficiency are more severe.[35] Foods that remedy the thiamin deficiency invariably also contain some riboflavin, so they clear up both deficiencies. People obtain as much as half of their riboflavin from milk and milk products. Leafy green vegetables,

thiamin (THIGH-uh-min) a B vitamin involved in the body's use of fuels.

beriberi the thiamin-deficiency disease; characterized by loss of sensation in the hands and feet, muscular weakness, advancing paralysis, and abnormal heart action.

riboflavin (RIBE-o-flay-vin) a B vitamin active in the body's energy-releasing mechanisms.

Table 7-6 on page 262 lists the symptoms of riboflavin deficiency.

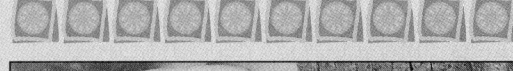

SNAPSHOT 7-5

THIAMIN

RDA for men: 1.5 mg/day
RDA for women: 1.1 mg/day

Green peas 0.23 mg per ½ c cooked

Pork chop 0.75 mg per 3 oz broiled chop

Black beans 0.21 mg per ½ c cooked

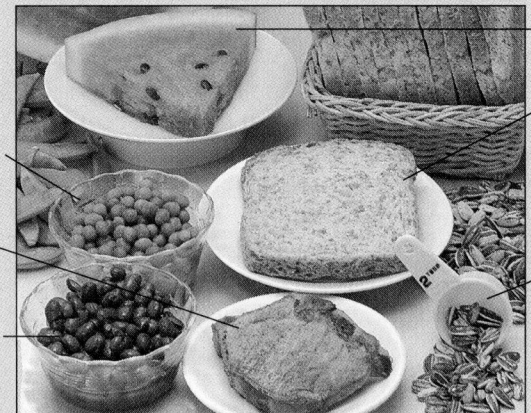

Watermelon 0.39 mg per melon wedge

Whole-wheat bread 0.12 mg per slice

Sunflower seeds (shelled) 0.1 mg per 2 tbs

niacin a B vitamin needed in energy metabolism. Niacin can be eaten preformed or can be made in the body from tryptophan, one of the amino acids. Other forms of niacin are *nicotinic acid, niacinamide,* and *nicotinamide.*

pellagra (pell-AY-gra) the niacin-deficiency disease (*pellis* means "skin"; *agra* means "rough"). Symptoms include the "4 Ds": diarrhea, dermatitis, dementia, and, ultimately, death.

niacin equivalents the amount of niacin present in food, including the niacin that can theoretically be made from its precursor tryptophan, present in the food.

folate (FOH-late) a B vitamin that acts as part of a coenzyme important in the manufacture of new cells. Other names for folate are *folacin* and *folic acid.*

whole-grain breads and cereals, and some meats contribute the rest of the riboflavin in people's diets (see Snapshot 7-6).

Niacin The vitamin **niacin,** like thiamin and riboflavin, participates in the energy metabolism of every body cell. The niacin-deficiency disease **pellagra** appeared in Europe in the 1700s when corn from the New World came into wide acceptance as a staple food. At about the turn of this century in the United States, pellagra was devastating people's lives throughout the South and Midwest. Hundreds of thousands of pellagra victims were thought to be suffering from a contagious disease until this dietary deficiency was pinned down. The disease still occurs among poorly nourished people living in today's urban slums and particularly in those with alcohol addiction. Pellagra is also still common in parts of Africa and Asia.

Early workers seeking the cause of pellagra observed that well-fed people never got it. From there they defined a diet that reliably produced the disease—one of cornmeal, salted pork fat, and molasses. Corn happens not only to be low in protein, but also to lack tryptophan, the amino acid from which niacin is made. Salt pork contains too little protein to compensate; and molasses is virtually protein-free.

Figure 7-6 shows the skin disorder associated with pellagra. For comparison, Figure 7-7 shows a skin disorder associated with vitamin B_6 deficiency, a reminder that any nutrient deficiency affects the skin and all other cells. The skin just happens to be the organ you can see.

The key nutrient that prevents pellagra is niacin, but any protein containing sufficient amounts of the amino acid tryptophan will serve in its place. Tryptophan, which is abundant in almost all proteins (but is unavailable from the protein of corn), is converted to niacin in the body. In fact, it is possible to cure pellagra by administering tryptophan alone. Thus a person eating more than adequate protein (as most people do) will not be deficient in niacin. The amount of niacin in a diet is therefore stated in terms of **niacin equivalents,** a

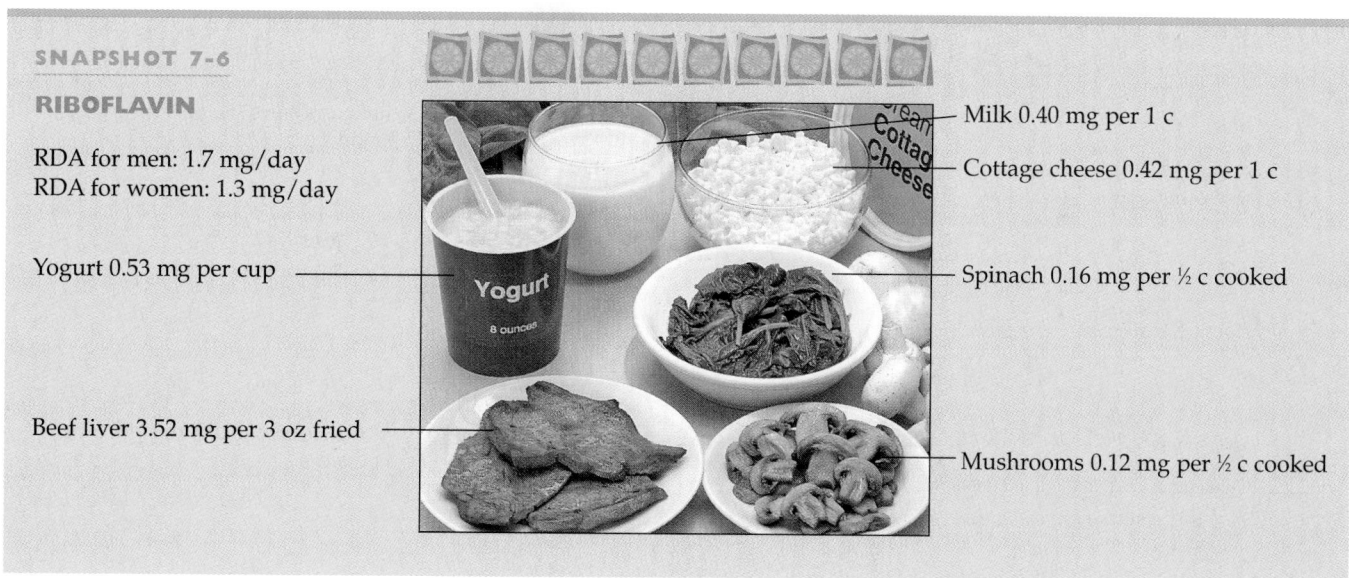

SNAPSHOT 7-6

RIBOFLAVIN

RDA for men: 1.7 mg/day
RDA for women: 1.3 mg/day

Yogurt 0.53 mg per cup

Beef liver 3.52 mg per 3 oz fried

Milk 0.40 mg per 1 c

Cottage cheese 0.42 mg per 1 c

Spinach 0.16 mg per ½ c cooked

Mushrooms 0.12 mg per ½ c cooked

measure that takes available tryptophan into account. Snapshot 7-7 shows some food sources of niacin.

Certain forms of niacin supplements in amounts ten times or more the RDA cause "niacin flush," a dilation of the capillaries of the skin with perceptible tingling that, if intense, can be painful. Some physicians administer large niacin doses as part of their arsenal of drugs against atherosclerosis.[36] Large doses of a form of niacin might also prove useful in preventing diabetes.[37] When used this way, niacin leaves the realm of nutrition to become a pharmacological agent, a drug. As with any drug, self-dosing with niacin is ill-advised; large doses may injure the liver, cause ulcers, and produce some symptoms of diabetes.[38]

Folate   The vitamin **folate** is required to make all new cells. Folate helps synthesize the DNA needed for the new cells. Deficiencies may result from an inadequate intake or from illnesses that impair folate's absorption or increase its excretion, or otherwise enlarge the need for folate.

Of all the vitamins, folate seems to be most likely to interact with medications. Ten major groups of drugs, including antacids and aspirin and its relatives, have been shown to interfere with the body's use of folate. Occasional use of these drugs to relieve headache or upset stomach presents no concern, but frequent users may need to attend to their folate intakes. These include people with chronic pain or ulcers who rely heavily on aspirin or antacids as well as those who smoke or take oral contraceptives or anticonvulsants.[39]

Because the blood cells and digestive tract cells divide most rapidly, they are most vulnerable to deficiency. As a result, deficiencies of folate cause anemia and abnormal digestive function. In the United States, a significant number of cases of folate-deficiency anemia occur yearly. Folate deficiency may also elevate a woman's risk for cervical cancer, a major health problem worldwide. A theory linking heart disease with folate deficiency is also gaining strength.[40] Along with deficiencies of several other B vitamins, a lack of folate may cause

FIGURE 7-6

PELLAGRA
The typical dermatitis of pellagra develops on skin that is exposed to light.

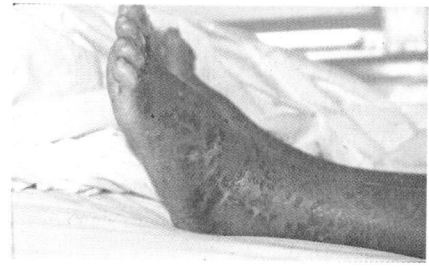

FIGURE 7-7

VITAMIN B₆ DEFICIENCY
In this dermatitis, the skin is greasy and flaky, unlike the skin affected by the dermatitis of pellagra.

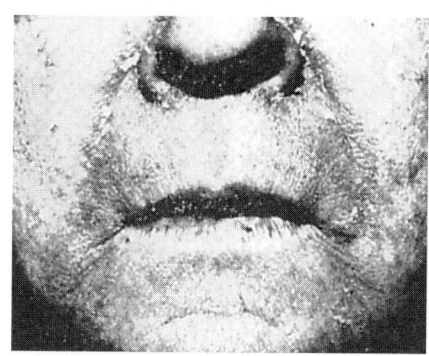

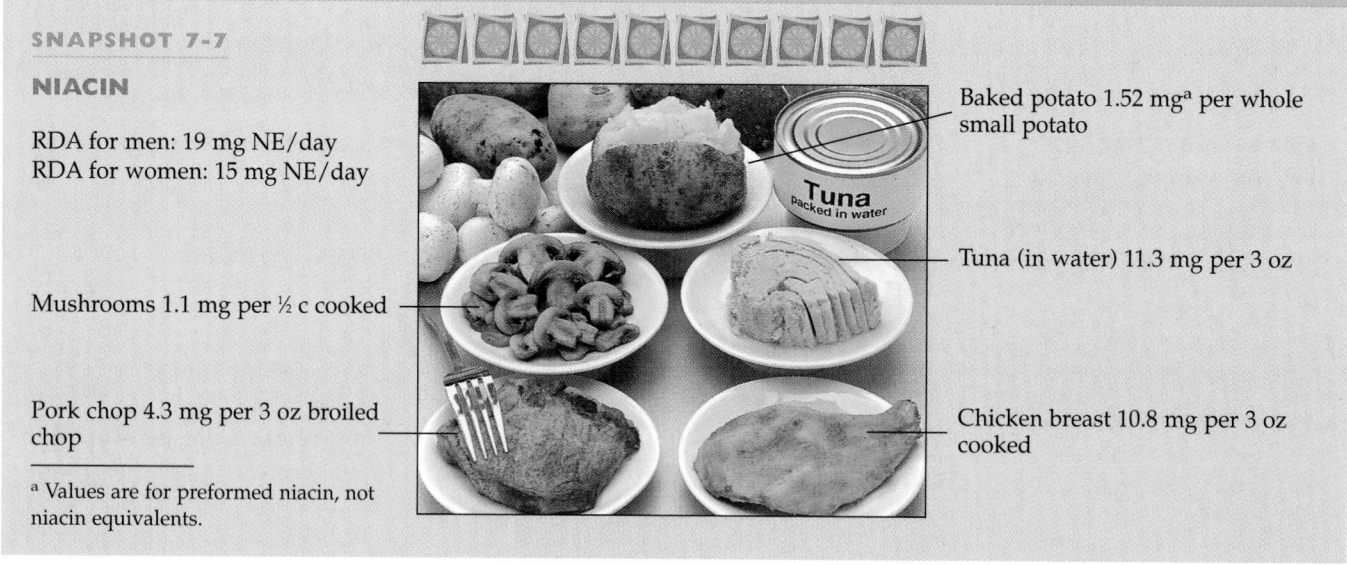

SNAPSHOT 7-7

NIACIN

RDA for men: 19 mg NE/day
RDA for women: 15 mg NE/day

Mushrooms 1.1 mg per ½ c cooked

Pork chop 4.3 mg per 3 oz broiled chop

_____

ª Values are for preformed niacin, not niacin equivalents.

Baked potato 1.52 mgª per whole small potato

Tuna (in water) 11.3 mg per 3 oz

Chicken breast 10.8 mg per 3 oz cooked

vitamin B₁₂ a B vitamin that enables folate to get into cells and also helps maintain the sheath around nerve cells. Vitamin B₁₂'s scientific name, not often used, is _cyanocobalamin._

Enrichment of grain foods was the topic of Chapter 4.

the buildup of an amino acid in the blood that seems somehow related to the development of heart disease.[41]

In 1992, the U.S. Public Health Service made an unprecedented recommendation. It advised all women of childbearing age to consume more than double the RDA for folate: 400 micrograms a day.[42] The reason is this: Folate deficiency is associated with a group of devastating birth defects known as neural tube defects. These defects affect 1 in every 1,000 births, making them the second most common form of birth defect after Down syndrome. Neural tube defects range from slight problems in the spine to mental retardation, severely diminished brain size, and death shortly after birth.[43]

Neural tube defects arise in the first days or weeks of pregnancy, long before most women even suspect that they are pregnant. By recommending that women obtain extra folate _before_ pregnancy, the Public Health Service hopes to prevent about half of all neural tube defects (the other half is attributable to causes other than folate deficiency).[44] Unfortunately, most women eat too few fruits and vegetables to supply even half the folate being recommended. The FDA has therefore ordered fortification of all enriched grain products with an especially absorbable form of folate.[45] Still unanswered are concerns about folate's ability to mask deficiencies of vitamin B₁₂ (more about this effect later).[46]

Folate's name is derived from the word _foliage,_ and as that implies, folate is abundant in leafy green vegetables such as spinach and turnip greens (see Snapshot 7-8). Fresh, uncooked vegetables and fruits are the best sources because the heat of cooking and the oxidation that occurs during storage destroy as much as half the folate in foods. Eggs also contain some folate. Orange juice and legumes are rich in folate, but they contain factors that may interfere with folate absorption, so their usefulness as folate contributors may be limited.[47] Milk, on the other hand, may enhance the absorption of folate, although it is unclear which constituent in milk may do so.[48]

Vitamin B₁₂   With the help of **vitamin B₁₂,** folate works to make red blood cells. Vitamin B₁₂ by itself also serves the body by helping to maintain the

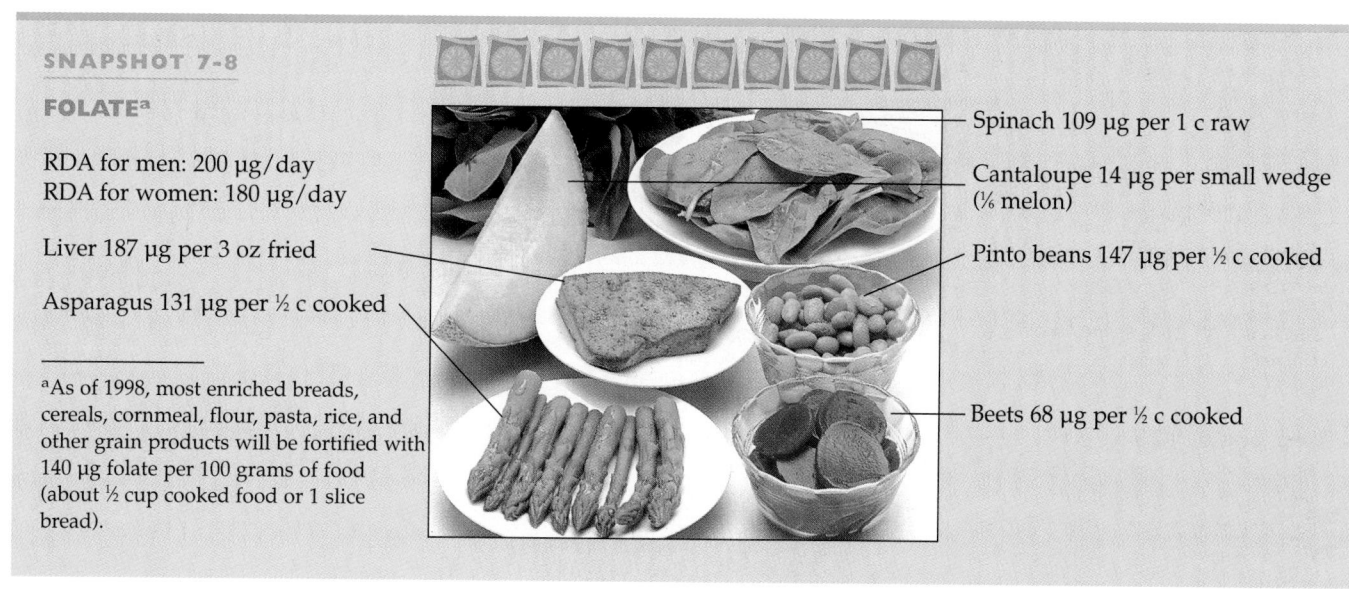

SNAPSHOT 7-8

FOLATE[a]

RDA for men: 200 µg/day
RDA for women: 180 µg/day

Liver 187 µg per 3 oz fried

Asparagus 131 µg per ½ c cooked

_____

[a]As of 1998, most enriched breads, cereals, cornmeal, flour, pasta, rice, and other grain products will be fortified with 140 µg folate per 100 grams of food (about ½ cup cooked food or 1 slice bread).

Spinach 109 µg per 1 c raw

Cantaloupe 14 µg per small wedge (⅙ melon)

Pinto beans 147 µg per ½ c cooked

Beets 68 µg per ½ c cooked

---

sheaths that surround and protect nerve fibers. It may also influence the cells that build bone tissue.

The absorption of vitamin B_{12} requires an **intrinsic factor,** a compound made inside the body. The design for this factor is carried in the genes. The intrinsic factor is synthesized in the stomach, where it attaches to the vitamin; the complex then passes to the small intestine and is absorbed into the bloodstream. A few people have an inherited defect in the gene for intrinsic factor, which makes vitamin B_{12} absorption abnormal, beginning in mid-adulthood. Without normal absorption of vitamin B_{12} from food, they develop deficiency symptoms. In this case or in the case of stomach injury that limits production of intrinsic factor, vitamin B_{12} must be supplied by injection to bypass the defective absorptive system. The vitamin B_{12} deficiency caused by lack of intrinsic factor is known as **pernicious anemia.**

Without sufficient vitamin B_{12}, nerves become damaged and folate fails to do its blood-building work, so vitamin B_{12} deficiency causes an anemia identical to that caused by folate deficiency. The blood symptoms of deficiencies of either folate or vitamin B_{12} include the presence of large, immature red blood cells. Giving extra folate will often clear up this blood condition, but it is a poor choice, because the deficiency of vitamin B_{12} can continue undetected. Vitamin B_{12}'s other functions then become compromised, and the results can be devastating: damaged nerve sheaths, creeping paralysis, and general malfunctioning of nerves and muscles.

A physician may notice signs of the B_{12} problem, but it is hard to diagnose correctly. More likely, the damage will proceed unchecked. This is why FDA's mandate to enrich foods with folate specifies exact amounts of folate allowed for addition to various foods—to prevent excessive folate intakes that could mask symptoms of a vitamin B_{12} deficiency.

As Snapshot 7-9 shows, vitamin B_{12} is present only in foods of animal origin, not in foods from plants. Consequently, the uninformed, strict vegetarian is at special risk. People who give up all foods of animal origin may not show signs of deficiency right away because up to five years' worth of vitamin B_{12}

intrinsic factor a factor found inside a system. The intrinsic factor necessary to prevent pernicious anemia is now known to be a compound that helps in the absorption of vitamin B_{12}.

pernicious (per-NISH-us) **anemia** a vitamin B_{12}–deficiency disease, caused by lack of intrinsic factor and characterized by large, immature red blood cells and damage to the nervous system (*pernicious* means "highly injurious or destructive").

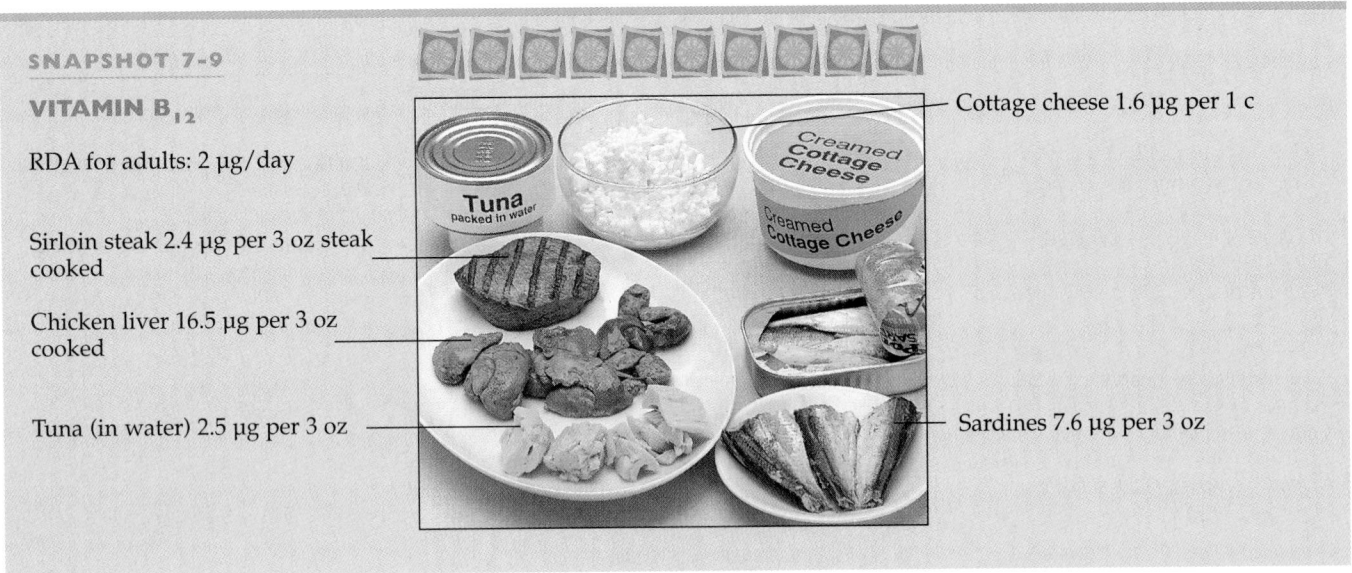

SNAPSHOT 7-9

VITAMIN B$_{12}$

RDA for adults: 2 µg/day

Sirloin steak 2.4 µg per 3 oz steak cooked

Chicken liver 16.5 µg per 3 oz cooked

Tuna (in water) 2.5 µg per 3 oz

Cottage cheese 1.6 µg per 1 c

Sardines 7.6 µg per 3 oz

---

vitamin B$_6$ a B vitamin needed in protein metabolism. Its three active forms are *pyridoxine, pyridoxal,* and *pyridoxamine.*

can be stored in the body; but eventually signs develop. A pregnant or lactating woman who is eating such a diet should be aware that her infant can develop a vitamin B$_{12}$ deficiency, even if the mother appears healthy. A deficiency of this vitamin can cause irreversible nervous system damage in the fetus. The birth of an infant with nerve problems can be the mother's first clue to the deficiency. All strict vegetarians, and especially pregnant women, must be sure to use vitamin B$_{12}$–fortified products, such as vitamin B$_{12}$–fortified soy "milk," or to take the appropriate supplements.

The way folate masks the anemia of vitamin B$_{12}$ deficiency underlines a point already made several times. It takes a skilled professional to correctly diagnose a nutrient deficiency or imbalance, and you clearly take a serious risk when you diagnose yourself or listen to would-be experts. A second point should also be underlined here. Since vitamin B$_{12}$ deficiency in the body may be caused by either a lack of the vitamin in the diet or a lack of the intrinsic factor necessary to absorb the vitamin, a change in diet alone may not correct the deficiency, another reason for seeking professional diagnosis of physical symptoms.

Vitamin B$_6$ In the cells, **vitamin B$_6$** helps to convert one kind of amino acid, of which cells have an abundance, to others that the cells need more of. It also aids in the conversion of tryptophan to niacin and plays important roles in the synthesis of hemoglobin. Vitamin B$_6$ also assists in releasing stored glucose from glycogen and thus contributes to regulation of blood glucose. During the last decade or so, vitamin B$_6$ research has revealed roles for the vitamin in immune function and steroid hormone activity.[49] In addition, vitamin B$_6$ is critical to the developing brain and nervous system of a fetus. Without enough of the vitamin during this stage, the child suffers behaviorally later on.[50]

Because of these diverse functions, vitamin B$_6$ deficiency is expressed in general symptoms, such as weakness, irritability, and insomnia. Other symptoms include the greasy dermatitis depicted in Figure 7-7 on page 245, anemia, and, in advanced cases of deficiency, convulsions. A shortage of vitamin B$_6$ also weakens the immune response.[51]

SNAPSHOT 7-10

VITAMIN B₆

RDA for men: 2.0 mg/day
RDA for women: 1.6 mg/day

Chicken breast 0.51 mg per 3 oz cooked

Spinach 0.22 mg per ½ c cooked

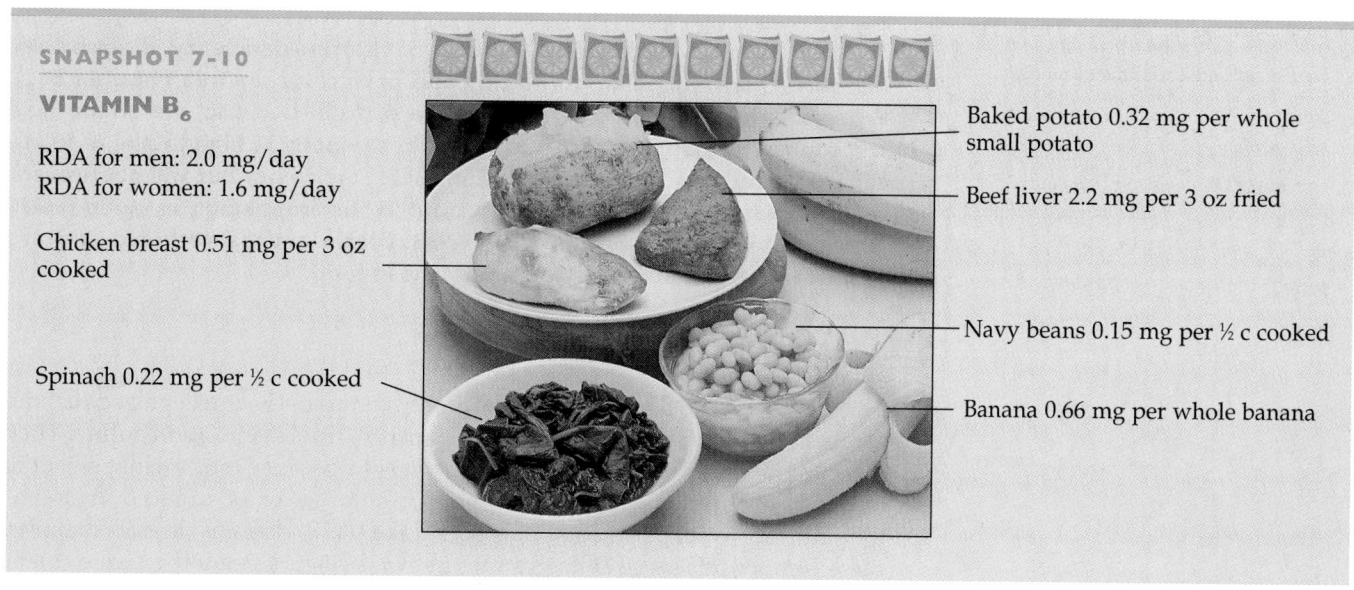

Baked potato 0.32 mg per whole small potato

Beef liver 2.2 mg per 3 oz fried

Navy beans 0.15 mg per ½ c cooked

Banana 0.66 mg per whole banana

Large doses of vitamin B₆ can be dangerous. Years ago it was generally believed that, like most of the other water-soluble vitamins, vitamin B₆ could not reach toxic concentrations in the body. This belief changed when a report told of women who took more than 2 grams of vitamin B₆ daily (the RDA for women is less than 2 *milligrams*) for two months or more in an attempt to cure the symptoms of premenstrual syndrome (PMS). The women developed numb feet, then lost sensation in their hands, and eventually became unable to work. Later, in some cases, their mouths became numb. Since the first report of vitamin B₆ toxicity, researchers have seen toxicity symptoms in more than 100 women who took vitamin B₆ supplements for more than five years. The women recovered after they stopped taking the supplements. The potential toxicity of vitamin B₆ is yet another reason why people should not self-diagnose and self-prescribe vitamins for their own illnesses. Table 7-6 on pages 262–265 lists common deficiency and toxicity symptoms of vitamin B₆ and other water-soluble vitamins.

Because vitamin B₆ plays many roles in protein metabolism, the RDA for vitamin B₆ is roughly proportional to protein intakes. Meats, fish, and poultry (protein-rich foods), potatoes, leafy green vegetables, and some fruits are good sources of vitamin B₆ (see Snapshot 7-10).

Biotin and Pantothenic Acid   Two other B vitamins, **biotin** and **pantothenic acid,** are, like thiamin, riboflavin, and niacin, important in energy metabolism. Biotin is a cofactor for several enzymes active in the metabolism of carbohydrate, fat, and protein. Pantothenic acid was first recognized as a substance that stimulates growth. Pantothenic acid is a component of a key coenzyme that makes possible the release of energy from the energy nutrients. It also participates in more than 100 different steps in the synthesis of lipids, neurotransmitters, steroid hormones, and hemoglobin.[52]

Although rare diseases may precipitate deficiencies of biotin and pantothenic acid, both vitamins are widespread in foods. Healthy people eating ordinary diets are not at risk for deficiencies.

biotin (BY-o-tin) a B vitamin; a coenzyme necessary for fat synthesis and other metabolic reactions.

pantothenic (PAN-to-THEN-ic) **acid** a B vitamin.

The links between PMS and vitamin B₆ are explored in Chapter 13.

inositol (in-OSS-ih-tall) a nonessential nutrient found in cell membranes.

lipoic (lip-OH-ic) **acid** a nonessential nutrient.

choline (KOH-leen) a nonessential nutrient used to make the phospholipid lecithin and other molecules.

scurvy the vitamin C–deficiency disease.

✔ **KEY POINT**   Historically, famous **B** vitamin–deficiency diseases are beriberi (thiamin), pellagra (niacin), and pernicious anemia (vitamin B_{12}). Pellagra can be prevented by adequate protein because the amino acid tryptophan can be converted to niacin in the body. A high intake of folate can mask the blood symptom of vitamin B_{12} deficiency but will not prevent the associated nerve damage. Vitamin B_6 is important in amino acid metabolism and can be toxic in excess. Biotin and pantothenic acid are important to the body and are abundant in food.

Non-B Vitamins

The section on the B vitamins has left a few compounds unrecognized that are sometimes *called* B vitamins. These are **inositol, lipoic acid,** and **choline.** They might more appropriately be called *nonvitamins* because they are not essential nutrients for human beings. Deficiencies can, however, be induced in laboratory animals for experimental purposes. Like the B vitamins described above, these compounds serve as coenzymes in metabolism. Even if they were essential in human nutrition, supplements would be unnecessary because they are abundant in foods.

In addition to inositol, lipoic acid, and choline, other substances have been mistakenly thought essential in human nutrition because they are needed for growth by bacteria or other life-forms. These substances include PABA (para-aminobenzoic acid), bioflavonoids ("vitamin P" or hesperidin), and ubiquinone (coenzyme Q). Other names you may hear are "vitamin B_{15}," or pangamic acid (a hoax); "vitamin B_{17}" (laetrile or amygdalin, not a cancer cure and not a vitamin by any stretch of the imagination); "vitamin B_T" (carnitine, an important piece of cell machinery but not a vitamin); and more.

Links between choline and brain function are discussed in Chapter 13.

✔ **KEY POINT**   Many substances that people claim are **B** vitamins are not. Among these substances are inositol, lipoic acid, and choline.

Vitamin C

Two hundred odd years ago, any man who joined the crew of a seagoing ship knew he had only half a chance of returning alive—not because he might be slain by pirates or die in a storm but because he might contract **scurvy,** a dreaded disease that might kill as many as two-thirds of a ship's men on a long voyage. Only ships that sailed on short voyages, especially around the Mediterranean Sea, were safe from this disease. It was not known at the time that the special hazard of long ocean voyages was that the ship's cook used up his fresh fruits and vegetables early and relied for the duration of the voyage on cereals and live animals.

The first nutrition experiment to be conducted on human beings was devised nearly 250 years ago to find a cure for scurvy. A British physician divided some sailors with scurvy into groups. Each group received a different test substance: vinegar, sulfuric acid, seawater, oranges, or lemons. Those receiving the citrus fruits were cured within a short time. Sadly, it was 50 years before the British Navy made use of the information and required all its vessels to provide lime juice to every sailor daily. The term *limey* was applied to

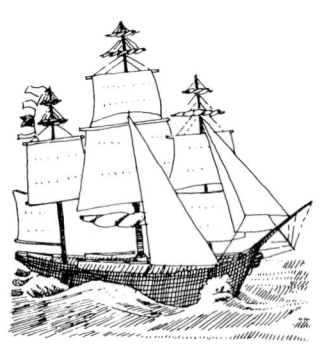

Long voyages without fresh fruits and vegetables spelled death by scurvy for the crew.

the British sailors in mockery because of this requirement. The name later given to the vitamin, **ascorbic acid,** literally means "no-scurvy acid."

The Work of Vitamin C   Since vitamin C is a water-soluble vitamin like the B vitamins, you might expect its mode of action to resemble that of the B vitamins. To some extent, in some situations, vitamin C does help a specific enzyme perform its job, just as the B vitamins do. In others, vitamin C acts in a more general way, as an antioxidant. Many substances found in foods and important in the body can be destroyed by oxidation. Vitamin C protects them from oxidation by being oxidized itself. In the intestines, vitamin C protects iron from oxidation and so promotes its absorption. The antioxidant roles of vitamin C are the focus of extensive study, especially in relation to disease prevention.

Vitamin C is required for the production and maintenance of **collagen,** a protein substance that forms the base for all connective tissues in the body: bones, teeth, skin, and tendons. Collagen forms the scar tissue that heals wounds, the reinforcing structure that mends fractures, and the supporting material of capillaries that prevents bruises.

Vitamin C also enhances the immune response and so protects against infection. The vitamin is also important to the production of thyroxine, the hormone that regulates basal metabolic rate and body temperature. The relationship between vitamin C and the common cold is the topic of the following Consumer Corner.

The Need for Vitamin C   The adult RDA for vitamin C of 60 milligrams is midway between two extremes. At one extreme is the requirement, 10 milligrams per day, which is enough to prevent the symptoms of scurvy from appearing. At the other extreme is the amount at which the body's pool of vitamin C is full to overflowing: about 100 milligrams per day.[53] The RDA for smokers is set at the high end, 100 milligrams, because this amount is needed to maintain blood levels comparable to those of nonsmokers.[54] Other authorities have set different standards. For example, Canada recommends 30 milligrams per day and Japan 100. The next RDA committee may change the RDA for vitamin C.[55]

Cigarette smoking, among its many harmful effects, interferes with the use of vitamin C. Smokers, and even "passive smokers" who live and work with smokers, therefore need more vitamin C than others.[56] Consumption of extra vitamin C can normalize blood levels but cannot protect against the damage caused by exposure to tobacco smoke.

Most of the symptoms of scurvy can be attributed to the breakdown of collagen in the absence of vitamin C: loss of appetite, growth cessation, tenderness to touch, weakness, bleeding gums (shown here in Figure 7-8), loose teeth, swollen ankles and wrists, and tiny red spots in the skin where blood has leaked out of capillaries. One symptom, anemia, reflects an important role already mentioned—that vitamin C helps the body to absorb and use iron.

In the United States, scurvy is seldom seen today except in infants who are fed only cow's milk, in the elderly, and in people addicted to alcohol or other drugs. Breast milk and infant formula supply enough vitamin C, but infants who are fed cow's milk and receive no vitamin C in formula, fruit juice, or other outside sources are at risk.[57] Low intakes of fruits and vegetables and a

ascorbic acid one of the active forms of vitamin C (the other is *dehydroascorbic acid*); an antioxidant nutrient.

collagen (COLL-a-jen) the chief protein of most connective tissues, including scars, ligaments, and tendons, and the underlying matrix on which bones and teeth are built.

FIGURE 7-8

SCURVY
Vitamin C deficiency causes breakdown of collagen, which supports the teeth.

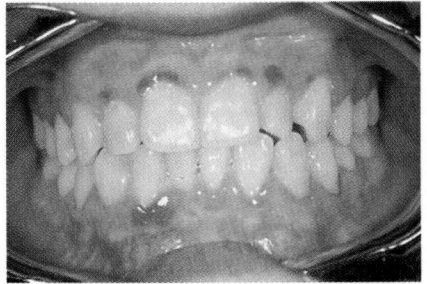

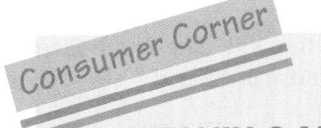

VITAMIN C AND THE COMMON COLD

For years, people have claimed that vitamin C can help cure colds, but researchers have found little, if any, support for such claims. A major review of the research on vitamin C in the treatment and prevention of the common cold revealed a significant difference of one-tenth of a cold per year and an average difference in duration of one-tenth of a day per cold in favor of those taking vitamin C. Is that enough savings to warrant taking supplements? Scientists think not; supplement users seem to think so.

Interestingly, subjects of one study who received a placebo but *thought* they were receiving vitamin C had fewer colds than the group who in reality had received vitamin C but thought they were receiving the placebo. At work was the powerful healing effect of faith—the placebo effect, first defined in Chapter 1.

One other role of vitamin C may link the vitamin with the common cold. Some research suggests that vitamin C (2 grams taken daily for two weeks) reduces blood histamine.[58] Anyone who has ever had a cold knows the effects of histamine: sneezing, a runny or stuffed-up nose, and swollen sinuses. A group of drugs used in cold medications, antihistamines, provide relief from just those symptoms. In druglike doses, vitamin C works like an antihistamine by deactivating histamine.[59] While the supplements do nothing to prevent or cure a cold, then, they may sooth it by relieving some of its symptoms.[60] No drug is risk-free, however, and large doses of vitamin C have side effects, described below.

2,000 —— Megavitamin recommendation

1,000

800

600

400

200

100 —— Maintains full body pool; RDA for cigarette smokers

75
60 —— RDA for nonsmokers
50
40 —— Canadian RNI for men
30 —— Supports metabolism;
20 Canadian RNI for women
10 —— Prevents scurvy
0

poor appetite for food in general lead to low vitamin C intakes and are not uncommon among people 65 years of age and older.[61]

Vitamin C Overdoses   The easy availability of vitamin C in pill form and the publication of books recommending vitamin C to prevent and cure colds and cancer have led thousands of people to take large doses of vitamin C. These "volunteer" subjects enabled researchers to study the toxic effects of large vitamin C doses. Effects that are theoretically possible (but that have not been seen with intakes as high as 3 grams a day) include formation of kidney stones, alteration of the acid-base balance, and interference with the action of vitamin E. One effect that has been observed with a 2-gram dose is alteration of the insulin response to carbohydrate in people with otherwise normal glucose tolerances.[62]

Other adverse effects are common, including nausea, abdominal cramps, excessive gas, and diarrhea. Several instances of interference with medical regimens are known. Large amounts of vitamin C excreted in the urine can obscure the results of tests used to detect diabetes, giving a false positive result in some instances and a false negative result in others. People taking medications to prevent blood clotting may unwittingly undo the effect if they also take massive doses of vitamin C.[63] Vitamin C supplements in any dosage are dan-

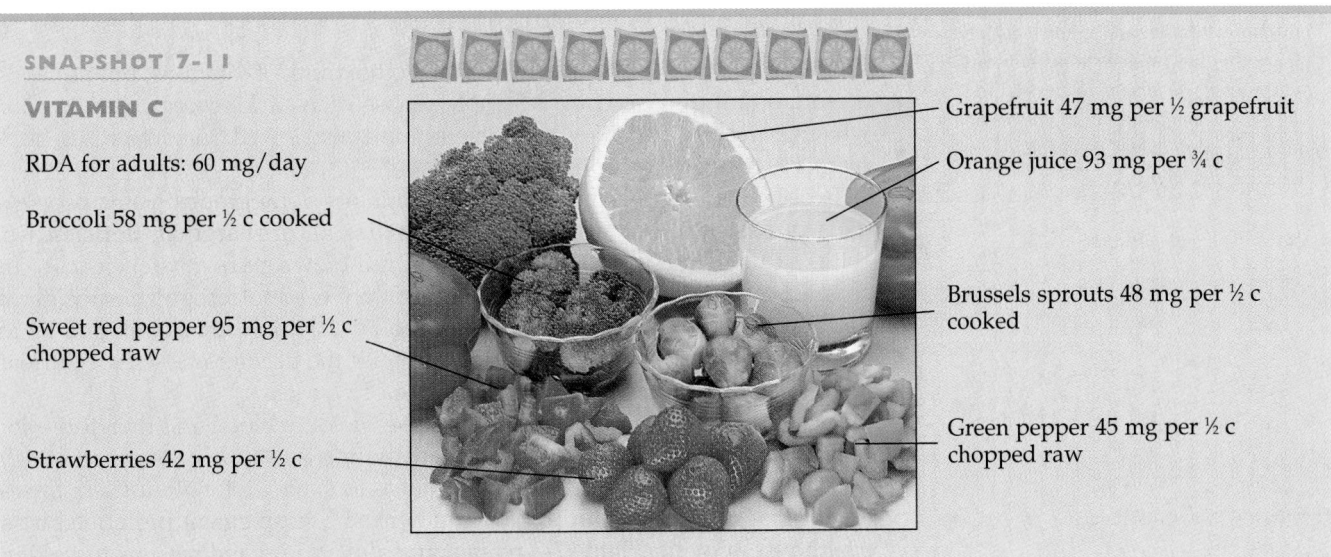

SNAPSHOT 7-11

VITAMIN C

RDA for adults: 60 mg/day

Broccoli 58 mg per ½ c cooked

Sweet red pepper 95 mg per ½ c chopped raw

Strawberries 42 mg per ½ c

Grapefruit 47 mg per ½ grapefruit

Orange juice 93 mg per ¾ c

Brussels sprouts 48 mg per ½ c cooked

Green pepper 45 mg per ½ c chopped raw

gerous for people with an overload of iron in the blood because vitamin C increases iron absorption from the intestine and releases iron from storage.[64]

The published research on large doses of vitamin C reveals few instances in which consuming more than 100 to 300 milligrams a day is beneficial. Adults may not be taking major risks if they dose themselves with a gram a day, but doses approaching 10 grams are clearly unsafe. In short, the range of safe vitamin C intakes seems to be broad. Between the absolute minimum of 10 milligrams a day and the reasonable maximum of 2,000 milligrams (2 grams), nearly everyone should be able to find a suitable intake. People who venture outside these limits do so at their own risk. Vitamin C from food sources such as those shown in Snapshot 7-11 is always safe.

When people dose themselves with supplements, they leave the realm of nutrition and enter that of pharmacology. Like drugs, large doses of nutrients can have medicinal effects on the body and can present serious side effects as well. The next section discusses supplements as sources of nutrients. The Controversy takes up topics of interest to those who would seek medicinal effects from nutrients, herbs, and foods.

✓ KEY POINT **Vitamin C, an antioxidant, helps to maintain the connective tissue protein collagen, protects against infection, and helps in iron absorption. The theory that vitamin C prevents or cures colds or cancer is not well supported by research. High vitamin C doses may be hazardous. Ample vitamin C can be obtained from foods.**

VITAMIN SUPPLEMENTS

Who should take supplements of vitamins? Almost 40 percent of the population do so regularly, collectively spending billions of dollars a year on them.[65] But who really needs supplements? No one? Everyone? Some people? Which people? And which supplements should they take? The answers are not always clear-cut.

Multivitamin-Mineral Supplements

When people think of supplements, they often think of vitamins, but minerals are important, too, of course. People whose diets lack several vitamins, for whatever reason, probably lack several minerals as well. In some cases, supplements may be appropriate.

People who may need supplements fall into several groups. Some people's diets put them at risk of developing **subclinical,** or **marginal, deficiencies:** states of unwellness shy of the classical, full-blown nutrient deficiencies. In contrast to the classical deficiencies, which are easy to recognize, subclinical deficiencies are subtle and easy to overlook.[66] The first remedy should be to attempt to improve the diet so that it supplies the needed nutrients. Nutrient supplements may also be appropriate in special cases.

Consider the case of the woman who loses a lot of blood and therefore a lot of iron and other blood-building nutrients in menstruation each month. Such a woman may be able to eat in such a way as to make up for all nutrient losses except that of iron, and for iron, she may need a supplement prescribed by a health-care provider. Table 7-2 points out valid and invalid reasons for taking supplements.

✔ KEY POINT **People who routinely fail to obtain the recommended amounts of vitamins and minerals from the diet and people with special needs, such as those who are pregnant or elderly, may be at risk for deficiencies and may benefit from a multivitamin-mineral supplement.**

Supplement Risks and Problems

When people self-prescribe supplements, they have to choose doses. "I'll take one of these a day," a person may say, or "I'll take two of these and three of those a day." Whatever the choice, the higher the dose, the greater the risk of toxicity. People's tolerances for high doses of nutrients vary. Amounts that some can tolerate may not be safe for others, and no one knows who falls into which category. Toxic overdoses of vitamins and minerals may be more common than we realize.*

Even more worrisome than short-term, acute overdose effects is chronic, low-level nutrient toxicity in which the subtle effects develop slowly and go unrecognized. An example is that of a woman who took just 1,000 RE (5,000 IU) of vitamin A a day, an amount typically found in vitamin-mineral supplements—but she took this dose daily for ten years. Then she was diagnosed with liver disease. Only when she discontinued the supplement did the condition clear up.[67] Vitamin A reliably produces hepatic injury at doses greater than 10,000 RE, and even at 5,000 RE, abnormal levels of liver enzymes are detectable in the blood.[68] In view of the potential hazards that supplements present, some authorities believe they should be required to bear warning labels, but such labels have not been seriously considered.

---

*One report estimates accidental nutrient overdoses in 1990 at more than 1,300. Centers for Disease Control, as cited in *Hype and Hope: The Cost of Vitamins,* 1992 (New York City Department of Consumer Affairs, 42 Broadway, New York, NY 10004), p. 2.

TABLE 7-2

Some Valid and Invalid Reasons for Taking Supplements

These People May Need Supplements:	These People Don't:
■ Pregnant or lactating women (they may need iron and folate). ■ Newborns (they are routinely given a vitamin K dose). ■ Infants (they may need various supplements, see Chapter 12). ■ Those who are lactose intolerant (they need calcium to forestall osteoporosis). ■ Habitual dieters (they may eat insufficient food). ■ Elderly people (they may eat less, have trouble chewing, choose poorly). ■ Victims of AIDS or other wasting illnesses (they lose nutrients faster than they can eat foods to supply nutrients). ■ Those addicted to drugs or alcohol (they absorb fewer and excrete more nutrients; they urgently need recovery programs, and nutrients cannot undo damage from drugs or alcohol). ■ Those recovering from surgery, burns, injury, or illness (they need extra nutrients to help regenerate tissues). ■ Strict vegetarians (they may need vitamin B_{12}, vitamin D, iron, and zinc). ■ People taking medications that interfere with the body's use of nutrients.	■ Those who feel insecure about the amounts of nutrients in the food supply. ■ Those who feel tired and falsely believe that supplements can provide energy. ■ Those who have faith that supplements will help them cope with stress. ■ Those who wish to build lean body tissue without physical work or wrongly believe that supplements will build muscles faster than work and diet alone. ■ Those who want to prevent or cure self-diagnosed conditions from the common cold to cancer. ■ Those who hope that excess nutrients will produce mysterious, though beneficial, reactions in the body. ■ Those who are taking certain medications because supplements may interfere with the action of the medications.

bioavailability absorbability; the individual differences in the proportion of a nutrient that is available for absorption from various sources.

It is impossible yet to say how much of a nutrient is too much although experts are wrestling with this problem.[69] Assuming, however, that it is best to err on the conservative side, Table 7-3 presents suggested limits for vitamin and mineral doses in supplements for daily use.

Also, supplements may lull their takers into a false sense of security. A person may eat irresponsibly, thinking, "My supplement will cover my needs." More often, supplements supply just the nutrients people need least—those that they consume in food—while failing to provide those missing from the diet.

Another problem is that of **bioavailability.** In general, nutrients are absorbed best from foods in which they are dispersed among other ingredients that facilitate their absorption. In contrast, nutrients taken in pure, concentrated form are likely to interfere with the absorption of other nutrients. Minerals provide examples: zinc hinders copper and calcium absorption, iron hinders zinc absorption, calcium hinders magnesium and iron absorption, and so on. Interactions between vitamins also exist.

TABLE 7-3

Vitamin and Mineral Doses for Supplements

Substance	Safe Range of Intakes	Average Multivitamin Pill	Average Single Supplement
Vitamins			
Vitamin A	75 to 750 RE[a]	5,000 IU	8,000 IU
Vitamin D	10 µg[a] (up to age 18)	400 IU	—
	5 µg[a] (adults)		
Vitamin E	6 to 800 mg[a, b]	30 mg	200 to 1,000 mg
Thiamin	1 to 2 mg	1.5 mg	100 mg
Riboflavin	1 to 2 mg	1.7 mg	25 mg
Niacin (as niacinamide)	10 to 20 mg	20 mg	100 mg
Vitamin B_6	1.5 to 2.5 mg	2 mg	100 mg
Folate	0.1 to 0.4 mg (in multivitamin form)	400 µg	400 µg
Vitamin B_{12}	3 to 10 µg	6 µg	100 µg
Pantothenic acid	5 to 20 mg (in multivitamin form)	10 mg	—
Biotin	Not recommended in supplement form	30 µg	—
Vitamin C	50 to 1,000[c] mg	60 mg	500 to 1,000 mg
Minerals			
Calcium	400 to 800 mg	160 mg	500 mg
Phosphorus	No need to supplement	110 mg	—
Magnesium	No need to supplement	100 mg	250 mg
Iron	10 to 39 mg (women)	18 mg	325 mg
Zinc	10 to 25 mg (adults)	15 mg	60 mg
Iodine	Not recommended in supplement form	150 µg	—

[a]Some supplements are measured in International Units (IU). To convert to RDA-compatible units, see Appendix C, Aids to Calculations.

[b]Upper limit for vitamin E from R. J. Sokol, Vitamin E in E. E. Ziegler and L. J. Filer, eds., *Present Knowledge in Nutrition* (Washington, D.C.: ILSI Press, 1996), pp. 130–136.

[c]Upper limit for vitamin C from M. Levine and coauthors, Vitamin C pharmacokinetics in healthy volunteers: Evidence for a Recommended Dietary Allowance, *Proceedings of the National Academy of Sciences* 93 (1996): 3704–3709.

dietary supplement a product, other than tobacco, added to the diet that contains one of the following ingredients: a vitamin, mineral, herb, botanical (plant extract), amino acid, metabolite, constituent, extract, or combination of any of these ingredients.

Another concern is not about known nutrients, but about the landslide of other substances legally sold in the United States as "dietary supplements" (Table 7-4 provides a sampling). A quirk of U.S. labeling laws allows almost any substance, including herbs, amino acids, dried animal organ tissues, microorganisms, or even concentrated hormones, to be sold freely over the counter, even though little is known about its effects or safety.

The Dietary Supplement Health and Education Act of 1994 defined the term **dietary supplement.**[70] The definition is so broad, however, that one concerned speaker on the topic concluded that producers could legally "manufacture dirt as a supplement" and it would be up to the FDA to prove the product unsafe.[71] This extreme example makes its point: no safety guarantee comes with dietary supplements. The point is underscored by the many hundreds of victims who have suffered ill effects, and more than 15 who died, from taking supplements containing the stimulant **ephedrine** (see Table 7-4) and related compounds. The effects range from headaches and vomiting to heart attacks and brain hemorrhage. Manufacturers are not legally required to prove that their supplements are safe; they must only state truthfully the contents of the package and refrain from making unapproved health claims on the label. FDA is charged with detecting hazards among supplements, but so many supplement ingredi-

TABLE 7-4

A Sample of Substances Sold as Dietary Supplements

According to new legal definitions all of these substances qualify as dietary supplements, even though some appear to have the effects of drugs, not nutrients.

- **DHEA**[a] a hormone secretion of the adrenal gland whose level falls with advancing age. DHEA may protect antioxidant nutrients; low blood levels are associated with elevated risk of diseases. Theories that DHEA might stimulate hormone-responsive cancers such as breast or prostate are unproved. Real DHEA is available only by prescription; herbal DHE imitator for sale in health food stores is not active in the body. No safety information exists for long-term consumption of DHEA or its herbal imitator.
- **desiccated liver** a powder sold in health-food stores and supposed to contain in concentrated form all the nutrients found in liver. Possibly not dangerous, this supplement has no particular nutritional merit, and grocery store liver is considerably less expensive (*desiccated* means "totally dried").
- **ephedrine** One of a chemically-related group of compounds with dangerous amphetamine-like stimulant effects; commonly added to herbal preparations such as Ma huang, to weight-loss products, and to products claimed to imitate the effects of illegal drugs of abuse. Side effects include heart attacks, strokes, seizures, psychoses, headaches, nausea, tremors, chest pains, insomnia, vomiting, fatigue, dizziness, and death. Ephedrine poses the greatest threat in combination with caffeine. FDA has issued a warning of ephedrine's dangers, and may soon restrict its use and require a label to warn consumers.
- **garlic oil** an extract of garlic; may or may not contain the chemicals associated with garlic; claims for health benefits unproved.
- **green pills, fruit pills** pills containing dehydrated, crushed vegetable or fruit matter. An advertisement may claim that each pill equals a *pound* of fresh produce, but in reality a pill may equal one small forkful—minus nutrient losses incurred in processing.
- **kelp tablets** tablets made from dehydrated kelp, a kind of seaweed used by the Japanese as a foodstuff.
- **Ma huang** an evergreen plant derivative that supposedly boosts energy and helps with weight control; Ma huang contains ephedrine (see above), especially dangerous in combination with kola nut or other caffeine-containing substances.
- **melatonin** a hormone of the pineal gland believed to help regulate the body's daily rhythms to reverse the effects of jet lag, and to promote sleep. Claims for life extension or enhancement of sexual prowess are without merit. Proof of melatonin's safety or effectiveness is lacking.
- **nutritional yeast** a preparation of yeast cells, often praised for its high nutrient content. Yeast is a source of B vitamins, as are many other foods. Also called *brewer's yeast*; not the yeast used in baking.
- 1,000 others

[a]Dehydroepiandrosterone
NOTE: Table 11-10 of Chapter 11 defines medicinal herbs.

ents continue to emerge that FDA resources are inadequate to test and remove them before they cause harm. As of this writing, FDA has issued a warning about ephedrine's dangers, especially when combined with caffeine; however, supplements containing ephedrine compounds remain on store shelves for purchase by unsuspecting consumers.[72]

One of the dietary supplements defined in Table 7-4 is **melatonin,** a hormone harvested from a light-sensitive gland of the brain and sold to those with insomnia as a sleep aid. Research supports the idea that a tiny (0.3 milligram) dose of melatonin induces normal sleep without the side effects of other sleep agents on the market. Melatonin is sold in health-food and other stores in doses ten or more times as great as the dose that promotes sleep. At this dosage, melatonin remains in the body for too long and can cause dizziness or drowsiness the next day. It may also interrupt other body cycles that follow the natural daily melatonin ebb and flow, with effects such as insomnia and abnormal body temperature swings.

In view of all the negatives associated with supplement taking, several nutrition societies have indicated that most people should not use supplements. These experts urge that whenever a person's diet is inadequate, the remedy is to improve food choices and eating patterns. Failing this, supplements rank a distant second choice.

✔ KEY POINT **Before you decide to take supplements, make sure to recognize the potential for toxicity as well as the associated limitations.**

Selection of a Multinutrient Supplement

Now the question is, do *you* need a supplement? As the foregoing section indicated, if you choose to take one, you do so at some risk. If you fall into one of the categories already noted, however, and if you cannot meet your nutrient needs from foods, a supplement may be in order.

The next question is, which supplement to choose? Do you need one—"For vitality!" "Infants only!" "Time release!" "Stress formula!"—as the ads claim? It doesn't take much time in front of a supplement counter to see that competition for consumer dollars is fierce, and not always highly ethical.[73]

The first step in escaping the clutches of the health hustlers is to use your imagination and simply white out the label picture of sexy people on the beach and the meaningless, glittering generalities like "new and improved." Now all you have left is the list of ingredients, what form they are in, and the price—the plain facts.

You have two basic questions to answer. The first question: What form do you want—chewable, liquid, or pills? If you'd rather drink your vitamins and minerals than chew them, fine. (If you choose chewables, be aware that vitamin C can erode tooth enamel. Swallow promptly and flush the teeth with a drink of water.) The second question: Who are you? What vitamins and minerals do you need? The RDA table (inside front cover) and the RNI Table for Canadians (Canadiana, Appendix B) are the standards appropriate for virtually all reasonably healthy people.

Generally, an appropriate supplement provides all the RDA nutrients in amounts smaller than, equal to, or very close to the RDA. Avoid any preparation that, in a daily dose, provides more than the RDA of vitamin A, vitamin D, or any mineral or more than ten times the RDA for any nutrient. A warning: Expect to reject about 80 percent of available preparations when you choose according to these criteria; be choosy where your health is concerned. Avoid these:

- High doses of iron (more than 10 milligrams per day) except for menstruating women. People who menstruate need more iron, but people who don't, don't.
- "Organic" or "natural" types of preparations with added substances. They are no better than standard types, but they cost much more.[74]
- "High-potency" or "therapeutic dose" supplements. More is not better.
- Items not needed in human nutrition, such as choline and inositol. These particular items won't harm you, but they reveal a marketing strategy that makes the whole mix suspect. The manufacturer wants you to believe that its pills contain the latest "new" nutrient that other brands omit, but, in fact, for every valid discovery of this kind, there are 999,999 frauds.
- "Stress formulas." Although the stress response depends on certain B vitamins and vitamin C, the RDA amount provides all that is needed of these. If you are under stress (and who isn't?), generous servings of fruits and vegetables will more than cover your need.
- Pills containing extracts of parsley, alfalfa, and other vegetable components. The Controversy section that follows this chapter makes clear that vegetables, not pills, supply chemical mixtures that benefit health.
- Geriatric "tonics." They are generally poor in vitamins and minerals and yet may be so high in alcohol as to threaten inebriation.

Ironically, people today are far more likely to suffer from overnutrition and poor lifestyle choices than from nutrient deficiencies. People wish they could just take vitamin pills to gain health. The truth—that they need to make efforts to improve their eating and exercise habits—is harder to swallow.

✓ **KEY POINT**   **If you feel a supplement is needed, then remember to examine the ingredients and choose one that satisfies *your* needs.**

This chapter has addressed all 13 of the vitamins. It sums up the basic facts about each one in Tables 7-5 and 7-6.

TABLE 7-5

The Fat-Soluble Vitamins—Functions, Deficiencies, and Toxicities

VITAMIN A

Other Names	Deficiency Symptoms	Toxicity Symptoms
Retinol, retinal, retinoic acid; main precursor is beta-carotene	**Blood/Circulatory System**	
	Anemia (small-cell types)[a]	Red blood cell breakage, nosebleeds
Chief Functions in the Body	**Bones/Teeth**	
Vision; health of cornea, epithelial cells, mucous membranes; skin health; bone and tooth growth; reproduction; hormone synthesis and regulation; immunity	Cessation of bone growth, painful joints; impaired enamel formation, cracks in teeth, tendency to decay	Bone pain; growth retardation; increase of pressure inside skull mimicking brain tumor; headaches
Beta-carotene: antioxidant	**Digestive System**	
	Diarrhea, changes in lining	Abdominal cramps and pain, nausea vomiting, diarrhea, weight loss
Deficiency Disease Name	**Immune System**	
Hypovitaminosis A	Depression; frequent respiratory, digestive, bladder, vaginal, and other infections	Overreactivity
Significant Sources	**Nervous/Muscular Systems**	
Retinol: fortified milk, cheese, cream, butter, fortified margarine, eggs, liver	Night blindness (retinal)	Blurred vision, pain in calves, fatigue, irritability, loss of appetite
Beta-carotene: spinach and other dark, leafy greens; broccoli; deep orange fruits (apricots, cantaloupe) and vegetables (squash, carrots, sweet potatoes, pumpkin)	**Skin and Cornea**	
	Keratinization, corneal degeneration leading to blindness,[b] rashes	Dry skin, rashes, loss of hair
	Other	
	Kidney stones, impaired growth	Cessation of menstruation, liver and spleen enlargement

VITAMIN D

Other Names	Deficiency Symptoms	Toxicity Symptoms
Calciferol, cholecalciferol, dihydroxy vitamin D; precursor is cholesterol	**Blood/Circulatory System**	
		Raised blood calcium
Chief Functions in the Body	**Bones/Teeth**	
Mineralization of bones (raises blood calcium and phosphorus via absorption from digestive tract, and by withdrawing calcium from bones and stimulating retention by kidneys)	Abnormal growth, misshapen bones (bowing of legs), soft bones, joint pain, malformed teeth	
	Nervous System	
	Muscle spasms	Excessive thirst, headaches, irritability, loss of appetite, weakness, nausea
Deficiency Disease Name	**Other**	
Rickets, osteomalacia		Kidney stones, stones in arteries, mental and physical retardation
Significant Sources		
Self-synthesis with sunlight; fortified milk or margarine, eggs, liver, sardines		

(continued on next page)

TABLE 7-5

The Fat-Soluble Vitamins—Functions, Deficiencies, and Toxicities continued

VITAMIN E

Other Names	Deficiency Symptoms	Toxicity Symptoms
Alpha-tocopherol, tocopherol	Blood/Circulatory System	
Chief Functions in the Body	Red blood cell breakage, anemia	Augments the effects of anticlotting medication
Antioxidant (detoxification of strong oxidants), stabilization of cell membranes, regulation of oxidation reactions, protection of PUFA and vitamin A	Digestive System	
		General discomfort
	Nervous/Muscular Systems	
	Degeneration, weakness, difficulty walking, leg cramps	
Deficiency Disease Name	Other	
(No name)	Fibrocystic breast disease	
Significant Sources		
Polyunsaturated plant oils (margarine, salad dressings, shortenings), green and leafy vegetables, wheat germ, whole-grain products, nuts, seeds		

VITAMIN K

Other Names	Deficiency Symptoms	Toxicity Symptoms
Phylloquinone, naphthoquinone	Blood/Circulatory System	
Chief Functions in the Body	Hemorrhaging	Interference with anticlotting medication; vitamin K analogues may cause jaundice.
Synthesis of blood-clotting proteins and a blood protein that regulates blood calcium		
Deficiency Disease Name		
(No name)		
Significant Sources		
Bacterial synthesis in the digestive tract; liver, green leafy vegetables, cabbage-type vegetables, milk		

[a]Small-cell anemia is termed *microcytic anemia*; large-cell type is *macrocytic* or *megaloblastic anemia*.

[b]Corneal degeneration progresses from *keratinization* (hardening) to *xerosis* (drying) to *xerophthalomia* (thickening, opacity, and irreversible blindness).

TABLE 7-6
The Water-Soluble Vitamins—Functions, Deficiencies, and Toxicities

THIAMIN

Other Names	Deficiency Symptoms	Toxicity Symptoms
Vitamin B$_1$	**Blood/Circulatory System**	
	Edema, enlarged heart, abnormal heart rhythms, heart failure	(No symptoms reported)
Chief Functions in the Body	**Nervous/Muscular Systems**	
Part of a coenzyme used in energy metabolism, supports normal appetite and nervous system function	Degeneration, wasting, weakness, pain, low morale, difficulty walking, loss of reflexes, mental confusion, paralysis	(No symptoms reported)
Deficiency Disease Name		
Beriberi		
Significant Sources		
Occurs in all nutritious foods in moderate amounts; pork, ham, bacon, liver, whole grains, legumes, nuts		

RIBOFLAVIN

Other Names	Deficiency Symptoms	Toxicity Symptoms
Vitamin B$_2$	**Mouth, Gums, Tongue**	
	Cracks at corners of mouth,[a] magenta tongue	(No symptoms reported)
Chief Functions in the Body	**Nervous System and Eyes**	
Part of a coenzyme used in energy metabolism, supports normal vision and skin health	Hypersensitivity to light,[b] reddening of cornea	(No symptoms reported)
Deficiency Disease Name	**Other**	
Ariboflavinosis	Skin rash	(No symptoms reported)
Significant Sources		
Milk, yogurt, cottage cheese, meat, leafy green vegetables, whole-grain or enriched breads and cereals		

(continued on next page)

TABLE 7-6

The Water-Soluble Vitamins—Functions, Deficiencies, and Toxicities continued

NIACIN		
Other Names	**Deficiency Symptoms**	**Toxicity Symptoms**
	Digestive System	
Nicotinic acid, nicotinamide, niacinamide, vitamin B$_3$; precursor is dietary tryptophan	Diarrhea	Diarrhea, heartburn, nausea, ulcer, irritation, vomiting
	Mouth, Gums, Tongue	
Chief Functions in the Body	Black, smooth tongue[c]	
	Nervous System	
Part of a coenzyme used in energy metabolism; supports health of skin, nervous system, and digestive system	Irritability, loss of appetite, weakness, dizziness, mental confusion progressing to psychosis or delirium	Fainting, dizziness
Deficiency Disease Name	*Skin*	
Pellagra	Flaky skin rash on areas exposed to sun	Painful flush and rash ("niacin rush"), sweating
Significant Sources	*Other*	
Milk, eggs, meat, poultry, fish, whole-grain and enriched breads and cereals, nuts, and all protein-containing foods		Abnormal liver function, low blood pressure

VITAMIN B$_6$		
Other Names	**Deficiency Symptoms**	**Toxicity Symptoms**
	Blood/Circulatory System	
Pyridoxine, pyridoxal, pyridoxamine	Anemia (small-cell type)[d]	Bloating
Chief Functions in the Body	*Mouth, Gums, Tongue*	
	Smooth tongue[c]	
Part of a coenzyme used in amino acid and fatty acid metabolism, helps convert tryptophan to niacin, helps make red blood cells	*Nervous/Muscular Systems*	
	Abnormal brain wave pattern, irritability, muscle twitching, convulsions	Depression, fatigue, impaired memory, irritability, headaches, numbness, damage to nerves, difficulty walking, loss of reflexes, weakness, restlessness
Deficiency Disease Name	*Skin*	
(No name)	Irritation of sweat glands, rashes, greasy dermatitis	
Significant Sources	*Other*	
Green and leafy vegetables, meats, fish, poultry, shellfish, legumes, fruits, whole grains	Kidney stones	

(*continued on next page*)

TABLE 7-6

The Water-Soluble Vitamins—Functions, Deficiencies, and Toxicities continued

FOLATE

Other Names	Deficiency Symptoms	Toxicity Symptoms
Folic acid, folacin, pteroylglutamic acid	**Blood/Circulatory System**	
	Anemia (large-cell type)[d]	
Chief Functions in the Body	**Digestive System**	
Part of a coenzyme needed for new cell synthesis	Heartburn, diarrhea, constipation	
Deficiency Disease	**Immune System**	
(No name)	Suppression, frequent infections	
Significant Sources	**Mouth, Gums, Tongue**	
Leafy green vegetables, legumes, seeds, liver	Smooth red tongue[c]	
	Nervous System	
	Depression, mental confusion, fainting	
	Other	
	Masks vitamin B_{12} deficiency	

VITAMIN B_{12}

Other Names	Deficiency Symptoms	Toxicity Symptoms
Cyanocobalamin	**Blood/Circulatory System**	
Chief Functions in the Body	Anemia (large-cell type)[d]	(No toxicity symptoms known)
Part of a coenzyme used in new cell synthesis, helps maintain nerve cells	**Mouth, Gums, Tongue**	
	Smooth tongue[c]	
Deficiency Disease	**Nervous System**	
(No name)[e]	Fatigue, degeneration progressing to paralysis	
Significant Sources	**Skin**	
Animal products (meat, fish, poultry, milk, cheese, eggs)	Hypersensitivity	

PANTOTHENIC ACID

Other Names	Deficiency Symptoms	Toxicity Symptoms
(None)	**Digestive System**	
Chief Functions in the Body	Vomiting, intestinal distress	
Part of a coenzyme used in energy metabolism	**Nervous System**	
	Insomnia, fatigue	
Deficiency Disease	**Other**	
(No name)		Water retention (infrequent)
Significant Sources		
Widespread in foods		

(continued on next page)

TABLE 7-6

The Water-Soluble Vitamins—Functions, Deficiencies, and Toxicities continued

BIOTIN

Other Names	Deficiency Symptoms	Toxicity Symptoms
(None)	**Blood/Circulatory System**	
Chief Functions in the Body	Abnormal heart action	(No toxicity symptoms reported)
Part of a coenzyme used in energy metabolism, fat synthesis, amino acid metabolism, and glycogen synthesis	**Digestive System**	
	Loss of appetite, nausea	
	Nervous/Muscular Systems	
	Depression, muscle pain, weakness, fatigue	
Deficiency Disease	**Skin**	
(No name)	Drying, rash, loss of hair	
Significant Sources		
Widespread in foods		

VITAMIN C

Other Names	Deficiency Symptoms	Toxicity Symptoms
Ascorbic acid	**Blood/Circulatory System**	
Chief Functions in the Body	Anemia (small-cell type),[d] atherosclerotic plaques, pinpoint hemorrhages	
Collagen synthesis (strengthens blood vessel walls, forms scar tissue, matrix for bone growth), antioxidant, thyroxine synthesis, amino acid metabolism, strengthens resistance to infection, helps in absorption of iron	**Digestive System**	
		Nausea, abdominal cramps, diarrhea, excessive urination
	Immune System	
	Suppression, frequent infections	
Deficiency Disease Name	**Mouth, Gums, Tongue**	
Scurvy	Bleeding gums, loosened teeth	
Significant Sources	**Nervous/Muscular Systems**	
Citrus fruits, cabbage-type vegetables, dark green vegetables, cantaloupe, strawberries, peppers, lettuce, tomatoes, potatoes, papayas, mangoes	Muscle degeneration and pain, hysteria, depression	Headache, fatigue, insomnia
	Skeletal System	
	Bone fragility, joint pain	
	Skin	
	Rough skin, blotchy bruises	Rashes
	Other	
	Failure of wounds to heal	Interference with medical tests; aggravation of gout symptoms; deficiency symptoms may appear at first on withdrawal of high doses

[a]Cracks at the corners of the mouth are termed *cheilosis* (kee-LOH-sis).

[b]Hypersensitivity to light is *photophobia*.

[c]Smoothness of the tongue is caused by loss of its surface structures and is termed *glossitis* (gloss-EYE-tis).

[d]Small-cell anemia is termed *microcytic anemia*; large-cell type is *macrocytic* or *megaloblastic anemia*.

[e]The name *pernicious anemia* refers to the vitamin B_{12} deficiency caused by lack of intrinsic factor, but not to that caused by inadequate dietary intake.

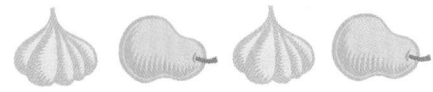

CHOOSING FOODS RICH IN VITAMINS

Most people, upon learning how important the vitamins are to their health, want to choose foods that are vitamin-rich. A way to identify such foods is to look at the vitamins and calories in single servings. This method is shown in Table 7-7.

The serving sizes in these figures are those recommended by the Food Guide Pyramid. For example, 3 ounces is used for most meats. The vegetable serving size is ½ cup. The colors of the bars represent the various food groups.

Some people, after viewing a figure such as this, believe that to meet their vitamin needs, they must memorize the richest sources of each vitamin and include those foods daily. This notion is false and can lead people to limit the variety of foods they choose while overemphasizing the components of a few foods. While it is reassuring to know that your carrot-raisin salad at lunch provided more than the entire Daily Value amount for vitamin A, it is a mistake to think that you must then select equally rich sources of all the other vitamins. Such rich sources do not exist for many vitamins. Rather, foods work in harmony to provide most nutrients. For example, a baked potato, though not a star performer among vitamin C providers, contributes substantially to a day's need for this nutrient and contributes some thiamin, too. By the end of the day, assuming that your food choices were made with reasonable care, the bits of thiamin, vitamin B6, and vitamin C from each serving of food have accumulated to make a more-than-adequate total diet.

With a few exceptions, nutritious foods generally provide small quantities of thiamin, as shown in Figure 7-9. A few meats are exceptionally good thiamin sources; these are members of the pork family. As you can see in the graph, one small pork chop (275 calories) provides over half of the Daily Value for thiamin, but again, this does not suggest that you eat pork every day. Legumes and grains are also good, low-fat sources, and they provide beneficial fiber and nutrients lacking from meats. On the other hand, beans lack the vitamin B_{12} provided by meats. Peanut butter is a good source of thiamin, as it is of most B vitamins, but its high fat and calorie contents call for moderation in its use.

The vitamin B_6 data provide another insight to support the argument for variety. From just the few foods listed here, you can see that no one source can provide the whole day's requirement, but that a variety of meats, fish, and poultry along with potatoes and a few other vegetables and fruits can work together to supply it.

Folate and vitamin C are represented in foods in the last two graphs of Figure 7-9. These nutrients are both richly supplied by fruits and vegetables. The richest source of either may be only a moderate source of the other, but the recommended servings of fruits and vegetables in food group plans cover both needs amply. As for vitamin E, vegetable oils are the richest sources. Some vegetables, nuts, and fruits contribute some vitamin E, too.

Are you ready to try out what you've learned about the food sources of vitamins? The Do It section that follows gives you a chance to test your skills.

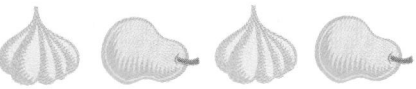

TABLE 7-7
Vitamin Contents of Restaurant Meals

	Energy (cal)	Vitamin A (RE)	Thiamin (mg)	Niacin (mg)	Vitamin C (mg)	Folate (µg)	Vitamin B₁₂ (µg)
Breakfast Foods							
Hotcakes with syrup and butter, scrambled egg and sausage patty	1,140	150	0.41	4	0	32	1.7
Egg, ham, and cheese muffin	290	100	0.49	3	0	30	0.7
Oatmeal, brown sugar	107	2	0.13	0	0	5	0
Corn flakes	110	375	0.87	5	15	100	0
Hashbrowned potatoes	130	0	0.08	1	3	8	0
2 small cinnamon sweet rolls	300	50	0.25	2	2	20	0.1
Large blueberry muffin	400	10	0.2	2	2	20	0.1
English muffin	130	0	0.25	2	0	20	0.1
Orange juice	80	40	0.17	1	90	60	0
Milk (low-fat)	120	140	0.1	0	2	10	0.8
Lunch Foods							
Homemade chili/crackers	350	150	0.26	5	25	40	0.5
Cold cut hoagie sandwich/chips	460	80	1.0	6	12	55	1.1
Peanut butter and jelly sandwich on whole wheat; fruit cocktail	450	30	0.3	7	3	62	0
Tuna sandwich on white; banana	470	40	0.32	6	11	49	0.6
Chef's salad with cheese, ham, turkey, and dressing/crackers	580	140	0.43	7	16	100	0.8
Nonfat milk	85	150	0.1	0	0	10	0.9
Apple juice	120	0	0.05	0	2	0	0
Supper Foods							
New England boiled dinner	440	150	0.27	5	80	70	1.4
Vegetable plate	400	680	0.26	2	53	120	0.1
Spaghetti and meatballs; small salad	600	220	0.38	6	25	50	1.3
Fried fish, tartar sauce, corn, and macaroni salad	510	70	0.26	3	6	83	1
Rolls	100	0	0.15	1	0	0	0
Garlic bread	190	4	0.4	3	0	0	0
Corn muffins	300	0	0.12	2	0	0	0
Lemon Pie	350	70	0.16	1	4	11	0.2
Chocolate cake	250	20	0.02	0	0	5	0.1

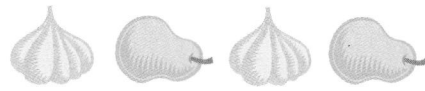

FIGURE 7-9

FOOD SOURCES OF VITAMINS SELECTED TO SHOW A RANGE OF VALUES

VITAMIN A

Food	Serving Size (Energy)	RE
Beef liver	3 oz fried (185 cal)	9,123
Sweet potato	1 whole boiled (158 cal)	2,574
Carrots	1/2 c boiled (35 cal)	1,914
Cantaloupe	1/2 melon (94 cal)	860
Spinach	1/2 c boiled (21 cal)	737
Butternut squash	1/2 c baked (41 cal)	718
Winter squash	1/2 c boiled (39 cal)	252
Milk, nonfat	1 c (85 cal)	149
Tomatoes	1/2 c boiled (33 cal)	89
Cheddar cheese	1 oz (114 cal)	86
Peach	1 fresh medium (37 cal)	47
Summer squash	1/2 c boiled (18 cal)	27
Apple	1 fresh medium (81 cal)	7
Sirloin steak	3 oz lean (165 cal)	0
Whole-wheat bread	1 slice (70 cal)	0
Baked potato	1 whole (220 cal)	0

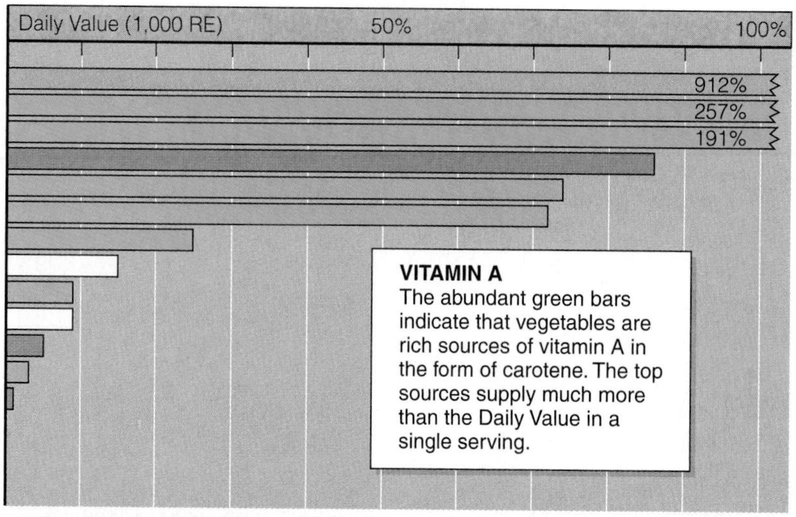

Daily Value (1,000 RE) — 50% — 100%
912%
257%
191%

VITAMIN A
The abundant green bars indicate that vegetables are rich sources of vitamin A in the form of carotene. The top sources supply much more than the Daily Value in a single serving.

VITAMIN E

Food	Serving Size (Energy)	mg
Sunflower seeds	1/4 c dry (186 cal)	10.0
Sweet potato	1 baked (117 cal)	7.0
Sunflower seed oil	1 tbs (120 cal)	6.5
Cottonseed oil	1 tbs (120 cal)	5.0
Safflower oil	1 tbs (120 cal)	4.5
Shrimp	3 oz boiled (84 cal)	3.0
Peanuts	1 oz dry roasted (166 cal)	3.0
Corn oil	1 tbs (120 cal)	2.5
Canola oil	1 tbs (120 cal)	2.5
Salmon	3 oz broiled/baked (184 cal)	2.0
Peanut butter	2 tbs (190 cal)	2.0
Apple	1 fresh medium (81 cal)	1.5
Parsley	1 tbs fresh chopped (1 cal)	1.0
Cheddar cheese	1 oz (114 cal)	0.5
Whole-wheat bread	1 slice (70 cal)	0.0

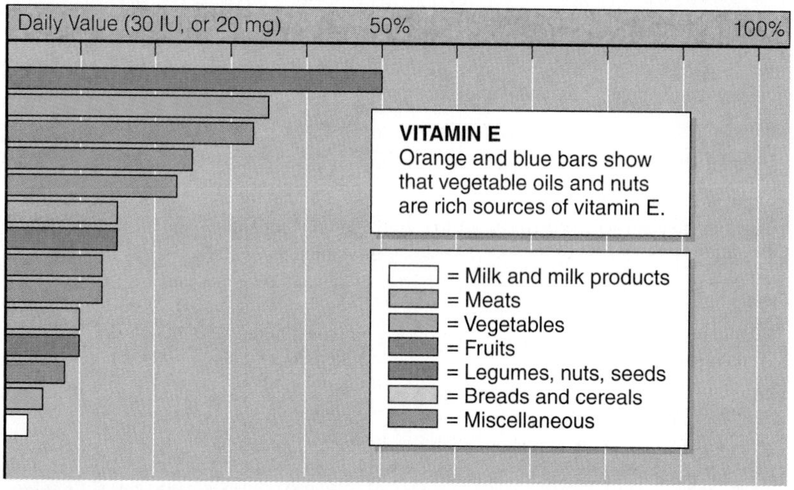

Daily Value (30 IU, or 20 mg) — 50% — 100%

VITAMIN E
Orange and blue bars show that vegetable oils and nuts are rich sources of vitamin E.

☐ = Milk and milk products
▨ = Meats
▨ = Vegetables
▨ = Fruits
▨ = Legumes, nuts, seeds
▨ = Breads and cereals
▨ = Miscellaneous

THIAMIN

Food	Serving Size (Energy)	mg
Pork chop	3 oz broiled (275 cal)	0.87
Black beans	1 c cooked (228 cal)	0.42
Watermelon	1 slice (154 cal)	0.39
Baked potato	1 whole (220 cal)	0.22
Green peas	1/2 c cooked (67 cal)	0.21
Orange juice	3/4 c fresh (84 cal)	0.17
Sirloin steak	3 oz lean (165 cal)	0.15
Oatmeal	1/2 c cooked (73 cal)	0.13
Whole-wheat bread	1 slice (70 cal)	0.10
Milk, nonfat	1 c (85 cal)	0.09
Oysters	3 oz (69 cal)	0.06
Summer squash	1/2 c cooked (18 cal)	0.04
Cabbage	1/2 c cooked (16 cal)	0.04
Sunflower seeds	1/4 c dry (186 cal)	0.03
Apple	1 fresh medium (81 cal)	0.02
Cheddar cheese	1 oz (114 cal)	0.01

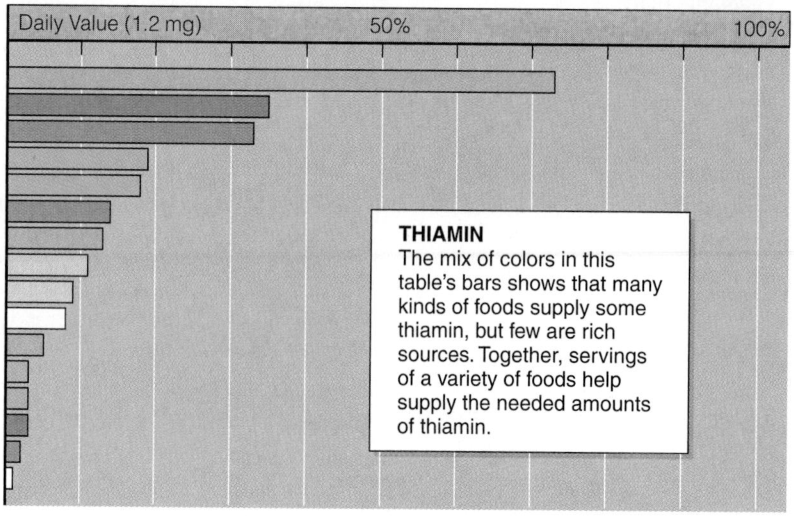

Daily Value (1.2 mg) — 50% — 100%

THIAMIN
The mix of colors in this table's bars shows that many kinds of foods supply some thiamin, but few are rich sources. Together, servings of a variety of foods help supply the needed amounts of thiamin.

(continued on next page)

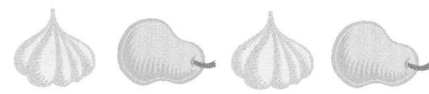

FIGURE 7-9

FOOD SOURCES OF VITAMINS SELECTED TO SHOW A RANGE OF VALUES (CONTINUED)

Food	Serving Size (Energy)	mg
VITAMIN B₆		
Baked potato	1 whole (220 cal)	0.70
Watermelon	1 slice (154 cal)	0.69
Banana	1 peeled (104 cal)	0.66
Turkey	3 oz (133 cal)	0.61
Sirloin steak	3 oz lean (165 cal)	0.51
Pork chop	3 oz broiled (275 cal)	0.35
Spinach	½ c cooked (21 cal)	0.22
Salmon	3 oz broiled/baked (184 cal)	0.19
Navy beans	½ c cooked (129 cal)	0.15
Broccoli	½ c cooked (22 cal)	0.11
Milk, nonfat	1 c (85 cal)	0.10
Apple	1 fresh medium (81 cal)	0.07
Orange juice	¾ c fresh (84 cal)	0.07
Summer squash	½ c boiled (18 cal)	0.06
Whole-wheat bread	1 slice (70 cal)	0.05
Cheddar cheese	1 oz (114 cal)	0.02

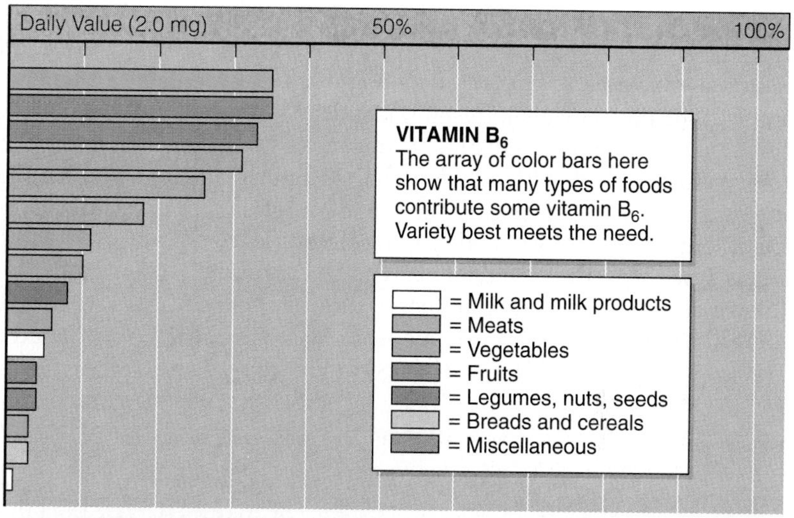

Daily Value (2.0 mg)   50%   100%

VITAMIN B₆
The array of color bars here show that many types of foods contribute some vitamin B₆. Variety best meets the need.

☐ = Milk and milk products
▨ = Meats
▨ = Vegetables
▨ = Fruits
▨ = Legumes, nuts, seeds
▨ = Breads and cereals
▨ = Miscellaneous

Food	Serving Size (Energy)	µg
FOLATE		
Beef liver	3 oz fried (185 cal)	187
Spinach	½ c cooked (21 cal)	131
Turnip greens	½ c cooked (15 cal)	85
Orange juice	¾ c fresh (84 cal)	57
Broccoli	½ c cooked (22 cal)	52
Cantaloupe	½ melon (94 cal)	46
Beets	½ c cooked (27 cal)	46
Asparagus	2 spears cooked (8 cal)	30
Lima beans	½ c cooked (105 cal)	23
Summer squash	½ c cooked (18 cal)	19
Whole-wheat bread	1 slice (70 cal)	14
Milk, nonfat	1 c (85 cal)	13
Winter squash	½ c cooked (39 cal)	13
Sirloin steak	3 oz lean (165 cal)	11
Cheddar cheese	1 oz (114 cal)	5
Apple	1 fresh medium (81 cal)	4

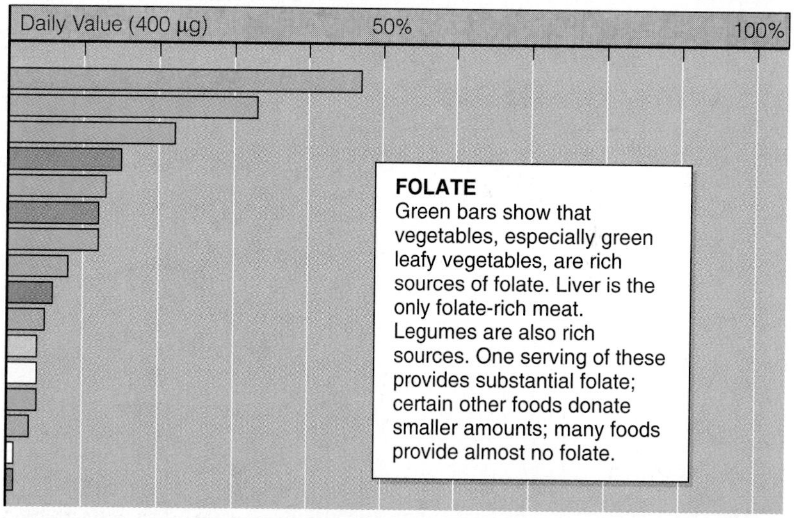

Daily Value (400 µg)   50%   100%

FOLATE
Green bars show that vegetables, especially green leafy vegetables, are rich sources of folate. Liver is the only folate-rich meat. Legumes are also rich sources. One serving of these provides substantial folate; certain other foods donate smaller amounts; many foods provide almost no folate.

Food	Serving Size (Energy)	mg
VITAMIN C		
Cantaloupe	½ melon (94 cal)	112
Orange juice	¾ c fresh (84 cal)	93
Broccoli	½ c cooked (22 cal)	58
Brussels sprouts	½ c cooked (31 cal)	49
Green peppers	½ c (14 cal)	45
Tomato juice	¾ c canned (32 cal)	34
Baked potato	1 whole (220 cal)	26
Cabbage	½ c cooked (16 cal)	19
Apple	1 fresh medium (81 cal)	8
Oysters	3 oz (69 cal)	7
Milk, nonfat	1 cup (85 cal)	2
Whole-wheat bread	1 slice (70 cal)	0
Sirloin steak	3 oz lean (165 cal)	0
Cheddar cheese	1 oz (114 cal)	0

Daily Value (60 mg)   50%   100%

187%
155%

VITAMIN C
Fruits (purple) and vegetables (green) head the list. One serving of any of the top suppliers exceeds the Daily Value; meeting vitamin C needs without fruits and vegetables is almost impossible.

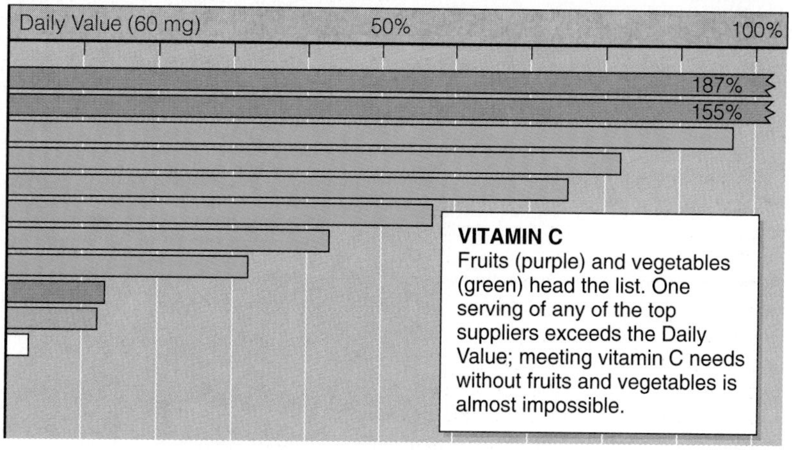

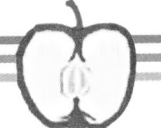

Do It!

FIND THE VITAMINS ON A MENU

Can you meet your vitamin needs when you eat in restaurants? One way is to learn to identify the foods on restaurant menus that are rich sources of vitamins. Assume you spent a day on the road and have to eat all three of the day's meals in restaurants. Read over the three menus in Figure 7-10 and create a meal from each one, using the foods offered. Note that, just like real menus, these menus lack serving size information. For this exercise, take for granted that the serving sizes of foods agree with those in the Food Guide Pyramid. (Never assume this about real menus, however—commercial serving sizes vary enormously.) Most vegetable and grain servings in the meals listed in Figure 7-10 are

one-half cup servings. Those identified as "large" are one-cup servings; meats are two- to three-ounce portions; milk is an eight-ounce serving, and so forth.

Step 1. On a copy of Form 7-1, record your food choices down the left-hand column.

Step 2. Consult Table 7-7 on page 267, earlier, to determine the values for calories and nutrients in the day's meals. Fill in the values for the foods you listed on Form 7-1. Coffee, tea, and water contribute negligible energy and vitamins; use zeros for their values on Form 7-1.

Step 3. Enter your RDA (inside front cover) or RNI (Canadian section, Appendix B) in the spaces provided on Form 7-1.

FIGURE 7-10

RESTAURANT MENUS

Welcome to
BURGER DOODLE
★   ★   ★

★ **BREAKFAST**
Hotcakes, eggs, and sausage ....

Egg, ham, and cheese muffin ....

Oatmeal with brown sugar ....

Cornflakes ....

★ **SIDES**
Hash browned potatoes ....

A pair of cinnamon sweetrolls ....

Large blueberry muffin ....

Plain English muffin ....

★ **BEVERAGES**
Orange juice ....

Low-fat milk ....

Coffee or tea ....

The Box Lunch
EXPRESS

Soups
Homemade chili with crackers ....

Sandwiches
Cold cut hoagie sandwich with chips ....

Peanut butter and jelly sandwich on whole wheat bread, served with fruit cocktail ....

Tuna sandwich on white bread, served with a fresh banana ....

Salads
Large chef's salad with cheese, ham, and turkey with crackers ....

Beverages
Nonfat milk ....

Apple juice...................................

Sparkling water........................

Elf's Cafeteria
Blue Plate Specials

Specials
New England boiled dinner: corned beef, large serving of potatoes, and brussels sprouts with margarine

Southern Style vegetable plate: steamed yellow squash, collard greens, fried okra, candied yams, and fried green tomatoes

Large spaghetti & meatballs with small salad

Fried fish, tartar sauce, macaroni, salad, and corn on the cob with margarine

Choice of 2 rolls, 1 slice garlic bread, or 2 corn muffins

Beverages
Tea or coffee

Desserts
Lemon pie or chocolate cake

FORM 7-1

Vitamin Tally

	Energy (cal)	Vitamin A (RE)	Thiamin (mg)	Niacin (mg)	Vitamin C (mg)	Folate (µg)	Vitamin B$_{12}$ (µg)
Breakfast							
Lunch							
Supper							
Day's totals							
Energy and vitamin goals							
% of recommendations							

Step 4. Divide the day's total intakes by the RDA/RNI amount and multiply by 100 to determine the percentages of your nutrient and energy needs contributed by the foods chosen this day.

Example, if total vitamin C intake equals 40 milligrams and your vitamin C RDA equals 60 milligrams, then $(40 \div 60) \times 100 = 67\%$. The meals met two thirds of the daily recommended amount of vitamin C.

Repeat this process for all 5 vitamins and for energy.

(continued on next page)

ANALYSIS

Answer the following questions:

1. How did the day's totals for calories and vitamins compare with your recommended amounts? Did the day's meals meet or exceed your need for energy or any of these vitamins? Which ones?

2. Did the meals present too little of energy or any of the nutrients listed here? Which ones? What changes in your choices among those foods would have improved the vitamin totals for the day?

3. Which foods listed on the menus contributed significant amounts of vitamin A? Remembering that brightly colored fruits and vegetables offer the vitamin A precursor beta-carotene, name any foods in your meal choices that provide beta-carotene (turn back to Snapshot 7-1 on page 232 for hints). Which foods contributed little or no vitamin A in any form?

4. Did your choices supply enough folate to meet your requirement? Remembering that young women are urged to obtain 400 micrograms of folate each day, what percentage of your folate need did the day's meals provide? Which individual foods were richest in folate? Turn to the Table of Food Composition, Appendix A, and look down the folate column of the fruits and vegetables sections. Identify some foods that, in a single serving, provide 10 percent or more of the 400 micrograms of folate recommended for women?

5. What are the sources of niacin in the day's meals? Rich sources are shown in Snapshot 7-7.

6. What about vitamin C? What percentage of vitamin C of your day's need did these meals provide? Which individual foods were the main contributors? To what food groups do they belong?

7. How did your total energy intake compare with your energy need? Express your answer as a percentage, and use it to answer the next two questions.

8. Which meals are vitamin "bargains"? Compare the vitamin contents (as percent of your need) with the energy contents of the chosen meals (also as percent of your need). Which are the most vitamin-dense, providing the most vitamins for the fewest calories?

9. Among breakfast choices, which one is highest in vitamin A? Which is highest in folate and niacin? What characteristics of this food makes its vitamin content so high?

10. Which foods on the menus, while low in vitamins, possess other valuable constituents that make them desirable as part of a health-promoting diet?

Should you wonder about the vitamins in other foods you choose, you can find their vitamin and other nutrient contents in several references in this book. First, the vitamin Snapshots appearing throughout this chapter depict the richest vitamin sources; second, the Daily Food Guide, on pages 44 and 45, notes which vitamins characterize foods of each group; and third, the Table of Food Composition, Appendix A, provides actual values for vitamins in about 2,000 foods. With these references, you can judge the vitamin values of foods on virtually any menu.

✔   **SELF-CHECK**

Answers to these Self-Check questions are in Appendix G.

1. Which of the following vitamins are fat-soluble?
   a. vitamins B, C, D, and E
   b. vitamins B, C, and E
   c. vitamins A, C, E, and K
   d. vitamins A, D, E, and K

2. A deficiency of vitamin D may result in which disease?
   a. rickets
   b. beriberi
   c. scurvy
   d. pellagra

3. Night blindness and xerophthalmia are the result of a deficiency of which vitamin?
   a. niacin
   b. vitamin C
   c. vitamin A
   d. vitamin K

4. Which of the following foods is (are) rich in beta-carotene?
   a. sweet potatoes
   b. pumpkin
   c. cantaloupe
   d. all of the above

5. Which vitamin(s) is (are) present only in foods of animal origin?
   a. the active form of vitamin A
   b. vitamin B_{12}
   c. riboflavin
   d. (a) and (b)

6. Which of the following describes the water-soluble vitamins?
   a. vitamins D and E
   b. frequently toxic
   c. stored extensively in tissues
   d. easily absorbed and excreted

7. Almost any substance, including herbs, amino acids, dried animal organ tissues, microorganisms, and hormones can be sold freely over the counter in the United States.   T   F

8. In general, nutrients are absorbed equally well from foods and supplements.   T   F

9. People today are more likely to suffer from overnutrition than from nutrition deficiencies.   T   F

10. The best way to consume a diet rich in vitamins is to eat a variety of foods every day.   T   F

11. The body's defenses against free-radical damage include vitamin E, vitamin C, beta-carotene, and phytochemicals. (Read about these in the upcoming Controversy.)   T   F

〜 **NOTES**

Notes are in Appendix F.

Antioxidant Vitamins: Magic Bullets?

What have you heard about the antioxidant vitamins? Some intriguing revelations have come to light concerning the activities of these metabolic busybodies. Knowledgeable people claim that *foods* rich in these vitamins help to prevent disease. Others claim that vitamin *supplements* are more reliable allies. Consumers can tell who is right by weighing the evidence on either side. This Controversy offers a way to score foods versus supplements as sources of these beneficial compounds. To anticipate the punch line, the antioxidant vitamins are only a few among thousands of health-promoting constituents of foods, about which Chapter 11 has much more to say. Still, these vitamins are of great interest in themselves.

Most of the results presented here are preliminary. More research is needed to confirm or deny their possible implications. Supplement makers rightly claim that

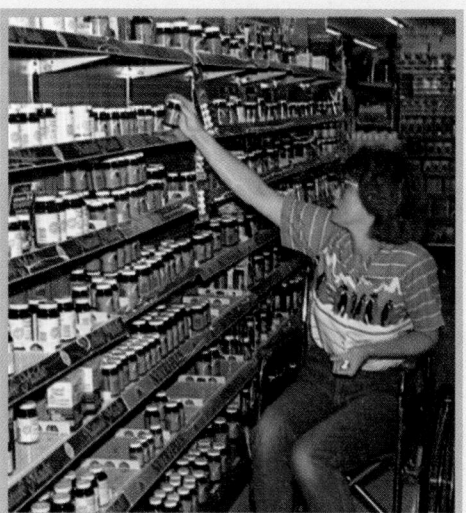

"scientific evidence backs up the claims we make for our products," but nearly all of the evidence is from epidemiological studies, that is, studies of large populations. These studies suggest interesting general trends, but have no specific implications for individuals. So proceed with caution and demand rigorous, repeated testing before you consider a finding confirmed—but do proceed. The evidence that lies before you holds secrets that will soon evolve into tomorrow's established nutrition concepts.

FREE RADICALS AND DISEASE

The body's cells user oxygen to produce energy. In the process, oxygen sometimes reacts with body compounds to produce highly unstable molecules known as **free radicals** (see Table C7-1 for the definition of this and related terms). In addition to normal body processes, environmental factors such as radiation, pollution, tobacco smoke, and others can cause free radical formation (see Table C7-2).[1]

A free radical is a molecule with one or more unpaired **electrons.*** An electron without a partner is unstable and highly reactive. To regain its stability, the free radical quickly finds a stable but vulnerable compound from which to steal an electron. With the loss of an electron, the formerly stable molecule becomes a free radical itself, and steals an electron from some other nearby molecule. Thus, an electron-snatching chain reaction is under way.

Often, free radicals are like sparks, starting wildfires that lead to widespread damage by **oxidative stress.** Free-radical damage commonly disrupts unsaturated fatty acids in cell membranes, damaging the membranes' ability to transport substances into and out of cells.[2] Free radicals also produce damage to cell pro-

TABLE C7-1
Antioxidant Terms

- **electron** part of an atom; a negatively charged particle. Stable atoms (and molecules, which are made of atoms) have even numbers of electrons in pairs. An atom or molecule with an unpaired electron is a *free radical*.
- **free radical** an atom or molecule with one or more unpaired electrons that make it unstable and highly reactive.
- **oxidative stress** damage inflicted on living systems by free radicals.
- **oxidant** a compound (such as oxygen itself) that oxidizes other compounds. Compounds that prevent oxidation are called *anti*oxidants, whereas those that promote it are called *pro*oxidants.

anti = against

pro = for

NOTE: The *antioxidant vitamins* are vitamin E, vitamin C, and beta-carotene, the plant precursor of vitamin A. Some internal enzyme systems also counteract oxidation, notably the *superoxide dismutase (SOD)* system. Certain mineral nutrients, notably iron, copper, and selenium, are also important in preventing oxidation, and often assist enzymes in this work. Chapter 8 offers more on these minerals.

---

*Oxygen-derived free radicals are common in the human body. Examples are superoxide radical ($O_2 \bullet^-$), hydroxyl radical ($OH\bullet$), and nitric oxide ($NO\bullet$). The dots in the symbols represent the unpaired electrons. Scientists sometimes use the term *reactive oxygen species* to describe all of these compounds.

TABLE C7-2

Factors That Increase Free-Radical Formation

Body Factors	Environmental Factors
Aerobic metabolism	Air pollution
Diabetes	Asbestos
Exercise	High levels of vitamin C
Illness	High levels of oxygen
Immune responses	Radioactive emissions (for
Injury	example, from radon gas)
Obesity	Some herbicides
Other diseases	Tobacco smoke
Other metabolic reactions	Trace minerals (iron,
	copper)
	Ultraviolet light rays

SOURCE: Data from B. N. Ames and coauthors, Oxidants, antioxidants, and the degenerative disease of aging, *Proceedings of the National Academy of Sciences* 90 (1993): 7915–7920.

teins, altering their functions; and to DNA, disrupting all cells that inherit the damaged DNA.

Scientists have proposed connections between oxidative stress and the development of over 200 diseases, among them diabetes, cancer, cataracts, age-related blindness, and cardiovascular disease.[3] In diabetes, oxidative stress both makes cell membranes less responsive to insulin and damages arteries, producing severe vascular disease.[4] Even the physical effects of aging are thought by some to be related to years of free-radical damage.

Free radicals are not all bad. In fact, their destructive properties are put to good use by some cells of the immune system. These cells make free radicals, when they are needed as ammunition, in an "oxidative burst" that lays waste to disease-causing viruses and bacteria. Partly for this reason, infections caused a detectable increase in free-radical activity all over the body.

THE BODY'S DEFENSES AGAINST FREE RADICALS

The body's natural defense and repair systems try to handle all free radicals, but these systems are not 100 percent effective. If insufficient disease-fighting agents are present in the body, or if disease initiators such as free radicals become excessive, health problems may develop.[5] Unrepaired damage accumulates with age. The body's two main systems of defense are its reserves of antioxidants; and its enzyme systems that oppose oxidation.

Antioxidation Vitamins   The body maintains pools of the antioxidant vitamins: vitamin E; vitamin C; and the Vitamin A precursor beta-carotene. These vitamins actively scavenge and quench free radicals, becoming oxidized (and inactive) themselves. Once oxidized, they can to some extent be regenerated to become active antioxidants again, but some are dismantled and discarded. Free radicals attack the body continuously, so to maintain defenses, a person's supplies of antioxidants must be replenished as rapidly as they are used up.

Among the antioxidant vitamins, vitamin E and beta-carotene defend the body's lipids. Vitamin E efficiently breaks the free radical chain reaction at a rate 200 times faster than BHT,* a commercial antioxidant added to baked goods to prevent rancidity from fat oxidation. Vitamin C protects the body's watery components, such as the fluid of the blood, against free radical attacks. Vitamin C seems especially adept at neutralizing free radicals from polluted air and cigarette smoke; it also has the knack of restoring oxidized vitamin E to its active state. An example of how these defenders prevent tissue damage from free radicals appear in Figure C7-1.

If extra antioxidants are present in the tissues, then free radicals are less likely to damage the cells (see Figure C7-2). This line of thinking is used to sell millions of dollars worth of antioxidant supplements to consumers each year, although in fact, protection may be conferred, not by these particular nutrients, but by as yet unidentified *other* factors in foods that contain them.

Phytochemicals   Some phytochemicals have antioxidant activity, although they work in many other ways, too. Scientists are buzzing about these fascinating compounds, and research is pursuing new lines of study which, 20 years ago, would have been dismissed as science fiction. One phytochemical filters incoming light, some act as hormones, some inhibit harmful chemical reactions, one slows blood clotting, some stimulate immunity, and many act by mechanisms as yet unknown. One enthusiastic researcher predicts that the phytochemicals will be "the vitamins of the next century."[6] The evidence on phytochemicals concludes the core chapters of this book, in Chapter 11, but even those who never read it can arrive at a conclusion based on what will be presented here. Foods or

---

*BHT is butylated hydroxytoluene.

FIGURE C7-1

THE THEORY OF ANTIOXIDANTS AND DISEASE

Free-radical formation occurs during metabolic processes, and it accelerates when diseases or other stresses strike.

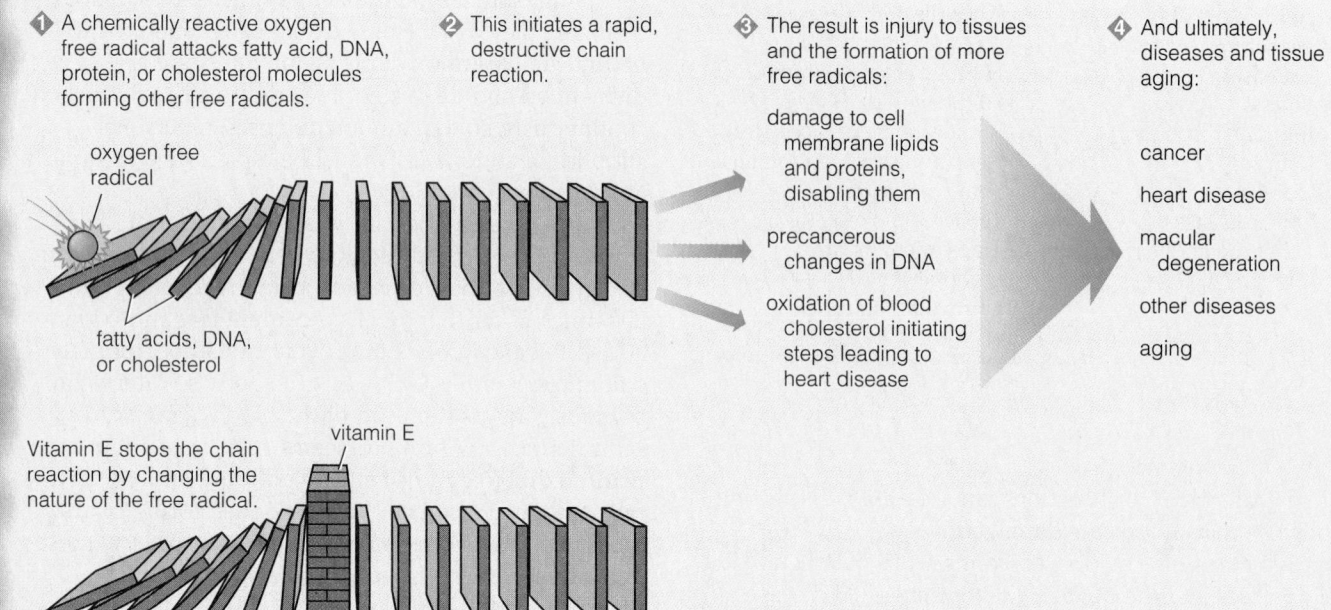

❶ A chemically reactive oxygen free radical attacks fatty acid, DNA, protein, or cholesterol molecules forming other free radicals.

oxygen free radical

fatty acids, DNA, or cholesterol

❷ This initiates a rapid, destructive chain reaction.

❸ The result is injury to tissues and the formation of more free radicals:

damage to cell membrane lipids and proteins, disabling them

precancerous changes in DNA

oxidation of blood cholesterol initiating steps leading to heart disease

❹ And ultimately, diseases and tissue aging:

cancer

heart disease

macular degeneration

other diseases

aging

Vitamin E stops the chain reaction by changing the nature of the free radical.

vitamin E

---

supplements: which is the better choice? Phytochemicals score a major point in favor of foods. Foods: 1. Supplements: 0.

The Internal Defense System   In addition to using antioxidant compounds from foods, the body defends itself against the free-radical threat by using a powerful system of cellular enzymes that neutralize the free radicals they encounter. These enzymes are proteins whose concentrations are controlled by inherited genes. One is *superoxide dismutase (SOD)*, which has been intensively studied and even purified for use as an anti-aging supplement. Because SOD is a protein, however, it is useless as a dietary supplement. Enzymes taken by mouth are digested in the stomach and small intestine long before they reach the bloodstream. In our tally of scores of foods versus supplements, then, supplements still score 0 points.

DO ANTIOXIDANTS PROTECT AGAINST CANCER?

Cancers arise when cellular DNA is damaged—sometimes by free-radical attacks.[7] If antioxidant nutrients protect DNA from this damage, then they probably reduce cancer risks. The strongest evidence that they do is found in studies of populations with high intakes of vegetables and fruits rich in antioxidant nutrients. They consistently are found to have low rates of cancer. Laboratory studies with animals and with cell cultures seem to support such findings.[8]

Beta-Carotene and Its Relatives   People with high cancer rates have been found to consumer the fewest vegetables and fruits, especially those containing beta-carotene and its relatives.[9] This evidence was strengthened by findings of researchers who collected human blood samples and found that low concentrations of beta-carotene consistently correlated with the development of both lung and breast cancers.[10] For a while, people were convinced that this evidence provided conclusive proof of beta-carotene's protective effect. In fact, many people bought and took beta-carotene supplements long before they were proved safe and effective.

Recently, however, support for beta-carotene supplements has crumbled. One study declared them useless in preventing a condition that leads to colon cancer.[11] A surprise result came from another study designed to determine the benefits of beta-carotene supplements on the incidence of lung cancer among smokers.[12] The researchers expected to see a beneficial effect, but instead found that smokers given beta-carotene supplements suffered a *greater* incidence of lung cancer than did smokers given placebos.[13] A major clinical trial of beta-carotene supplements had to be stopped when 28 percent more of the participants taking beta-carotene developed lung cancer than did the members of the control group who took placebos. The researchers are continuing to observe the experimental group to detect any possible long-term adverse effects of taking beta-carotene. Another long-term study reported no differences in disease rates between physicians who took beta-carotene for 14 years and a matched group who took placebos.[14] What, exactly, these results mean to the individual supplement taker is unknown, but overall, the studies seem to indicate no benefit, and a possible risk, from taking supplements of beta-carotene.

A contradiction exists in beta-carotene research. Beta-carotene in foods and elevated beta-carotene in the blood are associated with lower cancer incidence, but the taking of beta-carotene supplements is not. Researchers quickly discovered why, however. Beta-carotene itself was just one of many antioxidant nutri-ents present in the foods chosen for study. Many other essential nutrients were present with them, not only the vitamins named here, and not only antioxidants, but nutrients that fight cancer in other ways. These include vitamin A itself, vitamin B_6, pantothenic acid, vitamin B_{12}, zinc, iron, copper, selenium, and more.

Besides all of these nutrients, dozens or hundreds of phytochemicals are present in foods, too. Health effects attributed to beta-carotene may, in reality, be the work of one or a number of *nonnutrient* compounds in fruits and vegetables.[15] Beta-carotene may simply tag along, serving as a marker for one of its relatives or for one or more as-yet-unknown phytochemicals that are actually responsible for the effect. Foods now have 2 points in their favor; supplements still score 0.)

Vitamins C and E   When people's diets include foods rich in vitamin C, they seem to develop fewer cancers of the mouth, larynx, and esophagus.[16] A dozen or so studies have confirmed this relationship. However, like beta-carotene, vitamin C occurs in foods together with other cancer-fighting constituents. For example, broccoli, leafy greens, and citrus fruits, which are all vitamin C-rich foods, also contain powerful phytochemicals thought to be active against cancer. They are also fiber-rich and low in fat—two other diet

---

FIGURE C7-2

THE ANTIOXIDANT THEORY OF DISEASE PREVENTION

A. Normally, the body's antioxidant enzymes, vitamins, and other molecules are sufficient to neutralize free-radical molecules before they do much damage.

B. An increased free-radical load can overwhelm the body's antioxidant systems. Free radicals then damage the tissues.

C. The body stocked with extra antioxidants is best equipped to handle an increase in free radicals. The two ways to obtain more antioxidants are to build them into cells by exercising, which stimulates production of more antioxidant enzymes, and to eat them in foods or supplements, which supply antioxidant vitamins and phytochemicals.

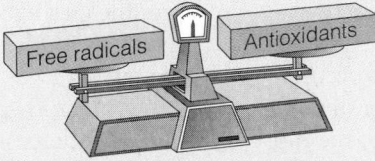

(a) Balanced system

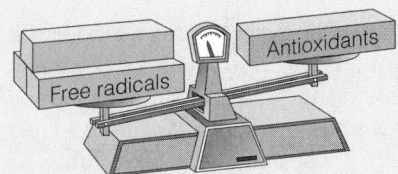

(b) Additional free-radical load—damage

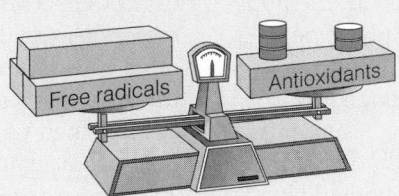

(c) Additional antioxidants added and balance restored

factors believed to reduce cancer risk. Like beta-carotene, then, Vitamin C may simply be a marker for a diet rich in fruits and vegetables. If so, the taking of vitamin C pills alone will do nothing to prevent cancer. Foods: 3. Supplements: still 0.

Last on the list of vitamins against cancer is vitamin E. A study reported a reduced risk of melanoma, a deadly skin cancer, in people with high intakes of *foods* rich in vitamin E.[17] Two studies have found vitamin E *supplements* useless against both colon and lung cancers.[18] Foods: 4. Supplements: still 0.

The FDA agrees that foods, not supplements, provide anticancer benefits. After reviewing the evidence, the agency concluded that *diets* high in fruits and vegetables, which are particularly good sources of beta-carotene and vitamin C, are strongly associated with reduced risks of several types of cancer. The reductions in risk could not be attributed solely to the named vitamins. Accordingly, the FDA rejected a request by the supplement industry to allow health claims on the labels of antioxidant supplements; and ruled that food labels may make health claims only in terms of fruits and vegetables and cancer. From the evidence so far, then, give supplements another zero, but score another point for foods. Foods: 5. Supplements: 0.

EVIDENCE CONCERNING AGE-RELATED BLINDNESS

The leading cause of age-related blindness in the United States is macular degeneration, already mentioned in Chapter 7. This form of blindness occurs when the macula, located at the focal center of the retina, loses integrity. This causes the loss of the most important field of vision, the area in focus (peripheral vision remains unimpaired). This blindness has, until now, been untreatable and unpreventable, but the hope of prevention has been suggested by a study of people's diets. Researchers have reported a 43-percent reduced incidence of macular degeneration in those consuming diets high in carotenoids.[19] Beta-carotene is not, however, the carotenoid credited with reducing risk. Other, nonnutritive carotenoids are more likely at work in this regard. These carotenoids, supplied by fruits and vegetables, have the ability to filter out damaging light rays before they can harm the macula. Foods now have 6 points. Supplements: still 0.

DO ANTIOXIDANTS NUTRIENTS PROTECT AGAINST HEART DISEASE?

Antioxidant nutrients, especially vitamin E, may help protect against cardiovascular disease.[20] A theory about how vitamin E might accomplish this concerns oxidation of blood cholesterol. Cholesterol carried in low-density lipoproteins (LDL) in the blood correlates directly with cardiovascular disease. Further, most of the cholesterol scientists have collected from damaged arteries has turned out to be oxidized cholesterol. The theory suggest that LDL undergo oxidation by free radicals inside the artery wall and promote the formation of artery-clogging plaques.[21]

Vitamin E and Heart Disease   Vitamin E may offer some protection against heart disease by protecting LDL from oxidation. Some research supports this possibility.[22] Scientists selected groups of men in 16 European regions where rates of death from heart disease varied sixfold. The researchers compared the plasma vitamin E, cholesterol, and blood pressure among the men from each region. The men with the lowest vitamin E values died more often from heart disease. The correlation of heart disease mortality with low vitamin E was even stronger than that with high cholesterol or high blood pressure, supporting the "antioxidant hypothesis" of heart disease. The authors cautioned, though, that although this evidence was suggestive, it was also indirect. The question remained whether the vitamin E in the blood was "the" agent to get the credit, or whether it came as part of a package (such as foods) that also contained an unknown active agent.

Evidence bearing on this question comes from two large epidemiological studies that used large-dose vitamin E supplements. The supplements appeared to be associated with a significantly reduced risk of heart disease.[23] This correlation remained strong after the researchers analyzed for heart disease risks and for other dietary antioxidants. In another study, researchers tracked changes in the arteries of men with heart disease. In men who were taking cholesterol-lowering drugs as well at least 100 milligrams of vitamin E a day and whose arteries were only mildly damaged, the disease progressed more slowly than in others. Men with advanced disease and those not talking cholesterol-lowering drugs gained no benefit from vitamin E.[24] A recent study on women suggests that a diet of foods rich in vitamin E is associated with fewer heart disease deaths.[25]

An elegant experimental study recently added another piece of evidence to the vitamin E-heart disease puzzle. Researchers at Cambridge University, England, who are conducting a long-term clinical experiment, have released data supporting the idea that vitamin E may prevent heart attacks in people with diagnosed advanced heart disease.[26] Ten months into the study, the researchers could already see that, given doses of 400 and 800 milligrams of vitamin E per day for 2 years, these people suffered fewer *heart attacks* than others like them who were not given vitamin E. Total *deaths* from heart disease were, however, unaffected by vitamin E.

Another theory exists concerning vitamin E's heart-defending effect. As mentioned earlier, active vitamin E (alpha tocopherol) is oxidized to other compounds. One such compound, vitamin E quinone, has physiological effects of its own, unrelated to the effects of an alph-tocophrol.[27] Vitamin E quinone is a powerful inhibitor of vitamin K activity, and therefore exerts an anticlotting effect on the blood. This anticlotting effect of vitamin E quinone might help ward off the blood clots that cause heart attacks. Vitamin E supplements have been found to be mixtures of both the active vitamin and the quinone, so there is no way of knowing whether benefits seen are due to vitamin E's antioxidant protection of LDL, or to the quinone's anticlotting activity.

By whatever mechanism, high doses of vitamin E, a nutrient, produce health effects like those of a drug. Because both supplements and foods have been observed to coincide with reduced heart disease, the rationale for taking supplements of vitamin E gains credibility. At last, we can give a point to supplements, specifically those of vitamin E, but vitamin E-rich foods must receive another point, too. Foods: 7. Supplements: 1.

Vitamin C and Heart Disease

Vitamin C may or may not affect susceptibility to heart disease; research results are mixed.[28] Logic suggests teamwork between vitamin C and vitamin E in defending LDL against oxidation: vitamin C defends against free radicals in the watery compartments of cells, vitamin E in lipid environments. Also, as mentioned, vitamin C regenerates vitamin E from its oxidized form, making it available to act again as an antioxidant.[29] Some studies also suggest that vitamin C may raise HDL, lower total

cholesterol, and improve blood pressure.[30] These findings might serve a point for vitamin C supplements, but it's easy to get vitamin C from foods. A few servings a day of vitamin C-rich foods can make high-dose vitamin C supplements, along with their associated risks, unnecessary.[31] Perhaps both could receive a point. Foods: now 8. Supplements: 2.

PERSONAL STRATEGY ON VITAMIN SUPPLEMENTS

To this point, foods have beaten vitamin supplements by a score of 8 to 2. Much more evidence in favor of foods over supplements arises from study of the phytochemicals, still to be discussed in Chapter 11. Still, a wrap-up can be based on what has been presented here.

Should We Take Supplements, Just to Be Safe?

Supplement manufacturers have proclaimed single antioxidant *pills* as the new magic bullets against aging, disease, and even death itself. Dr. Victor Herbert, renowned speaker in the science of nutrition, energetically opposes these claims. He points to a host of side effects that might endanger supplement takers' health. Among these effects are the following:

- Vitamin E supplements, taken over a period of time, may increase the risk of brain hemorrhage (a form of stroke).
- Vitamin E supplements delay blood clotting.
- Vitamin E supplements may worsen auto-immune diseases, such as asthma or rheumatoid arthritis.
- Vitamin C and other vitamin supplements act as *pro*oxidants (cause free radical formation) at high levels, especially when trace minerals such as iron are present.[32]
- Vitamin C supplements enhance iron absorption, making iron overload likely in some people.
- Daily supplements of vitamin E, beta-carotene, or both do not reduce the incidence of lung cancer among smokers, and beta-carotene may increase it.[33]
- Early reports warn that women who take beta-carotene supplements are more likely to develop a precancerous condition of the cervix* than women who abstain from supplement use.[34]

---

*The precancerous condition of the cervix mentioned here is *cervical dysplasia*.

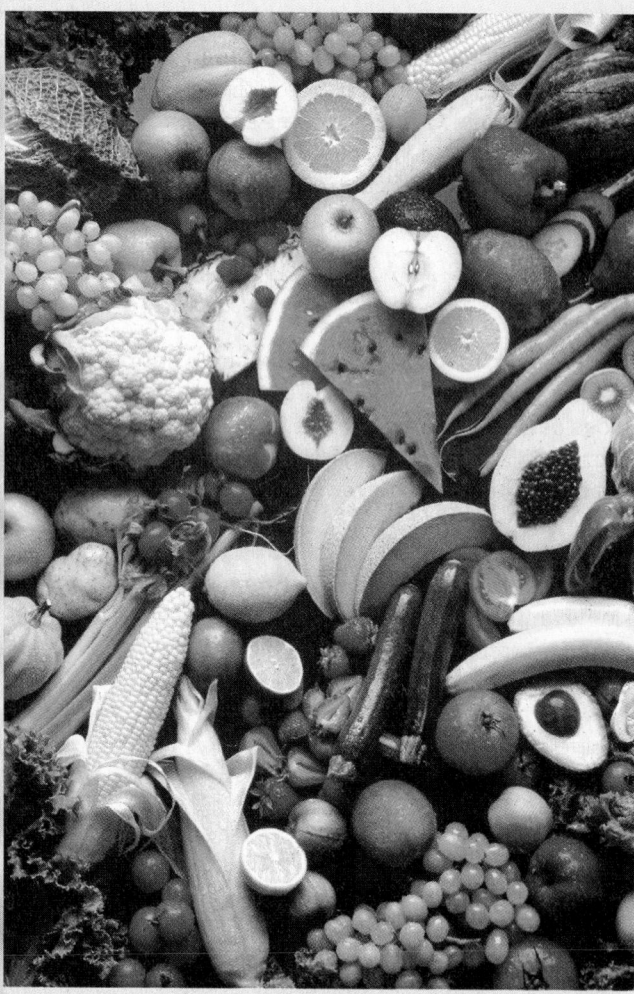

For the latest cancer fighters, visit your local produce counter.

Dr. Herbert makes the point that while orange juice and pills may both contain vitamin C, the orange juice presents a balancing array of chemicals that control vitamin C's effects. The pill provides only vitamin C, a lone chemical.[35] And in general, although fruits and vegetables rich in antioxidant nutrients have been associated with a diminished risk of many cancers, supplements of beta-carotene and vitamins C and E have not always proven beneficial.[36]

The struggle for truth continues. Members of the Food and Nutrition Board of the National Research Council are thinking about broadening the RDA, offering two values for each nutrient. One would be a recommended daily intake to prevent classic deficiency disesase. The other, a substantially higher recommended intake, would help protect against chronic diseases.[37] Before they do so, though, they must first weigh all of the evidence on high nutrient doses: not only the benefits, but also the risks. Meanwhile, most scientists agree that it is too early to recommend that people start taking antioxidant supplements now, even those of vitamin E or vitamin C. The risks are real, and clinical studies to quantify them and clarify the benefits will take several years to complete.

Should We Try to Eat More Vitamin-Rich Foods? Foods deliver thousands of chemicals other than the handful we call nutrients. Anyone judging a food purely by its nutrient content might score a turnip root or a radish because these foods appear almost devoid of nutrients in a nutrient-composition table such as the one in this book's Appendix A. But turnip roots and radishes are full of phytochemicals that enhance their value to the body. Researchers must be careful in crediting a particular health benefit to a nutrient when the source of that nutrient is whole food.

It seems reasonable, for now, to conclude by recommending this personal strategy. Don't try to single out only a few magic vitamins to take as supplements. Instead, eat a wide variety of fruits and vegetables in generous quantities every day. It is one of the most important favors you can do yourself, and the benefits are well backed by research.

NOTES

Notes are in Appendix F.

That a distinction is made between the major and the trace minerals doesn't mean that one group is more important in the body than the other. A daily deficiency of a few micrograms of iodine is just as serious as a deficiency of several hundred milligrams of calcium. Major minerals and trace minerals all play specific roles. Because the major minerals are present in larger total quantities, however, they influence the body fluids, thereby affecting the whole body in a general way.

A person can drink pure water, but in the body, that water mingles with minerals to become fluids in which all life processes take place. This chapter begins with a discussion of water—the most indispensable nutrient of all—and the major minerals that characterize the body's fluids and regulate their distribution within the body. Then the chapter discusses the specialized roles of the minerals.

WATER

You began as a single cell bathed in a nourishing fluid. As you became a beautifully organized, air-breathing body of trillions of cells, each of your cells had to remain next to water to remain alive. Water brings to each cell the exact ingredients the cell requires and carries away the end products of its life-sustaining reactions.

Water in the body is not simply a river coursing through the arteries, capillaries, and veins. Some of the water is part of the chemical structure of compounds that form the cells, tissues, and organs of the body. For example, proteins hold water molecules within them. This water is locked in and is not readily available for any other use. Water also participates actively in many chemical reactions.

Water's Work

As the medium for the body's traffic of nutrients and waste products, water is nearly a universal solvent. Luckily for our physical integrity, this is not quite the case, but water does dissolve amino acids, glucose, minerals, and many other substances needed by the cells. Fatty substances are specially packaged with water-soluble proteins so that they too can travel freely in the blood and lymph. The water of the body fluids is thus the transport vehicle for all the nutrients.

Water is also the body's cleansing agent. Small molecules, such as the nitrogen wastes generated during protein metabolism, dissolve in the watery blood and must be removed before they build up to toxic concentrations. The job of a healthy pair of kidneys is to filter these wastes from the blood and excrete them, mixed with water, as urine. When the kidneys become diseased, as can happen in diabetes, toxins can build to life-threatening levels. A machine must then take over the task of cleansing the blood by filtering wastes into water contained within the machine.

Another important characteristic of water is its incompressibility. Its molecules resist being crowded together. Thanks to this characteristic, water can act as a lubricant and a cushion for the joints. For the same reason, it can protect a sensitive tissue such as the spinal cord from shock. The fluid that fills the eye serves in a similar way to keep optimal pressure on the retina and lens. The

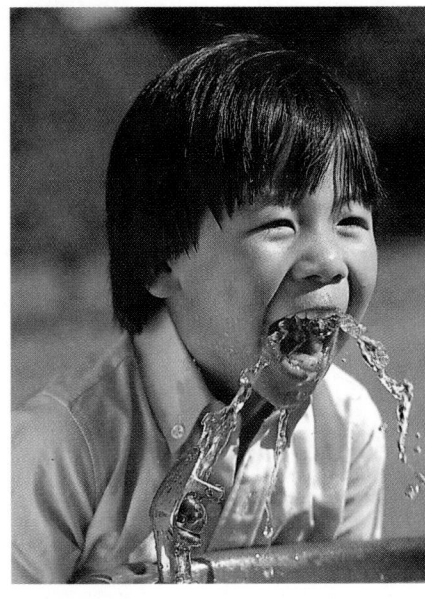

Water is the most indispensable nutrient.

Boasting scientist: "I'm working on discovering the universal solvent."

Skeptic: "Is that so? Well, when you've got it, what are you going to keep it in?"

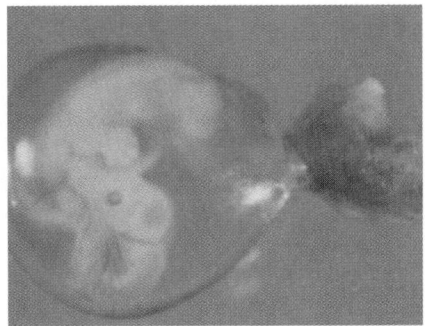

Human life begins in water.

unborn infant is cushioned against shock by the bag of amniotic fluid in which it develops. Water also lubricates the digestive tract and all tissues that are moistened with mucus.

Still another of water's special features is its heat-regulating capacity. This characteristic of water is familiar to coastal dwellers; who know that land surrounded by water is protected from wide variations in temperature from day to night. Water itself changes temperature slowly; at night, when the land cools, the water gives up its heat gradually to the air, moderating the coolness of the night. In contrast, the desert varies widely in temperature from day to night because it is dry. Similarly, water helps to maintain body temperature.

The water of sweat is the body's coolant. Heat, produced as a by-product of energy metabolism, can build up dangerously in the body. To rid itself of excess heat, the body routes its blood supply through the capillaries just under the skin. At the same time, the skin secretes sweat and its water evaporates, cooling the skin and the underlying blood. Converting water to vapor takes energy; as sweat evaporates, heat energy dissipates, cooling the skin. Cooled blood then flows back to cool the body's core. Sweat is constantly evaporating from the skin, usually in slight amounts that go unnoticed; thus the skin is a major organ through which water is lost from the body. To sum up, water:

- Carries nutrients throughout the body.
- Cleanses the blood of wastes.
- Serves as the solvent for minerals, vitamins, amino acids, glucose, and other small molecules.
- Actively participates in many chemical reactions.
- Acts as a lubricant around joints.
- Serves as a shock absorber inside the eyes, spinal cord, joints, and amniotic sac surrounding a fetus in the womb.
- Aids in maintaining the body's temperature.

An extra drink of water benefits both young and old.

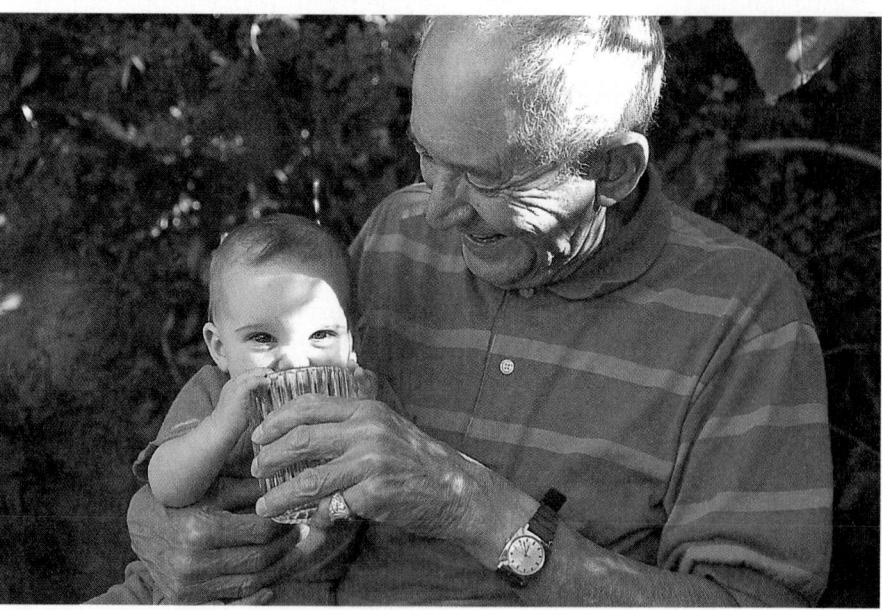

TABLE 8-1

Factors That Increase Water Needs

- Very young or old age
- Diseases that disturb water balance, such as diabetes
- Prolonged diarrhea, vomiting, or fever
- Forced air environments, such as airplanes or sealed buildings
- Heated environments
- Medications (diuretics)
- Hot weather
- Alcohol or caffeine consumption
- Pregnancy, breastfeeding (Chapter 12)
- Exercise (Chapter 10)
- Surgery, blood loss, burns

water balance the balance between water intake and water excretion, which keeps the body's water content constant.

dehydration loss of water. The symptoms progress rapidly, from thirst to weakness to exhaustion and delirium, and end in death.

water intoxication the rare condition in which body water content is too high. Symptoms are headache, muscular weakness, lack of concentration, poor memory, and loss of appetite.

✓ **KEY POINT**   **Water acts as a solvent, provides the medium for transportation, participates in chemical reactions, provides lubrication and shock protection, and aids in temperature regulation in the human body.**

The Body's Water Balance

Water makes up about 60 percent of the body's weight. It is such an integral part of us that people seldom are conscious of its importance, unless they are deprived of it. You can survive a deficiency of any of the other nutrients for a long time, in some cases even for months or years, but you can survive only a few days without water. Since the body must excrete at least a pint of water a day to cleanse its fluids, a person must consume at least a pint each day to avoid life-threatening losses, that is, to maintain **water balance.** Table 8-1 lists some factors that increase water needs.

The total amount of fluid in the body is kept constant by delicate balancing mechanisms. Imbalances can occur, such as **dehydration** and **water intoxication,** but the balances are restored to normal as promptly as the body can manage it. Both intake and excretion are controlled to maintain water balance.

The weight of the body's water varies by pounds at a time, especially in women who retain water at the menses. Anyone who eats a meal high in salt can temporarily increase the body's water content, which the body sheds over the next day or so as the sodium is excreted. These temporary fluctuations in body water also cause changes in body weight on the scales. People who gain or lose water weight may believe the change reflects a change in body fat, but fat weight takes days or weeks to change noticeably, while water weight can change overnight.

✓ **KEY POINT**   **Water makes up about 60 percent of the body's weight. A change in the body's water content can bring a change in body weight.**

Quenching Thirst and Balancing Losses

Thirst and satiety govern water intake. When the blood is too concentrated (having lost water but not salt and other dissolved substances), the molecules

FIGURE 8-2

WATER BALANCE

Water enters the body in liquids and foods, and some water is created in the body as a by-product of metabolic processes. Water leaves the body through the evaporation of sweat, in the moisture of exhaled breath, in the urine, and in the feces.

Water input (Total = 1,450–2,800 ml)

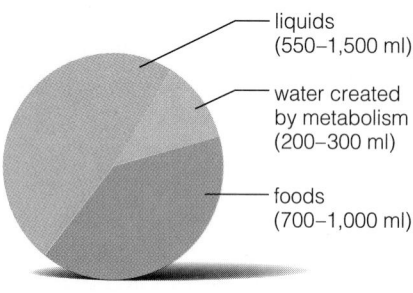

liquids
(550–1,500 ml)

water created
by metabolism
(200–300 ml)

foods
(700–1,000 ml)

Water output (Total = 1,450–2,800 ml)

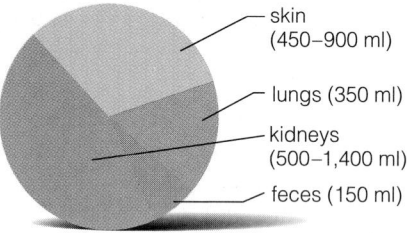

skin
(450–900 ml)

lungs (350 ml)

kidneys
(500–1,400 ml)

feces (150 ml)

diuretics (dye-you-RET-ics) compounds, usually medications, causing increased urinary water excretion; "water pills."

and particles in the blood attract water out of the salivary glands. The mouth becomes dry as a result, and you drink to wet your mouth. The brain center known as the hypothalamus (described in Chapter 3) also monitors the concentration of the blood. When the blood is too concentrated, or when the blood volume or pressure is too low, the hypothalamus initiates impulses that stimulate drinking behavior. The hypothalamus also calls forth a hormone from the pituitary gland that directs the kidneys to shift water back into the bloodstream from the pool destined for excretion. The kidneys themselves also respond to the sodium concentration in the blood passing through them and secrete regulatory substances of their own. The net result is that the more water the body needs, the less it excretes. Figure 8-2 shows how intake and excretion naturally balance out.

Thirst lags behind a lack of water. A water deficiency that develops slowly can switch on drinking behavior in time to prevent serious dehydration, but one that develops quickly may not. When too much water is lost from the body and is not replaced, dehydration can threaten survival. A first sign of dehydration is thirst, the signal that the body has lost up to 2 cups of its total fluid. Rather than waiting until thirst sets in, people should drink regularly throughout the day. But say a person is unable to obtain fluid or, as in many elderly people, fails to perceive the thirst message. With a loss of just 5 percent of body fluid, perceptible but general symptoms appear: headache, fatigue, confusion or forgetfulness, and an elevated heart rate. Instead of "wasting" any of its precious water in sweat, the dehydrated body diverts most of its water into the blood vessels to maintain the life-supporting blood pressure. Meanwhile, body heat builds up because sweating has ceased, creating the possibility of serious consequences (see Table 8-2).

✓ **KEY POINT** **Water losses from the body necessitate intake equal to output to maintain balance. The brain regulates water intake; the brain and kidneys regulate water excretion. Dehydration can have serious consequences.**

Water Recommendations and Sources

Water needs vary greatly depending on the foods a person eats, the environmental temperature and humidity, the person's activity level, and other factors. The committee on Recommended Dietary Allowances (RDA) recommends that under normal dietary and environmental conditions adults need between 1 and 1½ milliliters of water from all sources for each calorie spent in the day.[1] For the person who expends about 2,000 calories a day, this works out to a fluid intake of about 2 to 3 liters (about 7 to 11 cups). Sweating increases water needs.

In addition to water itself and other beverages made of water, nearly all foods contain water. Most fruits and vegetables contain large quantities of water, up to 95 percent; many meats and cheeses contain at least 50 percent. Also, the energy-yielding nutrients in foods release additional water as the body breaks them down. Beverages containing alcohol or caffeine have a negative effect on the body's water balance—they are **diuretics,** compounds that cause water excretion. The person who drinks beer or coffee, then, may end up with a net fluid loss rather than a gain, to the detriment of the body's fluid balance. Better choices are foods and beverages that present abundant water but

TABLE 8-2

Signs of Mild and Severe Dehydration

Mild	Severe
Thirst	Pale skin
Sudden weight loss	Bluish lips and fingertips
Rough dry skin	Confusion/disorientation
Dry mouth, throat, and internal body linings	Rapid shallow breathing
	Weak, rapid, irregular pulse
Rapid heart rate	Thickening of blood
Low blood pressure	Shock
Lack of energy	Seizures
Weakness	Coma
Impaired kidney function	Death
Highly concentrated urine, but low in volume	

hard water water with high calcium and magnesium concentrations.

soft water water with a high sodium concentration.

bottled water drinking water sold in bottles.

without unwanted alcohol or caffeine (see the list in the margin). The Table of Food Composition, Appendix A, lists the water contents of most other foods and beverages.

Water naturally occurs as **hard water** or **soft water,** a distinction that affects health with regard to three minerals. Hard water has high concentrations of calcium and magnesium. Soft water's principal mineral is sodium. In practical terms, soft water makes more bubbles with less soap; hard water leaves a ring on the tub, a jumble of rocklike crystals in the teakettle, and a gray residue in the wash. Soft water may seem more desirable, and homeowners even purchase water softeners that remove magnesium and calcium and replace them with sodium. However, soft water appears to aggravate hypertension and heart disease in areas where it is used. Hard water may oppose these conditions.

Soft water also more easily dissolves certain metals, such as cadmium and lead, from pipes. Cadmium is not an essential nutrient. In fact, it can harm the body, affecting enzymes by displacing zinc from its normal sites of action. Cadmium is also suspected of promoting hypertension. Lead is another toxic metal, and the body seems to absorb it more readily from soft water than from hard water, possibly because the calcium in hard water protects against its absorption. Old plumbing may contain cadmium or lead. People who live in old buildings should run the cold water tap a minute to flush out harmful minerals before drawing water for use at breakfast.

Many people turn to **bottled water** as an alternative to tap water. As the Consumer Corner points out, though, bottled water may or may not contain more health-promoting mineral arrays than ordinary tap water does.

Water content of various foods and beverages:

- 100% = water, diet soft drinks, seltzer (unflavored), plain tea
- 95–99% = sugar-free gelatin dessert, clear broth, Chinese cabbage, celery, cucumber, lettuce, summer squash, black coffee
- 90–94% = Gatorade, grapefruit, fresh strawberries, broccoli, tomato
- 80–89% = sugar-sweetened soft drinks, milk, yogurt, egg white, fruit juices, low-fat cottage cheese, fresh apple, carrot
- 60–79% = low-calorie mayonnaise, instant pudding, banana, shrimp, lean steak, pork chops, baked potato
- 40–59% = diet margarine, sausage, chicken, macaroni and cheese
- 20–39% = bread, cakes, cheddar cheese, bagel, cooked oatmeal
- 10–19% = butter, margarine, regular mayonnaise, cooked rice
- 5–9% = peanut butter, popcorn
- 1–4% = ready-to-eat cereals, pretzels
- 0% = cooking oils, meat fats, shortening, white sugar

✔ KEY POINT **Hard water is high in calcium and magnesium. Soft water is high in sodium, and it dissolves cadmium and lead from pipes.**

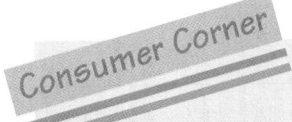

WHICH TYPE OF WATER IS SAFEST?

Many people, knowing that contaminated water can be injurious to health, are concerned about the safety of their water supplies. Households, traffic, industry, and agriculture all add pollutants to environmental water and thereby degrade its quality. Hundreds of contaminants, including disease-causing bacteria and viruses from human wastes, toxic pollutants from highway fuel runoff, spills and heavy metals from industry, and organic chemicals such as pesticides from agriculture, have been detected in public drinking water.

Treatment by public water systems can at least partly remove some of these hazards. The treatment includes the addition of a disinfectant (usually chlorine) to kill most microorganisms. Private well water is usually not chlorinated or cleansed, so the 40 million Americans who drink water from private wells are especially likely to encounter microorganisms in their water. All public drinking water must be tested regularly for contamination, and the Environmental Protection Agency (EPA) is responsible for ensuring that public water systems meet minimum standards for protection of public health.

A newly signed law mandates that local water authorities disclose results from water tests to consumers. Once a year, customers of public water utilities will receive a statement, written in plain language, that names the chemicals and bacteria found in local water. This document makes fascinating reading for those interested in how pure their tap water is. The law also requires public notice within 24 hours of discovering any dangerous contaminants in drinking water. An intent of the law is to focus efforts on the most harmful contaminants such as the parasite Cryptosporidium, common in lakes and rivers, that caused 400,000 people living in Milwaukee, Wisconsin to fall ill several years ago. Symptoms of infection ranged from digestive distress to death. Water authorities plan to monitor the water for this microbe, which often survives the killing effects of chlorine.

Some people fear that chlorine itself presents a danger to health, and several preliminary studies of tap water use have issued disturbing results. Researchers have noted a statistical correlation between consuming chlorinated surface water and the likelihood of developing bladder and rectal cancer.[2] Earlier experiments revealed that by-products in chlorinated water cause cancer in laboratory animals.

While most investigators acknowledge a connection between consumption of chlorinated drinking water and cancer incidence, they also passionately defend chlorination as a benefit to public health. In parts of the world without chlorination, 25,000 people are estimated to die *each day* from diseases caused by organisms carried by water and easily killed by chlorine.

While substitutes for chlorine exist, these may create their own by-products; no substitute that is practical has proved safer than chlorine. Under development is a treatment to destroy organic compounds in water by bombarding them with beams of high-energy electrons. This method destroys living organisms and some toxic chemicals, but it is years away from approval for use.[3] In the meanwhile, what is a consumer to drink?

One option may be to purify tap water with home purifying equipment. Ranging in price from about $20 to $800, home systems may succeed only in improving the water's taste or they may do an adequate job of removing lead. Many are not designed to remove dangerous microorganisms that are left unaffected by chlorine. Each system has advantages and drawbacks, and all require periodic maintenance or filter replacements that vary in price. Unfortunately, not all companies or representatives are legitimate. Some perform water tests that yield dramatic-appearing but meaningless results to sell unneeded systems. Verify all claims of contamination with local water agencies before buying any purifying system.

Many people seek an alternative water source. As a result, about 1 in 15 households uses bottled water as the main drinking water source, believing it to be safer than tap water and therefore worth its substantial price.

Unfortunately, bottled water is just as vulnerable to contamination as tap water is. After all, whether water comes from the tap or is poured from a bottle, all water comes from the same sources, **surface water** and **ground water.** Each of these sources supplies water for about half of the population.

Surface water comes from lakes, rivers, and reservoirs and provides drinking water for most of the nation's major cities. Surface water is easily contaminated. Acid rain; runoff from highways; pesticides, fertilizer, and animal waste from agricultural areas; and industrial wastes run directly from pavements, septic tanks, farmlands, and industrial areas into streams that feed surface water bodies.

Surface water generally moves faster than ground water and stays aboveground so it is cleansed somewhat by aeration and exposure to sunlight. It is also filtered by the plants and microorganisms that live in it. These processes can remove some contaminants, but others stay in the water.

Ground water comes from **aquifers,** underground rock formations saturated with water. People in rural areas rely mostly on ground water pumped up from private wells. Ground water is susceptible to contamination from hazardous waste sites, dumps, oil and gasoline pipelines, and landfills, as well as downward seepage from surface water bodies. Ground water moves slowly and lacks aeration and exposure to sunlight, so contaminants break down more slowly than in surface water. Ground water, however, must "percolate," or seep through soil, sand, and rock, to reach the aquifer. Percolation filters out some contaminants.

surface water water that comes from lakes, rivers, and reservoirs.

ground water water that comes from underground aquifers.

aquifers underground rock formations containing water that can be drawn to the surface for use.

Lead poisoning is especially harmful to children (see Chapter 13).

(continued on next page)

salts compounds composed of charged particles (ions). An example is potassium chloride (K^+Cl^-).

ions (EYE-ons) electrically charged particles, such as sodium (positively charged) or chloride (negatively charged).

electrolytes compounds that partly dissociate in water to form ions, such as the potassium ion (K^+) and the chloride ion (Cl^-).

Bottled water is classed as a food, so it is regulated by the Food and Drug Administration (FDA).[4] The FDA requires yearly tests of bottled water composition to ensure that it meets the same standards as those set for purity and sanitation of U.S. tap water.[5]

Overwhelmingly, the people who buy bottled water say that it simply tastes better than the water from their taps. Most water-bottling plants disinfect their products with ozone, a form of oxygen that, unlike chlorine, leaves no flavor or odor in the water. Another reason people choose bottled water is to avoid public water that consistently tests positive for one or more chemical or other contaminants.

As a consumer, what should you look for when buying bottled water? Look for the trademark of the International Bottled Water Association (IBWA). The IBWA supports the FDA's regulations and enforcement efforts. Determine the water's source. If the bottled water comes from a public source, what kind of treatment processes were used to remove contaminants? If the bottled water comes from a spring or stream, where is it located? Is the area agricultural, residential, industrial, or undeveloped? Bottled water from municipal sources must be labeled as such unless it has been distilled or otherwise purified. Table 8-3 provides some definitions for terms you may see on labels.

If your water is dispensed from a water cooler, disinfect the cooler once a month by running half a gallon of white vinegar through it. Remove the vinegar residue by rinsing the cooler with 4 or 5 gallons of tap water. The microbial content of water coolers has been found to be considerably higher than that recommended by the government. Bacterial and mold growths can cause serious infection and disease in those who ingest water contaminated with them.

Sales of bottled water show little sign of slowing down as more and more people question the safety of their water. Before you spend your money, though, be sure of what you are getting in return.

BODY FLUIDS AND MINERALS

Much of the body's water weight is contained inside the cells, and some also bathes the outsides of the cells. The remainder fills the blood vessels. Special provisions are needed to ensure that the cells do not collapse when water leaves them or swell up when too much water enters them. The cells cannot regulate the amount of water directly by pumping it in and out because water slips across membranes freely. They can, however, pump minerals across their membranes. The major minerals form **salts** that dissolve in the body fluids; the cells direct where the salts go; and this determines where the fluids flow, because water follows salt.

When mineral (or other) salts dissolve in water, they separate into single, electrically charged particles known as **ions.** Unlike pure water, which conducts electricity poorly, ions dissolved in water carry electrical current. For this reason, the electrically charged ions are called **electrolytes.** Figure 8-3 shows

TABLE 8-3

Water Terms That May Appear on Labels

- **artesian water** water drawn from a well that taps a confined aquifer in which the water is under pressure.
- **carbonated water** water that contains carbon dioxide gas, either naturally occurring or added, that bubbles from it; also called *bubbling* or *sparkling* water. Seltzer, soda, or tonic waters are legally soft drinks and are not regulated as water.
- **distilled water** water that has been vaporized and recondensed, leaving it free of dissolved minerals.
- **filtered water** water treated by filtration, usually through *activated carbon filters* that reduce the lead in tap water, or by *reverse osmosis* units that force pressurized water across a membrane removing lead, arsenic, and some microorganisms from tap water.
- **mineral water** water from a spring or well that typically contains 250 to 500 parts per million (ppm) of minerals. Minerals give water a distinctive flavor. Many mineral waters are high in sodium.
- **natural water** water obtained from a spring or well that is certified to be safe and sanitary. The mineral content may not be changed, but the water may be treated in other ways such as by filtration or ozonization.
- **public water** water from a municipal or county water system that has been treated and disinfected.
- **purified water** water that has been treated by distillation or other physical or chemical processes that remove dissolved solids. Because purified water contains no minerals or contaminants, it is useful for medical and research purposes.
- **spring water** water originating from an underground spring or well. It may be bubbly (carbonated) or "flat" or "still," meaning not carbonated. Brand names such as "Spring Pure" do not necessarily mean that the water comes from a spring.
- **well water** water drawn from ground water by tapping into an aquifer.

fluid and electrolyte balance maintenance of the proper amounts and kinds of fluids and minerals in each compartment of the body.

fluid and electrolyte imbalance failure to maintain the proper amount and kind of fluid in every body compartment; a medical emergency.

acid–base balance maintenance of the proper degree of acidity in each of the body's fluids.

how the body uses electrolytes to move its fluids around. Figure 6-11 of Chapter 6 showed that proteins form the pumps that move mineral ions across cell membranes. The successful result is **fluid and electrolyte balance,** the proper amount and kind of fluid in every body compartment.

If something happens to overwhelm the fluid balance, severe illness can result quickly, since fluid can shift rapidly from one compartment to another. For example, in vomiting or diarrhea, the loss of water from the intestinal tract pulls fluid from between the cells in every part of the body. Fluid then leaves the inside of the cells to restore balance. Meanwhile the kidneys detect the water loss and attempt to retrieve water from the pool destined for excretion. To do this, they raise the sodium concentration outside the cells, and this pulls still more water out of them. When this happens, the very serious condition of **fluid and electrolyte imbalance** occurs. Water and minerals lost in vomiting or diarrhea ultimately come from every body cell. This loss disrupts the heartbeat and threatens life. It is a cause of death among those with eating disorders.

Controversy 10 describes the problems of eating disorders.

FIGURE 8-3

FLUIDS AND ELECTROLYTES
Water flows in the direction of the more highly concentrated solution.

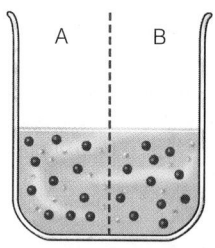

❶ With equal numbers of dissolved particles on both sides, water levels remain equal.

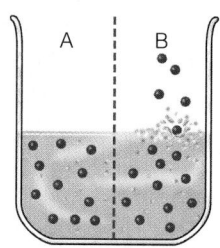

❷ Now additional particles are added to increase the concentration on side B. Particles cannot flow across the divider (in the case of a cell, the divider is a membrane).

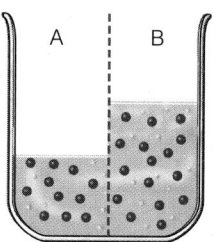

❸ Water can flow both ways across the divider, but tends to move from side A to side B, where there is a greater concentration of dissolved particles. The *volume* of water increases on side B, and the *concentrations* on sides A and B become equal.

---

buffers molecules that can help to keep the pH of a solution from changing by gathering or releasing H ions.

Figure 3-13 of Chapter 3 showed where common substances fall along the pH scale.

Major minerals
- Calcium
- Chloride
- Magnesium
- Phosphorus
- Potassium
- Sodium
- Sulfur

The minerals help manage still another balancing act, the **acid–base balance,** or pH, already mentioned in Chapters 3 and 6. When dissolved in water, some of the major minerals give rise to acids, some to bases. A small percentage of water molecules (H_2O) also exist as positive and negative ions, H (positive) and OH (negative). Excess H ions in a solution make it an acid; they lower the pH. Excess OH ions in a solution make it a base; they raise the pH.

The body's proteins and some of its mineral salts help prevent changes in the acid–base balance of its fluids by serving as **buffers**—molecules that gather up or release H ions as needed to maintain the correct pH. The kidneys help to control the pH balance by excreting more or less acid (H ions). The lungs help also by excreting more or less carbon dioxide. (In solution in the blood, carbon dioxide forms an acid, carbonic acid.) The tight control of the acid–base balance permits all other life processes to take place.

✔ KEY POINT **Electrolytes help keep fluids in their proper compartments and buffer these fluids, permitting all life processes to take place.**

THE MAJOR MINERALS

While all the major minerals help to maintain the balances just described, each also plays some special roles of its own. These roles are described in the following sections and are summarized in Table 8-13 on pages 320–321.

Calcium

As Figure 8-1 showed, calcium is by far the most abundant mineral in the body. Nearly all (99 percent) of the body's calcium is stored in the bones, where it plays two important roles. First, it is an integral part of bone structure. Second, bone calcium serves as a bank that can release calcium to the body fluids if even the slightest drop in blood calcium concentration occurs. Many people have the idea that, once deposited in bone, calcium (together with the other minerals of bone) stays there forever—that once a bone is built, it is inert, like a rock. Not so. The minerals of bones are in constant flux, with formation and dissolution taking place every minute of the day and night.

Calcium and phosphorus are essential to the formation of bone (see Figure 8-4). As bones begin to form, calcium phosphate salts crystallize on a foundation material composed of the protein collagen. The resulting **hydroxyapatite** crystals, invade the collagen and gradually lend more and more rigidity to the maturing bones until they are able to support the weight they will have to carry. During and after this bone-strengthening process, flouride may displace the "hydroxy" parts of these crystals, making **fluorapatite**, which is resistant to decay. Thus the long leg bones of children can support their weight by the time they have learned to walk.

The formation of teeth follows a pattern similar to that of bones. Hydroxyapatite crystals form on a collagen matrix to create the dentin that gives strength to the teeth (see Figure 8-5). Calcification of the "baby" teeth occurs in the gums during the latter half of the infant's time in the womb. The calcification of the permanent teeth takes place during early childhood, up to about the age of three; that of the "wisdom" teeth begins at about the age of ten. The turnover of minerals in teeth is not as rapid as in bone, but some withdrawal and redepositing do take place throughout life. As in bone, fluoride hardens and stabilizes the crystals of teeth, opposing the withdrawal of minerals from them.

hydroxyapatite (hi-DROX-ee-APP-uh-tight) the chief crystal of bone, formed from calcium and phosphorus.

fluorapatite (floor-APP-uh-tight) a crystal of bones and teeth, formed when fluoride displaces the hydroxy portion of hydroxyapatite. Fluorapatite resists being dissolved back into body fluid.

FIGURE 8-4

A BONE

Blood travels in capillaries throughout the bone. It brings nutrients to the cells that maintain the bone's structure, and carries away waste materials from those cells. It picks up and deposits minerals as instructed by hormones.

This bone derives its structural strength from the lacy network of crystals that lie along the bone's lines of stress. If minerals are withdrawn to cover deficits elsewhere in the body, the bone will grow weak, and ultimately will bend or crumble.

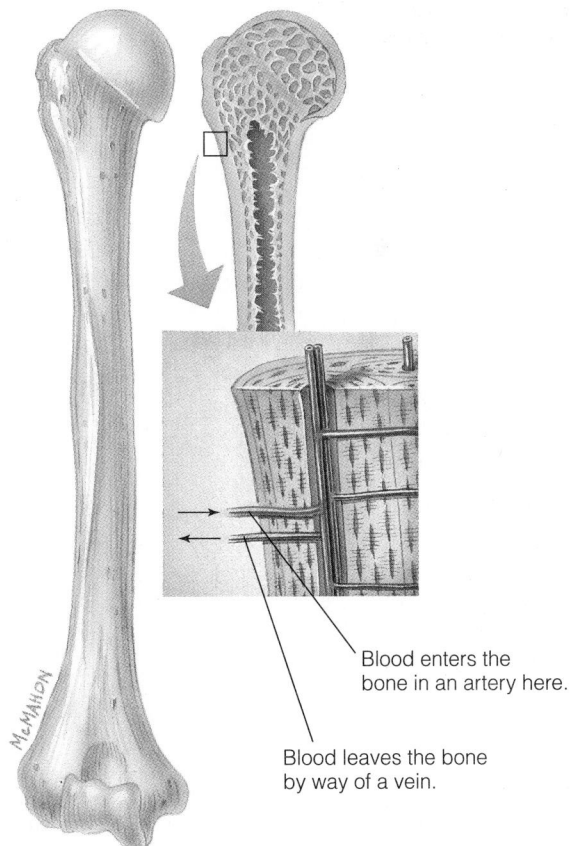

Blood enters the bone in an artery here.

Blood leaves the bone by way of a vein.

FIGURE 8-5

A TOOTH

The inner layer of dentin is bonelike material that forms on a protein (collagen) matrix. The outer layer of enamel is harder than bone. Both dentin and enamel contain hydroxyapatite crystals (made of calcium and phosphorus). The crystals of enamel may become even harder when exposed to the trace mineral fluoride.

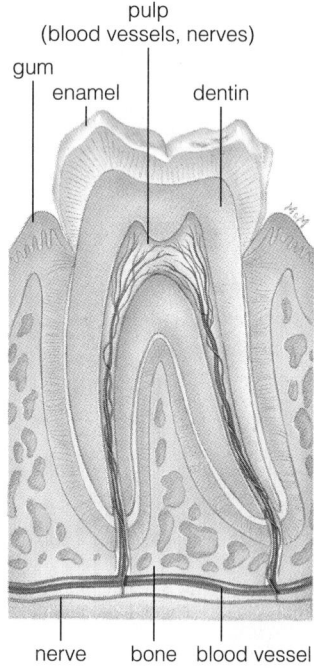

pulp
(blood vessels, nerves)

gum

enamel   dentin

nerve   bone   blood vessel

---

osteoporosis (OSS-tee-oh-pore-OH-sis) a condition of older persons in which the bones become porous and fragile (*osteo* means "bones"; *poros* means "porous"); also known as **adult bone loss.**

peak bone mass the highest attainable bone density for an individual; developed during the first three decades of life.

Calcium in Body Fluids   Only about 1 percent of the body's calcium is in the fluid that bathes and fills the cells, but this tiny amount plays major roles:

- It regulates the transport of ions across cell membranes and is particularly important in nerve transmission.
- It helps maintain normal blood pressure (see Chapter 11).
- It is essential for muscle contraction and therefore for the heartbeat.
- It allows secretion of hormones, digestive enzymes, and neurotransmitters.
- It plays an essential role in the clotting of blood.

Because of its importance, blood calcium is tightly controlled.

Calcium Balance   Cells need continuous access to calcium, so the body maintains a constant calcium concentration in the blood. The skeleton serves as a bank from which the blood can borrow and return calcium as needed. Blood calcium is regulated, not by a person's daily calcium intake, but by hormones sensitive to blood calcium.* This means that you can go without adequate dietary calcium for years and not suffer noticeable symptoms. Only later in life do you suddenly discover that your calcium savings account has dwindled to the point at which the integrity of your skeleton can no longer be maintained. This means that throughout your adult years you have been developing the fragile bones of **osteoporosis**, or **adult bone loss.** Osteoporosis constitutes a major health problem for many older people whose bones suddenly begin to shatter. The problem and its possible causes and prevention are the topics of this chapter's Controversy.

Calcium deficiencies are widespread, due largely to losses in adulthood. To protect against these losses, high calcium intakes early in life are recommended. A calcium-poor diet during the growing years may prevent achievement of maximum **peak bone mass** and density.[6] Too little calcium packed into the skeleton during childhood and young adulthood strongly predicts susceptibility to osteoporosis later in adulthood.[7] The body of an adolescent girl hungers for calcium, absorbing and retaining more calcium from each meal than does the body of an adult.[8]

The body is sensitive to an increased need for calcium, although it sends no signals to the conscious brain indicating calcium need. Instead, it quietly increases its absorption of the mineral from the intestine and prevents its loss from the kidneys, thus conserving it. For example, more calcium is needed for growth, so infants and children absorb up to 75 percent of ingested calcium; and pregnant women, about 50 percent. Other adults, who are not growing, absorb about 30 percent.[9] The body also absorbs a higher percentage of calcium when less total calcium is provided in the diet. Deprived of calcium for months or years, an adult may double the calcium absorbed; when supplied for years with abundant calcium, the same person may absorb only about one-third the normal amount. These adjustments take time. A person accustomed

---

*Calcitonin, made in the thyroid gland, is secreted whenever the calcium concentration in the blood rises too high. It acts to stop withdrawal from bone and to slow absorption somewhat from the intestine. Parathormone, from the parathyroid glands, has the opposite effect.

TABLE 8-4

Calcium Intake Recommendations

Healthy People 2000

■ Increase calcium intake, so that at least 50% of youth aged 12 years and 50% of pregnant and lactating women consume three or more servings of calcium-rich foods daily and at least 50% of people aged 25 years and older consume two or more servings of calcium-rich foods daily.

Recommended Dietary Allowances (RDA)[a]

■ Women and men (19–24 yr): 1,200 mg/day.
■ Women and men (25 yr and older): 800 mg/day.

National Institutes of Health[b]

■ Adolescents and young adults (11–24 yr): 1,200–1,500 mg/day.
■ Women (25–50 yr) and women past menopause taking estrogen: 1,000 mg/day.
■ Men (25–65 yr): 1,000 mg/day.
■ Women and men (>65 yr) and women past menopause not taking estrogen: 1,500 mg/day.

World Health Organization

■ 400 to 500 mg/day.

[a]For RDA values for other groups, see the inside front cover; Canadian values are listed in Appendix B.

[b]NIH Consensus Panel, Optimal calcium intake, *Journal of the American Medical Association* 272 (1994): 1942–1948.

---

to high calcium intakes who suddenly cuts back is likely to lose calcium from bone stores until the body adapts to the lower intake.

Calcium Recommendations and Sources   Because the human body can adjust its calcium absorption to varying levels of intake, setting recommended allowances is difficult. The U.S. and Canadian recommendations for calcium intake are high, especially for young people up to the age of 24 years. The high intake recommendations are perhaps appropriate because people develop their peak bone mass during their young years. After 30 years of age or so, the skeleton no longer adds significantly to bone density. After about 40 years of age, regardless of calcium intake, bones begin to lose density.[10] Thus obtaining enough calcium during the young years of life ensures that the skeleton will start out with enough mass to minimize bone losses through life. This is why the RDA for calcium has been set at 1,200 milligrams daily for young adults up to the age of 24 years. After 24 years, the RDA is lowered to 800 milligrams a day because the opportunity to build strong bones may have passed and the lower amount is sufficient to maintain bone tissue. Table 8-4 offers other calcium goals. Everyone needs to meet their calcium needs, and the Food Feature later in the chapter provides ways to do so. Snapshot 8-1 provides a look at some foods that supply calcium.

✔ **KEY POINT**   **Calcium makes up bone and tooth structure and plays roles in nerve transmission, muscle contraction, and blood clotting. Calcium absorption increases when there is a dietary deficiency or an increased need such as during growth.**

In vitamin D deficiency:
✔ Rickets causes the bones of children to be soft and malformed.
✔ Osteomalacia causes the bones of adults to soften and bend.

In osteoporosis:
✔ Bones of older adults become brittle and fragile.

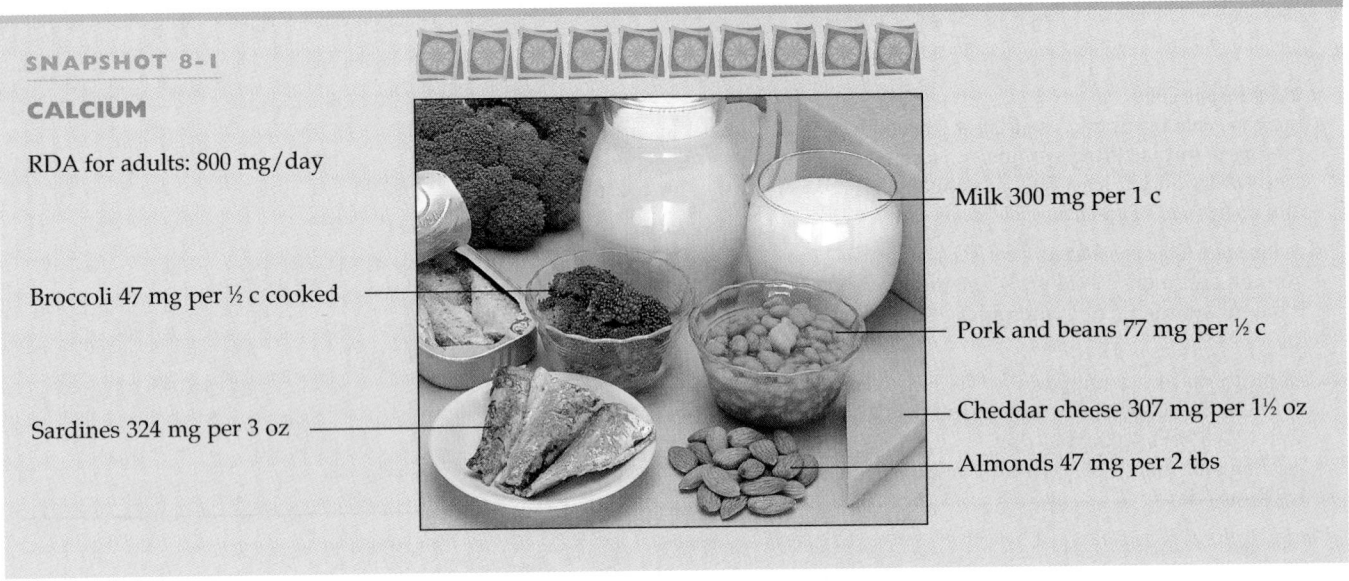

SNAPSHOT 8-1

CALCIUM

RDA for adults: 800 mg/day

Broccoli 47 mg per ½ c cooked

Sardines 324 mg per 3 oz

Milk 300 mg per 1 c

Pork and beans 77 mg per ½ c

Cheddar cheese 307 mg per 1½ oz

Almonds 47 mg per 2 tbs

Phosphorus

Note: The mineral is *phosphorus*. The adjective form is spelled with an -ous (as in *phosphorous salts*).

Phosphorus is the second most abundant mineral in the body. About 85 percent of it is found combined with calcium in the crystals of the bones and teeth.

The concentration of phosphorus in the blood is less than half that of calcium, but its functions are critical to life. Phosphorous salts buffer the acid–base balance of cellular fluids. Each cell also depends on phosphorus as part of its genetic material, thus making phosphorus essential for growth and renewal of tissues. In cells' metabolism of energy nutrients, phosphorous compounds handle energy and work with many enzymes and vitamins to extract the energy from nutrients. Recall from Chapter 5 that phosphorus forms part of the molecules of the phospholipids, lipids that are principal components of the membranes surrounding each cell and its parts.

As Snapshot 8-2 shows, animal protein is the best source of phosphorus. The reason is that phosphorus is abundant in the cells of animals. Recommended intakes for phosphorus are the same as those for calcium, except during infancy. Luckily, needs for phosphorus are easily met by almost any diet, and deficiencies are unknown.

✓ **KEY POINT   Most of the phosphorus in the body is in the bones and teeth. Phosphorus in the blood helps maintain acid–base balance, is part of the genetic material in cells, assists in energy metabolism, and is part of cell membranes. Under normal circumstances, deficiencies of phosphorus are unknown.**

Magnesium

Magnesium barely qualifies as a major mineral: only about 1¾ ounces are present in the body of a 130-pound person, over half of it in the bones. Most of the

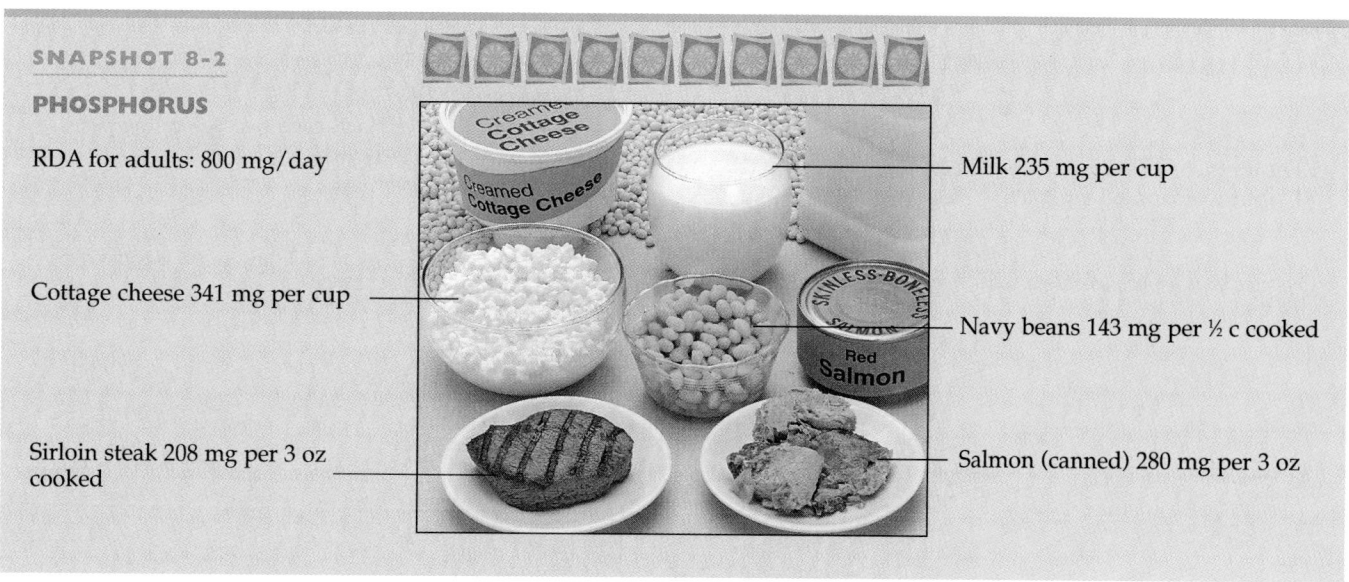

SNAPSHOT 8-2

PHOSPHORUS

RDA for adults: 800 mg/day

Cottage cheese 341 mg per cup

Sirloin steak 208 mg per 3 oz cooked

Milk 235 mg per cup

Navy beans 143 mg per ½ c cooked

Salmon (canned) 280 mg per 3 oz

rest is in the muscles, heart, liver, and other soft tissues, with only 1 percent in the body fluids. The supply of magnesium in the bones can be tapped to maintain a constant blood level whenever dietary intake falls too low. The kidneys can also act to conserve magnesium.

Magnesium is critical to the operation of hundreds of enzymes, and it directly affects the metabolism of potassium, calcium, and vitamin D. Magnesium acts in the cells of all the soft tissues, where it is part of the protein-making machinery and is necessary for the release of energy. Magnesium helps muscles relax after contraction and promotes resistance to tooth decay by holding calcium in tooth enamel.

Deficiency of magnesium may occur as a result of inadequate intake, vomiting, diarrhea, alcoholism, or protein malnutrition. It may also occur in hospital clients who have been fed magnesium-poor fluids into a vein for too long or in persons using diuretics. People whose drinking water has a high magnesium content experience a lower incidence of sudden death from heart failure than other people. It seems likely that magnesium deficiency makes the heart unable to stop itself from going into spasms once it starts. Magnesium deficiency may also be related to cardiovascular disease, heart attack, and high blood pressure.[11] A deficiency also causes hallucinations that can be mistaken for mental illness or drunkenness. Despite intakes below the RDA, overt deficiency symptoms in normal, healthy people are rare.[12]

Most people in the United States receive only about three-quarters of their magnesium RDA from their diets. In various parts of the country, water can contribute significantly to magnesium intakes, so people living in those regions need less from food. Snapshot 8-3 shows magnesium-rich foods. Magnesium is easily washed and peeled away from foods during processing, so slightly processed or unprocessed foods are the best choices.

Toxicities are most often reported in older people who abuse magnesium-containing laxatives, antacids, and other medications. The consequences can be severe: lack of coordination, confusion, coma, and, in extreme cases, death.[13]

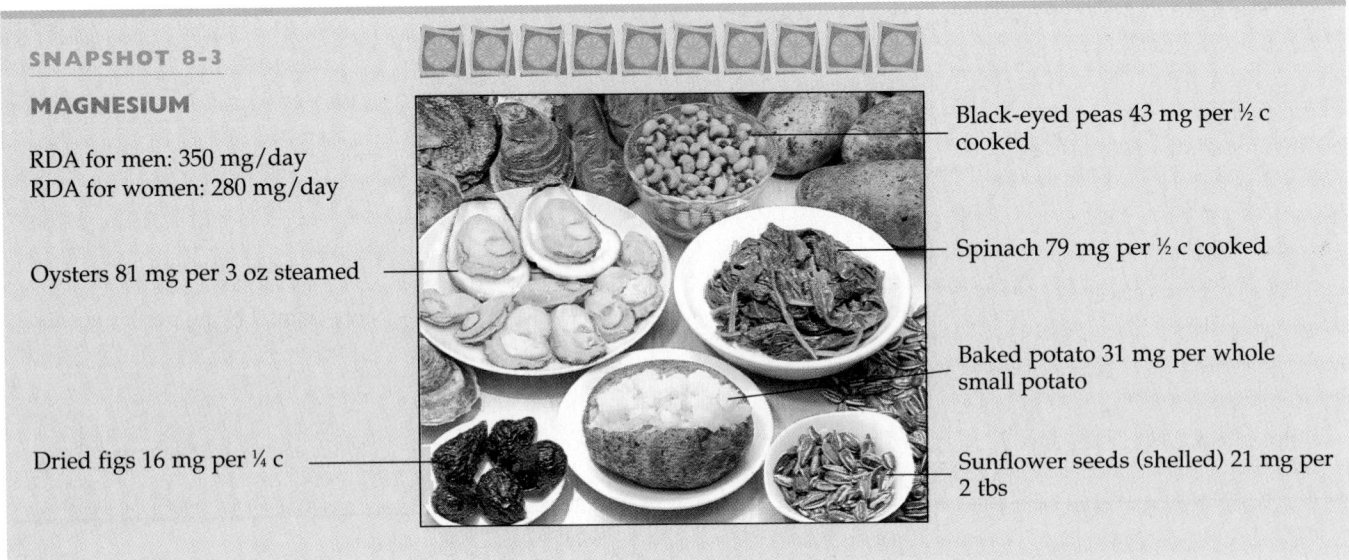

SNAPSHOT 8-3

MAGNESIUM

RDA for men: 350 mg/day
RDA for women: 280 mg/day

Oysters 81 mg per 3 oz steamed

Dried figs 16 mg per ¼ c

Black-eyed peas 43 mg per ½ c cooked

Spinach 79 mg per ½ c cooked

Baked potato 31 mg per whole small potato

Sunflower seeds (shelled) 21 mg per 2 tbs

✓ KEY POINT **Most of the body's magnesium is in the bones, and can be drawn out for all the cells to use in building protein and using energy. Most people in the United States fail to obtain enough magnesium from their food.**

Sodium

Salt has been known throughout recorded history. The biblical saying "You are the salt of the earth" means that a person is valuable. If, on the other hand, "you are not worth your salt," you are worthless. Even the word *salary* comes from the word *salt*. Sodium is the positive ion in the compound sodium chloride (table salt) and contributes 40 percent of its weight. Thus a person who consumes a gram of salt consumes 400 milligrams of sodium. As already mentioned, sodium is the chief ion used to maintain the volume of fluid outside cells. Sodium also helps maintain acid–base balance and is essential to muscle contraction and nerve transmission. About 30 to 40 percent of the body's sodium is thought to be stored on the surface of the bone crystals, where the body can easily draw upon it to replenish the blood concentration, if necessary.

Balancing Sodium A deficiency of sodium would be harmful, but few diets lack sodium. Foods usually include more salt than is needed, and the body absorbs it freely. The kidneys filter the surplus out of the blood into the urine. They can also sensitively conserve salt. In the rare event of a deficiency, they can return to the bloodstream the exact amount needed. Normally, the amount of sodium you excrete in a day equals the amount you have ingested that day.

If blood sodium rises, as it will after a person eats salted foods, thirst ensures that the person will drink water until the sodium-to-water ratio is restored. Then the kidneys excrete the extra water along with the extra sodium.

To the chemist, a salt results from neutralization of an acid and a base. Sodium chloride, table salt, results from the reaction between hydrochloric acid and the base sodium hydroxide. The positive sodium ion unites with the negative chloride ion to form the salt. The positive hydrogen ion unites with the negative hydroxide ion to form water.

    Base + acid = salt + water.
    Sodium hydroxide + hydrochloric acid
    = sodium chloride + water.

For a brief summary of the kidneys' actions, see Chapter 3.

Dieters sometimes think that eating too much salt or drinking too much water will make them gain weight, but they do not gain fat, of course. They gain water, but they excrete this excess water immediately. Excess salt is excreted as soon as enough water is drunk to carry the salt out of the body. From this perspective, then, the way to keep body salt (and "water weight") under control is to drink more, not less, water.

If blood sodium drops, body water is lost, and both water and sodium must be replenished to avert an emergency. Overly strict use of low-sodium diets in the treatment of hypertension, kidney disease, or heart disease can deplete the body of needed sodium; so can vomiting, diarrhea, or extremely heavy sweating. As Chapter 10 makes clear, the sodium lost by way of normal sweating due to exercise is easily replaced later in the day with ordinary foods.

Sodium Intakes   No known human diet lacks sodium.[14] For this reason, no RDA has been set. Instead, the RDA committee estimated the minimum sodium requirement for adults to be 500 milligrams, an amount provided by a diet of plain foods with no salt added.[15] The World Health Organization emphasizes moderation as its key concern about sodium (see Table 8-5).

Cultures vary in their use of salt. Men in the United States consume an average of 3,300 milligrams of sodium, or more than 8 grams of salt, a day.[16] Asian people, whose staple sauces and flavorings are based on soy sauce and monosodium glutamate (MSG or Accent), may consume the equivalent of about 30 to 40 grams of salt per day. Often, communities with high intakes of salt experience high rates of hypertension and cerebral hemorrhage (a hypertension-related form of stroke). In China, Japan, and Korea, the prevalence of high blood pressure is equal to or greater than in the United States.[17]

Controlling Salt Intake   Controlling salt is a major step toward controlling high blood pressure for people sensitive to salt's effects. The connection between salt and blood pressure in salt-sensitive people is direct: the more salt they eat, the higher their blood pressure goes. People tending toward salt sensitivity usually include those with kidney disease, those of African descent,

TABLE 8-5

Salt and Sodium Intake Guidelines

Estimated Safe and Adequate Daily Intakes
- Adolescents and adults: 500 milligrams per day.

World Health Organization
- Upper limit: 6 grams salt from mixed food sources per day. Lower limit: not defined.

Healthy People 2000
- Decrease salt and sodium intake so that at least 65% of home meal preparers prepare foods without adding salt, at least 80% of people avoid using salt at the table, and at least 40% of adults regularly purchase foods modified or lower in sodium.

Dietary Guidelines
- Choose a diet moderate in salt and sodium.

More on factors relating to hypertension and cancer in Chapter 11.

those whose parents had high blood pressure, and people over 50. Salt responders benefit from mild salt restriction, but others with hypertension may not.[18]

Other valid reasons exist for most people to hold their salt intakes below the recommended maximum. For example, excessive salt may directly stress a weakened heart.[19] Also, Asians' high salt intakes have been suggested as a possible cause for their greatly elevated rate of stomach cancer.[20] A study has aroused suspicion that dietary sodium may also worsen asthma in men (the researchers did not study women).[21] Men with asthma should take note: a moderate reduction in sodium intake is harmless and may bring some relief from asthma. Table 8-6 offers tips for cutting down on salt and sodium in the diet.

An obvious step in controlling salt intake is to control the saltshaker, but this source may contribute as little as 15 percent of the total salt consumed. A more productive step may be to cut down on processed and fast foods, the source of almost 75 percent of salt in the U.S. diet.[22] Notice, too, from Table 8-7, that in each food group the least processed foods are not only lowest in sodium but also highest in potassium, an added benefit. Figure 8-6 and this Chapter's Do It! section go on to identify some sodium sources in the U.S. diet.

✓ **KEY POINT** **Sodium is the main positively charged ion outside the body's cells. Sodium attracts water. Thus too much sodium (or salt) may aggravate hypertension. Diets rarely lack sodium.**

TABLE 8-6

How to Cut Salt Intake

Foods eaten without salt may seem less tasty at first, but with repetition, tastes adjust and the natural flavor becomes the preferred taste. Strategies to cut salt intake include:

- Cook with only small amounts of added salt; add little or no salt at the table.
- Prepare foods with sodium-free spices such as basil, bay leaves, curry, garlic, ginger, lemon, mint, oregano, pepper, rosemary, and thyme.
- Read labels with an eye open for salt. (See Table 2-8 on page 57 for terms used to describe the sodium contents of foods on labels.)
- Choose high-salt foods only rarely and in small portions; use low-salt or salt-free products regularly.

Use these foods sparingly:

- Foods prepared in brine, such as pickles, olives, and sauerkraut.
- Salty or smoked meats, such as bologna, corned or chipped beef, frankfurters, ham, lunch meats, salt pork, sausage, and smoked tongue.
- Salty or smoked fish, such as anchovies, caviar, salted and dried cod, herring, sardines, and smoked salmon.
- Snack items such as potato chips, pretzels, salted popcorn, salted nuts, and crackers.
- Fast foods, such as pizza, chicken nuggets, fish and chips, tacos, sausage biscuits, fried chicken, convenience dinners, frozen TV dinners, canned pastas (except versions of all these labeled *healthy* or *low-sodium*).
- Bouillon cubes; seasoned salts; soy, Worcestershire, and barbecue sauces.
- Cheeses, especially processed types.
- Canned and instant soups.
- Prepared horseradish, ketchup, and mustard.

TABLE 8-7

Processing Reduces Potassium, Increases Sodium in Foods

Food	Potassium (mg)	Sodium (mg)	Ratio
Milk Products			
Milk (whole), 1 c	371	120	3:1
Chocolate pudding, 1 c (home cooked)	506	274	2:1
Chocolate pudding, 1 c (instant)	488	834	1:2
Meats			
Beef Roast (cooked), 3 oz	336	53	6:1
Corned beef (canned), 3 oz	115	855	1:7
Frankfurter, 1 large	95	638	1:7
Chipped beef, 3 oz	377	2,953	1:8
Vegetables			
Corn (cooked), 1 c	228	8	28:1
Creamed corn (canned), 1 c	344	730	1:2
Cornflakes, 1 c	23	256	1:11
Fruits			
Peaches (fresh), 1	171	1	171:1
Peaches (canned), 1	149	10	15:1
Peach pie, 1 piece	158	340	1:2
Grains			
Whole-wheat flour, 1 c	486	6	81:1
Shredded wheat cereal, 1 c	155	4	39:1
Whole-wheat bread, 1 slice	88	184	1:2
Wheat crackers, 4	15	64	1:4

FIGURE 8-6

SOURCES OF SODIUM IN THE U.S. DIET

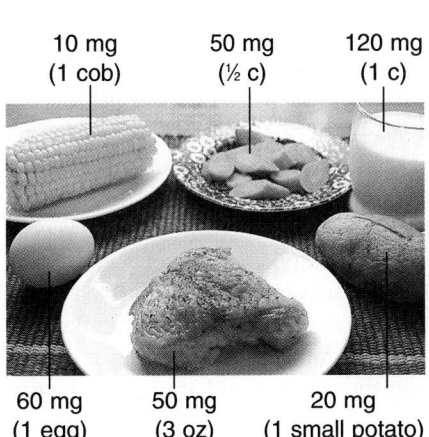

10 mg (1 cob)   50 mg (½ c)   120 mg (1 c)

60 mg (1 egg)   50 mg (3 oz)   20 mg (1 small potato)

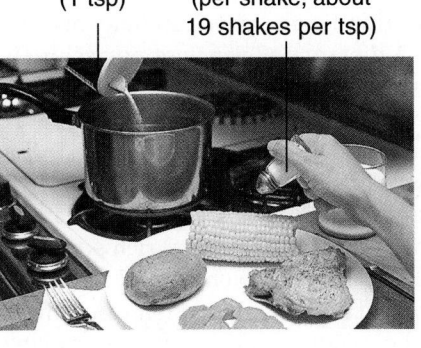

1,900 mg (1 tsp)   100 mg (per shake; about 19 shakes per tsp)

400 mg (½ c)   1,820 mg (1 TV dinner)   900 mg (½ c)   830 mg (1 pickle)

300 mg (½ c)   400 mg (1 oz slice)   1,280 mg (3 oz)   1,470 mg (1 fast-food breakfast biscuit)

725 mg (1 small cheeseburger)

Unprocessed foods that are low in sodium contribute less than 10 percent of the total sodium in the U.S. diet.

Salt added at home, in cooking or at the table, contributes 15 percent of the total sodium in the U.S. diet.

Processed foods such as these contribute 75 percent of the sodium in the U.S. diet.

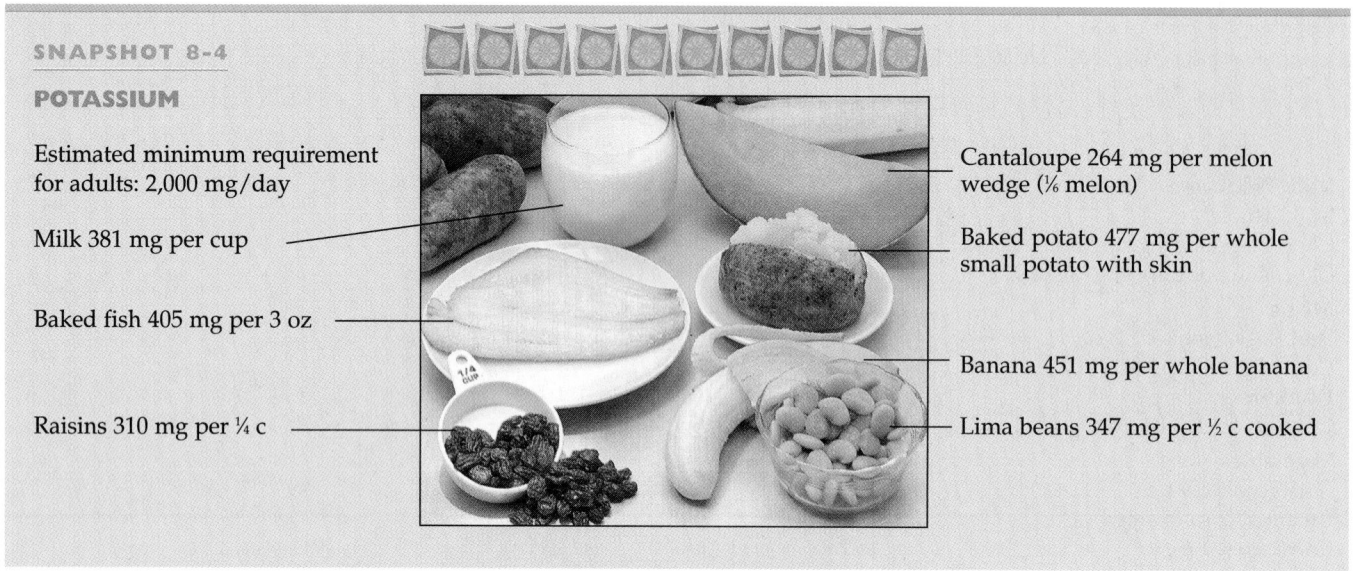

SNAPSHOT 8-4

POTASSIUM

Estimated minimum requirement for adults: 2,000 mg/day

Milk 381 mg per cup

Baked fish 405 mg per 3 oz

Raisins 310 mg per ¼ c

Cantaloupe 264 mg per melon wedge (⅙ melon)

Baked potato 477 mg per whole small potato with skin

Banana 451 mg per whole banana

Lima beans 347 mg per ½ c cooked

Kwashiorkor was described in Chapter 6.

Unlike sodium, potassium may exert a positive effect against hypertension and related ills. See Chapter 11 for details.

Potassium

Potassium is the principal positively charged ion inside body cells. It plays a major role in maintaining fluid and electrolyte balance and cell integrity. It is also critical to maintaining the heartbeat. The sudden deaths that occur during fasting or severe diarrhea and in kwashiorkor children or people with eating disorders are thought to be due to heart failure caused by potassium loss.

Dehydration leads to potassium loss from inside cells. It is especially dangerous because potassium loss from brain cells makes the victim unaware of the need for water. For this reason, adults are warned not to take diuretics (water pills) that cause potassium loss except under a physician's supervision. When taking such diuretics, a person should alert all other health-care providers to their use. Any physician prescribing such diuretics will tell the client to eat potassium-rich foods to compensate for the losses. Depending on the diuretic, the physician may also advise a lower sodium intake.

A dietary deficiency of potassium is unlikely in healthy people, although a low potassium intake is possible with a steady diet of highly processed foods. Because potassium is found inside all living cells and because cells remain intact unless foods are processed, the richest sources of potassium are *fresh* foods of all kinds (see Snapshot 8-4). Most whole vegetables and fruits are outstanding. Bananas, despite their fame as the richest potassium source, are just one choice among many rich sources. Bananas, however, are available everywhere, are easy to chew, and have a sweet taste that almost everyone likes, so health-care providers often recommend them to enhance potassium intake.

Potassium chloride pills are available over the counter and are sold in health food stores without a warning label, but they should not be used except on a physician's advice. People's lives are not normally threatened by potassium overdoses as long as they are taken by mouth because the presence of excess potassium in the stomach triggers a vomiting reflex that expels the unwanted substance. A person with a weak heart, however, should not be put through this trauma, and a baby may not be able to withstand it. Several infants have died when well-meaning parents overdosed them with potassium supplements.

☑ **KEY POINT**   **Potassium, the major positive ion inside cells, is important in many metabolic functions. Fresh foods are the best sources of potassium. Diuretics can deplete the potassium and so can be dangerous; potassium excess can also be dangerous.**

Chloride and Sulfur

The chloride ion is a major negative ion in the body. In the fluids outside the cells, it accompanies sodium; inside the cells, it occurs primarily in association with potassium. Thus it helps to maintain the crucial fluid balances (acid–base and electrolyte balances) mentioned earlier in the discussion of water. The chloride ion also plays a special role as part of the hydrochloric acid that maintains the strong acidity of the stomach. Its principal food source is salt, both added and naturally occurring in foods. In its elemental form, chlorine forms a deadly green gas; dissolved in fluid, chlorine can be useful as a disinfectant, but it must be handled carefully.

As for sulfur, the body does not use it by itself as a nutrient, but it is present in essential nutrients that the body does use, such as thiamin and all proteins. Sulfur plays its most important role in helping strands of protein to assume a particular shape. Skin, hair, and nails contain some of the body's more rigid proteins, which have high sulfur contents.

There is no recommended intake for sulfur, and deficiencies are unknown. The summary table at the end of this chapter presents the main facts about the major minerals.

☑ **KEY POINT**   **Chloride is the body's major negative ion inside and outside of cells. It is essential to the acid–base balance and is part of the stomach's hydrochloric acid necessary to digest protein. Sulfur is also considered a major mineral, although it occurs only as part of other compounds such as protein.**

THE TRACE MINERALS

An obstacle to determining the precise roles of the trace elements is the difficulty of providing an experimental diet lacking in the one element under study. Thus research in this area is limited mostly to the study of laboratory animals, which can be fed highly refined, purified diets in environments that are free of all contamination. Laboratory techniques developed in the last two decades have enabled scientists to detect minerals in smaller and smaller quantities in living cells and research is now rapidly expanding knowledge about them. Whole books have been published on the trace minerals alone. As Table 8-8 shows, the committee on RDA has established recommended dietary allowances for the best-known trace elements—iron, zinc, iodine, and selenium. Tentative ranges for safe and adequate daily intakes of others are also published. Still others are recognized as essential nutrients for some animals, but have not been proven to be required for human beings.

TABLE 8-8

Trace Minerals

RDA Nutrients
Iron Zinc Iodine Selenium
Safe and Adequate Daily Dietary Intakes Established
Copper Manganese Fluoride Chromium Molybdenum
Known Essential for Animals; Human Requirements under Study
Arsenic Nickel Silicon Boron
Known Essential for Some Animals; No Evidence That Intake by Humans Is Ever Limiting: No RDA Necessary
Cobalt

The evidence for requirements and essentiality is weak for the trace minerals cadmium, lead, lithium, tin, and vanadium.

goiter (GOY-ter) enlargement of the thyroid gland due to iodine deficiency is *simple goiter*; goiter due to an excess is *toxic goiter*.

cretinism (CREE-tin-ism) severe mental and physical retardation of an infant caused by the mother's iodine deficiency during her pregnancy.

Iodine

Iodine is needed by the body in an infinitesimally small quantity, but its principal role in human nutrition makes obtaining this amount critical. Iodine is a part of thyroxine, the hormone responsible for regulating the basal metabolic rate. Iodine must be available for thyroxine to be synthesized.

When the iodine concentration of the blood is low, the cells of the thyroid gland enlarge in an attempt to trap as many particles of iodine as possible. Sometimes the gland enlarges until it makes a visible lump in the neck, a **goiter.** People with iodine deficiency this severe suffer sluggishness and weight gain. In a pregnant woman, severe iodine deficiency causes extreme and irreversible mental and physical retardation of the infant known as **cretinism.** Much of the mental retardation can be averted if the pregnant woman's deficiency is detected and treated within the first six months of pregnancy, but if treatment comes too late or not at all, the child may live his or her whole life with an IQ as low as 20 (100 is average).[23] Iodine deficiency is one of the world's most common and most preventable causes of mental retardation.[24] In developing nations, both cretinism and goiter pose problems of enormous proportions.[25]

The iodine in food varies. Generally, it reflects the soil in which plants are grown or on which animals graze. Iodine is plentiful in the ocean, so seafood is a completely dependable source. In the central parts of the United States that were never under the ocean, the soil is poor in iodine. In those areas, the use of iodized salt and the consumption of foods shipped in from iodine-rich areas have been necessary to wipe out the iodine deficiency that once was widespread. Surprisingly, sea salt delivers little iodine to the eater because iodine becomes a gas and flies off into the air during the salt-drying process. In the United States, salt box labels state whether salt is iodized; in Canada all table salt is iodized.

A dramatic increase in iodine intakes in the United States concerns some observers. Excessive intakes of iodine can cause an enlargement of the thyroid gland resembling goiter, which in infants can block the airways and cause suffocation.[26] Intakes reached an all-time high of 800 micrograms per person per day in 1974; since then, intakes have declined somewhat but are still several times the RDA of 150 micrograms. The toxic level at which detectable harm results is thought to be over 2,000 micrograms per day for an adult, an amount only a few times higher than the amount most people receive daily. Like chlorine and fluorine, iodine is a deadly poison in large amounts.

Much of the excess iodine in U.S. diets today comes from bakery products and from milk. The baking industry uses iodine-containing dough conditioners, and most dairies feed cows iodine-containing medications and use iodine to disinfect milking equipment. One cup of milk supplies nearly the RDA of iodine, and so does less than a half teaspoon of iodized salt.[27] Both the dairy and bakery industries have been reducing their use of iodine compounds, but the emergence of this problem points to a need for continued surveillance of the food supply.

✓ **KEY POINT** **Iodine is part of the hormone thyroxine, which influences energy metabolism. The deficiency diseases are goiter and cretinism. Iodine occurs naturally in seafood and in foods grown on land that was once covered by oceans; it is an additive in milk and bakery products. Large amounts are poisonous.**

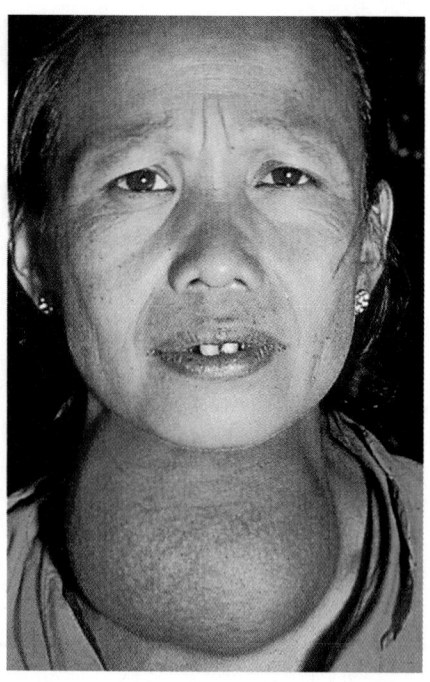

In iodine deficiency, the thyroid gland enlarges—a condition known as simple goiter.

Iron

Every living cell, whether plant or animal, contains iron. Most of the iron in the body is a component of the proteins **hemoglobin** in red blood cells and **myoglobin** in muscle cells. Hemoglobin in the blood carries oxygen from the lungs to tissues throughout the body. Myoglobin carries and stores oxygen for the muscles. Both hemoglobin and myoglobin contain iron, and the iron helps them to hold and carry oxygen and then release it.

All the body's cells need oxygen to help them handle the carbon and hydrogen atoms they release as they break down energy nutrients. The oxygen combines with these atoms to form the waste products carbon dioxide and water; thus the body constantly needs fresh oxygen and nutrients to keep the cells going. As cells use up and excrete their oxygen (as carbon dioxide and water), red blood cells shuttle between the metabolizing tissues and the lungs to bring in fresh oxygen supplies. Besides helping hemoglobin to carry oxygen around and myoglobin to hold it in muscles, iron helps many enzymes in energy pathways to use oxygen. Iron is also needed to make new cells, amino acids, hormones, and neurotransmitters.

Iron is clearly the body's gold, a precious mineral to be tightly hoarded. The liver packs iron sent from the bone marrow into new red blood cells and ships them out to the blood, where they live for about three to four months. When red blood cells die, the spleen and liver break them down, save their iron, and send it back to the bone marrow to be kept for reuse. Only tiny losses of iron occur in nail clippings, hair cuttings, and shed skin cells. If bleeding occurs, the loss of blood can cause significant iron loss from the body.

The body has special provisions for obtaining iron. Normally, only about 10 to 15 percent of dietary iron is absorbed; but if the body's supply is diminished or if the need increases for any reason (such as pregnancy), absorption increases.

When Iron Is Lacking If absorption cannot compensate for losses or low dietary intakes, then iron stores are used up and iron deficiency sets in. Iron deficiency and anemia are not one and the same, though they often go hand in hand. The distinction between **iron deficiency** and **iron-deficiency anemia** is a matter of degree. People may be iron deficient, meaning that they have depleted iron stores without being anemic or they may be iron deficient *and* anemic. With regard to iron, the term *anemia* refers to severe depletion of iron stores resulting in low blood hemoglobin.

The body that has been severely deprived of iron becomes unable to make enough hemoglobin to fill its new blood cells—anemia results. A sample of iron-deficient blood examined under the microscope shows smaller cells that are lighter red than normal (see Figure 8-7). The undersized cells contain too little hemoglobin and thus deliver too little oxygen to the tissues. This limits the cells' energy metabolism, so a person with iron-deficiency anemia lacks "get up and go." Tiredness, apathy, and a tendency to feel cold all reflect the energy deficiency of iron-deficiency anemia.

Long before the red blood cells are affected, though, people exhibit the impact of iron deficiency in their behavior. Even at slightly lowered iron levels, physical work capacity and productivity are impaired. With reduced energy available to work, play, think, or learn, people simply do these things less. Because they work and play less, they become less physically fit. Many of the

hemoglobin (HEEM-oh-globe-in) the oxygen-carrying protein of the blood; found in the red blood cells (*hemo* means "blood"; *globin* means spherical protein").

myoglobin (MYE-oh-globe-in) the oxygen-holding protein of the muscles (*myo* means "muscle").

iron deficiency the condition of having depleted iron stores, which, at the extreme, causes iron-deficiency anemia.

iron-deficiency anemia a form of anemia caused by iron deficiency and characterized by red blood cell shrinkage and color loss. Accompanying symptoms are weakness, apathy, headaches, pallor, intolerance to cold, and inability to pay attention. (For other anemias, see the index).

Feeling fatigued, weak, and apathetic is a sign that something is wrong. It is not a sign that you necessarily need iron or other supplements. Two actions are called for: first, get your diet in order; then, if symptoms persist for more than a week or two, consult a physician for a diagnosis.

FIGURE 8-7

NORMAL AND ANEMIC BLOOD CELLS

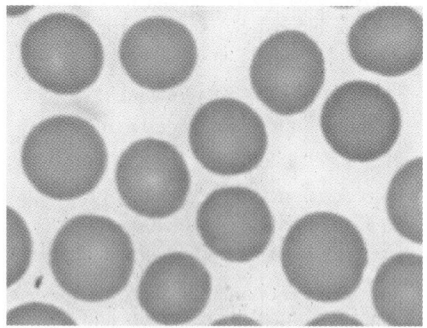

Normal red blood cells. Both size and color are normal.

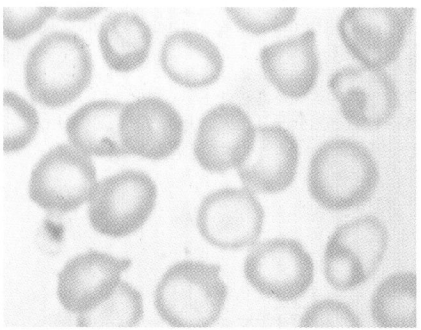

Blood cells in iron-deficiency anemia. These cells are small and pale because they contain less hemoglobin.

pica (PIE-ka) a craving for nonfood substances. Also known as *geophagia* (gee-oh-FAY-gee-uh) when referring to clay eating, and *pagophagia* (pag-oh-FAY-gee-uh) when referring to ice craving (*geo* means "earth"; *pago* means "frost"; *phagia* means "to eat").

iron overload the state of having more iron in the body than it needs or can handle. Too much iron is toxic and can damage the liver.

symptoms associated with iron deficiency are easily mistaken for behavioral or motivational problems. Children deprived of iron become restless, irritable, and unable to pay attention, and they fall behind their peers academically. Such symptoms disappear when iron intakes improve.

A curious symptom seen in some people with iron deficiency is an appetite for ice, clay, paste, and other nonnutritious substances. Such people have been known to eat as many as eight trays of ice in a day. This consumption of non-food substances, usually observed in poverty-stricken women and children, has been given the name **pica.** In many cases, pica clears up dramatically within days after iron is given, even before the red blood cells have had a chance to respond. Other times, pica is unresponsive to iron.

What Causes Iron Deficiency?   The cause of iron deficiency is usually mal-nutrition, that is, inadequate iron intake, either from sheer lack of food or from high consumption of the wrong foods. In the Western world, overconsuming foods rich in sugar and fat and poor in nutrients is often responsible for low iron intakes.

Among nonnutritional causes of anemia, blood loss is the primary one. About 80 percent of the iron in the body is in the blood, so iron losses are great whenever blood is lost. Women's menstrual losses make their iron needs one and a half times as great as men's needs. Anyone who loses blood loses iron. Women are especially vulnerable to iron deficiency because they not only lose more iron than men but also, on average, eat less food. The information about iron in foods, later in this section, is especially important for most women.

In developing countries, parasitic infections of the digestive tract cause people to lose blood daily. For their entire lives, they may feel tired and unener-getic but never know why. Ulcers and other sores of the digestive tract can also cause blood loss severe enough to cause anemia.[28]

Worldwide, iron deficiency is the most common nutrient deficiency.[29] Iron-deficiency anemia affects an estimated 40 percent of the world's population, with the highest prevalence in developing countries.[30] Older infants, young children, and pregnant women are especially vulnerable. Happily, the last decade has brought improvement in the iron status of U.S. infants and young children, thanks to more widespread breastfeeding, which promotes iron absorption, and to greater use of iron-fortified infant formula and cereals.[31] For low-income families, the Special Supplemental Food Program for Women, Infants, and Children (WIC), provides coupons redeemable for foods high in iron, giving another boost to the iron status of many U.S. children.[32]

The Danger of Iron Toxicity   Iron is toxic in large amounts, and once inside the body, it is difficult to excrete. The body's defense against iron poisoning is a control system: the intestinal cells trap some of the iron and hold it within their boundaries. When they are shed, these cells carry out of the intestinal tract the excess iron that they collected during their brief lives.

Some individuals, most often men, are poorly defended against iron toxic-ity. Once considered rare, **iron overload** has emerged as an important iron dis-order that seems to have increased in frequency over the last few decades.[33] Iron overload is caused by a hereditary defect that causes the intestine to help-lessly absorb excess iron. Tissue damage occurs, especially in iron-storing organs such as the liver. Infections are also likely because bacteria thrive on iron-rich blood. The effects are most severe in alcohol abusers because alcohol damages the intestine, impairing its defense against absorbing too much iron.

The body guards against iron's renegade nature. Left free, iron is a powerful oxidant that can start free-radical reactions that damage cellular structures.[34] Protein carriers guard the body's iron molecules and keep them away from vulnerable body compounds, thereby preventing damage. Iron's actions are thus tightly controlled.[35]

An interesting study of Finnish men suggested a link between increased risk of heart disease and elevated iron stores.[36] Among about 20 heart attack risk factors, including smoking, blood pressure, cholesterol, and serum ferritin (the protein that carries iron in the blood), researchers found high serum ferritin doubled the risk of heart attack. The only stronger predictor of heart attack was smoking.

A review of other studies concluded that the data available so far do not completely confirm that there is a link between iron and heart disease. More will be known as research progresses.[37]

Other links between iron and health are possible. Cancer of the colon may be affected by the iron in foods.[38] One report raises a suspicion that iron supplements may stunt normal growth in healthy, well-fed children.[39] Much more work is needed to clarify these associations.

An argument against widespread fortification of foods with iron is that it might put still more people at risk of iron overload. The U.S. population's love of vitamin C supplements may be worsening the problem because vitamin C greatly enhances iron absorption.[40] In any case, widespread iron fortification of foods makes it difficult for susceptible people to follow a low-iron diet.

Be forewarned against unnecessarily taking supplements that contain iron, and keep such pills safely out of children's reach. Iron supplements are the number one cause of fatal accidental poisonings among U.S. children under three years old.[41] The FDA has called for a label warning for parents that states "iron may be lethal to children."[42]

Iron Recommendations and Sources   The iron RDA is 10 milligrams a day for men and women past age 51. For women of childbearing age, the RDA is high, 15 milligrams, to replace menstrual losses. During pregnancy, a woman needs double this amount, 30 milligrams. Adult men rarely experience iron-deficiency anemia. Should a man have a low hemoglobin concentration, this alerts his health-care provider to examine him for a blood-loss site. Table 8-9 sums up iron recommendations.

To meet iron needs, it is best to rely on foods, since the iron from supplements is much less well absorbed than that from food. However, the usual Western mixed diet provides only about 5 to 6 milligrams of iron in each 1,000 calories, not enough for some people. An adult male who eats 2,500 calories or more a day has no trouble meeting his RDA of 10 milligrams, but a woman who eats fewer calories and needs more iron understandably does have trouble meeting her need. To meet it, she must select high-iron, low-calorie foods from each food group.

Iron occurs in two forms in foods. Some is bound into **heme,** the iron-containing part of hemoglobin and myoglobin in meat, poultry, and fish. Some is nonheme iron, the kind in foods from plants and the nonheme iron in meats. The form affects absorption.

Table 8-13, pp. 320–321, summarizes the effects of iron toxicity.

Dietary factors that increase iron absorption
- Vitamin C
- MFP factor

Factors that hinder iron absorption
- Tea
- Coffee
- Calcium and phosphorus
- Phytates and fiber

heme (HEEM) the iron-containing portion of the hemoglobin and myoglobin molecules.

MFP factor a factor (identity unknown) present in meat, fish, and poultry that enhances the absorption of nonheme iron present in the same foods or in other foods eaten at the same time.

phytates compounds present in plant foods (particularly whole grains) that bind iron and prevent its absorption.

tannins compounds in tea (especially black tea), and coffee that bind iron. Tannins also denature proteins.

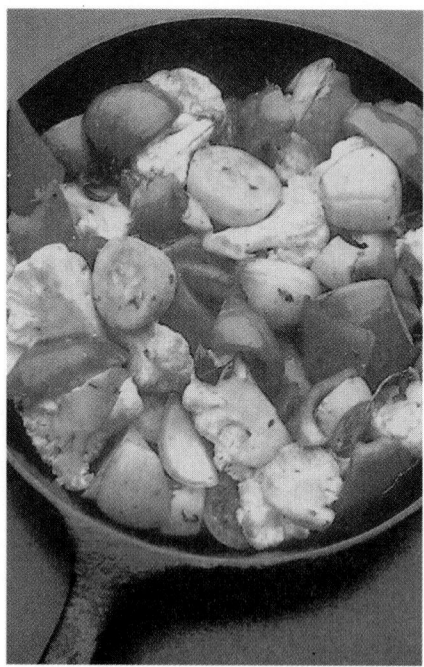

The old-fashioned iron skillet adds supplemental iron to foods.

TABLE 8-9

Iron Intake Recommendations

Recommended Dietary Allowances (RDA)[a]
- Men   (19–50 yr) 10 mg/day.
            (51 yr and older) 10 mg/day
- Women (19–50 yr) 15 mg/day
            (51 yr and older) 10 mg/day.

Healthy People 2000
- Reduce iron deficiency to less than 3% among children aged 1 to 4 and among women of childbearing age.

[a]Canadian values are listed in Canadiana, Appendix B.

Absorbing Iron   Heme iron is much more reliably absorbed than is nonheme iron. Healthy people with adequate iron stores absorb heme iron at a rate of about 23 percent over a wide range of meat intakes. People absorb nonheme iron at rates of 2 to 20 percent, depending on dietary factors and iron stores.

Meat, fish, and poultry contain a factor **(MFP factor)** other than heme that promotes the absorption of nonheme iron from other foods eaten with it. Vitamin C also proves to be a potent promoter of iron absorption and can triple nonheme iron absorption from foods eaten in the same meal.[43] A system of calculating the amount of iron absorbed from a meal, based on these factors, is presented in Table 8-10.

Some factors impair iron absorption. These include tea, coffee, the calcium and phosphorus in milk, and the **phytates** and **tannins** in fiber in whole-grain cereals. Ordinary black tea is so efficient at reducing absorption of iron that clinical dietitians advise people with iron overload to drink it with their meals. For those who need more iron, the opposite advice applies—don't drink tea with food. Snapshot 8-5 shows iron amounts in foods regarded as iron-rich sources.

The amount of iron ultimately absorbed from a meal depends on the interaction between promoters of iron absorption and inhibitors. When you eat meat with legumes (for example, ham and beans or chili with beans and meat), MFP factor enhances iron absorption from both. The vitamin C from a slice of tomato and a leaf of lettuce in a sandwich will enhance iron absorption from the bread. The meat and tomato in spaghetti sauce help the eater absorb the iron from the spaghetti. A sauce cooked in an iron pan draws iron from this source, too.

Foods cooked in iron pans contain iron salts somewhat like those in supplements. The iron content of 100 grams of spaghetti sauce simmered in a glass dish is 3 milligrams, but it is 87 milligrams when the sauce is cooked in a black iron skillet. Even in the short time it takes to scramble eggs, a cook can triple the eggs' iron content by scrambling them in an iron pan. Similarly, the reason dried peaches or raisins contain more iron than the fresh fruit is because they are dried in iron pans. This iron salt is not as well absorbed as iron from meat, but some does get into the body, especially if the meal also contains MFP factor or vitamin C.

TABLE 8-10

Calculation of Iron Absorbed from Meals

Three factors go into the calculation of the amount of iron absorbed from a meal: first, how much of the iron in the meal was heme iron and how much was nonheme iron; second, how much vitamin C was in the meal; and third, how much total meat, fish, and poultry (MFP factor) was consumed. (It is assumed your iron stores are moderate; otherwise, you'd have to take this into consideration, too.) Write down the foods you eat at a typical meal, look up their iron content in the Table of Food Composition, Appendix A, and then answer these questions:

1. How much iron was from animal tissues (MFP)? _____ mg.
2. 40% of (1), on the average, is heme iron: (1) _____ mg × 0.40 = _____ mg heme iron.
3. How much iron was from other sources? _____ mg.
4. This (3), plus 60% of (1), is nonheme iron: (3) _____ mg + 0.60 × (1) _____ mg = _____ mg nonheme iron.
5. How much vitamin C was in the meal? Less than 25 mg is low; 25 to 75 mg is medium; more than 75 mg is high. _____ mg.
6. How much MFP factor was in the meal? Less than 1 oz lean MFP is low; 1 to 3 oz is medium; more than 3 oz is high.[a] _____ oz.
7. Now calculate the heme iron absorbed. You absorbed 23% of the heme iron, or (2) _____ mg × 0.23 = _____ mg heme iron absorbed.
8. Now, take your best score from (5) and (6). If either vitamin C or MFP factor was high or if both were medium, the availability of your nonheme iron was high. If neither was high, but one was medium, the availability of your nonheme iron was medium. If both were low, your nonheme iron had poor availability. You absorbed:

   - High availability: 8% of the nonheme iron.
   - Medium availability: 5% of the nonheme iron.
   - Poor availability: 3% of the nonheme iron.

9. Now calculate the nonheme iron absorbed. You absorbed _____ % of the nonheme iron, or (4) _____ mg × _____ = _____ mg nonheme iron absorbed.
10. Add the heme and nonheme iron from (7) and (9) together:

    - _____ mg heme iron absorbed.
    - _____ mg nonheme iron absorbed.

    Total = _____ mg iron absorbed.

The RDA assumes you will absorb 10% of the iron you ingest. Thus, if you are a man over age 18 or a woman over age 50 (RDA 10 mg), you need to absorb 1 mg per day. If you are a woman 11 to 50 years old (RDA 15 mg), you need to absorb 1.5 mg per day. If you have higher menstrual losses than the average woman, you may need still more.

[a]We have adapted the calculation of Monsen and coauthors, stating it in ounces. Her actual numbers are less than 23 g cooked meat, low; 23 to 46 g, medium; and 69 g or more, high.

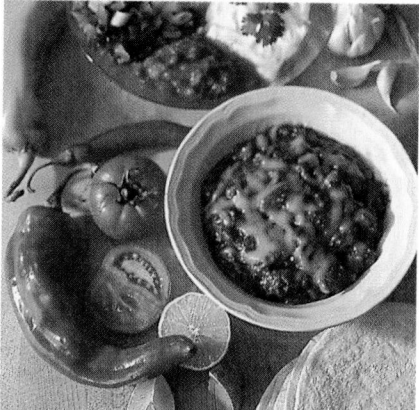

This chili dinner provides iron and MFP factor from meat, iron from legumes, and vitamin C from tomatoes. The combination of heme iron, nonheme iron, MFP factor, and vitamin C helps to achieve maximum iron absorption.

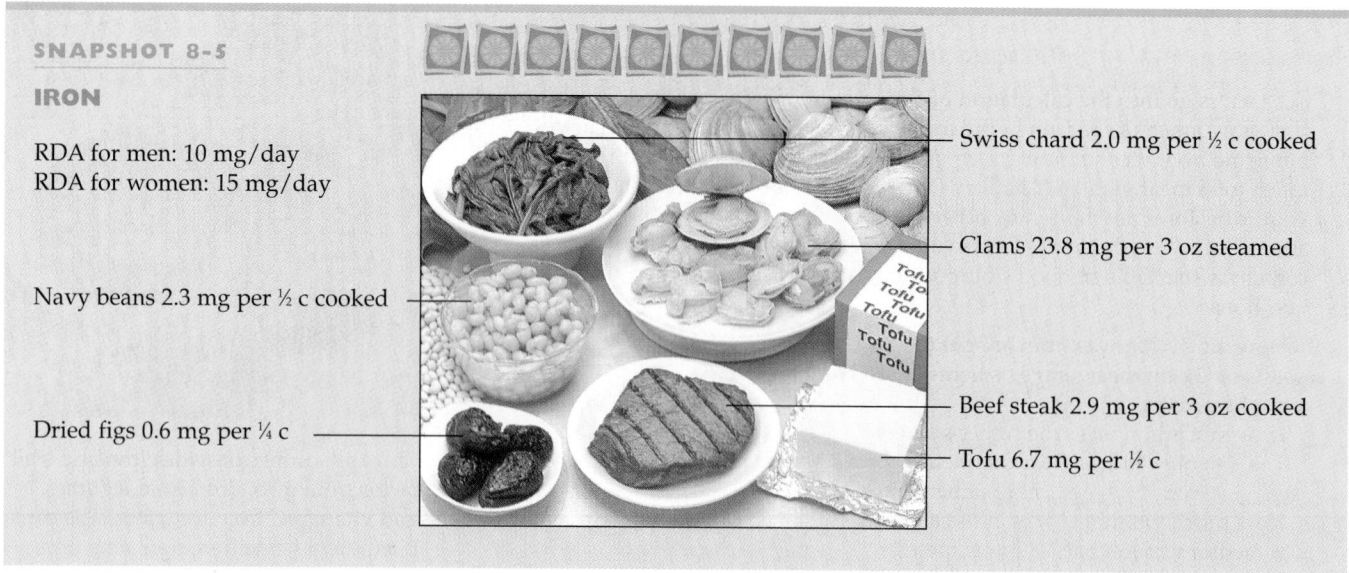

SNAPSHOT 8-5

IRON

RDA for men: 10 mg/day
RDA for women: 15 mg/day

Navy beans 2.3 mg per ½ c cooked

Dried figs 0.6 mg per ¼ c

Swiss chard 2.0 mg per ½ c cooked

Clams 23.8 mg per 3 oz steamed

Beef steak 2.9 mg per 3 oz cooked

Tofu 6.7 mg per ½ c

leavened (LEV-end): literally, "lightened" by yeast cells, which digest some carbohydrate components of the dough and leave behind bubbles of gas which make the bread rise.

✔ **KEY POINT** **Most iron in the body is contained in hemoglobin and myoglobin or occurs as part of enzymes in the energy-yielding pathways. Iron-deficiency anemia is a problem worldwide; too much iron is toxic. Iron is lost through menstruation and other bleeding; the shedding of intestinal cells protects against overload. For maximum iron absorption, use meat, other iron sources, and vitamin C together.**

Zinc

Zinc occurs in a very small quantity in the body, but works with proteins in every organ. It helps more than 100 enzymes to:

- Make parts of cells' genetic material.
- Make heme in hemoglobin.
- Help the pancreas with its digestive functions.
- Help metabolize carbohydrate, protein, and fat.
- Liberate vitamin A from storage in the liver.
- Dispose of damaging free radicals.

Zinc also affects behavior and learning, assists in immune function, and is essential to wound healing, sperm production, taste perception, fetal development, and growth and development in children. Zinc is needed to produce the active form of vitamin A in visual pigments. When zinc deficiency occurs, it impairs all these and other functions. Even a mild zinc deficiency can result in impaired immunity, abnormal taste, and abnormal vision in the dark.[44]

Problem: Too Little Zinc Zinc deficiency in human beings was first reported in the 1960s from studies with growing children and adolescent boys in the Middle East. The native diets were typically low in animal protein and high in whole grains and beans; consequently, they were high in fiber and phytates, which bind zinc as well as iron. Furthermore, the bread was not the **leavened** type; in leavened bread, yeast breaks down phytates.

Since the first reports, zinc deficiency has been recognized elsewhere, and it is known to affect much more than just growth. It alters digestive function profoundly and causes diarrhea, which worsens the malnutrition already present, with respect not only to zinc but to all nutrients. It drastically impairs the immune response, making infections likely. Infections of the intestinal tract worsen malnutrition, including zinc malnutrition. Normal vitamin metabolism depends on zinc, so zinc-deficiency symptoms often include vitamin-deficiency symptoms. Zinc deficiency also disturbs thyroid function and slows the body's energy metabolism. It causes loss of appetite and slows wound healing. In fact, its symptoms are so pervasive that when faced with it, physicians are more likely to diagnose it as general malnutrition and sickness than as zinc deficiency.

While severe zinc deficiencies are not widespread in developed countries, they occur among some groups, including pregnant women, young children, the elderly, and the poor. Among these people, poor growth, poor appetite, and impaired taste sensitivity may indicate zinc deficiency. When pediatricians or other health workers evaluating children's health note poor growth accompanied by poor appetite, they should think zinc.

Problem: Too Much Zinc   Zinc is toxic in large quantities, and zinc supplements can cause serious illness or even death in high enough doses. Doses of zinc only a few milligrams above the RDA, especially when taken regularly over time, block copper absorption and lower the body's copper content, an effect that, in animals, leads to degeneration of the heart muscle.[45] In high doses, zinc also alters cholesterol metabolism and appears to accelerate the development of atherosclerosis.

High doses of zinc can also inhibit iron absorption from the digestive tract.[46] In the blood, a protein that carries iron from the digestive tract to tissues that need it also carries some zinc. If this protein is burdened with excess zinc, little or no room is left for iron to be picked up from the intestine. The opposite is also true; too much iron leaves little room for zinc to be picked up, thus impairing zinc absorption. Zinc and iron are often found together in foods, but food sources are safe and never cause imbalances like these in the body. Supplements, though, can easily do so.

Unlike excess iron, excess zinc has a normal escape route from the body. The pancreas secretes zinc-rich juices into the digestive tract, and some of these are excreted. Still, overdoses from zinc supplements can overwhelm the escape route and cause toxicity. Thus zinc supplements should be avoided unless prescribed by a physician.

Meats, shellfish, and poultry are top providers of zinc (see Snapshot 8-6). Among plant sources, some legumes and whole grains are rich in zinc, but the zinc is not as well absorbed from them as from meat.[47] Most people probably do not meet the RDA of 15 milligrams per day for men and 12 milligrams per day for women; the average intake is probably closer to 10 milligrams. Vegetarians are advised to eat varied diets that include whole-grain breads well leavened with yeast, which helps make zinc available for absorption.

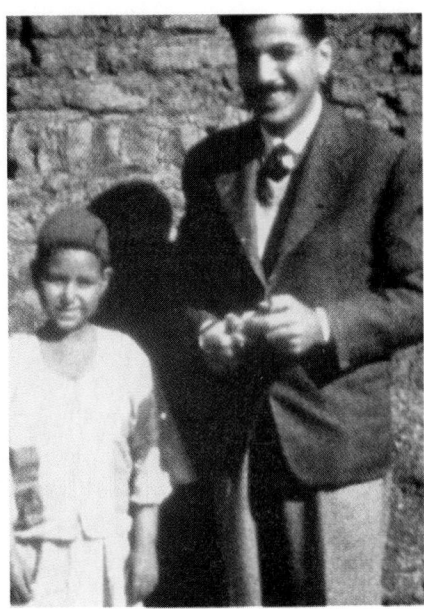

How old does the boy in the picture appear to be? He is 17 years old but is only 4 feet tall, the height of a seven-year-old in the United States. His genitalia are like those of a six-year-old. The retardation is rightly ascribed to zinc deficiency because it is partially reversible when zinc is restored to the diet. The photo was taken in Egypt.

✔ **KEY POINT** **Zinc assists enzymes in all cells. Deficiencies in children cause growth retardation with sexual immaturity. Zinc is toxic in large amounts. Animal foods are the best sources.**

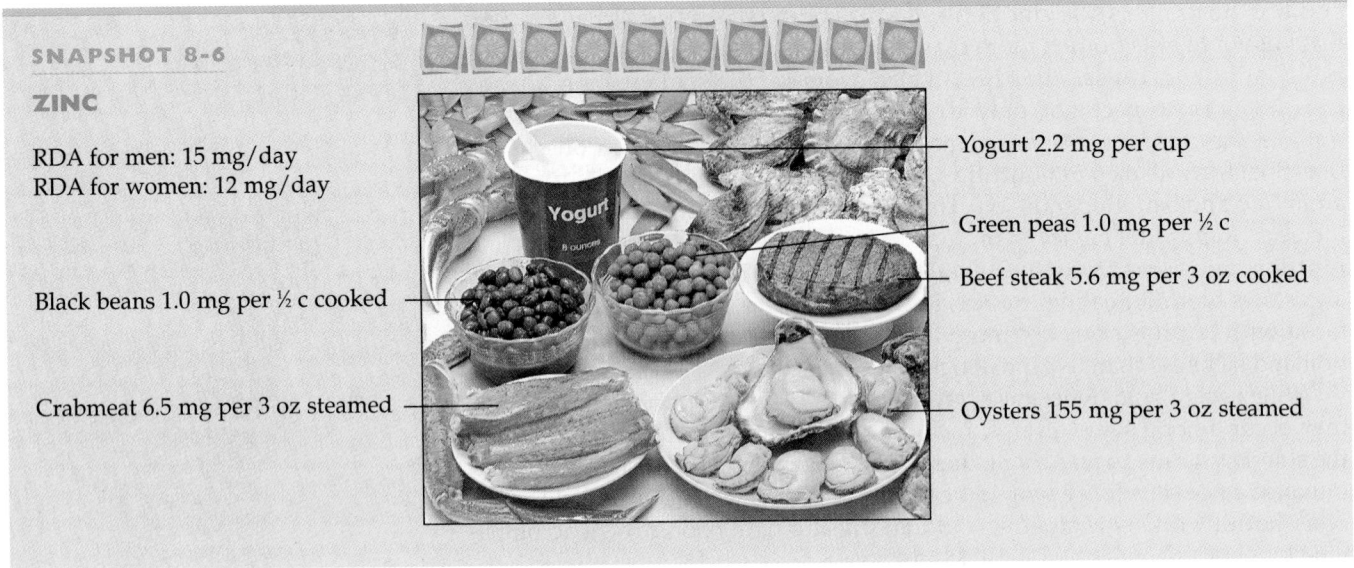

ZINC

RDA for men: 15 mg/day
RDA for women: 12 mg/day

Black beans 1.0 mg per ½ c cooked

Crabmeat 6.5 mg per 3 oz steamed

Yogurt 2.2 mg per cup

Green peas 1.0 mg per ½ c

Beef steak 5.6 mg per 3 oz cooked

Oysters 155 mg per 3 oz steamed

Selenium

Selenium has been attracting attention for its antioxidant activity in protecting vulnerable body chemicals from oxidation. Selenium assists an enzyme in preventing free-radical formation. If free radicals do form, vitamin E halts the destructive chain reaction. Thus selenium and vitamin E work in concert. The question of whether selenium protects against the development of cancers is currently under investigation. So far the results are inconclusive.[48] Among the most recent discoveries about selenium is that it plays a role in activating thyroid hormone, the hormone that regulates the body's rate of metabolism.[49]

A deficiency of selenium can open the way for a specific type of heart disease (unrelated to the heart disease discussed in Chapters 5 and 11). The condition, first identified in China among people from areas with selenium-deficient soils, prompted researchers to give this mineral its rightful place among the essential nutrients (see the inside front cover; page B lists selenium's RDA value). Foods grown on U.S. and Canadian soils supply plenty of selenium.

Anyone who eats a normal diet composed of mostly unprocessed foods need not worry about selenium. It is widely distributed in foods such as meats and shellfish and in vegetables and grains grown on selenium-rich soil. From current indications, it is likely that most people in the United States receive well over the RDA amount, partly because they eat supermarket foods transported from many regions, and partly because they eat meat, a rich source of selenium.[50]

Toxicity is possible, especially when people take selenium supplements over a long period. Selenium toxicity brings on symptoms such as hair loss, diarrhea, and nerve abnormalities. Selenium supplements taken inappropriately as an anticancer agent make selenium toxicity likely.[51]

✔ KEY POINT   **Selenium works with vitamin E to protect body compounds from oxidation. A deficiency induces a disease of the heart. Defi-**

ciencies in developed countries are rare, but toxicities occur from overuse of supplements.

fluorosis (floor-OH-sis) discoloration of the teeth due to ingestion of too much fluoride during tooth development.

Fluoride

Fluoride has not been proven to be an essential nutrient.[52] Only a trace of fluoride occurs in the human body, but with this amount the crystalline deposits in bones and teeth are larger and more perfectly formed. As mentioned earlier, fluoride replaces the hydroxy portion of hydroxyapatite, forming the more decay-resistant fluorapatite.

Drinking water is the usual source of fluoride. In communities in which the water contains too much—2 to 8 parts per million—discoloration of the teeth, or **fluorosis,** may occur. Where fluoride is lacking, the incidence of dental decay is very high. Fluoridation of water to raise its fluoride concentration to 1 part per million is recommended as an important public health measure. Those fortunate enough to have had sufficient fluoride during the tooth-forming years of infancy and childhood are protected from tooth decay throughout life.[53] Figure 8-8 shows the extent of fluoridation nationwide; states that have adopted fluoridation in more than half of their counties are shown in color.

Despite fluoride's value, violent disagreement often surrounds the decision to fluoridate community water. Proponents argue that fluoridation is an obvious, safe, and cost-effective measure to help prevent dental caries in the young.[54] Opponents argue that altering the community water supply is "unnatural" and deprives its consumers of the freedom to refuse to take fluoride. They may claim that communities using fluoridated water have an increased cancer rate, but studies show no connection.

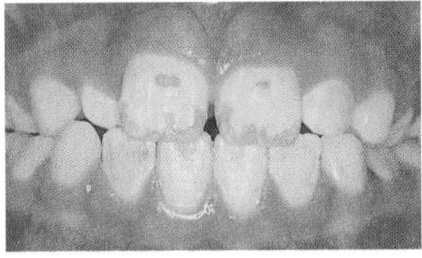

Fluorosis.

FIGURE 8-8

FLUORIDATION IN THE UNITED STATES

SOURCE: Fluoridation Census 1989 Summary, U.S. Department of Health and Human Services, Public Health Service, Centers for Disease Control and Prevention, National Center for Prevention Services, Division of Oral Health, Atlanta, GA, April 1993.

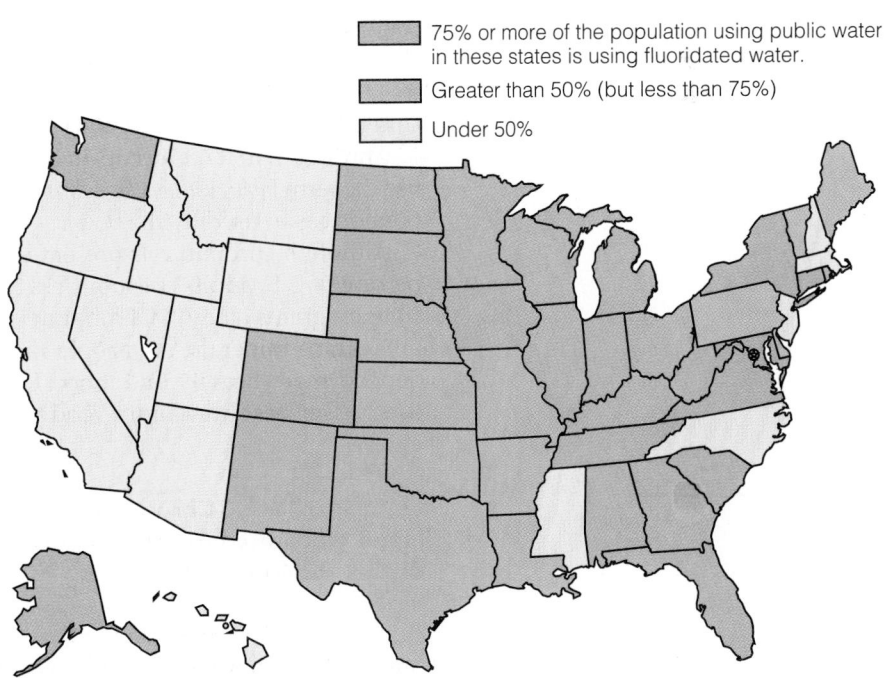

75% or more of the population using public water in these states is using fluoridated water.

Greater than 50% (but less than 75%)

Under 50%

Opponents of fluoridation also fear accidental overdoses. In fact, serious cases of fluoride poisoning have occurred when public water systems failed and allowed fluoride to reach toxic concentrations.[55] Such incidents make a strong case for vigorous monitoring of those responsible for public water supplies. Also, now that fluoride has been added to many water supplies, the amounts in foods processed with use of that water are increasing. The total fluoride consumed by certain populations may therefore be greater than expected. No hazard exists at present levels of fluoride consumption, but fluoride supplements are no longer recommended for children from birth, and recommended doses for older children have been reduced to prevent fluorosis.[56]

On the basis of the accumulated evidence of its beneficial effects, fluoridation has been endorsed by the National Institute of Dental Health, the American Dietetic Association, the American Medical Association, the National Cancer Institute, and the National Nutrition Consortium. The allegation that it causes cancer has no basis in fact and has been refuted by the National Cancer Institute, the American Cancer Society, and the National Institute of Dental Research.

✔ KEY POINT   **Fluoride stabilizes bones and makes teeth resistant to decay. Excess fluoride discolors teeth; large doses are toxic.**

Chromium

Chromium works closely with the hormone insulin to regulate and release energy from glucose. When chromium is lacking, insulin action is impaired, resulting in a diabeteslike condition of high blood glucose that resolves with chromium supplementation.[57] Supplements of chromium cannot cure the common forms of diabetes, of course, but people with diabetes who eat low-chromium diets make their condition worse.[58] Diets high in simple sugars deplete the body's supply of chromium.[59] People who take chromium-containing supplements in hopes of building extra muscle tissue or losing body fat are in for a disappointment. Chromium has no effect on body composition in well-nourished people.[60]

Chromium in foods occurs in complexes with other compounds. Researchers use the term *biologically active chromium** to describe chromium-containing compounds easily used by the body.

Although chromium is present in a variety of foods, it is estimated that 90 percent of U.S. adults consume less than the recommended minimum intake of 50 micrograms a day.[61] Chromium is easily lost during food processing, as are other trace minerals. As people find themselves more pressed for time and depend more heavily on refined foods, chromium deficiencies become more likely. The best chromium food sources are liver, whole grains, nuts, and cheeses.

✔ KEY POINT   **Chromium works with the hormone insulin to control blood glucose concentration. Many adults in the United States have low dietary intakes of chromium.**

---

*An older name for biologically active chromium is *glucose tolerance factor.*

Copper

Among copper's most vital roles are to help form hemoglobin and collagen. Many enzymes depend on copper for its oxygen-handling ability. Copper, like iron, assists in reactions leading to the release of energy. One enzyme that helps to control free-radical activity depends on copper for its activation.* Some researchers are investigating the possibility that a low-copper diet may contribute to heart disease by suppressing the activity of this enzyme.

Copper deficiency is rare but not unknown. It has been seen in children with protein deficiency and iron-deficiency anemia, and it can severely disturb growth and metabolism. In adults, it may impair immunity and blood flow through the arteries.[62] Excess zinc interferes with copper absorption and can cause deficiency.[63] Copper toxicity from foods is unlikely, but supplements can cause it. The best food sources of copper include organ meats, seafood, nuts, and seeds.

✔ KEY POINT   **Copper is needed to form hemoglobin and collagen and in many other body processes. Copper deficiency is rare.**

Other Trace Minerals and Some Candidates

In addition to fluoride, chromium, and copper, estimated safe and adequate daily dietary intakes have been established for two other trace minerals, molybdenum and manganese. Molybdenum functions as part of several metal-containing enzymes, some of which are giant proteins. Manganese works with dozens of different enzymes that facilitate many different body processes.

Several other trace minerals are now recognized as important to health. Research suggests that a low intake of boron may enhance susceptibility to osteoporosis by way of its effects on calcium metabolism.[64] The richest food sources of boron are noncitrus fruits, leafy vegetables, nuts, and legumes. Cobalt is recognized as the mineral in the large vitamin B_{12} molecule; the alternative name for vitamin B_{12}, cobalamin, reflects its presence. Nickel is important for the health of many body tissues; deficiencies harm the liver and other organs. Silicon is known to be involved in bone calcification, at least in animals. The future may reveal key roles played by many other trace minerals including barium, cadmium, lead, lithium, mercury, silver, tin, and vanadium. Even arsenic, a known poison and carcinogen, may turn out to be essential in tiny quantities.

All of the trace minerals are toxic in excess. The hazards of overdoses are among the chief risks faced by people who take multiple nutrient supplements. The way to obtain the trace minerals is from food, which is not hard to do. You need only eat a variety of whole foods in the amounts recommended in the Food Guide Pyramid. Some claim that organically grown foods contain more trace minerals than those grown with chemical fertilizers. Organic fertilizers do contain more trace minerals than do refined chemical fertilizers, and plants do take up some of the minerals they are given, so this claim may turn out to be valid.

---

*The enzyme is superoxide dismutase, first mentioned in Controversy 7.

As research on the trace minerals continues, many interactions among them are also coming to light. An excess of one may cause a deficiency of another. A slight manganese overload, for example, may aggravate an iron deficiency. A deficiency of one may open the way for another to cause a toxic reaction. Iron deficiency, for example, makes the body much more susceptible to lead poisoning than it normally is. Good food sources of one are poor food sources of another, and factors that cooperate with some trace elements oppose others. Vitamin C, for example, enhances the absorption of iron and depresses that of copper. The continuous outpouring of new information about the trace minerals is a sign that we have much more to learn. Table 8-13 on pages 320–321 sums up what this chapter has said about the minerals and fills in some additional information.

✓ KEY POINT　**Many different trace elements play important roles in the body. All of the trace minerals are toxic in excess.**

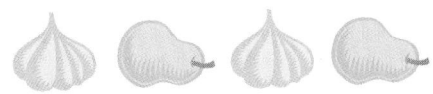

MEETING THE CALCIUM RDA

Label-reader's tip: To convert percent Daily Value for calcium to milligrams, drop the percent sign and add a zero.* Example: 40% Daily Value = 400 mg.

*Note: This tip works for calcium, but not for other minerals.

TABLE 8-11

Recommended Fluid Milk Intakes

Age	Recommended U.S. Daily Intake
Children	2 cups
Teenagers	3 cups
Adults	2 cups
Pregnant or lactating women	3 cups
Pregnant or lactating teens	4 cups

Most people consume far less than the RDA amount of calcium. The average woman meets just a third of her requirement; men do somewhat better, with intakes close to three-fourths of their needs. Low calcium intakes are associated with all sorts of major illnesses, including adult bone loss (see the following Controversy for details), high blood pressure and colon cancer (see Chapter 11), kidney stones, and even lead poisoning.[65] This Food Feature focuses attention on the sources of calcium in the diet.

MILK, YOGURT, AND CHEESE GROUP

Milk and milk products are traditional sources of calcium for people who can tolerate them. Table 8-11 shows the current milk recommendations that help to meet the RDA for various age groups. People who do not use milk because of lactose intolerance, dislike, or allergy must obtain calcium from other sources. Care is needed, though; *wise* substitutions must be made. Most of milk's many relatives are recommended choices: yogurt, **kefir,** buttermilk, cheese (especially the low-fat or nonfat varieties), and, for people who can afford the calories, ice milk. Cottage cheese and frozen yogurt desserts contain about half the calcium of milk, with 2 cups being equivalent in calcium to 1 cup of milk. Butter, cream, and cream cheese are almost pure fat and contain negligible calcium. If no milk product is acceptable as is, consider tinkering with it to make it work. Add cocoa to milk, fruit to yogurt, or nonfat milk powder to any dish.

VEGETABLES

Among vegetables, rutabaga, broccoli, beet greens, turnip greens, mustard greens, bok choy (a Chinese cabbage), and kale are good sources of available calcium. So are collard greens, green cabbage, kohlrabi, watercress and parsley,

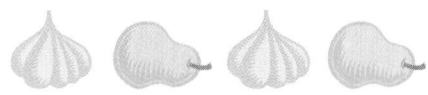

and probably some seaweeds, such as the **nori** popular in Japanese cookery. Certain other foods, including spinach, Swiss chard, and rhubarb, appear equal to milk in calcium content but actually provide no calcium, or very little, to the body because they contain binders that prevent calcium's absorption (see Figure 8-9). Of course, the presence of calcium binders does not make spinach an inferior food. Dark greens of all kinds are superb sources of riboflavin and virtually indispensable for the vegan or anyone else who does not drink milk. Spinach is also rich in iron, beta-carotene, and dozens of other essential nutrients. Just don't rely on it for calcium. Table 8-12 lists the calcium amounts that the body derives from foods various, compared with the calcium they contain.

CALCIUM IN OTHER FOODS

For the many people who cannot use milk and milk products, oysters are a rich source of calcium. So are small fish such as canned sardines or other canned fishes prepared with their bones. Stocks or extracts made from bones are another rich source. The Vietnamese people's tradition of making such a stock helps account for their adequate calcium intake without the use of milk. To make a high-calcium extract, soak cracked bones from chicken, turkey, pork, or fish in vinegar; then slowly boil them until the bones become soft, indicating that they have released their calcium into the acid medium. By this time, most of the vinegar taste will have boiled off. Use the stock in place of water to cook soup, vegetables, rice, or stew. One *tablespoon* of such stock may contain over 100 milligrams of calcium.

CALCIUM-FORTIFIED FOODS

Next in order of preference among nonmilk sources of calcium are foods that contain large amounts of calcium salts by an accident of processing or by intentional fortification. In the processed category are bean curd (tofu: calcium salt is often used to coagulate it); canned tomatoes (firming agents donate 63 milligrams per cup of tomatoes); **stone-ground flour** or self-rising flour; stone-ground whole or self-rising cornmeal; and blackstrap molasses.

Some food products available to U.S. consumers are specially fortified to add calcium to people's diets. The richest in calcium is high-calcium milk itself, that is, milk with extra calcium added, which provides more calcium per cup than any natural milk, 500 milligrams per 8 ounces. Then comes calcium-fortified orange juice, with 300 milligrams per 8 ounces, a good choice because the bioavailability of its calcium compares favorably with that of milk. Calcium-fortified soy milk can also be prepared so that it contains more calcium than whole cow's milk. Soy-based infant formula is fortified with calcium, and no law prevents adults from using it in cooking for themselves.

Finally, there are supplements intended to meet calcium needs without regard to needs for energy or other nutrients. Most people who take calcium supplements do so in hopes of warding off osteoporosis. As Controversy 8 points out, however, supplements are not magic bullets against bone loss.

kefir a yogurt-based beverage.

nori a type of seaweed popular in Asian, particularly Japanese, cooking.

stone-ground flour flour made by grinding kernels of grain between heavy wheels made of limestone a kind of rock derived from the shells and bones of marine animals. As the stones scrape together, bits of the limestone mix with the flour, enriching it with calcium.

FIGURE 8-9

CALCIUM ABSORPTION FROM FOOD SOURCES

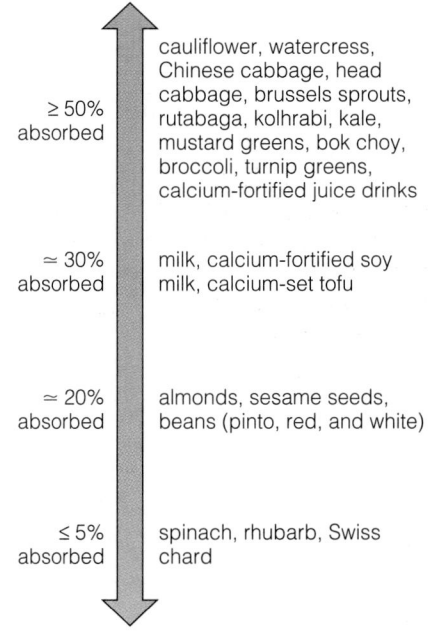

SOURCE: Data from C. M. Weaver and K. L. Plawecki, Dietary calcium: Adequacy of a vegetarian diet, *American Journal of Clinical Nutrition* 59 (1994): 1238S–1241S; R. P. Heaney and coauthors, Absorbability of calcium from *Brassica* vegetables: Broccoli, bok choy, and kale, *Journal of the American Dietetic Association* 58 (1993): 1378–1380.

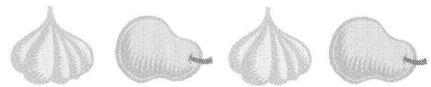

TABLE 8-12

Calcium Contents versus Calcium Absorbed

Food[a]	Total Calcium (mg)	Absorbable Calcium (mg)	Percent Absorption
Milk	300	96	32%
Citrus punch (calcium fortified)	300	150	50
Fruit punch (calcium fortified)	300	156	52
Tofu, calcium set	258	80	31
Rhubarb	174	9	5
Spinach	122	6	5
Beans, white	113	19	17
Turnip greens	99	51	52
Almonds, dry roasted	80	17	21
Cabbage, Chinese	79	43	54
Mustard greens	64	37	58
Kale	47	28	59
Beans, pinto	45	8	17
Beans, red	41	7	17
Sesame seeds, no hulls	37	8	21
Rutabaga	36	22	61
Broccoli	35	18	53
Cabbage, green	25	16	65
Kohlrabi	20	13	67
Watercress	20	13	67
Brussels sprouts	19	12	64
Cauliflower	17	12	69
Radish	14	10	74
Soy milk, unfortified	5	2	32

[a]Serving sizes are ½ cup, except for milk and juice punches (1 cup) and almonds and sesame seeds (1 ounce).

SOURCE: Data from C. M. Weaver and K. L. Plawecki, Dietary calcium: Adequacy of a vegetarian diet, *American Journal of Clinical Nutrition* 59 (1994): 1238S–1241S.

MAKING MEALS RICH IN CALCIUM

The following are some tips for including calcium-rich foods in your day's meals. Many cooks slip extra calcium into meals by sprinkling a tablespoon or two of nonfat dry milk into almost everything. The added calorie value is small, changes to taste and texture of the dish are practically nil, but each 2 tablespoons adds about 100 extra milligrams of calcium. Here are some related tips:

AT BREAKFAST

Serve tea or coffee with milk, hot or iced.

Choose cereals, hot or cold, with milk.

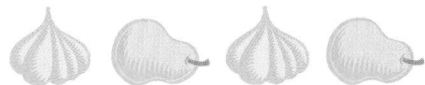

Cook hot cereals with milk instead of water; then mix in 2 tablespoons of nonfat dry milk.

Make muffin or quick bread mixes with milk and extra powdered milk.

Add milk to scrambled eggs.

Moisten cereals with flavored yogurt.

Choose calcium-fortified orange juice.

AT LUNCH

Add low-fat cheeses to sandwiches, burgers, or salads.

Use a variety of green vegetables, such as swiss chard or kale, in salads and on sandwiches.

Stuff potatoes with broccoli and low-fat cheese.

Try pasta such as ravioli stuffed with low-fat ricotta cheese instead of meat.

Sprinkle parmesan cheese on pasta salads.

Mix the mashed bones of canned salmon into salmon salad or patties.

Eat sardines with their bones.

Use nonfat milk or calcium-fortified soy milk as a beverage.

Marinate cabbage shreds or broccoli spears in low-fat Italian dressing for an interesting salad.

Choose coleslaw over potato and macaroni salads.

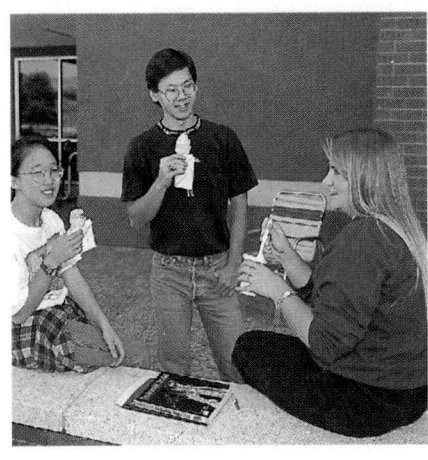

Calcium in a delicious form.

AT SUPPER

Add nonfat powdered milk to almost anything—meat loaf, sauces, gravies, soups, stuffings, casseroles, blended beverages, puddings, quick breads, cookies, brownies. Be creative.

Choose frozen yogurt, ice milk, or custards for dessert.

Toss a handful of thinly sliced green vegetables, such as kale or young turnip greens, with hot pasta dishes; the greens wilt pleasingly in the steam of the freshly cooked pasta.

Serve a green vegetable every night and try new ones—how about kohlrabi? It tastes delicious when boiled like broccoli.

Learn to stir-fry Chinese cabbage and other Asian foods.

Try some tofu (the calcium-set kind); this versatile food has inspired whole cookbooks devoted to creative uses.

People who learn to identify and regularly choose rich calcium sources among foods are rewarded with many benefits to their health. The Do It section that follows provides practice at finding calcium and other minerals in foods when you are in a hurry—from a convenience store.

TABLE 8-13

The Minerals—A Summary

Mineral and Chief Functions in the Body	Deficiency Symptoms	Toxicity Symptoms	Significant Sources
Major Minerals			
Calcium			
The principal mineral of bones and teeth. Also acts in normal muscle contraction and relaxation, nerve functioning, blood clotting, blood pressure, and immune defenses.	Stunted growth in children; adult bone loss (osteoporosis).	Excess calcium is excreted except in hormonal imbalance states (not caused by nutritional deficiency).	Milk and milk products, oysters, small fish (with bones), tofu (bean curd), greens, legumes.
Phosphorus			
Phosphorus is important in cells' genetic material, in cell membranes as phospholipids, in energy transfer, and in buffering systems.	Phosphorus deficiency unknown.	Excess phosphorus may cause calcium excretion.	All animal tissues.
Magnesium			
A factor involved in bone mineralization, the building of protein, enzyme action, normal muscular contraction, transmission of nerve impulses, and maintenance of teeth.	Weakness; confusion; depressed pancreatic hormone secretion; if extreme, convulsions, bizarre movements (especially of eyes and face), hallucinations, and difficulty in swallowing. In children, growth failure.[a]	Excess magnesium from abuse of laxatives and other medications by the elderly or those with kidney disease has caused confusion, lack of muscle coordination, coma, and death.	Nuts, legumes, whole grains, dark green vegetables, seafoods, chocolate, cocoa.
Sodium			
Sodium, chloride, and potassium (electrolytes) maintain cells' normal fluid balance and acid–base balance in the body. Sodium is critical to nerve impulse transmission.	Muscle cramps, mental apathy, loss of appetite.	Hypertension.	Salt, soy sauce, processed foods.
Chloride			
Chloride is also part of the hydrochloric acid found in the stomach, necessary for proper digestion.	Growth failure in children; muscle cramps, mental apathy, loss of appetite; can cause death (uncommon).	Normally harmless (the gas chlorine is a poison but evaporates from water); can cause vomiting.	Salt, soy sauce; moderate quantities in whole, unprocessed foods, large amounts in processed foods.
Potassium			
Potassium facilitates reactions, including the making of protein; the maintenance of fluid and electrolyte balance; the support of cell integrity; the transmission of nerve impulses; and the contraction of muscles, including the heart.	Deficiency accompanies dehydration; causes muscular weakness, paralysis, and confusion; can cause death.	Causes muscular weakness; triggers vomiting; if given into a vein, can stop the heart.	All whole foods: meats, milk, fruits, vegetables, grains, legumes.

(continued on next page)

[a]A still more severe deficiency causes tetany, an extreme, prolonged contraction of the muscles similar to that caused by low blood calcium.

TABLE 8-13

The Minerals—A Summary continued

Mineral and Chief Functions in the Body	Deficiency Symptoms	Toxicity Symptoms	Significant Sources
Major Minerals			
Sulfur			
A component of certain amino acids; part of the vitamins biotin and thiamin and the hormone insulin; combines with toxic substances to form harmless compounds; stabilizes protein shape by forming sulfur-sulfur bridges (see Figure 6-10 in Chapter 6).	None known; protein deficiency would occur first.	Would occur only if sulfur amino acids were eaten in excess; this (in animals) depresses growth.	All protein-containing foods.
Trace Minerals			
Iodine			
A component of the thyroid hormone thyroxine, which helps to regulate growth, development, and metabolic rate.	Goiter, cretinism.	Depressed thyroid activity; goiter-like thyroid enlargement.	Iodized salt; seafood; bread; plants grown in most parts of the country and animals fed those plants.
Iron			
Part of the protein hemoglobin, which carries oxygen in the blood; part of the protein myoglobin in muscles, which makes oxygen available for muscle contraction; necessary for the use of energy.	Anemia: weakness, pallor, headaches, reduced resistance to infection, inability to concentrate, lowered cold tolerance.	Iron overload: infections, liver injury, possible increased risk of colon cancer, growth retardation in children, acidosis, bloody stools, shock.	Red meats, fish, poultry, shellfish, eggs, legumes, dried fruits.
Zinc			
Part of insulin and many enzymes; involved in making genetic material and proteins, immune reactions, transport of vitamin A, taste perception, wound healing, the making of sperm, and normal fetal development.	Growth failure in children, sexual retardation, loss of taste, poor wound healing.	Fever, nausea, vomiting, diarrhea, muscle incoordination, dizziness, anemia, accelerated atherosclerosis, kidney failure.	Protein-containing foods: meats, fish, shellfish, poultry, grains, vegetables.
Selenium			
Part of an enzyme that breaks down reactive chemicals that harm cells; works with vitamin E.	Muscle discomfort, weakness, pancreas damage, heart disease (cardiomyopathy).	Nausea, abdominal pain, nail and hair changes, nerve damage.	Seafoods, organ meats; other meats, grains and vegetables depending on soil conditions.
Fluoride			
Helps form bones and teeth; confers decay resistance on teeth.	Susceptibility to tooth decay.	Fluorosis (discoloration) of teeth, nausea, vomiting, diarrhea, chest pain, itching.	Drinking water if fluoride containing or fluoridated; tea; seafood.
Chromium			
Associated with insulin; needed for energy release from glucose.	Abnormal glucose metabolism.	Unknown.	Meat, unrefined grains; vegetable oils.
Copper			
Helps form hemoglobin; part of several enzymes.	Anemia.	Vomiting, diarrhea.	Meat, drinking water.

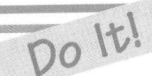

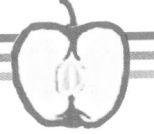

FIND THE MINERALS IN SNACK FOODS

In an ideal world, each person would set aside time each day for planning, shopping, and cooking nutritious meals. In the real world, you've had nothing to eat, your research papers are due, your room is topsy turvy, and your car needs fuel as you're rushing to class. A convenience store seems like a good idea; you can fill up your car and grab a bite to eat in one stop. What you grab makes a difference to your day's calorie and mineral intakes, however—to the benefit or detriment of your nutritional health.

The shelves of convenience stores are lined with all sorts of edible items, and luckily, their labels list their contents of energy, calcium, iron, and sodium. For the sake of learning, we've added two other minerals to this exercise: magnesium and zinc. The data in Table 8-14 was obtained from the Food Processor diet analysis program by ESHA Research, 1996.

LIST YOUR RDA AND CHOOSE SOME FOODS

Step 1. List your RDA or RNI values for energy and iron, zinc, and magnesium (see the inside front cover, or the Canadiana Appendix) as indicated on Form 8-1. For sodium, use the recommended upper limit of 2,400 mg as your target for the day.

Step 2. Scan the variety of items on the convenience store shelves represented in Figure 8-10. Choose a snack and enter your choices on Form 8-1. The portion sizes are those commonly used for such foods, and not those recommended in the Food Guide Pyramid. For example, a can of vienna sausages contains 5 ounces of sausages, not the recommended 3 ounces.

FORM 8-1

Energy and Mineral Tally

Your Snack Foods	Energy (cal)	Sodium (mg)	Potassium (mg)	Calcium (mg)	Iron (mg)	Zinc (mg)	Magnesium (mg)
Snack Totals							
Personal RDA/RNI Goals		2,400					
% of Recommendation							

FIGURE 8-10

SNACKS AT THE FUEL 'N' FEED

Snacks at the Fuel 'n' Feed

Sandwiches/Canned foods
Cheese pizza slice
Ham biscuit
Pork and beans
Roast beef sandwich
Sardines
Vienna sausage

Beverages
Milk, 1% fat
Chocolate milk, 2% fat
Cola
Pineapple orange juice

Snacks
Apple pie, packaged
Banana
Cheese slice
Chocolate candy bar
Dill pickle
Dried fruit mix
Fig bar cookies
Ice cream and sherbet bar
Potato chips, small bag
Pretzels, regular
Pretzels, unsalted
Roasted almonds
Sunflower seeds, shelled
Wheat crackers
Yogurt, low fat, with fruit

RECORD ENERGY AND MINERAL VALUES

Step 3. Obtain energy and mineral values for your snack choices from Table 8-14 and enter these values on Form 8-1. Total the six columns for energy and minerals.

Step 4. Calculate the percentages of energy and mineral requirements contributed by this snack. Divide each nutrient total by the recommendation for that nutrient, and multiply by 100. Example: a snack providing 40 mg calcium would meet 5 percent of an RDA of 800 mg (40 ÷ 800) × 100 = 5%.

TABLE 8-14

Energy and Mineral Contents of Selected Convenience Store Foods

	Energy (cal)	Calcium (mg)	Iron (mg)	Magnesium (mg)	Potassium (mg)	Sodium (mg)	Zinc (mg)
Cheese pizza, slice	243	184	0.7	16	209	467	0.8
Ham biscuit	386	160	2.7	23	210	1432	1.7
Vienna sausages, 5 oz	395	14	1.3	10	86	1347	2.3
Sardines, 3¾ oz	221	405	3.1	41	338	536	1.4
Pork and beans, 5 oz	139	80	4.7	50	425	624	8.4
Roast beef sandwich	318	47	3.1	22	367	1252	3.0
Ice cream and sherbet bar	92	62	0.1	7	102	43	0.4
Potato chips, small bag, 4¾ oz	152	7	0.5	19	361	168	0.3
Pretzels, unsalted, 1 oz	110	10	1.2	10	41	60	0.2
Pretzels, salted, 1 oz	108	10	1.2	10	41	486	0.2
Fig bar cookie, 4	195	36	1.3	15	116	214	0.2
Chocolate candy bar, 1½ oz	226	84	0.6	26	169	36	0.6
Wheat crackers, 1 oz	134	14	1.3	18	84	225	0.5
Apple pie, fast food type	225	6	1.0	6	67	179	0.2
Low-fat chocolate milk, 2% fat, 1 c	179	285	0.6	33	423	151	1.0
Pineapple orange drink, 12 oz	170	17	0.9	20	156	10	0.2
Cola, 12 oz	186	14	0.1	5	3	18	0.0
Milk, 1% fat, 1 c	102	300	0.1	34	381	123	1.0
Dill pickle	12	6	0.3	7	75	833	0.1
Low-fat yogurt, with fruit, 8 oz	232	345	0.2	33	478	133	1.7
Sunflower seeds, shelled, 3¾ oz	654	123	7.2	375	513	3	5.4
Dried fruit mix, 3¾ oz	258	40	2.9	41	846	19	0.5
Banana	105	7	0.4	33	451	1	0.2
Cheese slice, 1 oz	69	121	0.2	6	59	250	0.6
Roasted almonds, salted, 3¾ oz	660	326	4.0	273	629	828	3.3

ANALYSIS

Now answer these questions:

1. What percentage of your energy need did the snack contribute? Did the snack also contribute a proportional amount of calcium, iron, magnesium, or zinc?

2. What about sodium? Did the sodium in this snack exceed 10 percent of the maximum of 2,400 milligrams? Did it exceed 30 percent? If so, look for low-sodium supper choices to round out the day. Consult Figure 8-6 to review high- and low-sodium foods.

3. From foods listed in Table 8-14, which are the best "bargains" in terms of sodium and other minerals? For example, a food that supplies much of the daily sodium allowance and few other nutrients may support nutrition goals less well than a similar food with less sodium. List some high-sodium and low-sodium choices from among the foods.

4. Did you find any "bargains" in terms of energy and minerals among the foods? For example, calcium and potassium are delivered by many foods of varying calorie values. List snack food rich in needed minerals, yet relatively low in calories.

5. Where is the calcium in your snack foods? List the snack foods you chose that supply substantial calcium (10% of recommendation). If your choices lack calcium, look back to the menu and list some calcium sources you find there.

6. Can a person looking for iron do well in a convenience store? Which foods or ingredients contribute iron? See Snapshot 8-5 for good iron sources.

7. Is the iron in some of these snack foods more absorbable than in others? Explain. What constituents of these foods can enhance iron's absorption?

8. Did any of your choices provide 10% or more of your need for magnesium? Magnesium is easily lost in processing of foods and so is difficult to obtain from highly processed snacks.

9. Consider the zinc in your snack. Did any foods provide 10% or more of the daily recommendation? If so, which ones? If not, consult Snapshot 8-6 for ideas about the kinds of foods that are good sources of zinc, and list some snack foods likely to contain significant amounts.

10. What might a whole day's mineral intake look like if a person ate convenience foods at every meal?

Americans are snacking more as the pace of life quickens. Snacks, if well chosen, can enhance a person's nutritional health; chosen carelessly, they can detract from it. The next chapter makes clear that your choices among foods to snack on can make a difference to calorie intakes of several hundred calories a day.

SELF-CHECK

Answers to these Self-Check questions are in Appendix G.

1. Water excretion is governed by the:
   a. liver
   b. kidneys
   c. brain
   d. (b) and (c)

2. Compared with hard water, soft water:
   a. better supports the health of the heart.
   b. contains fewer harmful dissolved minerals.
   c. is higher in sodium.
   d. leaves a grey residue in the wash.

3. Which two minerals are the major constituents of bone?
   a. calcium and zinc
   b. phosphorus and calcium
   c. sodium and magnesium
   d. selenium and calcium

4. A deficiency of _____ is one of the world's most common preventable causes of mental retardation.
   a. zinc
   b. magnesium
   c. selenium
   d. iodine

5. Which mineral in excess is the number one cause of fatal accidental poisonings of U.S. children under three years old?
   a. iron
   b. sodium
   c. chloride
   d. potassium

6. Bottled water must meet higher standards for purity and sanitation than U.S. tap water.   T   F

7. You can survive being deprived of water for about a week.   T   F

8. The best way to control salt intake is to cut down on processed and fast foods.   T   F

9. Electrolytes help keep fluids in their proper compartments in the body.   T   F

10. The dairy foods butter, cream, and cream cheese are good sources of calcium whereas vegetables such as broccoli are poor sources.   T   F

11. Actions to prevent osteoporosis are best begun in middle age, when the bones are ceasing their growth. True or false? (This is addressed in the upcoming Controversy)   T   F

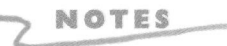

NOTES

Notes are in Appendix F.

Osteoporosis and Calcium

Last year two and a half million people in the United States suffered bone breaks attributable to osteoporosis, which is one of the most prevalent of the degenerative diseases.[1] Half of all women over age 45 and 90 percent of those over 75 suffer the effects of this disease.[2]

Osteoporosis sets in silently, producing no symptoms until late in life. Then, suddenly, dramatically, symptoms emerge. The causes are tangled, and although evidence is mounting that abundant dietary calcium influences development of osteoporosis, other factors are also major potential players. This Controversy addresses several questions about osteoporosis: What is it? Who gets it? What factors increase the risk? What can people do to reduce their risks? And where does calcium fit into the picture?

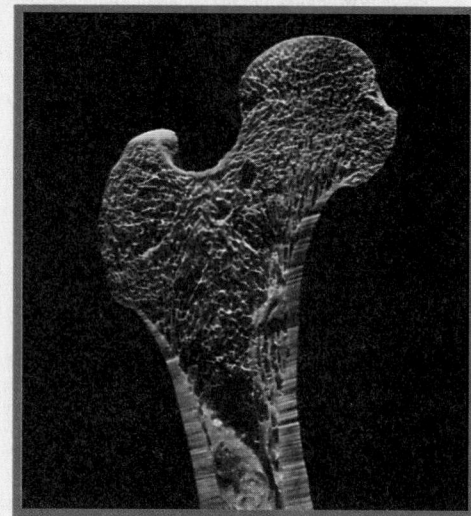

THE PROBLEM OF OSTEOPOROSIS

Often osteoporosis first becomes apparent when someone's hip suddenly gives way. People say, "She fell and broke her hip," but in fact the hip may have been so fragile that it broke *before* she fell. Just stepping off a curb may jar a bone enough to shatter it, if the bone is already porous from loss of minerals. The break is not clean; it is an explosion into fragments so numerous and scattered that they cannot be reassembled. Just to remove them is a struggle, and to replace them with an artificial joint requires major surgery. Such a fracture condemns many older people to wheelchairs for the rest of their lives. About a third die of complications within a year.

To understand how the skeleton loses minerals in later years, you must first know a few things about bones. Table C8-1 offers definitions of relevant terms. The photograph on this page shows a human leg bone sliced lengthwise, exposing the lattice of calcium-containing crystals (the **trabecular bone**) inside. These lacy crystals, part of the body's calcium bank, are tapped to raise blood calcium when the supply from the day's diet runs short; they are redeposited in bone when dietary calcium is plentiful. Invested as savings during the milk-drinking

years of childhood and young adulthood, these deposits provide a nearly inexhaustible fund of calcium.

In contrast to trabecular bone, **cortical bone** is the dense, ivory-like bone that forms the exterior shell of a bone and the shaft of a long bone (look closely at the photograph). Both types of bone are crucial to overall bone strength. Cortical bone forms a sturdy outer wall, and trabecular bone provides strength along the lines of stress.

The differences between the two types of bone are meaningful with regard to osteoporosis. Trabecular bone is generously supplied with blood vessels and is more metabolically active than is cortical bone. Trabecular bone is also more sensitive to hormones that govern calcium deposits and withdrawals from day to day. Cortical bone's calcium can be withdrawn, but slowly. Trabecular bone, on the other hand, readily gives up its minerals at the necessary rate whenever blood calcium needs replenishing. Losses of trabecular bone begin to be significant for men and women in their twenties, although losses can occur anytime calcium withdrawals exceed calcium deposits. Cortical

TABLE C8-1

Osteoporosis Terms

- **bone density** a measure of bone strength; the degree of mineralization of the bone matrix.
- **cortical bone** the ivorylike outer bone layer that forms a shell surrounding trabecular bone and that comprises the shaft of a long bone.
- **trabecular** (tra-BECK-you-lar) **bone** the weblike structure composed of calcium-containing crystals inside a bone's solid outer shell. It provides strength and acts as a calcium storage bank.
- **type I osteoporosis** osteoporosis characterized by rapid bone losses, primarily of trabecular bone.
- **type II osteoporosis** osteoporosis characterized by gradual losses of both trabecular and cortical bone.

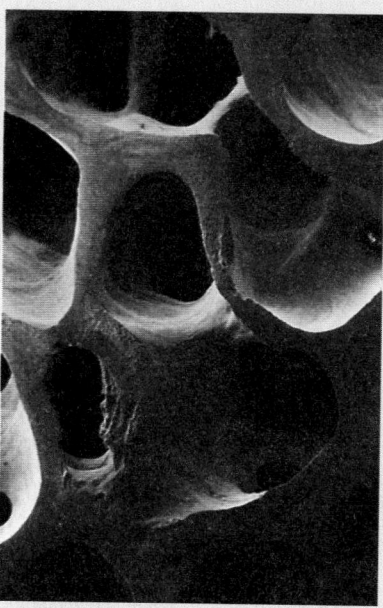

Electron micrograph of healthy trabeculae.

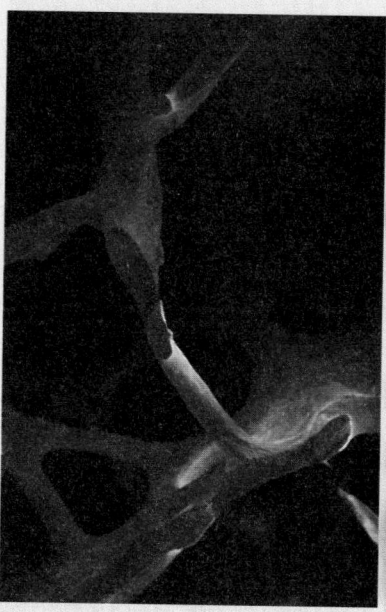

Electron micrograph of trabecular bone affected by osteoporosis.

bone loss begins at about age 40; bone tissue dwindles steadily thereafter.

Menopause, a period in which a woman's estrogen secretion sharply declines and menstruation ceases, makes bone losses surge. This surge tapers off after a few years so that, once again, women's losses equal those sustained by men of the same age. Losses of bone minerals continue throughout the rest of a woman's life, but not at the free-fall pace of the menopause years.

As age advances and losses compound, the later symptoms of osteoporosis can become dramatic. Researchers have associated the losses of trabecular and cortical bone with two types of osteoporosis, types I and II, identified by the bone breaks they produce. People with **type I osteoporosis** lose mostly trabecular bone (see Figure C8-1), sometimes at three times the expected rate or even faster, and bone breaks may suddenly become frequent when the victim passes the age of 65 years. In this condition trabecular bones become so fragile that the body's weight can overburden the spine; vertebrae may suddenly disintegrate and crush down, painfully pinching major nerves. Wrists may break as trabecula-rich bone ends weaken, and teeth may loosen or fall out as the trabecular bone of the jaw

recedes. Women are most often the victims of type I osteoporosis, six to one over men.

In **type II osteoporosis,** the calcium of both cortical and trabecular bone is drawn out of storage, but slowly over the years. As old age approaches, the vertebrae may compress into wedge shapes, usually painlessly, forming what is insensitively called "dowager's hump," the posture seen in many older people as they "grow shorter." Figure C8-2 shows the effect of the compression of spinal bone on a woman's height and posture. Because the cortical shell as well as the trabecular interior weaken, breaks most often occur in the hip, as in the opening example. A woman is twice as likely as a man to suffer type II osteoporosis, probably due to the process set in motion years before at menopause.

Scientists searching for ways to prevent osteoporosis must first discover its causes. So far, many findings seem to conflict with each other, and others simply lead to more questions. Nevertheless, some areas of agreement have been reached. Whether a person develops osteoporosis seems to depend partly on heredity and partly on the environment, including nutrition. The sections that follow discuss the factors thought to be the main determinants of **bone density.**

FIGURE C8-2

LOSS OF HEIGHT IN A WOMAN CAUSED BY OSTEOPOROSIS

The woman on the left is about 50 years old. On the right, she is 80 years old. Her legs have not grown shorter; only her back has lost length, due to collapse of her spinal bones (vertebrae). Collapsed vertebrae cannot protect the spinal nerves from pressure that causes excruciating pain.

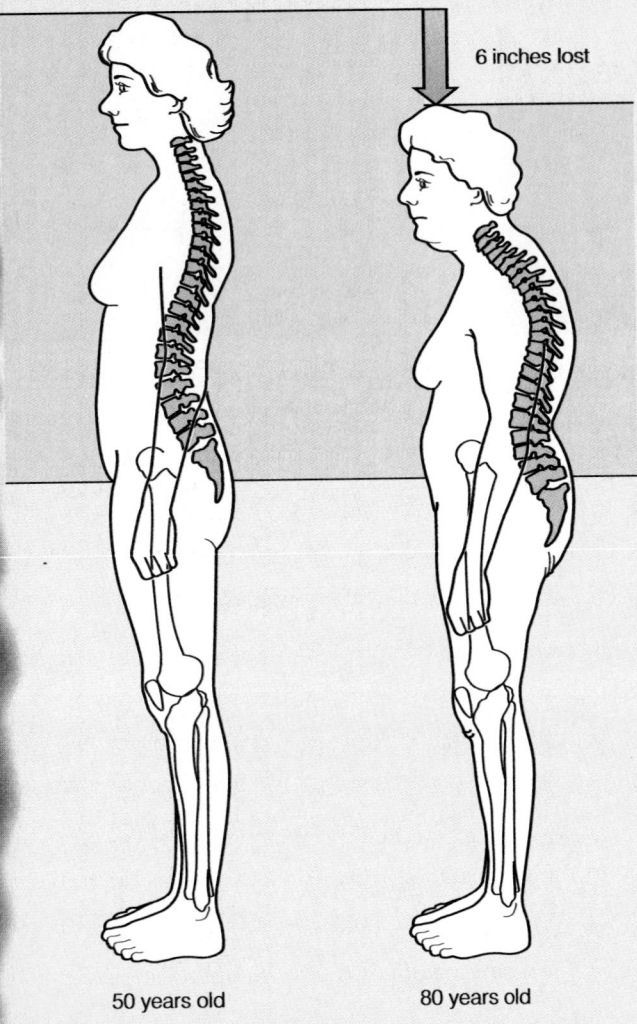

6 inches lost

50 years old   80 years old

AGE, CALCIUM, FLUORIDE, AND VITAMIN D

The bones gain strength and density all through the growing years and into young adulthood. As the mid-thirties approach, bones stop growing, and as years pass, bone tissue is lost and bones lose strength and density. With advancing age, the cells that build bone gradually become less active, while those that dismantle bone continue working.

One likely factor to weigh in the balance of bone withdrawal and deposition is calcium nutrition during childhood and early adult life. Preteen children who consume extra calcium together with adequate vitamin D lay more calcium into the structure of their bones than children with less adequate intakes.[3] In addition to calcium and vitamin D, fluoride taken during the bone-building years may increase bone density. (Fluoride supplements are not effective, however, in treating osteoporosis.)

Another factor, which becomes important in later life, is calcium absorption. Absorption declines after about the age of 65 years, probably because the kidneys do not activate vitamin D as well as they did earlier. Also, sunlight is needed to form vitamin D, and many older people fail to go outdoors into the sunshine. Some of the hormones that regulate bone maintenance and calcium metabolism also change with age and accelerate bone mineral withdrawal.*

When people reach the bone-losing years of middle age, those who formed dense bones during youth have the advantage. They simply have more bone tissue starting out and can lose more before beginning to suffer ill effects. Therefore, whatever factors contribute to the building of strong bones in youth, these same factors become protective against osteoporosis much later. One of these factors may be calcium nutrition. A new line of research is investigating a possible link between bone loss and sodium intakes. A group of researchers found that women who kept sodium intakes low did not lose bone tissue from their hips, but those who consumed more sodium did lose bone.[4] It may turn out that a twofold diet plan for the bones include both increasing calcium intakes in the early years and reducing sodium intakes in the later years.

GENDER AND HORMONES

After age itself, experiencing menopause is, for women, the next-strongest predictor of loss of bone density with aging. As mentioned, as estrogen secretion declines at menopause in women at about age 50, but cases exist in which *young* women's ovaries fail to produce enough estrogen to maintain menstruation. These young women also undergo rapid bone losses. In some, dis-

---

*Among the hormones suggested as influential in governing calcium balance are parathyroid hormone and calcitonin.

eased ovaries have had to be removed; in others, the ovaries produce inadequate estrogen because the women overexercise and restrict their body weights unreasonably, and so develop athletic amenorrhea (discussed in Controversy 10). Estrogen taken as a prescription drug can help nonmenstruating women to prevent further bone loss, and current therapy regimens carry little risk to health. For those who take them, the drugs do indeed reduce the incidence of bone fractures.[5]

If estrogen deficiency is a major cause of osteoporosis in women, what is the case in men? Men produce only a little estrogen, yet they are normally more resistant to osteoporosis than are women. Do male sex hormones play roles in osteoporosis? Perhaps so, because men do suffer more fractures after undergoing removal of diseased testes or when their testes lose function with aging.

Even in women, estrogen is clearly only one of several factors affecting bone. Some women lose bone tissue in middle age before menopause, as though they were predisposed to do so.

INHERITED BONE DIFFERENCES

Studies of mothers and daughters confirm that heredity plays a role in bone density.[6] Most likely, inheritance influences both the maximum bone mass possible during growth and the extent of bone loss during menopause. The extent to which a given genetic potential is realized, however, depends on individual life experiences. Those who attend to nutrition and physical activity, for example, maximize their peak bone density during growth, whereas those who overuse alcohol or use tobacco accelerate their bone losses.

Risks of osteoporosis run along racial lines. People of African extraction have denser bones than do those of Northern European descent, and these differences are dramatically evident even before birth in X-ray images of fetuses.[7] This holds true for both sexes of all ages and expresses itself in a much lower total rate of osteoporosis among Africans. Hip fractures, for example, are reported to be about three times more likely in 80-year-old Northern European women than in African women of the same age.

Other ethnic groups have lower bone densities than do Northern Europeans. Asians from China and Japan, Mexican-Americans, Hispanic people from Central and South America, and Inuit people from St. Lawrence Island all have lower bone density than do people with Northern European background. Knowing this might

lead to the prediction that these groups would suffer more bone fractures, but the picture is not that tidy. Chinese people living in Singapore have low bone density, but have hip fracture rates among the lowest in the world. Researchers in former Yugoslavia found bone fracture rates were tied to locations despite racial similarities. The lower fracture rates occurred in areas where calcium intakes were high, and higher rates were found in areas where calcium intakes were lower.

These studies of populations demonstrate that although a person's genes may lay the groundwork for a likely outcome, environmental factors influence the genes' ultimate expression. From the findings reported from former Yugoslavia, it appears that calcium nutrition may be one of those environmental factors, but there are others, such as physical activity, body weight, smoking, alcohol use, and protein intake. It is worth noting that all of these factors are under people's own control.

PHYSICAL ACTIVITY

While you can't do much about your genetic inheritance, you can control your physical activity. It has long been known that when people lie idle—for example, when they are confined to bed—the bones lose strength just as the muscles do. Astronauts who live without gravity for days or weeks at a time also experience remarkably rapid and extensive bone losses.

Muscle strength and bone strength usually go together, and muscle use seems to promote bone strength. When cross sections of bones of sedentary and active people are compared, the active bones are denser by far.[8] The hormones that promote synthesis of new muscle tissue also favor the building of bone. To keep the bones healthy, then, include weight-bearing exercises such as walking, dancing, jogging, sports, gardening, or calisthenics every day. Even swimming may build bone strength, although exactly how it does so is not known.[9]

As mentioned, exercise can be overdone to the detriment of bone tissue, as evidence presented in Controversy 10 shows. Female athletes who have extremely low body fat contents and have ceased menstruating are especially at risk for bone loss.[10] Bone density in such athletes in their twenties may be as low as that of nonathlete women in their seventies. No amount of calcium can completely protect against bone loss in this condition, but athletes who suffer these disturbances and also take in too little calcium put themselves at a special disadvantage.

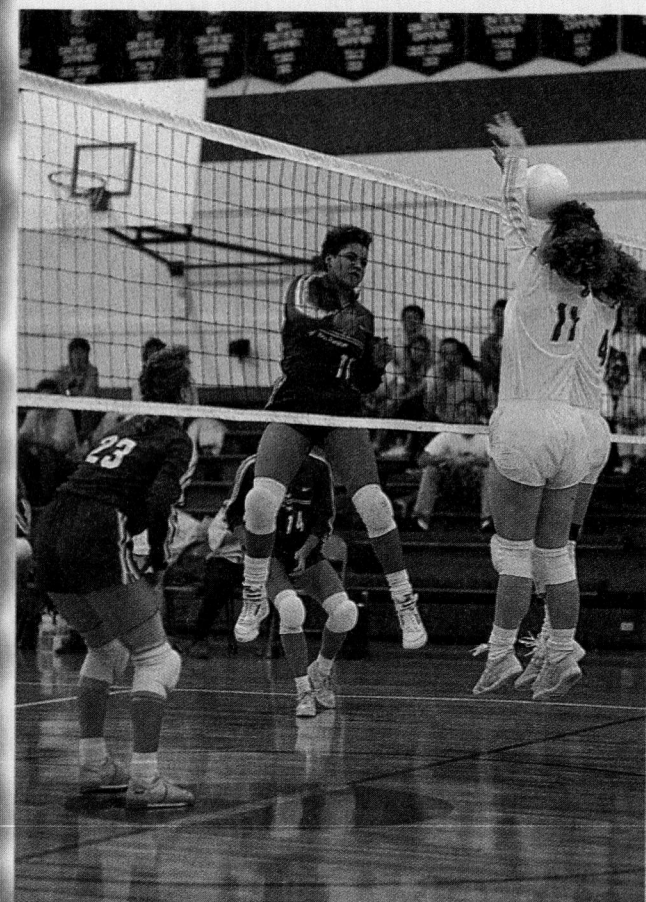

These college women are putting bone in the bank.

BODY WEIGHT

Heavier body weights, and to some degree higher body fatness, stress bones and promote their maintenance; osteoporosis is most often associated with under-weight.[11] Women who are thin through life, and especially those who lose 10 percent or more of their body weight after the age of menopause, face a hip fracture rate twice as high as that of most other women.[12] Also, the type of diabetes associated with slender body structure alters the body's handling of calcium and magnesium with possible harmful effects on the health of the bones.[13]

SMOKING, ALCOHOL, AND CAFFEINE

Smokers experience more fractures from slight injury than do nonsmokers. Women who smoke lose 5 to 10 percent more of their bone density than nonsmokers by the time they reach menopause.[14] Researchers speculate that the lower body weights of smokers may be one causal factor; early menopause in female smokers may be another.[15]

People who are addicted to alcohol also experience relatively more frequent fractures. It may be that because alcohol (a diuretic) causes fluid excretion, it induces excessive calcium losses through the urine. Also, women's ovaries are sensitive to the effects of alcohol, and heavy drinking may upset the hormonal balance required for healthy bones.

Heavy users of caffeinated beverages, such as coffee, tea, or colas, should be aware that while some evidence suggests a link between caffeine use and osteoporosis, other results are inconclusive. It may be that caffeine exerts an effect only when calcium intakes are low.[16]

Table C8-2 summarizes the risk factors covered so far and includes some others, among them, high protein and low calcium intakes, discussed next. The more risk factors that apply to you, the greater your chances of developing osteoporosis in the future and the more seriously you should take the advice offered in a later section of this Controversy.

A ROLE FOR PROTEIN

Researchers have discovered that extra dietary protein causes the body to excrete calcium in the urine. The finding has often been repeated, leading to the suspicion that a lifetime of consuming excess dietary protein may accelerate bone loss.[17] One study showed that even when calcium intakes were very high (1,400 milligrams a day in this experiment), excess protein intake caused a negative calcium balance.

The converse is also true: that is, diets low in protein help to conserve bone density. This is seen both in laboratory animals and in strict vegetarians, who consume a lower than average amount of protein. Vegetarians who center meals on eggs and dairy products, however, have been observed to take in as much protein and to lose bone just as rapidly as do meat eaters.[18] A tentative link has been suggested between the hormone insulin, released in response to dietary protein, and increased calcium losses in the urine.[19]

There is a limit to how low the protein intake can safely be, of course. Below that limit, too little protein is as harmful as too much. In fact, protein deprivation also stimulates calcium losses.[20] These facts seem to conflict at first glance, but they really just demonstrate a sound nutrition principle—that a happy medium is best.

TABLE C8-2

Risk and Protective Factors That Correlate with Osteoporosis

Risk Factors	Protective Factors
High Correlation	
Advanced age	Black race
Alcoholism	Estrogens,
Chronic steroid use	long-term use
Female gender	
Rheumatoid arthritis	
Surgical removal of ovaries or testes	
Thinness or weight loss	
White race	
Moderate Correlation	
Chronic thyroid hormone use	Having given birth
Cigarette smoking	High body weight
Diabetes (insulin-dependent type)	
Early menopause	
Excessive antacid use	
Low-calcium diet	
Sedentary lifestyle	
Vitamin D deficiency	
Probably Important but Not Yet Proved	
Alcohol taken in moderation	High-calcium diet
Caffeine use	Regular physical activity
Family history of osteoporosis	
High-fiber diet	
High-protein diet	

SOURCE: Adapted from C. D. Arnaud and S. D. Sanchez, The role of calcium in osteoporosis, *Annual Review of Nutrition* 10 (1990): 397–414.

CALCIUM RECOMMENDATIONS

The RDA committee recommends 1,200 milligrams of calcium, the amount in about 4 cups of milk, each day for everyone 11 through 24 years of age. After age 24, throughout life, other factors can either hasten or slow the bone loss that occurs in everyone. Once a person reaches middle age and bone loss has begun, however, the person can still do a few things to maintain the bones, as discussed earlier.

Unfortunately, few girls meet the RDA for calcium during their bone-forming years. (Boys generally obtain intakes close to those recommended because they eat more food.) Even if girls do meet the RDA, this amount may not be enough to achieve the maximum bone den-

sity.[21] As for adults, women rarely meet the RDA of 800 to 1,200 milligrams from food within their energy allowances. Furthermore, evidence is accumulating that calcium recommendations should be higher still, especially for postmenopausal women.[22] As Table 8-4 of this chapter showed, some authorities suggest 1,500 milligrams of calcium for postmenopausal women who are not receiving estrogen. As a rule, women taking estrogen need no more calcium than the RDA.

And how should all of this calcium be obtained? Consider a bit of hard-won advice: use foods if at all possible, not supplements. People can best support their bones' health by following the recommendations of Table C8-3.

Calcium supplements cannot equal any of the actions listed in the table. No one should be led to think that popping pills can take the place of sound food choices and other healthy habits. For those who desire details on supplements, however, a discussion follows.

TABLE C8-3

A Lifetime Plan for Healthy Bones

Age	Action
0–18	Use milk as the primary beverage to meet the RDA for calcium within a balanced diet that provides all nutrients; play actively in sports or other activities; limit television; do not start smoking or drinking alcohol; drink fluoridated water.
19–25	Choose milk as the primary beverage, or if milk causes distress, include other calcium sources to meet the RDA; commit to a lifelong program of physical activity; do not smoke or drink alcohol—if you have started, quit; drink fluoridated water.
26–50	Continue as for 19- to 25-year-olds. At menopause, women should be evaluated for possible estrogen replacement therapy. Obtain the RDA for calcium from food. Take calcium and fluoride supplements only if prescribed by physician.
51 and above	Continue as for 19- to 25-year-olds; continue following physician's advice concerning estrogen and supplements. Continue striving to meet the calcium RDA from diet, and continue bone-strengthening exercises.

A PERSPECTIVE ON CALCIUM SUPPLEMENTS

As important as calcium intake may be, bone loss is not a calcium-deficiency disease comparable to iron-deficiency anemia. In iron-deficiency anemia, high iron intakes reliably reverse the condition. With respect to calcium balance, though, high calcium intakes alone do little or nothing to reverse bone loss. During the menopausal years, calcium supplements of 1 gram may slow, but cannot fully prevent, the inevitable bone loss.[23]

Calcium supplements are part of standard therapy for already developed osteoporosis. Taking self-prescribed calcium supplements entails problems, though (see Table C8-4). Nutrition-minded people who cannot consume milk products or other calcium-rich foods are forced to consider calcium supplements. Regular vitamin-mineral pills contain little or no calcium. The label may list a few milligrams of calcium, but remember that the RDA is close to a gram (1,000 milligrams) for adults.

Supplements are available in three forms. Simplest are the purified calcium compounds, such as calcium carbonate, citrate, gluconate, lactate, malate, or phosphate, and compounds of calcium with amino acids (called **amino acid chelates**). Then there are mixtures of calcium with other compounds, such as calcium carbonate with magnesium carbonate, with aluminum salts (as in some **antacids**), or with vitamin D. Then there are powdered, calcium-rich materials such as **bone meal, powdered bone, oyster shell,** or **dolomite** (limestone). See Table C8-5 for supplement terms.

The first question to ask is how well the body absorbs and uses the calcium from various supplements. Based on research to date, it seems that many people absorb calcium reasonably well—and about as well as from milk—from amino acids chelated with calcium, calcium phosphate dibasic, calcium acetate, calcium carbonate, **calcium citrate,** calcium gluconate, and calcium lactate. People absorb calcium less well from a mixture of calcium and magnesium carbonates, from oyster shell calcium fortified with inorganic magnesium, from a chelated calcium-magnesium combination, or from calcium carbonate fortified with vitamins and iron. Some people absorb calcium better from milk and milk products than from even the most absorbable supplements named above.

The next question to ask is how much calcium the supplement provides. Healthy people have consumed over 2 grams daily of calcium without problems. To be safe, though, supplements should provide less than

TABLE C8-4

Calcium Supplement Pitfalls to Avoid

Calcium supplements may cause:

- *Impaired iron or zinc status.* This is due to the change in stomach pH caused by calcium, which interferes with mineral absorption. Calcium taken with meals impairs absorption of other minerals, but taking it between meals limits absorption of calcium itself.
- *Accelerated calcium loss.* Calcium-containing antacids that also contain aluminum and magnesium hydroxide cause a net calcium loss.
- *Other nutrient interactions.* Calcium phosphate dibasic inhibits magnesium absorption.
- *Exposure to contaminants.* Some preparations of bone meal and dolomites are contaminated with hazardous amounts of arsenic, cadmium, mercury, and lead.
- *Vitamin D toxicity.* Vitamin D is needed to enhance calcium absorption, but continued high intakes of vitamin D, which is present in many calcium supplements, can be toxic.
- *Excess blood calcium.* This complication is seen only with doses of calcium fourfold or more greater than customarily prescribed.
- *Urinary tract stones or kidney damage in susceptible individuals.* People who have a history of kidney stones should be monitored by a physician; calcium citrate supplements may be the safest type in this regard.
- *Milk alkali syndrome.* This alkalosis (that is, a disturbance of the acid–base balance of the blood) is seen only with doses of calcium of 4 to 10 grams/day. This condition disappears when supplementation is discontinued.
- *Drug interactions.* Calcium and tetracycline form an insoluble complex that impairs both mineral and drug absorption.
- *Constipation, intestinal bloating, and excess gas.* These symptoms are reported most often with calcium carbonate, least often with calcium citrate.

SELECTED REFERENCES: V. Argiratos and S. Samman, The effect of calcium carbonate and calcium citrate on the absorption of zinc in healthy female subjects, *European Journal of Clinical Nutrition* 48 (1994): 198–204; The inhibitory effect of dietary calcium on iron bioavailability: A cause for concern? *Nutrition Reviews* 53 (1995): 77–80; B. S. Levine and coauthors, Effect of calcium citrate supplementation on urinary calcium oxalate saturation in female stone formers, *American Journal of Clinical Nutrition* 60 (1994): 592–596; Safety of some calcium supplements questioned, *Nutrition Reviews* 52 (1994): 95–105.

TABLE C8-5

Calcium Supplements Terms

- **amino acid chelates** compounds of minerals (such as calcium) combined with amino acids in a form that favors their absorption. Absorption approximates that of calcium from milk.
- **antacids** acid-buffering agents used to counter excess acidity in the stomach. Some preparations (such as Tums) contain calcium, but others do not.
- **bone meal, powdered bone** crushed or ground bone preparations intended to supply calcium to the diet, but not well absorbed and often contaminated with toxic materials.
- **calcium citrate** a calcium salt reported to have high absorbability. Other absorbable forms are calcium malate and calcium phosphate dibasic.
- **dolomite** a compound of minerals (calcium magnesium carbonate) found in limestone and marble. Dolomite is powdered and is sold as a calcium-magnesium supplement, but may be contaminated with toxic minerals such as arsenic, cadmium, mercury, and lead and is not well absorbed.
- **elemental calcium** a term on supplement labels referring to the amount of calcium present among other constituents. For example, an antacid may contain 1,200 milligrams of calcium carbonate, but just 500 milligrams of calcium itself; the rest is made up of carbonate.
- **oyster shell** a product made from the powdered shells of oysters; sold as a calcium supplement, but not well absorbed by the digestive system.

this, since foods also provide calcium. Read the label to fine out how much a dose supplies. Calcium carbonate is 40 percent **elemental calcium,** whereas calcium gluconate is only 9 percent. The user should select a low-dose supplement and take it several times a day rather than taking a large-dose supplement all at once.[24] Divided doses can improve a day's total absorption by up to 20 percent.

Then consider that when manufacturers compress large quantities of calcium into small pills, the stomach acid has difficulty penetrating the pill. To test a supplement's absorbability, drop it into a 6-ounce cup of vinegar, and stir occasionally. A high-quality formulation will dissolve within half an hour.

Think one more time, then, before you commit yourself to taking supplements for calcium. The Consensus Conference on Osteoporosis recommends milk. The American Society for Bone and Mineral Research recommends foods as a source of calcium in preference to supplements. The *Diet and Health* report from the National Academy of Sciences concludes that foods are best.[25] The authors of this book are so impressed with the importance of using abundant, calcium-rich foods that they have worked out ways to do so at every meal. Seldom do nutritionists agree so unanimously.

NOTES

Notes are in Appendix F.

ENERGY BALANCE AND WEIGHT CONTROL

9

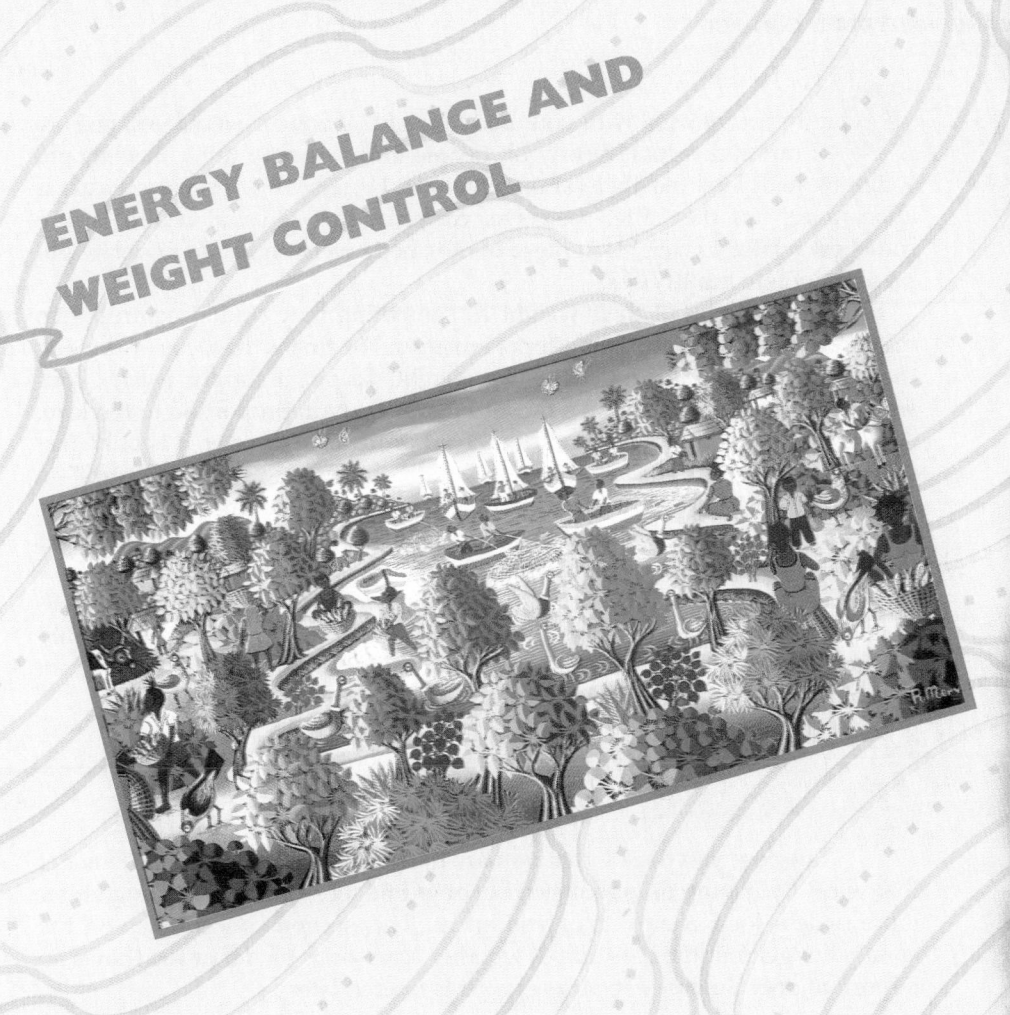

CONTENTS

R. Mervilus, *Tree Landscape with Sailing Boats,* © SuperStock.

body composition the proportions of muscle, bone, fat, and other tissue that make up a person's total body weight.

Are you pleased with your body weight? If you answered yes, you are a rare individual. Nearly all people in our society think they should weigh more or less (mostly less) than they do. Usually, their primary reason is appearance, but they often perceive, correctly, that physical health is also somehow related to weight. At the extremes, both overweight and underweight present definite health risks.

People also think of their weight as something they should control. Two misconceptions frustrate their efforts, however. The first is the focus on weight; the second is the focus on *controlling* weight. To put it simply, it isn't your weight you need to control; it's the fat in your body in proportion to the lean. And it isn't possible to control either the fat or the lean directly; it is only possible to control your *behavior*. In other words, the words "Weight Control" in this chapter's title are wrong; they should be replaced with the words "Behavior to Promote Appropriate Body Composition." If the chapter bore that name, though, hardly anyone would read it.

This chapter's missions are to present the problems associated with deficient and excessive body fatness, to present strategies for solving these problems, and to point out how appropriate **body composition,** once achieved, can be maintained. First, consider how the body manages its energy budget.

ENERGY BALANCE

Suppose you decide that you are too fat or too thin. How did you get that way? By having an unbalanced energy budget—that is, by eating either more or less food energy than you spent. This section concentrates on the energy budget, but the question of whether a person is too fat or too thin is an important one. Guidance in answering it is offered later.

Energy In

As made clear, excess fat enters the fat cells for storage, and stored fat is withdrawn when energy supplies run low. A day's energy balance can therefore be stated like this:

Change in energy stores equals food energy taken in minus energy spent on metabolism and muscle activities.

More simply:

Change in energy stores = energy in − energy out.

The energy in foods and beverages is the only contributor to the "energy in" side of the energy balance equation. Before you can decide how much food energy you need in a day, you must first become familiar with the amounts of energy in foods and beverages. One way to do this is to look up calorie amounts associated with foods and beverages in the Table of Food Composition (Appendix A). Some people may have access to computers programmed to provide this information in the blink of an eye. Still another way is to estimate calories using the exchange system, presented in full in Appendix D. However they are derived, the numbers are always fascinating to those concerned with managing body weight.

As examples of the numbers of calories associated with food portions, an apple gives you 125 calories from carbohydrate; a regular-size candy bar gives you 425 calories mostly from fat and carbohydrate. You may already know that for each 3,500 calories you eat in excess of expenditures, you store approximately 1 pound of body fat.*

✔ KEY POINT **The "energy in" side of the body's energy budget is measured in calories taken in each day in the form of foods and beverages. Calories in foods and beverages can be estimated using the exchange system or obtained from published tables or computer diet analysis programs.**

Energy Out

While it is easy to estimate the energy present in a serving of food or in a day's meals, it is not easy to determine the energy an individual spends or needs. The committee on Recommended Dietary Allowances (RDA) and Health and Welfare Canada have published recommended energy intakes for various age-sex groups in their populations. These recommendations are useful for population studies, but the range of energy needs among individuals in a group is so broad that it is impossible to guess any individual person's need without knowing something about the person's lifestyle and metabolism.

The RDA for energy are based on average people. For example, the energy RDA for a woman is for a 20-year-old woman who is 5 feet 5 inches tall, weighs about 128 pounds, is of average body fatness, and engages in light activity. This woman needs 2,200 calories of energy a day. The RDA for a man is for a healthy 20-year-old man of average body fatness who stands 5 feet 10 inches tall, weighs 160 pounds, and is lightly active. He needs 2,900 calories a day. Taller people need proportionately more energy than shorter people to balance their energy budgets because their greater surface area allows more energy to escape as heat. Older people generally need less than younger people due to slowed metabolism, reduced muscle mass, and reduced activity. The energy need diminishes by 5 percent per decade on average beyond the age of 30 years.

In reality, though, no one is average and people's energy needs vary widely. In any group of 20 similar people with similar activity levels, one may expend twice as much energy per day as another. Clearly, with such a wide range of variation, a necessary step in determining any person's energy need is to study that person.

One way to estimate your energy needs is to monitor your food intake and body weight over a period of time in which your activities are typical of your lifestyle. If you keep an accurate record of all the foods and beverages you consume for a week or two and if your weight has not changed during the past few months, you can conclude that your energy budget is balanced. At least three days of record keeping are necessary because intakes fluctuate from day to day. A week or two is better still. (On about half the days, you eat less food energy than the average; on the other half, more.)

---

*Pure fat is worth 9 calories per gram. A pound of it (450 grams), then, would store 4,050 calories. A pound of *body* fat is not pure fat, though; it contains water, protein, and other materials—hence the lower calorie value.

1 lb body fat = 3,500 cal.

The energy RDA are presented in the inside front cover; Canadian energy allowances are presented in Appendix B.

For both women and men, *light activity* means sleeping or lying down for eight hours a day, sitting for seven hours, standing for five, walking for two, and spending too hours a day in light physical activity.

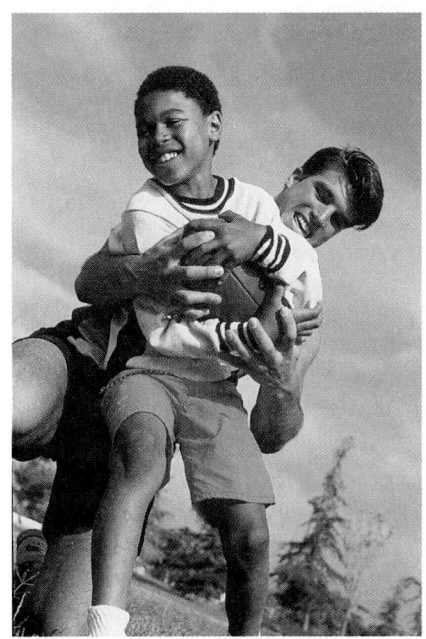

Balancing food energy intake with physical activity can add to life's enjoyment.

FIGURE 9-1

COMPONENTS OF ENERGY EXPENDITURE

Generally, basal metabolism represents a person's largest expenditure of energy, followed by exercise and the thermic effect of foods. Of these categories, energy spent in physical activity is most responsive to voluntary control.

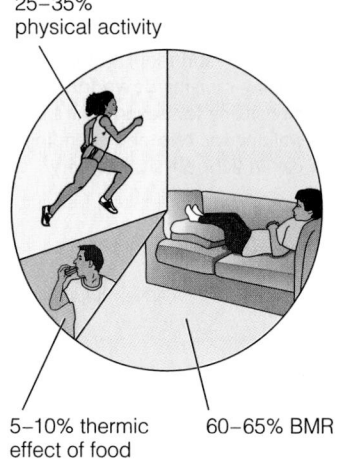

25–35% physical activity

5–10% thermic effect of food

60–65% BMR

thermic effect of food (TEF) the body's speeded-up metabolism in response to having eaten a meal. Also called *diet-induced thermogenesis.*

basal metabolism the sum total of all the involuntary activities that are necessary to sustain life, including circulation, respiration, temperature maintenance, hormone secretion, nerve activity, and new tissue synthesis, but excluding digestion and voluntary activities. Basal metabolism is the largest component of the average person's daily energy expenditure.

voluntary activities intentional activities (such as walking, sitting, running) conducted by voluntary muscles.

basal metabolic rate (BMR) the rate at which the body uses energy to support its basal metabolism.

An alternative method of determining energy output is to look up data for, and compute, the two major components of energy expenditure and then add them together. This method leaves out a third energy component, the body's metabolic response to food, first mentioned in Controversy 5. About 5 to 10 percent of a meal's energy value is used up in stepped-up metabolism in the five or so hours following each meal; this category of energy expenditure is called the **thermic effect of food.** This amount of energy could affect expenditures over the long run, but most experts believe its effects are negligible.[1] For our purposes here, it can be ignored.

The two major ways in which the body spends energy are (1) to fuel its **basal metabolism** and (2) to fuel its **voluntary activities** (see Figure 9-1). Basal metabolism generates energy to support the body's work that goes on all the time without our conscious awareness.

The **basal metabolic rate (BMR)** is surprisingly fast and varies from person to person.[2] A person whose total energy needs are 2,000 calories a day spends as many as 1,200 to 1,400 of them to support basal metabolism. The hormone thyroxine directly controls basal metabolism—the less secreted, the lower the energy requirements for basal functions. Many other factors also affect the BMR (see Table 9-1).

People often want to know how they can speed up their metabolism to promote fat loss. You cannot speed up your BMR much today. You can, however, amplify the second component of your energy expenditure, your voluntary activities. If you do this, you will spend more calories today, and if you keep doing this day after day, your BMR will gradually increase. Lean tissue is more metabolically active than fat tissue, so a way to speed up your BMR to the maximum possible rate is to make endurance and strength-building exercise a daily habit, so that your body composition becomes as lean as possible.[3] A warning: some ads for weight-loss diets claim that eating certain foods can elevate the BMR and thus promote weight loss. This claim is false. Any meal

TABLE 9-1

Factors That Affect the BMR

Factor	Effect on BMR
Age	The BMR is higher in youth; as lean body mass declines with age, the BMR slows.
Height	Tall people have a larger surface area, so their BMRs are higher.
Growth	Children and pregnant women have higher BMRs.
Body composition	The more lean tissue, the higher the BMR.
Fever	Fever raises the BMR.
Stress	Stress hormones raise the BMR.
Environmental temperature	Adjusting to either heat and cold raises the BMR.
Fasting/starvation	Fasting/starvation hormones lower the BMR.
Malnutrition	Malnutrition lowers the BMR.
Thyroxine	The thyroid hormone thyroxine is a key BMR regulator; the more thyroxine produced, the higher the BMR.

TABLE 9-2

Activity Equivalents of Food-Energy Values

FOOD	ENERGY (CAL)	ACTIVITY EQUIVALENT FOR A 150-POUND PERSON TO WORK OFF THE CALORIES (MINUTES)		
		Walk[a]	Run[b]	Wait[c]
Apple, large	125	24	8	75
Regular beer, 1 glass (8 oz)	100	19	6	61
Cookie, chocolate chip (10 g)	50	10	3	30
Ice cream, ½ c (10 g)	175	34	11	106
Steak, T-bone (6 oz)	475	91	31	288

[a]Energy cost of walking at 3.5 miles per hour—5.2 calories per minute.
[b]Energy cost of running at 9 miles per hour—15.5 calories per minute.
[c]Energy cost of sitting—1.65 calories per minute.

promotes a temporary stepped-up energy expenditure in the form of the thermic effect of food; in the context of a mixed diet, the differences among foods are not large enough to be worth notice.

As for fuel for voluntary activities, the amount of energy you spend in exercise depends somewhat on your personal style. In general, the heavier the weight of the body parts you move in your activity and the longer the time you invest, the more calories you spend. So important to energy balance is physical activity that much of Chapter 10 is devoted to presenting details of how the body spends its energy during activity. For fun right now, Table 9-2 translates some activity values into food-energy terms.

Long periods of vigorous activity, engaged in frequently, can place great demands on energy supplies. During football or basketball season, a player may need 5,000 calories a day or even more to play well and to maintain weight. To avoid gaining unwanted fat after the season, it is equally important for an athlete to cut back to an energy intake that suits the off-season activity. The next section shows how to calculate an approximation of your daily energy output.

✔ **KEY POINT**   **Two major components of the "energy out" side of the body's energy budget are basal metabolism and voluntary activities. A third component of energy expenditure is the thermic effect of food.**

Estimation of Energy Needs

To estimate total energy expenditure, first estimate the two major components separately, then add them together. The first component is the energy spent in basal metabolism. Follow these steps. Use the BMR factor 1.0 calorie per kilogram of body weight per hour for men or 0.9 for women (men usually have more muscles (metabolically active tissue) than women do). Example (for a 150-pound man):

1. Change pounds to kilograms:

    150 pounds ÷ 2.2 pounds per kilogram = 68 kilograms.

2. Multiply weight in kilograms by the BMR factor:

68 kilograms $\times$ 1 calorie per kilogram per hour = 68 calories per hour.

3. Multiply the calories used in one hour by the hours in a day:

68 calories per hour $\times$ 24 hours per day = 1,632 calories per day.

The second major component of energy expenditure, physical activity, has been mentioned previously. It is calculated by multiplying the BMR calories by a percentage that varies by activity level. These percentages are estimates or approximations of energy expenditure based on the amount of muscular work a person typically performs in a day:

- Sedentary lifestyle: Men 25 to 40 percent; women 25 to 35 percent.
- Light activity: Men 50 to 70 percent; women 40 to 60 percent.
- Moderate activity: Men 65 to 80 percent; women 50 to 70 percent.
- Heavy activity: Men 90 to 120 percent; women 80 to 100 percent.
- Exceptional activity: Men 130 to 145 percent; women 110 to 130 percent.[*]

To select the activity level appropriate for you, remember to think in terms of the amount of *muscular* work performed; don't confuse being *busy* with being *active*. If you sit down most of the day and drive or ride whenever possible, use the values for a sedentary person. If you move around some of the time, as a teacher might during working hours, use the light activity values. If you do some amount of intentional exercise, such as an hour of jogging four or five times a week, or if your occupation calls for some physical work, consider yourself moderately active. A person whose job requires much physical labor, such as a roofer or a carpenter, would be in the heavy activity range. The exceptional category is reserved for those few who spend many hours a day in intense physical training, such as professional or college athletes during their seasons. A table in Chapter 10 provides more exact energy costs per minute of activities based on body weight.

Calculate your energy expenditure using both the upper and lower ends of the range of percentages given for your gender and activity level. Suppose the 150-pound man used as an example earlier is a student who bikes about ten minutes a day and walks to classes but otherwise sits and studies. He falls into the light activity category, so we can estimate the range of energy he needs by multiplying his BMR calories per day by both 50 and 70 percent:

1,632 calories per day $\times$ 0.50 = 816 calories per day.

1,632 calories per day $\times$ 0.70 = 1,142 calories per day.

The man needs from 816 to 1,142 calories per day for his activities. Now total the metabolic and activity components, first using the lower number for activity energy, then using the higher number. In a day, the man in our example spends either:

1,632 calories per day + 816 calories per day = 2,448 calories per day

or

1,632 calories per day + 1,142 calories per day = 2,774 calories per day.

Voluntary activity for control of body fatness is a topic of Chapter 10.

*Percentages are derived from the RDA (1989) formula for energy expenditure, allowing a 15 to 30 percent range.

Express the man's needs as a range of rounded values: 2,400 to 2,800 calories per day.

> ✔️ KEY POINT   **To estimate the energy spent on basal metabolism, use the factor (for men) 1.0 calories per kilogram of body weight per hour (or for women, 0.9 calories per kilogram per hour) for a 24-hour period. Then add a percentage of this amount depending on how much daily muscular activity the person engages in.**

THE PROBLEMS OF TOO MUCH OR TOO LITTLE BODY FAT

Both deficient and excessive body fat present health risks. It has long been known that thin people will die first during a siege or in a famine. A fact not always recognized, even by health-care providers, is that overly thin people are also at a disadvantage in the hospital, where they may have to go for days without food so that they can undergo tests or surgery. Underweight also increases the risk for any person fighting a **wasting** disease. In fact, people with cancer often die, not from the cancer itself, but from starvation. Thus excessively underweight people are urged to gain body fat as an energy reserve and as protection for the bones, and to acquire protective amounts of all the nutrients that can be stored.

As for excessive body fat, it too, is associated with increased risks of disease.[4] For example, even a modest weight gain during adulthood brings an increased risk of diabetes among women.[5] Excess weight has been named as the cause of up to half of all cases of hypertension, and thus increases the risk of stroke.[6] Often weight loss alone can normalize the blood pressure of an overfat person; some people with hypertension can tell you exactly at what weight their blood pressure begins to rise. Being overfat also triples a person's risk of developing diabetes and all of its associated ills. If hypertension or diabetes runs in your family, you urgently need to attend to controlling body fatness.

The health risks of overfatness are so many that it has been declared a disease: **obesity.** In addition to diabetes and hypertension, other risks threaten obese adults. Among them are high blood lipids, cardiovascular disease, sleep apnea (abnormal pauses in breathing during sleep), osteoarthritis, abdominal hernias, some cancers, varicose veins, gout, gallbladder disease, arthritis, respiratory problems (including Pickwickian syndrome, a breathing blockage linked with sudden death), liver malfunction, complications in pregnancy and surgery, flat feet, and even a high accident rate. Moreover, after the effects of diagnosed diseases are taken into account, the risk of death from other causes remains almost twice as high for people with lifelong obesity as for others.[7]

As Figure 9-2 shows, more and more people are gaining enough body fat to slip into the weight range that incurs such risks. One out of three adults and one out of five children and teenagers in the United States are now obese.[8] The Healthy People 2000 goals include mandates to reduce obesity prevalence (see Table 9-3). Sadly, prospects of reaching these goals by the year 2000 are remote, as the incidence of overfatness is currently on the rise.

People want to know exactly how fat is too fat for health, but research results vary on this point. Some evidence indicates that being even mildly or moderately overweight increases the risk of heart disease. This implies, of

wasting the progressive, relentless loss of the body's tissues that accompanies certain diseases and shortens survival time.

obesity overfatness with adverse health effects, as determined by reliable measures and interpreted with good medical judgment. Obesity is sometimes defined as a body mass index over 30 (see p. 344).

FIGURE 9-2

PREVALENCE OF OBESITY AMONG ADULTS IN THE UNITED STATES

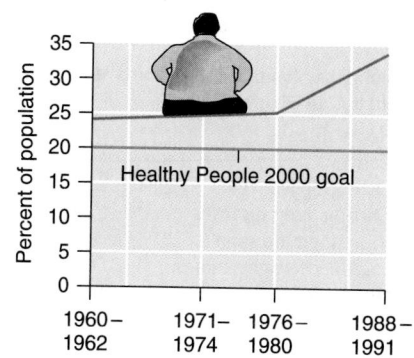

visceral fat fat stored within the abdominal cavity in association with the internal abdominal organs. Also called *intraabdominal fat*.

central obesity excess fat in the abdomen and around the trunk.

subcutaneous fat fat stored directly under the skin (*sub* means "beneath"; *cutaneous* refers to the skin).

TABLE 9-3

Guidelines for Weight Control

Healthy People 2000:

- Increase to at least 50% the proportion of overweight people aged 12 years and older who have adopted sound dietary practices combined with regular physical activity to attain an appropriate body weight.
- Reduce overweight to a prevalence of no more than 20% among people aged 20 years and older and maintain prevalence at no more than 15% among adolescents aged 12 through 19 years.

Dietary Guidelines:

- Balance the food you eat with physical activity—maintain or improve your weight.

Smoking may keep some people's weight down, but at what cost?

- ✓ Heart disease
- ✓ Cancer
- ✓ Osteoporosis
- ✓ Chronic lung diseases
- ✓ Shortened life span
- ✓ Low-birthweight babies
- ✓ Miscarriage
- ✓ Sudden infant death
- ✓ Many others

course, that excess weight is composed of fat, not muscle. Even lean adults who were 20 pounds or more overweight as teenagers may be at increased risk of dying of heart disease.[9] On the other hand, some obese people seem to remain healthy and live long despite their excess body fatness. Body composition may have an effect. In some populations of the world, the longest-lived people seem to be those on the heavy end of the normal weight range; whether their high weights are due to extra fat or muscle is not known. Genetics may also determine who among the overweight are most susceptible to diseases and who are likely to stay well. Still, the majority of obese people do develop health problems.

Even more than total fatness, fat that collects deep within the central abdominal area of the body, called **visceral fat,** may be especially dangerous with regard to risks of diabetes, stroke, hypertension, and coronary artery disease. In fact, the risk of death from all causes may be higher in those with **central obesity** than in those whose fat accumulates elsewhere in the body (see Figure 9-3). The health risks of obesity seem to run on a continuum: normal weight brings no extra risk, central obesity carries severe risks, and other forms of obesity fall somewhere in between.[10]

Researchers theorize that, unlike the fat layers lying just beneath the skin **(subcutaneous fat)** of the abdomen and elsewhere, the visceral fat, when mobilized, goes directly to the liver. There, it is made into cholesterol-carrying low-density lipoprotein (LDL). Fat from elsewhere may arrive in the liver eventually, but it takes a circuitous route that gives other tissues the chance to pull it from circulation and metabolize it.

Some people are more prone to develop the "apple" profile of central obesity while others develop more of a "pear" profile (fat around the hips and thighs). Men of all ages and women past menopause are more likely to be "apples" than are women in their reproductive years, who are more often "pears."[11] Some women change profile at menopause, and lifelong "pears" may suddenly face increased risks of diseases that accompany the apple profile. Smokers, too, may carry more of their body fat centrally. Whereas a smoker may weigh less than the average nonsmoker, the smoker's waist-to-hip ratio may be greater, leading researchers to think that smoking may directly affect body fat distribution.[12] Two other factors may affect body fat distribution. High intakes of alcohol have a positive association with central adiposity and high exercise levels have a negative association.

A further word about smoking seems in order. Smokers tend to weigh less than nonsmokers, and many gain weight when they stop smoking.[13] Smoking a cigarette eases feelings of hunger. A smoker who receives a hunger signal can quiet it with a cigarette instead of food. Smoking may also stimulate the release of fat from fat cells and its subsequent use by body tissues. Weight gain is often a concern for people who are thinking of quitting smoking. Whether the weight gained is excessive seems to be partly determined by the genetic makeup of the quitter.[14] The best advice to smokers wanting to quit seems to be to adjust diet and exercise habits to maintain weight during and after cessation.

While some overfat people seem to escape health problems, no one who is fat in our society quite escapes the social and economic handicaps. Our society places enormous value on thinness, especially for women, and fat people are less sought after for romance, less often hired, and less often admitted to college.[15] They pay higher insurance premiums, and they pay more for clothing.

Psychologically, too, fat people are made to feel rejected and embarrassed, and this diminishes self-esteem.

Traditional medical advice urges all obese people to reduce their fatness to reduce associated risks. This advice stems from concern for their health and, indeed, may be lifesaving for some. Lately, though, experts are divided on whether this advice applies equally to all obese people or whether some may be more at risk from the process of losing weight than from the obesity itself. This chapter's Controversy explores this debate from both points of view.

✔ **KEY POINT** **Both deficient and excessive body fatness present health risks, and overfatness presents social and economic handicaps as well. Central obesity may be more hazardous to health than other forms of obesity.**

BODY WEIGHT VERSUS BODY FATNESS

Once upon a time the definition of appropriate body fatness was simple. A person's weight could be compared with that in the "ideal weight" tables. If the actual weight was 20 percent or more above the table weight, then the person was obese; if it was 10 percent under, the person was underweight. Now (to tell a long story in a few words), the term *ideal weight* is no longer in use, and the definition of obesity is no longer simple.

The Weight-for-Height Tables

A problem of using weight as an indicator of health or risk status is that body weight says so little about body composition. A person whose weight seems right according to suggested weights for heights may still carry too much of that weight as body fat, especially when lean muscle tissue is minimal due to lack of exercise. Conversely, a person who seems to weigh too much may not be too fat. People tend to shrink in height and gain fat as they age, making the height and weight charts meaningless in later years. A dancer or an athlete, whose muscles are well developed and whose bones are well mineralized thanks to consistent exercise, may weigh above the suggested weight range, but still be at a healthy weight. An example of incorrectly relying on height-weight tables to determine obesity occurred with a group of football players. They were rejected from the armed forces for being obese according to the table, but their *muscle* weight was actually responsible for the elevated scale weights.

Over the years, standard weight tables have steadily added pounds to the recommended weights for U.S. citizens. For example, the 1990 version allowed people over 35 years old to gain a few pounds as they aged. Then came research findings indicating increased cardiovascular disease risk in women who gained weight while remaining within the suggested range.[16] New tables issued in 1995 restrict body weight for all adults with no variation by age. Not every nutrition authority is pleased with the new tables, and they may change again as more becomes known about the correlations between body weight and health.

Despite problems with their use, the weight tables have three undeniable advantages in assessing obesity—they are available, cheap, and easy to use. If

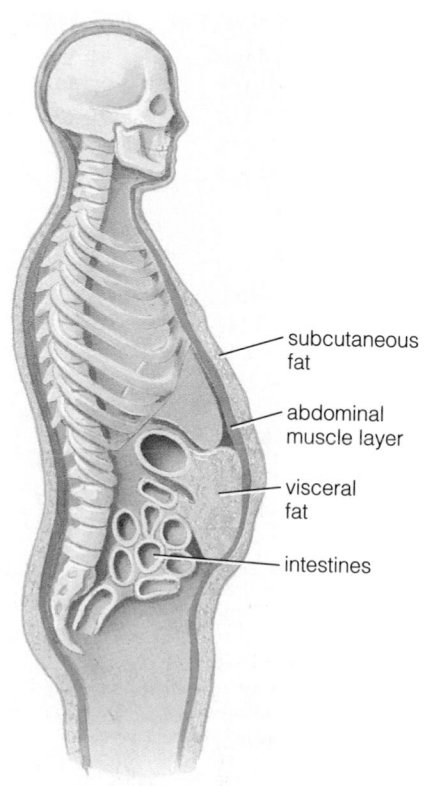

FIGURE 9-3

VISCERAL FAT AND SUBCUTANEOUS FAT
The fat lying deep within the body's abdominal cavity may pose an especially high risk to health.

subcutaneous fat

abdominal muscle layer

visceral fat

intestines

TABLE 9-4

Suggested Weights for Adults of All Ages: 1995 Guidelines

HEIGHT[a]	WEIGHT (LB)[a]	
	Midpoint	Range[b]
4'10"	105	91–119
4'11"	109	94–124
5'0"	112	97–128
5'1"	116	101–132
5'2"	120	104–137
5'3"	124	107–141
5'4"	128	111–146
5'5"	132	114–150
5'6"	136	118–155
5'7"	140	121–160
5'8"	144	125–164
5'9"	149	129–169
5'10"	153	132–174
5'11"	157	136–179
6'0"	162	140–184
6'1"	166	144–189
6'2"	171	148–195
6'3"	176	152–200
6'4"	180	156–205
6'5"	185	160–211
6'6"	190	164–216

[a]Without shoes or clothes.

[b]Higher weights within the ranges generally apply to men, and lower weights to women, because men tend to have more muscle and bone.

SOURCE: Report of the Dietary Guidelines Advisory Committee on the Dietary Guidelines for Americans, 1995.

Find Your BMI:

$$BMI = \frac{weight\ (kg)}{height\ (m)^2}$$

or

$$BMI = \frac{weight\ (lb)}{height\ (in)^2} \times 705$$

Example: A 5'10" person weighing 150 lb has a BMI of 21.6

$$BMI = \frac{150}{70^2} \times 705$$

$$BMI = \frac{150}{4,900} \times 705$$

$$BMI = .0306 \times 705$$

$$BMI = 21.6\ (rounded)$$

you choose to use Table 9-4, be sure to use your barefoot height, and if you wear clothing while weighing, adjust the numbers. Add three pounds to the table weight for light summer clothing, five pounds for heavier winter apparel. If you have medical conditions, disease risk factors, or central obesity, the table data are null and void; a physical examination with interview, body measurements, and lab tests is the route to assessing your risk from overweight.

While weight measurements have advantages, they also have the two major drawbacks already mentioned: they fail to indicate how much of the weight is fat and where that fat is located. To find out, one must measure body composition and fat distribution. There is no easy way to look inside a person to measure bones and muscles, but some indirect approximations can reveal clues about health risks associated with overfatness or underweight.

✓ KEY POINT **Defining both ideal weight and obesity based on standard weight tables is beset with problems for many people.**

Body Mass Index

To define healthy weight and obesity, nutritionists often prefer to use a standard derived from height and weight measures, but manipulated mathematically—the **body mass index (BMI).** BMI values correlate fairly well with health risk with underweight or overweight as Table 9-5 shows. The inside back cover of this book provides an easy way to find and evaluate BMI.

The BMI values are probably most valuable for evaluating degrees of obesity and are less useful for evaluating nonobese people's body fatness. BMI values do not reflect fat distribution, however, so other measures are also needed.[17]

✓ KEY POINT **The body mass index mathematically correlates heights and weights with risks to health. It is especially useful for evaluating health risks of obesity but fails to measure body fat distribution.**

Estimating Body Fatness

Several laboratory techniques for estimating body fatness have also been used for years. These include, among others:

TABLE 9-5

BMI Values for Men and Women

BMI		RISK
Men	Women	
<20.7	<19.1	Underweight. The lower the BMI, the greater the risk.
20.7 to 26.4	19.1 to 25.8	Normal, very low risk
26.4 to 27.8	25.8 to 27.3	Marginally overweight, some risk
27.8 to 31.1	27.3 to 32.2	Overweight, moderate risk
31.1 to 45.4	32.3 to 44.8	Severe overweight, high risk
>45.4	>44.8	Morbid obesity, very high risk

FIGURE 9-4

THREE METHODS OF ASSESSING BODY FATNESS

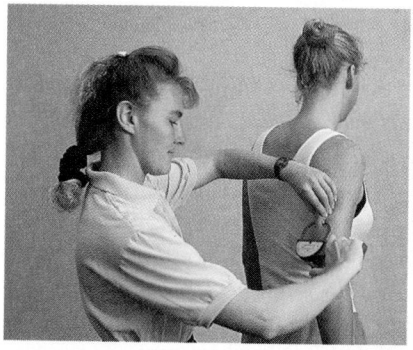

A. A fatfold measure can yield accurate results when taken by a trained technician using a calibrated metal caliper.

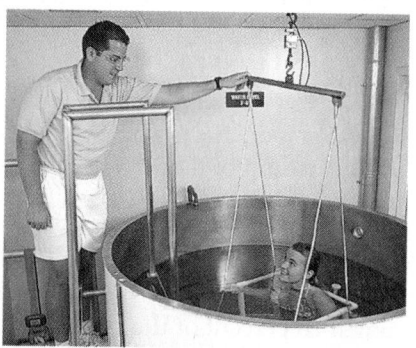

B. Underwater weighing determines body volume and density, measurements reflecting the percentage of body fat in experimental subjects.

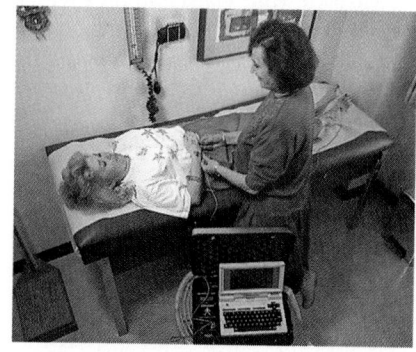

C. Bioelectrical impedance is simple, painless, and accurate when properly administered; the method determines body fatness by measuring conductivity.

- *Anthropometry.* Measurements such as the **fatfold test** or body circumferences can be taken (see Figure 9-4).[18]
- *Density* (the measurement of body weight compared with volume). Lean tissue is denser than fat tissue, so the denser a person's body is, the more lean tissue it must contain. Density can be determined by **underwater weighing.**
- *Conductivity.* Only lean tissue and water conduct electrical current; **bioelectrical impedance** measures how well a tiny harmless electrical charge is conducted through the lean tissue of the body and so reflects the body's contents of lean tissue, including water. A drawback is that temporary changes in body water content can produce changes in the measurement.

Other sophisticated techniques are available. Some can not only estimate lean versus fat tissue but also determine where the fat is located. Even these methods do not provide perfect analyses of some people, however. For example, the body fat of African-American women may be underestimated in laboratory studies because standard methods do not account for variability of body composition among ethnic groups.[19]

Fatfold measurements provide an accurate estimate of total body fat and a fair assessment of the fat's location.[20] About half of the fat in the body lies directly beneath the skin, so the thickness of this subcutaneous fat is assumed to reflect total body fat. Measures taken from central-body sites (around the abdomen) better reflect changes in fatness than those taken from upper sites (arm and back). Fatfold measurements taken without skill and training are often inaccurate, however. For a fair indication of whether you develop fat centrally, try the simple method of comparing waist and hip measurements presented in Figure 9-5.

body mass index (BMI) an indicator of obesity, calculated by dividing the weight of a person by the square of the person's height.

fatfold test measurement of the thickness of a fold of skin on the back of the arm (over the triceps muscle), below the shoulder blade (subscapular), or in other places, using a caliper (depicted in Figure 9-4). Also called *skinfold test.*

underwater weighing a measure of density and volume used to determine body fat content.

bioelectrical impedance a technique to measure body fatness by measuring the body's electrical conductivity.

FIGURE 9-5

DETERMINING YOUR WAIST-TO-HIP
CIRCUMFERENCE RATIO

1. Measure your waist and hips with a
   measuring tape. For your hips, use
   the largest circumference you find.
2. Calculate your waist-to-hip circumference ratio:

   Waist-to-hip ratio = waist
   circumference ÷ hip circumference

   Example: a woman with a 28-inch
   waist and 38-inch hips:

   28 ÷ 38 = 0.74 ratio

3. Evaluate your ratio. A ratio over .95
   for males or .80 for females indicates
   a need to reduce body fatness to
   reduce health risks. Our example
   woman's ratio of 0.74 is in the range
   considered healthy.

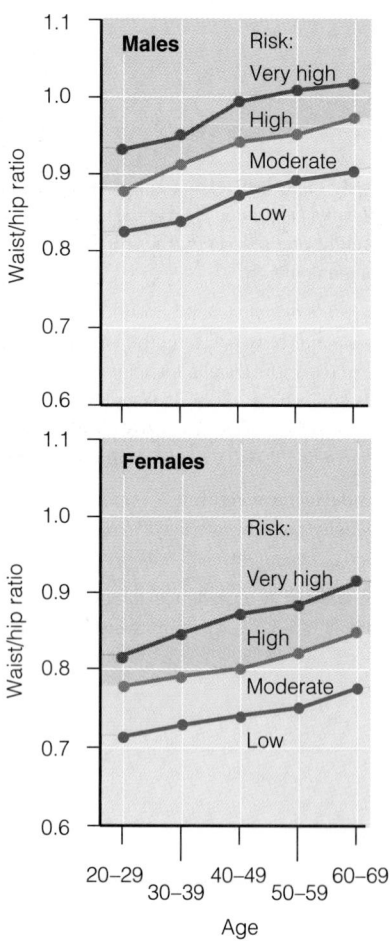

SOURCE: Percentile scales from National Research
Council, *Diet and Health: Implications for Reducing
Chronic Disease Risks* (Washington, D.C.: National
Academy Press, 1989), p. 566.

✔ **KEY POINT** **An assessor can determine the percentage of fat in a person's body by measuring fatfolds, body density, or other parameters. Distribution of fat can be estimated by determining the waist-to-hip ratio.**

Defining Priorities

Even after you have a body fatness estimate, questions arise. What is the
"ideal" amount of fat for a body to have? The question, ideal for what? has to
be answered first. If the answer is "society's approval," be aware that fashion
is fickle. Body shapes valued for looks may have little to do with health.

If the answer is "health," the ideal depends partly on who you are. A man
of normal body composition may have, on the average, 15 percent and a
woman 20 percent of the body weight as fat. Researchers draw the line when
body fat exceeds 22 percent in young men, 25 percent in older men, 32 percent
in younger women, and 35 percent in older women; these are the values used
to define obesity, with age 40 as the dividing line between younger and older.[21]

Lifestyles and stages necessitate using different standards for different people, that is, applying judgment. For example, competitive endurance athletes
need just enough body fat to provide fuel, insulate the body, and permit normal fat-soluble hormone activity, but not so much as to weigh them down. An
Alaskan fisherman, in contrast, needs a blanket of extra fat to insulate against
the cold. For a woman starting pregnancy, the ideal percentage of body fat may
be different again; the outcome of pregnancy is compromised if the woman
begins it with too little body fat. Below a threshold for body fat content set by
heredity, some individuals become infertile, develop depression or abnormal
hunger regulation, or become unable to keep warm. These thresholds are not
the same for each function or in all individuals, and much remains to be
learned about them.

Beyond the basic needs for body fat, you should strive to keep body fat low.
Blood pressure and other disease risk indicators—blood glucose and blood
cholesterol, for example—also rise and fall with body fatness. For those in
whom these signs appear with added fat, weight reduction may be critical. For
now, professionals are still seeking a method of pinpointing the amount of fatness that poses dangers to any individual.

The person seeking a single, authoritative answer to the question "How
much should I weigh?" is bound to be disappointed. No one can tell you
exactly how much you should weigh; but with health as a value, at least you
have a starting framework. Your weight should fall within the range that best
supports your health.

✔ **KEY POINT** **No single body weight suits everyone; different people
have different needs and goals.**

THE MYSTERY OF OBESITY

Why do some people get fat? Why do some get thin? And most amaz-
ingly, why do some people stay at the same weight year after year? Is weight
controlled by hereditary, metabolic factors? Or is it controlled by environmental

influences? Is it a matter of behavior—and if so, is behavior controlled by the environment, or by heredity, or both? The next two sections sort the peices of the puzzle into inside-the-body and outside-the-body factors, but no law says that only one type of cause must prevail. In all likelihood, internal and external factors operate together, and in different combinations in different people.

Inside-the-Body Causes of Obesity

Researchers have attempted to study what makes people consume more energy (calories) than they spend by investigating **hunger, appetite,** and **satiety** (see Figure 9-6). Hunger is a drive programmed into us by our heredity. Appetite, which is learned, can teach us to ignore hunger or to overrespond to it. Hunger is physiological, while appetite is psychological, and the two do not always coincide. Satiety (feeling full) signals that no more food is needed, most likely as a result of communication to the brain, especially to the hypothalamus, about the presence or absence of food or nutrients in the mouth, stomach, or intestines, or in the blood.[22] Some overeaters claim they never feel full, indicating that these sensations may not always convey need perfectly. A sampling of other lines of study follows.

Genetic Inheritance Theory   For a person who has one parent with obesity, the chance of becoming obese is 60 percent; if both parents have obesity, the probability may rise to as high as 90 percent.[23] This suggests that a person's genetic makeup may influence the tendency of the body to consume or store too much energy or burn too little. Recently, researchers have discovered a gene in humans, the *ob (obese)* gene.[24] Mice with defective versions of such genes weigh up to three times as much as normal mice.[25]

Two findings creating great excitement among obesity researchers are the isolation of a protein hormone, **leptin,** made by the *ob* gene in fat cells, and the discovery of its responding sites in the human brain.[26] In mice, leptin stimulates the brain's hypothalamus to suppress appetite and to speed up metabolism; together, appetite and metabolism play a large role in maintaining body fat stores. Mice like the round one pictured in the margin have long been used in laboratory obesity research because they are genetically obese—they lack the ability to produce leptin. The thin mouse is of the same strain—it is also genetically obese—but has received injections of leptin, so its weight remains normal.

Oddly, in people, high body fatness seems to correlate *positively* with leptin in the blood. In obese people, the more fat tissue, the *higher* the leptin concentrations.[27] Just a small percentage of obese people are exceptions: they fail to produce leptin at all.

Logically, it would seem that obese people, with their large amounts of fat tissue and so greater concentrations of leptin, should feel *less* hungry than people of normal fatness. This is not the case, however. Fat people feel hungry and stay fat despite their elevated leptin levels. Researchers speculate that the brain cells of obese people may be unresponsive to leptin in much the same way as the body cells of people with the common type of diabetes are unresponsive to insulin. Potentially, harnessing the activities of the *ob* gene and leptin could lead to new effective therapies for obesity—an outcome much desired, but so far not rendered feasible by research.

hunger the physiological need to eat, experienced as a drive for obtaining food, an unpleasant sensation that demands relief.

appetite the psychological desire to eat; a learned motivation and a positive sensation that accompanies the sight, smell, or thought of appealing foods.

satiety a feeling of satisfaction that sends the signal to stop eating.

leptin an appetite-suppressing hormone produced in the fat cells that conveys information about body fatness to the brain; believed to be involved in the maintenance of body composition (*leptos* means "slender").

Chapter 3 described the brain's hypothalamus.

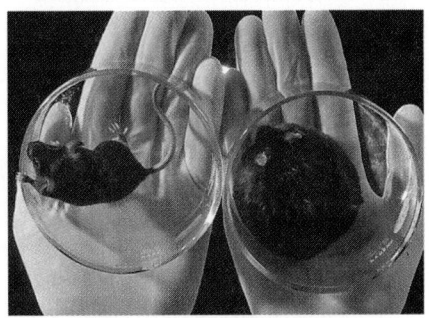

The mouse on the right is genetically obese—it lacks the gene for producing leptin. The mouse on the left is *also* genetically obese but remains lean because it receives leptin.

FIGURE 9-6

HUNGER AND APPETITE

This is a partial list of the factors that are thought to affect hunger and appetite.

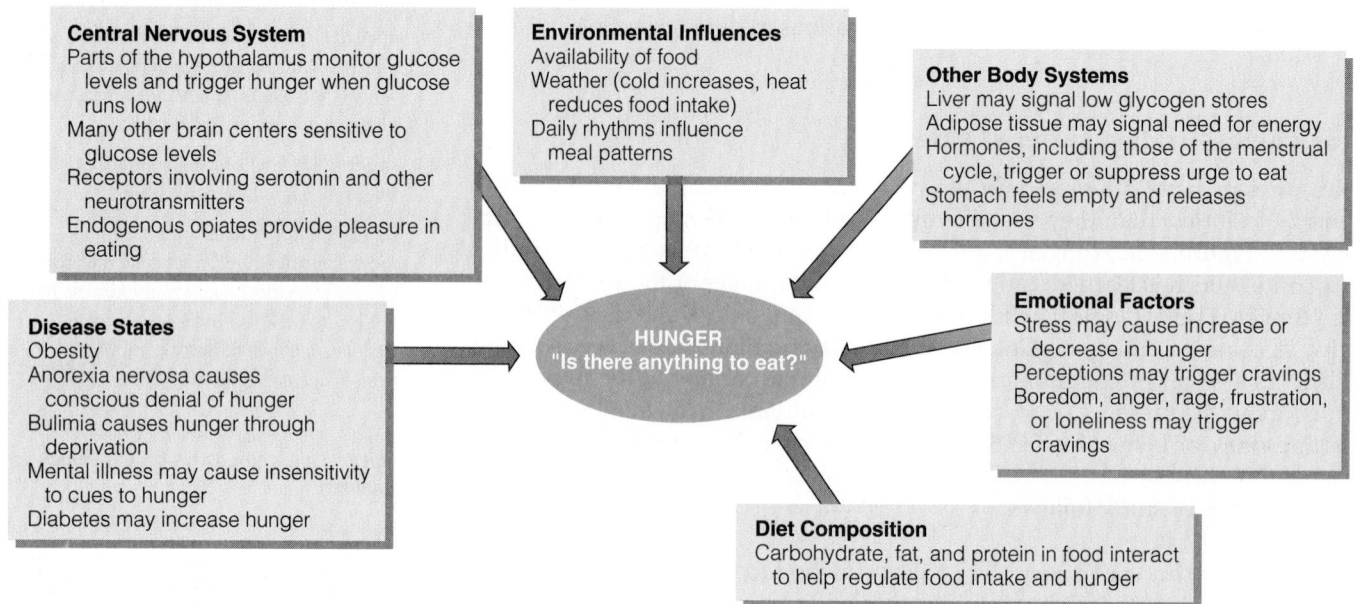

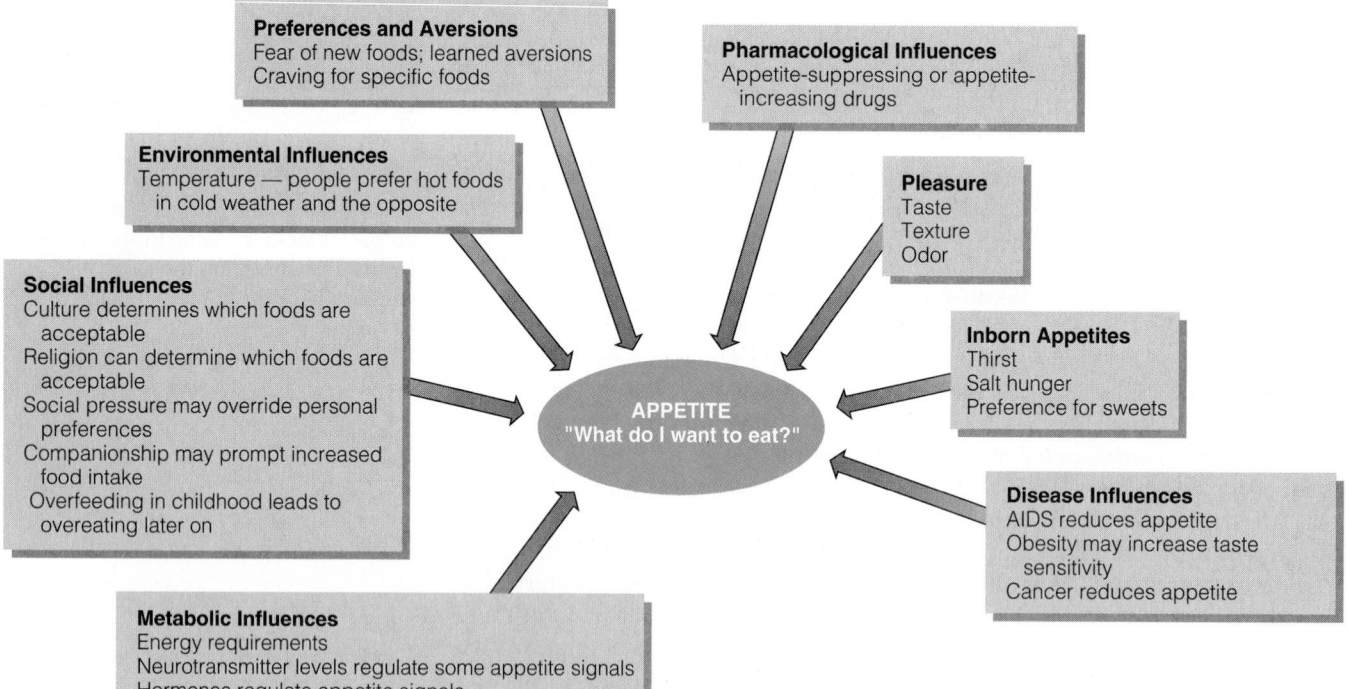

SOURCE: Adapted from the classic model of T. W. Castonguay and coauthors, Hunger and appetite: Old concepts/new distinctions, *Nutrition Reviews* 41 (1983): 101–110.

Set-Point Theory   The discovery of the leptin regulating system may help to support the long-popular theory of why the obese person's body may store too much fat, the **set-point theory.** Most people who lose weight on reducing diets later quickly regain all the lost weight. This phenomenon seems to suggest that somehow the body chooses a weight that it wants to be and defends that weight by regulating eating behaviors and hormonal actions.[28]

Unfortunately for those trying to lose weight or maintain weight loss, evidence is piling up to support the idea that biological systems, and not human will, determine a body weight set point. Just as a thermostat setting triggers a heater to run when air temperature falls and to turn off when warmth is restored, whenever weight is lost or gained, the set point mechanism seems to trigger a change in metabolic rate in the direction that restores the initial body weight: energy expenditure increases with weight gain and decreases with weight loss.[29] These changes in energy expenditure are greater than those predicted based on body composition and may help to explain why it is so difficult for obese people to maintain weight losses.

Enzyme Theory   Strong evidence also links fat storage with elevated concentrations of the enzyme that enables fat cells to store triglycerides. Concentrations of this enzyme, **LPL** or **lipoprotein lipase,** increase as cells become enlarged with fat. The more LPL, the more easily fat cells store lipid, and the more likely the body will remain obese.[30] An interesting question relating to the set-point theory just described is whether some people's fat cells contain elevated concentrations of LPL *before* the onset of obesity. If so, this situation might partly explain why obesity tends to run in families, for the making of all enzymes including LPL is governed by the genes.

Fat Cell Theory   Another cause of obesity may be the development of excess fat cells during childhood. The amount of fat on a person's body reflects both the *number* and the *size* of fat cells. The number of fat cells increases during the growing years and then levels off during adulthood. Fat cell number increases more rapidly in obese children than in lean children, and obese children entering their teen years may already have as many fat cells as do adults of normal weight.

A fat cell can expand eight to tenfold in size. Once a cell reaches some critical size, it may also divide. Fat cells of obese people also contain more LPL, so they are likely to reach a large size quickly.[31] Therefore, obesity reflects not only more and larger fat cells, but more efficient ones, too. With fat loss, the fat cells shrink in size, but not in number and perhaps not in their LPL enzyme numbers, either.[32] For this reason, people with extra fat cells may encounter extra difficulty in trying to lose weight. They may also tend to regain lost weight rapidly. Obesity-fighting measures may therefore be most effective during the growing years when fat cell number is increasing and prevention of not-yet-developed obesity may be more effective in the long term than efforts to cure already-established obesity.

The Theory of Thermogenesis   A theory about the body's manufacturing of heat, **thermogenesis,** and its relation to obesity concerns a tissue that specializes in converting energy to heat—**brown fat.** Regular white fat cells store energy in fat's chemical bonds and have a slow metabolic rate; brown fat cells

set-point theory the theory that the body tends to maintain a certain weight by means of its own internal controls.

LPL (lipoprotein lipase) an enzyme mounted on the surfaces of fat cells that splits triglycerides in the blood into fatty acids and glycerol to be absorbed into the cells for reassembly and storage.

thermogenesis the generation and release of body heat associated with the breakdown of body fuels.

brown fat adipose tissue abundant in hibernating animals and human infants. Brown fat cells are packed with pigmented, energy-burning enzymes that release heat rather than manufacturing fuels from fat. These enzymes give the cells a darkened appearance under a microscope.

arousal heightened activity of certain brain centers associated with attention, excitement, and anxiety.

stress eating eating in response to stress, an inappropriate activity.

break those bonds and actively release their stored energy as heat. Brown fat is more abundant and more active in lean animals than in fat ones. It is theorized that a person whose fat burns off too little energy or a person who has less than the normal amount of brown fat would tend to store more white fat than other people store. No one yet knows how much brown fat tissue normally occurs in adults.

New evidence supports the idea that the fat cells, both brown and white, of obese people may burn off less heat energy than normal. A group of genetic researchers found that the fat cells of some obese people inherit a regulatory mechanism that slows the rate of fat breakdown and thermogenesis. The researchers suggest that people with the tendency to metabolize fat more slowly and to generate less heat may store body fat efficiently.[33]

Thermic Effect of Food   Another form of thermogenesis, the thermic effect of food (TEF) mentioned earlier, varies between obese and nonobese people. In lean people who have just eaten a meal, energy use speeds up for a while and then drops back to normal. In many obese people, no change in energy use occurs after eating. While TEF costs little energy, some researchers believe this amount of energy adds up over a lifetime and may contribute to leanness.

So far no one has shown conclusively that overweight people expend less energy overall than normal-weight people, and in fact, the opposite seems to hold true. Overweight people seem to spend more energy each day, not less, than do people of normal weight.[34] This is probably because heavier bodies require more energy to move and to maintain themselves.

✔ **KEY POINT**   **Inside-the-body theories about causes of obesity include the genetic inheritance theory, set-point theory, enzyme theory, fat cell theory, and theories centered around thermogenesis.**

Outside-the-Body Causes of Obesity

A different line of research pursues the question whether obesity is determined by behavioral responses to environmental stimuli. These researchers ask what external forces might cause people to eat more food than they need.

Eating behavior seems to occur not only in response to internal hunger and appetite, but also to complex human sensations such as yearning, craving, addiction, or compulsion. For an emotionally insecure person, eating when lonely may be less threatening than calling a friend and risking rejection. Often people eat to relieve boredom or depression. Some people experience food cravings when feeling down or depressed.[35] Food picks them up for a while.

Any kind of **arousal** can cause overeating, perhaps because arousal feelings are mistaken for hunger. The eating done in response to arousal is **stress eating.** While some people overeat in response to stress, however, others under-eat or cannot eat at all. It is not yet known why people react differently. Obese people do not seem especially likely to feel anxiety or depression.

External Cue Theory   Proponents of this view hold that people overeat as a response to stimuli in their surroundings—foremost among them, the availability of a multitude of delectable foods.[36] This theory cannot fully explain obesity development because almost everyone, not just obese people, can be enticed to overeat when choosing from an abundance of rich and appetizing foods. A classic experiment showed that even animals respond in this way. Normal-weight rats rapidly became obese when fed "cafeteria style" on a variety of rich, palatable foods. Rats are known to maintain a precise, healthy weight when fed a standard rat-chow diet.

It may be that obese people are supersensitive to delicious tastes, and that this sensitivity may lead them to consume more of whatever food they perceive as delicious. The overweight subjects of one study more often sought the foods they found most palatable and ate them more quickly.[37] These ideas may bear on the kinds and quantities of foods overweight people eat in a day.

One food constituent stands out among others in being perceived as palatable—fat.[38] Controversy 5 made clear that not only does fat deliver more than twice the calories, gram for gram, as protein and carbohydrate, it also seems to be stored preferentially by the body and with great efficiency. Of the three energy nutrients, fat stimulates the least energy expenditure in diet-induced thermogenesis and may be least powerful in signalling satiety.[39] Carbohydrate and protein, on the other hand, stimulate much larger responses. A person whose diet contains much fat, even when total calories are reasonable, is often one who battles against overweight. Total calories still matter, though, as evidenced by recent increases in both intakes of carbohydrate calories and incidence of obesity in the United States.

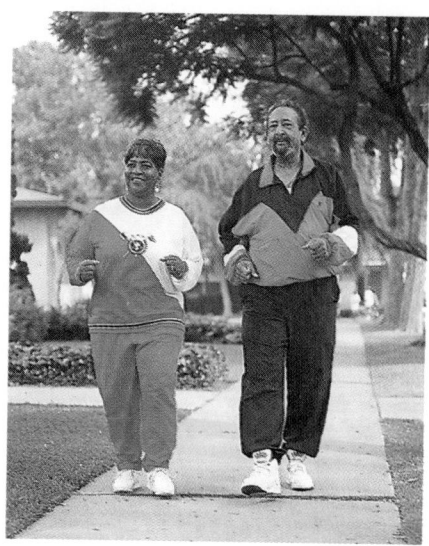

Physical activity can help to regulate the appetite.

Exercise   Although, as mentioned, overweight people may spend more energy than normal-weight people in their regular daily activities, they may engage in less exercise.[40] For many people, television watching has all but replaced outdoor work and play as the major spare-time activity. In addition, sponsors run advertisements for delicious, high-fat (and low-nutrient) foods designed to trigger the appetites of viewers. One study showed that in children, obesity increases by 2 percent per hour of television watching per day. Another reports that watching television costs *less* energy than simply doing nothing.[41] Another factor in obesity development, described in Chapter 2, is widespread consumer demand for ever-increasing food portion sizes.[42]

✓ **KEY POINT**   **Among the theories of behavioral causes of obesity are inappropriate eating in response to stress, arousal, or the sight, smell, and taste of foods. Two major contributors to obesity are believed to be the fattening power of fat in foods and the sedentary lives of some obese people.**

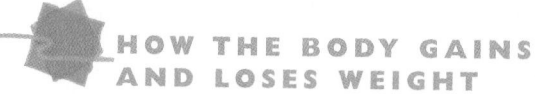

HOW THE BODY GAINS AND LOSES WEIGHT

The balance between the energy you take in and the energy you spend determines whether you will gain, lose, or maintain body *fat*. When you step on the scale and note a change in *weight* of a pound or two, however, this may not indicate a change in body fat. A change in weight can reflect shifts in body fluid content, in bone minerals, in lean tissues such as muscles, or in the contents of the digestive tract. It often correlates with the time of day: people generally weigh the least before breakfast. It is important for people concerned with weight control to realize that quick, large changes in weight are usually not changes in fat alone, or even at all.

A person who stands about 5 feet 10 inches tall and weighs 150 pounds carries about 90 of those pounds as water and 30 as fat. The other 30 pounds are the so-called lean tissues: muscles; organs such as the heart, brain, and liver; and the bones of the skeleton. Stripped of water and fat, then, the person weighs only 30 pounds!* This lean tissue is vital to health. The person who seeks to lose weight wants, of course, to lose fat, not this precious lean tissue. And for someone who wants to gain weight, it is desirable to gain lean and fat in proportion, not just fat.

The type of tissue gained or lost depends on how the person goes about losing or gaining it. To lose fluid, for example, one can take a "water pill" (diuretic), causing the kidneys to siphon extra water from the blood into the urine. Or one can engage in heavy exercise while wearing thick clothing in the heat, losing abundant fluid in sweat. (Both practices are dangerous, incidentally, and are not being recommended here.) To gain water weight, a person can overconsume salt and water; for a few hours, the body will retain water until it manages to excrete the salt. (This, too, is not recommended.) Most quick weight-change schemes promote large changes in body fluids that register temporary, dramatic changes on the scale but accomplish little weight change in the long run. It is important to stress physical activity as a means of gaining and maintaining lean tissue during weight adjustments.

Gain of Body Weight

Weight gain comes from spending less food energy than is taken in. Weight may be gained as body fat or as lean tissue, depending largely upon whether the eater is also exercising. Those who begin weight training and dieting to gain lean tissue may be disappointed when body weight on the scales doesn't change much. Muscle, however, does develop quickly with the right kind of regular exercise. If muscle is growing while fat is shrinking, the desired changes are happening, even if the scale reflects no change in weight.

Chapter 10 comes back to muscle gains in response to exercise.

What happens inside the body when a person does not use up all of the food energy taken in? What does the body do with it? Previous chapters have already provided the answer; the energy-yielding nutrients contribute to body stores as follows:

- Carbohydrate (other than fiber) is broken down to sugars for absorption. In the body tissues, excesses of these may be built up to *glycogen* and stored, burned off as heat, or converted to *fat* and stored.
- Fat is broken down to glycerol and fatty acids for absorption. Inside the body, these are especially easy for the body to store as body *fat*.
- Protein is broken down to amino acids for absorption. Inside the body, these may be used to replace lost body *protein* and, in a person who is exercising, to build new muscle and other lean tissue. This protein must be functioning protein; excess protein is not passively stored. Excess amino acids can have their nitrogen removed and be used for energy or be converted to *glucose* or *fat*, mostly fat.

---

*For a healthy person 5 feet tall and weighing 100 pounds, the comparable figures would be 60 pounds of water, 20 pounds of fat, 20 pounds of lean.

Note that although three kinds of energy-yielding nutrients enter the body, they become only two kinds of energy stores: glycogen and fat. Glycogen stores amount to about three-fourths of a pound; fat stores can, of course, amount to many pounds. Note, too, that when excess protein is converted to fat, it cannot be recovered later as protein because the nitrogen is stripped from the amino acids and excreted in the urine. No matter whether you are eating steak, brownies, or baked beans, then, if you eat enough of them, any excess will be turned to fat within hours.

Alcohol, too, becomes fat if it isn't burned off, and may also make fat storage likely. Ethanol, the alcohol of alcoholic beverages, has been shown to slow down the body's use of fat for fuel by as much as a third, causing more fat to be stored, primarily in the visceral fat tissue of the "beer-drinker's belly" and also on the thighs, legs, or anywhere the person tends to store surplus fat.[43] Alcohol therefore is fattening, both through the calories it provides and through its effects on fat metabolism.*

It is worth emphasizing these points by repeating them:

- Any food can make you fat if you eat enough of it. A net excess of energy is almost all stored in the body as fat in fat tissue.
- Fat, as opposed to carbohydrate or protein, from food is especially easy for the body to store as fat tissue.
- Protein is not stored in the body except in response to exercise; it is present only as working tissue. Excess protein is stored mostly as fat.
- Alcohol both delivers calories and encourages fat storage.
- Too little physical activity encourages body fat accumulation.

✓ **KEY POINT**   **When energy balance is positive, carbohydrate is converted to glycogen or fat, protein is converted to fat, and food fat is stored as fat. Alcohol delivers calories and encourages fat storage.**

Moderate Weight Loss versus Rapid Weight Loss

When you eat less food energy than you need, your body draws on its stored fuel to keep going. It is a great advantage to be able to eat periodically, store fuel, and then use up that fuel between meals. The between-meal interval is normally about 4 to 6 waking hours—about the length of time it takes to use up most of the available liver glycogen—or 12 to 14 hours at night, when body systems are slowed down and the need is less.

When you moderately restrict your calories and consume an otherwise balanced diet that meets your protein and carbohydrate needs, your body will be forced to use up its stored fat for energy. Gradual weight loss will occur. This is preferred to rapid weight loss because lean body mass is spared and fat is lost.

If a person doesn't eat for, say, three whole days or a week, then the body makes one adjustment after another. Soon, the liver's glycogen is essentially exhausted. Where, then, can the body obtain *glucose* to keep its nervous system going? Not from the muscles' glycogen because that is reserved for the

---

*People addicted to alcohol are often overly thin because of diseased organs, depressed appetite, and subsequent malnutrition.

ketone bodies acidic compounds derived from fat and certain amino acids. Normally rare in the blood, they help to feed the brain during times when too little carbohydrate is available. Also defined in Chapter 4.

In Early Food Deprivation:

The nervous system cannot use fat as fuel; it can use only glucose.

Body fat cannot be converted to glucose.

Body protein can be converted to glucose.

In Later Food Deprivation:

Ketone bodies help feed the nervous system and so help spare tissue proteins.

muscles' own use. The underfed body must turn to the protein in its own lean tissues.

An alternative source of *energy* might be the abundant fat stores most people carry, but these are of no use to the nervous system. The muscles, heart, and other organs use fat as fuel, but at this stage the nervous system needs glucose. Most importantly, the body's major fuel, fat, cannot be converted to glucose—the body lacks enzymes for this conversion.* The body does, however, possess enzymes that can convert protein to glucose. Therefore, body proteins are sacrificed to supply raw materials from which to make glucose.

If the body were to continue to consume its lean tissue unchecked, death would ensue within about ten days. After all, not only skeletal muscle but also the blood proteins, the liver, the heart muscle, and the lung tissue—all vital tissues—are being burned as fuel. (In fact, fasting or starving people remain alive only until their stores of fat are gone or until half their lean tissue is gone, whichever comes first.) To prevent this, the body plays its last ace: it begins converting fat into compounds that the nervous system can adapt to use and so forestall the end. This is ketosis, which was first mentioned in Chapter 4 as an adaptation to prolonged fasting or carbohydrate deprivation.

In ketosis, instead of breaking down fat molecules to carbon dioxide and water as it normally does, the body takes partially broken-down fat fragments and combines them to make **ketone bodies,** compounds that are normally rare in the blood. It converts some amino acids to ketone bodies, too—those that cannot be used to make glucose. These ketone bodies circulate in the bloodstream and help to feed the brain, since about half of the brain's cells can make the enzymes needed to use them for energy. Within about ten days of fasting, the brain and nervous system can meet most of their energy needs using ketone bodies.

Thus indirectly the nervous system begins to feed on the body's fat stores. Ketosis reduces the nervous system's need for glucose, it spares the muscle and other lean tissue from being devoured quickly, and it prolongs the starving person's life. Thanks to ketosis, a healthy person starting with average body fat content can live totally deprived of food for as long as six to eight weeks. Figure 9-7 reviews how energy is used during both feasting and fasting.

Fasting has been practiced as a periodic discipline by respected, wise people in many cultures. Clearly, the body tolerates short-term fasting, although there is no evidence that the body becomes internally "cleansed," as some believe. Ketosis may harm the body by upsetting the acid-base balance of the blood and by promoting mineral losses in the urine. Strong evidence also indicates that food deprivation produces a tendency to overeat or even binge on food when food becomes available.[44] The effect seems to last beyond the point when weight is restored to normal. In addition, people with eating disorders (see Chapter 10's Controversy section) often report that a fast or a severely restrictive diet heralded the beginning of their loss of control over eating.

For the person who wants to lose weight, fasting is not the best way. The body's lean tissues continue to be degraded. The body is deprived of nutrients it needs to assemble new enzymes, red and white blood cells, and other vital components. The body also slows its metabolism to conserve energy. A diet

---

*Glycerol, 5 percent of fat, can yield glucose but is a negligible source.

FIGURE 9-7

FEASTING AND FASTING

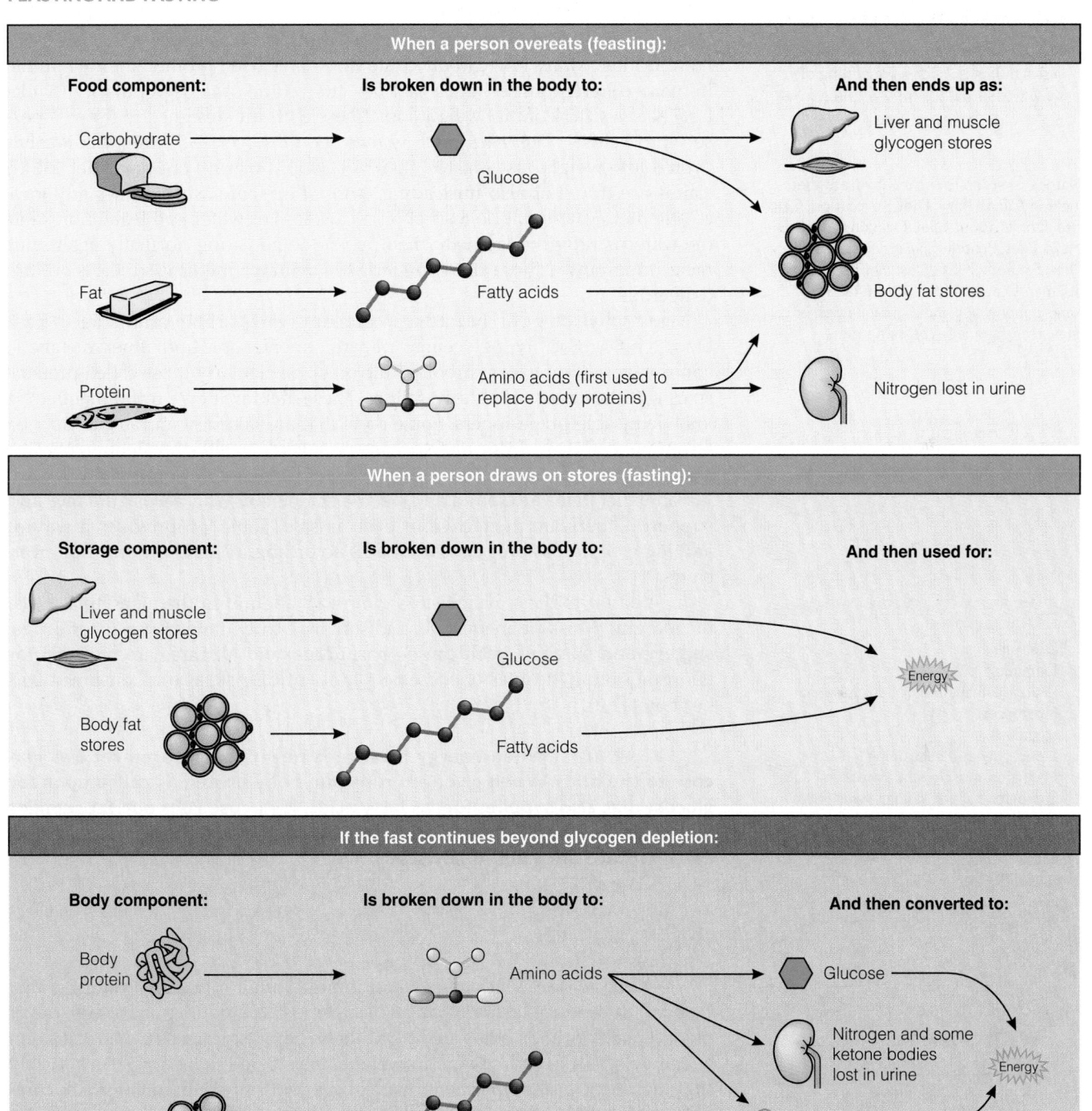

lapse a falling back into a former condition. In weight maintenance, a temporary backslide into old habits.

relapse the outcome of an uncontrolled series of lapses, such as regaining of weight after successful loss and returning to old patterns of eating.

Names of some low-carbohydrate diets include Atkins New Diet Revolution, Calories Don't Count Diet, Drinking Man's Diet, Mayo Diet, Protein-Sparing Fast, Scarsdale Diet, Simeons HCG Diet, Ski Team Diet, Stillman Diet and the Zone Diet. New ones keep coming out under new names, but they are essentially the same diet.

Ineffective or Dangerous Weight-Loss Gimmicks:

Diet pills
Expanding pills
Glucomannan, bee pollen, spirulina
Hormones
Laxatives
Lipectomy and suctioning
Massages, muscle stimulators
Spa belts, rollers, saunas, whirlpools
Stomach stapling, surgery, balloons

only moderately restricted in calories has actually been observed to promote a greater rate of *weight* loss, a faster rate of *fat* loss, and the retention of more lean tissue than a severely restricted fast.[45]

Any diet too low in carbohydrate will bring about responses that are similar to fasting. Many low-carbohydrate diets have been promoted to the public in many different guises. Each diet has enjoyed a surge of popularity thanks largely to a sizable initial weight loss. These diets are designed to throw a person into ketosis. The sales pitch is that "you'll never feel hungry" and that "you'll lose weight fast—faster than you would on any ordinary diet." Both claims are true, but also misleading. Loss of appetite accompanies any low-calorie diet. Severe calorie restriction means loss of water and lean tissue, and the water is rapidly regained when people begin eating normally again. But most importantly, these diets, undertaken without medical supervision, are dangerous.

Many physiological hazards accompany low-carbohydrate diets: high blood cholesterol, hypoglycemia, mineral imbalances, and other metabolic abnormalities. Some low-carbohydrate diets, particularly those called protein-sparing fasts, have caused heart failure. These diets are never recommended by knowledgeable practitioners. Some diets that are very low in calories may be recommended by physicians to correct severe, health-threatening obesity. These are the very-low-calorie diets (VLCD) discussed in Controversy 9.

Some diet plans are sound and can assist a person who needs guidance and support. Others are ineffective or even unsafe. Table 9-6 provides a way of judging weight-loss programs and diets according to standard nutrition principles.

In addition to diets, weight-loss gimmicks abound in the marketplace (see the margin). Most are ineffective, and some are truly dangerous. As for drugs, surgery, and stapling, each can be hazardous, and all three are reserved for efforts at saving the lives of obese people at critical risk, as the Consumer Corner points out.

✓ **KEY POINT** **When energy balance is negative, glycogen returns glucose to the body. When glycogen runs out, body protein is called upon for glucose. Fat also supplies fuel as fatty acids. If glucose runs out, fat supplies fuel as ketone bodies, but ketosis can be dangerous. Both fasts and low-carbohydrate diets are ill advised.**

WEIGHT MAINTENANCE

One reason why gadgets and gimmicks fail in weight control is that they fail to produce lasting change. "I have lost 200 pounds, but I was never more than 20 pounds overweight." Millions have experienced the frustration of achieving a desired change in weight only to see their hard work visibly slipping away. Disappointment, frustration, and self-condemnation are common in dieters who find themselves in a **lapse;** they fear sliding toward a **relapse.** Whether the goal is to lose or gain, weight cycling with periodic losses and gains often becomes a lifelong pattern. What makes the difference between a successful, long-term weight-control program and one that doesn't stick?

People who maintain their weight losses have some things in common. Women are most likely to keep weight goals over the years. Also, people of both genders who develop social support systems seem most successful; they

TABLE 9-6

Rating Sound and Unsound Weight-Loss Schemes

Start by giving each diet or program 160 points. Subtract points as instructed, whenever a plan falls short of ideals. A plan that loses more than 20 points might still be of value, but deserves careful scrutiny.

Does the diet or program:

1. Provide a reasonable number of calories (not fewer than 1,200 calories for an average-size person)? If not, give it a minus 10.
2. Provide enough, but not too much, protein (at least the recommended intake or RDA, but not more than twice that much)? If no, minus 10.
3. Provide enough fat for balance but not so much fat as to go against current recommendations (about 30% of calories from fat)? If no, minus 10.
4. Provide enough carbohydrate to spare protein and prevent ketosis (100 g of carbohydrate for the average-size person)? Is it mostly complex carbohydrate (not more than 10% of the calories as concentrated sugar)? If no to either or both, minus 10.
5. Offer a balanced assortment of vitamins and minerals by including foods from all food groups? If it omits a food group (for example, meats), does it provide a suitable substitute? Count five food groups in all: milk/milk products, meat/fish/poultry/eggs/legumes, fruits, vegetables, and breads/cereals/grains. For *each* food group omitted and not adequately substituted for, subtract 10 points.
6. Offer variety, in the sense that different foods can be selected each day? If you'd class it as boring or monotonous, give it a minus 10.
7. Consist of ordinary foods that are available locally (for example, in the main grocery stores) at the prices people normally pay? Or does the dieter have to buy special, expensive, or unusual foods to adhere to the diet? If you would class it as "bizarre" or "requiring special foods," minus 10.
8. Promise dramatic, rapid weight loss (substantially more than 1% of total body weight per week)? If yes, minus 10.
9. Encourage permanent, realistic lifestyle changes, including regular exercise and the behavioral changes needed for weight maintenance? If not, minus 10.
10. Misrepresent salespeople as "counselors" supposedly qualified to give guidance in nutrition and/or general health without a profit motive, or collect large sums of money at the start, or require that clients sign contracts for expensive, long-term programs? If so, minus 10.
11. Fail to inform clients about the risks associated with weight loss in general or the specific program being promoted? If so, minus 10.
12. Promote unproven or spurious weight-loss aids such as human chorionicgonadotrophin hormone (HCG), starch blockers, diuretics, sauna belts, body wraps, passive exercise, ear stapling, acupuncture, electric muscle stimulating (EMS) devices, spirulina, amino acid supplements (e.g., arginine, ornithine), glucomannan, appetite suppressants, "unique" ingredients, and so forth? If so, minus 10.

attend support groups or create supportive relationships with others. Another key factor is physical activity. Successful weight maintainers exercise regularly. Still another factor is planning and the ability to carry a plan through. Those who maintain weight:

- Follow written diet plans and keep records.
- Eat three meals a day of controlled portions at planned times, and eat them at a leisurely pace.

gastric bypass surgery that reroutes food from the stomach to the lower part of the small intestine, creating a chronic, lifelong state of malabsorption by preventing normal digestion and absorption of nutrients.

gastroplasty surgery involving partitioning of the stomach by stapling off a "pouch" or otherwise constricting the volume of food the stomach can accept at a meal, and thereby reducing total food intake.

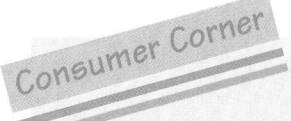

SURGERY AND DRUGS FOR WEIGHT LOSS

People who suffer from obesity may seek help from surgery, prescription or over-the-counter pills, and other products. Medical interventions can indeed help, but only rarely.

Weight-loss help from surgery is available only to those facing serious risks of disease and early death from severe obesity. Two surgical procedures performed today—**gastric bypass** and **gastroplasty**—seem to offer some hope. Bypass surgery, the shortening of the digestive tract by joining a section of the small intestine directly to the stomach, has proved to reduce risks associated with coronary artery disease.[46] Gastroplasty, the constricting of the stomach's volume (sometimes called stomach stapling), can also reverse a trend toward worsening health as a result of obesity. About half of those who undergo these two procedures achieve long-term success, defined as five to ten years of reduced weight and lasting improvements in medical and other conditions arising from obesity.[47] The other half of surgical patients, though, fail to lose or fail to maintain their losses.

Surgeons carefully screen obesity candidates for surgery because the risks can be severe. During surgery, obese people face more infections, more respiratory problems, more blood clots, more difficulties in anesthesia, and slower wound healing than do normal-weight surgery patients. In addition to immediate risks of surgery, the person may face lifelong problems of severe diarrhea, frequent vomiting, intolerance to sweets and milk, dehydration, limited dietary intake, and multiple nutrient deficiencies even with medical follow-up care.[48] Staples pull out, stomach pouches enlarge, and surgeries must sometimes be repeated with repeated risks. Lifelong medical supervision is critical for those who choose the surgical route, but for up to half of those who choose it, the benefits of weight loss prove worth the risks.

Somewhat less risky than surgery for help in weight loss are prescription drugs. Most prescription drugs either cause a drop in food intake by suppressing appetite or they increase the use of fat for fuel by speeding up energy metabolism. A drug currently under testing acts on the small intestine's fat-digesting enzymes to prevent digestion and absorption of about a third of the fat consumed. The drug, tetrahydrolipostatin, faces years of rigorous study before it can be approved by the Food and Drug Administration (FDA). Government regulations restrict the use of prescription drugs for obesity to a three-month maximum time limit. While some drugs have proved effective in promoting initial weight loss, the long-term effects of their use are unknown.[49]

Years ago physicians routinely prescribed amphetamines (speed) to reduce the appetite. Not only did amphetamines prove of little value in weight loss; they are also highly addictive. Many dieters who used them remained overweight and were left addicted to the drugs. The FDA no longer approves amphetamines for weight loss.

phenylpropanolamine (PPA) a stimulant of the sympathetic nervous system used as a weight-loss agent and available in over-the-counter medications.

Another drug, dexfenfluramine,* is not addicting; it curbs the appetite and may also stimulate metabolism. The drug works by prolonging the action of the brain's neurotransmitter serotonin, which in turn depresses the appetite and produces mood changes. Its possible side effects are many, with the most serious being a dangerous form of hypertension that damages the lungs and heart. Uncertainty also exists about the possibility of brain tissue changes from long-term use. Another drug treatment involves administering two drugs, phentermine and fenfluramine (phen-fen for short); the drugs seem to augment each other's appetite-suppressing effects while opposing adverse mood swings that are likely with either drug alone. Several other appetite-suppressing drugs are also under study and may one day prove their worth.

For most people with just a few pounds to lose, prescription drugs are not the answer. What about over-the-counter (OTC) weight-loss pills? Are they safe? Some people who have tried OTC pills that they assumed to be safe have ended up on a surgeon's table, and one person died from a complication of the surgery.[50] The pills they took contained soluble fiber (guar gum) that swelled in their systems. The intent was to make them feel full and eat less, but the result was a dangerous intestinal blockage that required surgical removal. This weight-loss product and most others sold over the counter were swept from the shelves when the FDA reviewed their ingredients and found the pills to be both unsafe and ineffective. Some preparations, such as chromium picolinate, are still available as supplements but because no scientific evidence exists to support their effectiveness, their labels cannot make weight loss claims.

Two OTC drug ingredients remain lawfully for sale today in weight-loss preparation drugs. One, **phenylpropanolamine (PPA)** also found in cold medications, carries a side effect of elevated blood pressure.[51] It makes some people feel jumpy because one of the drug's actions is to trigger the body's stress response. The other ingredient, the anesthetic benzocaine (usually in gum or candy form), numbs the taste buds and supposedly reduces the desire to taste food. These two drugs are still under study by the FDA and may be removed from shelves if they prove ineffective or unsafe.

As for water pills, they do nothing to solve a fat problem. Excess water in the body can add to body weight and taking a water pill (diuretic) can get rid of it, but the weight lost is only water weight. Inappropriate diuretic use threatens the taker with dehydration and mineral imbalances.

A new "thigh cream" also recently hit the market. The cream contains an asthma medication that two obesity researchers, citing two small

---

*Dexfenfluramine's trade name is Redux.

(*continued on next page*)

weight cycling repeated rounds of weight loss and subsequent regain, with reduced ability to lose weight with each attempt. Also called *yo-yo dieting.*

unpublished studies, claim shrinks fat on women's thighs. This cream is considered a cosmetic, not a drug, and so needs no proof of effectiveness before marketing.

In the end, the only means of reducing body fat is to shift the energy budget from positive to negative, to take less energy in and put more energy out. Nonprescription diet pills, diuretics, illegal hormones, fat-melting creams, and use of jiggle machines at spas are useless. They enjoy brisk sales only because the lifelong effort required for weight control is difficult and people can be lured by seemingly easy cures.

- Follow the rule of no eating after a certain time in the evening (usually about 6:00 to 8:00 P.M.).
- Plan high-fiber foods into their diets, along with 8 glasses or more of water a day.

They also cultivate positive attitudes and beliefs and use techniques such as positive self-talk: "You can do it," "You're a success." They believe in their ability to succeed, even if they haven't in the past. Also important are realistic expectations regarding body size and shape. Acceptance of how slowly weight loss proceeds and how long it takes prepares the mind for the task ahead.

An interesting discovery was made regarding the role of exercise in weight maintenance. At the end of a study of the effects of a low-calorie diet and exercise on weight loss, some subjects gave up exercise along with the experimental diet. The researchers continued tracking their body weights. Predictably, the subjects quickly regained all the weight they had lost. The outcome was dramatically different for subjects who continued exercising after the diet period. The group kept their weight off even after abandoning the diet.

Those who endeavor to lose weight without exercise often become trapped in **weight cycling,** endless repeating rounds of weight loss and regain from "yo-yo" dieting. When people repeatedly lose weight only to regain it, their bodies become very efficient at making and storing fat. This increased efficiency shows itself in a way familiar to dieters who have lost and gained—and lost and gained again. With each attempt, it becomes harder and takes longer to lose weight and easier and quicker to gain it back. In fact, previous weight-cycling history can predict a person's success (or lack thereof) in maintaining weight loss.[52]

The next chapter provides details about exercising and weight maintenance.

Another key to success is a sense of ownership of and responsibility for the weight loss. People must grasp the reality that they alone are ultimately responsible for their weight control. No other person can control their weight for them. Many unsuccessful dieters place the responsibility for their weight control outside themselves, on weight-loss programs, on health-care professionals, or on pills and potions. This attitude weakens people's self-confidence and predicts failure.

Ownership is learnable. Successful dieters report coming to a turning point at which they accept responsibility for their own body weights. Only then can they develop workable solutions to barriers. The lesson is, expect success but also know that you alone can make it happen.

Self-acceptance predicts success, while self-hate predicts failure. When people feel disgusted with their appearance and hate themselves when they get on the scale, they erode the positive mental environment needed to maintain weight once it is lost. A paradox of behavior change is that it takes self-acceptance (loving the overweight self) to lay the foundation for change. Self-acceptance leads to an unshakable self-worth that does not depend on body weight.

✓ KEY POINT **People who succeed at maintaining lost weight keep to their eating routines, keep exercising, and take responsibility for their weight. The more traits related to positive self-image a person possesses or cultivates, the more likely that person will succeed.**

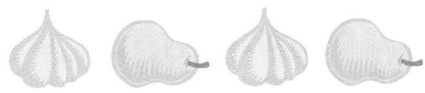

At the start of this chapter, the point was made that *behavior* is the only piece of the weight-control puzzle that is truly under voluntary control. The following sections therefore present a series of strategies for shaping eating-related behavior to promote a change in body weight. Keep in mind that this section presents just one side of the weight-change equation—diet. The other, equally important component to weight change is exercise, the topic of the next chapter.

DIET STRATEGIES FOR BODY FAT LOSS

Whether a person wants to lose 10 pounds or 50 pounds of body fat, the techniques of diet, physical activity, and **behavior modification** discussed here apply equally. The following sections are written in terms of advice to "you," not to put you under pressure to take it personally, but to give you the illusion of listening in on a conversation in which an overweight person (with, say, 50 pounds to lose) is being competently counseled by someone familiar with techniques known to be safe and effective.

An important concept is that habits direct behaviors. Habits are like the "auto pilot" feature of a plane—they'll always take you somewhere, but to arrive at your desired destination, you must consciously plan the route ahead of time. Table 9-7 applies behavior modification principles to helping you plan and adjust your habits concerning diet and exercise.

No particular food plan is magical, and no particular food must be either included or avoided. You are the one who will have to live with the plan, so you had better be involved in designing it. Don't think of yourself as going "on" a *diet* because then you may be tempted to go "off." Think of yourself as adopting an eating *plan* for life. It must consist of foods that you like or can learn to like, that are available to you, and that are affordable.

Choose an energy level you can live with. For the person wanting to lose weight, a deficit of 500 calories a day for seven days (3,500 calories a week) is enough to lose a pound a week of body fat. It is urgent not to try to cut calories too far for all the reasons already mentioned. A rule of thumb is that you

FOOD FEATURE

BEHAVIORS TO PROMOTE WEIGHT CONTROL

behavior modification alteration of behavior using methods based on the theory that actions can be controlled by manipulating the environmental factors that cue, or trigger, the actions.

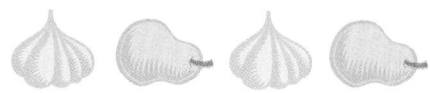

TABLE 9-7

Six Behaviors to Promote Control of Body Fatness[a]

1. Eliminate inappropriate eating cues:

   - Don't buy problem foods.
   - Eat only in one room at the designated time.
   - Shop when not hungry.
   - Turn off television food commercials.
   - Avoid vending machines, fast-food restaurants, and convenience stores.

2. Suppress the cues you cannot eliminate:

   - Serve individual plates; don't serve "family style."
   - Make small portions look large by spreading them over the plate.
   - Create obstacles to consuming problem foods—wrap them and freeze them, making them less quickly accessible.
   - Control deprivation; plan and eat regular meals.

3. Strengthen cues to appropriate behaviors:

   - Share appropriate foods with others.
   - Store appropriate foods in convenient spots in the refrigerator.
   - Learn appropriate portion sizes.
   - Plan appropriate snacks.
   - Keep sports and play equipment by the door.

4. Repeat desired behaviors:

   - Slow down eating—put down utensils between bites.
   - Always use utensils.
   - Leave some food on your plate.
   - Move more—shake a leg, pace, stretch often.
   - Join groups of active people and participate.

5. Arrange negative consequences for negative behavior:

   - Ask that others respond neutrally to your deviations (make no comments—even negative attention is a reward).
   - If you slip, don't punish yourself.

6. Reward yourself personally and immediately:

   - Buy tickets to sports events, movies, concerts, or other nonfood amusement.
   - Indulge in a new small purchase.
   - Get a massage; buy some flowers.
   - Take a bubble bath; read a good book.
   - Join a card game; listen to music.
   - Praise yourself; visit friends.
   - Nap; relax.

[a]These behaviors are based on the *behavior modification* technique of controlling actions by controlling the environment.

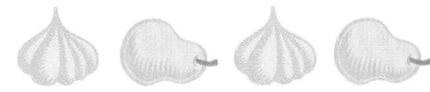

need to eat at least 10 calories per pound of current body weight each day to lose fat efficiently while retaining lean tissue.

There is no point in hurrying. You will never go off the plan; you will only modify it slightly when you have reached your goal. Nutritional adequacy is hard to achieve on a low-calorie diet, and even a small person should not try to get by on fewer than 1,200 calories. A larger person should adjust the calories upward; some people can lose weight steadily on diets of 1,600 calories or more. When planning meals, follow a pattern that includes at least the minimum servings suggested in the Daily Food Guide (Chapter 2) without frills. Making the diet adequate is a way of putting yourself first. For the lower calorie ranges, say, below 1,600 calories, it is appropriate to take a balanced vitamin-mineral supplement; see Chapter 7 for how to choose one.

If you plan resolutely to include a certain number of servings of food that you enjoy from each food group each day, you will find that after eating all the servings of the foods you need, you will have little appetite left for high-fat or empty-calorie foods. Foods such as fruits, vegetables, and whole grains are high in carbohydrates and fiber, low in fat, and take a lot of chewing, too. Crunchy, wholesome foods offer bulk and satiety for far fewer calories than smooth, refined foods. Limit your meats: an ounce of ham contains more calories than an ounce of bread, and many of them are from fat. Remember to pay attention to portion sizes.

Especially don't lose track of the fat you add. Remember that fat calories probably contribute more to body fat stores than do carbohydrate calories, and fat has so many calories per bite that it is easy to overload quickly. Just a few bites of fatty food can use up the whole allowance of calories for a meal long before the diner feels full.

People lose weight fastest when they restrict both calories and fats. Beware, therefore, of overdoing some of the foods that are manufactured to be low in fat but compensate by being high in sugar. For example, a nonfat fig bar contains almost the same number of calories as the regular bar. Fat-free frozen yogurt may be pumped so full of sugar that its calorie value exceeds that of regular yogurt, and so forth. In contrast, some low-fat items, such as salad dressings, are truly low in calories, making them useful substitutes for the regular products they replace.

Three meals a day is standard for our society, but no law says you shouldn't have four or five—only be sure they are smaller, of course. Make sure that hunger, not appetite, is prompting you to eat. Eat regularly and, if at all possible, eat before you become extremely hungry. When you do decide to eat, eat the entire meal you have carefully planned for yourself. Then don't eat again until the next meal. Save calorie-free or favorite foods or beverages for a planned snack at the end of the day if you need insurance against late-evening hunger.

One meal you should strive to include is breakfast. Much evidence supports the health effects of breakfast, and people who eat breakfast seem to need fewer snacks and consume less fat all day long.[53]

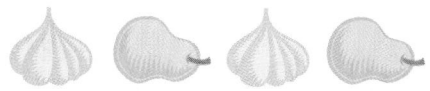

DIET STRATEGIES FOR WEIGHT GAIN

Should an underweight person try to gain weight? Not necessarily: the question is whether the underweight affects health. If you are healthy at your present weight, stay there. If your physician has advised you to gain, if you are excessively tired, if you are unable to keep warm, if you are 15 percent below the expected weight, or if, for women, you have missed at least three consecutive menstrual periods, you may be in danger from a too-low body weight.

Weight gain is an individual matter. In deciding whether to undertake it, be as aware as you can be of what your body will permit and tolerate, and be willing to accept what you cannot change. Some people are unalterably thin by reasons of heredity or early physical influences. Those who wish to gain weight for appearance's sake or to improve athletic performance should be aware that a healthful weight gain can be achieved only through physical activity, particularly strength training (see Chapter 10 for details), combined with eating a high-calorie diet. Eating more calories of food can bring about weight gain, but it will be mostly fat, and this can be as detrimental to health as being slightly underweight. In an athlete, such a weight gain can impair performance. Therefore, in weight gain, as in weight loss, physical activity is an essential component of a sound plan.

As important to weight gain as exercise are the calories to support that activity—otherwise you will lose weight (body fat). If you eat just enough to fuel the activity, you will build muscle, but at the expense of body fat; that is, fat will be burned to support the muscle building. If you eat more, you will gain both muscle and fat.

It takes an excess of about 2,000 to 2,500 calories, in theory, to support the gain of a pound of pure lean tissue, and about 3,500 calories to gain a pound of fat.[54] To gain both, then, which is the goal, requires about 3,000 calories. The rate at which a person can build muscle tissue also depends on the person. Both men and women have both male and female hormones; those with more male hormones build muscle more easily than others, but the limits are not known. (Chapter 10 provides cautions on the abuse of steroid hormone drugs.) Conventional advice on diet to the person building muscle is to eat about 700 to 1,000 calories a day above normal energy needs; this is enough to support both the added activity and the formation of new muscle.

It is as hard for a person who tends to be underweight to gain a pound as it is for a person who tends to be overweight to lose one. Like the weight loser, the person who wants to gain must learn new habits and learn to eat new foods. No matter how many sticks of celery you consume, you won't gain weight very fast because celery simply doesn't offer enough calories. The person who cannot eat much volume is encouraged to use calorie-dense foods in meals (the very ones the dieter is trying to stay away from). These foods are high in fat, but if they are contributing energy that will be spent building new tissue, and if their fat is mostly unsaturated, they will not contribute to heart disease. Choose nutritious foods, but choose peanut butter instead of lean meat, avocado instead of cucumber, olives instead of pickles, whole-wheat muffins instead of whole-wheat bread, milkshakes instead of milk. When you do eat celery, stuff it with tuna salad (use oil-packed tuna); add creamer and

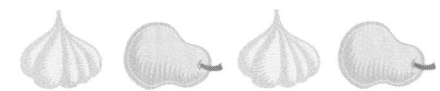

sugar to coffee; use olive oil or canola oil dressings on salads, whipped top-pings on fruit, soft margarine on potatoes, and the like. Because fat contains twice as many calories per teaspoon as sugar, it adds calories without adding much bulk, and its energy is in a form that is easy for the body to store.

Expect to feel full, sometimes even uncomfortably so. Most underweight individuals are accustomed to small quantities of food. When they begin eat-ing significantly more food, they complain of uncomfortable fullness. This is normal, and it passes over time.

Eat frequently. Make three sandwiches in the morning and eat them between classes in addition to the day's three regular meals. Spend time mak-ing foods appealing—the more varied and palatable, the better. If you fill up fast during a meal, eat the highest-calorie items first. Start with the main course or a meat- or cheese-filled appetizer. Drink between meals, not with them, to save space for higher-calorie foods. Make milkshakes of milk, frozen bananas, and flavorings to drink between meals. Always finish with dessert. Many an underweight person has simply been too busy (for months) to eat or to exer-cise enough to gain or to maintain weight.

LIVING WITH BEHAVIOR CHANGE

If you stop making progress, you may have to get tough with yourself. Ask yourself honestly, "What am I doing to undermine my weight control plan?" (no one is listening in). Seldom does an unpredicted weight plateau of any duration occur without an explanation of the person's own choices.

Also, if you stop making progress, be aware that this may be a good time to stop. Your weight may be at a point that you can accept, at least for the pres-ent. In fact, you may come to realize that your original goal weight was unre-alistic or not worth the effort it would take to get there. You may decide to join the ranks of people who have rejected the magazine-cover physical ideal and opt to work on other facets of your life leading to self-acceptance. Hold your head high and take the attitude, "This is the way I am."

Should you choose to continue weight-loss or weight-gain efforts, you may find help in a group; such as Weight Watchers or other groups. Or you may benefit from individual nutrition counseling with a registered dietitian (RD). RDs are trained to assist with changes in food behavior. Obtaining some assertiveness training may also help. For those striving to lose weight, learning to say "No, thank you" might be one of your first objectives. Learning not to "clean your plate" might be another.

From all the available behavior changes, you choose the ones to begin with. Don't try to master them all at once. No one who attempts too many changes at one time is successful. Set your own priorities. Pick one behavior you can handle, start with that, and practice it until it is habitual and automatic. Then select another.

As you progress in physical activity and behavior change, enjoy your new, emerging self. Get in touch with—reach out your hand to—your fit and healthy self, and help that self to feel welcome in the light of day.

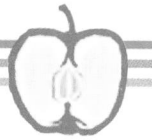

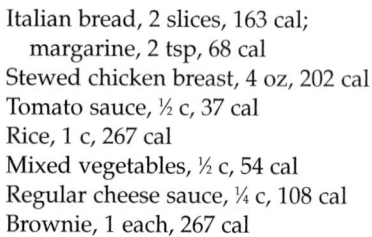

CONTROL THE CALORIES IN A DAY'S MEALS

This exercise speaks to the person who wants to control calorie intakes to control body fatness. To choose foods to meet nutrient needs while staying within a calorie limit, a diet planner can choose any or all of these four lines of action:

- *Cut down food portions,* if they are significantly larger than those recommended in the Food Guide Pyramid.
- *Eliminate* high-calorie, low-nutrient foods from the everyday diet (save for special treats).

- *Remove the high-calorie constituents* from most foods (trim fat from meat, choose nonfat milk).
- *Replace* high-calorie foods with lower-calorie versions, either naturally occurring or manufactured.

Fat is a main target for cutting calories because of its high calorie density. When using manufactured low-fat and nonfat items, the consumer must read labels carefully, however. These products may be lower in *fat,* but some contain as many *calories* as the originals.

FIGURE 9-8

CALORIES IN TWO SETS OF MEALS

About 3,200 cal
2% Milk, 1 c, 121 cal
Orange juice, 1 c 112 cal
Waffles, 2 each, 185 cal;
    margarine, 2 tsp, 68 cal;
    syrup, 4 T, 210 cal
Banana slices, ½ c, 69 cal

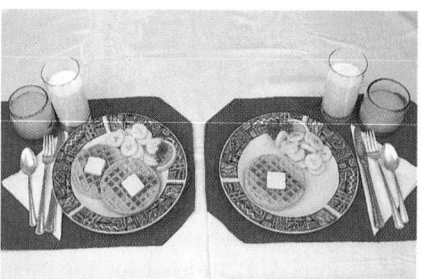

About 2,300 cal
2% Milk, 1 c, 121 cal
Orange juice, ¾ c, 84 cal
Waffle, 1 each, 93 cal;
    Margarine, 1 tsp, 34 cal;
    Syrup, 2 T, 105 cal
Banana slices, ½ c, 69 cal

2% Milk, 1 c, 121 cal
Hamburger, quarterpound, 415 cal
French fries, large (about 50), 448 cal
Ketchup, 2 tbs, 32 cal
Apple pie, 1 each, 225 cal

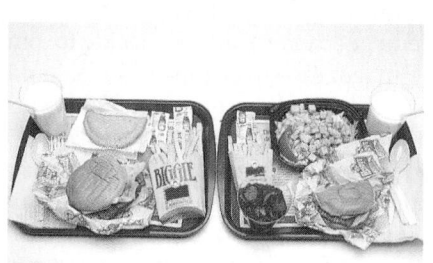

2% Milk, 1 c, 121 cal
Hamburger, small, 266 cal
Green salad, 1 c, with light dressing, 1 tbs,
    67 cal; croutons, ½ c, 50 cal
French fries, regular serving, 207 cal
Ketchup, 1 tbs, 16 cal
gelatin dessert with fruit, 73 cal

Italian bread, 2 slices, 163 cal;
    margarine, 2 tsp, 68 cal
Stewed chicken breast, 4 oz, 202 cal
Tomato sauce, ½ c, 37 cal
Rice, 1 c, 267 cal
Mixed vegetables, ½ c, 54 cal
Regular cheese sauce, ¼ c, 108 cal
Brownie, 1 each, 267 cal

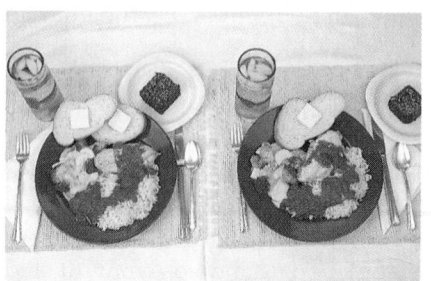

Italian bread, 1 slice, 82 cal;
    margarine, 1 pat, 34 cal
Stewed chicken breast, 4 oz, 202 cal
Tomato sauce, ½ c, 37 cal
Rice, 1 c, 267 cal
Mixed vegetables, ½ c, 54 cal
Low-fat cheese sauce, ¼ c, 85 cal
Brownie, 1 each, 267 cal

READ FIGURE 9-8

The meals shown in Figure 9-8 represent one person's attempt to control calories. Shown on the left are the meals this person started with; the number of calories was too large to permit weight maintenance. On the right side of Figure 9-8, the meals have been modified to reduce their calories while still presenting the minimum number of servings from each food group recommended in the *Food Guide Pyramid*. Note that through these changes, the person has already reduced calories by almost a thousand. To reduce calories further, however, takes more careful thought. The person must cut calories while still meeting the minimum number of servings from the food groups to maintain nutrient adequacy.

The three top contributors of both calories and fat in the high-calorie meals are:

french fries > large hamburger > brownie

FORM 9-1

Try Your Hand: Reduce Calories Further

2,300 Calorie Day	Suggested Changes	Calories Saved	Food Group Servings	
			Name of Group	Number of Servings
Breakfast				
2% Milk, 1 c, 121 cal				
Orange juice, ¾ c, 84 cal				
Waffle, 1 each, 93 cal;				
Margarine, 1 tsp, 34 cal;				
Syrup, 2 T, 105 cal				
Banana slices, ½ c, 69 cal				
Lunch				
2% Milk, 1 c, 121 cal				
Hamburger, small, 2 oz, 266 cal				
Green salad, 1 c,				
with 1 tbs light dressing, 67 cal				
croutons, ½ c, 50 cal				
French fries, regular, 207 cal (about 30)				
Ketchup, 1 tbs, 16 cal				
Gelatin dessert with fruit, 73 cal				
Dinner				
Italian bread, 1 slice, 82 cal;				
margarine, 1 pat, 34 cal				
Stewed chicken breast, 4 oz, 202 cal				
Tomato sauce, ½ c, 37 cal				
Rice, 1 c, 267 cal				
Mixed vegetables, ½ c, 54 cal				
Low-fat cheese sauce, ¼ c, 85 cal				
Brownie, 1 each, 267 cal				

Total Calories Saved: _____

2,300 − _____ = _____
(calories saved) (new day's total calories)

Food Group Totals:
Milk, yogurt, cheese _____ Fruit _____ Vegetables _____ Meats and alternates _____
Bread, cereal, rice, pasta _____

These foods are worth considering when cutting calories. Also, remember from Chapter 5's Food Feature that breads, cereals, baked goods, rice, and pasta also vary in their fat and sugar contents, and therefore in calories. For example, the waffles depicted in the breakfast of Figure 9-8 contribute more calories than plain bread does because waffle mix contains fat; and the syrup served on top presents more calories than the waffles do.

Some 400 calories were trimmed from the 3,200-calorie meals by reducing sweets—reducing syrup served at breakfast and eliminating apple pie from lunch. (The planner kept the brownie, however—pleasure matters, too!) These two actions alone, repeated each day for one month, produce a calorie reduction more than sufficient to make a 3½-pound difference in the person's body weight.

REDUCE CALORIES FURTHER

Try your hand at cutting calories further to 1,800 or even 1,600 calories for the day. The only "must" in cutting calories is to make the diet adequate. Make substitutions with an eye for adequacy: for example, substituting diet cola for one of the two milk servings would compromise calcium adequacy and so is not allowable.

Step 1. Use Form 9-1, the column marked *Suggested Changes,* to record your changes in the 2,300-calorie day's meals (already listed for convenience at the left of the form).

Step 2. Record the calorie savings. As you make changes, turn to the Table of Food Composition, Appendix A, to find calorie values for foods you propose as substitutions for the originals. Subtract the calorie value of the new food from that of the original and write the calorie differences in the column marked *Calories Saved.* There is no need to look up every food on the menu—just the substitutes for those you choose to change.

Step 3. Add the *Calories Saved* column to obtain your total calorie savings for the day.

Step 4. Subtract the total savings from the original total of 2,300 calories to find the calorie value of the new day's meals.

Step 5. Assign each food from the new menu to its appropriate food group, and estimate the number of servings it represents. (Tips on how to estimate servings were given in Chapter 2's Do It section.) Write the food group names down the left-hand side of the column of

Form 9-1 entitled "Food Group Servings." On the right-hand side of the same column write in your estimates of the numbers of servings each food item represents. Total the day's servings from each group and write the totals in the spaces provided at the bottom of the form.

ANALYSIS

Answer the following questions:

1. How many total calories did your changes save?
2. Assuming that a pound of body weight is worth 3,500 calories, how much weight would a dieter theoretically lose in a month by cutting every day's calories to this extent?
3. By what methods (see the 4-item list in the first paragraph of this Do It) did you reduce calories?
4. Did you remove high-calorie constituents from any foods? Which ones?
5. Which high-calorie foods did you replace with lower-calorie ones? Did this substantially affect the saturated fat, vitamin, mineral, or fiber content of the meals? How?
6. Which of the changes most significantly reduced calories in the meals? Which changed calories least?
7. Did you find it necessary to replace the fast-food lunch in the diet? Why or why not?
8. Were you able to cut calories significantly while still meeting the minimum number of servings from each food group? If not, which groups fell short? List ways of adjusting your choices to include the missing foods.
9. Are the reduced-calorie meals appealing? If not, how can you include more appealing foods without increasing the calorie values?
10. Did your meals include any sweets or other treats? If so, which ones? If not, why not?

When you develop skill in making these sorts of changes, they tend to come to mind whenever the opportunity arises. Then, choosing foods with an eye for their contributions of calories and nutrients becomes a natural part of living. In case you are curious about how the authors might reduce calories, Table 9-8 shows our ideas for changes.

TABLE 9-8

Our Answers to Figure 9-8
New Calorie Level: about 1,900 cal

Food	Changes	Calories Saved
orange juice	same	0
milk	replace with skim	35
waffle	same	0
margarine/syrup	replace with light margarine	12
banana	same	0
milk	replace with skim	35
hamburger	same	0
french fries	omit	207
ketchup	same	0
salad	same	0
croutons	same	0
gelatin	omit	73
Italian bread with margarine	same	0
chicken	same	0
rice	same	0
tomato sauce	same	0
mixed vegetables	same	0
low-fat cheese sauce	omit	85
brownie	same	0
Total Calories Saved	447	

Food Group Totals

Milk, yogurt, cheese ___2___   Fruit ___2___
   Vegetables ___4___   Meats and alternates ___2___
   Bread, cereal, rice, pasta ___7___

SELF-CHECK

Answers to these Self-Check questions are in Appendix G.

1. Which of the following statements about basal metabolic rate (BMR) is correct?
   a. The more fat tissue, the higher the BMR.
   b. The more thyroxine produced, the higher the BMR.
   c. Fever lowers the BMR.
   d. Pregnant women have lower BMRs.

2. Which of the following is a health risk associated with excessive body fat?
   a. high blood lipids
   b. diabetes
   c. gallbladder disease
   d. all of the above.

3. Body density (the measurement of body weight compared with volume) is determined by which technique?
   a. fatfold test
   b. bioelectrical impedance
   c. underwater weighing
   d. all of the above

4. The obesity theory that suggests that the body chooses to be at a specific weight is the:
   a. set-point theory
   b. enzyme theory
   c. fat cell theory
   d. external cue theory

5. Which of the following is a recommended weight-loss strategy?
   a. muscle stimulators
   b. stomach stapling
   c. hormones and bee pollen
   d. none of the above

6. Which of the following is a possible physical consequence of a very-low-calorie diet?
   a. loss of lean body tissues
   b. sudden death
   c. menstrual irregularity
   d. all of the above

7. The thermic effect of food plays a major role in energy expenditure. True or false?   T   F

8. If you bike about ten minutes a day and walk to classes but otherwise sit and study, you are considered lightly active. True or false?   T   F

9. People tend to shrink in height and gain fat as they age, making the height and weight charts meaningless in later years. True or false?   T   F

10. In ketosis, the body cleanses itself and loses body fat rapidly due to an increase in metabolic rate. True or false?   T   F

NOTES

Notes are in Appendix F.

Some leaders in obesity research are questioning the very foundations of obesity treatment. The issues dividing the experts center on how, when, or even whether to advise weight-loss dieting for overfat clients.

Do all obese clients benefit from routine advice to lose weight? The question comes on the heels of research that suggests that diets almost always fail in the long term. Right away, it should be said that weight loss is possible and that the techniques explained in Chapter 9 are valid. The chapter also made clear, however, that controlling body composition is a lifelong effort that involves more than diet alone. Lost fat can be regained when overweight people "go on a diet," lose weight, but then return to old eating patterns and sedentary lifestyles. Another problem is unrealistic expectations. Practically no dieters will end up looking like fashion models despite sales pitches from diet programs. A more attainable and sustainable goal would be losing enough body fat to prevent diseases or regain health. This Controversy centers on the question of who, exactly, should lose body fat for health's sake; it also introduces an alternative for healthy overfat people: self-acceptance.

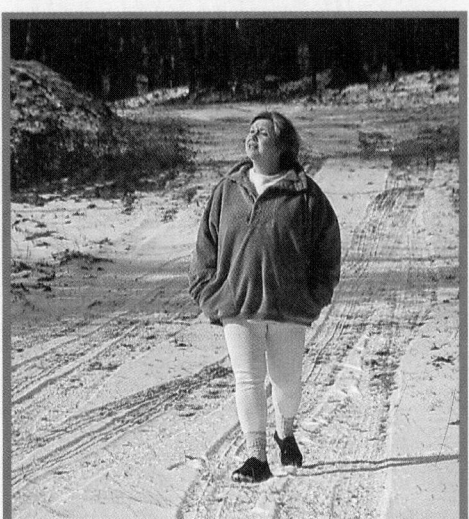

THE DECISION TO TREAT OBESITY

Those in favor of aggressive treatment of obesity are still in the majority. All major government dietary guidelines mention weight control as a health-supporting ideal. The experts cite many studies showing that with obesity come increased disease risks and that weight loss reduces those risks.[1] What good would it do to treat a person's diabetes, say researchers, without treating the obesity underlying the disorder? The treatment may reduce the ravages of the present symptoms, but more symptoms will surely develop unless truly effective and lasting treatment for the predisposing condition is offered. According to one estimate, prevention of obesity could have saved over $45 billion in medical costs in 1990 alone.[2] The definition of obesity is important in

this regard. Who should be told to lose weight? At what point does extra fat present a health risk?

An experiment was designed that followed the weights, health status, and mortality rates of women over a period of 16 years.[3] By the end of the study, the researchers had determined that women who had gained 22 pounds or more since age 18 were nearly twice as likely to die from heart disease as women who gained little or no weight. This risk tripled for women gaining more than 44 pounds during the study period. The women with a body mass index below 19 who weighed at least 15 percent *below* the average U.S. weights had the lowest risk of death from all causes. A related study found similar trends in men.

The women's study findings are presented in Figure C9-1, graph A. Observe that the correlation is direct: the higher the body mass index, the higher the mortality rate. An interesting note about the data represented is that they exclude smokers. Typical results of data not excluding smokers are shown in graph B of the figure. Because smoking contributes to both low body weight and early death, inclusion of smoker's data elevates the risk of mortality at the lowest BMI values. These researchers concluded that thinness itself is not a risk factor for early death, but that smoking is. Opposing these views is a recent study analyzing the very same findings. When smoking is excluded from the data, the mortality risks of being underweight still appear as severe as the risks of extreme obesity.[4]

The opposing view also points out that, in science, correlation is not cause. Yes, obesity is often found in those who suffer from the conditions mentioned in the chapter, but this does not prove that obesity *causes* those conditions. It is as likely that a high-fat diet, excess caloric intake, or lack of exercise cause both the diseases and obesity. Or it may be that a hereditary factor predisposes people to developing both the diseases and the obesity (some evidence exists to support this idea). To say that obesity is a direct cause of disease, and that it must be reversed to prevent disease, is to

FIGURE C9-1

MORTALITY DATA: THE EFFECTS OF BODY WEIGHT AND SMOKING

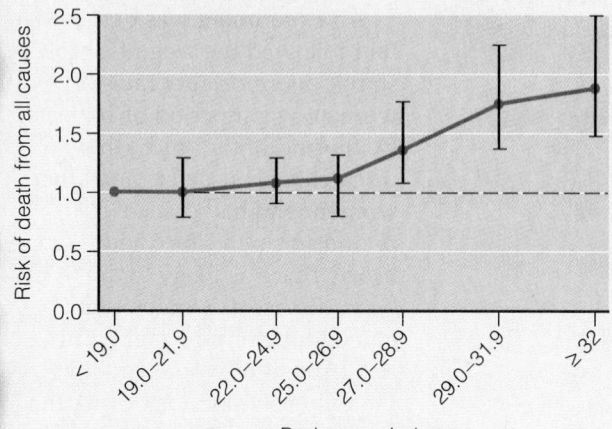

A. Women who never smoked (1,499 deaths)

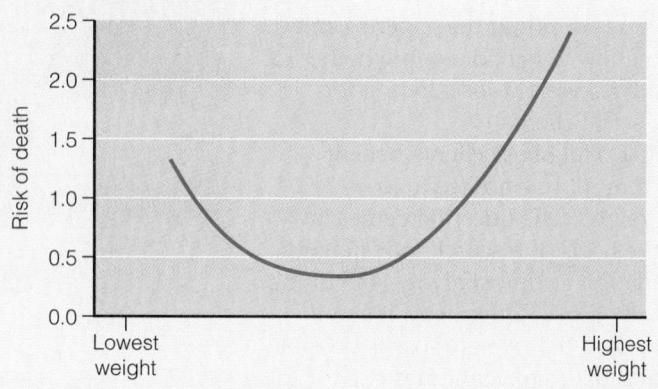

B. Data that include smokers

A. These are actual data for mortality and body mass index (BMI) that exclude smokers. There is a direct linear relationship between higher BMI and higher mortality.

B. Data for mortality and body weight that include smokers often generate a J-shaped graph like this one. Smokers weigh less, but they die sooner than others, so their deaths may elevate the left-hand side of the curve.

SOURCE: Adapted from J. E. Manson and coauthors, *New England Journal of Medicine*, 1995, vol. 333, pp. 677–685. Copyright 1995. Massachusetts Medical Society. All rights reserved.

---

disobey the laws of scientific reasoning. An interesting correlation to support this view is that cardiovascular disease incidence *declined* during a period when obesity was on the *rise*.[5]

Other medical authorities counter these arguments by pointing to proved benefits from even 10 to 20 pounds of weight loss in obese patients.[6] They report rapid improvement in many of the complications of obesity such as glucose tolerance and insulin resistance, hypertension, hyperlipidemia, and sleep disturbances. The practical effects accompanying weight loss in the obese who suffer these conditions are proved beneficial, and whether they are brought about by reduction in body fatness or adoption of healthy lifestyle habits seems immaterial.

Other researchers point out, however, that a large subset of the obese population, termed "healthy obese," is not at increased risk of disease. For these people, the risks associated with weight-loss dieting may far outweigh any health benefits they can expect from weight loss.

A larger question may be whether the weight loss and benefit correlation holds as true for slightly obese as for very obese people. Obese people may carry 80,

100, or even more pounds of excess fat and suffer health hazards, but is a seemingly healthy person who carries 20 or 30 extra pounds also inviting those hazards? Should such a person be advised by medical and nutrition experts to lose weight? A blanket weight-loss recommendation to all overweight people, based on health, may or may not be warranted.

DIET SAFETY—PROVED OR JUST IMPLIED?

When consumers are offered a medical treatment, they expect to be fully informed of any risks involved in undertaking it. This expectation is reasonable because the FDA requires proof that treatments such as medicines and surgery not only work, but are safe. This is not true of many diets, which pose risks but do not inform users about them, a practice that many believe to be unethical. An expert witness to a Senate subcommittee investigating weight-loss fraud said that, overall, "the unregulated multibillion dollar weight-loss industry is placing our citizens at significant health risk."[7]

The risks associated with weight loss are more serious than most dieters would suspect. Linked with fluctuations in body weight, but not specific to any one mode of achieving weight loss, may be an increased risk of death from heart disease.[8] Also, anyone who undertakes to restrict caloric intake invites the risk of losing control of dieting and developing an eating disorder such as anorexia nervosa or bulimia (more about this link in Controversy 10).

New York City has adopted a "Truth-in-Dieting" regulation that calls for voluntary steps on the part of the weight-loss businesses in that city to disclose safety risks to clients before they sign up. The regulation resulted from an undercover investigation of diet programs that revealed that weight-loss centers intentionally hid risks and costs associated with the programs while exaggerating their efficacy. What is true of weight-loss businesses in New York City is probably true across the country, and a movement to standardize and regulate the weight-loss industry is gaining support.[9] Table C9-1 presents a list of guidelines for weight-management programs recommended by the American Heart Association.

If most diet programs are unsafe, very-low-calorie diets (VLCD) can be even more so, even when medically supervised (see Table C9-2). The fewer the calories a diet provides or the more out of balance it is, the greater the risks it presents. In an effort to find a diet to promote rapid weight loss safely, many commercially prepared VLCD formulas were developed in the 1980s. Most VLCD formulas provide about 400 to 800 calories per day and are available by prescription only. They also provide the RDA of all vitamins and minerals but fall short of the minimum for fiber and energy-yielding nutrients.

At first, these plans appealed to millions of people who wanted to lose 10 or 20 pounds. Many hospitals and clinics met this need by establishing centers to administer VLCD and to monitor their use. Today, most clinics and hospitals have stopped using VLCD except in cases of extreme, life-threatening obesity because, although the diets successfully produce large initial weight losses, the long-term outlook for those who use them is bleak. More than 90 percent of clients who lost weight using the diets alone regained all of it, and many ended up fatter than before they started.

MEDICAL ETHICS, WEIGHT LOSS, AND PROFITS

Obesity is classified as a disease. Most physicians feel compelled by medical ethics to offer treatment for all diseases. One conscientious weight-control expert believes obesity carries medical risks so severe that for a physician to delay offering treatment would be a form of malpractice.[10] Not only do obese people who lose weight experience reversal of disease risks, he says, but they may acquire a new sense of self-esteem and improved quality of life. Certainly, to give people of the opportunity to achieve these benefits would be desirable.

TABLE C9-1

American Heart Association Weight-Management Program Guidelines

Properly constructed weight-loss programs provide:

- Participant information about the program format, its costs, and potential risks; the qualifications of its professionals, the expected results, and the time frame both for reaching goals and for follow-up.
- Qualified experts with credentials in nutrition, exercise, and behavior change.
- Medical screening for conditions that may make weight loss risky, and physician evaluation of those identified as having such conditions.
- Reasonable weight-loss goals to support specific health targets, such as reduced risk from cardiovascular disease.
- Nutrition, exercise, and behavior components, specifically designed by experts to meet individual needs.
- A maintenance program of at least 2 years.
- Follow-up at 2 and 5 years.

SOURCE: Adapted from AHA Medical/Scientific Statement, *American Heart Association Guidelines for Weight Management Programs for Healthy Adults,* available from Office of Scientific Affairs, AHA, 7272 Greenville Ave., Dallas, TX 75231–4596.

TABLE C9-2

Possible Physical Consequences of Very-Low-Calorie Diets

Blood	Immunity
▪ Blood carotene concentrations increase ▪ Blood cholesterol concentrations increase ▪ Blood urea concentrations increase	▪ Immune response diminishes ▪ White blood cells decrease in number

Cardiovascular/Respiratory	Metabolic
▪ Blood pressure declines ▪ Carbon dioxide production declines ▪ Cardiac output declines ▪ Heart muscle atrophies ▪ Heartbeat becomes irregular ▪ Low blood pressure develops ▪ Oxygen consumption declines ▪ Pulse rate declines ▪ Respiratory rate declines	▪ Basal metabolism declines ▪ Bone mineral content shifts ▪ Cold intolerance occurs ▪ Dehydration may occur ▪ Gout may occur ▪ Ketosis develops ▪ Lean body tissues are lost ▪ Mineral and electrolyte imbalances occur ▪ Nitrogen balance becomes negative.

Digestive	Other
▪ Gallstones and kidney stones form ▪ GI tract motility declines ▪ Liver inflammation and fibrosis develop ▪ Nausea, vomiting, diarrhea, abdominal discomfort, and constipation occur	▪ Body and breath odor (from ketone excretion) may become apparent ▪ Hair falls out ▪ Headaches occur ▪ Lethargy, fatigue, and loss of stamina set in ▪ Skin dries out ▪ Sleeplessness may occur ▪ Sudden death becomes possible

Hormonal	
▪ Menstrual irregularity develops ▪ Sex drive is lost	

SOURCES: Evidence on metabolic rate, lean body tissue, liver, gallstone, heartbeat, bones, nitrogen balance from various authors in *American Journal of Clinical Nutrition* 56 (1992): supplement; immune failure reported in C. J. Field, R. Gougeon, and E. B. Marliss, *American Journal of Clinical Nutrition* 54 (1991): 123–129; reduced oxygen consumption reported in K. N. Pavlou and coauthors, Exercise as an adjunct to weight loss and maintenance in moderately obese subjects, *American Journal of Clinical Nutrition* 49 (1989): 1115–1123; low blood pressure, headache, atrophy of heart muscle, and hormonal effects from R. L. Atkinson, Low calorie diets and obesity, in D. D. Bills and S. D. Kung, *Biotechnology and Nutrition* (Boston: Butterworth-Heinemann, 1992), pp. 29–45.

Besides, weight-loss advocates argue, if doctors withdraw their medical support for weight control, quacks will rush to fill the void in the multibillion-dollar diet industry. Physicians may not be able to dictate to society or even to individuals what an ideal weight should be, but they should stay involved with weight control and strive to guide their clients toward healthy habits.

While no one can argue against treating a disease that causes misery and illness, questioners point out that weight-loss efforts involving dietary changes are not effective—they almost always fail to produce long-term results.[11] This makes it unethical and misleading to promote them as effective treatments. If the FDA was asked to approve the sale of a medical drug with the failure record of weight-loss programs, the agency would declare the drug ineffective. If obesity is treated as a medical problem, shouldn't prescribed treatments be required to meet the criteria that other treatments must meet?

Unquestionably, the huge potential for profit drives many programs.[12] An estimated 30 to 40 percent of all adult U.S. women (and 20 to 25 percent of U.S. men) are trying to lose weight at any given time and spending $30 to $40 billion each year to do so. Such income potentials are bound to attract an army of "get-rich-quick" scammers. In fact, the FDA names weight-loss schemes as one of the leading forms of fraud in the United States. People have come to attach so many unproved benefits to weight loss that they are willing to risk huge sums for the slightest chance of success. These factors—a hard-to-change condition, a willingness to believe in unproved benefits, and the ability to pay—create a fertile field for profiteers who continue, year after year, to rake in huge sums while hiding the improbable odds of success.[13]

ATTITUDES TOWARD BODY FATNESS

People in the United States today value slenderness highly. The image of successful, healthy, well-adjusted people almost invariably includes a slender body form. Irrationally, many people equate slenderness with happiness, intelligence, psychological stability, harmony in relationships, success in the workplace, and many other valued attributes that have little if anything to do with body size or weight. Some claim we place emphasis on a slender appearance, especially for women, not for the sake of their health, but for other people's viewing pleasure.

A widespread misconception holds that obese people are to blame for their overfatness; they face unspoken accusations of laziness, slothfulness, and self-indulgence. Prejudice and discrimination against overweight people, especially overweight women, cause them great psychological stress. Overweight people in our society readily assume the burden of responsibility for their fatness and feel personally guilty when weight-loss diets fail to produce promised results.[14]

Especially damaging are the attitudes of some physicians and other health professionals toward the overweight. A story is told of a woman who had this problem:

> The woman had complained to her family physician for years about her indigestion and diarrhea. He always reminded her that she was overweight and if she wouldn't eat so much, her digestion would be fine. Finally, she was diagnosed by a specialist as having a gluten [wheat] intolerance. Although her health is better today, she is still overweight and is embarrassed to see her family doctor for her regular checkup.[15]

Not only physicians, but other health-care providers including dietitians who run weight-loss clinics can be moralistic in their approach to the obese.[16] They present weight loss as an easily achievable goal, a grossly misleading message. They may consider those who do not become slender as "deviant" and as failures. In reality, such people are among the overwhelming majority who have repeatedly proved that it is really the weight-loss diet schemes that are the failures.

TOWARD DEVELOPING ANSWERS

In searching for appropriate future solutions to the problem of obesity, researchers have looked back 100 years to the population of the time. In those days, significantly fewer people were overweight, and dieting was practically unknown. Physical activity was necessarily a part of life, for elevators, automobiles, and other labor-saving devices were yet to be invented.

With the advent of fast food, obesity gained prevalence in the U.S. population. It is known that adopting a calorie-controlled low-fat, high-carbohydrate eating plan for life can significantly push body composition toward the lean. Equally important, though, is an active lifestyle. Our forebears worked hard physically.

Should obese people make efforts to lose weight? "Yes," if risks of illness are present (see Figure C9-2 to

FIGURE C9-2

DO I NEED TO LOSE WEIGHT?

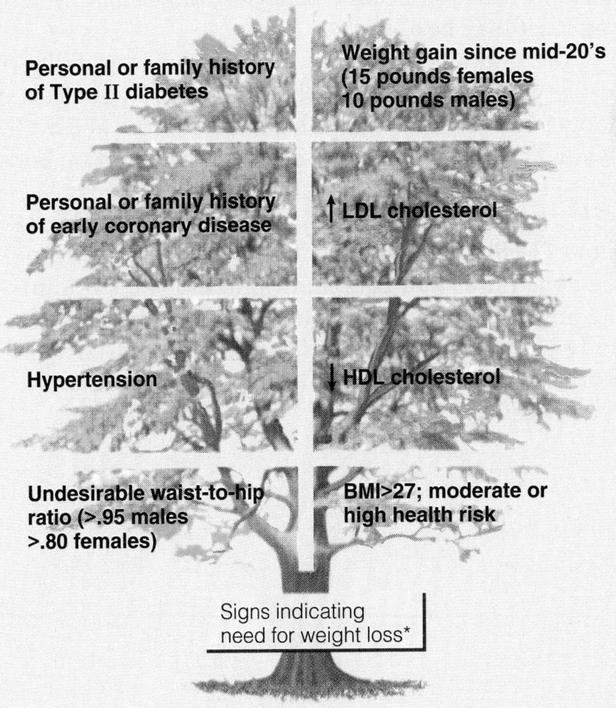

Personal or family history of Type II diabetes

Weight gain since mid-20's (15 pounds females 10 pounds males)

Personal or family history of early coronary disease

↑ LDL cholesterol

Hypertension

↓ HDL cholesterol

Undesirable waist-to-hip ratio (>.95 males >.80 females)

BMI>27; moderate or high health risk

Signs indicating need for weight loss*

* The more factors that are present, the higher the risk of developing health problems in the future.

TABLE C9-3

Tips for Accepting a Healthy Body Weight

- Adopt a new value system. Value yourself and others for human attributes other than body weight. Realize that prejudging people by weight is as harmful as prejudging them by race, religion, or gender.
- Use supportive, nonjudgmental descriptions of your body; never use degrading negative descriptions.
- Take compliments seriously. Positive comments from others probably reflect an objective viewpoint.
- Avoid frequent checking of your weight or appearance; focus on your whole self including your intelligence, social grace, and professional and scholastic accomplishments.
- Accept that no magic diet can help anyone lose weight, and that it is *diets* that fail, not the people who try to employ them.
- Stop dieting to lose weight. Adopt healthy eating and exercise habits.
- Memorize and employ the Food Guide Pyramid. Never restrict food intake beyond the minimum levels that meet nutrient needs.

- Become physically active, not because it will help you get thin but because it will enhance your health. Use all the tips suggested in the next chapter for doing so.
- Seek support from loved ones. Explain what you have learned about the mysteries of why people become overweight. Tell them of your plan for a healthy life in the body you have been given.
- Seek professional counseling, *not* from a weight-loss counselor, but from someone who can help you make gains in self-esteem without weight as a factor.
- Join with others to fight weight discrimination and fashion stereotypes. (Search your local paper, or see the Nutrition Resources Appendix for names of groups.)
- Become politically active. Tell your representative that you support efforts to end the misleading and false claims made by the weight-loss industry. Ask them to lobby for full disclosure by diet peddlers of the risks of dieting. Write and ask the FDA to establish safety and effectiveness criteria for diets and weight-loss programs.

evaluate the risks). What weight to aim for is a trickier question. An immediate goal might be to stop gaining. Then, focusing on healthy behaviors rather than weight loss itself may be a key.

Others should seriously question the desirability of losing weight. People who hold to thin ideals face a danger to their own and others' self-esteem and well-being. Fashion models whose careers depend on body shape often suffer from eating disorders. Teenage girls across the country feel compelled to diet, ignorant of their peril. To break free from these dangerous ideals requires that people revamp old ways of thinking and accept themselves and others regardless of body weight. Table C9-3 offers tips to people who are working to accept their body weights rather than to change them.

A safe option exists for those who would like to improve their body composition without attempting weight loss. The low-fat, adequate diet advocated by the *Dietary Guidelines* and the Daily Food Guide can make a difference for those who are accustomed to eating high-fat diets. Taken with the routine of behavior modification and physical activity described in Chapter 9, the change can help produce fitness while removing the issue of weight from the realm of success or failure. This course of action is not only life-changing for the people who adopt it, but it also sends an important message of self-acceptance to a younger generation.

NOTES

Notes are in Appendix F.

NUTRIENTS, PHYSICAL ACTIVITY, AND THE BODY'S RESPONSES

10

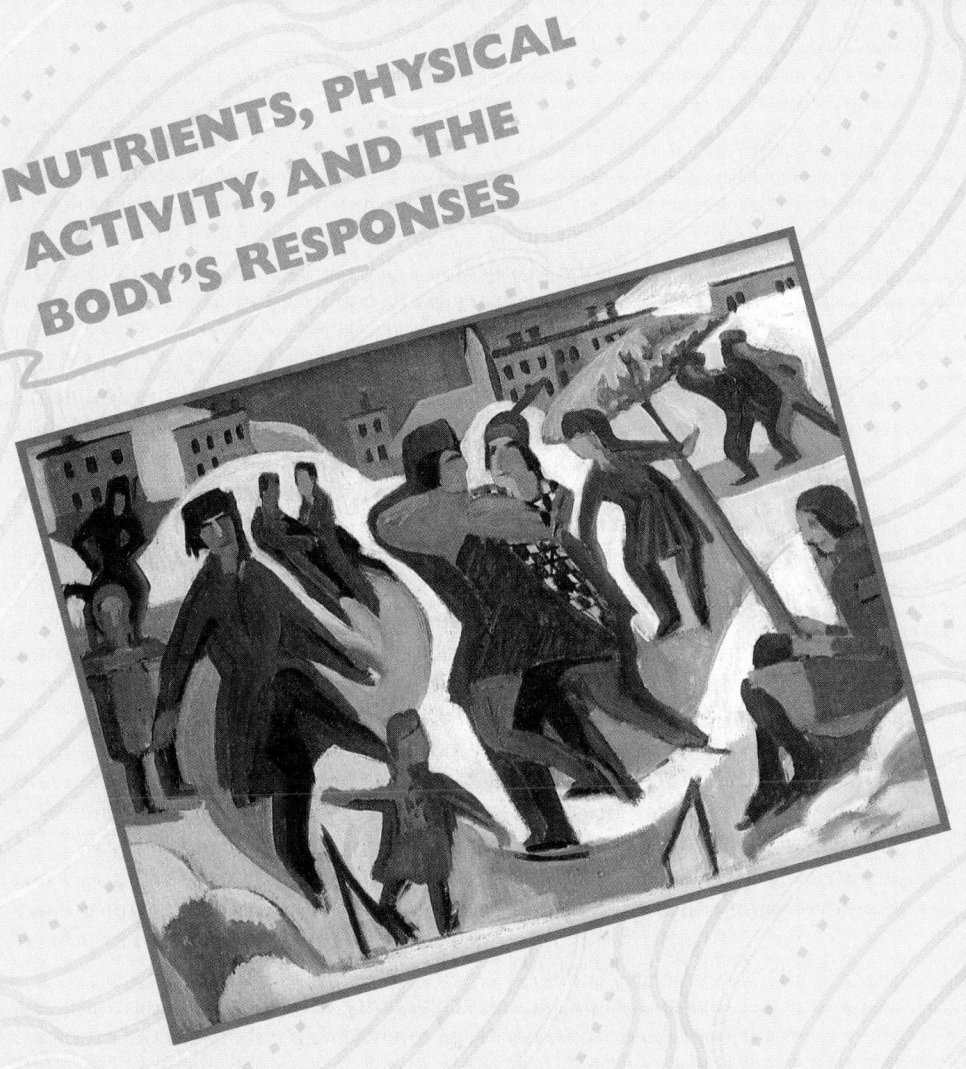

CONTENTS

Ernst Ludwig Kirchner, 1880–1938, *Eisbahn Mit Schlittschulaufern*, © SuperStock.

Ways to include physical activity in a day:

Work out at a fitness club.

Work out with friends who help one another stay fit.

Play a sport.

Take classes for credit in dancing, sports, conditioning, or swimming.

Hike, bike, or walk to nearby stores.

Park a block from your destination and walk.

Take the stairs, not the elevator.

Give two labor-saving devices to charity.

Stretch often during the day.

Lift small hand weights while talking on the phone or watching TV.

Garden.

Play with children.

Walk a dog.

Coach a sport.

Mow, trim, and rake by hand.

Wash your car with extra vigor, or bend and stretch to wash your toes in the bath.

Many others—be imaginative.

In the body, nutrition and physical activity go hand in hand. The working body demands all three energy-yielding nutrients to fuel activity; it also needs protein and a host of supporting nutrients with which to build lean tissue. In addition, it needs stores of fuel in the form of fat and glycogen for physical activity. Physical activity uses up fat and stimulates the building of lean tissue, and so pushes body composition toward the lean, a change that benefits health.

People don't have to run marathons to reap the health rewards of physical activity. In fact, people who regularly engage in just moderate physical activity live longer on average than those who fail to exercise.[1] A sedentary lifestyle ranks with such powerful risk factors as smoking and obesity for developing the major killer diseases of our time—cardiovascular disease, some forms of cancer, stroke, diabetes, and hypertension.[2]

The American College of Sports Medicine (ACSM) made two sets of recommendations concerning physical activity (see Table 10-1).[3] One set of recommendations is for the person wanting to obtain *health* benefits from activity. The other is aimed at the person hoping for improved *physical fitness*. An expert panel has concluded that for health's sake, people should spend an accumulated minimum of 30 minutes in some sort of physical activity on most days of each week.[4] A 1996 Surgeon General's report agreed that 30 minutes of physical activity a day brings benefits and that the activity need not be sports. A few minutes spent climbing up stairs, another few spent pulling weeds, and several more spent walking the dog all contribute to the day's total. Even the health seeker would do well to strive to meet the more demanding guidelines for developing fitness, though, because improved fitness brings still greater health benefits (further reduction of cardiovascular disease risk and improved body composition, for example).[5]

No one yet knows whether too much activity can compromise health. For the vast majority of Americans, however, too much activity is not the problem.

Though scientists are still working out details about how much of what activities are best, they generally agree that people who exercise regularly with a degree of vigor live longer than do sedentary people.[6] Active people may also receive these benefits:

TABLE 10-1

Physical Activity Guidelines

Guidelines for obtaining *health* benefits:

- Frequency of activity: every day.
- Intensity of activity: any level (can be minimal).
- Duration of activity: at least 30 minutes total of activity (can be intermittent).
- Mode of activity: any activity.

Guidelines for developing and maintaining *physical fitness*:

- Frequency of activity: three to five days per week.
- Intensity of activity: 50 to 90% of maximum heart rate.
- Duration of activity: 20 to 60 minutes of continuous activity.
- Mode of activity: any activity that uses large muscle groups.
- Resistance activity: strength training of moderate intensity at least two times per week.

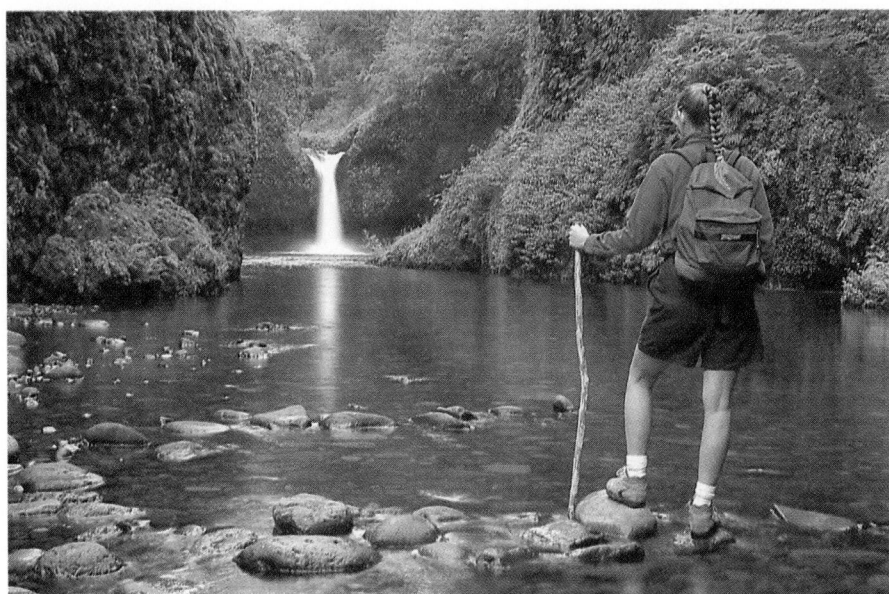

Physical activity benefits both mind and body.

- Improved mental outlook and capacity.
- Feeling of vigor.
- Feeling of belonging—the fun and companionship of sports.
- Strong self-image and self-confidence.
- Reduced body fatness and increased lean body tissue.
- Greater bone density—better protection against osteoporosis.[7]
- Improved circulation, heart capacity, and lung function.
- Sound, beneficial sleep.
- A youthful appearance, healthy skin, and improved muscle tone.
- Reduced risk of cardiovascular disease—normalized blood pressure and slowed resting pulse rate.
- Reduced low-density lipoprotein (LDL) cholesterol and raised high-density lipoprotein (HDL), indicators of low heart disease risk.
- Improvement of symptoms of diabetes.
- Reduced risk of some types of cancer (colon cancer, breast cancer, and others).[8]
- Fast wound healing.
- Improvement or elimination of menstrual cramps.
- Improved resistance to colds and infections.[9]*

Science cannot promise that you will receive all of these benefits if you exercise, but almost everyone who is physically active reaps at least some of them. If even half of these rewards were yours for the asking, wouldn't you step up to claim them? Despite evidence of the benefits, more than two-thirds of U.S. adults are either irregularly active or completely inactive. Perhaps this is because they think of exercise as another task to add to their already work-

---

*Moderate physical activity can stimulate immune function. Intense, vigorous activity such as marathon running, however, may compromise immune function.[10]

training regular practice of an activity, which leads to physical adaptations of the body, with improvements in flexibility, strength, or endurance.

flexibility the capacity of the joints to move through a full range of motion; the ability to bend and recover without injury.

strength the ability of muscles to work against resistance.

muscle endurance the ability of a muscle to contract repeatedly within a given time without becoming exhausted.

cardiovascular endurance the ability of the lungs and cardiovascular system to sustain effort over a period of time.

overload an extra physical demand placed on the body; an increase in the frequency, duration, or intensity of an activity. A principle of training is that for a body system to improve, it must be worked at frequencies, durations, or intensities that increase by increments.

hypertrophy (high-PURR-tro-fee) an increase in size (for example, of a muscle) in response to use.

atrophy (AT-tro-fee) a decrease in size of a muscle because of disuse.

aerobic (air-ROE-bic) requiring oxygen. Aerobic activity requires the heart and lungs to work harder than normal to deliver oxygen to the tissues, and therefore strengthens them.

myoglobin the muscles' iron-containing protein that stores and releases oxygen in response to the muscles' energy needs.

filled days. We'd like them to think, instead, in terms of enjoyable physical activities that will meet their needs for both relaxation and the maintenance of fitness.

This chapter is written for "you," whoever you are—the athlete, the health seeker, the sports player, the weight-loss seeker, or the person who has yet to become physically active. To understand the interactions between physical activity and nutrition, you must first know a few things about **training.**

✔ KEY POINT **Physical activity benefits people's physical, psychological, and social well-being and improves their resistance to disease. A certain minimum amount of physical activity is necessary to produce these benefits.**

THE ESSENTIALS OF TRAINING

Training doesn't require that you develop a Ms. Olympia or Mr. Universe body; rather, you need to develop your own potential along several lines. You need to achieve enough of the four components of fitness—**flexibility, strength, muscle endurance,** and **cardiovascular endurance**—to allow you to meet the everyday demands of life, plus some to spare and to achieve a reasonable body composition.

The Body's Response to Activity People shape their bodies by what they choose to do and not do. Muscle cells and tissues respond to an **overload** of physical activity by gaining strength and size, a response called **hypertrophy.** The opposite is also true: if not called on to perform, muscles dwindle and weaken, a response called **atrophy.** Thus cyclists often have well-developed legs but little arm or chest strength; a tennis player may have one arm that is superbly strong, while the other may be just average. A variety of physical activities will produce the best overall fitness. To this end, people are told to work different muscle groups from day to day. For balanced fitness, stretching enhances flexibility, weight training and calisthenics develop muscle strength and endurance, and **aerobic** activity improves cardiovascular endurance. It makes sense to give muscles a rest, too, because it takes a day or two to replenish muscle fuel supplies and to repair wear and tear incurred through physical activity.

Periodic rest also gives muscles time to adapt to an activity. During rest, muscles build more of the equipment required to perform the activity that preceded the rest. The muscle cells of a superbly trained weight lifter, for example, store extra granules of glycogen, build up strong connective tissues, and add bulk to the special proteins that contract the muscle, thereby increasing the muscle's ability to perform.* In the same way, the muscle cells of a distance swimmer develop huge stocks of **myoglobin,** the muscle's oxygen-storing protein, and other equipment needed to burn fat and to sustain prolonged exertion. Therefore, if you wish to become a better jogger, swimmer, or biker, you

---

*All muscles contain a variety of muscle fibers, but there are two main types—slow-twitch (also called *red fibers*) and fast-twitch (also called *white fibers*). Slow-twitch fibers contain extra metabolic equipment to perform fat-burning aerobic work, while the fast-twitch type store extra glycogen for anaerobic work. Muscle fibers of one type take on some of the characteristics of the other as an adaption to exercise.

FIGURE 10-1

DELIVERY OF OXYGEN BY THE HEART AND LUNGS TO THE MUSCLES

The more fit a muscle is, the more oxygen it draws from the blood. This oxygen comes from the lungs, so the person with more fit muscles extracts oxygen from inhaled air more efficiently than a person with less fit muscles. The cardiovascular system responds to increased demand for oxygen by building up its capacity to deliver oxygen. Researchers can measure cardiovascular fitness by measuring the amount of oxygen a person consumes per minute while working out. This measure of fitness is called **VO₂ max.**

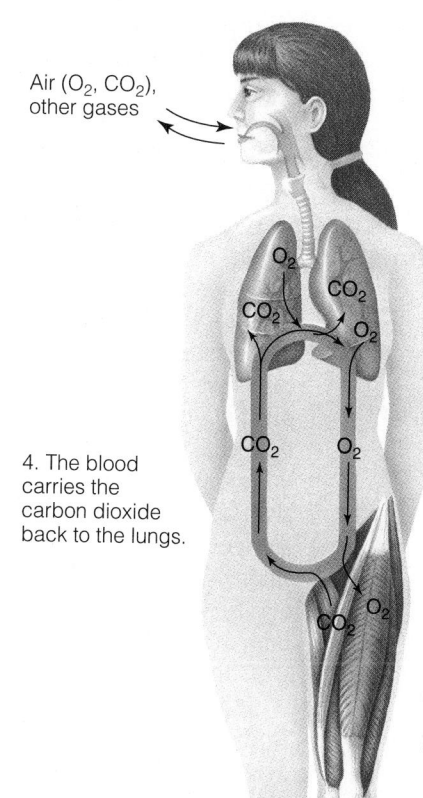

Air (O_2, CO_2), other gases

1. The respiratory system delivers oxygen to the blood.

2. The circulatory system carries oxygenated blood throughout the body.

4. The blood carries the carbon dioxide back to the lungs.

3. The muscles and other tissues obtain oxygen from the blood and release carbon dioxide into it.

should train mostly by jogging, swimming, or biking. Your performance will improve as the muscles develop the specific equipment they need to do the activity. Keep in mind that while everyone's muscles adapt to physical activity to some degree, true champions in sports are born with the genetic potential to excel while others are not.[11] This fact cannot be changed even through hard work.

Aerobic Activity and the Heart Aerobic activity builds cardiovascular endurance: a healthy condition of the heart, lungs, and arteries. With cardiovascular endurance, the total blood volume and number of red blood cells increase, so the blood can carry more oxygen. The heart muscle becomes stronger and larger, and each beat empties the heart's chambers more completely, so the heart pumps more blood per beat. This makes fewer beats necessary, so the pulse rate falls. The muscles that inflate and deflate the lungs gain strength and endurance, and this allows breathing to become more efficient. Blood moves easily through the blood vessels because the muscles of the heart contract powerfully, and contraction of the skeletal muscles pushes the blood through the veins. Such improvements keep resting blood pressure normal. They also raise blood HDL, the beneficial lipoprotein. Figure 10-1 shows the major relationships among the heart, lungs, and muscles.

Which activities produce these beneficial changes? Recall from page 378 that the advice for obtaining health benefits was to spend 30 *collective* minutes on

VO₂ max the maximum rate of oxygen consumption by an individual (measured at sea level).

The importance of HDL to heart health is a topic of the next chapter.

anaerobic (AN-air-ROE-bic) not requiring oxygen. Anaerobic activity may require strength but does not work the heart and lungs very hard for a sustained period.

cardiac output the volume of blood discharged by the heart each minute.

stroke volume the amount of oxygenated blood ejected from the heart toward body tissues at each beat.

Cardiovascular endurance is characterized by:

✓ Increased **cardiac output** and oxygen delivery.
✓ Increased heart strength and **stroke volume.**
✓ Slowed resting pulse.
✓ Increased breathing efficiency.
✓ Improved circulation.
✓ Reduced blood pressure.

most days each week in various activities. In contrast, training for cardiovascular endurance requires *sustained* activity—that is, activity performed for certain time periods. Effective activities elevate the heart rate, are sustained for longer than 20 minutes, and use most of the large muscle groups of the body (legs, buttocks, and abdomen). Examples are swimming, cross-country skiing, rowing, fast walking, jogging, fast bicycling, soccer, hockey, basketball, water polo, lacrosse, and rugby.

An informal pulse check can give you some indication of how conditioned your heart is. The average resting pulse rate for adults is around 70 beats per minute, but the rate can be higher or lower. Active people can have resting pulse rates of 50 or even lower. To take your pulse, place your finger over a pulse point (under the jawbone at the side of the Adam's apple of the throat, for instance), and count the number of beats in 30 seconds. Multiply by two to get beats per minute.

Anaerobic activity generally brings about less cardiovascular conditioning than aerobic activity does, but it superbly develops muscle strength and bulk. It involves sudden, all-out exertions of muscles that last for fewer than 90 seconds. This form of activity develops lean tissue and so improves overall body composition. Examples include sprinting (100 meter dash), serving a tennis ball, jumping a fence, doing pushups, or lifting weights.

After learning the ways activity affects the body, people often want to know whether their own activity levels meet their body needs. Complex ways of finding this out are available, but a group of researchers devised a quicker way. They asked this single question: "Do you currently participate in any regular activity or program (either on your own or in a formal class) designed to improve or maintain your physical fitness?" The researchers discovered that positive answers correlated closely with healthy body mass index, high blood HDL, and efficient use of oxygen, all indicators of health-promoting physical activity levels.[12] If your honest answer to their question is "yes," chances are good that you are physically active enough to enhance your own health.

The person who wishes to develop a fit body for health or sports performance must also master nutrition. The rest of this chapter provides detailed descriptions of interactions between nutrients and physical activity. Nutrition alone cannot endow you with fitness or athletic ability, but along with the right mental attitude, it can complement the effort you put forth to obtain them. Conversely, unwise food selections can stand in your way.

✓ **KEY POINT** **The components of fitness are flexibility, strength, muscle endurance, and cardiovascular endurance. To build fitness, a person must engage in physical activity. Muscles adapt to activities they are called upon to perform.**

USING GLUCOSE TO FUEL ACTIVITY

The body responds to physical activity by adjusting its fuel mix. During rest, the body derives a little more than half of its energy from fatty acids, most of the rest from glucose, and a little from amino acids. Of the fuels mentioned, carbohydrate is of major interest to physically active people. The stored glucose of muscle glycogen is a major fuel for physical activity. In the early minutes of an activity, muscle glycogen provides the majority of energy the muscles use to go into action. As activity continues, messenger molecules, including the hormone epinephrine flow into the bloodstream to signal the liver and fat cells to liberate their stored energy nutrients, primarily fatty acids and glucose. Thus hormones set the table for the muscles' energy feast, and the muscles help themselves to the fuels passing by in the blood.

Glucose Use and Storage

Both the liver and muscles store glucose as glycogen, a fuel considered vital for physical activity; the liver can also make glucose from fragments of other nutrients. It has been said that muscles hoard their glycogen stores—they do not release their glucose into the bloodstream to share with other body tissues, as the liver does. This is fortunate. A muscle that shared its glycogen reserves with other tissues might lack glucose at critical times, say, when running from danger. A muscle that conserves its glycogen is prepared to act in emergencies because muscle glucose is the fuel for quick action. Later on, as activity continues, glucose from the liver's stored glycogen and dietary glucose absorbed from the digestive tract also become important sources of fuel for muscle activity.

Muscle glycogen also supports long-duration endurance activity; and the more glycogen muscles store, the longer the stores will last to support this activity. A classic report compared fuel use during physical activity among three groups of runners, each on a different diet.[13] For several days before testing, one of the groups ate a normal mixed diet (55 percent of calories from carbohydrate); a second group ate a high-carbohydrate diet (83 percent of calories from carbohydrate); and the third group ate a high-fat diet (94 percent of calories from fat). As Figure 10-2 shows, the high-carbohydrate diet enabled the athletes

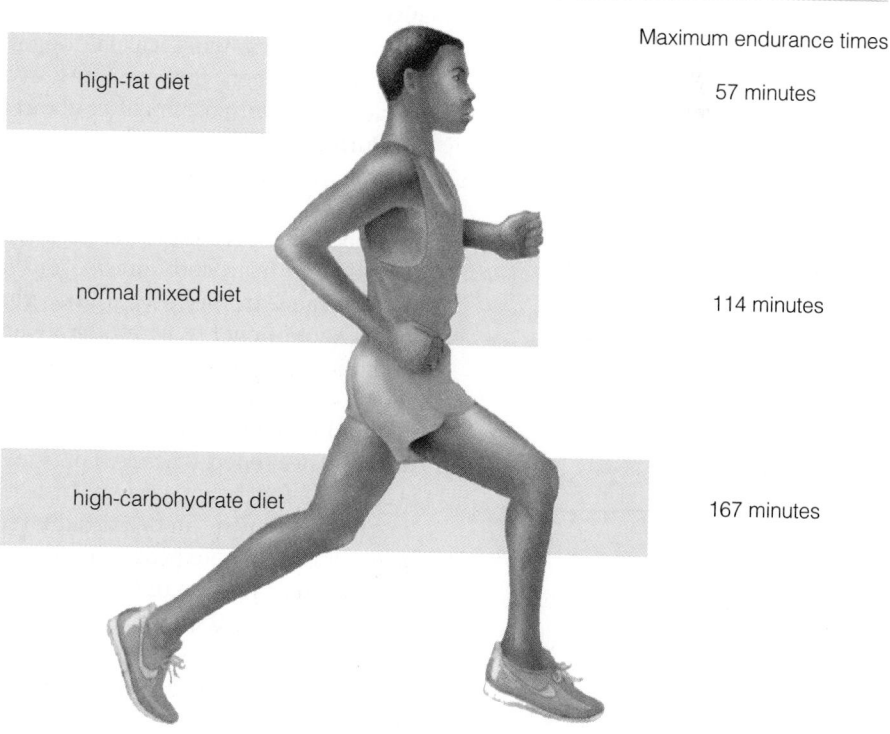

FIGURE 10-2

THE EFFECT OF DIET ON PHYSICAL ENDURANCE
A high-carbohydrate diet can triple an athlete's endurance.

high-fat diet

normal mixed diet

high-carbohydrate diet

Maximum endurance times

57 minutes

114 minutes

167 minutes

to work longer before exhaustion. This study and many others that followed established that a high-carbohydrate diet enhances an athlete's endurance by ensuring ample glycogen stores.

When a high-carbohydrate diet is consumed, glycogen storage is speeded up, as is the body's use of carbohydrate for fuel.[14] These two actions are especially important because the body ordinarily has such limited carbohydrate storage capacity. The body stores what glucose it can as glycogen and uses up much of the remainder as fuel. Any excess must be converted to fat before storage, an inefficient process.

The amount of glycogen that muscles use and store is affected by training as well as diet. When muscles work hard enough one time to deplete their glycogen stores, they adapt to store more glycogen the next time.

✔ KEY POINT **Glucose is supplied by dietary carbohydrate or made by the liver. It is stored in both liver and muscle tissue as glycogen. Total glycogen stores affect an athlete's endurance. Both storage and use of glycogen increase with increasing carbohydrate intakes and with glycogen-depleting physical activity.**

Activity Intensity, Glucose Use, and Glycogen Stores

Compared with the body's fat, its glycogen stores are much more limited. A person with 30 pounds of body fat to spare may have only a pound or so of muscle and liver glycogen to draw on. How long an exercising person's glycogen will last depends not only on diet but also on the intensity of the activity. The most intense activities—the kind that make it difficult "to catch your breath," such as a quarter-mile run—use glycogen quickly. Other, less intense activities, such as jogging, during which breathing is steady and easy, use glycogen more slowly. Thus competitive athletes place large demands on their glycogen stores, while casual joggers demand less from their stores. Joggers still use glycogen, however, and eventually they can run out of it. Glycogen depletion usually occurs after about two hours of vigorous exercise.[15*]

During *moderate* physical activity, the lungs and circulatory system have no trouble keeping up with the muscles' need for oxygen. The individual breathes easily, and the heart beats at a faster pace than at rest but steadily—the activity is aerobic. As Figure 10-3 shows, during aerobic activity muscles extract their energy from both glucose and fatty acids when both are present together with oxygen. In this way, a little glucose helps to metabolize a lot of fat. Fat yields a lot of energy, so moderate aerobic activity conserves glycogen stores.

Intense activity presents a different picture. The heart and lungs can provide only so much oxygen only so fast. When muscle exertion is so great that the demand for energy outstrips the oxygen supply, aerobic metabolism cannot sufficiently meet energy needs. This means that fat cannot be used, because oxygen is required for its breakdown. Instead muscles must begin to rely more heavily on glucose, which can be partially broken down *anaerobically*. Thus the muscles begin drawing more heavily on their limited glycogen supply.

The upper portion of Figure 10-3 shows that glucose can yield some energy in anaerobic metabolism, but not as much as in aerobic metabolism. Anaerobic

---

*Here "vigorous exercise" means exercise at 75 percent of VO_2 max.

FIGURE 10-3

GLUCOSE AND FATTY ACIDS IN THEIR ENERGY-RELEASING PATHWAYS

Glucose is partially broken down under anaerobic conditions. It yields some quick energy and leaves behind some fragments which must await the renewed availability of oxygen (aerobic conditions) to be broken down completely to carbon dioxide, water, and energy. Fat can enter the energy cycle only in the presence of oxygen.

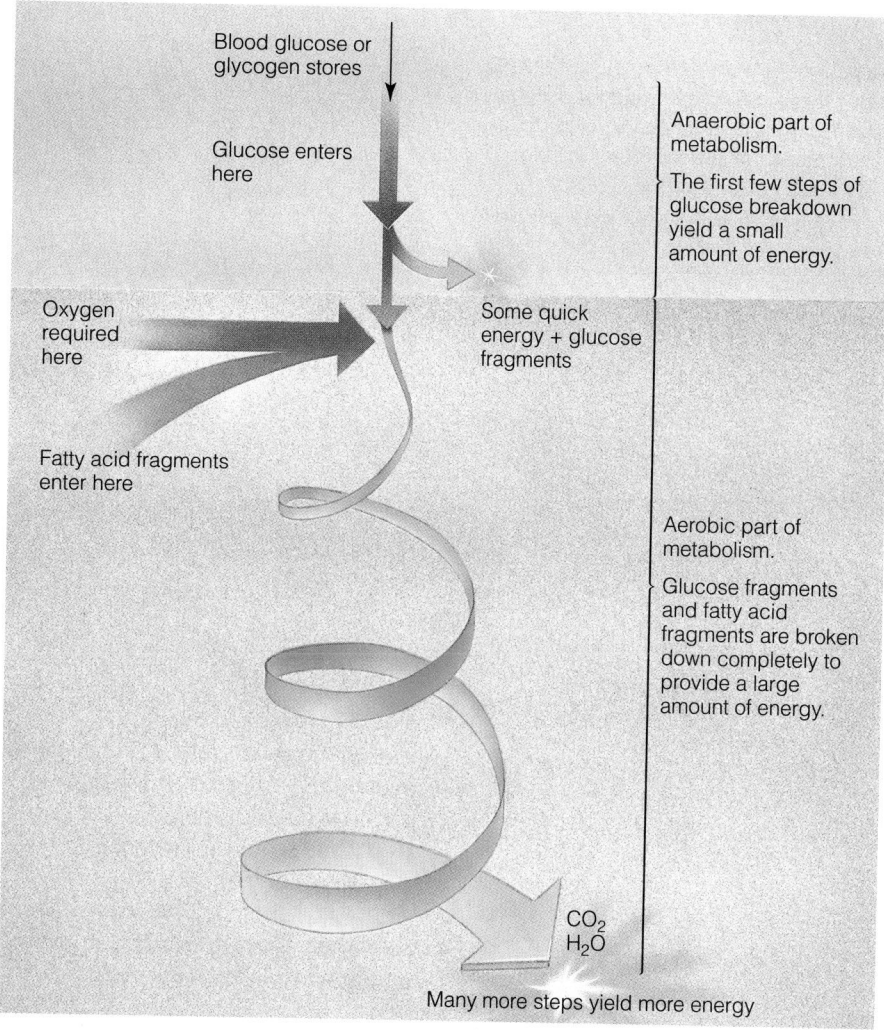

Blood glucose or glycogen stores

Glucose enters here

Oxygen required here

Fatty acid fragments enter here

Some quick energy + glucose fragments

Anaerobic part of metabolism.

The first few steps of glucose breakdown yield a small amount of energy.

Aerobic part of metabolism.

Glucose fragments and fatty acid fragments are broken down completely to provide a large amount of energy.

CO_2
H_2O

Many more steps yield more energy

breakdown of glycogen yields energy to muscle tissue when energy demands are so large as to outstrip the ability to provide energy aerobically, for example, during intense activity. Thus anaerobic metabolism supplies energy, but it does so by lavishly spending the muscles' glycogen reserves.

Anaerobic glucose breakdown produces **lactic acid,** fragments of glucose molecules that accumulate in the tissues and blood. When the nervous and hormonal systems detect these fragments in the blood, they respond by speeding up the heart and lungs to draw in more oxygen and break down the fragments. At some point, however, the heart and lungs are no longer able to keep up, and lactic acid accumulates. If you exercise intensely, you may have to slow down or even stop to "catch your breath" (replenish your oxygen supply). Then your body begins relying on aerobic metabolism once more. At this point lactic acid is burned for fuel or used by the liver to regenerate glucose.

Lactic acid causes burning muscle pain, followed within seconds by a type of muscle fatigue. A strategy for dealing with lactic acid is to relax the muscles

lactic acid a product of the incomplete breakdown of glucose during anaerobic metabolism. When oxygen becomes available, lactic acid can be completely broken down for energy or converted back to glucose.

FIGURE 10-4

GLYCOGEN DEPLETION IN CYCLISTS

After three and a half hours of constant cycling, muscle glycogen is used up, but the demand for glucose fuel declines only slightly (dotted line).

SOURCE: Adapted from E. F. Coyle and S. J. Montain, Carbohydrate and fluid ingestion during exercise: Are there trade-offs? *Medicine and Science in Sports and Exercise* 24 (1992): 671–678.

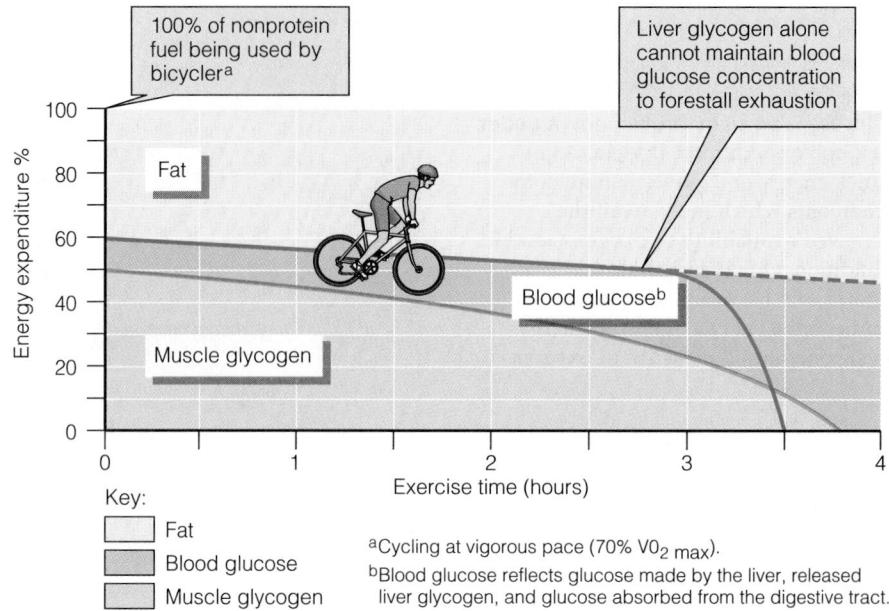

at every opportunity during activity so that the circulating blood can carry away the lactic acid and bring in more oxygen to sustain aerobic metabolism. This is what mountaineers are doing when they relax their leg muscles at each step (the "mountain rest step").

✓ KEY POINT **The more intense an activity, the more glucose it demands. During anaerobic metabolism, the body spends glucose rapidly and accumulates lactic acid.**

Activity Duration, Glucose Use, and Glycogen Stores

Glucose use during physical activity depends on the *duration* of the activity as well as on its *intensity*. In the first 10 minutes or so of an activity, the active muscles rely almost completely on their own stores of glycogen. Within the first 20 minutes or so of moderate activity, a person uses up about one-fifth of the available glycogen. As the muscles devour their own glycogen, they become ravenous for more glucose and increase their uptake of blood glucose 30-fold or more.[16] If you tested a person's blood glucose during moderate activity, you would see it decline slightly, reflecting the muscles' use of blood glucose.

A person who continues exercising moderately for longer than 20 minutes begins to use less glucose and more fat for fuel. Still, glucose use continues, and if the activity goes on for long enough and at a high enough intensity, muscle and liver glycogen stores will run out almost completely (see Figure 10-4). Physical activity can continue for a short time thereafter only because the liver scrambles to produce some glucose from available lactic acid and certain amino acids.[17] This minimum amount of glucose may briefly forestall exhaustion, but when hypoglycemia accompanies glycogen depletion, it brings nervous system function almost to a halt, making activity impossible. This is what "hitting the wall" means to runners of a marathon.[18]

To postpone exhaustion, endurance athletes must try to maintain their blood glucose concentrations for as long as they can. Three dietary strategies and one training strategy may help maintain glucose concentrations. One diet strategy is to eat a high-carbohydrate diet on a day-to-day basis (see this chapter's Food Feature). Another is to take in some glucose during the activity, usually in fluid (see next paragraph). The third is to eat carbohydrate-rich foods following activity to boost the storage of glycogen. As for training, the strategy involves training the muscles to store as much glycogen as they can, while supplying enough dietary glucose to do so (carbohydrate loading, as described in the next section).

During a long-duration competition, glucose ingested before or during the event makes its way from the digestive tract to the working muscles to augment dwindling glucose supplies from the muscle and liver glycogen stores.[19] Especially during games such as soccer or hockey, which last for hours and demand repeated bouts of intense activity, athletes may benefit from carbohydrate-containing drinks taken during the activity.

Before concluding that sugar might be good for your own performance, consider first whether you engage in *endurance* activity. That is, do you run, swim, bike, or ski nonstop at a rapid pace for more than 1 hour at a time, or do you compete in games lasting for hours? If not, the sugar picture changes. For an everyday jog or swim lasting less than 60 minutes, sugar probably won't help performance. The body's glycogen stores are not limited by carbohydrate availability, so more will not be better. Even among athletes, extra carbohydrate does not benefit those who engage in sports in which fatigue is unrelated to blood glucose, such as 100-meter sprinting, baseball, casual basketball, and weight lifting.[20]

Four strategies can help to maintain blood glucose to support sports performance (for endurance athletes only):

1. Eat a high-carbohydrate diet regularly.
2. Take glucose (usually in diluted fruit juice or other sweet beverages) during endurance activity.
3. Eat carbohydrate-rich foods after performance.
4. Train the muscles to maximize glycogen stores.

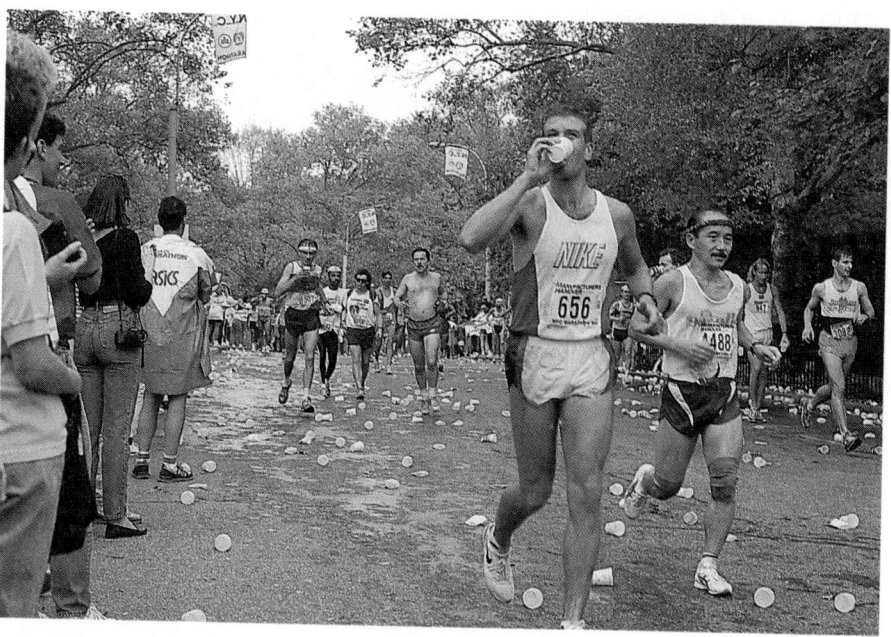

Those who compete in endurance activities require fluid and carbohydrate fuel.

carbohydrate loading a regimen of performing exhausting exercise, followed by eating a high-carbohydrate diet, that enables muscles to store glycogen beyond their normal capacity; also called *glycogen loading* or *glycogen super-compensation*.

Casual exercisers who want small amounts of sugary foods or beverages during their workouts probably do themselves no harm by partaking of them. Some specific recommendations for athletes concerning carbohydrate intakes before, during, and after activity appear later on.

✔ KEY POINT **Physical activity of long duration places demands on the body's glycogen stores. Carbohydrate ingested before and during long-duration activity may help to forestall hypoglycemia and fatigue.**

Carbohydrate Loading

Athletes whose sports exhaust their glycogen stores sometimes use a technique called **carbohydrate loading** to trick their muscles into storing extra glycogen before competition. At one time athletes were taught to severely restrict carbohydrates and to exercise heavily to empty their muscles of glycogen. Then they would cut back on exercise and eat an extremely high-carbohydrate diet. This older method of carbohydrate loading can have serious side effects such as abnormal heartbeats and swollen muscles. Today athletes use a safer plan. During the first 4 days of the week before competition, the athlete trains moderately hard (1 to 2 hours per day) and eats a diet that is moderate in carbohydrate. During the 3 days before competition, the athlete gradually cuts back on activity and eats a very-high-carbohydrate diet. By manipulating activity and carbohydrate, the athlete packs in extra glycogen to fuel activity lasting 90 minutes or longer at a stretch. In a hot climate, extra stored glycogen confers an additional advantage on the endurance athlete. As glycogen breaks down, it releases water, which helps to meet the athlete's fluid needs.

A simpler measure is possible. The athlete can eat a high-carbohydrate meal, such as a glass of orange juice and some crackers, toast, or cereal, within two hours after physical activity. This accelerates the rate of glycogen storage by 300 percent.[21] Timing is important—eating the meal after two hours has passed reduces the glycogen synthesis rate by almost half.

To make glycogen, muscles need carbohydrate, but they also need rest. Vary daily activity routines to work different muscles on different days.

Casual exercisers need not make an effort to load up on extra carbohydrate. They need only eat a regular high-carbohydrate diet.

✔ KEY POINT **Carbohydrate loading is a regime of physical activity and diet that enables an athlete's muscles to store larger-than-normal amounts of glycogen to extend endurance.**

Degree of Training and Carbohydrate Use

Factors that affect glucose use during physical activity:
✔ Carbohydrate intake.
✔ Intensity and duration of activity.
✔ Degree of training.

The degree of training of the muscles affects glycogen use during activity. Trained muscles can burn more fat, and at higher intensities, than untrained muscles, so they require less glucose to perform the same amount of work. A person attempting an activity for the first time uses up much more glucose per minute than an athlete who is trained to perform it. A trained person can work at high intensities longer than an untrained person while using the same amount of glycogen.

Chapter 4 described the action of insulin on blood sugar.

People with diabetes should know that the moderating effect of physical training on glucose metabolism may have implications for them. Those who must take insulin or insulin-eliciting drugs sometimes find that as their muscles adapt to physical activity, they can reduce their daily drug doses. Another benefit to those with diabetes: physical activity helps the body lose excess fat, and this also helps to improve Type II diabetes.

✔ **KEY POINT**   **Highly trained muscles use less glucose and more fat than do untrained muscles to perform the same work, so their glycogen lasts longer.**

USING FAT AND FATTY ACIDS TO FUEL ACTIVITY

If a person should regularly eat mostly fat and protein with little measurable carbohydrate, that person would burn more fat than normal during physical activity. However, that person might also sacrifice athletic performance, as Figure 10-2 showed, and could incur a major risk of cardiovascular disease. Not even physically active people are immune to heart attacks and strokes, so it is no wonder that every reliable source speaks out against high-fat diets for athletes.

Body fat stores are more important as fuel for activity than is fat in the diet. Unlike the body's glycogen stores, which are limited, fat stores can fuel hours of activity without running out; body fat is (theoretically) an unlimited source of energy. Even the lean bodies of elite runners carry enough fat to fuel several marathon runs.

Early in activity, muscles begin to draw on fatty acids from two sources—fats stored within the working muscles and fats from fat deposits such as the fat under the skin. Areas that have the most fat to spare donate the greatest amounts of fatty acids to the blood (although they may not be the areas that you would choose to lose fat from). This is why "spot reducing" doesn't work: muscles do not own the fat that surrounds them. Fat cells release fatty acids into the blood for all the muscles to share. Proof of this is found in a tennis player's arms: the fatfolds measure the same in both arms, even though one arm has better-developed muscles than the other.

Intensity and Duration Affect Fat Use   The *intensity* of physical activity also affects the percentage of energy contributed by fat. Figure 10-3 showed that fat can be broken down for energy in only one way, by aerobic metabolism. When the intensity of activity becomes so great that energy demands surpass the ability to provide energy aerobically, the body cannot burn more fat. Instead, it burns more glucose.

The *duration* of activity also matters to fat use. At the start of activity, the blood fatty acid concentration falls, but a few minutes into an activity, the neurotransmitter norepinephrine signals the fat cells to break apart their stored triglycerides and to liberate fatty acids into the blood. After about 20 minutes of activity, the blood fatty acid concentration rises above the normal resting concentration. It is during this phase of sustained, submaximal activity, beyond the first 20 minutes, that the fat cells begin to shrink in size as they empty out their fat stores.

Degree of Training Affects Fat Use   It is training—repeated aerobic activity—that stimulates the muscles to develop more fat-burning enzymes. Aerobically trained muscles burn fat more readily than untrained muscles. Another

Factors that affect fat use during physical activity:
✔ Fat intake.
✔ Intensity and duration of the activity.
✔ Degree of training.

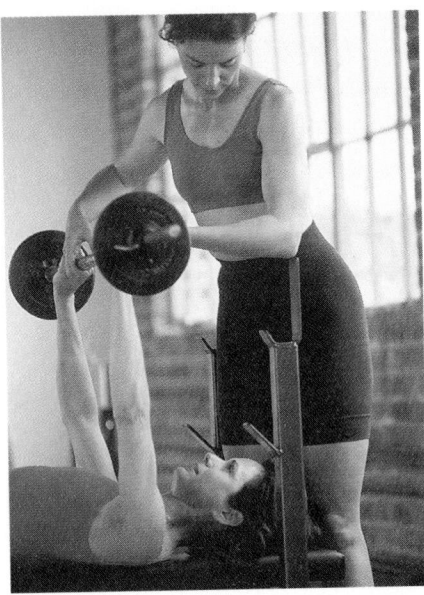

Physical activity itself triggers the building of muscle proteins.

outcome of aerobic training: the heart and lungs become stronger and better able to deliver oxygen to muscles at high-activity intensities.

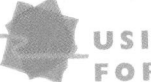

USING PROTEIN AND AMINO ACIDS FOR BUILDING MUSCLES AND TO FUEL ACTIVITY

If a high-fat diet is ill advised for athletes, what about a high-protein diet? Physically active people need protein to build muscle and other lean tissue structures and, to a small extent, for fuel.

Protein for Building Muscle Tissue

In the hours of rest that follow physical activity, muscles speed up their rate of protein synthesis—they build more of the proteins they need to perform the activity. Additionally, whenever the body rebuilds a part of itself, it must tear down the old structures to make way for the new ones. Physical activity, with just a slight overload, calls into action both the protein-dismantling and the protein-synthesizing equipment of each muscle cell.

Dietary protein provides the needed amino acids for synthesis of new muscle proteins. The true director of synthesis of muscle protein, however, is physical activity itself. Repeated activity sends the signal to the muscle cells' genetic material to begin producing more of the proteins needed to perform the work at hand.

The genetic protein-making equipment inside the nuclei of muscle cells seems to "know" when proteins are needed. Furthermore, it knows *which* proteins are needed to support each type of physical activity. The key communicator seems to be the activity itself—the intensity and pattern of muscle contractions initiate signals that direct the muscles' genetic material to make particular proteins. For example, a weight lifter's workout sends the information that muscle fibers need added bulk for strength and more enzymes for making and using glycogen. A jogger's workout stimulates production of proteins needed for aerobic oxidation of fat and glucose. Muscle cells are exquisitely responsive to the need for proteins, and they build them conservatively.

Finally, after muscle cells have made all the decisions about when to build proteins and which proteins are needed, protein nutrition comes into play. During active muscle-building phases of training, a weight lifter might add to existing muscle mass between ¼ ounce and 1 ounce (between 7 and 28 grams) of protein each day. This extra protein comes from ordinary food.

✓ KEY POINT **Physical activity stimulates muscle cells to break down and synthesize protein, resulting in muscle adaptation to activity.**

Protein Used for Fuel

Not only do athletes retain more protein, but they also use a little more protein as fuel.[22] Studies of nitrogen balance show that the body speeds up its use of amino acids for energy during physical activity, just as it speeds up its use of glucose and fatty acids. Protein contributes about 10 percent of the total fuel used, both during activity and during rest. Endurance athletes use up enormous amounts of all energy fuels during performance, so they break down more protein. Moderate exercisers use less. However, all who eat enough total calories of a balanced, high-carbohydrate diet also consume enough protein.

The factors that regulate how much protein is used during activity seem to be the same three that regulate the use of glucose and fat. One factor is diet—a carbohydrate-rich diet spares protein from being used as fuel. Some amino acids can be converted into glucose when need be. Others, the **branched-chain amino acids,** can stand in for glucose in energy pathways. If the diet is low in carbohydrate, much more protein will be used in place of glucose.

Second, the intensity and duration of the activity also modify protein use.[23] Casual exercisers, those who engage in moderate activity for less than an hour, seem to show no increased need for protein.

Finally, the degree of training also modifies the use of protein. The better trained the athlete, the less protein used during activity at a given intensity.

How much protein should an athlete consume? A joint position paper from the American Dietetic Association (ADA) and the Canadian Dietetic Association (CDA)[a] recommends 1 to 1.5 grams of protein per kilogram of body weight each day, an amount somewhat higher than the 0.8 g/kg/day recommended for sedentary people.[24] Another authority suggests different protein intakes for different athletes.[25] Table 10-2 lists some recommendations and translates them into daily intakes for an athlete who weighs 70 kilograms (154 pounds).

After considering these recommendations, athletes may still wonder whether the diet they choose provides the protein they need. This chapter's Food Feature answers questions about choosing a performance diet. Meanwhile, relax. Most people's protein intakes are already within the highest ranges recommended for athletes by any knowledgeable source.[26]

☑ **KEY POINT**   **Athletes use some protein both for building muscle tissue and for energy, but they need not strive to consume more protein than is present in the average U.S. diet.**

---

[a]The Canadian Dietetic Association now uses the name Dietitians of Canada (DC).

> **branched-chain amino acids** amino acids that, unlike the others, can provide energy directly to muscle tissue: leucine, isoleucine, and valine.

> **Factors that affect protein use during physical activity:**
> ✓ Carbohydrate intake.
> ✓ Intensity and duration of the activity.
> ✓ Degree of training.

TABLE 10-2

Total Daily Protein Needs of a 70-Kilogram (154-Pound) Athlete

Authority	Recommendation (g/kg/day)	Protein/Day (g)
Food and Nutrition Board (RDA)	0.8	56
ADA/CDA	1.0–1.5	70–105
Lemon, P. W. R. (endurance athletes)	1.2–1.4	84–98
Lemon, P. W. R. (strength-speed athletes)	1.2–1.7	84–119

SOURCES: Position of the American Dietetic Association and the Canadian Dietetic Association: Nutrition for physical fitness and athletic performance for adults, *Journal of the American Dietetic Association* 93 (1993): 691–695; P. W. R. Lemon, Effect of exercise on protein requirements, in C. Williams and J. T. Devlin, eds., *Foods, Nutrition and Sports Performance: An International Scientific Consensus* (London: E & FN Spon, 1992), pp. 65–86.

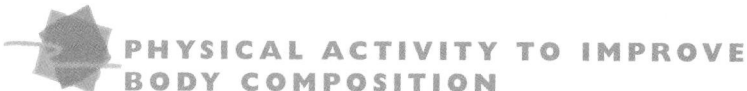

PHYSICAL ACTIVITY TO IMPROVE BODY COMPOSITION

Physical activity can shift body composition toward more lean and less fat tissue. It can ensure that weight loss is mostly fat loss, and that weight gain is mostly muscle gain. People trying to lose body fat or maintain a loss of fat find it difficult to do without physical activity.[27] People trying to slim down, maintain weight, or gain weight (and isn't that all people?) can rely on physical activity to help them achieve their goals.

Trimming Down

A long-held nutrition truth states that physical activity contributes to a healthy body composition. Physical activity offers all of the benefits listed at this chapter's start, and for the weight-reducer, it:

- increases energy expenditure.
- increases resting metabolic rate (slightly) over the long term.
- accelerates loss of body fat.
- helps regulate appetite.
- helps control stress and stress-induced overeating or undereating.
- enhances self-esteem.

Strategies for using physical activity for weight control:
1. Choose active exercise.
2. Move large muscle groups.
3. Expand the time you spend exercising.
4. Incorporate exercise into informal daily routines.

Keep in mind that if physical activity is to help with fat loss, it must involve the voluntary moving of muscles, not passive motion such as being jiggled by a machine at a health spa or being massaged. Passive activity does not increase energy expenditure or build muscles, but active activity does. The more muscles you move actively, and the more time you spend doing it, the more calories you spend and the more muscle tissue you build. Table 10-3 shows the approximate numbers of calories people of various weights spend on activities.

Some people have the impression that to aid in fat loss, physical activity must be of long duration; others think it must be intense. Actually, both types of exercise are effective. Health-care professionals often recommend activities of low-to-moderate intensity for long duration, such as fast-paced, hour-long walks, for those who want to lose body fat. They emphasize that activity of low-to-moderate intensity burns more fat than high-intensity activity, because more fat than carbohydrate is used to fuel activity at low intensities. The greater the intensity, the less contribution fat makes to the total fuel used. Within a given time period, however, although the *proportion* of fat used for energy is greater at lower intensities, more *total energy* will be expended at higher intensities, and so more *total energy from fat* will be used. Thus, in a given time frame, total energy spent, as well as total energy from fat, is greater with higher-intensity activity.[28]

Good news: Both working slowly for *long* times and working fast for *short* times will burn fat.

The bottom line on how much fat loss physical activity will promote seems to be total energy expenditure, regardless of how you do it. To lose fat, expend as much energy as your time and stamina allow.

Activities of low-to-moderate intensity are often recommended for those who are overweight or habitually sedentary. People whose motivation is shaky are more likely to stick with such activities and are less likely to injure themselves. People who are overweight or have been sedentary have to gain confidence in their ability to be active. The more confident they become, the more likely they will continue to be active. Whether a person's initial motivation to

TABLE 10-3

Energy Demands of Activities

Activity	Energy per Pound of Body Weight per Minute	Body Weight (lb)				
	cal/lb/min[a]	110	125	150	175	200
		cal/min[b]				
Aerobic dance (vigorous)	.062	6.8	7.8	9.3	10.9	12.4
Basketball (vigorous, full court)	.097	10.7	12.1	14.6	17.0	19.4
Bicycling						
13 miles per hour	.045	5.0	5.6	6.8	7.9	9.0
15 miles per hour	.049	5.4	6.1	7.4	8.6	9.8
17 miles per hour	.057	6.3	7.1	8.6	10.0	11.4
19 miles per hour	.076	8.4	9.5	11.4	13.3	15.2
21 miles per hour	.090	9.9	11.3	13.5	15.8	18.0
23 miles per hour	.109	12.0	13.6	16.4	19.0	21.8
25 miles per hour	.139	15.3	17.4	20.9	24.3	27.8
Canoeing (flat water, moderate pace)	.045	5.0	5.6	6.8	7.9	9.0
Cross-country skiing (8 miles per hour)	.104	11.4	13.0	15.6	18.2	20.8
Golf (carrying clubs)	.045	5.0	5.6	6.8	7.9	9.0
Handball	.078	8.6	9.8	11.7	13.7	15.6
Horseback riding (trot)	.052	5.7	6.5	7.8	9.1	10.4
Rowing (vigorous)	.097	10.7	12.1	14.6	17.0	19.4
Running						
5 miles per hour	.061	6.7	7.6	9.2	10.7	12.2
6 miles per hour	.074	8.1	9.2	11.1	13.0	14.8
7.5 miles per hour	.094	10.3	11.8	14.1	16.4	18.8
9 miles per hour	.103	11.3	12.9	15.5	18.0	20.6
10 miles per hour	.114	12.5	14.3	17.1	20.0	22.9
11 miles per hour	.131	14.4	16.4	19.7	22.9	26.2
Soccer (vigorous)	.097	10.7	12.1	14.6	17.0	19.4
Studying	.011	1.2	1.4	1.7	1.9	2.2
Swimming						
20 yards per minute	.032	3.5	4.0	4.8	5.6	6.4
45 yards per minute	.058	6.4	7.3	8.7	10.2	11.6
50 yards per minute	.070	7.7	8.8	10.5	12.3	14.0
Table tennis (skilled)	.045	5.0	5.6	6.8	7.9	9.0
Tennis (beginner)	.032	3.5	4.0	4.8	5.6	6.4
Walking (brisk pace)						
3.5 miles per hour	.035	3.9	4.4	5.2	6.1	7.0
4.5 miles per hour	.048	5.3	6.0	7.2	8.4	9.6

[a]Use this column if you want to calculate calories spent for your own exact body weight. Multiply cal/lb/min by your exact weight and then multiply that number by the number of minutes spent in the activity. For example, if you weigh 142 pounds, and you want to know how many calories you spent doing 30 minutes of vigorous aerobic dance: .062 × 142 = 8.8 calories per minute. 8.8 x 30 (minutes) = 264 total calories spent.

[b]Use this column if you weigh 110, 125, 150, 175, or 200 pounds. This eliminates the need to calculate from column 1.

SOURCE: Values for swimming, bicycling, and running have been adapted with permission of Ross Laboratories, Columbus, Ohio 43216, from G. P. Town and K. B. Wheeler, Nutrition concerns for the endurance athlete, *Dietetic Currents* 13 (1986): 7–12. Copyright 1986 Ross Laboratories. Values for all other activities have been adapted from *Physical Fitness for Practically Everybody: The Consumers Union Report on Exercise.* Copyright 1983 by Consumers Union of U.S., Inc., Yonkers, NY 10703–1057. Reprinted by permission from CONSUMER REPORTS BOOKS, 1983.

be more physically active is fat loss, weight maintenance, or improved fitness, the ultimate goal is to sustain a lifetime of physical activity. Starting out too fast and too hard invites failure.

For fat loss, choose an activity that you enjoy. Choose an activity that you can eventually sustain for 45 minutes or more at least 3 days a week. Some people love walking; others want to dance or ride bikes. If you want to be stronger and firmer as well, lift weights or do push-ups, pull-ups, and stomach crunches. And remember this benefit: muscle is more metabolically active than fat, so the more muscle you build, the more energy you'll burn in a given time.

Another strategy is to incorporate more physical activity into your daily schedule in many simple, small-scale ways. Park the car at the far end of the parking lot; use the stairs instead of the elevator; work in a garden; work your abdominal muscles while you stand in line; tighten your buttocks each time you get up from your chair. These activities burn only a few calories each, but over a year's time the total becomes significant.

✔ KEY POINT Physical activity favors a lean body composition, important in weight loss and maintenance. To be effective, the activity needs to be active, not passive.

Building Up

Some of the principles of physical activity offered to the weight-loss seeker apply to those who wish to gain as well. For one thing, no special machine that electrifies, vibrates, or moves muscles around will do anything to build them up. The activities you choose must be active and undertaken regularly, at least every other day. They must also present the demands of overload if they are to help build muscles.

You may experience a depression of appetite when you first begin a training program. This is normal. Don't be concerned—within a few days, your appetite will probably exceed your normal appetite. A word about smoking and appetite: Nicotine depresses the appetite and smoking makes taste buds and olfactory (smelling) organs less sensitive. A person who smokes should quit before trying to gain weight. Quitters find that appetite picks up, food tastes and smells better, and the body reaps additional benefits too numerous to mention.

Also, be aware that most "weight-gain" supplements designed to add body weight are useless without physical activity and confer no special benefits on the taker. Of body weight gained in a day, only a half ounce to an ounce is protein tissue, so no special protein supplements can help speed weight gain faster than an ordinary high-calorie balanced diet. Ordinary food in abundance along with exercise to work the nutrients into place supports efforts to gain weight.

Once you have succeeded in changing your body composition, will you maintain the change? This may be even more difficult than achieving the change in the first place, but some people do succeed.

✔ KEY POINT High-intensity exercise can strengthen muscles, add lean tissue to the body, and increase body weight.

More on the effects of nicotine and other drugs on nutrition in Controversy 12.

Strategies for using physical activity to build up body mass:
1. Choose strength-building exercises.
2. Think in terms of activity intensity.
3. Expect appetite changes; follow your hunger signals.

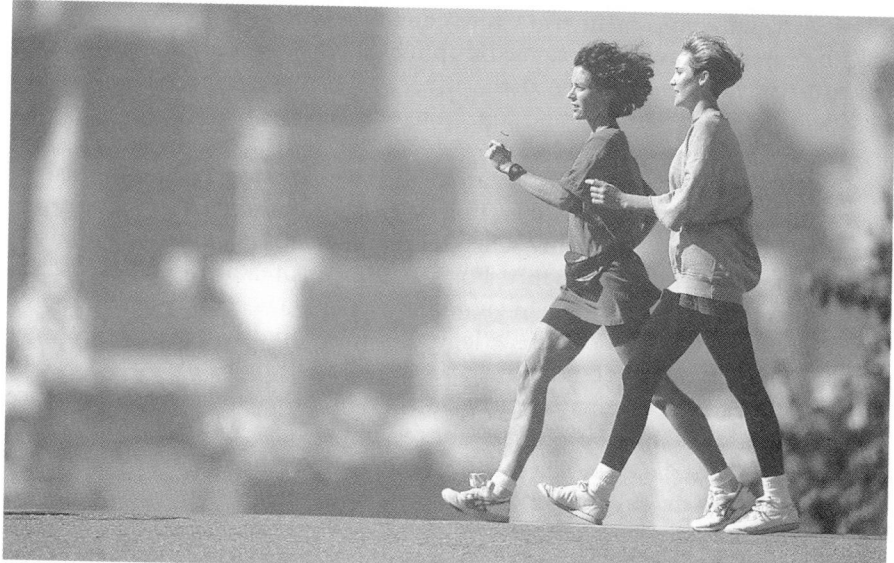

Physical activity can help overweight people to lose fat and underweight people to gain muscle mass.

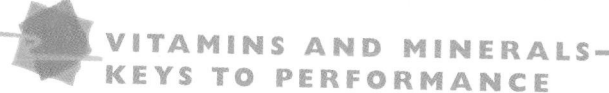

VITAMINS AND MINERALS—
KEYS TO PERFORMANCE

Many vitamins and minerals assist in releasing energy from fuels and transporting oxygen. In addition, vitamin C is needed for the formation of the protein collagen, the foundation material of bones and the cartilage that forms the linings of the joints, and other connective tissues. Folate and vitamin B_{12} help build the red blood cells that carry oxygen to working muscles. Calcium and magnesium help make muscles contract, and so on. Do active people need extra nutrients to support their work? Do they need supplements?

Vitamins and Performance

An estimated 84 percent of world-class athletes take nutrient supplements. Many other athletes and even casual exercisers also take supplements in the hope of improving their performance. Do they benefit from supplements?

Thiamin, Riboflavin, and Niacin   This vitamin trio plays key roles in energy release. Scientists have concluded, however, that extra amounts of these vitamins from supplements do not benefit performance.[29] An adequate diet supplies all the thiamin, riboflavin, and niacin an active person needs, even an athlete. Athletes, with their greater energy needs, eat more food, so most athletes' diets are adequate in these vitamins. Extra amounts provide no competitive advantage.

Indeed, niacin in excess of the RDA may affect performance adversely: excess niacin suppresses the release of fatty acids and thus forces muscles to use extra glycogen during physical activity. This may shorten the time to glycogen depletion and make the work seem more difficult.

These comments should not be interpreted to mean that thiamin, riboflavin, niacin, or any other vitamins are not important. The words *adequate diet* are weighty in this regard. They mean that athletes should obtain most of the extra energy they need from nutrient-dense foods, not fats, sweets, or highly refined

The summary tables listing functions of vitamins and minerals begin on pages 260 and 320.

foods. Anyone who consumes a "junk" diet of relatively empty-calorie foods risks becoming vitamin deficient. But athletes who use only nutrient-dense foods to provide energy exceed the RDA by far, not only for thiamin and riboflavin, but for vitamin C and four minerals as well.[30]*

Vitamin B_6 and Vitamin B_{12}   Vitamin B_6 plays key roles in the release of energy from nutrients, in the liberation of glucose from glycogen, and in the formation of hemoglobin. Thus sellers of supplements claim that vitamin B_6 pills promote athletic performance, but scientific research proves otherwise. To ensure that the diet is adequate in vitamin B_6, a person need only include some green leafy vegetables, meats, fish, legumes, fruits, and whole grains. Megadoses of vitamin B_6 can do no more, and large doses can be toxic.

The belief that vitamin B_{12} supplementation will enhance performance stems from its role in the production of red blood cells. Anemias of all kinds reduce the number and impair the function of circulating red blood cells and rob the blood of its oxygen-carrying capacity. Vitamin B_{12} deficiency causes anemia, but so do iron and folate deficiencies (and others, see the margin). Chances are that a diet low enough in vitamin B_{12} to bring on anemia will be low in other nutrients as well. A person with so poor a diet does not need to take pills; the person needs to eat right. For a well-nourished athlete, any perceived benefits from vitamin B_{12} supplements or shots taken before competition are based on psychology, not physiology.

Vitamin C   Years ago evidence that physical activity enhanced the excretion of vitamin C led some to think that two to three times the RDA of vitamin C might best serve the needs of physically active people. Since that time the great bulk of work designed to explore this theory has opposed it.[31] In one study, even severe *restriction* of vitamin C intakes caused no measurable changes in athletes' aerobic power.[32] Most experiments show that athletes perform no better when taking vitamin C supplements than when they receive the RDA from food. Even so, athletes are often told by "advisers" in health food stores to ingest huge quantities of vitamin C, measured in multiples of a gram.

For people who eat a reasonable diet, it is almost impossible not to receive enough vitamin C. A person who drinks a small glass of orange juice and eats a baked potato and a serving of broccoli in a day receives two to three times the RDA for vitamin C from these foods alone. When shown the full array of vitamins, minerals, and phytochemicals in foods such as these, people have been known to throw away their pills and learn to cook broccoli.

Vitamins A, D, and E   Of the fat-soluble vitamins, supplemental A, D, and E have been shown not to benefit athletic performance, and they are toxic in excess. Vitamin E, however, is important, especially to endurance athletes. During endurance events, the cells use great quantities of oxygen to process fuels, and vitamin E vigorously defends the cell membranes against oxidative damage.[33] In hopes of preventing oxidative damage to muscles, many athletes and active people take megadoses of vitamin E. One study showed that 300 milligrams of vitamin E a day reduced oxidative damage in cyclists.[34] Other kinds of muscle damage, for example from overwork, are unaffected by vitamin E.[35] Before you conclude that vitamin E supplements

Nutrients necessary to ward off anemias include vitamins A, B_6, B_{12}, and folate, and the minerals iron, zinc, copper, and magnesium along with protein—in short, the perfect mix of nutrients that occurs naturally in whole, nutrient-dense foods.

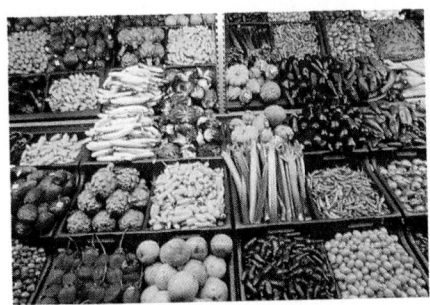

Foods like these are packed with the nutrients that active people need.

See Chapter 11 for details about the effects of phytochemicals in foods.

*The four minerals are calcium, magnesium, iron, and zinc.

might be a good idea, recall from Controversy 7 that some health risks may accompany their use.

So far, then, research indicates that, with the possible exception of vitamin E, no benefit to the working body is gained from taking vitamin supplements. Athletes need only to meet the RDA for vitamins from food—and they certainly can do this. Other athletes who must lose weight to meet low body weight requirements may consume so little food that they fail to obtain all the nutrients they need. For them, a single daily multivitamin-mineral tablet that provides no more than the RDA of nutrients may be beneficial.

✔ KEY POINT   **Vitamins are essential for releasing the energy trapped in energy-yielding nutrients and for other functions that support physical activity. Active people can meet their vitamin needs if they eat enough nutrient-dense foods to meet their energy needs.**

Physical Activity and Bone Loss

Osteoporosis, the condition of reduced bone mass, increases susceptibility to bone damage, including **stress fractures.** Controversy 8 pointed out that moderate physical activity and adequate calcium intakes protect against bone loss. Extremes in physical activity, however, may be detrimental to bone health, at least in some young women and especially in adolescent girls.[36] Many young women athletes restrict energy intakes to meet the weight guidelines of their sport and thus have calcium intakes below the RDA.[37] Such athletes risk developing a potentially fatal triad of medical problems: abnormal eating behaviors, **amenorrhea,** and osteoporosis.[38] These three associated disorders, named "the female athlete triad," are discussed in Controversy 10.

✔ KEY POINT   **Moderate physical activity strengthens the bones, but young women athletes who train strenuously, become amenorrheic, and practice abnormal eating behaviors are susceptible to stress fractures and osteoporosis.**

Iron and Performance

Endurance athletes, and especially women athletes, are prone to iron deficiency. Physical activity may impair iron status in any of several ways. One possibility is that iron lost in sweat contributes to the deficiency. Another possible route to iron loss is red blood cell destruction; blood cells are squashed when body tissues (such as the soles of the feet) make high-impact contact with an unyielding surface (such as the ground). In addition, physical activity may cause small blood losses through the digestive tract, at least in some athletes. Perhaps more significant than losses are the high iron demands by muscles to make the iron-containing molecules of aerobic metabolism.

Studies often find women athletes have low iron intakes. One study of adolescent girl gymnasts found 95 percent had iron intakes below the RDA.[39] Habitually low intakes of iron-rich foods as well as increased losses may contribute to iron deficiency in young women athletes.[40] Vegetarian women athletes may be especially vulnerable to iron insufficiency.[41]

Iron deficiency impairs performance because iron helps deliver the muscles' oxygen. Iron reduced oxygen delivery reduces aerobic work capacity, so the person tires easily. Whether marginal deficiency without clinical signs of anemia hinders physical performance is a point of debate among researchers.[42]

stress fracture a bone injury or break caused by the stress of exercise on the bone surface.

amenorrhea the absence or cessation of menstruation.

Chapter 7 can guide an athlete in selecting an appropriate supplement.

Stringent weight requirements pose a risk of developing eating disorders. See this chapter's Controversy.

Female athlete triad:
✔ Disordered eating.
✔ Amenorrhea.
✔ Osteoporosis.

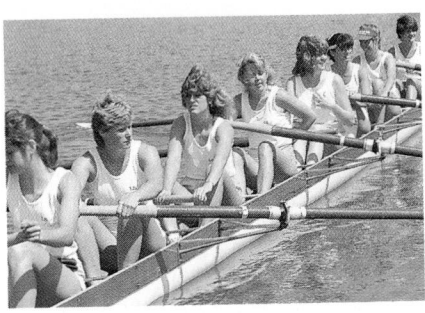

Women athletes may be at special risk of iron deficiency.

Early in training, athletes may develop low blood hemoglobin for a while. This condition, sometimes called "sports anemia," probably reflects a normal adaptation to physical activity. Aerobic training promotes increases in the fluid of the blood; with more fluid, the red blood cell count in a unit of blood drops. True iron-deficiency anemia requires treatment with prescribed iron supplements, but sports anemia goes away by itself, even with continued training.

The best strategy concerning iron may be to determine individual needs. Many menstruating women probably border on iron deficiency even without the additional iron losses incurred by physical activity.[43] Teens of both sexes, because they are growing, have high iron needs, too. Especially for women and teens, then, prescribed supplements may be needed to correct a deficiency of iron as determined by tests to detect iron deficiency. (Medical testing is needed to eliminate nondietary causes of anemia, such as internal bleeding or cancer.)

✔ KEY POINT **Iron-deficiency anemia impairs physical performance because iron is the blood's oxygen handler. Sports anemia is probably a harmless temporary adaptation to physical activity.**

Other Minerals

Three trace minerals—chromium, zinc, and copper—have specific roles in physical activity. The excretion of all three accelerates during physical training.[44] So far it is too early to pinpoint the nutrition implications of this finding.

Electrolytes, the minerals sodium, potassium, chloride, and magnesium, are lost from the body in sweat. Beginners lose the first three of these (but not magnesium) to a much greater extent than do trained athletes. As the body adapts to physical activity, it becomes better at conserving these electrolytes.

Magnesium losses in sweat are not greater for trained than for untrained individuals. More magnesium is lost from the body in urine than in sweat.[45] Some studies suggest that physical activity accelerates magnesium excretion; perhaps working muscles take the mineral from storage for their use and then release it; then the kidneys exrete it.

Wise athletes plan to obtain enough magnesium. They know that a deficiency of magnesium has been shown to cut by *half* the muscle gains associated with a given amount of training.[46] Magnesium is abundant in leafy vegetables, legumes, and whole-wheat products. Other foods offer small but significant amounts. Convenience and highly processed snack foods lack magnesium.

Normally, potassium remains safely inside the cells where it does its work. In prolonged dehydration from profuse sweating, it may migrate outside the cells and be lost by excretion in the urine. Even so, potassium is easily replaced with just a few servings of fresh fruits and vegetables. Avoid potassium supplements unless prescribed by a physician because while they improve some conditions, they worsen others. Most times, a regular diet supplies all the electrolytes athletes need.

Athletes comprise a huge and favorable market for the supplement industry, and they are one of the groups most often victimized by frauds. The following Consumer Corner touches some of the most common schemes aimed at athletes and warns of the dangers of using steroid and other drugs.

✔ KEY POINT **The body adapts to compensate for sweat losses of electrolytes, but urinary magnesium and potassium losses may persist. Athletes are advised to use foods, not supplements, to make up for these losses.**

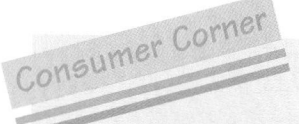

STEROIDS AND "ERGOGENIC" AIDS

Athletes can be sitting ducks for quacks. An endless array of scams are aimed at them: protein supplements, vitamin or mineral supplements, steroid replacers, "muscle-building" powders, electrolyte pills, and many other so-called **ergogenic** aids. Some athletes take dangerous, illegal drugs to try to gain a competitive edge. Others use sodium bicarbonate, caffeine, or other products (see Table 10-4). The term *ergogenic* implies that such products have special work-enhancing powers, but no food or supplement is really ergogenic.

An athlete who takes a nutrient supplement or other substance to improve performance cannot be sure that it will deliver on the promises made for it. A variety of supplements make claims based on misunderstood or misinterpreted nutrition principles. The claims may sound good, but they have no factual basis. In some cases the supplements contain ingredients for which little or no information is available. In other cases, dosage levels for listed ingredients are not given, or the suggested doses are extremely high. Rarely, if ever, do the products mention possible side effects or offer warnings to pregnant women or people with hypertension or other conditions that might contraindicate their use. The findings of a survey of advertisements in a dozen popular health and bodybuilding magazines underscore these points.[47] Researchers identified over 300 products containing 235 different ingredients advertised as beneficial, mostly for muscle growth. None was scientifically proven effective.

Even worse, someone considering using illegal drugs such as steroids should be aware that such drugs can contain anything, even poisons, because no one tests them. Among the most dangerous products sold to athletes are steroids, other hormones, amphetamines, cocaine, muscle relaxants, tranquilizers, barbiturates, diuretics, and even veterinary drugs.

Of the hormones, **anabolic steroid hormones** are made naturally by the testes and adrenal cortex in men and by the adrenal cortex in women. The steroid drugs some athletes take are synthetic varieties that combine the masculinizing effects of male hormones and growth stimulation of the adrenal steroids. In the body, the steroids produce accelerated muscle bulking in response to physical activity in both men and women. Injections of these hormones produce muscle size and strength far beyond that attainable by training alone, but at the price of great risks to health as Figure 10-5 demonstrates.

Though not a steroid, **growth hormone** can induce huge body size and is less readily detected in drug tests than steroids. Its abuse can result in a condition known as acromegaly, characterized by a widened jawline, widened nose, protruding brow, buck teeth, weakened heart walls, and an increased likelihood of death before age 50. Athletes who have paid the price of hormone abuse, even some for whom the drugs made careers

ergogenic the term implies "energy giving," but, in fact, no products impart such a quality (*ergo* means "work"; *genic* means "gives rise to").

anabolic steroid hormones chemical messengers related to the male sex hormone, testosterone, that stimulate building up of body tissues. *Anabolic* means *promoting growth; sterol* refers to compounds chemically related to cholesterol.

growth hormone a hormone produced by the brain's pituitary gland that regulates normal growth and development. Also called *somatotropin*.

(continued on next page)

TABLE 10-4

Products Athletes Use

- **bee pollen** a product consisting of bee saliva, plant nectar, and pollen that confers no benefit on athletes and may cause an allergic reaction in individuals sensitive to it.
- **boron** a nonessential mineral that is promoted as a "natural" steroid replacement.
- **branched-chain amino acids** see text, page 391.
- **caffeine** a stimulant that in small amounts may produce alertness and reduced reaction time in some people, but that also creates fluid losses. Overdoses cause headaches, trembling, an abnormally fast heart rate, and other undesirable effects. More about caffeine appears later in this chapter and in Controversy 12.
- **calcium pangamate** a compound once thought to enhance aerobic metabolism, but now known to have no such effect.
- **carnitine** a nitrogen-containing compound formed in the body from glutamine and methionine that helps transport fatty acids across the mitochrondrial membrane. Carnitine supposedly "burns" fat and spares glycogen during endurance events, but it does neither.
- **cell salts** a mineral preparation supposedly prepared from living cells.
- **chaparral** an herb, promoted as an antioxidant (see also Table 11-10, page 452).
- **chromium picolinate** a trace element supplement; falsely promoted to increase lean body mass, enhance energy, and burn fat.
- **coenzyme Q10** a lipid found in cells (mitochondria) that has been shown to improve exercise performance in heart disease patients, but is not effective in improving performance of healthy athletes.
- **creatine** a nitrogen-containing compound that combines with phosphate to burn a high-energy compound stored in muscle. Claims that creatine enhances energy and stimulates muscle growth need further confirmation.
- **DNA and RNA (deoxyribonucleic acid and ribonucleic acid)** the genetic materials of cells necessary in protein synthesis; falsely promoted as ergogenic aids.
- **ginseng** a plant whose extract supposedly boosts energy (see also Table 11-10, page 452).
- **glycine** a nonessential amino acid, promoted as an ergogenic aid because it is a precursor of the high-energy compound phosphocreatine. Other amino acids that are commonly packaged for athletes but are equally useless include ornithine, arginine, lysine, and the branched-chain amino acids.
- **growth hormone releasers** herbs or pills that supposedly regulate hormones; falsely promoted for enhancing athletic performance.
- **guarana** a reddish berry found in Brazil's Amazon valley that contains seven times as much caffeine as its relative the coffee bean. It is used as an ingredient in carbonated sodas and taken in powder or tablet form to enhance speed and endurance and serve as an aphrodisiac, a "cardiac tonic," an "intestinal disinfectant," and a smart drug that supposedly improves memory and concentration and wards off senility. High doses may stress the heart and can cause panic attacks.

TABLE 10-4

Products Athletes Use continued

- **inosine** an organic chemical that is falsely said to "activate cells, produce energy, and facilitate exercise." Studies have shown that it actually reduces the endurance of runners.
- **Ma huang** an herbal preparation sold with promises of weight loss and increased energy, but that contains ephedrine, a cardiac stimulant with serious adverse effects (see Table 7-4, page 257).
- **octacosanol** an alcohol extracted from wheat germ, often falsely promoted as enhancing athletic performance.
- **phosphate salt** a salt that has been demonstrated to raise the concentration of a metabolically important compound (diphosphoglycerate) in red blood cells and enhance the cells' potential to deliver oxygen to muscle cells. The salts may cause calcium losses from the bones if taken in excess.
- **plant sterols** lipid extracts of plants, called ferulic acid, oryzanol, phytosterols, or "adaptogens," marketed with false claims that they contain hormones or enhance hormonal activity.
- **royal jelly** a substance produced by worker bees and fed to the queen bee; often falsely promoted as enhancing athletic performance.
- **sodium bicarbonate** baking soda; an alkaline salt believed to neutralize blood lactic acid and thereby reduce pain and enhance possible workload. "Soda loading" may cause intestinal bloating and diarrhea.
- **superoxide dismutase (SOD)** an enzyme that protects cells from oxidation. When it is taken orally, the body digests and inactivates this protein; it is useless to athletes.

in sports possible, have come forward to warn young athletes away from growth hormones. They say that even the rewards of success in sports don't make the drug use worth it.

Growth hormone "stimulators," such as the amino acids ornithine and arginine, are useless in the form sold to athletes. In laboratory studies, huge doses of these amino acids do stimulate growth hormone release, but the effective dose would be too dangerous to take. There are safe ways to maximize growth hormone production, however. One is rest. Growth hormone is released during sleep, especially after physical activity, so getting enough rest and adequate training are effective.

Extracted herb and insect sterols are hawked as legal substitutes for steroid drugs.[48] Sellers falsely claim that these substances contain hormones or that they enhance the body's natural ability to make anabolic hormones. In some cases, the substances actually are plant or insect

(continued on next page)

FIGURE 10-5

PHYSICAL RISKS OF TAKING EXCESS STEROID HORMONE DRUGS

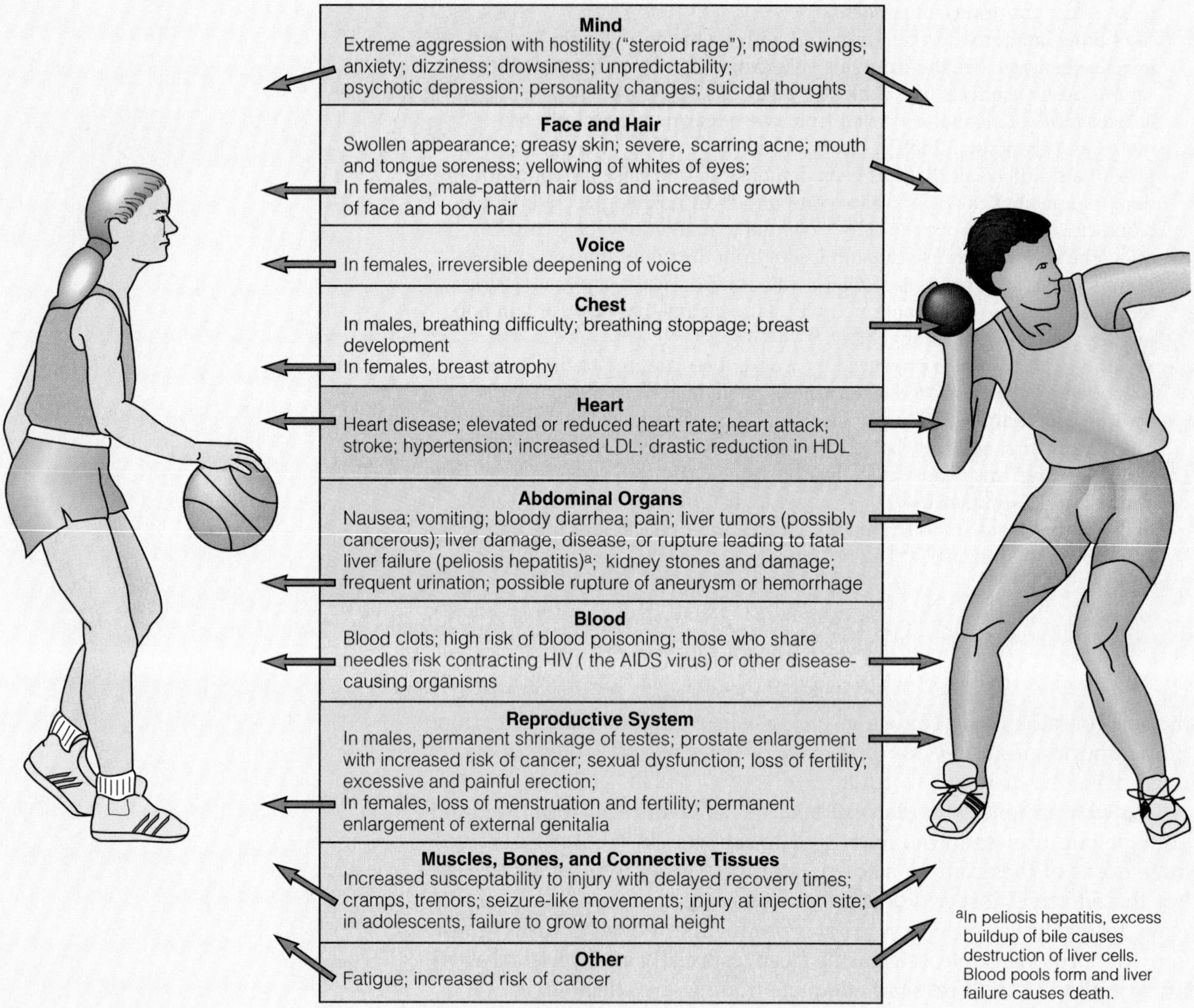

Mind
Extreme aggression with hostility ("steroid rage"); mood swings; anxiety; dizziness; drowsiness; unpredictability; psychotic depression; personality changes; suicidal thoughts

Face and Hair
Swollen appearance; greasy skin; severe, scarring acne; mouth and tongue soreness; yellowing of whites of eyes; In females, male-pattern hair loss and increased growth of face and body hair

Voice
In females, irreversible deepening of voice

Chest
In males, breathing difficulty; breathing stoppage; breast development
In females, breast atrophy

Heart
Heart disease; elevated or reduced heart rate; heart attack; stroke; hypertension; increased LDL; drastic reduction in HDL

Abdominal Organs
Nausea; vomiting; bloody diarrhea; pain; liver tumors (possibly cancerous); liver damage, disease, or rupture leading to fatal liver failure (peliosis hepatitis)[a]; kidney stones and damage; frequent urination; possible rupture of aneurysm or hemorrhage

Blood
Blood clots; high risk of blood poisoning; those who share needles risk contracting HIV (the AIDS virus) or other disease-causing organisms

Reproductive System
In males, permanent shrinkage of testes; prostate enlargement with increased risk of cancer; sexual dysfunction; loss of fertility; excessive and painful erection;
In females, loss of menstruation and fertility; permanent enlargement of external genitalia

Muscles, Bones, and Connective Tissues
Increased susceptibility to injury with delayed recovery times; cramps, tremors; seizure-like movements; injury at injection site; in adolescents, failure to grow to normal height

Other
Fatigue; increased risk of cancer

[a]In peliosis hepatitis, excess buildup of bile causes destruction of liver cells. Blood pools form and liver failure causes death.

sterols, but, the body cannot convert them to human steroids. None of these products has any proven anabolic activity, nor can they strengthen muscles; in fact, they may contain natural toxins. Controversy 7 first made this point, but it is worth repeating: Don't make the mistake of equating "natural" with "harmless."

It also bears repeating that amino acid supplements can be dangerous (see the Consumer Corner at Chapter 6). Healthy athletes never need them. Advertisers point to research that identifies the branched-chain amino acids as a source of fuel for the exercising body but fail to mention that when amino acids are needed, the muscles have plenty on hand. Any diet low in carbohydrate or calories seems to activate or assist an enzyme that breaks down branched-chain amino acids for energy.[49] Otherwise, branched-chain amino acids are conserved. The wise athlete, then, takes no amino acid supplements, but eats a diet adequate in carbohydrate and energy.

The overwhelming majority of schemes touted for athletes are frauds.* The placebo effect is strongly at work, however. When you hear reports of a performance boost from a new concoction, give it time. Chances are that the effect came from the power of the mind over the body. Incidentally, don't discount that power—it is formidable. You can use it by visualizing yourself as a winner in your sport. You don't have to rely on magic for an extra edge because you already have a real one— your mind.

---

*If you have questions about a fitness product, book, or program, write to the American College of Sports Medicine at the address in the Nutrition Resources, Appendix E.

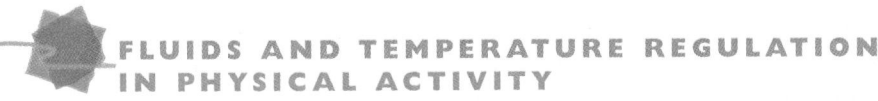

FLUIDS AND TEMPERATURE REGULATION IN PHYSICAL ACTIVITY

The body's need for water far surpasses that for any other nutrient. If the body loses too much water, as in dehydration, its life-supporting chemistry is compromised.

The body loses water primarily via sweat; second to that, breathing costs water, exhaled as vapor. During physical activity, both routes can be significant, and dehydration is a real threat. The first symptom of dehydration is

heat exhaustion a fluid-depleted state with slightly elevated body temperature (below 104° Fahrenheit) that, while usually not dangerous, requires intake of fluid and rest in a cool place to avoid heat stroke.

heat stroke an acute and life-threatening reaction to heat buildup in the body.

hypothermia a below-normal body temperature.

Symptoms of heat exhaustion: weak, rapid pulse, low blood pressure, sweating, headache, dizziness, weakness, and somewhat elevated body temperature.

Symptoms of heat stroke: headache, nausea, dizziness, clumsiness, stumbling, sudden cessation of sweating (hot, dry skin), internal (rectal) temperature above 104° Fahrenheit, and confusion or loss of consciousness.

fatigue. A water loss of even 1 to 2 percent of body weight can reduce a person's capacity to do muscular work. A person with a water loss of about 7 percent is likely to collapse.[50] The athlete who arrives at an event even slightly dehydrated starts out at a disadvantage.

Temperature Regulation

Chapter 8 pointed out that sweat cools the body. The conversion of water to vapor uses up a great deal of heat, so as sweat evaporates, it cools the skin's surface and the blood flowing beneath it.

In hot, humid weather, sweat may fail to evaporate because the surrounding air is already laden with water. Little cooling takes place and body heat builds up, triggering thermal injuries—**heat exhaustion** or its more severe cousin, **heat stroke.** Heat stroke is an especially dangerous accumulation of body heat with accompanying loss of body fluid. A triad of measures to prevent heat stroke are to drink enough fluid before and during the activity, to rest in the shade when tired, and to wear lightweight clothing that encourages evaporation. Hence the rubber or heavy suits sold with promises of weight loss during physical activity are dangerous because they promote profuse sweating, prevent sweat evaporation, and invite heat stroke. If you experience any of the symptoms of heat exhaustion or heat stroke listed in the margin, stop your activity, sip cold fluids, seek shade, and ask for help. The condition demands medical attention; it can kill.

In cold weather, **hypothermia,** or loss of body heat, can pose as serious a threat as heat stroke does in hot weather. Inexperienced runners participating in long races on cold or wet, chilly days are especially vulnerable to hypothermia. Slow runners can produce too little heat to keep warm, especially if their clothing is inadequate. Early symptoms of hypothermia include shivering and euphoria. As body temperature continues to fall, shivering may stop, and weakness, disorientation, and apathy may set in. Persons with these symptoms soon become helpless to protect themselves from further body heat losses. Even in cold weather, the body still sweats and needs fluids, but the fluids should be warm or at room temperature, not cold.

✔ **KEY POINT** **Evaporation of sweat cools the body. Heat exhaustion and heat stroke are common threats to physically active people in hot, humid weather. Hypothermia threatens those who exercise in the cold.**

Fluid Needs during Physical Activity

Endurance athletes can lose 2 or more quarts of fluid in every hour of activity, but the digestive system can absorb only about a quart or so an hour.[51] Hence the athlete must hydrate before and rehydrate during and after activity to replace it all. Even then, in hot weather the digestive tract may not be able to absorb enough water fast enough to keep up with an athlete's sweat losses, and some degree of dehydration becomes inevitable. Wise athletes preparing for competition drink extra fluids in the few days of training before the event. The extra fluid is not stored in the body, but drinking extra ensures maximum tissue hydration at the start of the event. Any coach or athlete who withholds fluids during practice for any reason takes a great risk and is subject to sanctions by the American College of Sports Medicine.

TABLE 10-5

Schedule of Hydration before, during, and after Physical Activity

When to Drink	Total Amount of Fluid (Consume in 1 cup Servings)
2 hr before exercise	About 3 c
10 to 15 min before exercise	About 2 c
Every 15 to 30 min during exercise	4–8 oz (about 1 qt in 60 to 90 min)
After exercise	Replace each pound of body weight lost with 2 c fluid

Casual exercisers should be aware that activity blunts the thirst mechanism. Active people who rely on thirst to govern fluid intake can easily become dehydrated. During activity thirst becomes detectable only *after* fluid stores are depleted. Don't wait to feel thirsty before drinking. Table 10-5 presents one schedule of hydration for physical activity. To find out how much water you need to replenish losses, weigh yourself before and after the activity. The difference is all water. Two cups (16 ounces) of fluid weigh about a pound.

What is the best fluid to support physical activity? Surprisingly, the best drink for most active bodies is just plain cool water, for two reasons: (1) water rapidly leaves the digestive tract to enter the tissues, and (2) it cools the body from the inside out. As mentioned earlier, however, endurance athletes are an exception: they need more from their fluids than water alone. The first priority for endurance athletes should always be to replace fluids to prevent life-threatening heat stroke.[52] But they also need carbohydrate to supplement their limited glycogen stores, so glucose is important, too.

Many good-tasting drinks are marketed for active people. Manufacturers reason that if a drink tastes good, people will drink more, thereby ensuring adequate hydration. The drinks also can provide a psychological edge to people who associate them with success in sports. Keep in mind that while you may hear much promotion of these drinks from their manufacturers, no company is likely to run ads about the possible advantages of water because they aren't selling water. The next section compares these two drink options objectively.

✓ **KEY POINT   Physically active people lose fluids and must replace them to avoid dehydration. Thirst indicates that water loss has already occurred.**

Sports Drinks

Physically active people sweat. Sweat contains minerals. So do active people need special mineral-containing drinks to replace those lost in sweat? Most authorities agree that active people and athletes normally need not replace minerals lost in sweat until after the activity when they resume eating normal food.

In strenuous world-class competitions lasting for many hot, humid days, heavy sweating coupled with drinking large amounts of plain water has been reported to dangerously dilute blood sodium. If an athlete works up a drenching sweat, exceeding 5 to 10 pounds a day (or 3 percent of body weight) for several consecutive days, electrolyte replacement is advised. Athletes who *compete* for longer than six to eight hours each day may especially need to replace sodium.[53]

Sports drinks supply glucose. A beverage that supplies glucose in some form can be useful during endurance activity lasting longer than 60 minutes or during prolonged competitive games that demand repeated intermittent activity. Not just any sweet beverage can meet this need, however, because a carbohydrate concentration greater than 10 percent can delay fluid emptying from the stomach and thereby slow down the delivery of water to the tissues. Most sports drinks contain about 7 percent glucose—a safe level for fluid transport.

No evidence supports the old idea that electrolytes taken during activity prevent muscle cramping, but small amounts of sodium in sports drinks seem to accelerate water and glucose absorption from the digestive tract. Sodium also enhances fluid retention after physical activity, an effect that may or may not be of value.

Equally as effective as commercial sports drinks but much less expensive is a homemade mixture of one-third teaspoon of salt (to provide sodium chloride) and 1 cup of sugar-sweetened fruit juice (to provide potassium and glucose) per quart of water. Avoid electrolyte or salt tablets; they increase potassium losses, can irritate the stomach, cause vomiting, and always pull water out of the tissues into the digestive tract at first.

✔ **KEY POINT** **For most athletes, electrolyte and mineral repletion is best accomplished by eating a balanced diet, not by taking mineral-containing drinks. In the heat, however, electrolyte-containing fluids may benefit athletes who are training or competing.**

Other Beverage Choices

Some drinks, such as iced tea, deliver caffeine along with fluid. Moderate doses of caffeine (2 milligrams per pound of body weight or about 2 cups of coffee) one hour prior to activity seem to assist some people's athletic performance.[54] Theoretically, caffeine may stimulate the release of fatty acids into the blood early in activity, thus conserving glycogen. Better than caffeine for this purpose, though, is a warm-up activity. Light activity initiates fat release, but unlike caffeine, it also warms the muscles and connective tissues, making them flexible and resistant to injury.

Caffeine also has adverse effects, including stomach upset, nervousness, sleeplessness, irritability, headaches, and diarrhea. It has been shown to constrict the arteries and raise some exercisers' blood pressure above normal.[55] Constricted arteries make the heart's work harder pumping blood to working muscles, an effect detrimental to sports performance.

In a hot environment, caffeine's diuretic effect is potentially hazardous, too. Exercise slows the excretion of caffeine, prolonging its effects, so beverages containing caffeine should be used in moderation and in addition to other fluids, not as a substitute for them.[56] In college, national, and international athletic competitions, the use of caffeine is forbidden in amounts greater than about 800 milligrams, the equivalent of 5 or 6 cups of strong, brewed coffee drunk within an hour or two.

Athletes, like others, sometimes drink beverages that contain alcohol, but these beverages are inappropriate as fluid replacements. Like caffeine, alcohol

Controversy 12 provides a discussion of caffeine's effects and sources.

Beer facts:

✔ Beer is not carbohydrate-rich. Beer is calorie-rich, but only one-third of its calories are from carbohydrates. The other two-thirds are from alcohol.

✔ Beer is mineral-poor. Beer contains a few minerals, but to replace those lost in sweat, athletes need good sources such as fruit juices.

✔ Beer is vitamin-poor. Beer contains tiny traces of some B vitamins, but it cannot compete with rich food sources.

✔ Beer causes fluid losses. Beer is a fluid, but alcohol is a diuretic and causes the body to lose more fluid in urine than is provided by the beer.

is a diuretic. Both substances promote the excretion of water; of vitamins such as thiamin, riboflavin, and folate; and of minerals such as calcium, magnesium, and potassium—exactly the wrong effects for fluid balance and nutrition. It is hard to overstate alcohol's detrimental effects on physical activity. It impairs temperature regulation, making hypothermia or heat stroke much more likely. It alters perceptions and slows reaction time. It depletes strength and endurance and deprives people of their judgment, thereby compromising their safety in sports. Many sports-related fatalities and injuries each year involve alcohol or other drugs.

KEY POINT **Caffeine-containing drinks within limits may not impair performance but water and fruit juice are preferred. Alcohol use can impair performance in many ways and is not recommended.**

Read about alcohol's effects on the brain in Controversy 11.

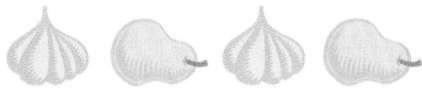

No particular diet supports an athlete's performance perfectly; many different diets can be excellent for athletes. However, food choices must obey the rules for diet planning.

NUTRIENT DENSITY

First, athletes and active people need a diet composed mostly of nutrient-dense foods, the kind that supply a maximum of vitamins and minerals for the energy they provide. When athletes eat mostly refined, processed foods that have suffered nutrient losses and that contain added sugar and fat, nutrition status suffers.[57] Even if foods are fortified or enriched, manufacturers cannot replace the whole range of nutrients and nonnutrients lost in refining. Consider, for example, that manufacturers mill out much of a food's original magnesium and chromium but do not replace them. This doesn't mean that athletes can never choose a white bread, bologna, and mayonnaise sandwich but only that later they should eat a large, fresh salad or big portions of vegetables and whole grains and drink a glass of milk to compensate. The nutrient-dense foods will provide the magnesium and chromium; the bologna sandwich provided extra energy, mostly from fat.

BALANCE

Athletes must eat for energy, and their energy needs may be immense. Athletes need full glycogen stores, and they need to strive to prevent heart disease and cancer by limiting fat and saturated fat. Simply stated, a diet that is high in carbohydrate (60 to 70 percent of total calories), low in fat (20 to 25 percent), and adequate in protein (12 to 15 percent) is best for all these purposes. Even if the athlete does not compete in glycogen-depleting events, such a diet will provide adequate fiber while supplying abundant nutrients and energy.

With these principles in mind, compare the two 500-calorie sandwich meals in the margin. The trick to getting enough carbohydrate energy is easy,

FOOD FEATURE

CHOOSING A PERFORMANCE DIET

Compare and decide which best meets your needs:

1 sandwich of 2 slices bologna, 2 slices white bread, 2 tbs mayonnaise (525 calories, 9% protein, 23% carbohydrate, 69% fat)

OR

2 sandwiches of 2 slices lean ham, 4 slices whole-wheat bread, 2 tsp mayonnaise

(503 calories, 20% protein, 51% carbohydrate, 29% fat)

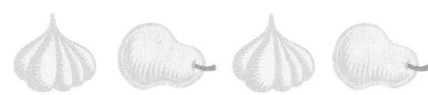

Small daily choices, when made consistently, enhance an athlete's nutritional health.

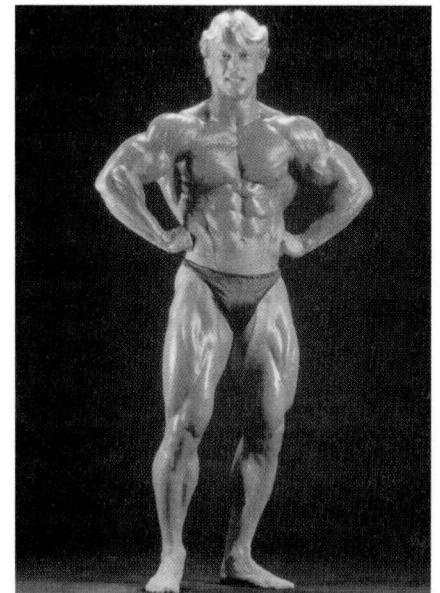

This is a body that vegetables built: Andreas Cahling, a vegetarian.

at least in theory: just reduce the amount of fat and meat in a meal and let carbohydrate-rich foods fill in for them.

Adding carbohydrate-rich foods is a sound and reasonable option for increasing energy intake, up to a point. The point at which it becomes unreasonable is when the person cannot eat enough food to meet energy needs. At that point the person can cram more food energy into the diet only by using refined sugars and fats or liquid meals. Still, these energy-rich additions must be superimposed on nutrient-rich choices; energy alone is not enough.

PROTEIN

In addition to carbohydrate, athletes need protein. What quantities of what kinds of foods supply enough protein to meet the needs of athletes? Meats and milk products head the list of protein-rich foods, but suggesting that athletes eat more than the recommended servings of meat would be short-sighted advice for many reasons. Athletes must protect themselves from heart disease, and even lean meats contain fat, much of it saturated fat. Besides, the extra servings of carbohydrate-rich foods such as legumes, grains, and vegetables that an athlete needs to meet energy requirements also boost protein intakes.

Earlier in this chapter, Table 10-2 showed some possible protein intakes for a 70-kilogram athlete based on recommendations of various authorities. It is likely that an athlete weighing 70 kilograms who engages in vigorous physical activity on a daily basis could require 3,000 to 5,000 calories per day. As a rule of thumb, endurance athletes should aim for an intake of 50 calories per kilogram (2.2 pounds) of body weight, on average.[58] Others may need more. To meet such an energy requirement, an athlete could select from a variety of nutrient-dense foods. Figure 10-6 provides one example; it itemizes foods that provide the extra nutrients an athlete needs beyond regular meal selections to attain a 3,000-calorie diet. These meals supply 124 grams of protein, an amount greater than all but the highest recommended level of 140 grams per day for such a person. For those with reasonable diets, protein is rarely a problem.

The meals in Figure 10-6 provide 61 percent of their calories from carbohydrate. Athletes who train exhaustively for endurance events may want to aim for somewhat higher carbohydrate levels—from 65 to 75 percent. Notice that breakfast, though light in fat, is filling and hearty. Current thinking supports the idea that athletes benefit from such a morning start.[59] If you train early in the morning, try splitting breakfast into two parts. An hour or so before training eat just some toast, juice, and fruit. Later, after your workout, come back for the cereal and milk.

PLANNING AN ATHLETE'S MEALS

Table 10-6 shows some sample food intake patterns for athletes at various high energy and carbohydrate intakes. These plans are effective only if the user chooses foods to provide nutrients as well as energy—extra milk for calcium

FIGURE 10-6

AN ATHLETE'S MEALS

This figure shows how to modify regular meals to meet an athlete's needs.

Regular Meals	Modifications	Athlete's Meals

1 c coffee   8 oz nonfat milk

½ c strawberries

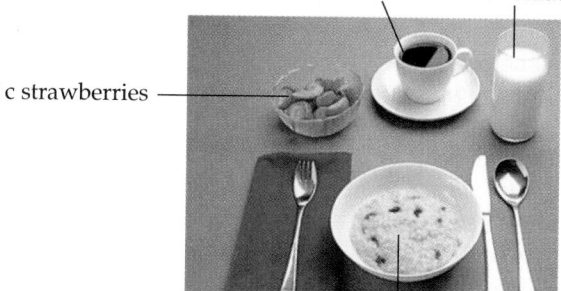

1 c oatmeal and raisins

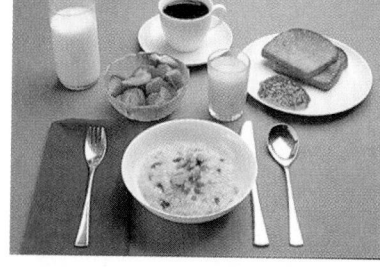

The regular breakfast *plus:*
- 2 pieces whole-wheat toast
- 4 tsp jelly
- ½ c orange juice
- 2 tsp brown sugar on the oatmeal
- low-fat milk instead of nonfat

The regular morning snack

4 tbs trail mix

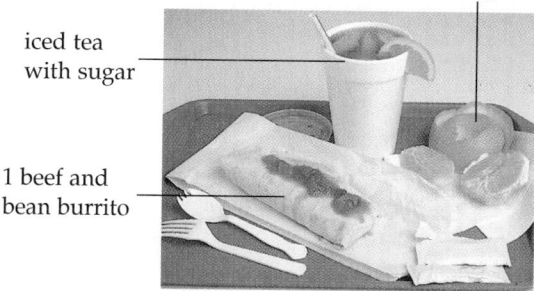

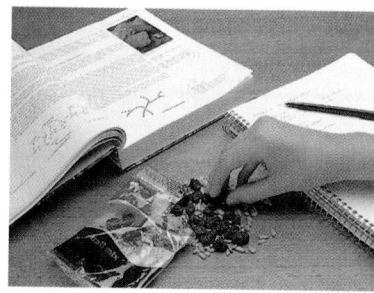

1 orange

iced tea with sugar

1 beef and bean burrito

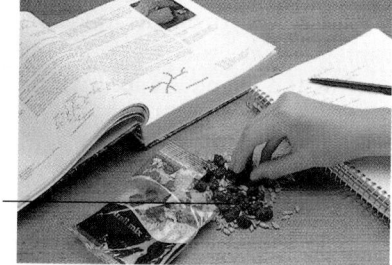

The regular lunch *plus:*
- 1 beef and bean burrito
- 1 banana

Plus an afternoon snack:
- 1 c low-fat milk
- 1 piece angel-food cake

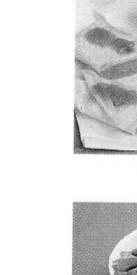

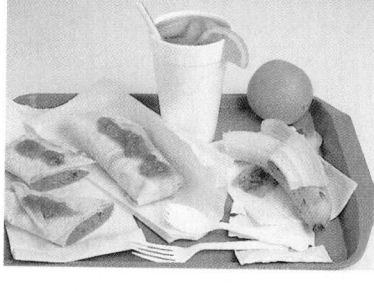

½ c sherbet   8 oz nonfat milk

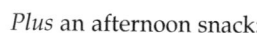

spinach salad with 1 tbs dressing

¼ tomato

½ c noodles with parsley and 2 tsp butter

4 oz salmon   1 c broccoli

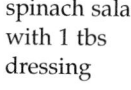

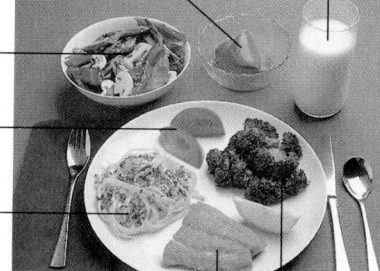

The regular dinner *plus:*
- 1 dinner roll
- 2 tsp butter
- ¼ c noodles
- ½ c sherbet
- low-fat milk instead of nonfat

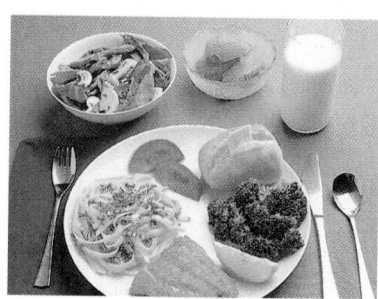

Total cal: 1,759
57% cal from carbohydrate
24% cal from fat
19% cal from protein

Total cal: 3,119
61% cal from carbohydrate
24% cal from fat
15% cal from protein

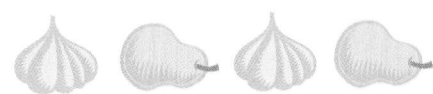

pregame meal a meal eaten three to four hours before athletic competition.

and riboflavin, many servings of fruit for folate and vitamin C, energy-rich vegetables such as sweet potatoes, peas, and legumes, modest portions of lean meat, and especially red meat for iron and other vitamins and minerals, and whole grains for B vitamins, magnesium, zinc, and chromium. In addition, these foods provide plenty of electrolytes.

A trick used by professional sports nutritionists to maximize athletes' intakes of energy and carbohydrates is to make sure that vegetable and fruit choices are as dense as possible in both nutrients and energy. A whole cupful of iceberg lettuce supplies few calories or nutrients, but a half-cup portion of cooked sweet potatoes is a powerhouse of vitamins, minerals, and carbohydrate energy. Similarly, it takes a whole cup of cubed melon to equal the calories and carbohydrate in a half-cup of canned fruit. Small choices like these, made consistently, can contribute significantly to nutrient, energy, and carbohydrate intakes.

Before competition athletes may eat particular foods or practice rituals that convey psychological advantages. One eats steak the night before; another spoons up honey at the start of the event. As long as these foods or rituals remain harmless, they should be respected. Still, science has recommendations for the **pregame meal**. The foods should be carbohydrate-rich and the meal light (300 to 800 calories). It should be easy to digest and should contain fluids. Breads, potatoes, pasta, and fruit juices, carbohydrate-rich foods low in fat, protein, and fiber, form the basis of the pregame meal. Bulky, fiber-rich foods such as raw vegetables or high-fiber cereals, although usually desirable, are best avoided just before competition. Such foods can cause stomach discomfort

TABLE 10-6

High-Carbohydrate Food Patterns for Athletes

| Food Group | Number of Servings for a Daily Energy Intake of: | | | | | |
	1,500 cal	2,000 cal	2,500 cal	3,000 cal	3,500 cal	4,000[a] cal
Milk	3	3	4	4	4	4
Fruit	5	6	7	9	10	12
Vegetable	3	3	3	5	6	7
Grain	7	11	16	18	20	24
Fat[b]	2	3	5	6	8	10
Meat (ounces)	5	5	5	5	6	6
Percent carbohydrate:	58%	58%	63%	64%	60%	62%

[a]A way to add more energy to the diet without adding much bulk is to snack on milkshakes or "complete meal" liquid supplements (see text).
[b]A fat serving is one teaspoon of butter, margarine, oil, or the equivalent.

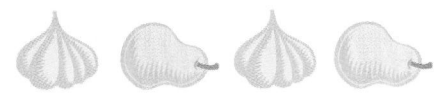

TABLE 10-7

Commercial and Homemade Meal Replacers Compared

	Energy (cal)	Protein (g)	Carbohydrate (g)	Fat (g)
12-ounce commercial liquid meal replacer[a] Cost: about $2 per serving	360	15 (17% of calories)	55 (61%)	9 (22%)
12-ounce homemade milkshake[b] Cost: about 50¢ per serving	330	15 (18% of calories)	53 (63%)	7 (19%)

[a]Average values for three commercial formulas.

[b]Home recipe: 8 oz nonfat milk, 4 oz ice milk, 3 heaping tsp malted milk powder. For even higher carbohydrate and calorie values, blend in 1/2 mashed banana or ½ c other fruit. For athletes with lactose intolerance, use lactose-reduced milk or soy milk and chocolate or other flavored syrup, with mashed banana or other fruit blended in.

during performance. The competitor should finish eating three to four hours before competition to allow time for the stomach to empty before exertion.

What about drinks or candylike sport bars claiming to provide "complete" nutrition? These mixtures of carbohydrate, protein (usually amino acids), fat, some fiber, and certain vitamins and minerals usually taste good and provide additional food energy before a game or for those needing to gain weight. Many of them fall short of providing "complete" nutrition, however, since they lack many of real food's nutrients and the nonnutrients that benefit health. These products provide no special advantage for active people except one— they are easy to eat in the hours before competition. However, they are expensive. As Table 10-7 demonstrates, there is no point in paying high prices for fancy brand-name drinks. Homemade shakes are inexpensive and easy to prepare, and they perform every bit as well as do commercial products. Don't drop a raw egg in the blender, though, because raw eggs often carry bacteria that cause food poisoning.[60]

The person who wants to excel physically will apply the most accurate nutrition knowledge along with dedication to rigorous training. A diet that provides ample fluid and consists of a variety of nutrient-dense foods in quantities to meet energy needs will enhance not only athletic performance but overall health as well. Training and genetics being equal, who would win a competition—the person who habitually consumes less than the amounts of nutrients needed or one who arrives at the event with a long history of full nutrient stores and well-met metabolic needs?

Good choices for pregame meals:

Apricot nectar, pineapple juice, grape juice, Jello, sherbet, popsicles, jams, jellies, honey, toast, pancakes with syrup, baked white or sweet potatoes, pasta with steamed vegetables, lentils or other peas or beans, raisins, figs, dates, frozen yogurt, graham crackers, sponge cake, angel-food cake.

Not recommended:

Stuffing, muffins, biscuits, croissants, french fries, onion rings, potato chips, meats, cheese, pies, ice cream, eggnog, creams, nuts, butter, gravy, mayonnaise, salad dressing, frosted cakes.

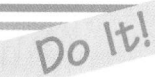
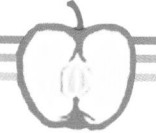

Do It!

DETECT FITNESS DECEPTION

Chapter 1 and Controversy 1 offered ways to distinguish between valid nutrition information and nutrition fraud, and the Consumer Corner in this chapter warned you about ergogenic products and the deceptive tactics some advertisers use to sell the products. Here is another chance to practice your deception detection skills, Browse the aisles of your local health food store or flip through the pages of any popular bodybuilding or fitness magazine. Look for products or ads for products that claim to provide amazing health or fitness benefits (see Figure 10-7). Then answer these questions:

1. What kinds of product descriptors are used on the labels or in the advertisements? Turn back to Figure C1-1 to get some ideas. What information do you gain from phrases such as "most scientifically advanced fat-burning formula" or "new cutting-edge formula" or "puts more meat in your muscle"?

2. Are you familiar with the ingredients in fitness products? Read the ingredient lists or descriptions, if shown. Do you know the health effects of each ingredient? For example, many product advertisements or labels boast that they contain steroid-like ingredients to enhance muscle growth and strength. The "steroid-like" ingredients are either plant or insect steroids whose effects on human beings, if any, are unknown. Such ingredients may contain toxins as well.

3. Do some products contain amino acids? Are these needed by healthy athletes?

4. Are the dosage levels for the ingredients given? If you are thinking about using a product, how much of each ingredient is appropriate? Compare vitamin and mineral amounts with the RDA; amounts between 50 and 150 percent of the RDA for each nutrient reflect ranges commonly found in foods. Such amounts are compatible with the body's normal handling of nutrients. For other ingredients, call the National Institute of Health Information Center, Office of Alternative Medicine: (301) 402-2466.

FIGURE 10-7

DECEPTIVE FITNESS CLAIMS

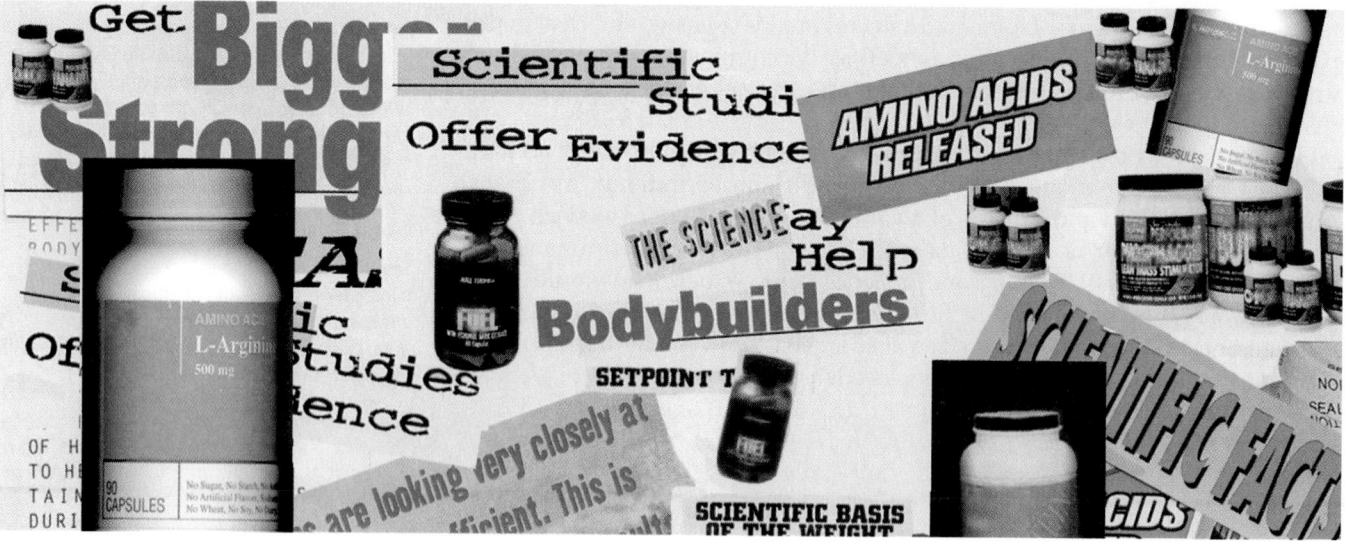

SELF-CHECK

Answers to these Self-Check questions are in Appendix G.

1. Which of the following provides most of the energy the muscles use in the early minutes of activity?
   a. fat
   b. protein
   c. glycogen
   d. (b) and (c)

2. Which diet has been shown to increase an athlete's endurance?
   a. high-fat diet
   b. high-carbohydrate diet
   c. normal mixed diet
   d. Diet has not been shown to have any effect.

3. Which of the following has been proved to impart work-enhancing powers to healthy athletes?
   a. chromium picolinate
   b. DNA and RNA supplements
   c. vitamin E
   d. none of the above

4. What effect does alcohol have on the exercising body?
   a. impairs temperature regulation
   b. acts as a diuretic
   c. enhances performance
   d. (a) and (b)

5. Which of the following stimulates synthesis of muscle cell protein?
   a. physical activity
   b. a high-carbohydrate diet
   c. a high-protein diet
   d. amino acid supplementation

6. The guidelines for developing and maintaining physical fitness are the same as the guidelines for obtaining health benefits.   T   F

7. The average resting pulse rate for adults is around 70 beats per minute, but the rate is higher in people who are physically fit.   T   F

8. It is best for an athlete to drink extra fluids in the few days of training before an event to ensure proper hydration.   T   F

9. Research does not support the idea that active people need supplements of vitamins to perform their best.   T   F

10. Anorexia nervosa occurs only in women. (Read about this in the upcoming Controversy.)   T   F

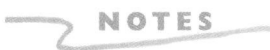

NOTES

Notes are in Appendix F.

What Causes Eating Disorders?

An estimated 2 million people in the United States, primarily girls and women, suffer from the **eating disorders, anorexia nervosa** and **bulimia nervosa.** Many more suffer from related conditions that do not meet the strict criteria for anorexia nervosa or bulimia nervosa but still imperil sufferers' well-being. This category of eating disorders is known among psychologists as **unspecified eating disorders.**[1] Some evidence indicates that certain characteristics of disordered eating such as restrained eating, binge eating, purging, fear of fatness, and distortion of body image may be extraordinarily common among young middle-class girls.[2] Two-thirds of adolescent girls and one-third of adolescent boys are dissatisfied with their body weight.[3] In most other societies, these behaviors and attitudes are much less prevalent.

Why do so many people in our society suffer from eating disorders? Excessive pressure to be thin is at least partly to blame. When low body weight becomes an important goal, people begin to view normal healthy body weight as being too fat, and they take unhealthy actions to lose weight. Overly severe restriction of food intake may create intense hunger that leads to binges. Research confirms this theory, showing that unhealthy or dangerous diets predict binge eating in adolescent girls.[4] Energy restriction followed by binge-ing can set in motion a pattern of repeated weight losses and gains—weight cycling. Worsening the situation further, weight cycling may make weight loss and maintenance more difficult over time.[5]

Young girls who attempt extreme weight loss are dissatisfied with their bodies to begin with; they may also be depressed or suffer social anxiety. As weight loss and maintenance become more and more difficult, psychological problems worsen and the likelihood of developing full-blown eating disorders intensifies.

Athletes are at special risk for eating disorders. Many women athletes appear healthy but in fact may easily develop the three associated medical problems of the **female athlete triad:** disordered eating, amenor-

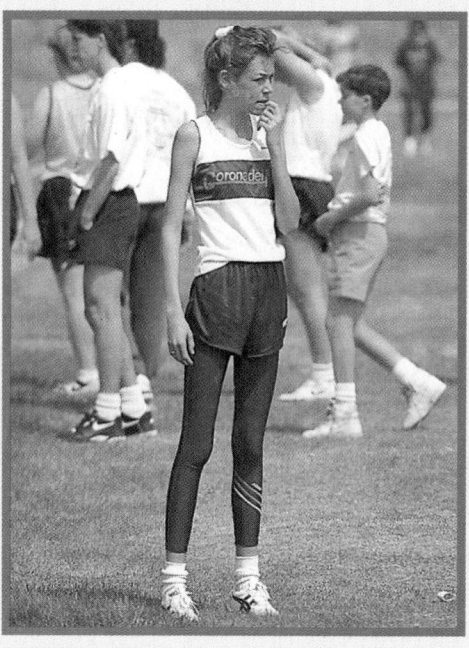

rhea, and osteoporosis.[6] Table C10-1 defines some eating disorder terms.

THE FEMALE ATHLETE TRIAD

At age 14, Suzanne was a top contender for a spot on the state gymnastics team. Each day her coach reminded team members that they must weigh no more than a few ounces above their assigned weights in order to qualify for competition. The coach chastised gymnasts who gained weight, and Suzanne was terrified of being singled out. She was convinced that the less she weighed, the better she would perform. She weighed herself several times a day to confirm that she had not exceeded her 80-pound limit. Driven to excel in her sport, Suzanne kept her weight down by eating very little and training very hard. Unlike many of her friends at school, Suzanne never began menstruating. A few months before her 15th birthday, Suzanne's coach dropped her back to the second-level team. Suzanne blamed her poor performance on a slow-healing stress fracture. Mentally stressed and physically exhausted, she quit gymnastics and began overeating between her periods of self-starvation. Suzanne had developed the dangerous combination of problems—disordered eating, amenorrhea, and osteoporosis—collectively known as the female athlete triad.

Disordered Eating Some authorities have suggested that at least part of the reason many athletic women engage in disordered eating behaviors is that they and their coaches have embraced unsuitable weight standards. An athlete's body must be heavier for weight than a nonathlete's body because the athlete's body is denser; it contains more healthy muscle and bone tissue and less fat than a nonathlete's body. Athletes consulting standard weight-for-height tables and seeing that they are on the heavy side for their heights can easily be misled into believing that they are too fat. Weight standards that may work well

TABLE C10-1

Eating Disorder Terms

- **anorexia nervosa** an eating disorder characterized by a refusal to maintain a minimally normal body weight, self-starvation to the extreme, and a disturbed perception of body weight and shape; seen (usually) in teenage girls and young women (*anorexia* means "without appetite"; *nervos* means "of nervous origin").

- **binge eating disorder** a new eating disorder whose criteria are similar to those of bulimia nervosa, excluding purging or other compensatory behaviors.

- **bulimia** (byoo-LEEM-ee-uh) **nervosa** recurring episodes of binge eating combined with a morbid fear of becoming fat; usually followed by self-induced vomiting or purging.

- **cathartic** a strong laxative.

- **eating disorder** a disturbance in eating behavior that jeopardizes a person's physical or psychological health.

- **emetic** (em-ETT-ic) an agent that causes vomiting.

- **endogenous opiates, endorphins** compounds made in the brain whose actions mimic those of opiate drugs (morphine, heroin) in reducing pain and producing pleasure.

- **female athlete triad** a potentially fatal triad of medical problems seen in women athletes: disordered eating, amenorrhea, and osteoporosis.

- **limbic system** a group of tissues at the center of the brain responsible for feelings of pleasure and involved in the addiction process.

- **naloxone** a drug used in the treatment of narcotic addictions.

- **neurotransmitter** a substance released from the end of a nerve cell in response to a nerve impulse. The neurotransmitter diffuses across the gap to the next nerve cell, and alters that cell's membrane to make the cell more or less likely to fire.

- **unspecified eating disorders** eating disorders that do not meet the criteria for specific eating disorders previously defined. See Table C10-6.

for others are inappropriate for athletes. Body composition measures such as fatfold measures yield more useable information.

Many young athletes severely restrict their eating, attempting to improve performance, enhance the aesthetic appeal of their performance, or meet sport-related weight guidelines.[7] The increasing incidence of abnormal eating habits among athletes, especially young women athletes, is causing concern. Male

athletes, especially wrestlers and gymnasts, may be affected by these disorders as well, but research shows that female athletes, especially young ones, are most at risk.[8] Possible risk factors for this triad of disorders include the following:

- Young age (adolescence).

- Pressure to excel at a chosen sport.

- Focus on achieving or maintaining an "ideal" body weight or body fat percentage.

- Participation in endurance sports or competitions where performance is judged on aesthetic appeal such as gymnastics, figure skating, or dance.

- Dieting at an early age.

- Unsupervised dieting.

Amenorrhea   The prevalence of amenorrhea among premenopausal women in the United States is about 2 to 5 percent overall, but among female athletes, it may be as high as 66 percent.[9] Contrary to previous notions, amenorrhea is *not* a normal adaptation to strenuous physical training: it is a symptom of something going wrong.[10] Amenorrhea is characterized by low blood estrogen, infertility, and often bone mineral losses. Some research seems to indicate that depleted body fat contributes to amenorrhea. One study of ballet dancers found that those with extremely low body fat suffered more from amenorrhea and bone injuries than did those with more normal body fatness.[11] Other studies indicate that percentage of body fat is not critical for normal menstruation in athletes.[12] However amenorrhea develops, amenorrheic athletes are more likely to suffer bone loss than other women.

Osteoporosis   Osteoporosis, in which bone mass is reduced, increases susceptibility to stress fractures and bone breakage during physical activity. In general, weight-bearing physical activity, dietary calcium, and the hormone estrogen protect against bone loss, but in women with disordered eating and amenorrhea, strenuous activity may impair bone health. One study found that dancers with recent stress fractures had low body weights and a high incidence of eating disorders.[13] Vigorous training combined with low food energy intakes and other life stresses seems to trigger amenorrhea and promote bone loss. Low estrogen leads to diminished bone mass and increased bone fragility. Many amenorrheic athletes have bones like those of 50- to 60-year-old women when they should have dense,

TABLE C10-2

Tips for Combating Eating Disorders

General Guidelines

- Never restrict food servings to below the numbers suggested for adequacy by the Daily Food Guide.
- Eat frequently. People often do not eat frequent meals because of time constraints, but eating can be incorporated into other activities, such as snacking while studying or commuting. The person who eats frequently never gets so hungry as to allow hunger to dictate food choices.
- If not at a healthy weight, establish a reasonable weight goal based on a healthy body composition. (Chapter 9 provides help in doing so.)
- Allow a reasonable time to achieve the goal. A reasonable loss of excess fat can be achieved at the rate of about 1 percent of body weight per week.
- Establish a weight-maintenance support group with people who share interests.

Specific Guidelines for Athletes and Dancers

- Remember that eating disorders impair physical performance. Seek confidential help in obtaining treatment if needed.
- Restrict weight-loss activities to the off season.
- Focus on proper nutrition as an important facet of your training, as important as proper technique.

strong, bones. Amenorrheic athletes should be encouraged to consume at least 1,500 milligrams of calcium each day, to optimize their nutrient intakes, and to modify activity so that they expend no more energy than they consume. Future research will focus on the question of hormone replacement therapy for these women.

Preventing Eating Disorders in Athletes To prevent eating disorders in athletes and dancers, both the performers and their coaches must be educated about links between inappropriate body weight ideals, improper weight-loss techniques, eating disorder development, proper nutrition, and safe weight-control methods. Coaches and dance instructors should never encourage unhealthy weight loss to qualify for competition or to conform to distorted artistic ideals. Frequent weighings can push young people who are striving to lose weight into a cycle of starving to confront the scale, then binge eating uncontrollably afterward. The erosion of self-esteem that accompanies these events can interfere with the normal development

of identity and self esteem in the teen years and set the stage for serious problems later on. Perhaps the time has come to question old standards that involve appearance or body weight and to replace them with more performance-based standards.

Table C10-2 provides some suggestions to help athletes and dancers protect themselves against developing eating disorders. The next sections describe eating disorders that anyone, athlete or nonathlete, may experience.

ANOREXIA NERVOSA

Julie is 18 years old and is a superachiever in school. She watches her diet with great care, and she exercises daily, maintaining a heroic schedule of self-discipline. She is thin, but she is determined to lose more weight. She is 5 feet 6 inches tall and weighs 85 pounds. She has anorexia nervosa.

Julie is unaware that she is undernourished, and she sees no need to obtain treatment. She stopped menstruating several months ago and is moody and chronically depressed. She insists that she is too fat, although her eyes are sunk in deep hollows in her face. Although she is close to physical exhaustion, she no longer sleeps easily. Her family is concerned, and although reluctant to push her, they have finally insisted that she see a psychiatrist. Julie's psychiatrist has diagnosed anorexia nervosa and has prescribed group therapy as a start, but warns that if Julie does not begin to gain weight soon, she will need to be hospitalized.

Most anorexia nervosa victims come from middle- or upper-class families. Men account for only about 1 in 20 cases in the general population, but eating disorders among male athletes and dancers are much more common, possibly equaling the incidence among their female peers.[14] Male teenagers normally average about 15 percent of body weight as fat, but some high school athletes strive to carry only 5 percent or so of their body weight as fat.

Certain attitudes among coaches, trainers, and especially parents contribute to eating disorders.[15] Such authority figures are likely to be critical and to overvalue outward appearances while undervaluing inner self-esteem. Family patterns often include parents who oppose one another's authority, and who vacillate between defending the anorexic child's behavior and condemning it, confusing the child and disrupting normal parental control.[16] In the extreme, parents may even be abusive. Julie is a perfectionist, and her parents expect perfection: she identifies so strongly with her parents' ideals and goals that she cannot get in touch with her own identity. She sometimes feels like a robot, and she may act that way, too: polite but controlled, rigid, and unspontaneous. For Julie, rejecting food is a way of gaining control. While some of her behaviors appear out of control, they are a part of her plan. She smokes cigarettes and drinks coffee incessantly because she believes these substances reduce her sensations of starvation.

How can a person as thin as Julie continue to starve herself? Julie uses tremendous discipline to strictly limit her portions of low-calorie foods. She will deny her hunger, saying she is full after having eaten only a half-dozen carrot sticks. She can recite the calorie contents of dozens of foods and the calorie costs of as many exercises. If she feels that she has gained an ounce of weight, she runs or jumps rope until she is sure she has exercised it off. If she fears that the food energy she has eaten exceeds the exercise she has done, she takes laxatives to hasten the passage of food from her system. Her other methods of staying thin are so effective that she is unaware that laxatives have no effect on body fat. She is desperately hungry. In fact, she is starving, but she doesn't eat because her need for self-control dominates.

Many people, on learning of this disorder, say they wish they had "a touch" of it to get thin. They mistakenly think that people with anorexia nervosa feel no hunger. They also fail to recognize the pain of the associated psychological and physical trauma.

Central to the diagnosis of anorexia nervosa is a distorted body image that overestimates body fatness. When Julie looks at herself in the mirror, she sees her 85-pound body as fat. The more Julie overestimates her body size, the more resistant she is to treatment, and the more unwilling to examine her faulty values and misconceptions. Malnutrition itself is known to affect brain functioning and judgment in this way. People with anorexia nervosa cannot recognize it in themselves; only professionals can diagnose it. Table C10-3 shows the criteria that experts use.

Anorexia nervosa damages the body much as starvation does. Victims are dying to be thin, quite literally. In young people, growth ceases and normal development falters. They lose so much lean tissue that basal metabolic rate slows, an effect that may remain even after treatment and regain of weight.[17] In athletes, the loss of lean tissue handicaps physical performance. The heart pumps inefficiently and irregularly, the heart muscle becomes weak and thin, the chambers diminish in size, and the blood pressure falls. Electrolytes that help to

TABLE C10-3

Criteria for Diagnosis of Anorexia Nervosa

A person with anorexia nervosa demonstrates the following:

A. Refusal to maintain body weight at or above a minimal normal weight for age and height, e.g., weight loss leading to maintenance of body weight less than 85% of that expected; or failure to make expected weight gain during period of growth, leading to body weight less than 85% of that expected.

B. Intense fear of gaining weight or becoming fat, even though underweight.

C. Disturbance in the way in which one's body weight or shape is experienced; undue influence of body weight or shape on self-evaluation, or denial of the seriousness of the current low body weight.

D. In females past puberty, amenorrhea, i.e., the absence of at least three consecutive menstrual cycles. (A woman is considered to have amenorrhea if her periods occur only following hormone, e.g., estrogen, administration.)

Two types:

■ **Restricting type:** during the episode of anorexia nervosa, the person does not regularly engage in binge eating or purging behavior (i.e., self-induced vomiting or the misuse of laxatives, diuretics, or enemas).

■ **Binge eating/purging type:** during the episode of anorexia nervosa, the person regularly engages in binge eating or purging behavior (i.e., self-induced vomiting or the misuse of laxatives, diuretics, or enemas).

SOURCE: Reprinted with permission from American Psychiatric Association, *Diagnostic and Statistical Manual of Mental Disorders*, 4th ed. (Washington, D.C.: American Psychiatric Association, 1994).

regulate heartbeat go out of balance. Many deaths in people with anorexia are due to heart failure.

Starvation brings other physical consequences as well: impaired immune response, anemia, and a loss of digestive functions that worsens malnutrition. Digestive functioning becomes sluggish, the stomach empties slowly, and the lining of the intestinal tract shrinks. The ailing digestive tract fails to digest food adequately, even if the victim does eat. The pancreas slows its production of digestive enzymes. Diarrhea sets in, further worsening malnutrition.

Starvation also brings altered blood lipids, high concentrations of vitamin A and vitamin E in the blood, low blood proteins, dry skin, abnormal nerve functioning, low body temperature, and the development of

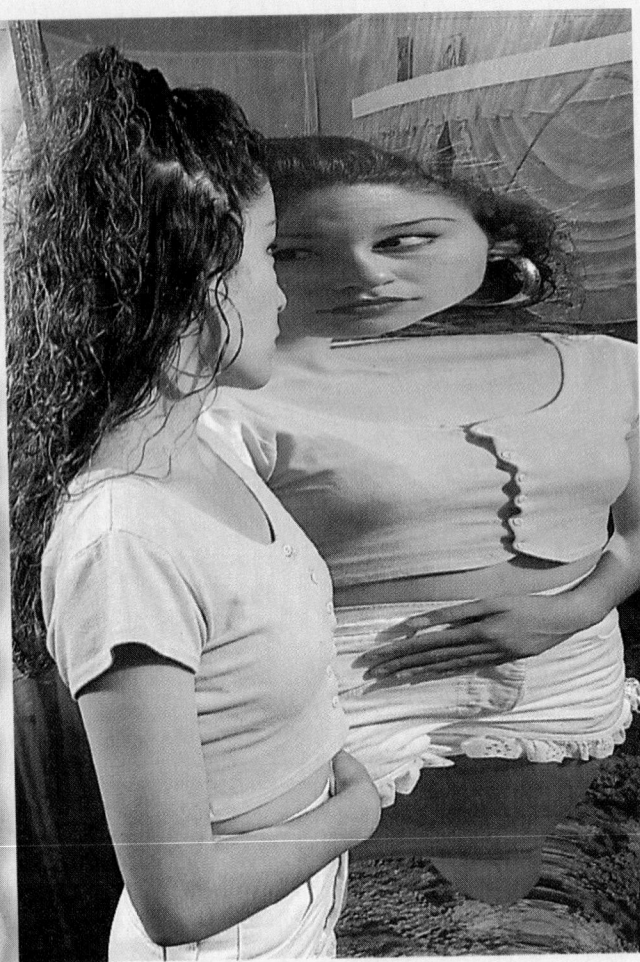

Women with anorexia nervosa see themselves as fat, even when they are dangerously underweight.

fine body hair (the body's attempt to keep warm). The electrical activity of the brain becomes abnormal, and insomnia is common. Both women and men lose their sex drives.

TREATMENT OF ANOREXIA NERVOSA

Treatment of anorexia nervosa requires a multidisciplinary approach that addresses two sets of issues and behaviors: those relating to food and weight and those involving relationships with oneself and others.[18] Teams of physicians, nurses, psychiatrists, family therapists, and dietitians work together to treat people with anorexia nervosa. Appropriate diet is crucial and must be tailored individually to each client's needs. Seldom are clients willing to eat for themselves, but if

they are, chances are they can recover without other interventions.

High-risk clients may require hospitalization and may need to be force-fed by tube at first to forestall death. This step causes psychological trauma.[19] Drugs are commonly prescribed, but to date, they play a limited role in treatment.[20]

Denial runs high among those with anorexia nervosa. Few seek treatment on their own. Almost half of the women who are treated can maintain their body weight within 15 percent of a healthy weight; at that weight, many of them begin menstruating again. The other half have poor or fair outcomes of treatment, and two-thirds of those treated continue a mental battle with recurring morbid thoughts about food and body weight.[21] Many relapse into abnormal eating behaviors to some extent. About 5 percent die during treatment, 1 percent by suicide.

Before drawing conclusions about someone who is extremely thin or who eats very little, remember that diagnosis of anorexia nervosa requires professional assessment. People who are seeking help with anorexia nervosa, either for themselves or for others, can contact any of a number of organizations for information.*

BULIMIA NERVOSA

Sophia is a charming, intelligent, 20-year-old airline stewardess of normal weight who thinks constantly about food. She alternately starves herself and then secretly binges; when she has eaten too much, she vomits. Few people would fail to recognize that these symptoms signify bulimia nervosa.

Bulimia nervosa is distinct from anorexia nervosa and is more prevalent, although the true incidence is difficult to establish because denial runs high in people with bulimia nervosa.[22] More men suffer from bulimia nervosa than from anorexia nervosa; but bulimia nervosa is still most common in women. The secretive nature of bulimic behaviors makes recognition of the problem difficult, but once it is recognized, diagnosis is based on the criteria listed in Table C10-4.

Families of bulimic people often establish unusually close emotional ties between members, and they may be overcontrolling and intermeshed in ways that stifle individual growth and development.[23] Should the member with bulimia nervosa begin taking steps

---

*Phone numbers and addresses are listed in Nutrition Resources, Appendix E.

TABLE C10-4

Criteria for Diagnosis of Bulimia Nervosa

A person with bulimia nervosa demonstrates the following:

A. Recurrent episodes of binge eating. An episode of binge eating is characterized by both of the following:

  1. eating, in a discrete period of time (e.g., within any two-hour period), an amount of food that is definitely larger than most people would eat during a similar period of time and under similar circumstances, and,

  2. a sense of lack of control over eating during the episode (e.g., a feeling that one cannot stop eating or control what or how much one is eating).

B. Recurrent inappropriate compensatory behavior in order to prevent weight gain, such as self-induced vomiting; misuse of laxatives, diuretics, enemas, or other medications; fasting; or excessive exercise.

C. Binge eating and inappropriate compensatory behaviors that both occur, on average, at least twice a week for three months.

D. Self-evaluation unduly influenced by body shape and weight.

E. The disturbance does not occur exclusively during episodes of anorexia nervosa.

Two types:

■ **Purging type:** the person regularly engages in self-induced vomiting or the misuse of laxatives, diuretics, or enemas.

■ **Nonpurging type:** the person uses other inappropriate compensatory behaviors, such as fasting or excessive exercise, but does not regularly engage in self-induced vomiting or the misuse of laxatives, diuretics, or enemas.

SOURCE: Reprinted with permission from American Psychiatric Association, *Diagnostic and Statistical Manual of Mental Disorders*, 4th ed. (Washington, D.C.: American Psychiatric Association, 1994).

weeks. As a flight attendant, she is required to "make weight," that is, to weigh no more than a certain cutoff weight slightly below the weight that her body maintains naturally.

Sophia seldom lets her bulimia nervosa interfere with her work or other activities, although a third of all bingers do so. From early childhood she has been a high achiever, emotionally dependent on her parents. As a young teen, Sophia cycled on and off crash diets. Sophia feels anxious at social events and cannot easily establish close relationships. She is usually depressed, is often impulsive, and has low self-esteem.

A bulimic binge is unlike normal eating, and the food is not consumed for its nutritional value. During a binge, Sophia's eating is accelerated by her hunger from previous calorie restriction. She may take in anywhere from 1,000 to many thousands of calories of easy-to-eat, low-fiber, smooth-textured, high-fat, and, especially, high-carbohydrate foods. Typically, she chooses cookies, cakes, and ice cream; and she eats the entire bag of cookies, the whole cake, and every spoonful in a carton of ice cream.

The binge is a compulsion and usually occurs in several stages: "anticipation and planning, anxiety, urgency to begin, rapid and uncontrollable consumption of food, relief and relaxation, disappointment, and finally shame or disgust." Then, to purge the food from her body, she may use a **cathartic**—a strong laxative that can injure the lower intestinal tract. Or she may induce vomiting, using an **emetic**—a drug intended as first aid for poisoning. After the binge she pays the

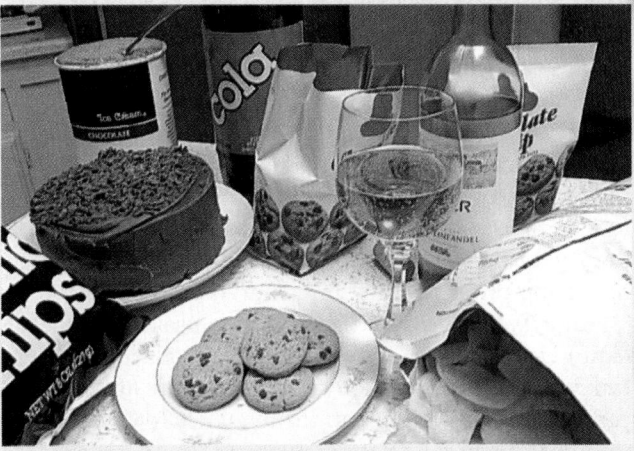

A person may consume up to 10,000 calories during an eating binge.

toward recovery, others in the family may feel threatened. Often any changes in the familial structure meet with resistance, even if such change would greatly benefit the person with bulimia nervosa. Typically, the family has "secrets" that are hidden from outsiders. Many bulimic women report having been abused sexually or physically by family members or family friends.

Like the typical person with bulimia nervosa, Sophia is single, female, and white. She is well educated and close to her ideal body weight, although her weight fluctuates over a range of 10 pounds or so every few price with hands scraped raw against the teeth during induced vomiting, swollen neck glands and reddened eyes from straining to vomit, and bloating, fatigue, headache, nausea, and pain that follow.

On first glance, purging seems to offer a quick and easy solution to the problems of unwanted calories and body weight. Many people perceive such behavior as neutral or even positive, when, in fact, bingeing and purging have serious physical consequences.[24] Fluid and electrolyte imbalances caused by vomiting or diarrhea can lead to abnormal heart rhythms and injury to the kidneys. Urinary tract infections can lead to kidney failure. Vomiting causes irritation and infection of the pharynx, esophagus, and salivary glands; erosion of the teeth; and dental caries. The esophagus or stomach may rupture or tear. Overuse of emetics can lead to death by heart failure.

Unlike Julie, Sophia is aware that her behavior is abnormal, and she is deeply ashamed of it. She wants to recover, and this makes recovery more likely for her than for Julie, who clings to denial. Feeling inadequate ("I can't even control my eating"), Sophia tends to be passive and to look to others, primarily men, for confirmation of her sense of worth. When she experiences rejection, either in reality or in her imagination, her bulimia nervosa becomes worse. If Sophia's depression deepens, she may seek solace in drug or alcohol abuse or other addictive behaviors. As many as 50 percent of women with bulimia nervosa are alcohol dependent.[25]

TREATMENT OF BULIMIA NERVOSA

To help clients gain control over food and establish regular eating patterns requires adherence to a structured eating plan. Restrictive weight-loss dieting almost always precedes and may even trigger bingeing. Weight maintenance, rather than cyclic gains and losses, is the goal for the person who has recovered. Many a former bulimia nervosa victim has taken a major step toward recovery by learning to eat enough food to satisfy hunger needs (at least 1,600 calories a day). Table C10-5 offers some ways to begin correcting the eating problems of bulimia nervosa.

Anorexia nervosa and bulimia nervosa are distinct eating disorders, yet they sometimes overlap in important ways. Victims of both conditions share an overconcern with body weight and the tendency to drastically undereat. Victims of both may purge. The two disorders can also appear in the same person, or one can lead to the other.

Societal pressure to be thin is no doubt a factor in the development of eating disorders. Most experts, agree, however, that the disorders are multifactorial: sociocultural, psychological, and perhaps neurochemical.

OTHER EATING DISORDERS

Many people with eating disorders fall short of the diagnostic criteria for either anorexia nervosa or bulimia nervosa and may have "unspecified" eating disorders. Disordered eating, fear of body fatness, distorted body image, purging, or bingeing pose risks of the same consequences that the more well-defined eating disorders present. About one-third of obese people regularly engage in binge eating. The 1994 American Psychiatric Association manual includes **binge eating disorder** under the category "eating disorders not otherwise specified." Table C10-6 lists the official diagnostic criteria for binge eating disorder.

Clinicians note differences between people with bulimia nervosa and those with binge eating disorder.[26] For example, binge eaters rarely purge or restrict eating too much during dieting. Similarities also exist, including feeling out of control; feeling disgusted, depressed, embarrassed, or guilty; and feeling distress caused by bingeing.[27]

Treatment of binge eating is a helpful complement to weight-control programs. It also improves physical

TABLE C10-5

Diet Strategies for Combating Bulimia Nervosa

- Avoid finger foods; eat foods that require the use of utensils.
- Enhance satiety by eating warm foods.
- Include vegetables, salad, and/or fruit at meals to prolong eating time.
- Choose whole-grain and high-fiber breads and cereals to maximize bulk.
- Eat a well-balanced diet and meals consisting of a variety of foods.
- Use foods that are naturally divided into portions, such as potatoes (rather than rice or pasta); 4 and 8 oz containers of yogurt, ice cream, or cottage cheese; precut steak or chicken parts; and frozen entrees.
- Include foods containing ample complex carbohydrates (for satiety) and some fat (to slow gastric emptying).
- Eat meals and snacks sitting down.
- Plan meals and snacks, and record plans in a food diary prior to eating.

TABLE C10-6

Criteria for Diagnosis of Binge Eating Disorder

A person with a binge eating disorder demonstrates the following:

A. Recurrent episodes of binge eating. An episode of binge eating is characterized by both of the following:

  1. Eating, in a discrete period of time (e.g., within any two-hour period) an amount of food that is definitely larger than most people would eat in a similar period of time under similar circumstances.

  2. A sense of lack of control over eating during the episode (e.g., a feeling that one cannot stop eating or control what or how much one is eating).

B. Binge eating episodes are associated with at least three of the following:

  1. Eating much more rapidly than normal.

  2. Eating until feeling uncomfortably full.

  3. Eating large amounts of food when not feeling physically hungry.

  4. Eating alone because of being embarrassed by how much one is eating.

  5. Feeling disgusted with oneself, depressed, or very guilty after overeating.

C. The binge eating causes marked distress.

D. The binge eating occurs, on average, at least twice a week for six months.

E. The binge eating is not associated with the regular use of inappropriate compensatory behaviors (e.g., purging, fasting, excessive exercise) and does not occur exclusively during the course of anorexia nervosa or bulimia nervosa.

SOURCE: Reprinted with permission from American Psychiatric Association, *Diagnostic and Statistical Manual of Mental Disorders*, 4th ed., (Washington, D.C.: American Psychiatric Association, 1994).

health, mental health, and the chances of success in breaking the cycle of rapid weight losses and gains.

EATING DISORDERS IN SOCIETY

Eating disorders seem to have complex causes. Some may have hereditary components; some may have psychological components that our society brings out. Proof that society plays a role in eating disorders is found in their demographic distribution: they are known only in developed nations, and they become more prevalent as wealth increases and food becomes plentiful.

A food-centered society that favors thinness puts people in a bind. Families may encourage hearty eating and socializing around the dinner table. Party hosts take pride in the delicacies they serve, and guests are obliged to indulge. A child raised in such a setting may see little alternative but to celebrate with the family; indulge in vast quantities of food; and then vomit, crash diet, or fast to "undo" possible weight gain. Then, starving and guilty, the child may begin bingeing in secret to relieve a desperate hunger.

No doubt our society sets unrealistic ideals for body weight, especially in women, and devalues those who do not conform to them. Even professionals, including physicians and dietitians, can suffer from these disorders or tend to praise people for losing weight and to suggest weight loss to people who do not need it. As a result, at so tender an age as 11 or 12, beautifully growing, normal-weight girls fear that they are too fat. Most are "on diets," and many are poorly nourished. Some eat too little food to support normal growth; thus they miss out on their adolescent growth spurts and may never catch up.

Perhaps a young person's best defense against these disorders is to learn to appreciate his or her own uniqueness. When people discover and honor the body's real needs, they become unwilling to sacrifice health for conformity. The author Eda LeShan, once a slave to bulimic behavior, achieved this inner ideal and described her recovery from overeating: "Deep inside there had always been a small child begging for my attention. . . . All I gave her was food. Now I give her love."[28]

NOTES

Notes are in Appendix F.

NUTRITION AND DISEASE PREVENTION

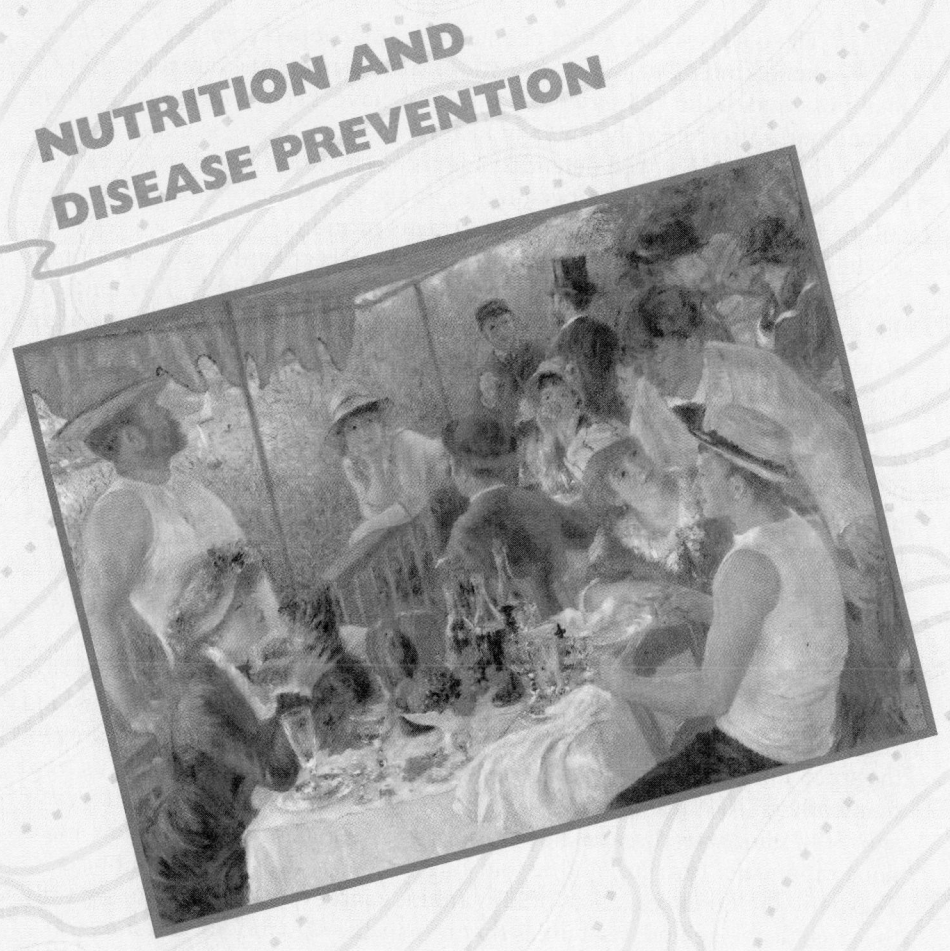

CONTENTS

Renoir, *The Luncheon of the Boating Party,* © The Philips Collection, Washington, D.C.

infectious diseases diseases caused by bacteria, viruses, parasites, and other microbes, which can be transmitted from one person to another through air, water, or food; by contact; or through vector organisms such as mosquitoes or fleas.

degenerative disease chronic, irreversible disease characterized by degeneration of body organs due in part to such personal lifestyle elements as poor food choices, smoking, alcohol use, and lack of physical activity. Also called *lifestyle diseases, chronic diseases,* or the *disease of old age.*

11 The diseases that afflict people in the developed countries are of two main kinds. One kind is **infectious disease;** examples are tuberculoses, smallpox, and polio. Diseases of this kind have been widespread among humankind since before the dawn of history, and they strike people of all ages. In any civilization not well defended against them, infectious diseases can cut life so short that the average person dies at age 20, 30, or 40, instead of living out the full potential lifespan of 70 or 80 years or more.

The other kind, **degenerative disease,** has long been with us, too; examples are diabetes, cancer, heart disease, and osteoporosis. Ironically, it is long life that opens the way for these diseases to take their toll. They become prevalent in a population only when infectious disease is kept firmly enough in control so that people can live to older ages.

Degenerative diseases set in, not from simple infection, but from a mixture of three sets of factors: hereditary susceptibility and prior disease, which people cannot control, and life circumstances, which people themselves can control. Young people can choose whether to nourish their bodies well, to smoke, to exercise, or to abuse alcohol. As people age, their bodies accumulate impacts from these choices, which in the later years can add up to make the difference between a life of health or one of chronic disability. In fact, degenerative diseases are often called the *chronic* diseases.

Today, we are fighting both kinds of diseases, and medical science has gained some ground against both. We have both preventive measures and cures for many infectious diseases. Our water supply is disinfected to prevent the spread of many infections. Immunizations and antibiotics protect us from many others. As a result, life expectancy is much longer than it was 100 years ago. Still, infectious diseases never go away. They gain ground as new infectious organisms turn up, and as old ones develop resistance to antibiotics.[1] They still remain major killers of humankind, and even if treated successfully, they may leave behind disabilities that impair life's quality for decades.

FIGURE 11-1

TEN LEADING CAUSES OF DEATH
The causes identified with the red bars are topics of this chapter; those with green bars are discussed in its Controversy section.

SOURCE: Data from G. K. Singh and coauthors, Annual summary of births, marriages, divorces, and deaths: United States, 1994, *Monthly Vital Statistics Report* 23 October 1995, p. 7.

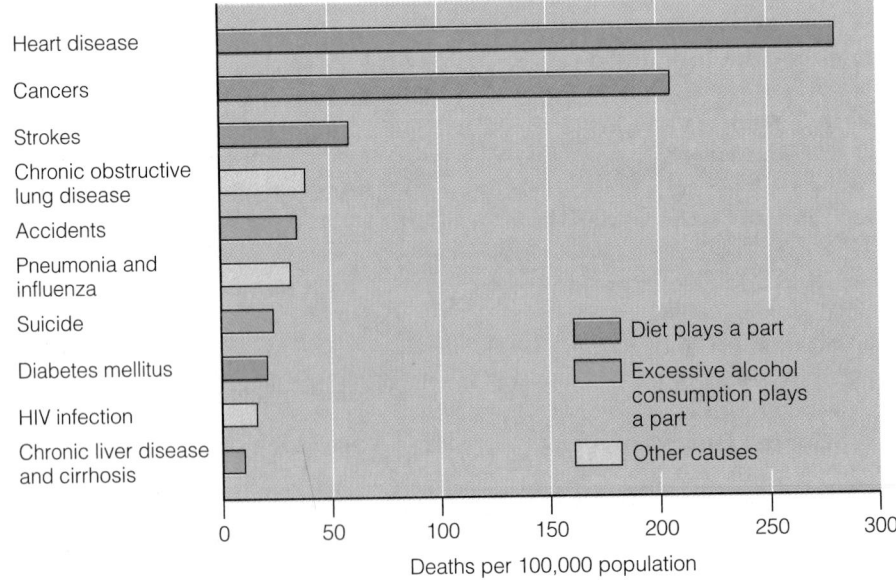

As for chronic diseases, medical research today is piecing together the many elements that influence them and devising ways to prevent, forestall, and cure them. Nutrition is turning out to be an important piece in many of these puzzles. Figure 11-1 shows today's top ten killers of adults, and this chapter is devoted to those in which nutrition plays important roles.

Nutrition can help *prevent* infectious diseases by supporting a healthy enough immune system to fend off some infections and help keep others from becoming major problems. A section of this chapter reveals the roles nutrition plays in immunity.

Nutrition *treatment* can exert major impacts on the course of both types of disease. It can support the body's immune responses; prevent wasting; help the body to withstand drug, surgical, or other treatments; and improve the quality and length of life. A section of this chapter describes nutrition in treatment of **AIDS** as an example.

With respect to prevention of chronic diseases, choices people make about their nutrition can help at least to postpone them and sometimes to avoid them altogether.[2] Most of this chapter presents what is now known of nutrition's relationships with chronic diseases.

AIDS acquired immune deficiency syndrome, caused by infection with HIV, a virus that is transmitted primarily by sexual contact, by contact with infected blood, by needles shared among drug users, or by materials transferred from an infected mother to her fetus or infant.

Wasting poses a severe threat to life by causing major losses of active body tissue in diseases such as some cancers, tuberculosis, or AIDS. People with wasting diseases often die from malnutrition rather than from the disease itself. See also page 341 of Chapter 9.

NUTRITION AND IMMUNITY

Without your awareness, your immune system guards continuously against thousands of enemy attacks mounted against you by microorganisms and cancer cells. If your immune system falters, you become vulnerable to disease-causing agents, and disease invariably follows.

Nutrients and the Immune System

Among the body's systems, the immune system responds most sensitively to subtle changes in nutrition status. When people do not eat well for whatever reason, malnutrition often sets in, compromising immunity. Impaired immunity opens the way for diseases, diseases impair food assimilation, and nutrition status suffers further. Drugs become necessary and most of them impair nutrition status (see Controversy 12). Other treatments, such as surgery, take a further toll. Thus disease and poor nutrition together form a downward spiral that must be broken for recovery to occur (see Figure 11-2).

Certain groups of people are especially likely to be caught in the downward spiral of malnutrition and weakened immunity. Among them are people who restrict their food intakes, whether for lack of appetite, because of eating disorders, for weight loss, or for any other reason.[3] Also susceptible are those who fit one or more, or even all four, of these descriptions: they are old, poor, hospitalized, or malnourished.[4]

Protein-energy malnutrition (PEM) is especially destructive to various immune-system organs and tissues. Table 11-1 shows PEM's effects on body defenses. Listed first are the body's initial barriers to infection—the skin and the mucous membranes. The digestive system is an especially active defense force. The mucous membranes of the digestive system are heavily laced with active immune tissues. These tissues both work at the absorptive site and form cells that travel to other organs, such as the liver, pancreas, mammary glands, and uterus.

FIGURE 11-2

NUTRITION AND IMMUNITY

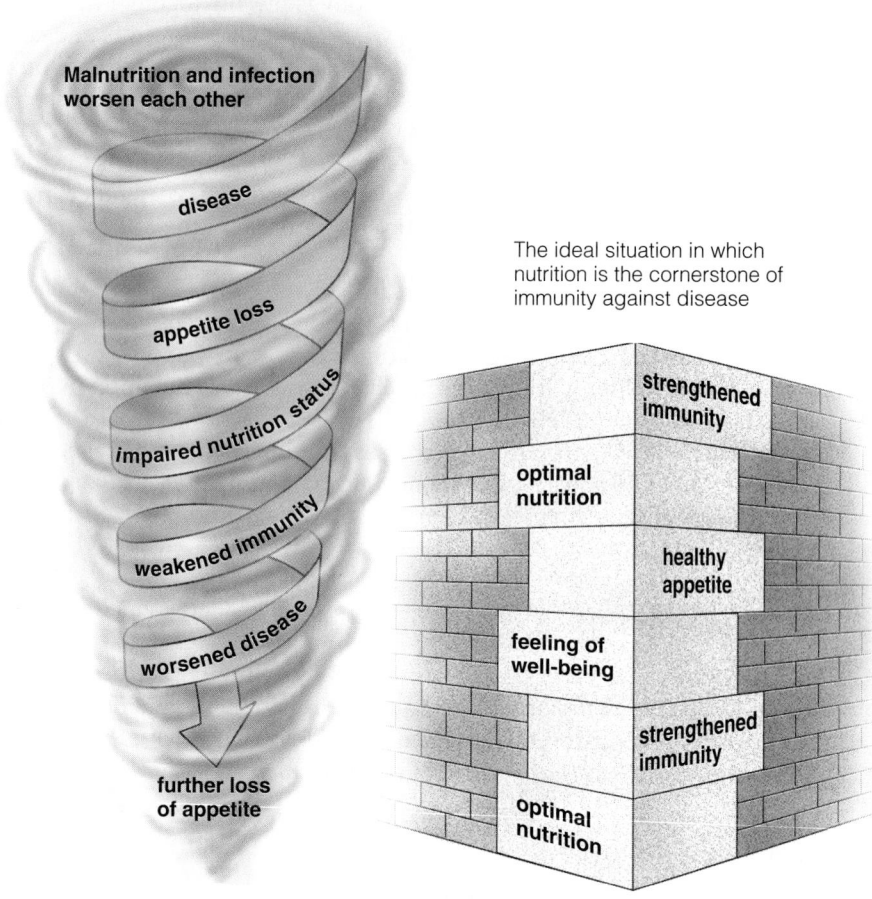

Malnutrition and infection worsen each other

disease

appetite loss

impaired nutrition status

weakened immunity

worsened disease

further loss of appetite

The ideal situation in which nutrition is the cornerstone of immunity against disease

strengthened immunity

optimal nutrition

healthy appetite

feeling of well-being

strengthened immunity

optimal nutrition

In PEM, indispensable tissues and cells of the immune system dwindle in size and number, opening the whole body to infection. Also the skin becomes thinner as its connective tissue is broken down, and so becomes less of a barrier to agents of disease. The number of antibodies normally present in secretions of the lungs and digestive tract diminish, opening the way for repeated lung and digestive tract infections. Normally barred from the body, infectious agents are allowed to enter, and the defensive responses to them, once they are inside, is weak.

A deficiency or toxicity of even a single nutrient can seriously weaken the body's defenses. For example, in vitamin A deficiency, the body's skin and membranous linings become unhealthy, and unable to ward off infectious organisms. A vitamin C deficiency robs white blood cells of their killing power. A copper or zinc deficiency reduces immune cell number. Table 11-2 lists the single-nutrient deficiencies and excesses known to weaken the immune response.[5]

Medical advances such as vaccines and antibiotics have lulled many people into complacency concerning infectious diseases. This is a serious error. New antibiotic-resistant bacterial strains threaten health and life across the globe. For example, tuberculosis, formerly declared a controlled disease, has now overpowered once-reliable treatment methods, producing a world-wide epidemic that some have called a modern-day plague.[6] While nutrition cannot

TABLE 11-1

Effects of Protein-Energy Malnutrition (PEM) on the Body's Defense Systems

System Component	Effects of PEM
Skin	Thinned, with less connective tissue to serve as a barrier for protection of underlying tissues; delayed skin sensitivity reaction to antigens
Digestive tract and other body linings	Antibody secretions and immune cell number reduced
Lymph tissues	Immune system organs[a] reduced in size; cells of immune defense depleted
General response	Invader kill time prolonged; circulating immune cells reduced; antibody response impaired

[a]Thymus gland, lymph nodes, and spleen.

TABLE 11-2

Single Nutrients That Affect Immunity

✔ Vitamin A deficiency/excess
✔ Vitamin B deficiency
✔ Vitamin B_{12} deficiency
✔ Vitamin C deficiency
✔ Vitamin D deficiency (rickets)
✔ Vitamin E deficiency/excess
✔ Folate deficiency (even mild)
✔ Copper deficiency/excess
✔ Magnesium deficiency/excess
✔ Zinc deficiency/excess
✔ Protein deficiency

directly prevent or cure infectious diseases, it can strengthen or weaken the body's ability to fight them off. One effective defense is to meet but not exceed protein and energy needs. Another is to meet the minimum need for each nutrient while not ingesting supplement doses so large as to cause harm.

✔ **KEY POINT** **Adequate nutrition is a key player in maintaining a healthy immune system to defend against infectious diseases.**

Nutrition in the Treatment of a Wasting Disease—AIDS

More and more people are finding that someone they know has been diagnosed with the human immunodeficiency virus (HIV) infection of AIDS. People with HIV infection frequently experience severe PEM and wasting which often begins early in the disease and becomes progressively worse. People with AIDS lose a lot of weight in the four to five months before death, not unlike those who die from starvation, and the wasting itself often causes death. Preventing and treating malnutrition and wasting should be a high priority in the care of HIV-infected people.[7] Weight loss, reduced body fat, and a low body mass index are early signs of deterioration in people with HIV infection.

Inadequate nutrient intake is the prime determinant of the wasting and malnutrition associated with HIV.[8] Different factors contribute in different cases: excessive nutrient losses, accelerated metabolism, and drug-nutrient interactions among them. Repeated infections and cancer attack with more and more vigor as immunity declines and wasting accelerates.

Adequate nutrition, while offering nothing in the way of cure, can help maintain body tissues and improve life's quality for the person infected with HIV.[9] People wishing to help someone with AIDS can do no better than to tend intelligently to the person's nutrition, which is often overlooked in medical treatment. People with AIDS suffer anorexia and may refuse food. They may more readily accept small, frequent snacks than large meals.

Supplements containing RDA amounts of vitamins and minerals can be helpful and will do no harm. Liquid meal supplements were originally developed to

Nutrition sometimes makes the difference between living independently and being confined to a nursing home or hospital.

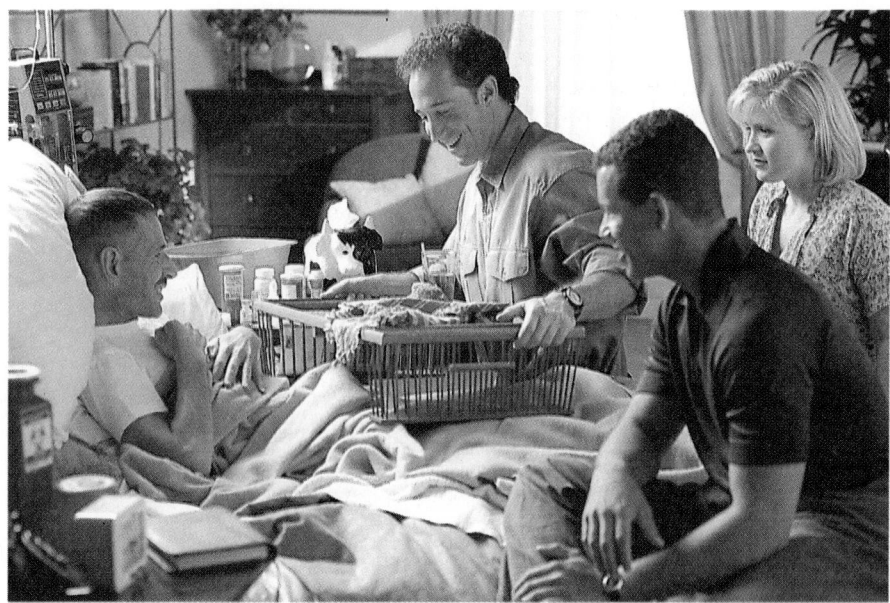

help sick persons to obtain their vitamins and minerals, along with the carbohydrate, fat, and protein that they need for energy and building materials. These supplements are excellent for these purposes, they taste good, and they are easy to swallow.*

Whatever foods are served, food safety is extremely important. A common bacterium in food, *Salmonella*, can kill people with compromised immunity.[10] Cleanliness and thorough cooking are protective. If AIDS complications progress, the caring attitude shown through attention to nutrition can still lend emotional support to the sick person, a powerful medicine in itself.

Family, friends, and victims may, out of desperation, try special diet regimens or supplements in hopes of finding a cure or adding days to life, but no diet regimen or supplement has been shown helpful beyond providing the nutrients needed to support the body's defenses. Unfortunately, though, frauds and charlatans eagerly profit by selling useless products to those desperate for help.[11] Faced with such practices, professionals must choose whether or not to expose them. In some cases, to extinguish hope might serve no purpose, and unproved dietary "remedies" might best be allowed if they do no harm.

The great majority of HIV infections are preventable. The authors urge you to seek out information about AIDS prevention and to heed it.

✔ KEY POINT   **Adequate nutrition cannot prevent or cure AIDS, but can minimize wasting and bolster the quality of life for the person with AIDS.**

_____

*Brand names of nutritious supplements include Ensure, Sustacal, and others.

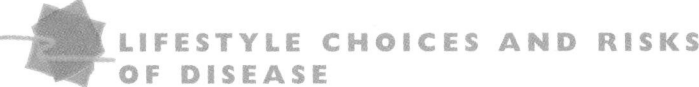

LIFESTYLE CHOICES AND RISKS OF DISEASE

In contrast to the infectious diseases, each of which has a distinct microbial cause such as a bacterium or virus, the degenerative diseases of adulthood tend to have clusters of suspected causes known as **risk factors.** Among them are environmental, behavioral, social, and genetic factors that tend to occur in clusters and interact with each other. In many cases one disease or condition intensifies the risk of another.

People's behaviors, including food behaviors, underlie many risk factors. The choice to eat a diet high in fat and calories, for example, is a choice to risk becoming obese and contracting cancer, hypertension, diabetes, atherosclerosis, diverticulosis, or other diseases. Figure 11-3 shows connections among some of the risk factors associated with today's major degenerative diseases and highlights the diet-related behaviors that contribute to them.

The exact contribution diet makes to each disease is hard to estimate. Many experts believe that diet accounts for about a third of all cases of coronary heart

> **risk factors** factors known to be related to (or correlated with) diseases but not proven to be causal.

FIGURE 11-3

DIET/LIFESTYLE RISK FACTORS AND DEGENERATIVE DISEASES

The chart at the top shows that the same risk factors affect many chronic conditions. For example, genetic risk factors and high-fat diets affect many diseases; smoking affects fewer; and environmental contaminants affect fewer still. This does not mean that people who smoke or are exposed to environmental contaminants become less often or less severely ill than those who eat a high-fat diet, but just that the fat-eaters may become ill from a larger variety of conditions.

The flow chart at the bottom shows that some conditions are themselves risk factors for others. For example, atherosclerosis and hypertension are known to worsen each other.

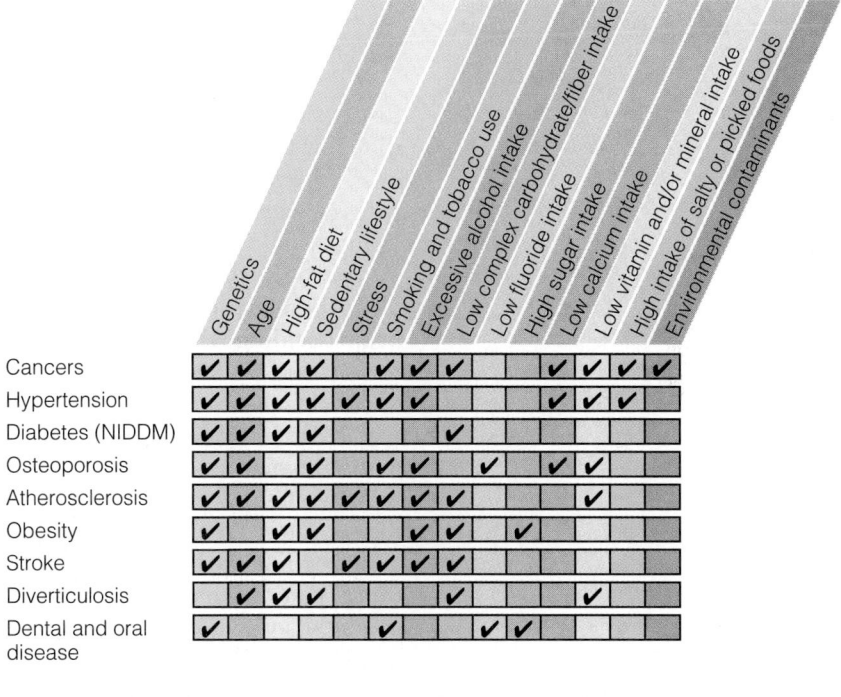

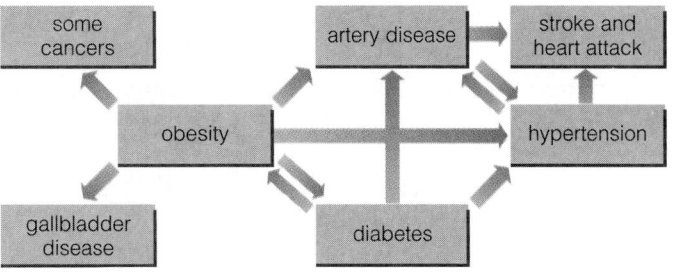

TABLE 11-3

Family and Medical Indicators for Increased Disease Risk

Nutrition Changes Recommended for All People	This Is Especially Important If Your Family History Indicates:	And/or If Your Medical History Indicates:
Reduce consumption of fat (especially saturated fat) and cholesterol. Achieve and maintain a desirable body weight. Increase consumption of complex carbohydrates and fiber.	Diabetes, obesity, cancer, or any form of cardiovascular disease (atherosclerosis, hypertension, heart attacks, strokes)	Glucose intolerance, high blood cholesterol or triglycerides, hypertension
Reduce intake of salt/sodium.	Hypertension, diabetes, or any form of cardiovascular disease (atherosclerosis, hypertension, heart attacks, strokes)	Hypertension
Drink alcohol in moderation, if at all.	Liver disease (cirrhosis), cancer, any form of cardiovascular disease (atherosclerosis, hypertension, heart attacks, strokes),[a] osteoporosis	Glucose intolerance, high blood cholesterol or triglycerides, hypertension, any sign of adult bone loss

[a]Moderate alcohol intakes may reduce cardiovascular disease risks in some people. Alcohol excesses injure the heart.

disease. Diet's link to cancer incidence is harder to pin down because cancer's different forms associate with different dietary factors. General trends, however, support many links between diet and cancer, and the evidence in some cases is overwhelming.* People can control their own food choices. If a dietary change can't hurt and might help, why not make it?

Making such choices is doubtless more important for some people than for others because some people are genetically predisposed to certain diseases. To begin deciding whether certain diet recommendations are especially important to you, you should search your family's medical history for diseases common to your forebears. Any condition that shows up in several close blood relatives may be a special concern for you. Also find out, after your next physical examination, which test results are out of line. Family history and lab test results together are powerful predictors of disease. Table 11-3 presents a summary of the signs to watch for in both categories.

Accepting that you have certain unchangeable "givens," you can look to the things you can change and choose the most influential among them. For example, a person whose parents, grandparents, or other close blood relatives suffered with diabetes and heart disease is urgently advised to avoid becoming obese. A person who has hypertension is urged to control weight, to exercise regularly, to eat a nutritious diet, to control salt intake, and not to smoke. The guidelines presented in the Food Feature of this chapter can benefit most people, while presenting the smallest possible risk to health.[12]

Diabetes and obesity may be the two conditions that are most important to prevent. Figure 11-3 already showed the relationship of diabetes to the major killer diseases. Both hasten the progression of degenerative diseases and each also worsens the other.

See Chapter 4 for a review of diabetes and its relationship to obesity.

---

*Other important risk factors for cancer include tobacco use, alcohol abuse, exposure to radiation and to environmental and other contamination, and advanced age.

✓ KEY POINT   **The same diet and lifestyle risk factors may contribute to several degenerative diseases. Diabetes and obesity also contribute to several other diseases.**

NUTRITION AND ATHEROSCLEROSIS

Currently, our major cause of death in men and women over 50 is disease of the heart and blood vessels (cardiovascular disease, henceforth abbreviated, CVD). CVD accounts for more of the world's deaths each year than any other single cause, mostly by way of heart attacks and strokes. Efforts to fight CVD have led to valuable discoveries and public education. We now know that smoking, high blood pressure, and high blood cholesterol are the three major risk factors for CVD, and many people have changed their lifestyles accordingly. Many have quit smoking or have refrained from starting. Many have been willing to change their diets, consuming less fat, less saturated fat, less cholesterol, less salt, more fruits and vegetables, and more fiber. The rate of CVD has fallen somewhat in recent years, but it still remains high. How can people minimize their risks? How can we improve our chances of leading long and healthy lives?

The twin demons that lead to most CVD are **atherosclerosis** and **hypertension.** Atherosclerosis is the common form of hardening of the arteries; hypertension is high blood pressure; and each makes the other worse. The remainder of this section and the next on hypertension describe these relationships.

How Atherosclerosis Develops

No one is free of atherosclerosis. The question is not whether you have it but how far advanced it is and what you can do to retard or reverse it. Atherosclerosis usually begins with the accumulation of soft, fatty streaks along the inner walls of the arteries, especially at branch points.[13] These gradually enlarge and become hardened **plaques** that damage artery walls, making them inelastic and narrowing the passage through them (see Figure 11-4). Most people have well-developed plaques by the time they reach age 30.

Normally, the arteries expand with each heartbeat to accommodate the pulses of blood that flow through them. Arteries hardened and narrowed by plaques cannot expand, however, so the blood pressure rises. The increased pressure damages the artery walls further and strains the heart. Damage sites make plaques especially likely to form, so the development of atherosclerosis becomes a self-accelerating process.

As pressure builds up in an artery, the arterial wall may become weakened and balloon out, forming an **aneurysm.** An aneurysm can burst, and in a major artery such as the **aorta,** this leads to massive bleeding and death.

Abnormal blood clotting can also threaten life. Clots form and dissolve in the blood all the time, and the balance between these processes ensures that clots do no harm. That balance is disturbed in atherosclerosis. Small, cell-like bodies in the blood, known as **platelets,** normally cause clots to form whenever they encounter injuries in blood vessels. In atherosclerosis, the platelets respond to plaques as they do to injuries and form unneeded clots. Platelets also release substances that enlarge plaques. Opposing platelet action are the active products of omega-3 fatty acids. A diet lacking the seafoods that contain these essential fatty acids may contribute to clot formation.[14]

A clot, once formed, may remain attached to a plaque in an artery and gradually grow until it shuts off the blood supply to the surrounding tissue. That

atherosclerosis (ath-er-oh-scler-OH-sis) the most common form of cardiovascular disease, characterized by plaques along the inner walls of the arteries (*athero* means "porridge" or "soft"; *scleros* means "hard"; *osis* means "too much"). The related term *arteriosclerosis* refers to all forms of hardening of the arteries and includes some rare diseases.

hypertension high blood pressure (see the next major section of this chapter).

plaques (PLACKS) mounds of lipid material, mixed with smooth muscle cells and calcium, that develop in the artery walls in atherosclerosis (*placken* means "patch"). The same word is also used to describe the accumulation of a different kind of deposits on teeth, which promote dental caries.

aneurysm (AN-you-rism) the ballooning out of an artery wall at a point that is weakened by deterioration.

aorta (ay-OR-tuh) the large, primary artery that conducts blood from the heart to the body's smaller arteries.

platelets tiny cell-like fragments in the blood, important in blood clot formation (*platelet* means "little plate").

Healthy People 2000: Reduce coronary heart disease deaths to no more than 100 per 100,000 people.

Chapter 5 described the effects of omega-6 and omega-3 fatty acids on heart health and identified some food sources of each.

FIGURE 11-4

THE FORMATION OF PLAQUES IN ATHEROSCLEROSIS

When plaques have covered 60 percent of the coronary artery walls, the critical phase of heart disease begins.

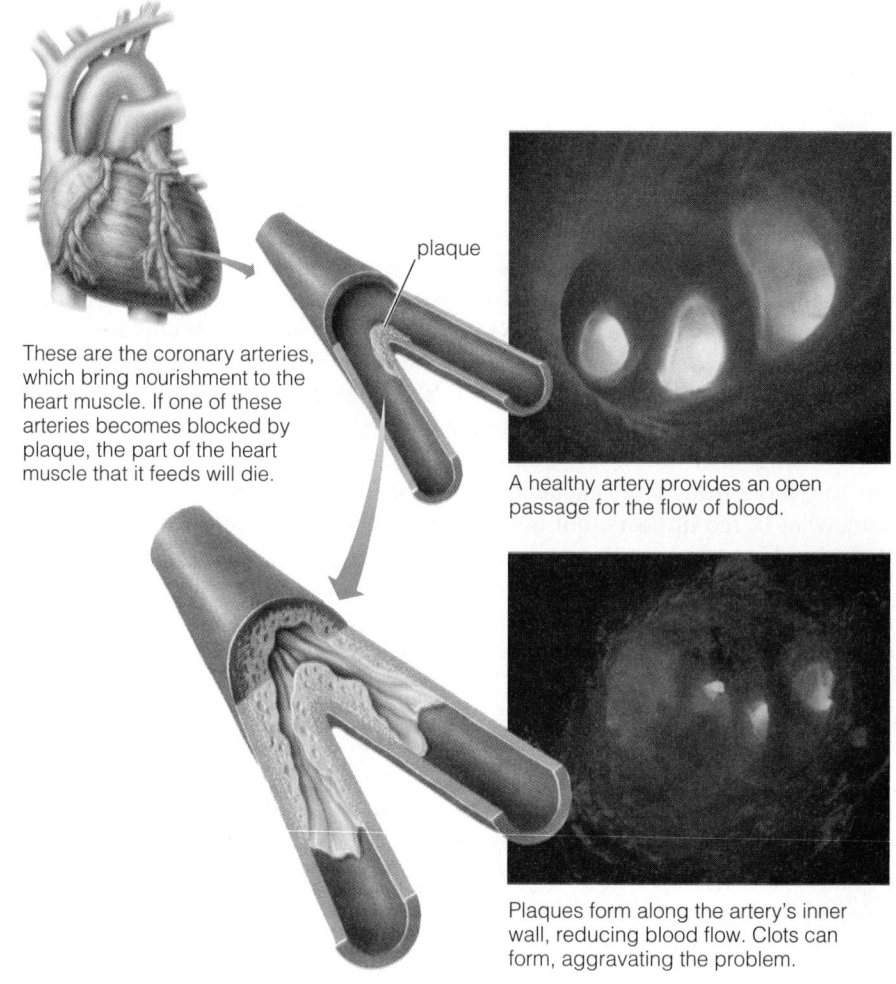

These are the coronary arteries, which bring nourishment to the heart muscle. If one of these arteries becomes blocked by plaque, the part of the heart muscle that it feeds will die.

plaque

A healthy artery provides an open passage for the flow of blood.

Plaques form along the artery's inner wall, reducing blood flow. Clots can form, aggravating the problem.

thrombus a stationary clot.

thrombosis a thrombus that has grown enough to close off a blood vessel. A *coronary thrombosis* is the closing off of a vessel that feeds the heart muscle. A *cerebral thrombosis* is the closing off of a vessel that feeds the brain (*coronary* means "crowning" [the heart]; *thrombo* means "clot"; the cerebrum is part of the brain).

embolus (EM-boh-luss) a thrombus that breaks loose (*embol* means "to insert").

embolism an embolus that causes sudden closure of a blood vessel.

tissue may die slowly and be replaced by nonfunctional scar tissue. The stationary clot is called a **thrombus.** When it has grown large enough to close off a blood vessel, it is a **thrombosis.** A clot can also break loose, becoming an **embolus,** and travel along the system until it reaches an artery too small to allow its passage. Then the tissues fed by this artery will be robbed of oxygen and nutrients and will die suddenly **(embolism).** Such a clot can lodge in an artery of the heart, causing sudden death of part of the heart muscle, a **heart attack.** The clot may also lodge in an artery of the brain, killing a portion of brain tissue, a **stroke.**

On many occasions heart attacks and strokes occur with no apparent blockage. An artery may go into spasms, restricting or cutting off the blood supply to a portion of the heart muscle or brain. Much research today is devoted to finding out what causes plaques to form, what causes arteries to go into spasms, what governs the activities of platelets, and why the body allows clots to form unopposed by clot-dissolving cleanup activity.

Hypertension worsens atherosclerosis. A stiffened artery, already strained by each pulse of blood surging through it, is still more stressed by high internal pressure. Injuries multiply, more plaques grow, and more weakened vessels become likely to burst and bleed.

Atherosclerosis also worsens hypertension. Since hardened arteries cannot expand, the heart's beats raise the blood pressure. Hardened arteries also fail to let blood flow freely through the kidneys, which control blood pressure. The kidneys sense the reduced flow of blood and respond as if the blood pressure were too low; they take steps to raise it further (see "How Hypertension Develops," later in the chapter).

✔ KEY POINT **Plaques of atherosclerosis induce hypertension and trigger abnormal blood clotting, leading to heart attacks or strokes. Abnormal vessel spasms can also cause heart attacks and strokes.**

Risk Factors for CVD

Table 11-4 lists the risk factors for CVD. Most people reaching middle age exhibit at least one of these factors, and many have several factors silently increasing their risks of CVD.[15] Figure 11-5 shows how rates of heart attacks for both men and women rise with the number of risk factors. It befits a nutrition book to focus on dietary strategies to reduce these risks. It should be noted, though, that diet is not the only, and perhaps not even the most important, factor in CVD causation. Still, as more people adopt dietary and other lifestyle habits to reduce their risks, the choices seem to be paying off. Since 1960, both blood cholesterol and CVD mortality have shown continuous downward trends.[16]

The big *diet-related* risk factors for CVD are glucose intolerance and obesity (subjects of Chapters 4 and 9), high blood cholesterol (discussed next), and hypertension (discussed after cholesterol). In diabetes, blood vessels often become blocked and circulation diminishes. More than 80 percent of people with diabetes die of CVD, usually from heart attacks. A woman with diabetes faces double the normal risk of heart attack death.[17] Even people without diabetes whose insulin values are high may face an elevated risk of heart disease.[18] About a third of middle-aged men may have a type of insulin resistance

heart attack the event in which the vessels that feed the heart muscle become closed off by an embolism, thrombus, or other cause with resulting sudden tissue death. A heart attack is also called a *myocardial infarction* (*myo* means "muscle"; *cardial* means "of the heart"; *infarct* means "tissue death").

stroke the sudden shutting off of the blood flow to the brain by a thrombus, embolism, or the bursting of a vessel (hemorrhage).

TABLE 11-4

CVD Risk Factors

- Smoking
- Hypertension
- High LDL cholesterol
- Low HDL cholesterol
- Obesity, especially central obesity, as described in Chapter 9[a]
- Glucose intolerance (diabetes)
- Lack of exercise[a]
- Heredity (history of CVD in family members younger than age 55 for males, 65 for females)
- Male gender (after age 45)
- Menopause in women

[a]The American Heart Association includes these factors; other organizations consider them to be contributors to other risk factors.

FIGURE 11-5

RISK FACTORS FOR HEART ATTACKS
This graph shows how the risk of heart disease rises dramatically in people who have high cholesterol, have high blood pressure, and/or smoke cigarettes. In the graph, "high cholesterol" is 260 or above, and "high blood pressure" is 150 or above (systolic pressure—the first figure in a blood pressure reading).

SOURCE: Framingham Heart Study. Personal communication, Thomas Thom, National Heart, Lung and Blood Institute.

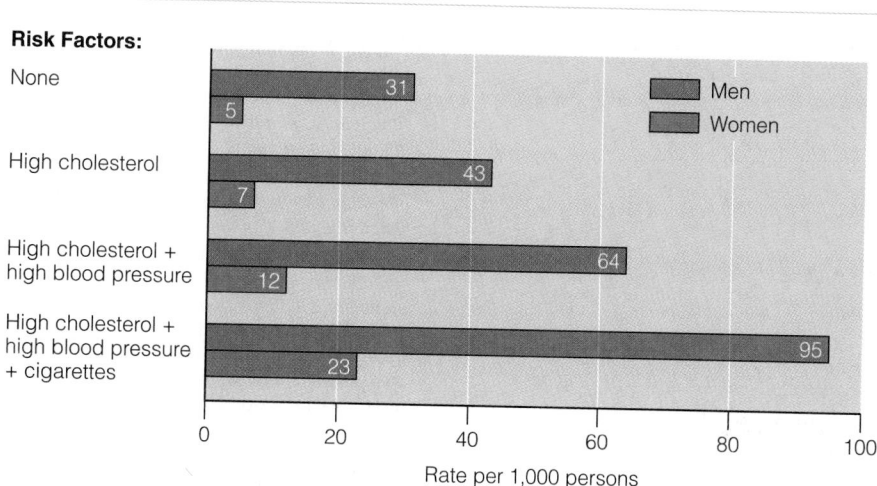

Risk Factors:

None — Men 31, Women 5
High cholesterol — Men 43, Women 7
High cholesterol + high blood pressure — Men 64, Women 12
High cholesterol + high blood pressure + cigarettes — Men 95, Women 23

Rate per 1,000 persons

that puts them at risk for heart attack.[19] When tested, the men's cholesterol values are within the normal range, but heart disease is still progressing. Without high cholesterol to warn them, the men take no steps to prevent the coming heart attacks. Whether such insulin resistance elevates risks for women is unknown.

Table 11-5 shows the standards by which blood lipids, blood pressure, and obesity are evaluated. Almost half of all deaths from CVD occur among men with blood cholesterol in the borderline-high range, so clearly only the lowest values, if any, are "safe." The moral of the story: everyone, even those with normal cholesterol values, should take seriously diet and exercise advice for reducing CVD risk.

As for triglycerides, this measurement is often elevated in people with CVD. By themselves, elevated triglycerides are not considered causal in CVD, but in

TABLE 11-5

U.S. Standards for CVD Risk Factors

Blood Pressure	Obesity
Diastolic pressure:[a] 85 or lower = normal. 85 to 89 = high normal. 90 to 99 = mild hypertension. 100 to 109 = moderate hypertension. 110 to 119 = severe hypertension. 120 or higher = very severe hypertension.	Body mass index: Men: greater than 27.8. Women: greater than 27.3.

Total Cholesterol	HDL and LDL
Below 200 mg/dL = desirable. 200 to 239 mg/dL = borderline high.[b] 240 mg/dL or higher = high.	HDL: 35 mg/dL or lower indicates risk.[c] LDL to HDL ratio above 5 for men or above 4.5 for women indicates risk.

LDL Cholesterol	Triglycerides (Fasting)[d]
Below 130 mg/dL = desirable. 130 to 159 mg/dL = borderline high. 160 mg/dL or higher = high.	Above 200 mg/dL may indicate risk in those with other risk factors (see text).

[a]The diastolic pressure is the lower of the two numbers in the blood pressure reading—for example, the 70 in 105/70; recently, systolic pressure has also been identified as predictive of heart attack and stroke.

[b]210–215 = average (U.S.).

[c]According to the 1993 NIH consensus conference on triglyceride, high-density lipoprotein, and CHD, this value may be too low for women; no alternative value has yet been proposed.

[d]High triglycerides do not normally indicate direct risk, but may reflect lipoprotein abnormalities associated with CVD. High triglycerides also occur in conditions such as kidney disease and diabetes, which suggest a high CVD risk.

SOURCES: Blood lipid standards adapted from summary of the second report of the National Cholesterol Education Program (NCEP), Expert Panel on Detection, Evaluation, and Treatment of High Blood Cholesterol in Adults (Adult Treatment Panel), *Journal of the American Medical Association* 269 (1993): 3015–3023. Hypertension standards adapted from the fifth report of the Joint National Committee on Detection, Evaluation, and Treatment of High Blood Pressure, National High Blood Pressure Education Program, National Heart, Lung, and Blood Institute, National Institutes of Health , October 30, 1992, p. 5.

association with other risk factors, elevated triglycerides may accelerate atherosclerosis and clotting activity while slowing clot destruction in the blood. To people with other risk factors for CVD, such as diabetes, central obesity, artery disease, hypertension, or kidney disease, triglyceride measures become meaningful.[20]

Other factors now beginning to take on importance in CVD research are the antioxidant nutrients, such as vitamin E. Detailed information about these was presented in Controversy 7.

The Significance of Blood Cholesterol   High *blood* cholesterol, particularly when the ratio of LDL to HDL is high, predicts CVD. Generally, cholesterol carried in LDL correlates *directly* with risk of heart disease, whereas that carried in HDL correlates *inversely* with risk (see Figure 11-6).[21] High total cholesterol generally reflects elevated LDL. Even in young men, high cholesterol seems to correlate strongly with high heart disease risks as they get older.[22] A population whose average blood cholesterol is 10 percent lower than another population's will suffer one-third less CVD; a 30 percent difference in blood cholesterol predicts a CVD rate that is four times lower.[23]

Diet and Blood Cholesterol   Now, how does *diet* relate to high blood cholesterol? In two ways: first, a diet high in saturated fat contributes to high blood cholesterol, and second, reducing the saturated fat in the diet lowers blood cholesterol and may reduce the rate of CVD.

Worldwide, generally, wherever diets are high in saturated fat and low in fish, fruits, and vegetables, blood cholesterol is high and heart disease takes a great toll on health and life.[24] Conversely, wherever dietary fat consists mostly of monounsaturated fats with abundant fish, fruits, and vegetables, blood cholesterol and the rate of death from heart disease are low.

The bulk of research supports the idea that lowering saturated fat intakes will lead to lower blood cholesterol and reduced heart disease risks.[25] Most authorities agree that for people living in the United States and Canada, the percentage of calories from saturated fat in the diet should be no more than 10 percent.[26]

Recommendations for U.S. and Canadian citizens also urge that total fat be held to no more than 30 percent of calories, and that the cholesterol intake from food be limited to 300 milligrams a day. These measures may be important for some people, but perhaps not for all. The links between intakes of dietary fat, dietary cholesterol, and high blood cholesterol are not as firm as the links between saturated fat, blood cholesterol, and CVD. Data on the people of Mediterranean countries illustrate that diets high in total fat can coexist with low rates of heart disease so long as the diet is rich in fish, fruits, and vegetables and the fat is of the monounsaturated type (Controversy 2 provided details).[27]

On the other hand, most people in this country eat diets rich in meats and hydrogenated fats, so if they reduce the *total* fat in their diets, the *saturated* fat may be significantly reduced as well. Table 11-6 presents diet adjustments to lower blood cholesterol in two steps. Step 1 is to reduce risk in everyone over age 2 years; step 2 is for people with high risks or already-diagnosed CVD.

Previous chapters have already mentioned other dietary factors that can lower blood cholesterol, including the fibers of cereals, fruits, legumes, and other vegetables.[28] Omega-3 fatty acids also seem to play a role, as they do in

FIGURE 11-6

LDL TO HDL RATIO AND RISK OF HEART DISEASE

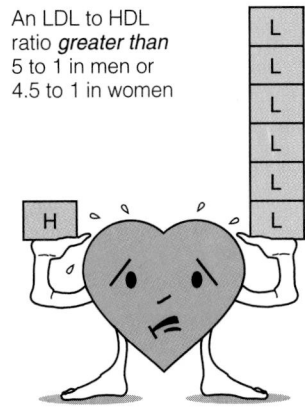

An LDL to HDL ratio *greater than* 5 to 1 in men or 4.5 to 1 in women

Increased risk of heart disease

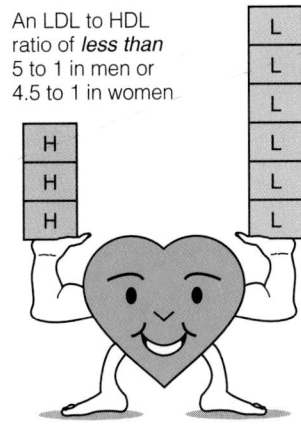

An LDL to HDL ratio of *less than* 5 to 1 in men or 4.5 to 1 in women

Reduced risk of heart disease

LDL and HDL were described in Chapter 5.

More about the Mediterranean diet in Controversy 2; food sources of saturated fat were listed in Chapter 5.

TABLE 11-6

LDL-Lowering Diet

	Step 1	Step 2
Energy	Energy should be adequate to achieve or maintain desirable weight in both step 1 and step 2.	
Total fat[a]	<30%	<30%
Saturated fat[a]	8–10%	<7%
Polyunsaturated fat[a]	<10%	<10%
Monounsaturated fat[a]	10–15%	10–15%
Cholesterol	<300 mg/day	<200 mg/day

[a]Fat amounts are expressed as percentages of total food energy, assuming energy intake is adequate to achieve and maintain desirable weight.

SOURCE: Adapted from The Expert Panel, Summary of the second report of the National Cholesterol Education Program (NCEP) Expert Panel on Detection, Evaluation, and Treatment of High Blood Cholesterol in Adults (Adult Treatment Panel II), *Journal of the American Medical Association* 269 (1993): 3015–3023.

Controversy 7 explores the link between disease risks and antioxidant nutrients and phytochemicals in foods.

helping prevent blood clots. With weight loss in the overweight, heart disease risk factors improve: blood pressure falls and blood lipid values decline.[29] Researchers are hopeful that the vitamin folate, along with vitamin B$_6$ and B$_{12}$, may also turn out to fight heart disease. These vitamins play roles in clearing from the blood an amino acid derivative* that scientists suspect may promote both the plaques of atherosclerosis and blood clots.[30] Also, a diet that includes foods rich in antioxidant nutrients such as vitamin E and phytochemicals—that is, one based upon legumes, vegetables, and fruits—repeatedly turns up in research as related to low risk for CVD and many other diseases.

Many aspects of life probably affect heart health but the focus of this section was on blood cholesterol. To return to the main points: (1) high blood cholesterol indicates a risk of heart disease, and (2) it is possible to lower blood cholesterol, in part, by controlling dietary saturated fat. If people lower their blood cholesterol, they will reduce their risk of heart disease.

✔ **KEY POINT** **Dietary measures to reduce fat, saturated fat, and cholesterol intakes are part of the first line of treatment for high blood cholesterol. Diets rich in fruits and vegetables are also important.**

Other Strategies for Reducing Risk of CVD

Diet alone may not be enough to reduce CVD risk. Physical activity can amplify a low-fat diet's benefits, and moderation in alcohol use may also play a role.

Physical Activity In addition to diet, some types of exercise are effective in lowering LDL and raising HDL concentrations. *Aerobic* exercise in particular, when combined with a low-fat diet, may help to reverse atherosclerosis. Some forms of weight training, if undertaken regularly, may also elevate blood HDL concentrations somewhat. If consistently pursued, even light exercise, such as

*The factor is homocysteine, derived from the amino acid methionine.

walking and gardening at intervals throughout the day, improves the odds against heart disease considerably.

The beneficial effects of exercise are manifold. In addition to helping normalize blood lipids, regular exercise can strengthen the heart and blood vessels, alter body composition in favor of lean over fat tissue, lower blood pressure, improve insulin response, and expand the volume of blood the heart can pump to the tissues at each beat and so reduce the heart's workload. Physical activity also stimulates development of new arteries to nourish the heart muscle, and this may be a factor in the excellent recovery seen in some heart attack victims who exercise. These changes are so beneficial that some experts believe that physical activity should be the primary focus of cardiovascular disease prevention efforts.[31]

Both exercise itself and the weight loss it induces raise HDL concentrations, and the effects of these two factors are additive. If exercise also brings about reduction of central obesity, the result is exceptionally beneficial.[32] Many experts think central obesity is the most important single determinant of CVD risk.[33]

Diet helps a little, physical activity helps more, and the combination is better still. People in a clinical setting have been able to reduce plaque buildup in their arteries by following a strict plan combining an extremely low-fat vegan diet (less than 10 percent of calories from fat), no smoking, stress management, and exercise.[34] Without this program, atherosclerosis would likely have progressed; instead, it regressed and did so without the use of lipid-lowering drugs. Some people do not respond favorably to such lifestyle changes, however, and for them, medication to bring their cholesterol values into line with recommendations can be life-saving.

Alcohol Consumption People ask whether moderate alcohol intakes may reduce CVD risk. When moderate drinkers (one or two drinks a day with no binge drinking) are compared with alcohol abstainers, the moderate drinkers have a reduced incidence of heart disease. Moderate alcohol intakes seem to elevate a form of HDL in the blood and reduce the blood's tendency to clot.[35] These benefits are most apparent in people over age 50, in those with one or more risk factors, and in those with elevated LDL cholesterol values.[36]

Heavy alcohol use and abuse is known to elevate blood pressure, to damage the heart muscle, and to have many other deleterious effects on the body's organs. More details about all of these effects are in this chapter's Controversy. Heavy drinking (three or more drinks a day) also increases the risk of death from other causes.[37] A later section in this chapter describes its link with cancer.

Other Strategies Drug therapy brings benefits in terms of lowering blood cholesterol, but it also presents risks and side effects that accumulate during years of therapy.[38] Cholesterol-lowering drugs seem to work best in association with other efforts, such as diet and exercise.

Periodically, the media repopularize the idea that the vitamin niacin can lower blood cholesterol. Experimentally, pharmaceutical doses of a form of niacin act like a drug in lowering blood cholesterol and prolonging life, but other drugs effective for this purpose have fewer side effects.[39] Ordinary niacin supplements are useless in lowering blood cholesterol, and high doses may sometimes cause side effects such as skin flushing, abnormal liver function, and some symptoms of diabetes.

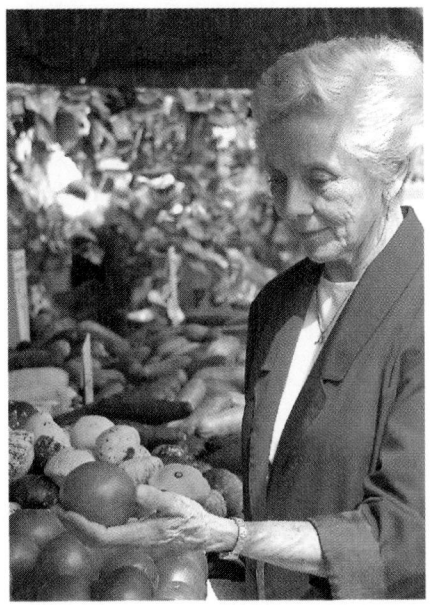

When diets are rich in vegetables and fruits, life expectancies are long.

Obesity worsens many disease risks (Chapter 9). Chapter 10 specified exercise guidelines for health.

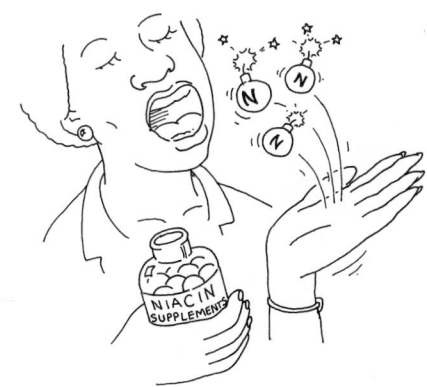

High doses of niacin may cause unexpected side effects.

systolic (sis-TOL-ik) **pressure** the first figure in a blood pressure reading (the "dub" of the heartbeat), which reflects arterial pressure caused by the contraction of the heart's left ventricle.

diastolic (dye-as-TOL-ik) **pressure** the second figure in a blood pressure reading (the "lub" of the heartbeat), which reflects the arterial pressure when the heart is between beats.

While diet and exercise are not the easy route to heart health that everyone hopes for, the combination is powerful for improving health. Weight control may not lower blood cholesterol, but it may reduce blood pressure (see the next section). So will eating a low-fat, restricted-cholesterol, high–complex carbohydrate diet with lots of fruits and vegetables. And even if the high–complex carbohydrate diet does not help by way of lowering cholesterol or blood pressure, it will help by normalizing blood glucose (diabetes). Remember, diabetes is a major risk factor for CVD. A meal of fish each week may help by favoring the right fatty acid balance so that clot formation is unlikely. The pattern of protection from the recommended diet and exercise regimen becomes clear—the effects of each small choice add to the beneficial whole. While you are at it, don't smoke. Relax. Meditate or pray. Play. Happy people have lower blood cholesterol levels.

✔ **KEY POINT** **Physical activity can reduce CVD risk. Moderate alcohol intake is also associated with reduced risk, but its use can be problematic.**

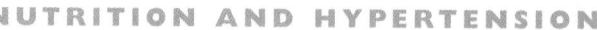

NUTRITION AND HYPERTENSION

Low blood pressure is generally a sign of long life expectancy and low heart disease risk, unless it is extreme. High blood pressure, in contrast, threatens to impair the quality of your life and even strike you down before your time. Chronic high blood pressure, or hypertension, remains one of the most prevalent forms of cardiovascular disease, affecting almost a quarter of the entire U.S. adult population.[40] It contributes to half a million strokes and to over a million heart attacks each year. The higher above normal the blood pressure, the greater the risk of heart disease. Paired with atherosclerosis, as it often is, hypertension is especially threatening.

You cannot tell if you have high pressure; it presents no symptoms you can feel. Because it is so prevalent, the most effective single step you can take toward protecting yourself from hypertension is to find out whether you have it. At checkup time, a health-care professional can take an accurate resting blood pressure reading. Self-test machines in drugstores and other places are often inaccurate. If your resting blood pressure is above normal, the reading should be repeated before confirming the diagnosis of hypertension. Thereafter it should be checked at regular intervals.

When blood pressure is measured, two numbers are important: the pressure during contraction of the heart's ventricles (large pumping chambers) and the pressure during their relaxation. The numbers are given as a fraction, with the top number representing the **systolic pressure** (ventricular contraction) and the bottom number the **diastolic pressure** (relaxation). Return to Table 11-5 to see how to interpret your resting diastolic pressure.

Resting blood pressure should ideally be 120 over 80 or lower, but less than 140 over 90 is also considered normal. Above this level the risks of heart attacks and strokes increase in direct proportion to increasing blood pressure.

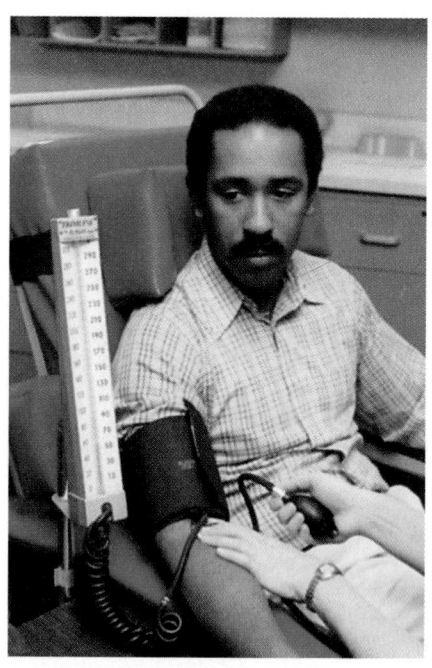

The most effective single step you can take against hypertension is to learn your own blood pressure.

✔ **KEY POINT** **Hypertension is silent, progressively worsens atherosclerosis, and makes heart attacks and strokes likely. All adults should know their blood pressure.**

How Hypertension Develops

Blood pressure is vital to life. It pushes the blood through the major arteries into smaller arteries and finally into tiny capillaries whose thin walls permit exchange of fluids between the blood and the tissues (see Figure 11-7). When the pressure is right, the cells receive a constant supply of nutrients and oxygen and can release their wastes.

The Role of the Kidneys   The kidneys depend on the blood pressure to help them filter waste materials out of the blood into the urine. (The pressure has to be high enough to force the blood's fluid out of the capillaries into the kidneys' filtering networks.) If the blood pressure is too low, the kidneys set in motion actions to increase it; they send hormones to constrict the peripheral blood vessels and bring about the retention of water and salt in the body.

Dehydration sets these actions in motion, and in this case they are beneficial because when the blood volume is low, higher blood pressure is needed to deliver substances to the tissues. By constricting the blood vessels and conserving water and sodium, the kidneys ensure that normal blood pressure is maintained until the dehydrated person can drink water. As mentioned in an earlier section, atherosclerosis also sets this process in motion, however, and this is not beneficial. By obstructing blood vessels, atherosclerosis fools the kidneys: they react as if there were a water deficiency. The kidneys raise the blood

FIGURE 11-7

THE BLOOD PRESSURE

Three major factors contribute to the pressure inside an artery. For one, the heart pushes blood into the artery. For another, the small-diameter arteries and capillaries at the other end resist the blood's flow (peripheral resistance). Third, the volume of fluid in the circulatory system, which depends on the number of dissolved particles in that fluid, adds pressure.

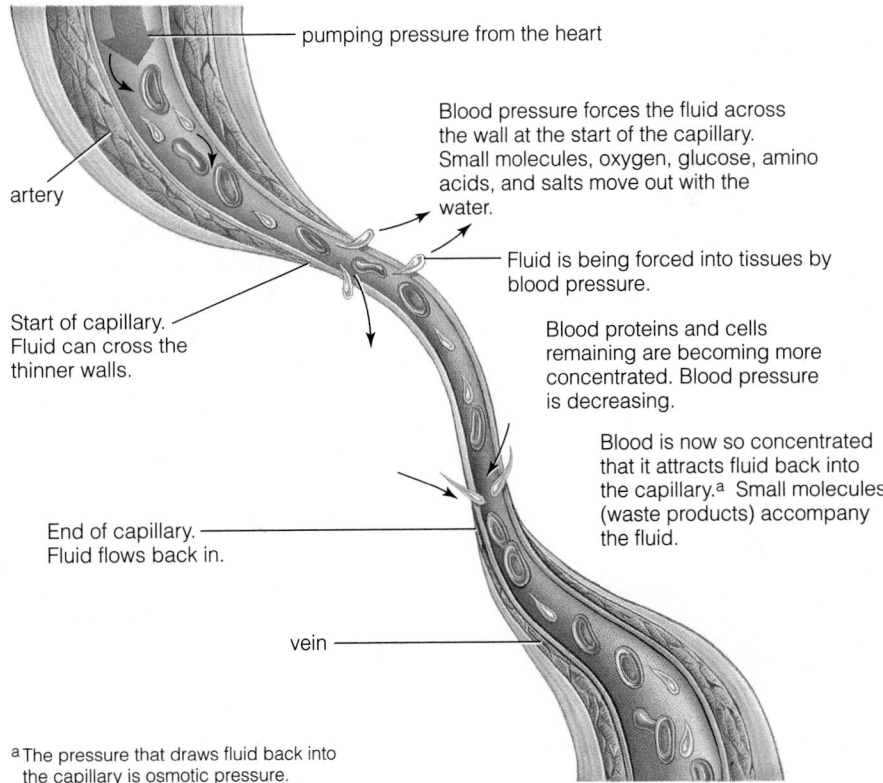

pumping pressure from the heart

Blood pressure forces the fluid across the wall at the start of the capillary. Small molecules, oxygen, glucose, amino acids, and salts move out with the water.

artery

Fluid is being forced into tissues by blood pressure.

Start of capillary. Fluid can cross the thinner walls.

Blood proteins and cells remaining are becoming more concentrated. Blood pressure is decreasing.

Blood is now so concentrated that it attracts fluid back into the capillary.[a] Small molecules (waste products) accompany the fluid.

End of capillary. Fluid flows back in.

vein

[a] The pressure that draws fluid back into the capillary is osmotic pressure.

pressure high enough so that they will get the blood they need, but in the process they may make the pressure too high for the arteries and heart to withstand. Hypertension also aggravates atherosclerosis by mechanically injuring the artery linings, making plaques likely to form; plaques restrict blood flow to the kidneys; this may raise the blood pressure still further; and the problem snowballs.

The Roles of Risk Factors   Primary among the risk factors that precipitate or aggravate hypertension are atherosclerosis, obesity, and insulin resistance (which leads to type II diabetes). These conditions cluster together frequently and put a severe strain on the heart and arteries, leading to many forms of cardiovascular disease.[41] Excess adipose tissue means miles of extra capillaries through which the blood must be pumped. Strain on the heart's pump, the left ventricle, can enlarge and weaken it, until it finally fails (heart failure). Pressure in the aorta may cause it to balloon out and burst (aneurysm). Pressure in the small arteries of the brain may make them burst and bleed (hemorrhage, a form of stroke). The kidneys can also be damaged when the heart cannot pump enough blood through them (kidney failure). Fluid may then accumulate in the body, straining the heart further and making it hard to breathe (congestive heart failure).

Epidemiological studies have identified several other risk factors that predict hypertension. One is age: people who develop hypertension do so in their 50s and 60s. Another is heredity: a family history of hypertension and heart disease raises the risk of developing hypertension two to five times, and people of African-American descent are likely to develop more severe hypertension, and earlier in life, than those of European or Asian descent. Other, perhaps unidentified environmental factors in the United States may also favor its development, because African Americans living in the United States have higher rates than Africans living in Africa.[42] Hypertension has also been observed to bear some relation to insulin resistance, and measures to prevent diabetes no doubt also protect against hypertension.

The rate of hypertension has been rising steadily over the past four decades.[43] While researchers continue looking for the cause or causes, clearly it is urgent to do what we can to prevent it. Failing in that, we must make every effort to detect and treat it. Even mild hypertension can be dangerous; but individuals who are treated are less likely to suffer illness or early death.

✔ KEY POINT   **Atherosclerosis, obesity, insulin resistance, age, family background, and race contribute to hypertension risks. Prevention and treatment both deserve high-priority effort.**

Nutrition in Hypertension Prevention and Treatment

Some people need blood pressure medications to bring their pressure down, but diet and exercise alone can bring improvements for many. For some, both drugs and diet and exercise are suggested at first until some progress has been made; then the drugs can be stopped. This section focuses on diet.

Salt (Sodium) and Prevention   The benefit from reducing salt intake in *treatment* of hypertension is not questioned. For about half of people with hypertension a reduction of blood pressure accompanies a lower salt (or sodium) intake.

As for diet in *prevention* of hypertension, there is less agreement, but many professionals and agencies believe that enough evidence is available to warrant a recommendation for everyone to moderately restrict salt intake (Chapter 8 showed how). They reason that, at worst, such a diet cannot be harmful.

As mentioned, salt (or sodium) plays a large role in about half of all hypertension cases, that is, in those who are sensitive to its effects. Most likely to be salt sensitive are people with chronic renal disease, those whose parents (one or both) have hypertension, African Americans, and persons over 50 years of age. For these people, salt avoidance prevents hypertension. For the other half of all people with hypertension, other nutrition-related factors are important, most notably, obesity and alcohol abuse. Lack of exercise and some dietary factors other than salt also play roles. A blanket recommendation for prevention of hypertension, then, would center on weight control, exercise, and reduced intakes of alcohol and salt.

Details concerning sodium, salt-sensitivity, and hypertension were presented in Chapter 8.

Weight Control and Exercise These factors are important in both prevention and treatment. For people who are obese and hypertensive, a weight loss of as little as 10 pounds may significantly lower blood pressure.[44] Those who are using drugs to control their blood pressure can often cut down their doses if they lose weight.[45]

Moderate physical activity helps in weight loss and also helps to reduce hypertension directly.[46] The right kind of physical activity, regularly undertaken, can lower blood pressure in almost everyone, even in those without hypertension.[47] The "right kind" of activity is the same kind observed to increase blood HDL and lower LDL, that is, the aerobic kind recommended for cardiovascular endurance (Chapter 10 provides details). Physical activity also changes the hormonal climate in which the body does its work. It reduces stress, and thereby stress hormone secretion, and this lowers blood pressure. It redistributes body water, and it eases transit of the blood through the peripheral arteries.

Alcohol In moderate doses, alcohol initially relaxes the peripheral arteries and so reduces blood pressure, but high doses clearly raise blood pressure. Hypertension is common among people with alcoholism. The hypertension is apparently caused directly by the alcohol, and it leads to cardiovascular disease, the same as hypertension caused by any other factor. Furthermore, alcohol causes strokes—even *without* hypertension. The *Dietary Guidelines* urge moderation for those who drink alcohol. *Moderation* means no more than a drink a day for women, or two drinks a day for men, an amount that seems safe relative to blood pressure.[48]

Other Nutrients Other dietary factors may help to regulate blood pressure.[49] Adequate diet certainly is one: evidence for calcium's reducing blood pressure in normal people as well as in those with hypertension has been called "compelling."[50] Adequate potassium* and magnesium also appear to help prevent and treat hypertension in certain populations. Similarly, vitamin C adequacy seems to help normalize blood pressure, while vitamin C deficiency may tend to raise it. Other dietary factors may affect blood pressure in

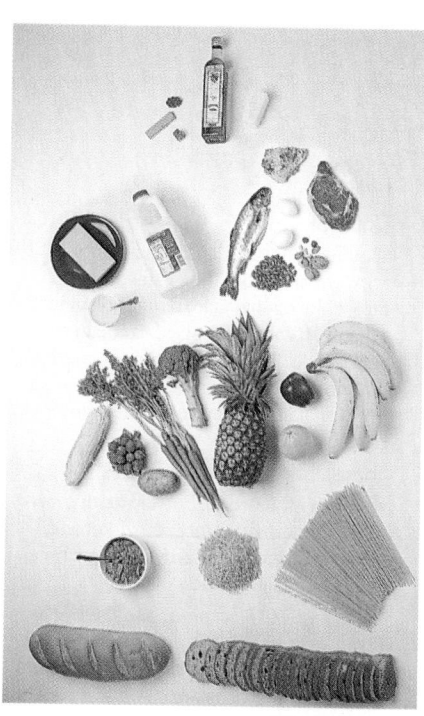

Simple advice can be powerful. Think Food Guide Pyramid.

---

*People using diuretics to control hypertension should know that some cause potassium excretion and can induce a deficiency. Those using these drugs must be particularly careful to include rich sources of potassium in their daily diets.

cancer a disease in which cells multiply out of control and disrupt normal functioning of one or more organs.

carcinogen (car-SIN-oh-jen) a cancer-causing substance (*carcin* means "cancer"; *gen* means "gives rise to").

initiation an event, probably in the cell's genetic material, caused by radiation or by a chemical carcinogen that can give rise to cancer.

promoters factors that do not initiate cancer but speed up its development once initiation has taken place.

Selected chemicals and carcinogens occurring naturally in breakfast foods:

Coffee:

acetaldehyde, acetic acid, acetone, atractylosides, butanol, cafestol palmitate, chlorogenic acid, dimethyl sulfide, ethanol, furan, furfural, guaiacol, hydrogen sulfide, isoprene, methanol, methyl butanol, methyl formate, methyl glyoxal, propionaldehyde, pyridine, 1,3,7-trimethylxanthine.

Toast and coffee cake:

acetic acid, acetone, butyric acid, caprionic acid, ethyl acetate, ethyl ketone, ethyl lactate, methyl ethyl ketone, propionic acid, valeric acid.

NOTE: Although some of the chemicals listed here are known carcinogens, the body is equipped to handle them safely, so consuming coffee, toast, and coffee cake does not elevate a person's risk of developing cancer.

one way or another. Roles for cadmium, selenium, lead, caffeine, protein, and fat are currently under study. The Food Feature of this chapter provides more detail on dietary measures that help support normal blood pressure.

✔ **KEY POINT** **For most people, weight reduction, exercise, restricted alcohol use, and a diet that provides adequate nutrients work to keep blood pressure normal. For some, salt restriction is also required.**

NUTRITION AND CANCER

In this country, one out of every four people will eventually contract **cancer,** and an estimated 20 to 50 percent of these cancers are attributable to diet.[51] Dietary fat, alcohol, and excess calories are thought to be especially important in relation to cancer causation, but diet relates to cancer in several ways. It is important to get them all in perspective. Constituents in foods may be cancer causing, cancer promoting, or protective against cancer. Also, for the person who has cancer, diet can make a crucial difference in recovery.

Of course, nondiet factors are also important in relation to cancer. A very few cancers are genetic and will appear regardless of lifestyle choices. Other cancers are related to environmental factors other than diet, including smoking, sun exposure, and water and air pollution. To give some idea about the extent of these relationships, Table 11-7 lists some of the factors linked to particular kinds of cancers. The emphasis here is on diet, of course.

How Cancer Develops

The steps in cancer development are thought to be as follows:

1. Exposure to a **carcinogen.**
2. Entry of the carcinogen into a cell.
3. **Initiation.** The carcinogen probably alters the cell's genetic material somehow.
4. Acceleration by other carcinogens, called **promoters,** so that the cell begins to multiply out of control.
5. Disruption of normal body functions.

Researchers think that the first three steps, which culminate with initiation, are the key ones. Many people therefore believe that they should avoid eating all foods that contain carcinogens. This would be impossible, however, because most carcinogens occur naturally among thousands of other chemicals and nutrients the body needs. Luckily, the body is well equipped to deal with the minute amounts of carcinogens naturally occurring in foods.

Many people suspect food additives of being carcinogenic. However, food additives are held to strict standards, and no additive legally present in food can cause cancer. (Details concerning saccharin are found in Controversy 4.) Contaminants that enter foods by accident or toxins that arise naturally, on the other hand, may be powerful carcinogens, or they may be converted to carcinogens by the body's attempts to metabolize them.[52] Luckily, these constituents, both synthetic and naturally occurring, are present in foods in low enough doses that they are believed unlikely to pose any significant cancer risk to consumers.[53] Chapter 14 comes back to the topic of accidental industrial contamination of foods, but you should know now that legal pesticides, when

TABLE 11-7

Some Factors Associated with Cancer

Cancer Sites	Incidence Associated with:	Protective Effect Associated with:
Bladder cancer	Weak associations with coffee, artificial sweeteners, and alcohol; stronger associations with cigarette smoking, chlorinated drinking water	Fruits and vegetables, especially green and yellow ones
Breast cancer	High intakes of food energy and possibly alcohol; sedentary lifestyle; probably not associated with dietary fat	Fruits and vegetables, especially green and yellow ones; soybeans and soy products; physical activity
Cervical cancer	Folate deficiency	Adequate folate intake
Colorectal cancer	High intakes of fat (particularly saturated fat), meat, and alcohol (especially beer); low intakes of fiber, folate, and vegetables; inactivity	Vegetables; calcium, vitamin D, and dairy intake; whole grains and other fiber-rich foods; physical activity
Endometrial cancer	No dietary risk factors established; associated with estrogen therapy, obesity, hypertension, and diabetes (NIDDM)	
Esophageal and mouth cancers	High alcohol, tobacco, and especially combined use; use of preserved foods (such as pickles); low intakes of vitamins and minerals; high intakes of vitamin A supplements	
Liver cancer	Infection with hepatitis virus; high intakes of alcohol; iron overload or other toxicity	
Ovarian cancer	No dietary risk factors established; inversely correlated with oral contraceptive use	Fruits and vegetables, especially green
Pancreatic and lung cancer	No dietary risk factors established; correlated with cigarette smoking and air pollution	Fruits and vegetables, especially green and yellow ones
Prostate cancer	High intakes of fats, especially saturated fats from meats	Fruits and vegetables, especially green and yellow ones; soybeans; flax seed
Stomach cancer	High intakes of smoke- or salt-preserved foods (such as dried, salted fish); low intakes of fresh fruits and vegetables; possibly, infection with ulcer-causing bacteria	Fresh fruits and vegetables, especially tomatoes

NOTE: Findings based on epidemiological studies.

SOURCES: National Research Council, *Diet and Health: Implications for Reducing Chronic Disease Risk* (Washington, D.C.: National Academy Press, 1989), pp. 594–600; J. H. Weisburger, Nutritional approach to cancer prevention with emphasis on vitamins, antioxidants, and carotenoids, *American Journal of Clinical Nutrition* (supplement) 53 (1991): 226–237; R. G. Ziegler, Vegetables, fruits, and carotenoids and the risk of cancer, *American Journal of Clinical Nutrition* (supplement) 53 (1991): 251–259; Potential mechanisms for food-related carcinogens and anticarcinogens: A scientific status summary by the Institute of Food Technologists' Expert Panel on Food Safety and Nutrition, *Food Technology* 47 (1993): 105–118; D. J. Hunter and coauthors, Cohort studies of fat intake and the risk of breast cancer—a pooled analysis, *New England Journal of Medicine* 334 (1996): 356–361; E. Giovannucci and coauthors, Intake of carotenoids and retinol in relation to risk of prostate cancer, *Journal of the National Cancer Institute* 87 (1995): 1767–1776.

used according to established guidelines, are believed to pose few risks to healthy adults.[54] Prudence dictates, however, that consumers should wash produce thoroughly before cooking or eating it.

The incidence of certain cancers varies both by region and by racial group. For example, Japanese citizens develop more stomach cancers and fewer colon cancers than do U.S. citizens. When Japanese people move to the United States, however, their children develop both stomach and colon cancers at the same rates as do native-born U.S. children. Japan and the United States are both

FIGURE 11-8

NEW CASES OF CANCER
IN WOMEN, 1995

In 1995, 180,000 women were diagnosed
with breast cancer, which has been
rising steadily in incidence since 1940.
(About 55,000 women were diagnosed
with breast cancer in 1940.)

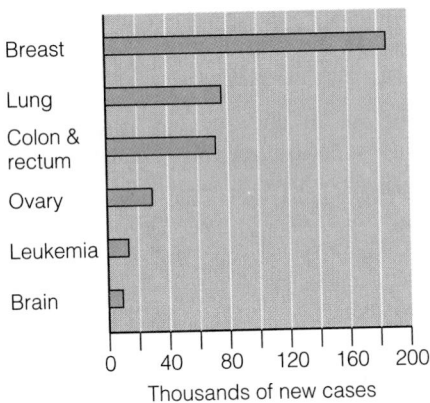

SOURCE: Data from American Cancer Society, *Cancer Facts and Figures—1996* (New York: National Media Office: American Cancer Society, 1995), pp. 7, 11.

industrial countries, and their environmental pollution rates are similar. Even so, something in the environment must account for the changed cancer pattern in immigrants, and an obvious candidate is diet. The traditional Japanese diet is rich in vegetables and low in fat, two characteristics of diets associated with low rates of colon cancer. The Japanese diet also contains many salted and pickled foods associated with stomach cancer. Traditional Japanese foods are not widely available in the United States, so immigrants largely adopt U.S.-style food choices.

Significantly, studies of populations suggest that low cancer rates correlate with high vegetable and grain intakes. Case-control studies, in which researchers can control some of the variables, support the population studies and implicate fat in cancer causation. A related finding is that vegetarians have lower mortality rates from cancer than the rest of the population, even when cancers linked to smoking and alcohol are taken out of the picture.

✓ **KEY POINT**   **Cancer develops in steps that include initiation and promotion, thought to be influenced by diet. The body is equipped to handle tiny doses of carcinogens that occur naturally in foods. Populations with high vegetable and grain intakes generally have low rates of cancer.**

Cancer and the Diet

From the evidence presented so far, it appears likely that diet affects cancer rates in the world's people both for the worse and for the better. The paragraphs that follow describe what is known about the effects of food constituents on cancer development. Later, this chapter's Consumer Corner addresses the marketing of products to consumers for cancer prevention and cure.

Fat and Fatty Acids   Laboratory studies using animals confirm suspicions that high fat intakes correlate with some forms of cancer. In human beings, diets high in fat and cholesterol associate positively with lung, prostate, and colon cancer risk and with the risk of developing precancerous lesions of the skin.[55] A diet high in meat, and therefore in fat, was recently associated with cancer of the lymph organs.[56] Overall, research indicates that breast cancer is probably unrelated to dietary fat.[57] An emerging explanation for rising breast cancer rates (see Figure 11-8) is that they are related to environmental pollutants, such as pesticides, that mimic estrogen in the body.[58]

Fat does not initiate the cancers. To get tumors started, an experimenter has to expose animals to a known carcinogen. After that exposure, the high-fat diet makes more cancers develop, and faster, than in animals fed low-fat diets. Thus fat appears to be a cancer promoter rather than an initiator. A high-fat diet may promote cancer in any of three ways. It may elicit the secretion of certain hormones that favor development of certain cancers. It may stimulate bile secretion, and organisms in the colon may then convert the bile into cancer-causing compounds. Or the fat may be incorporated into cell membranes and weaken their defenses against cancer-causing invaders.

It may not be fat in general but certain forms of fat that have these effects. The details from research can be hard to follow. For example, some findings point to linoleic acid, the essential omega-6 fatty acid of vegetable oils, as particularly implicated in promotion of cancer.[59] At the same time, a modified form of linoleic acid found only in food from animal sources seems protective against cancers.[60]* Importantly, it seems that omega-3 fatty acids from fish and monounsaturated fatty acids from olives and other sources may not promote cancer, and some preliminary evidence suggests they may protect against it.[61] In any case, moderation remains a sound principle concerning fat intakes.

Chapter 5's Food Feature offers suggestions for cutting fat from the diet, and Figure 5-5 shows the fatty acid breakdown of common fats.

Alcohol and Smoked Foods   Cancers of the head and neck seem to correlate best with the combination of alcohol and tobacco use and with low intakes of green and yellow fruits and vegetables. Alcohol intake alone is associated with cancers of the mouth, throat, and breast, and alcoholism often damages the liver and increases the risk of liver cancer. Controversy 11 comes back to the topic of alcoholic beverages and cancer risks.

Smoke generated from burning wood or charcoal, just like smoke from burning tobacco, is made up of a multitude of chemical substances, some of which initiate cancer.[†] Some carcinogens from smoke settle on food during cooking; some form when meat fats or added oils land on the coals and then vaporize, creating carcinogens that rise and stick to the food. Eating smoked, grilled, or charbroiled food introduces the carcinogens into the body, but once inside, the compounds are captured and detoxified by the body's competent detoxifying system. No studies to date link the eating of smoked or grilled foods with increased cancer risk. This is probably because detoxification speed up in the bodies of people who eat such foods and successfully defends them against the kinds of carcinogens produced.[62]

Food Energy   When calorie intakes are reduced, cancer rates fall. This **caloric effect** holds true regardless of the energy source; excess calories from carbohydrates, fat, or protein all raise cancer rates.[63] When researchers restrict the energy in laboratory animals' feed, the onset of cancer in the restricted animals is delayed beyond the time when animals on normal feed have died. At the moment, no experimental evidence exists showing this effect in human subjects, but some population observations seem to imply that the effect seen in animals may hold true for human beings as well.

The processes by which excess calories may promote cancer development remain obscure, but some researchers have a hunch that the hormones produced by the kidney's adrenal gland may be involved. High calorie intakes stimulate the release of these hormones, which cause inflammation, and inflammation stimulates the growth of tumors. Restricting energy intakes inhibits adrenal hormone release. Other theories about mechanisms also exist. Importantly, a high-calorie diet can potentiate the damaging actions of other carcinogens that may be present in the tissues, making the advice to consume diets moderate in energy particularly important.

Fiber   A diet with ample high-fiber foods also helps protect against some forms of cancer.[64] It may do so by promoting the excretion of bile from the body, by absorbing toxins and carrying them out of the body, or by generating beneficial hormone-like fragments within the colon. Whereas fiber is especially

---

*The linoleic compound referred to here is known by the acronym CLA for Conjugated (dienoic) Linoleic Acid.

†The carcinogens of greatest concern are some of those called polycyclic aromatic hydrocarbons.

important for preventing cancers of the colon, rectum, and possibly breast, some features of a high-fiber diet other than fiber itself may help fight other forms of cancer.[65] High-fiber diets that are also high in both fat and calories seem not to protect against cancer risks.

It may be that the source of fiber also plays a role. In a critical review of studies on high-fiber diets and colon cancer, one research group determined that colon cancer risk was reduced by 40 percent in people with high intakes of grains and vegetables.[66] Controversy 7 mentioned some phytochemicals that occur in these foods along with fiber; researchers are finding strong statistical associations between these constituents and cancer risks.

If a fat-rich, calorie-dense diet is implicated in causation of certain cancers and if a vegetable-rich diet is associated with prevention, then one would expect vegetarians to have a lower incidence of those cancers. They do, as the many studies cited in Controversy 6 have shown.

Folate and Other Vitamins   The vitamins E, C, and beta-carotene received close attention in Controversy 7, which included a section on their antioxidant roles and cancer-fighting effects. Other vitamins may fight against cancer in other ways, for example, as antipromoters. These include vitamins B_6 and B_{12} and pantothenic acid. Vitamin A regulates aspects of cell division and communication that go awry in cancer. It also helps to maintain the immune system.[67] Immune cells can often identify cancerous cells and destroy them before cancer can develop.

Folate is known to play a special role with respect to cervical cancer and may fight other cancers as well. Cervical cancer presents a major health threat for women worldwide.[68] In this country, 50,000 new cases of cervical cancer are diagnosed and many more cases of early precancerous changes known as cell dysplasia are treated each year. The underlying cause of this ailment is an often symptomless sexually transmitted virus, human papilloma virus (HPV), but inadequate dietary folate seems necessary for activation of the virus. For this reason alone, all sexually active women should attend to their folate needs. Many other reasons have appeared in previous chapters.

Calcium and Other Minerals   Some evidence suggests that a high-calcium diet may help to prevent colon cancer. In a large, long-term study, people who developed colon cancer were found to have consumed slightly less calcium and vitamin D than people who did not develop the cancer. Other studies attempting to confirm the finding have obtained mixed results, but when calcium intakes of populations are compared, the trend appears consistent. Populations consuming more calcium are seen to develop less colon cancer even after researchers subtract the effects of dietary fat out of their analysis.[69] In animal studies, calcium seems to protect the colon lining from some of the effects of a high-fat diet. These studies have not yet proved that dietary calcium prevents colon cancer, but with all the other points in calcium's favor, prudence dictates that everyone should arrange to meet calcium needs every day.

Other minerals are thought to play roles in cancer prevention, perhaps by helping antioxidant enzymes. These include zinc, iron, copper, selenium, and probably more.

Phytochemicals in Foods   More than 100 studies now confirm that the phytochemicals in plant foods play special roles in cancer resistance.[70] Not all of

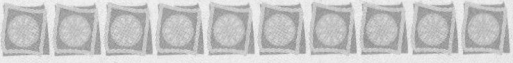

SOME FOODS CONTAINING PHYTOCHEMICALS UNDER STUDY FOR DISEASE PREVENTION

Get to know some of these players in the phytochemical game. The ones depicted in the photo appear in bold print in the list to the right.

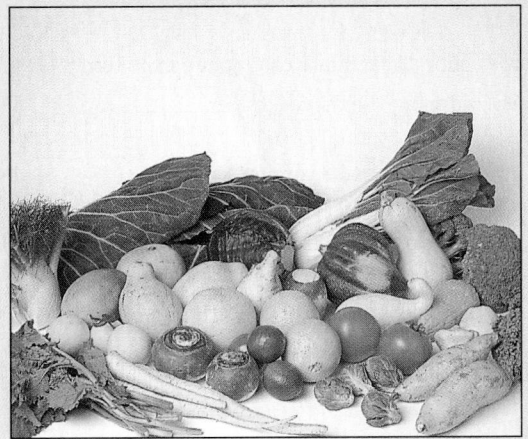

apricot, asparagus, barley, basil, berries, **bok choy, broccoli, broccoli rabe,** brown rice, **Brussels sprouts, cabbage** (all types), cantaloupe, carrots, cauliflower, celery, chives, **citrus fruit,** cucumber, **fennel,** flax seed, garlic, ginger, green onions, guava, **kale,** kohlrabi, **leafy greens, lemon,** lettuce (dark green), **mango,** oats, onion, orange, oregano, **papaya,** parsley, **parsnip,** potato (white), **rutabaga,** soybeans, soy products, spinach, **squash (winter), squash (summer), sweet potato,** tangerine, tarragon, tea (green and black), thyme, **tomato,** turmeric, **turnip roots,** whole wheat

the phytochemicals' effects have been pinned down as yet, nor can evidence on the specific chemicals be teased out of the evidence on foods themselves. A single tomato contains hundreds of phytochemicals, and tomato-based foods seem to be especially beneficial against prostate cancer, but no one knows exactly what chemical in tomatoes deserves the credit.[71]

Among the groups of phytochemicals active against cancer are beta-carotene's 50 or so relatives, the **carotenoids,** which are abundant in dark green and deep orange vegetables and fruits. Another group is the **flavonoids,** active antioxidants in vegetables, fruits, beverages such as tea and wine, and many herbs and spices.[72] Another class of possible anticancer compounds are the **protease inhibitors** found in soybeans, chick peas, lima beans, and potatoes. These are thought to inhibit enzymes associated with the spreading of tumors. Another group, the **phytosterols,** act like the hormones estrogen and progesterone in the human body; these occur abundantly in soybeans and soy products. One of them is **genistein,*** one of the most powerful antioxidants found in foods.[73]

Genistein is readily absorbed from foods. Combined with a protein, it travels in the bloodstream until cells that recognize it, such as those of the breast, prostate, brain, or uterus, selectively harvest it from the blood. Such cells can collect genistein because they are "estrogen-sensitive" cells, that is, they are equipped to recognize the hormone estrogen, and genistein chemically mimics estrogen. Genistein reduces mammary gland cancers in laboratory animals, and together with its chemical relatives also affect a woman's hormones in ways that may reduce her risk of breast cancer.[74]

At some concentrations, genistein acts just like estrogen, triggering rapid division in breast cancer cells in a laboratory dish. At higher levels, the opposite is true—it prevents cancer cell proliferation, as if it were an *anti*estrogen compound. From observations in Asian women, researchers are inclined to guess that genistein works both ways to confer estrogen's benefits, producing

protease inhibitors compounds that inhibit the action of protein-digesting enzymes.

---
*One of the isoflavones.

TABLE 11-8

Phytochemicals and Their Known Anticancer Effects

Phytochemicals and Their Effects		Known Food Sources
Allyl Sulfides	Trigger enzyme production to facilitate carcinogen excretion.	Chives, garlic, leeks, onions
Bioflavonoids	Acts as antioxidants, reducing the risk of cancer.	Fruits, oregano, spices, tea, vegetables, wine
Caffeic acid	Triggers enzyme production to make carcinogens water soluble facilitating excretion.	Fruits (blueberries, prunes, grapes), oats, soybeans
Capsaicin	Modulates blood clotting, possibly reducing the risk of fatal clots in heart and artery disease.	Hot peppers
Carotenoids[a] (including beta-carotene)	Acts as antioxidants, reducing the risk of cancer.	Deeply pigmented fruits and vegetables (carrots, sweet potatoes, tomatoes, spinach, broccoli, cantaloupe, pumpkin, apricots
Dithiolthiones	Probably protects against cancer.	Broccoli and other cruciferous vegetables, cauliflower, cabbage, brussels sprouts), horseradish, mustard greens
Ellegic acid	Scavenges carcinogens.	Grapes
Ferulic acid	Binds to nitrates in stomach, preventing the conversion to nitrosamines.	
Indoles[b]	Trigger enzymes to inhibit estrogen action, possibly reducing risk of breast cancer.	
Isothiocyanates	Trigger enzyme production to block carcinogen damage to cells' DNA.	
Lignans[c]	Block estrogen activity in cells, reducing the risk of breast, colon, ovarian, and prostate cancer.	
Limonene	Triggers enzyme production to facilitate carcinogen excretion.	Citrus fruits
Phenols	Inhibit lipid oxidation; block formation of carcinogenic nitrosamines in the body.	
Phytic acid	Binds to minerals, preventing cancer-causing free-radical formation.	Grains
Phytosterols[d]	Inhibit cell reproduction in GI tract, preventing colon cancer; posses estrogenic and antiestrogenic properties believed to reduce risks of breast cancer, ovarian cancer, and osteoporosis.	
Protease inhibitors	Suppress enzyme production in cancer cells, slowing tumor growth.	Soybeans, soy milk, tofu, other legumes and legume products, herbs, spices
Saponins	Interfere with DNA reproduction, preventing cancer cell multiplication; stimulate the immune response.	
Sulforaphane	Triggers enzyme production to block carcinogen damage to cells' DNA.	Broccoli and other cruciferous vegetables (cauliflower, cabbage, brussels sprouts), horseradish, mustard greens

[a]Other carotenoids include alpha-carotene, beta-cryptoxanthin, lectein, zeaxanthin, and lycopene.
[b]Indoles include dithiolthiones, isothiocyanates, sulforaphane, and others.
[c]Lignans are formed by colonic bacterial breakdown of lignin, a type of fiber.
[d]Phytosterols include phytoestrogens (one in genistein), phytoprogestin, and others.

low rates of osteoporosis and symptomatic menopause in Asian women, and also preventing estrogen-related cancers. Perhaps these diverse outcomes are a reflection of genistein's dual personality—its antiestrogenic and estrogenic nature. Geni-stein's anticancer effect may also be due in part to its antioxidant activity.

Table 11-8 identifies many other single phytochemicals and groups of them, credited with anticancer activity. Notice that these are only anti*cancer* compounds; other diseases are not included. Focus on the right-hand column, the food sources, and note what a tremendous argument they make for emphasizing plant foods in the diet. Note that they represent a great variety of foods. In no way could consumers ever combine dietary supplements into a feast like the one that plant foods provide.

Of course, ignoring this observation, many manufacturers have been trying to collect phytochemicals from foods and concentrate them into supplements they can sell. Presently on the market are broccoli extracts, spinach chemical pills, and vegetable or fruit pills and powders as supplements. Such products imply that they will deliver the nutrients and phytochemicals in many servings of vegetables, but fall far short—they contain just a few spoonfuls. Manufacturers have coined the term "nutraceuticals" to give the impression that the chemicals derived from foods not only can replace the foods that comprise a healthy diet, but also can act as drugs in disease treatment.

Commercial ventures also are creating "designer foods"—ordinary foods that carry extra-strength doses of one or another of the nutrients or phytochemicals. A problem concerning bioavailability may exist, however. For example, research shows that beta-carotene competes with other carotenes for absorption from the digestive tract and interferes with their use by the tissues.[75] It is likely that other such interactions among phytochemicals also occur, so if you consume a food too high in one phytochemical, you may miss out on benefits from others eaten with it.

Another problems exists, and it is even more serious. The small quantities of the combinations of phytochemicals occuring in whole *foods* present a variety of health benefits and can be consumed safely everyday. Large doses of purified phytochemicals, on the other hand, produce only single effects and may be as potentially toxic as medicinal herbs, another reason to award top honors to foods as deliverers of health. Table 11-9 lists tips for gaining the benefits of phytochemicals without risks and suggests some foods especially likely to be beneficial.[76]

TABLE 11-9

Tips for Consuming Phytochemicals

- Eat more fruit. The average U.S. diet provides only one serving a day. Remember to choose juices and raw or cooked fruits and vegetables at mealtimes as well as for snacks.
- Use herbs and spices in cooking. Cookbooks offer ways to include parsley, basil, garlic, hot peppers, oregano, and other beneficial seasonings.
- Replace some of the meat in the diet with grains, legumes, and vegetables. Oatmeal, soy meat replacer, or grated carrots mixed with ground meat and seasonings, make a luscious, nutritious meat loaf, for example.
- Try a new food each week. Walk through vegetable aisles and visit farmers' markets. Read recipes. Try tofu, soy milk, or soybeans in cooking.

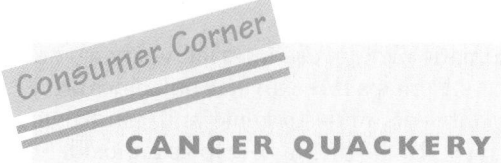

CANCER QUACKERY

What if a product existed that could prevent or cure cancer, but people in the medical sciences were unaware of it or labeled it a hoax? Would you use this product if someone you trusted suggested it? What if your personal health or recovery hung in the balance? If its cost was low, its use simple, and the people selling it presented many testimonials to its safety and effectiveness—would you try it? This is the dilemma that many people face when they strive for control over cancer.

Unsound products for prevention and cure of cancer comprise a large segment of today's medical fraud. Controversy 1 spelled out warning signs of nutrition quackery and drew distinctions between legitimate science and sales scams. This section offers some scientific evidence concerning a few unconventional diet-related cancer prevention and cure schemes. Later, the Food Feature offers legitimate and safe avenues to reduced cancer risks.

Understandably, when people hear of exciting research reports that hint at cancer prevention, they want to apply the findings right away. Preliminary findings, however, rarely apply to real life. For example, a tidal wave of vitamin sales followed the earliest reports of a possible role for beta-carotene in cancer prevention. Consumers who had read the news hastened to buy and start taking beta-carotene. Researchers, however, had established only a correlation between diets of *foods* rich in beta-carotene and a reduced cancer risk. They had not identified an exact mechanism by which beta-carotene might prevent cancer, nor had they tested the safety or efficacy of beta-carotene *supplements* against cancer.

Soon the scientists began having doubts. One study had to be prematurely terminated when lung cancer incidence increased among subjects taking experimental doses of beta-carotene.[77] Other studies found no effect of the supplements on cancer rates. Nevertheless, beta-carotene supplements are still being sold as anticancer agents. Many consumers buy and take them, expecting them to prevent cancer. They probably do not increase the risk of lung cancer, either, but without more research no one can be certain.

Other supplements maybe more risky. As more and more researchers shift their focus to phytochemicals, more and more bottles of concentrated phytochemicals will surely pop up on store shelves as dietary supplements.

Like beta-carotene, isolated phytochemicals removed from their food sources may well turn out to be ineffective or even harmful, especially if taken in concentrated doses over time. Many of the phytochemicals are brand-new to science, and their interactions with body systems are not understood. Some seem to act as extremely weak carcinogens. Others mimic steroid hormones. Sadly, no law prevents the sale of unproven ingredients as dietary supplements, and the maxim "let the buyer beware" rules the day.

kombucha a fermented tea drink of questionable safety; purported to bestow health benefits on the drinker. Not made from mushrooms, but often called *mushroom tea*.

A different sort of product is currently spreading across the nation as a cancer preventer, arthritis reliever, and baldness cure. People are brewing **kombucha,** by incubating a sort of mat formed by several species of yeast and bacteria, in sugar-sweetened black tea. The tea becomes highly acidic as the microorganisms ferment the sugar and release wastes into the fluid. People who drink it may be taking a chance with their health. The tea is easily contaminated with illness-causing organisms. Wild molds can enter the brew, and molds produce some of the most potent carcinogens known. Serious scientific studies of the effects of drinking kombucha are lacking.

Some real-world evidence raises doubts about the safety of kombucha, however. A report in a recent medical journal told of two women who drank it and had to be rushed to the emergency room with a life-threatening acid condition of the blood. One woman died; the other's heart stopped but was restarted, and she recovered. Both women had adopted a "more is better" attitude toward kombucha, brewing extra strong tea or doubling their dosages. The Center for Disease Control has asked physicians to be on the lookout for serious side effects in their patients who make and drink kombucha.

So many other cancer hoaxes fill the markets that just naming them all would take many pages. Coffee enemas (claimed to purge "bile" from the body), "living enzymes" from fresh juices (made especially by a $200 juice machine), and laetrile or amygdalin (a fake cancer cure falsely claimed to be a vitamin) are just a few. All of them capitalize on people's fear of cancer and distrust of the medical community. The sellers claim that a sinister medical establishment has suppressed these wonder marvels unethically. "The doctors don't care if you die," they say, "so long as you pay huge sums for their services." In fact they are describing themselves. The desire for control over cancer makes consumers vulnerable to those who would victimize them for profit.

Medicinal Herbs The presence of phytochemicals in herbs (among other plant foods) may explain why some herbs have long been given status as medicine. The bioflavonoids in tea and wine may help explain why people who drink moderately of these beverages have reduced risks of heart disease.[78] Similarly, the bioflavonoids and other active constituents in herbs may help explain why primitive folk medicine has survived amidst conventional medicine's technological advances. The secrets of herbs as medicines are as often as not based on the placebo effect, but some real effects are also revealed by science. Anyone who doubts that plants can cure illnesses should be convinced after learning that about 25 percent of the medicines prescribed by physicians in this country today are based on active ingredients in plants. Also, 80 percent

TABLE 11-10

Medicinal Herbs and Their Effects

- **aloe** a tropical plant with widely claimed value as a topical treatment for minor skin injury. Some scientific evidence supports this claim; evidence against its use in severe wounds also exists.
- **belladonna** any part of the deadly nightshade plant; a fatal poison.
- **cat's claw** an herb from the rain forests of Brazil and Peru, claimed, but not proved, to be an "all-purpose" remedy.
- **chamomile** flowers that may provide some limited medical value in soothing menstrual, intestinal, and stomach discomforts.
- **chaparral** an herbal product made from ground leaves of the creosote bush, and sold in tea or capsule form; supposedly this herb has antioxidant effects, delays aging, cleanses the bloodstream, and treats skin conditions—all unproven claims. Chaparral has been found to cause acute toxic hepatitis, a severe liver illness.
- **comfrey** leaves and roots of the comfrey plant; believed, but not proved, to have drug effects. Comfrey contains cancer-causing chemicals.
- **echinacea** an herb popular before the advent of antibiotics for its assumed "anti-infectious" properties and as an all-purpose remedy, especially for colds and allergy and for healing of wounds. A small body of research from the 1970s seems to lend preliminary support for some of the claims, but also points to an insecticidal property, leading to questions about safety. Also called *cone-flower*.
- **feverfew** an herb sold as a migraine headache preventive. Some evidence exists to support this claim.
- **foxglove** a plant that contains a substance used in the heart medicine digoxin.

- **ginkgo biloba** an extract of a tree of the same name, claimed to enhance mental alertness, but not proved to be effective or safe.
- **ginseng** (JIN-seng) a plant containing chemicals that have stimulant drug effects. *Ginseng abuse syndrome* is a group of symptoms associated with the overuse of ginseng, including high blood pressure, insomnia, nervousness, confusion, and depression.
- **hemlock** any part of the hemlock plant, which causes severe pain, convulsions, and death within 15 minutes.
- **kombucha** a product of fermentation of sugar-sweetened tea by various yeasts and bacteria. Proclaimed as a treatment for everything from AIDS to cancer but lacking scientific evidence and FDA approval. Microorganisms in home-brewed teas have caused serious illnesses in people with weakened immunity. Also known as *Manchurian tea*, *mushroom tea*, or *Kargasok tea*.
- **kudzu** a weedy vine, whose roots are harvested and used by Chinese herbalists as a treatment for alcoholism. Kudzu reportedly reduces alcohol absorption by up to 50 percent in rats.
- **medicinal herbs** nonwoody plants, plant parts, or extracts valued by some people for their medicinal qualities, both proved and unproved.
- **sassafras** root bark from the sassafras tree, once used in beverages but now banned as an ingredient in foods or beverages because it contains cancer-causing chemicals.
- **witch hazel** leaves or bark of a witch hazel tree; not proved to have healing powers.

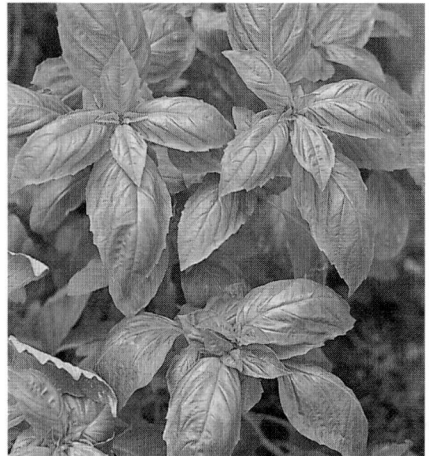

Herbs offer compounds that may provide health benefits.

of the world's people rely on plant-based medicine as their primary form of health care, although many such people have no access to modern medicines. Some plant-based medicines may not be effective against illnesses, and some may even be harmful, but some may be life saving. Some practitioners have given the name **medicinal herbs** to plants with biological effects (see Table 11-10).

If you choose to dabble in herbal medicine, however, be forewarned: harmful side effects are likely. A product that contains useful constituents is likely to contain some harmful ones as well and concentrations of all constituents vary widely from harvest to harvest. Some 700 plant species have caused serious illness or deaths in this part of the world; Table 11-10 includes some infamous poisonsous herbs to make the point that just because something is "natural" doesn't mean it is "safe."

Foods Themselves Table 11-8 provided abundant evidence in favor of eating a great variety of plant foods, but the phytochemicals listed there are only some of the ones known today. Hundreds of others are turning up as research proceeds. No one knows where the trail will end. Some facts are known about the single chemical genistein in soy products, described earlier, but many more are known about its food vehicle, soybeans and their relatives, which are known to contain several active compounds. Observations of women in Asia, for whome soybean products are staple foods, reveal that their blood genistein values are high, and that their estrogen values are just half of those typical in this country. Asian women also have low rates of osteoporosis and breast cancer; and the symptoms of menopause that are so common here are practically unheard of there. Yet, the fertility and reproductive health of Asian women is normal, as it is in Asian men. Other chemicals in soy products besides genistein may well deserve credit for some of these benefits; and other legumes doubtless possess such properties, too. Thus soybeans and other legumes, although lacking vitamin C, vitamin A, vitamin E, and others, should be highly prized as a health-promoting food.

In the same way, it is foods, not single chemicals, that hold credit for cancer prevention. They are known to contain combinations of **antipromoters,** substances that oppose cancer. Almost without exception, studies find that infrequent use of green and yellow fruits and vegetables and citrus fruits correlates with cancers of many types.[79] Specifically, infrequent use of **cruciferous vegetables**—cabbage, cauliflower, broccoli, brussels sprouts, turnips and the like—is common in colon cancer victims. Stomach cancer, too, correlates with low intakes of vegetables: in one study, vegetables in general; in another, fresh vegetables; in others, lettuce and other fresh greens or vegetables containing vitamin C.

Fruits and vegetables that contribute beta-carotene (and other members of the carotene family) seem to be especially active as cancer preventers.[80] Controversy 7 provided details. Even the exact types of cancers that foods prevent is being defined (see Table 11-11). Still largely a mystery, though, is which chemicals in these foods do what.

Nutrition is often associated with promoting health; and medicine with fighting disease, but if we ever believed that a real line separated the two, we surely can do so no longer.[81] Even the National Academy of Sciences now recognizes the medicinal power of some foods. The academy defines a **functional food** as any food that "encompass potentially healthful products [including] any modified food or food ingredient that may provide a health benefit beyond the traditional nutrients it contains."[82]

Important differences still remain, however. Medicines as we know them are measures employed only after health has deteriorated into illness. Foods are eaten every day, and they act over a lifetime quietly promoting health, usually in ways that scientists are only just beginning to appreciate. Medicines, medicinal herbs, and concentrated phytochemical preparations may offer important benefits, but foods offer more: protein; energy, as carbohydrate and fat; and fiber. It must be clear by now that we cannot know the identity and action of every chemical in every food. Even if we did, why take a supplement to try to replicate the effects of a food? Why not eat foods and enjoy the pleasure, nourishment, and health benefits they provide.[83]

✔ **KEY POINTS**   **High-fat diets are associated with cancer development. Fiber, vitamin C, *foods* containing beta-carotene and many other vitamins and minerals, and the phytochemicals found in cruciferous vegetables, greens, soybeans, tomatoes, and other vegetables are thought to be protective.**

antipromoters compounds in foods that act in several ways to oppose the formation of cancer.

cruciferous vegetables vegetables with cross-shaped blossoms. Their intake is associated with low cancer rates in human populations. Examples are cauliflower, cabbage, brussels sprouts, broccoli, turnips, and rutabagas.

TABLE II-II

Foods Known to Help Prevent Specific Kinds of Cancer

Green and Yellow Vegetables Prevent These Cancers

✔ bladder
✔ breast
✔ cervix
✔ lung
✔ mouth and throat
✔ ovaries
✔ prostrate
✔ stomach

Foods Rich in Antioxidant Vitamins Prevent These Cancers

✔ head
✔ neck
✔ lungs
✔ cervix
✔ pancreas
✔ stomach
✔ rectum
✔ colon
✔ ovary
✔ uterus
✔ breast
✔ bladder

Often it is foods like these, not individual chemicals, that lower people's cancer rates.

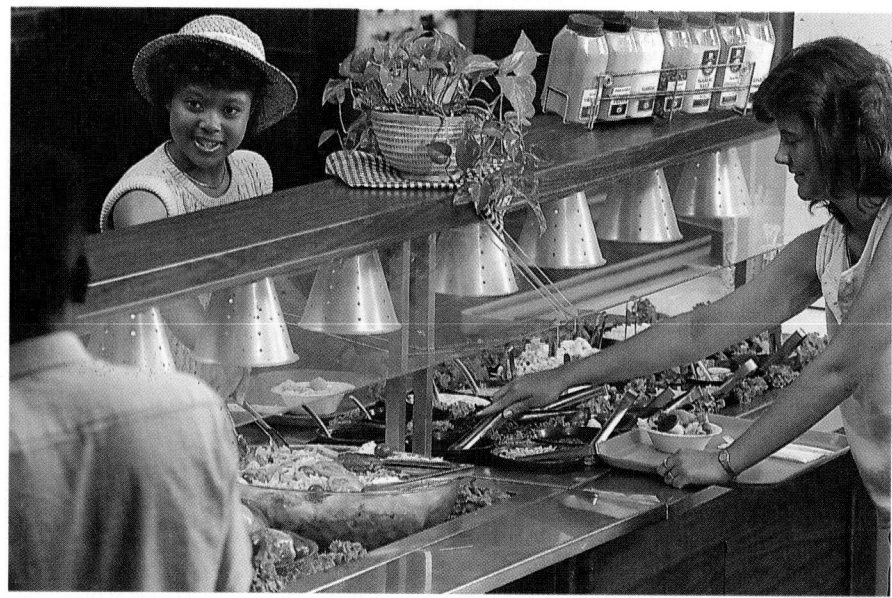

This chapter has summarized the major forms of disease and their links with nutrition. You may have noticed a philosophical shift from previous chapters. There, it was possible to say "a deficiency of nutrient X causes disease Y." Here is it possible only to quote theories and discuss research that illuminates current thinking. We can say with certainty, for example, that "a diet lacking vitamin C causes scurvy," but to say that a low-fiber diet that lacks vegetables causes cancer would be inaccurate.[84] We can say only that, as a general trend, people who eat few vegetables suffer more often from cancer. We can, however, recommend behaviors that are prudent and reduce the likelihood of illness. The Food Feature presents these recommendations.

This chapter concludes this book's treatment of normal adult nutrition. The next two chapters are about nutrition's contribution to health in each stage of the lifecycle from pregnancy and infancy to old age.

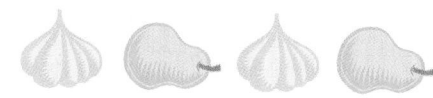

A remark by the Surgeon General is worth repeating: for the two of three Americans who do not smoke or drink excessively, "your choice of diet can influence your long-term health prospects more than any other action you might take."[85] Indeed, healthy young adults today are privileged to be the first generation in history who can know enough to lay the foundation for healthy later years through a lifetime of proper nutrition. Figure 11-9 illustrates this point.

An early chapter of this book presented dietary guidelines for the prevention of diseases. Chapters that followed focus on the "whys" and "hows" of those guidelines. This Food Feature comes full circle to revisit the guidelines with a broader and deeper understanding of their significance. As is already clear, not all of the diet recommendations that follow apply equally to all of the diseases, but fortunately for the consumer, most of the recommendations made to help prevent individual diseases support one another.

The American Heart Association and American Cancer Society offer suggestions specifically for disease prevention. Table 11-12 shows how very similar the bits of advice from the two sources are and clinches the argument that it's time to get busy putting them into practice. The following paragraphs review the specifics.

Primary among the recommendations is to reduce fat intake. The Food Feature of Chapter 5 showed how to keep total fat down by selecting low-fat foods. If the percentage of calories from fat is to be less than 30 percent, then it is especially important to limit pure fat foods such as sour cream, butter, and margarine; high-fat foods such as mayonnaise, cheese, and cream cheese; and foods high in hidden fat such as convenience foods with sauces, fried foods, fat-marbled meat cuts, sausages, ground beef, whole milk, and others. For each

FOOD FEATURE

DIET AS PREVENTIVE MEDICINE

"Knowledge about the causes of chronic diseases is now sufficiently strong to support the view that changes in dietary practices . . . can do much to prevent the premature death and disability caused by these diseases."*

*World Health Organization, 1991.

TABLE 11-12

Dietary Guidelines for Disease Prevention

American Heart Association Dietary Guidelines for Healthy American Adults, 1996a	American Cancer Society Guidelines on Diet, Nutrition, and Cancer Prevention, 1996
■ Eat a variety of foods. ■ Balance food intake with physical activity and maintain or reduce weight. ■ Choose a diet low in fat, saturated fatty acids, and cholesterol. ■ Choose a diet with plenty of vegetables, fruits, and whole-grain products. ■ Choose a diet moderate in sugar. ■ Use salt and sodium in moderation. ■ If you drink alcohol, do so in moderation.	■ Choose most of the foods you eat from plant sources. Eat five or more servings of fruits and vegetables each day. Eat other foods from plant sources, such as breads, cereals, grain products, rice, pasta, or beans several times each day. ■ Limit your intake of high-fat foods, particularly from animal sources. Choose foods low in fat. Limit consumption of meats, especially high-fat meats. ■ Be physically active: achieve and maintain a healthy weight. Be at least moderately active for 30 minutes or more on most days of the week. Stay within your healthy weight range. ■ Limit consumption of alcoholic beverages, if you drink at all.

aThe American Heart Association also recommends stopping smoking, and reducing weight in those who are overweight.

SOURCE: Adapted from American Heart Association Nutrition Committee, Dietary Guidelines for healthy American adults, *Circulation* 94 (1996): 1795–1800.

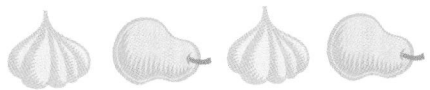

FIGURE II-9

PROPER NUTRITION SHIELDS AGAINST DISEASES

A well-chosen diet can protect your health.

SOURCE: Adapted from an idea in R. K. Chandra, 1990 McCollum Award Lecture: Nutrition and immunity: Lessons from the past and new insights into the future, *American Journal of Clinical Nutrition* 53 (1991): 1087–1101.

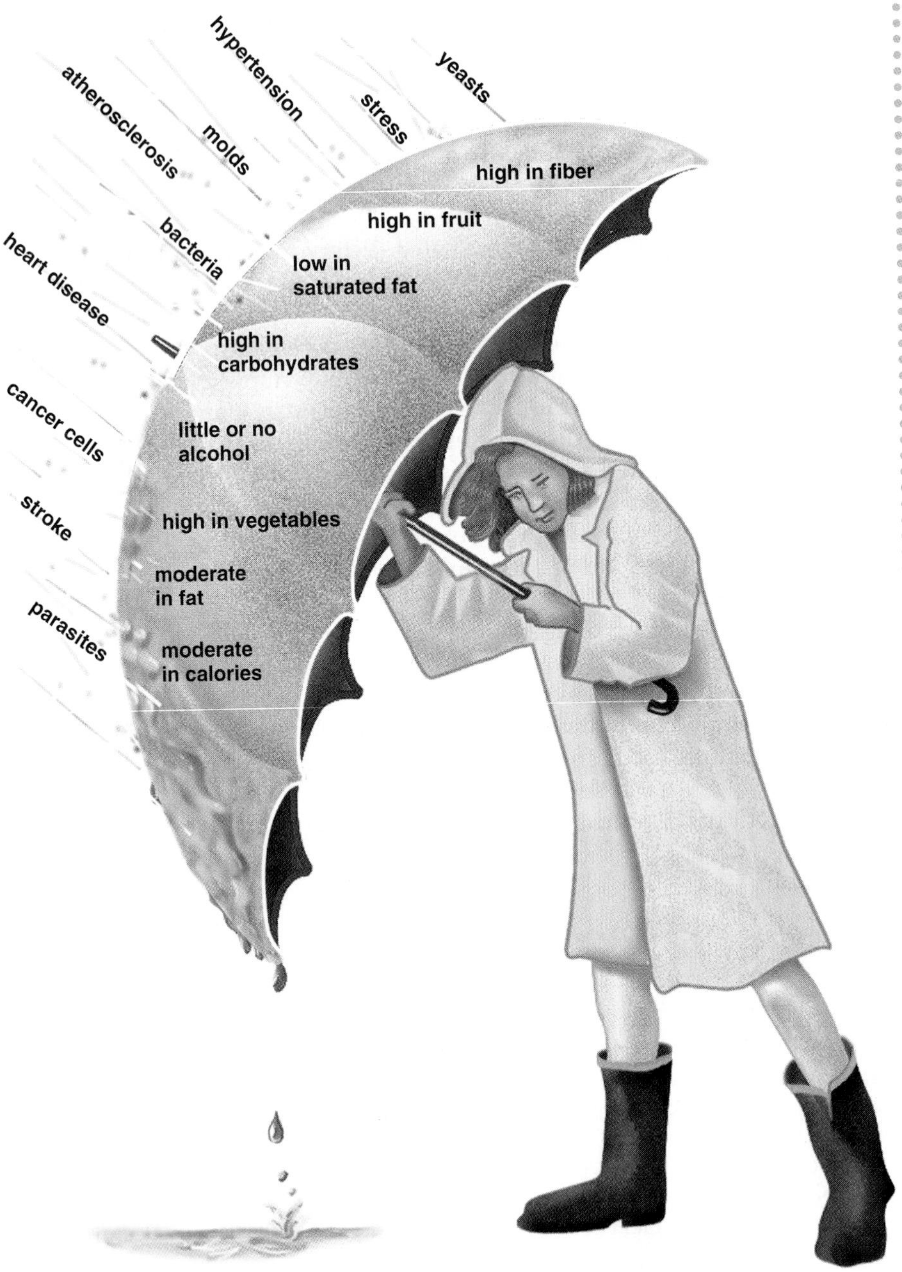

hypertension

atherosclerosis

molds

stress

yeasts

bacteria

heart disease

cancer cells

stroke

parasites

high in fiber

high in fruit

low in saturated fat

high in carbohydrates

little or no alcohol

high in vegetables

moderate in fat

moderate in calories

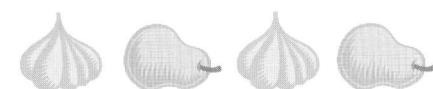

1,000 calories of food, about 30 grams of fat should be the maximum allowed. Shop for foods whose labels indicate no more than 3 grams of fat per 100 calories.

When you must add fat, use olive oil or canola oil, since these are high in monounsaturated fatty acids, but use them, like all fats, sparingly. Eat meals of fish regularly, especially fatty fish such as salmon, to balance your intakes of omega-6 fatty acids with the omega-3 type. Consult the Table of Food Composition, Appendix A for further details about the fatty acid contents of your favorite foods.

Every legitimate source of dietary advice urges people to include a variety of fruits and vegetables in the diet, not just for nutrients but also for the phytochemicals that promote health. Vow to try a new fruit or vegetable each week. Who knows? Some of the foods still waiting for you on the produce shelves may soon be your top favorites. An adventurous spirit is a plus in this regard. For example, soybeans and soy products are unfamiliar foods to most people, but soy milk is a natural addition to cereals, casseroles, or hot beverages; textured soy protein products can replace part of the hamburger in any recipe; tofu makes delicious puddings; and soybeans themselves are good in any recipe calling for beans. Read some cookbooks for ideas on incorporating other new foods into the diet.

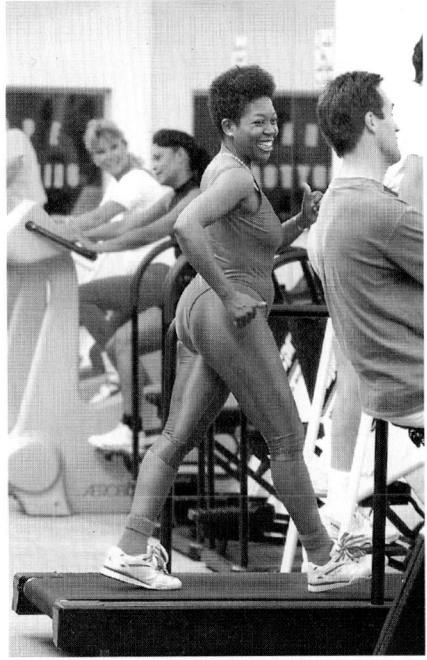

Exercise regularly, all your life.

The authorities of Table 11-12 advise people who are prone to hypertension to eat less salt, but it is probably best to follow all of the recommendations listed in the table. Maintain a proven program of weight control. Expend energy, so as to earn the right to eat more nutrient-dense foods; that is, be physically active. If the threat of CVD doesn't motivate you, then exercise to improve your self-image, to improve your morale, or to make friends—but do exercise. Eat foods high in potassium (whole foods), high in calcium and magnesium (milk products and appropriate substitutes), low in fat, and high in fiber (whole grains, legumes, vegetables, and fruits).

The advice not to let your diet become monotonous is also based on an important concept in the prevention of cancer initiation—dilution. Whenever you switch from food to food, you are diluting whatever is in one food with what is in the others. It is safe to eat *some* salt-cured foods or smoked or grilled meats, but don't eat them all the time. One recent study found that omission of several food groups from the diet brought extra risks of both cancer and cardiovascular disease.[86]

In the end, people's choices are based on their own likes and dislikes within the limits that their own lives impose on them. Whoever you are, we encourage you to take the time to work out ways of making your diet meet the guidelines known to support health, at least on most days. If you include fruits, vegetables, and high-fiber grains and control your fat intake, you can feel confident that you are supporting your health. Take time to enjoy your meals, too: the sights, smells, and tastes of good foods are among life's greatest pleasures. Joy, even the simple joy of eating, contributes to a healthy life.

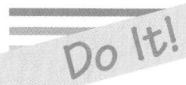

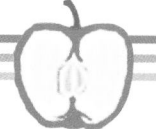

PRACTICE EYEBALLING A MEAL

Selecting nutritious foods from among pictures in a textbook is easy when the nutrient values of the foods appear on the page. More difficult is the task of selecting foods in the real world with nothing to go on but appearance. This Do It section offers the chance to hone your "eyeballing" skills for judging meals according to nutrient ideals such as the *Dietary Guidelines*.

Step 1. Study the suppers shown in Figure 11-10.

Step 2. Consider each dietary goal of Form 11-1 individually, and judge each of the suppers according to that goal.

Step 3. Write into the blanks on Form 11-1 the letters that identify the three meals that you think are highest or lowest in the characteristics named. (For example, for "Lowest in calories," you might write in "A B C.") Instructions and hints follow.

Calories List the three meals *lowest* in calories (or if you need to gain weight, list those highest in calories). Without nutrient data, this question might stump even the most skilled eyeballer. The person who can identify fats in foods (see Chapter 5's Food Feature) can "see" excess calories in foods right away. Added sugar adds calories, too (Chapter 4's Food Feature can help). Don't forget about portion sizes—too much of almost anything pushes the calories of a meal into the high ranges.

Fat, Saturated Fat, and Cholesterol Select the three meals likely to be *lowest* in fat, those lowest in saturated fat, and those lowest in cholesterol. These ingredients can be as obvious on the plate as pats of margarine and added salad dressings, or they can be hidden in dishes with fat–laden sauces, cheeses, high–fat meats, creamy

FORM 11-1

Dietary Recommendations Scoreboard

Write into the blanks the letters that identify the three meals that you judge to be highest or lowest in each characteristic.

The Three Meals	Your Score
Lowest in calories _____ _____ _____	_____
Lowest in fat _____ _____ _____	_____
Lowest in saturated fat _____ _____ _____	_____
Lowest in cholesterol _____ _____ _____	_____
Lowest in salt (sodium) _____ _____ _____	_____
Highest in vitamin A _____ _____ _____	_____
Highest in calcium _____ _____ _____	_____
Highest in fiber _____ _____ _____	_____
Highest in variety _____ _____ _____	_____
Total:	_____

Compare each of your responses with the ranking of meals in the charts of Table 11-10. To score, you must have identified meals listed among the top three for their chart. If you correctly identified the top three meals (in any order) for the category, give yourself three points. If you correctly identified two of the top-ranking meals, give yourself two points. For one meal, you get one point. If you scored:

- 22 or more points—you have excellent eyeballing skills
- 12–21 points—you are well on your way to developing your skills
- 11 or fewer—you should identify your weakest areas and reread the corresponding material, especially the Food Features, in previous chapters. Then retry this exercise.

FIGURE 11-10

SIX SUPPERS

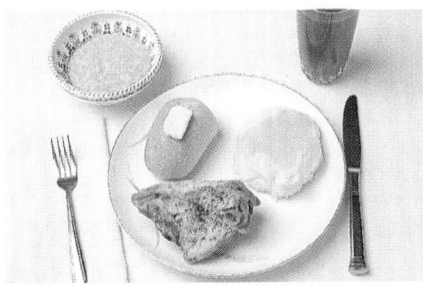

Meal A
roasted chicken breast with skin,
  1 average
creamed corn, ½ c
mashed potatoes, 1 c, with ¼ c gravy
dinner roll with 1 tsp margarine
fruit punch, 10 oz

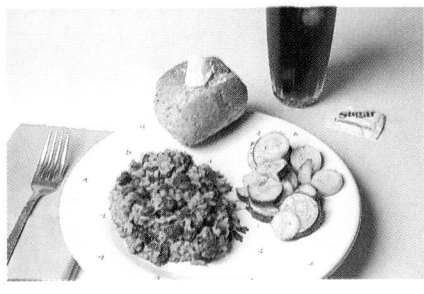

Meal B
red beans and rice, 1 c
zucchini and yellow squash mix, ½ c
whole wheat roll with 1 tsp margarine
sweetened iced tea, 10 oz

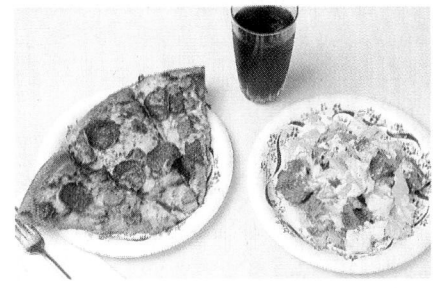

Meal C
extra cheese, sausage, and pepperoni
  pizza, 3 slices
lettuce and tomato salad, 1½ c with 2 tbs
  dressing
cola, 10 oz

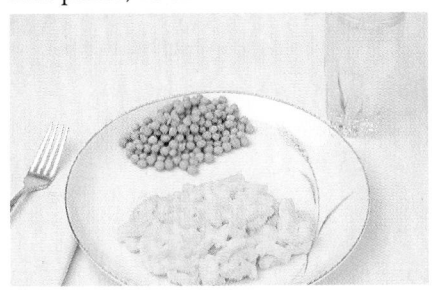

Meal D
macaroni and cheese, 1½ c
green peas, canned, ½ c
iced water

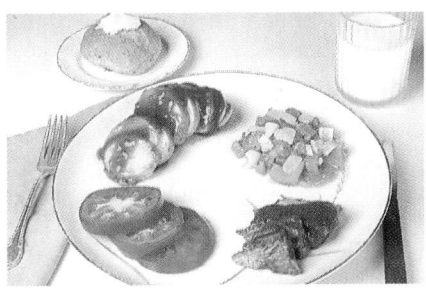

Meal E
pot roast, 2½ oz, with ½ c gravy
potatoes, 1 c
onions and celery mix, 1 c
whole wheat roll with 1 tsp margarine
tomato, ½ c
nonfat milk, 1 c

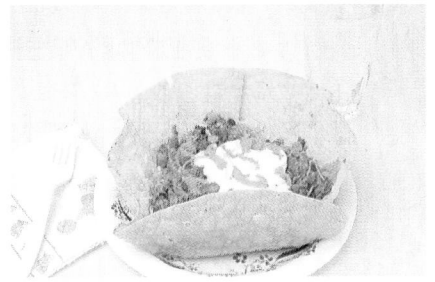

Meal F
taco salad, fast food
lemon-lime soda pop, 10 oz

sauces, baked goods, toppings, and crusts. Chapter 5's Food Feature identifies the lipids in common fatty foods.

Sodium   Select the meals you think are lowest in sodium. As mentioned in Chapter 8 (page 301), foods that contain the most salt, and therefore are highest in sodium, are often the most processed foods such as lunch meats, canned soups, chips, and condiments. It isn't always possible to guess which foods contain salt, but it's a safe best that most farm-fresh, unprocessed foods are low in salt, unless salt was added during preparation.

Vitamin A and Calcium   Pick out the three meals highest in vitamin A and the three highest in calcium. Foods rich in these nutrients are shown in the Snapshots on pages 232 and 296.

TABLE 11-13

Ranking Meals According to Dietary Recommendations

Important: The meal that comes closest to meeting each dietary ideal ranks highest on that chart; in other words, the meal *highest* in fiber is at the top of its list, as is the meal *lowest* in sodium, because both meals come closest to their ideals.

IDEAL: MODERATE IN CALORIES[a]		IDEAL: 30% OR FEWER CALORIES FROM FAT		IDEAL: 10% OR FEWER CALORIES FROM SATURATED FAT	
Meal		Meal		Meal	
B	Lowest in calories	B	lowest in fat	B	lowest in saturated fat
E	↕	A	↕	A	↕
D		E		E	
A		D		F	
F		C		C	
C	highest in calories	F	highest in fat	D	higest in saturated fat

IDEAL: MODERATE IN CHOLESTEROL[b]		IDEAL: MODERATE IN SODIUM[c]		IDEAL: 25g OR MORE OF FIBER	
MEAL		MEAL		MEAL	
B	lowest in cholesterol	B	lowest in sodium	B	highest in fiber
E	↕	F	↕	F	↕
A		A		E	
D		D		C	
F		E		A	
C	highest in cholesterol	C	highest in sodium	D	lowest in fiber

IDEAL: PROVIDES SIGNIFICANT VITAMIN A[d]		IDEAL: PROVIDES SIGNIFICANT CALCIUM[e]		IDEAL: MORE VARIETY	
Meal		Meal		Meal	
F	highest in vitamin A	C	highest in calcium	E	highest in variety
C	↕	D	↕	C	↕
D		E		A	
E		F		B	
A		A		F	
B	lowest in vitamin A	B	lowest in calcium	D	lowest in variety

[a] This ranking reflects a need to reduce calorie intakes. A person needing to increase calorie intakes might want to change the order of this list to give higher ranks to higher-calorie meals that also meet other guidelines.
[b] Ideal for cholesterol: a day's meals should contain 300 mg or fewer of cholesterol.
[c] Ideal for sodium: a day's meals should contain 2,400 mg or fewer of sodium.
[d] Ideal for vitamin A: a day's meals should contain 800 to 1,000 RE vitamin A.
[e] Ideal for calcium: a day's meals should contain 800 to 1,200 mg calcium.

Fiber   Select the three meals highest in fiber. Fiber follows fruits, vegetables, and whole grains.

Variety   Choose the meals that provide the *greatest* variety of foods. Of all the nutrition recommendations, the one concerning variety of foods may be hardest to measure. Chapter 2 suggested a minimum of eight different types of food in a day, as in the U.S. government's *Healthy Eating Index*. Other experts believe that more variety best supports health.

Step 4. Score yourself. Compare your answers with the actual ranking of the meals as shown in Table 11-13. Add to obtain a total score. Then interpret your score as suggested on Form 11-1, bottom.

ANALYSIS

Answer the following questions.

I. Did you guess which meals were highest in calories, fats, salt, and the rest? For example, logic might predict that a Taco Salad, because of the name salad, would be low in fat and calories, but high-fat ingredients such as sour cream, cheddar cheese, and commercial ground beef change the nutrient picture dramatically.

2. Which areas did you find to be the hardest to judge? How can you hone your eyeballing skills in these problem areas? What information are you lacking?

3. What do you notice about meals that are lowest in fat? Do they often meet more than one of the nutrition goals of this exercise?

4. On Table 11-13, which meal fell into the top three most often? What were the flaws in that meal?

5. Look at the meal that fell at the very bottom of each of the lists. Give some reasons why the meals fell so far from the nutrition goals in terms of the foods they included or lacked.

6. Does any meal rank at the top of the list for one goal and at the bottom of the list for another? Which one? What does this mean to the eater? Should you avoid such a meal, or might it bring benefits when used in moderation?

Keep in mind that not all the *Dietary Guidelines* focus on food, but also mention that being physically active and limiting alcohol are crucial to overall health. As you learn to identify meals that best meet your needs, choosing them will become second nature.

SELF-CHECK

Answer to these Self-Check questions are in Appendix G.

1. Most people have well-developed plaques in their arteries by the time they reach the age of _____.
    a. 20 years
    b. 30 years
    c. 40 years
    d. 50 years

2. Which of the following dietary factors may help to regulate blood pressure?
    a. calcium
    b. magnesium
    c. potassium
    d. all of the above.

3. Which of the following dietary factors appears to influence heart disease risk the most?
   a. sodium
   b. cholesterol
   c. saturated fat
   d. total fat

4. Which type of cancer is associated with overuse of alcohol?
   a. mouth
   b. breast
   c. throat
   d. all of the above

5. Which of the following constitutes a serving of alcohol delivering ½ ounce of pure ethanol? (Read about alcohol in the upcoming Controversy.)
   a. 12 ounces of beer
   b. 10 ounces of wine cooler
   c. 3 to 4 ounces of wine
   d. all of the above

6. The best way to plan a diet to support the immune system is to exceed the Recommended Dietary Allowances for each nutrient. T F

7. Vegetarians and meat eaters have the same mortality rates from cancer. T F

8. Resting blood pressure should ideally be 120 over 80 or lower. T F

9. The main diet-related risk factors for cardiovascular disease are glucose intolerance, obesity, high blood cholesterol, and hypertension. T F

10. Hypertension is more severe and occurs earlier in life among people of European or Asian descent than among African Americans. T F

NOTES

Notes are in Appendix F.

People naturally congregate to enjoy conversation and companionship, and it is only natural to offer beverages to companions. All beverages ease conversation, whether they contain alcohol or not. Still, some people in most of the world's cultures choose alcohol over cola, juice, milk, or coffee as a pleasant accompaniment to a meal, a drink of celebration, or a way to relax with friends. For some number of these people, alcohol use becomes a life-shattering addiction, **alcoholism,** that leads to severe malnutrition, physical illness, and demoralizing erosion of self-esteem. (Alcohol terms are defined in Table C11-1.)

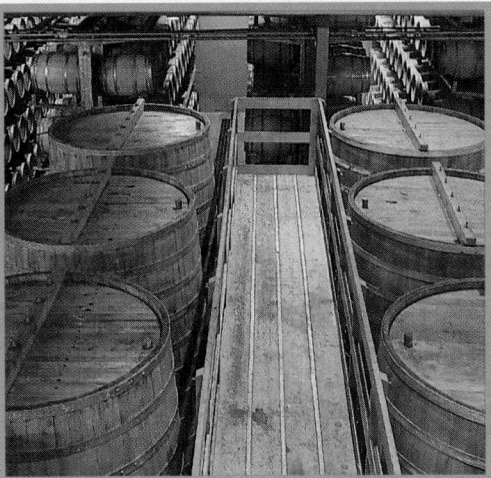

A serving of alcohol, commonly called a **drink,** delivers ½ ounce of pure **ethanol:**

3 to 4 ounces wine.
10 ounces wine cooler.
12 ounces beer.
1 ounce hard liquor (whiskey, gin, brandy, rum, vodka).

These standard measures may have little in common with the drinks served by enthusiastic bartenders, however. Many wine glasses easily hold 6 to 8 ounces of wine; a large beer stein can hold 16, 20, or even more ounces; a strong liquor drink may contain 2 or 3 ounces of various liquors. A liquor's **proof,** its percentage of alcohol, defines its strength: 100-proof liquor is 50 percent alcohol; 90-proof is 45 percent, and so forth. Compared with hard liquor, beer and wine have relatively low percentages of alcohol.

BENEFITS OF MODERATE ALCOHOL USE

Taken in moderation, alcohol relaxes people, reduces their inhibitions, encourages social interactions and produces feelings of **euphoria.** The term *moderation* is important in the statement just made. Just what is moderation in the use of alcohol? No single amount of alcohol per day is appropriate for everyone because people differ in their tolerances to alcohol. But authorities have attempted to set limits that are appropriate for most healthy people: not more than two drinks a day for the

average-sized, healthy man, and not more than one drink a day for the average-sized, healthy woman. This amount is supposed to be enough to elevate mood without incurring any long-term harm to health. An interesting side note: the nonalcoholic beers and wines now on the market also elevate mood and encourage social interaction, a testimony to the placebo effect at work.

Doubtless some people could safely consume slightly more than the alcohol dose called moderate; others, especially those prone to alcohol addiction, could definitely not handle nearly so much without significant risk. If you think your own drinking might not be moderate or normal, if it has caused problems in your life, or if you feel guilty about your drinking, you may want to seek a professional evaluation.*

Wine is credited with some special effects. The high potassium content of grape juice lowers high blood pressure, and this effect persists when the grape juice is made into wine. In fact, since alcohol raises blood pressure, the grape juice is more suitable than the wine for people with hypertension. Dealcoholized wine also facilitates the absorption of potassium, calcium, phosphorus, magnesium, and zinc. So does wine, but the alcohol in it promotes the *excretion* of these minerals, so again the dealcoholized version is preferred.

In addition to alcohol, wine contains phenols and other phytochemicals that may protect against cardiovascular disease.[1] These substances may act as antioxidants, opposing LDL oxidation, and may alter prostaglandin metabolism, reducing blood clot formation. A recent review of literature suggests that it may be the alcohol of alcoholic beverages that reduces heart disease risk.[2] These protective effects may explain the so-called French paradox: even though the French have many of the same risk factors as people in the United States, the wine-drinking population of France enjoys a lower incidence of heart disease. In general, though,

---

*The U.S. center for facts on alcohol is the National Clearinghouse for Alcohol and Drug Information: 1-800-729-6686.

TABLE C11-1

Alcohol Terms

- **acetaldehyde** (ass-et-AL-deh-hide) a substance to which ethanol is metabolized on its way to becoming harmless waste products that can be excreted.
- **alcohol dehydrogenase (ADH)** an enzyme system that breaks down alcohol. The antidiuretic hormone listed below is also abbreviated ADH.
- **alcoholism** a dependency on alcohol marked by compulsive uncontrollable drinking with negative effects on physical health, family relationships, and social health.
- **antidiuretic hormone (ADH)** a hormone produced by the pituitary gland in response to dehydration (or a high sodium concentration in the blood). It stimulates the kidneys to reabsorb more water and so to excrete less. (This hormone should not be confused with alcohol dehydrogenase, which is also abbreviated ADH.)
- **beer belly** central body fatness associated with alcohol consumption.
- **cirrhosis** (seer-OH-sis) advanced liver disease, often associated with alcoholism, in which liver cells have died, hardened, turned an orange color, and permanently lost their function.
- **congeners** (CON-jen-ers) chemical substances other than alcohol that account for some of the physiological effects of alcoholic beverages, such as taste and aftereffects.
- **drink** a dose of any alcoholic beverage that delivers ½ ounce of pure ethanol.

- **ethanol** the alcohol of alcoholic beverages, produced by the action of microorganisms on the carbohydrates of grape juice or other carbohydrate-containing fluids.
- **euphoria** an inflated sense of well-being and pleasure brought on by a moderate dose of alcohol and some other drugs.
- **fatty liver** an early stage of liver deterioration seen in several diseases, including kwashiorkor and alcoholic liver disease in which fat accumulates in the liver cells.
- **fibrosis** (fye-BROH-sis) an intermediate stage of alcoholic liver deterioration in which liver cells lose their function and assume the characteristics of connective tissue cells (fibers).
- **formaldehyde** a substance to which methanol is metabolized on the way to being converted to harmless waste products that can be excreted.
- **gout** (GOWT) accumulation of crystals of uric acid in the joints.
- **MEOS** (microsomal ethanol oxidizing system) a system of enzymes in the liver that oxidize not only alcohol but also several classes of drugs.
- **methanol** an alcohol produced in the body continually by all cells.
- **proof** a statement of the percentage of alcohol in an alcoholic beverage. Liquor that is 100 proof is 50% alcohol; 90 proof is 45%; and so forth.
- **urethane** a carcinogenic compound that commonly forms in alcoholic beverages.

most experts hesitate to recommend taking alcohol to benefit health.[3]

Alcoholic beverages affect the appetite. Usually, they reduce it, making people unaware that they are hungry. But in people who are tense and unable to eat, or in the elderly who have lost interest in food, small doses of wine taken 20 minutes before meals improve appetite. Certain compounds in the wine known as **congeners** are credited with this effect. For undernourished people and for people with severely depressed appetites, wine may facilitate eating even when psychotherapy fails to do so. Congeners are also involved in producing a hangover, as a later section notes.

Another example of the beneficial use of alcohol comes from research showing that moderate use of wine in later life improves morale, stimulates social interaction, and promotes restful sleep. In nursing homes, improved patient and staff relations have been attributed to greater self-esteem among elderly patients who drink moderate amounts of wine. Researchers

hypothesize that chronic fatigue may be responsible for some behaviors associated with old age. The positive effects of wine on sleep may alleviate the fatigue, easing social interactions.

The decision whether to drink alcohol to obtain its benefits must also take the risks into account. An individual's age and health history are critical to the decision of whether to drink alcohol. The numbers of deaths attributed to alcohol are greatest for people between the ages of 15 and 44—and their risks of heart disease are relatively minor. Clearly, for these people, the risks outweigh the benefits.

For people who choose to drink, a valid goal is learning to drink moderately. The next sections address that goal in the context of alcohol's physical effects.

ALCOHOL ENTERS THE BODY

From the moment an alcoholic beverage is swallowed, the body pays special attention to it. Unlike foods,

FIGURE C11-1

**FOOD SLOWS ALCOHOL'S
ABSORPTION**
The alcohol in a stomach filled with
food has a low probability of touching
the walls and diffusing through. Food
also holds alcohol in the stomach
longer, slowing its entry into the highly
absorptive small intestine.

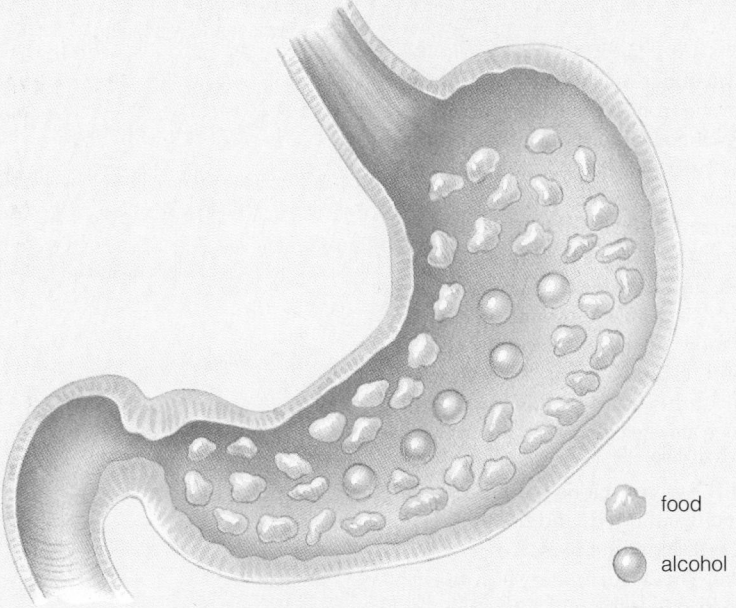

food

alcohol

which require digestion before they can be absorbed,
the tiny alcohol molecules can diffuse right through the
stomach walls and reach the brain within a minute.
Ethanol is a toxin, and a too-high dose of alcohol triggers one of the body's primary defenses against poison—vomiting. Many times, though, alcohol arrives
gradually and in a beverage dilute enough so that the
vomiting reflex is delayed and the alcohol is absorbed.

A person can become intoxicated almost immediately when drinking, especially if the stomach is
empty. When the stomach is full of food, molecules of
alcohol have less chance of touching the stomach walls
and diffusing through, so alcohol reaches the brain
more gradually (see Figure C11-1). By the time the
stomach contents are emptied into the small intestine,
however, alcohol is absorbed rapidly whether or not
food is present.

A person who wants to drink socially and not
become intoxicated should eat the snacks provided by
the host (avoid the salty ones; they make you thirstier).
Carbohydrate snacks slow alcohol absorption and high-
fat snacks help too because they slow peristalsis, keeping the alcohol in the stomach longer. Other tips
include adding ice or water to drinks to dilute them,
and choosing nonalcoholic beverages first and then
every other round to quench thirst.

If one drinks slowly enough, the alcohol, after
absorption, will be collected by the liver and processed
without affecting other parts of the body much. If one

drinks more rapidly, however, some of the alcohol
bypasses the liver and flows for a while through the
rest of the body and the brain.

ALCOHOL ARRIVES IN THE BRAIN

Some people use alcohol as a kind of social anesthetic
to help them relax or to relieve anxiety. One drink
relieves inhibitions, and this gives people the impression that alcohol is a stimulant. Actually, it gives this
impression by sedating *inhibitory* nerves, allowing exci-
tatory nerves to take over. This effect is temporary. Ultimately, alcohol acts as a depressant and sedates all the
nerve cells. Figure C11-2 presents alcohol's effects on
the brain.

It is lucky that the brain centers respond to rising
blood alcohol in the order shown, because a person
usually passes out before managing to drink a lethal
dose. It is possible, though, for a person to drink fast
enough so that the alcohol continues to be absorbed
and its effects continue to accelerate after the person
has gone to sleep. Every year, deaths take place during
drinking contests that are attributed to this effect. The
drinker drinks fast enough, before passing out, to
receive a lethal dose. Table C11-2 shows the blood alcohol levels that correspond with progressively greater
intoxication, and Table C11-3 shows the brain responses
that occur at these blood levels.

FIGURE C11-2

ALCOHOL'S EFFECTS ON THE BRAIN

When alcohol flows to the brain, it first sedates the frontal lobe, the reasoning part. As the alcohol molecules diffuse into the cells of this lobe, they interfere with reasoning and judgment.

With continued drinking, the speech and vision centers of the brain become sedated, and the area that governs reasoning becomes more incapacitated.

Still more drinking affects the cells of the brain responsible for large-muscle control; at this point people under the influence stagger or weave when they try to walk.

Finally, the conscious brain becomes completely subdued, and the person passes out. Now the person can drink no more. This is fortunate because a higher dose would anesthetize the deepest brain centers that control breathing and heartbeat, causing death.

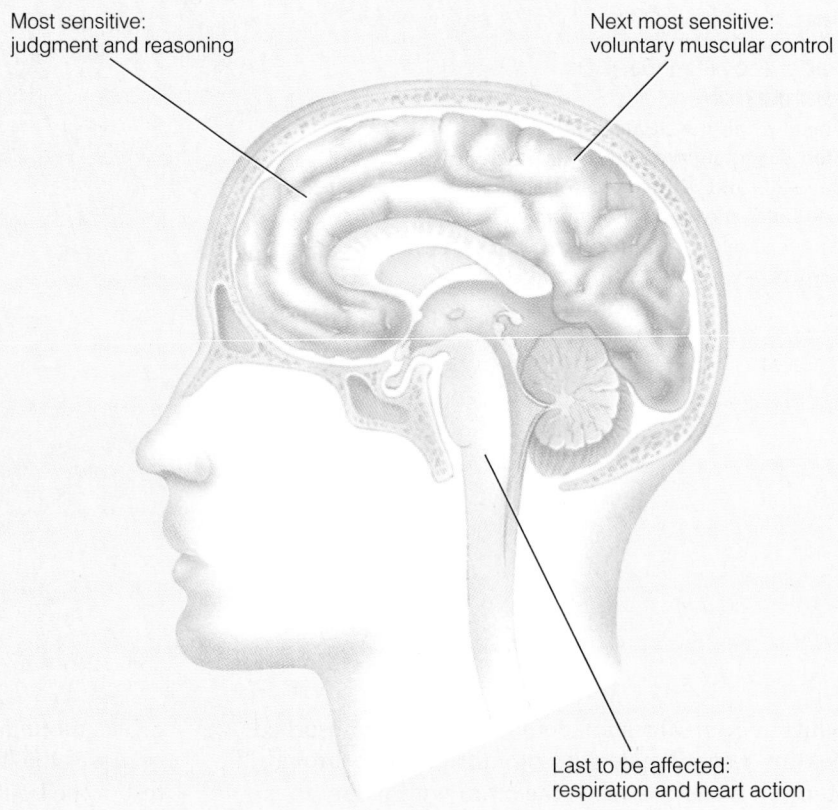

Most sensitive: judgment and reasoning

Next most sensitive: voluntary muscular control

Last to be affected: respiration and heart action

Binge Drinking Binge drinking (consuming 4 or more drinks in a short time) poses a serious health threat to college students, to others who engage in it, and to nearby nondrinkers.[4] A binge is most likely to occur at a party, a sporting event, or another social occasion. Compared with nondrinkers or moderate drinkers, bingers are more likely to damage property, to assault other people, to cause fatal automobile accidents, and to engage in risky unprotected and unplanned sexual intercourse. Bingers rarely identify themselves as problem drinkers until their drinking behavior causes a crisis, for example, a car crash, or until they've binged long enough to have caused substantial damage to their health. One target of such damage is the brain.

TABLE C11-2

Alcohol Doses and Blood Levels

Number of Drinks[a]	PERCENT BLOOD ALCOHOL BY BODY WEIGHT				
	100 lb	120 lb	150 lb	180 lb	200 lb
2	0.08	0.06	0.05	0.04	0.04
4	0.15	0.13	0.10	0.08	0.08
6	0.23	0.19	0.15	0.13	0.11
8	0.30	0.25	0.20	0.17	0.15
12	0.45	0.36	0.30	0.25	0.23
14	0.52	0.42	0.35	0.34	0.27

[a]Taken within an hour or so; each drink equal to ½ ounce pure ethanol.

Alcohol's Effects on the Brain Brain cells are particularly sensitive to excessive exposure to alcohol. The brain shrinks, even in people who drink only moderately. The extent of the shrinkage is proportional to the amount drunk. Abstinence, together with good nutrition, reverses some of the brain damage, and possibly all of it, if heavy drinking has not continued for more than a few years. However, prolonged drinking beyond an individual's capacity to recover can do severe and irreversible harm to vision, memory, learning ability, and other functions.

Anyone who has had an alcoholic drink has experienced one of alcohol's physical effects: alcohol increases

TABLE C11-3

Alcohol Blood Levels and Brain Responses

Blood Level (%)	Brain Response
0.05	Judgment impaired
0.10[a]	Emotional control impaired
0.15	Muscle coordination and reflexes impaired
0.20	Vision impaired
0.30	Drunk, totally out of control
0.35	In a stupor
0.50–0.60	Unconscious, then dead

[a]The 0.10 percent level is the legal limit for intoxication according to most states' highway safety ordinances; however, driving ability is already impaired at blood alcohol levels lower than 0.10 percent.

urine output. This is because alcohol depresses the brain's production of **antidiuretic hormone.** Loss of body water leads to thirst. The only fluid that will relieve dehydration is water, but if the only drinks available contain alcohol, each drink may worsen the thirst. The smart drinker, then, alternates alcoholic beverages with nonalcoholic choices and uses only the latter to quench thirst.

The water lost due to hormone depression takes with it important minerals, such as magnesium, potassium, calcium, and zinc, depleting the body's reserves. These minerals are vital to fluid balance and to nerve and muscle coordination. When drinking incurs mineral losses, the losses must be made up the next day if deficiencies are not to advance.

ALCOHOL ARRIVES IN THE LIVER

The capillaries that surround the digestive tract merge into veins that carry the alcohol-laden blood to the liver. Here the veins branch and rebranch into capillaries that touch every liver cell. The liver cells make nearly all of the body's alcohol-processing machinery, and the routing of blood through the liver allows the cells to go right to work on the alcohol. The liver's location at this point along the circulatory system enables it to remove toxic substances before they reach other body organs such as the heart and brain.

The Liver Metabolizes Alcohol The liver makes and maintains two sets of equipment for metabolizing alcohol. One is an enzyme that removes hydrogens from alcohol to break it down; the name, **alcohol dehydrogenase (ADH),** almost says what it does.* This enzyme handles about 80 percent or more of the alcohol in the body. The other set of alcohol-metabolizing equipment is a chain of enzymes known as the **MEOS** (listed in Table C11-1) thought to handle about 10 percent of alcohol. The remaining 10 percent is excreted through the breath and in the urine. Because the alcohol in the breath is directly proportional to the alcohol in the blood, the breathalyzer test that law enforcement officers administer when someone may be driving under the influence of alcohol accurately reveals how intoxicated they are.

The amount of alcohol a person's body can process in a given time is limited by the number of ADH enzymes that reside in the liver. If more molecules of alcohol arrive at the liver cells than the enzymes can handle, the extra alcohol must wait. It circulates again and again through the brain, liver, and other organs until enzymes are available to degrade it.

Some ADH enzymes reside in the stomach and break down some alcohol before it enters the blood. Research shows that people with alcoholism make less stomach ADH than others, and that women make less than men. Women may absorb about one-third more alcohol than do men, even when they are the same size and drink the same amount of alcohol.[5]

The number of ADH enzymes present is also affected by whether or not a person eats. Fasting for as little as a day causes degradation of body proteins, including the ADH enzymes, and this can reduce the rate of alcohol metabolism by half. Prudent drinkers drink slowly, with food in their stomachs, to allow the alcohol molecules to move to the liver cells gradually enough for the enzymes to handle the load. It takes about an hour and a half to metabolize one drink, depending on a person's body size, on previous drinking experience, on how recently the person has eaten, and on the person's current state of health. The liver is the only organ that can dispose of significant quantities of alcohol, and its maximum rate of alcohol clearance cannot be speeded up. This explains why only time will restore sobriety. Walking will not; muscles cannot metabolize alcohol. It is a myth that drinking a cup of coffee will help. Caffeine is a stimulant, but it won't speed up the metabolism of alcohol. The police say, ruefully, that a cup of coffee only makes a sleepy drunk

---

*There are actually two ADH enzymes, each performing a specific task in alcohol breakdown.

TABLE C11-4

Myths and Truths Concerning Alcohol

Myth:	A shot of alcohol warms you up.
Truth:	Alcohol diverts blood flow to the skin making you *feel* warmer, but it actually cools the body.
Myth:	Wine and beer are mild; they do not lead to addiction.
Truth:	Wine and beer drinkers worldwide have high rates of death from alcohol-related illnesses. It's not what you drink, but how much, that makes the difference.
Myth:	Mixing drinks is what gives you a hangover.
Truth:	Too much alcohol in any form produces a hangover.
Myth:	Alcohol is a stimulant.
Truth:	Alcohol depresses the brain's activity.
Myth:	Alcohol is legal, and therefore not a drug.
Truth:	Alcohol is legal, but it alters body functions and is medically defined as a depressant drug.

into a wide-awake drunk. Table C11-4 presents other alcohol myths.

A suggestion has been made that alcohol calories should be counted as fat in the diet because of the way fat and alcohol interact in the body.[6] Presented with both fat and alcohol, the body burns the alcohol for energy and stores the fat. Alcohol also promotes fat storage in the central abdominal area—the "**beer belly**" effect whose risks to the heart were already described in Chapter 9.[7] Alcohol yields 7 calories of energy per gram to the body, so many alcoholic drinks are much more fattening than their nonalcoholic counterparts.

Alcohol Affects Body Functions Upon exposure to alcohol, the liver speeds up its synthesis of fatty acids. Fat is known to accumulate in the livers of young men after a single night of heavy drinking and to remain there for more than a day. The first stage of liver deterioration seen in heavy drinkers, is therefore known as **fatty liver,** and it interferes with the distribution of nutrients and oxygen to the liver cells. If the condition lasts long enough, fibrous scar tissue invades the liver. This is the second stage of liver deterioration, called **fibrosis.** Fibrosis is reversible with good nutrition and abstinence from alcohol, but the next (last) stage, **cirrhosis,** is not. In cirrhosis, the liver

cells harden, turn orange, and die, losing function forever. All of this points to the importance of moderation in the use of alcohol.

The presence of alcohol alters amino acid metabolism in the liver cells. Synthesis of some proteins important in the immune system slows down, weakening the body's defenses against infection. Synthesis of lipoproteins speeds up, increasing blood triglyceride and HDL levels. In addition, excess alcohol adds to the body's acid burden and interferes with normal uric acid metabolism, causing symptoms like those of **gout.**

THE HANGOVER

The hangover—the awful feeling of headache pain, unpleasant sensations in the mouth, and nausea that one has the morning after drinking too much—is a mild form of drug withdrawal. (The worse form is a delirium with severe tremors that presents a danger of death and demands medical management.) Hangovers are caused by several factors. One is the toxic effects of congeners, already mentioned, that accompany the alcohol in alcoholic beverages. The congeners in gin are different from those in vodka, which in turn are different from those in bourbon or rye whiskey. One particular kind of liquor may produce a hangover and another may not. Congeners are only one of several factors that produce hangovers, however, and mixing or switching drinks will not prevent them if too much is drunk.

Dehydration of the brain is a second factor: alcohol not only causes the body to lose water, but actually reduces the brain cells' water content. When they rehydrate the morning after, nerve pain accompanies their swelling back to their normal size. Another contributor to the hangover is **formaldehyde,** the same chemical that medical laboratories use to preserve dead animals. Formaldehyde comes from **methanol,** an alcohol produced constantly by normal chemical processes in all the cells. Normally, a set of liver enzymes converts this methanol to formaldehyde, and then a second set immediately converts the formaldehyde to carbon dioxide and water, harmless waste products that can be excreted. But the same two sets of liver enzymes that do this are also used to process ethanol to its own intermediate waste product, **acetaldehyde,** and then to carbon dioxide and water. The enzymes prefer ethanol 20 times over methanol. Both alcohols are metabolized without delay until the excess acetaldehyde monopolizes the enzymes, leaving formaldehyde to wait for later detoxification. At that point, formaldehyde starts accumulating and the hangover begins.

Time alone is the cure for a hangover. Simple-minded remedies clearly will not work: vitamins, tranquilizers, aspirin, drinking more alcohol, breathing pure oxygen, exercising, eating, or drinking something awful are all useless. Fluid replacement can help to normalize the body's chemistry. The headache pain, unpleasantness in the mouth, and nausea of a hangover come simply from drinking too much.

ALCOHOL'S LONG-TERM EFFECTS

By far the longest-term effects of alcohol are those felt by the child of a woman who drinks during pregnancy. When a pregnant woman takes a drink, her fetus takes the same drink within minutes, and its body is defenseless against the effects. This is a topic so important that it is given a space of its own in Chapter 12, where the recommendation is made that pregnant women should not drink at all. For nonpregnant adults, however, what are the effects of alcohol over the long term?

A couple of drinks sets in motion many destructive processes in the body. The next day's abstinence can reverse them only if the doses taken are moderate, the time between them is ample, and nutrition is adequate meanwhile.

If the dose of alcohol are heavy, however, and the time between them short, complete recovery cannot take place, and repeated onslaughts of alcohol gradually take a toll on the body. For example, alcohol is directly toxic to skeletal and cardiac muscle, causing weakness and deterioration that is greater, the larger the dose.[8] Alcoholism makes heart disease likely, probably because chronic alcohol use raises blood pressure.[9] At autopsy, the heart of a person with alcoholism appears bloated and weighs twice as much as a normal heart.

Alcohol attacks brain cells directly, and alcoholism causes irreversible brain disorders that cost society an estimated $90 billion every year in medical services, lost wages, criminal costs, and other losses.[10] Cirrhosis also develops after 10 to 20 years from the cumulative effects of frequent heavy episodes of drinking.

Alcohol abuse also leads to cancers of the breast, mouth, throat, esophagus, rectum, and lungs. A reliable source tentatively ranks daily human exposure to ethanol high among possible carcinogenic hazards.[11]

A debated point is whether moderate alcohol intakes over many years increase cancer risks. Some studies link moderate alcohol intakes with breast cancer, but later studies have challenged these results. Cancer of the rectum occurs more often in those who drink more

than 15 ounces of beer each day than in others. It is unknown whether cancer's association with beer results from alcohol itself or from other compounds formed during brewing. One compound, **urethane,** is often found in some alcoholic beverages, especially flavored imported brandy. Urethane is known to cause cancer in animals, but the risk to human beings is unknown.[12]

Other long-term effects of alcohol abuse include the following:

- Diabetes (noninsulin-dependent).[13]
- Ulcers of the stomach and intestines.
- Severe psychological depression.
- Kidney, bladder, prostate, and pancreas damage.
- Skin rashes and sores.
- Impaired immune response.
- Deterioration of the testicles and adrenal glands.
- Feminization and sexual impotence in men.
- Central nervous system damage.
- Impaired memory and balance.
- Malnutrition.
- Bone deterioration and osteoporosis.
- Increased risks of death from all causes.[14]

This list is by no means all-inclusive. Alcohol abuse exerts direct toxic effects on all body organs.

ALCOHOL'S EFFECT ON NUTRITION

Alcohol abuse also does damage indirectly, via malnutrition. The more alcohol a person drinks, the less likely that he or she will eat enough food to obtain adequate nutrients. Alcohol is empty calories, like pure sugar and pure fat; it displaces nutrients. In a sense, each 150 calories spent on alcohol are going for a luxury item: the drinker receives no nutritional value in return. The more calories spent this way, the fewer are left to spend on nutritious foods. Table C11-5 shows the calorie amounts of typical alcoholic beverages.

Alcohol abuse also disrupts every tissue's metabolism of nutrients. Stomach cells oversecrete both acid and histamine, an agent of the immune system that produces inflammation. Beer in particular can irritate the stomach by stimulating it to release extra acid, opening the way for ulcers of the stomach and esophagus linings.[15] Intestinal cells fail to absorb thiamin, folate, vitamin B_6, and other vitamins. Liver cells lose efficiency in activating vitamin D and alter their production and excretion of bile. Rod cells in the retina, which normally process vitamin A alcohol (retinol) to

TABLE C11-5

Calories in Alcohol Beverages and Mixers

Beverage	Amount (oz)	Energy (cal)
Beer	12	150
Light beer	12	100
Gin, rum, vodka, whiskey (86 proof)	1½	105
Dessert wine	3½	140
Table wine	3½	85
Tonic, ginger ale	8	80
Cola, root beer	8	100
Fruit-flavored soda, Tom Collins mix	8	115
Club soda, plain seltzer, diet drinks	8	1

the form needed in vision, find themselves processing drinking alcohol instead. The kidneys excrete magnesium, calcium, potassium, and zinc.

Alcohol's intermediate products interfere with vitamin B_6 metabolism, too. They dislodge the vitamin from its protective protein so that it is destroyed, leading to a deficiency that reduces production of red blood cells.

Most dramatic is alcohol's effect on folate. When an excess of alcohol is present, the body actively expels folate from all of its sites of action and storage. The liver, which normally contains enough folate to meet all needs, leaks its folate into the blood. As blood folate rises, the kidneys are deceived into excreting it, as if it were in excess. The intestine normally releases and retrieves folate continuously, but becomes so damaged by folate deficiency and alcohol toxicity that it fails to retrieve its own folate and misses out on any that may trickle in from food as well. Alcohol also interferes with the action of what little folate is left. This inhibits the production of new cells, especially the rapidly dividing cells of the intestine and the blood.

Nutrient deficiencies are thus a virtually inevitable consequence of alcohol abuse, not only because alcohol displaces food but also because alcohol directly interferes with the body's use of nutrients, making them ineffective even if they are present. Over a lifetime, excessive drinking brings about deficits of all the nutrients. People treated for alcohol addiction also need nutrition therapy to reverse deficiencies, and even deficiency diseases rarely seen in others: night blindness, beriberi, pellagra, scurvy, and protein-energy malnutrition.

This discussion has touched on some of the ways alcohol affects health and nutrition. In contrast to some possible benefits of moderate alcohol consumption, excessive alcohol consumption presents a great potential for harm. Alcohol is guilty of contributing not only to deaths from health problems, but also to most of the other deaths of young people, including car crashes, falls, suicides, homicides, drownings, and other accidents.[16] The surest way to escape the harmful effects of alcohol is, of course, to refuse alcohol altogether. If you do drink, do so with care and in moderation.

NOTES

Notes are in Appendix F.

LIFE CYCLE NUTRITION: MOTHER AND INFANT

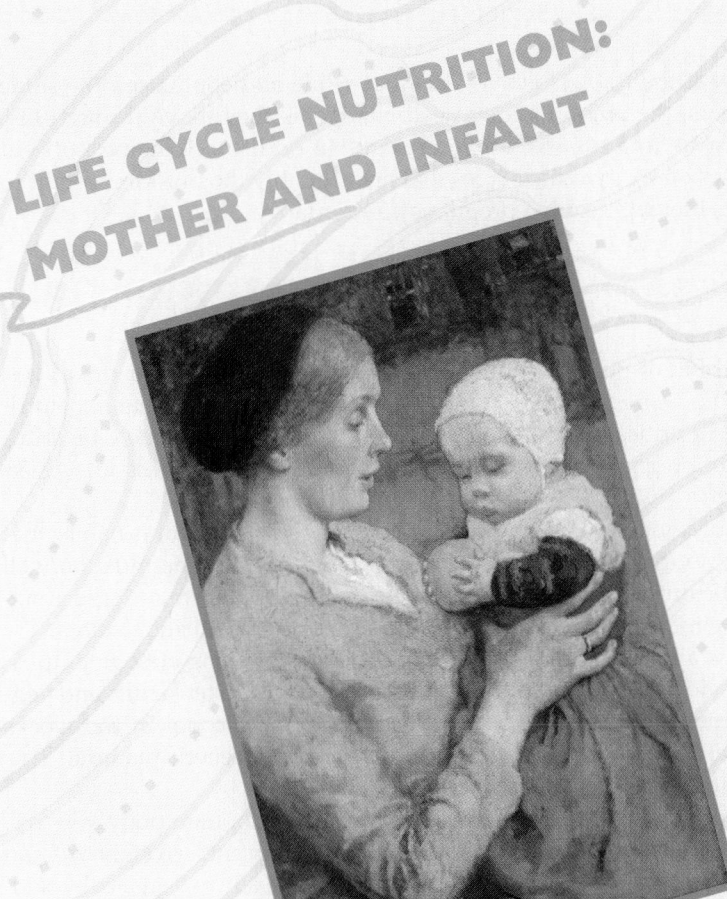

CONTENTS

Gari Melchers, *Mother and Child with Orange;* Peter Harboldt, Corbis.

gestation the period of about 40 weeks (three trimesters) from conception to birth; the term of a pregnancy.

low birthweight a birthweight of less than 5½ pounds (2,500 grams); used as a predictor of probable health problems in the newborn and as a probable indicator of poor nutrition status of the mother before and/or during pregnancy. Low-birthweight infants are of two different types. Some are *premature;* they are born early and are the right size for their gestational age. Others have suffered growth failure in the uterus; they may or may not be born early, but they are *small for gestational age (small for date).*

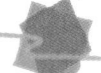

A look at the RDA tables reveals that while all people need the same nutrients, the amounts they need change as they move through life. This chapter is the first of a two-chapter segment on life's changing nutrient needs. It focuses on the two life stages that are arguably the most important to an individual's lifelong health—pregnancy and infancy.

PREGNANCY: THE IMPACT OF NUTRITION ON THE FUTURE

We normally think of our nutrition as personal, affecting only our own lives. The woman who is pregnant, or who will be, must understand that her nutrition today will be critical to the health of her child for years to come. The nutrition demands of pregnancy are extraordinary because the growth of a new person requires every nutrient, and extra amounts of most of them.

Before she becomes pregnant, a woman must establish eating habits that will optimally nourish both the growing fetus and herself. She must be well nourished at the outset because early in pregnancy the embryo undergoes significant developmental changes that depend on her prior nutrition status.

Fathers-to-be also are wise to place emphasis on obtaining adequate nutrients. Limited evidence suggests that men who consume too few fruits and vegetables containing vitamin C or who drink too much alcohol in the weeks before conception may sustain damage to their sperm's genetic material. This damage can cause birth defects in future children.

Prior to pregnancy, all women should strive for appropriate body weights. This is especially important for underweight women. An underweight woman who fails to gain adequately during pregnancy is most likely to bear a baby with a dangerously low birthweight. Infant birthweight is the most potent single indicator of an infant's future health status. Some researchers now suspect that poor nutrition during **gestation** may even set the stage for developing cardiovascular disease and a weak immune system in the future person's later life.[1]

A **low-birthweight** baby, defined as one who weighs less than 5½ pounds (2,500 grams), is nearly 40 times more likely to die in the first year of life than is a normal-weight baby.[2] Such a baby is also likely to be unable to do its job of obtaining nourishment by sucking or to win its mother's attention by energetic, vigorous cries and other healthy behavior. The low-birthweight baby may therefore become an apathetic, neglected baby, and this compounds the original malnutrition problem and leads to illnesses. For these reasons, underweight women are advised to try to gain weight before becoming pregnant or to strive to gain adequately during pregnancy.

Nutritional deficiency, coupled with low birthweight, is the underlying cause of more than half of all the deaths worldwide of children under five years of age. In 1994, the U.S. infant mortality rate was the lowest the nation has ever recorded: 7.9 deaths per 1,000 live births.[3] This rate remains higher than that of some other developed countries, but as part of a significant steady decline for over a decade, it stands as a tribute to public health efforts aimed at reducing infant deaths.

Second to underweight women, obese women are urged to attain healthy weights before pregnancy. The infant of an obese mother may be larger than normal and born late, or it may be large in size even if born prematurely. In the latter case, a large premature baby may not be recognized as such and may not

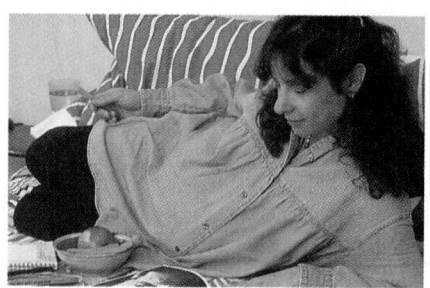

Nourishment for two.

receive the special care it requires from medical staff. Also, obese pregnant women more often suffer gestational diabetes (explained later), hypertension, and infections after the birth than do women of healthy weight. The birth itself may be more likely to require drugs to induce labor or require surgical intervention. An appropriate goal for the obese woman who wishes to become pregnant is to attain a body weight low enough to minimize her medical risks.

A major reason why the mother's nutrition before pregnancy is so crucial is that it determines whether her **uterus** will be able to support the growth of a healthy **placenta** during the first month of pregnancy. If the placenta works perfectly, the fetus wants for nothing; if it doesn't, no alternative source of sustenance is available and the fetus will fail to thrive.[4] The placenta is shown in Figure 12-1; it is a sort of cushion of tissue in which the mother's and baby's blood vessels intertwine and exchange materials. The two bloods never mix, but nutrients and oxygen cross from the mother's blood into the baby's blood while wastes move out of the baby's blood, ultimately to be excreted by the mother. The **amniotic sac** forms to cradle the baby, cushioning it with fluids.

Far from being passive in its transport of molecules, the placenta is a highly metabolic organ with some 60 sets of enzymes of its own. It actively gathers up hormones, nutrients, and protein molecules such as antibodies and transfers them into the fetal bloodstream. It also produces hormones that maintain pregnancy and prepare the mother's breasts for **lactation.**

If the mother's nutrient stores are inadequate during the period when the body is preparing to develop the placenta, then the placenta will never develop properly. As a consequence, no matter how well she eats later, the woman's unborn baby will not receive optimal nourishment. The infant is likely to be a low-birthweight baby with all of the associated risks. After getting such a poor

uterus (YOO-ter-us) the womb, the muscular organ within which the infant develops before birth.

placenta (pla-SEN-tuh) the organ that develops inside the uterus in early pregnancy in which the mother's and fetus's circulatory systems intertwine and in which exchange of materials between maternal and fetal blood takes place. The fetus receives nutrients and oxygen across the placenta; the mother's blood picks up carbon dioxide and other waste materials to be excreted via her lungs and kidneys.

amniotic (am-nee-OTT-ic) **sac** the "bag of water" in the uterus in which the fetus floats.

lactation production and secretion of breast milk for the purpose of nourishing an infant.

FIGURE 12-1

THE PLACENTA

The placenta is a sort of pillow of tissue in which maternal blood vessels lie side by side with fetal blood vessels entering it through the umbilical cord. This close association between the two circulatory systems permits the mother's bloodstream to deliver nutrients and oxygen to the fetus and to carry away fetal waste products.

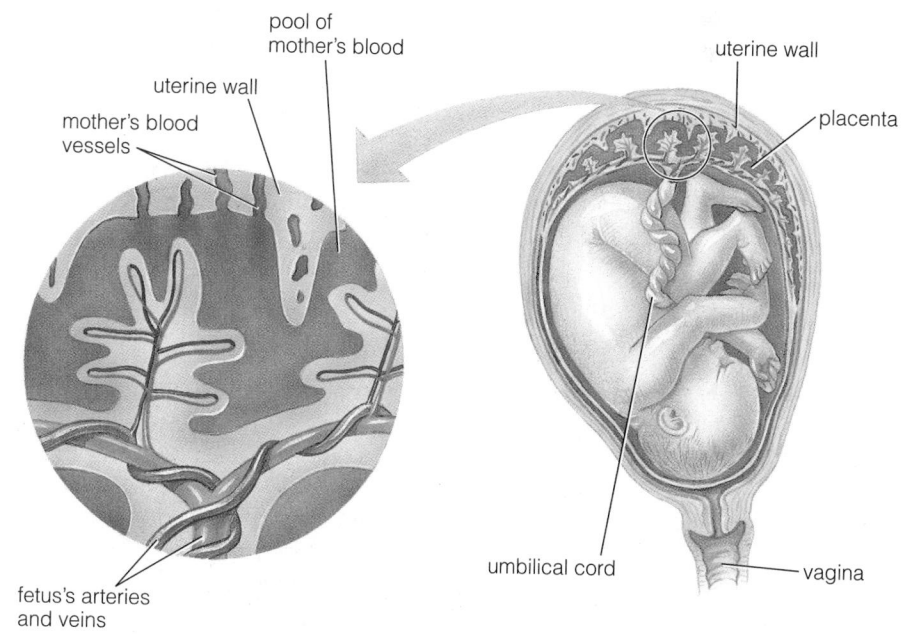

implantation the stage of development, during the first two weeks after conception, in which the fertilized egg embeds itself in the wall of the uterus and begins to develop.

ovum the egg, produced by the mother, that unites with a sperm from the father to produce a new individual.

zygote (ZYE-goat) the term that describes the product of the union of ovum and sperm during the first two weeks after fertilization.

critical period a finite period during development in which certain events may occur that will have irreversible effects on later developmental stages. A critical period is usually a period of cell division in a body organ.

embryo (EM-bree-oh) the stage of human gestation from the third to eighth week after conception.

fetus (FEET-us) the stage of human gestation from eight weeks after conception until birth of an infant.

start on life, children may be ill equipped, even as adults, to store sufficient nutrients, and a girl may also be unable to grow an adequate placenta. In turn, she may bear an infant who is unable to reach full potential.

Not all cases of low birthweight reflect poor nutrition. Other factors associated with low birthweight are heredity, disease conditions, smoking, and drug (including alcohol) use during pregnancy. Even with optimal nutrition and health during pregnancy, some women give birth to small infants for reasons unknown. Still, poor nutrition is the major factor in low birthweight, and, ideally, it is an avoidable one as later sections make clear.

✓ KEY POINT **Adequate nutrition before pregnancy establishes physical readiness and nutrient stores to support fetal growth. Babies who weigh less than 5½ pounds at birth face greater health risks than normal-weight babies.**

The Events of Pregnancy

On **implantation** of the newly fertilized **ovum** (or **zygote**) in the uterine wall, a placenta begins to grow inside the uterus. During the two weeks following fertilization, the zygote divides into many cells, and these cells sort themselves into three layers. Minimal growth in size takes place at this time, but it is a **critical period** developmentally. Adverse influences such as smoking, drug abuse, and malnutrition at this time lead to failure to implant or to abnormalities that can cause loss of the zygote, possibly even before the woman knows she is pregnant. Both mother and child will benefit most from an optimal supply of nutrients uncontaminated by other materials.

The next six weeks of the development of the **embryo** register astonishing physical changes (see Figure 12-2). At eight weeks, the **fetus** has a complete

FIGURE 12-2

STAGES OF EMBRYONIC AND FETAL DEVELOPMENT

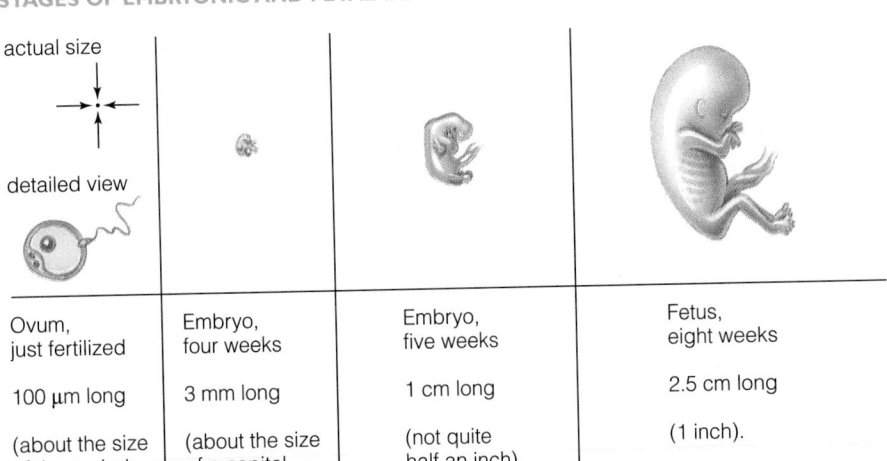
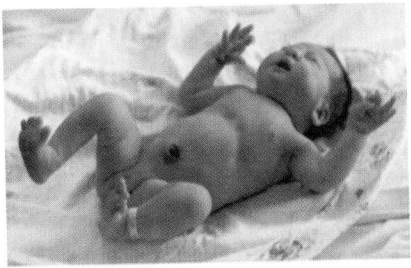

Ovum, just fertilized	Embryo, four weeks	Embryo, five weeks	Fetus, eight weeks	Newborn, nine months
100 μm long	3 mm long	1 cm long	2.5 cm long	50 cm long
(about the size of the period at the end of this phrase).	(about the size of a capital letter A).	(not quite half an inch).	(1 inch).	(20 inches, 5,000 times as long as the ovum, depicted in the first frame of this figure).

central nervous system, a beating heart, a fully formed digestive system, and the beginnings of facial features.

Each organ and tissue type grows with its own characteristic pattern and timing. Each organ depends most on its supply of nutrients during its own intensive growth period. For example, the fetus's heart and brain are well developed at 14 weeks; the lungs, ten weeks later. Therefore early malnutrition impairs the heart and brain; late malnutrition impairs the lungs.

Events during a critical period can occur only at that time and at no other. Whatever nutrients and other environmental conditions are necessary during this period must be supplied on time if the organ is to reach its full potential. If the development of an organ is limited during a critical period, recovery is impossible. Thus early malnutrition often does irreversible damage, although this may not become fully apparent until maturity and may never be attributed to events of pregnancy. Table 12-1 provides a list of factors that make nutrient deficiencies likely during pregnancy. Notice that young age heads the list; a later section explains why pregnant adolescents are especially prone to malnutrition.

The effects of malnutrition during critical periods are seen in neural tube defects of the nervous system (explained later), in the short height of people who were undernourished in their early years, and in the poor dental health of children whose mothers were malnourished during pregnancy.[5] As mentioned, when they reach adulthood, people having such a poor start on life may be vulnerable to infections, and some may have high risks of stroke or heart disease.[6] Clearly, the effects of malnutrition during critical periods are irreversible. There is no second chance to provide nutrients. No matter how abundant and nourishing the food, if it is fed after the critical time, it fails to remedy harm already done.

The last seven months of pregnancy, the fetal period, bring about a tremendous increase in the size of the fetus. Critical periods of cell division and development occur in organ after organ. The amniotic sac fills with fluid and the mother's body changes. The uterus and its supporting muscles increase in size, the breasts may become tender and full, the nipples may darken in preparation for lactation, and the mother's blood volume increases by half to accommodate the added load of materials it must carry. Gestation lasts approximately 40 weeks and ends with the birth of the infant.

✔ **KEY POINT** **Maternal nutrition before and during pregnancy affects both present and future development of the infant. Placental development, implantation, and early critical periods depend on nutrient supply and determine future growth and developmental events.**

Increased Nutrient Needs

Nutrient needs during periods of intensive growth are greater than at any other time and are greater for certain nutrients than for others. The nutrient needs of pregnancy are shown in Figure 12-3.

Energy, Protein, and Fat One of the smallest increases recommended is for energy: pregnancy requires only 300 extra calories a day, or somewhat more

TABLE 12-1

Factors Placing Pregnant Women at Nutritional Risk

Women likely to develop nutrient deficiencies include those who:

- Are young (adolescents).
- Have had many recent previous pregnancies. (This depletes maternal nutrient stores, but may not affect infant birthweight.)
- Lack nutrition knowledge, have too little money to purchase adequate food, or have too little family support.
- Ordinarily consume an inadequate diet due to food faddism, preferences, weight-loss "dieting," uninformed vegetarianism, other limited food choices, or other reasons.
- Smoke cigarettes or abuse alcohol or drugs.
- Are lactose intolerant or suffer chronic health conditions requiring special diets.
- Are underweight or overweight at conception.
- Are carrying twins or triplets.
- Gain insufficient or excessive weight during pregnancy.
- Have a low level of education.

Neural tube defects were first defined in Chapter 7.

FIGURE 12-3

COMPARISON OF NUTRIENT RDA OF NONPREGNANT, PREGNANT, AND LACTATING WOMEN
For actual values, turn to the RDA tables on the inside front cover.

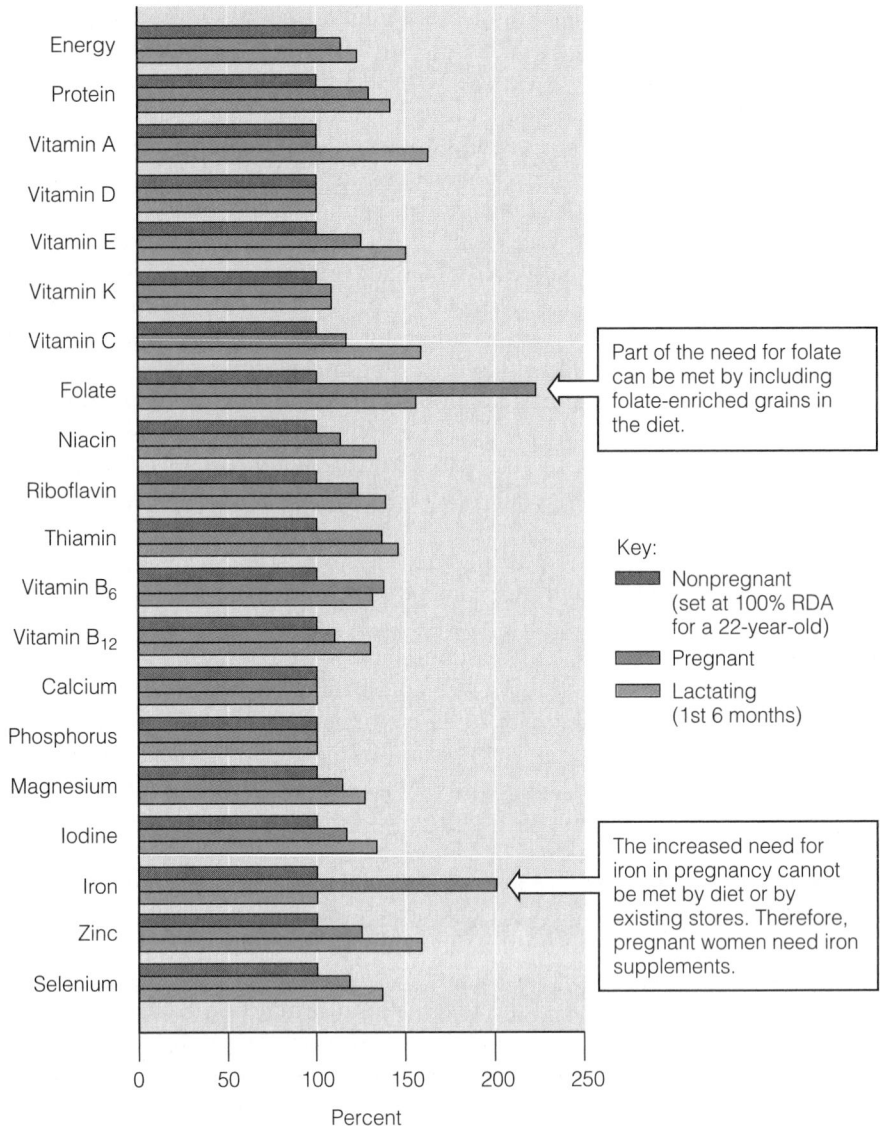

Part of the need for folate can be met by including folate-enriched grains in the diet.

Key:
■ Nonpregnant (set at 100% RDA for a 22-year-old)
■ Pregnant
■ Lactating (1st 6 months)

The increased need for iron in pregnancy cannot be met by diet or by existing stores. Therefore, pregnant women need iron supplements.

in the case of a teenager or a physically active pregnant woman. No additional energy is required in the first few weeks of pregnancy. The greatest energy need begins about week 10 and lasts about five months, with needs tapering off in pregnancy's final weeks.[7] This increment of extra energy is needed to spare protein for its all-important tissue-building work.

The increase recommended for protein is greater than for energy: from about 45 to 50 grams in a nonpregnant woman to about 60 grams per day for a pregnant woman. Many women in the United States, however, need not add protein-rich foods to their diets because they already exceed the recommended protein intake for pregnancy. Excess protein may have adverse effects, as Chapter 6 explained.

Some vegetarian women limit or omit protein-rich meats, eggs, and dairy products from their diets. For them, meeting the RDA for food energy each day

Recommended protein intake: 60 grams/day.

Recommended carbohydrate intake: about 50 percent of energy intake. In a 2,000 calorie/day intake, this represents 1,000 calories of carbohydrate, or about 250 grams.

and including several generous servings of plant-protein foods such as legumes, whole grains, nuts, and seeds are imperative steps. All pregnant women need generous amounts of carbohydrate-rich foods to spare their protein and to provide energy.

The high nutrient requirements of pregnancy leave little room in the diet for excess energy from added purified fats such as oil, margarine, and butter. Some lipids, especially the essential fatty acids, are important to the growth of the fetus and are regarded by some as "essential nutrients in early human development."[8] The brain is largely made of lipid material, and it depends heavily on products of both omega-3 and omega-6 fatty acids for its growth, function, and structure. If a mother-to-be regularly eats a diet that includes seafood, she receives a balance of the essential fatty acids and their derivatives. This benefits both her pregnancy, and afterward her infant, by way of her milk. Supplements of fish oil are not recommended, however, both because they may carry concentrated toxins and because high fish oil intakes seem to alter the course of pregnancy and labor with unknown effects.[9]

Vitamins and Minerals The growing fetus, the altered hormonal activity, and the increased protein metabolism of pregnancy increase the metabolic demand for vitamin B_6. A vitamin B_6 shift occurs during pregnancy, shunting the vitamin from the woman's blood to the tissues of pregnancy where it is needed. This shift causes most pregnant women to test low in blood indicators of vitamin B_6. While this might seem to indicate that supplements are needed, no one knows if supplementation would harm or help. The depressed blood vitamin B_6 in the woman seems not to be harmful. If she took excess vitamin B_6, it might be forced into the fetal tissue, causing a buildup with unknown consequences. No consistent benefit has been shown to result from supplements of vitamin B_6 in amounts greater than the RDA.

Of Special Interest: Folate and Vitamin B_{12} The pregnant woman's RDA for folate is twice that of the nonpregnant woman due to the great increase in her blood volume and the rapid growth of the fetus. Chapter 7 has already described one consequence of entering pregnancy without adequate folate stores and the RDA committee's unprecedented doubling of the folate recommendation for women of reproductive age. In review, the early weeks are a critical period for the **neural tube,** an open tube of tissue that will later develop to form the brain and spinal cord and then will close, sealing itself off from the body and the outside. Nearly 400,000 infants each year are born with **neural tube defects,** and half of these are believed to be related to inadequate maternal folate during the earliest weeks of pregnancy.

By the time a woman suspects she is pregnant, usually around the sixth week, the embryo's neural tube is supposed to have closed. If folate is inadequate before pregnancy, however, the tube may not close fully, and **spina bifida** may result (see Figure 12-4). Mild cases can go unnoticed, but in the worst cases the brain may fail to develop at all, and the infant soon dies of the condition, called **anencephaly.** More common problems include club foot, dislocated hip, kidney disorders, curvature of the spine, muscle weakness, mental retardation, and others.

Not every folate-deficient woman will give birth to a child with neural tube defects, but all fertile women of childbearing age should make sure to eat the

neural tube the embryonic tissue that later forms the brain and spinal cord.

neural tube defects a group of nervous system abnormalities caused by interruption of the normal early development of the neural tube.

spina bifida (SPEE-na BIFF-ih-duh) a birth defect: the infant is born with gaps in the bones of the spine, leaving the spinal cord protected only by a sheath of skin in those spots, or with no protection at all. The spinal cord may bulge and protrude through the gaps in the vertebral column.

anencephaly (an-en-SEFF-ah-lee) a severe neural tube defect that causes the brain not to form and leads to death soon after birth.

The general functions of folate appear in Chapter 7, along with more about folate supplements.

FIGURE 12-4

SPINA BIFIDA—A NEURAL TUBE DEFECT

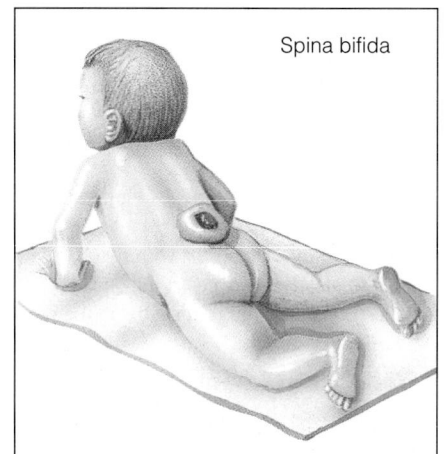

Spina bifida

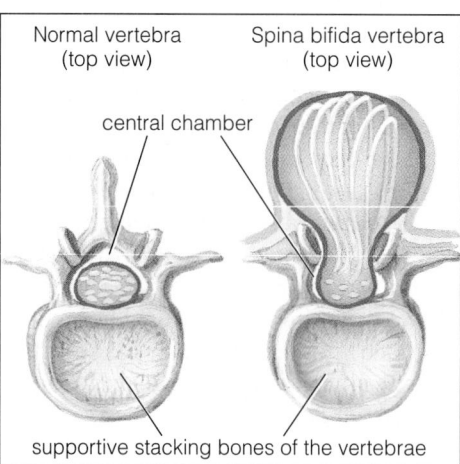

Normal vertebra (top view)   Spina bifida vertebra (top view)

central chamber

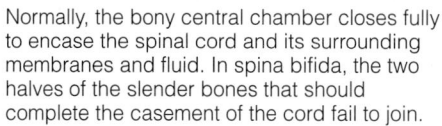

supportive stacking bones of the vertebrae

Normally, the bony central chamber closes fully to encase the spinal cord and its surrounding membranes and fluid. In spina bifida, the two halves of the slender bones that should complete the casement of the cord fail to join.

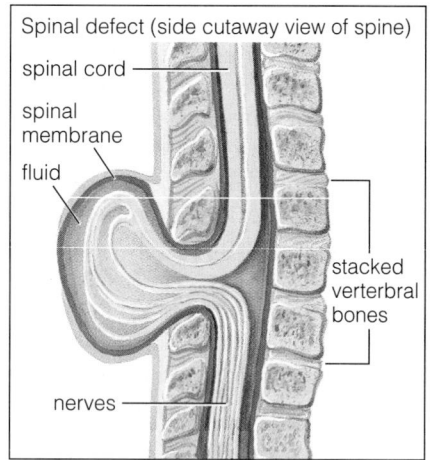

Spinal defect (side cutaway view of spine)

spinal cord

spinal membrane

fluid

stacked verterbral bones

nerves

In the serious form shown here, membranes and fluid have bulged through the gap and nerves are exposed, invariably leading to some degree of paralysis and often to mental retardation.

TABLE 12-2

Rich Folate Sources[a]

Asparagus	Liver
Beets	Orange Juice
Fortified cereals	Oranges
and enriched	Spinach and
grain products	other leafy
Legumes	greens

[a]Folate amounts for these and 2,000 other foods are listed in the Table of Food Composition in Appendix A.

needed folate-rich foods every day (see Table 12-2). It is possible but not easy to obtain enough folate for pregnancy from unfortified foods alone.[10] For this reason, folate has been added to the list of U.S. enrichment nutrients so that, as of 1998, all foods made of refined grains can be assumed to contribute significantly to the day's folate need. This way, most women will take in adequate folate *before* the onset of pregnancy. Folate supplements also provide a convenient way to ensure sufficient folate intake during pregnancy. Prenatal supplements that include sufficient folate and other nutrients of concern are probably the best type for the pregnant woman; other types may not meet her needs.

The pregnant woman also needs greater amounts of the B vitamin that assists folate in the manufacture of new cells, vitamin B_{12}. People who eat meat, eggs, or dairy products receive all they need, even for pregnancy. Those who exclude all animal products from the diet, however, need vitamin B_{12}–fortified soy milk or supplements.

Calcium and Other Minerals   Among the minerals, calcium, phosphorus, and magnesium are in great demand during pregnancy because they are involved in building the skeleton. Intestinal absorption of calcium doubles early in pregnancy and the mineral is stored in the mother's bones. Later, when the fetal bones begin to calcify, the mother's bone stores are drawn upon, and there is a dramatic shift of calcium across the placenta. Women's diets are notoriously low in calcium, so these withdrawals from the mother's skeletal reserves may weaken her bones. Thus the increases in calcium intake required for pregnancy may be large. The RDA for calcium and phosphorus is 1,200 milligrams per day each. Magnesium for bone and tissue growth, is needed during pregnancy in amounts slightly higher than the regular RDA.

The body conserves iron even more than usual during pregnancy. Menstruation ceases, and absorption of iron increases up to threefold. Despite these conservation measures, iron stores dwindle because the developing fetus draws on its mother's iron stores to create stores of its own to carry it through the first three to six months of life. In addition, maternal blood volume increases by as much as 50 percent, and this can give the blood the appearance of anemia in blood tests. The same amount of iron is still in the blood, but it has been diluted. Add to these factors that few women enter pregnancy with adequate stores to meet pregnancy demands, and the wisdom of the committee on RDA in recommending that women take prescribed iron supplements throughout pregnancy becomes evident. Supplements intended for use during pregnancy provide iron along with other needed nutrients (see Table 12-3). Ideally, supplements plus food intakes will cover the needs of all pregnant women, even pregnant vegetarians who most often lack iron.

Pregnancy is clearly a time of increased nutrient needs. A woman of limited financial means may need help in obtaining the needed food and counseling that women of greater means can afford. At the federal level, an underprivileged woman can turn to the **Special Supplemental Food Program for Women, Infants, and Children (WIC)** to receive nutrition counseling and vouchers redeemable for nutritious foods. Federal food stamps can also help to stretch her grocery dollars. Her own community may provide educational services and materials, including nutrition, food budgeting, and shopping information, through the local agricultural extension service. Organizations such as the American Diabetes Association and local hospitals may also provide nutrition information.

✔ **KEY POINT** **Pregnancy induces maternal physiological adjustments that demand increases in intakes of energy and even greater increases in intakes of nutrients.**

Weight Gain

The pregnant woman must gain a certain amount of weight during pregnancy as a defense against bearing a low-birthweight baby. Ideally, she will have begun her pregnancy at the appropriate weight for her height, but even more importantly, she will gain enough weight based on her prepregnancy body mass index (BMI; see Table 12-4). The ideal pattern is thought to be about 2 to 4 pounds during the first **trimester** and a pound per week thereafter.

Dieting during pregnancy is not recommended. Even an obese woman should gain about 15 pounds for the best chances of delivering a healthy infant.[11] Weight gain must be especially generous to meet the needs of a teenager who is still growing herself and to support women who are carrying twins or triplets. Women have been known to exceed or undershoot the recommended limits in pregnancy without ill effects, but the best chances of health are predicted by recommended weight gains. A sudden, large weight gain is always a danger signal: it may indicate the onset of pregnancy-induced hypertension. See the section entitled "Troubleshooting" later on.

Special Supplemental Food Program for Women, Infants, and Children (WIC) a USDA program to provide nutrition support to low-income women who are pregnant or who have infants or preschool children. WIC offers coupons redeemable for specific foods to supply the nutrients deemed most needed for growth and development.

trimester one-third of gestation, about 13 to 14 weeks.

Ordinarily, a hemoglobin below 13 grams/100 milliliters is considered low for a woman. In mid-pregnancy, values dipping below 12 grams are not unusual, and 10.5 grams is where the line defining anemia is often drawn.

SOURCE: National Academy of Sciences, Food and Nutrition Board, *Nutrition during Pregnancy* (Washington, D.C.: National Academy Press, 1990), pp. 274–275.

TABLE 12-3

Nutrient Supplements for Pregnancy

Nutrient	Amount
Folate	300 μg
Vitamin B_6	2 mg
Vitamin C	50 mg
Vitamin D	5 μg
Calcium	250 mg
Copper	2 mg
Iron	30 mg
Zinc	15 mg

SOURCE: Reprinted with permission from *Nutrition during Pregnancy* © 1990 by the National Academy of Sciences. Published by National Academy Press, Washington, D.C.

TABLE 12-4

Recommended Weight Gains for Pregnancy

- Underweight women: 28 to 40 lb
- Normal-weight women: 25 to 35 lb
- Overweight women: 15 to 25 lb
- Obese women: 13 lb minimum

NOTE: Underweight is defined as BMI <19.8; normal weight, as BMI 19.8 to 26.0; overweight as BMI 26.0 to 29.0; and obese as BMI >29.0 (BMI standards are on the inside back cover).

The weight the pregnant woman puts on is nearly all lean tissue: placenta, uterus, blood, milk-producing glands, and, of course, the baby itself (see Table 12-5). The fat she gains is needed later for lactation. Some weight is lost at delivery, but many women retain a pound or two from each pregnancy.

✔ KEY POINT   **Weight gain is essential for a healthy pregnancy. A woman's prepregnancy BMI, her own nutrient needs, and whether or not she is carrying multiple fetuses help to determine an appropriate weight gain.**

Physical Activity

Physical activity is important to the pregnant woman, not only to help her carry the extra weight of pregnancy without strain, but also to help ease her upcoming childbirth. In the old days, pregnant women were admonished to "stay off their feet" and to "take it easy." Taking it too easy, however, may be as detrimental to a pregnancy as overexertion. Staying active can improve the fitness of the mother-to-be, prevent complications in pregnancy, facilitate labor, and reduce psychological stress.[12] Pregnant women should take care in choosing their exercise programs, for some work-related physical activity, such as standing for many hours or working strenuously at fatiguing tasks, has been associated with a risk of preterm birth.[13] A pregnant woman should consult her health care provider before embarking on an exercise plan and should follow the rules listed in Table 12-6.

✔ KEY POINT   **Wisely chosen physical activity helps the pregnant woman stay fit and reduces risks of complications during the pregnancy.**

Teen Pregnancy

A pregnant adolescent presents a special case of intense nutrient needs. One in every five babies is born to a teenage mother, and more than one-tenth of these mothers are under age 15. Even when not pregnant, a teenage girl is hard put

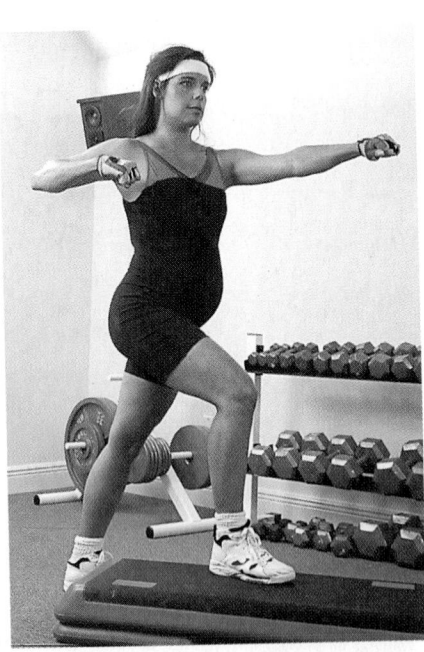

Pregnant women can enjoy the benefits of exercise.

TABLE 12-5

Components of Weight Gain during Pregnancy

Development	Weight Gain (lb)
Infant at birth	7½
Placenta	1½
Extra blood volume	4
Extra fluid volume	4
Growth of uterus	2
Growth of breasts	2
Amniotic fluid	2
Mother's fat stores	7
Total	30

SOURCE: The American College of Obstetricians and Gynecologists, *ACOG Guide to Planning for Pregnancy, Birth, and Beyond* (Washington, D.C.: The American College of Obstetricians and Gynecologists, 1990), p. 109.

TABLE 12-6

Rules for Exercising During and After Pregnancy

- Exercise regularly. Physical activity at least three times per week is preferable to intermittent activity.
- Do not exercise while lying on your back after about the fourth month of pregnancy. Such a position diverts blood from the uterus and fetus.
- Avoid prolonged periods of motionless standing.
- Reduce the intensity of exercise because pregnancy diminishes aerobic power.
- Stop the activity when feeling fatigued and do not exercise to exhaustion.
- Choose swimming, bicycling, or other weight-supporting activities as the weight of pregnancy increases.
- Protect against accidental injury.
- Eat sufficient energy and nutrients to fuel both the activity and the pregnancy.
- Avoid becoming overheated, especially in the first trimester: drink sufficiently, dress appropriately, and exercise lightly in hot, humid weather. Do not sit in hot tubs, steam rooms, or saunas.
- Continue these precautions for four to six weeks following delivery, or until prepregnancy abilities are gradually regained.

SOURCE: Adapted from American College of Obstetricians and Gynecologists, *Exercise during pregnancy and the postpartum period*, ACOG Technical Bulletin 189, February 1994.

to meet her own nutrient needs, but when pregnant, she is likely to be deficient in many vitamins and minerals, including vitamins A and C, niacin, iron, calcium, and chromium. Nourishing a growing fetus adds to her burden. Her own high nutrient requirements can compete with those of her fetus, especially if she is going through her most rapid growth phase. To support the needs of both mother and fetus, a pregnant teenager with a body mass index in the normal range is encouraged to gain 35 pounds or so. Teenagers who gain less have smaller newborns with associated risks.

Complications are common in teenage pregnancies. The greatest risk of a teen pregnancy is death of the infant. The infant mortality rate for mothers under the age of 20 years is high, and mothers under 15 have the highest rate of all. It seems that youth alone, without other negative factors, increases the risks of serious problems including stillbirths, preterm births, low-birthweight infants, and medical problems.[14] Poor nutrition compounds these risks.

A pregnant teenager's needs for many nutrients increase greatly, although her energy allowance increases by only a few percent. If a young woman starts pregnancy already malnourished or lacks education, resources, and support, she may develop serious nutrient deficiencies. Table 12-7 provides a guide to the number of food servings recommended to provide nutrients needed by teenagers, by pregnant and lactating teenagers, and by pregnant or lactating adult women according to the Daily Food Guide.

Teens are notorious for their poor eating habits. They skip meals, snack on chips and colas, or grab doughnuts for breakfast, and many continue on this path to malnutrition even after becoming pregnant. Luckily, some make at least some effort to eat well, but even those with the best intentions usually fall short of obtaining RDA amounts of at least some nutrients.[15]

In 1992, girls aged 15 to 17 gave birth to almost 190,000 babies.

TABLE 12-7

Daily Food Guide for Teenagers, Pregnant and Lactating Teenagers, and Adult Pregnant and Lactating Women

	NUMBER OF SERVINGS[a]		
FOOD GROUP	**Teenagers**	**Pregnant or Lactating Teenagers**	**Pregnant or Lactating Women**
Meat and meat alternates	2 to 3	3	3
Milk and milk products	3	4	3 to 4
Vegetables	3 to 5	4 to 5	4 to 5
Fruits	2 to 4	3 to 4	3 to 4
Breads/cereals/rice, pasta	6 to 11	9 to 12	7 to 11

[a]Figure 2-4 provided details concerning serving sizes and foods within the groups listed here.

A teenager's psychological development may affect her pregnancy and later motherhood as much as any economic or physical vulnerability.[16] Developing an individual identity is an important developmental task for each teenager.[17] The search for identity, though critical to later emotional health, can cause pregnant teens to reject most advice, including nutrition advice, from adults. Most teens do care about their future infants' health, and they may accept advice from respected school coaches or counselors or other people they trust.

✔ KEY POINT   **Of all the population groups, pregnant teenage girls have the highest nutrient needs.**

Cravings, Nausea, and Other Hobgoblins of Pregnancy

Does pregnancy give a woman the right to demand pickles and ice cream at 2 A.M.? Perhaps not for nutrition's sake. Food cravings and aversions during pregnancy, though common, do not seem to reflect real physiological needs. In other words, a woman who craves pickles is not likely to be in need of salt. Food cravings and aversions that arise during pregnancy are usually due to changes in taste and smell sensitivities, and they quickly disappear after the baby's birth.

Sometimes cravings may occur in women with nutrient-poor diets. A pregnant woman who is deficient in iron, zinc, or other nutrients may crave and eat clay, ice, cornstarch, and other nonnutritious substances, but this does not prove that the deficiency caused the craving. The practice is pica (first mentioned in Chapter 8). Such cravings are not adaptive; the substances the woman craves do not deliver the nutrients she needs. In fact, clay and other substances can cling to the intestinal wall and form a barrier that interferes with normal nutrient absorption.

The nausea of "morning" (actually, anytime) sickness seems unavoidable because it arises from the hormonal changes of early pregnancy. Nausea can sometimes be alleviated by sipping on carbonated drinks or lemonade and nibbling soda crackers or other salty snack foods before getting out of bed.[18] Other times women may do as well to simply eat what they desire whenever they feel hungry. Table 12-8 offers some other suggestions, but morning sickness can be stubborn. If morning sickness interferes with normal eating for more than a week or two, the woman should seek medical advice to prevent nutrient deficiencies.

Later, as the hormones of pregnancy alter her muscle tone and the thriving fetus crowds her intestinal organs, an expectant mother may complain of heartburn or constipation. Many women find that raising the head of the bed with two or three pillows helps to relieve nighttime heartburn. A high-fiber diet and a plentiful water intake help relieve constipation. Exercise may also help, and it should be a daily practice. The woman should use laxatives or heartburn medication only if her physician prescribes them.

✔ KEY POINT **Food cravings usually do not reflect physiological needs, and some may interfere with nutrition. Nausea arises from normal hormonal changes of pregnancy. Laxatives and heartburn medication should be taken only on a physician's advice.**

Practices to Avoid

Some substances in a woman's diet and environment can be harmful, and their potential impact is too great to ignore. Of these, alcohol predominates and is the topic of the next section. A few others also deserve some discussion.

A clearly harmful practice is smoking. Smoking restricts the blood supply to the growing fetus and so limits the delivery of oxygen and nutrients and the

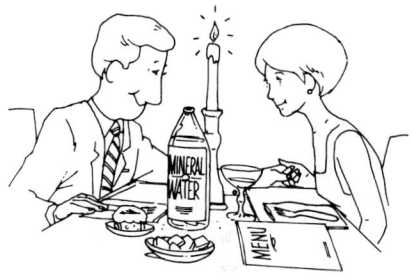

To plan a healthy pregnancy, both parents must make wise choices in advance.

TABLE 12-8

Tips for Relieving Common Discomforts of Pregnancy

To alleviate the nausea of pregnancy:

- On waking, arise slowly.
- Eat dry toast or crackers.
- Chew gum or suck hard candies.
- Eat small, frequent meals whenever hunger strikes.
- Avoid foods with offensive odors.
- When nauseated, drink no citrus juice, water, milk, coffee, or tea.

To prevent or alleviate constipation:

- Eat foods high in fiber.
- Exercise daily.
- Drink at least 8 glasses of liquids a day.
- Respond promptly to the urge to defecate.
- Use laxatives only as prescribed by a physician; avoid mineral oil—it carries needed fat-soluble vitamins out of the body.

To prevent or relieve heartburn:

- Eat small, frequent meals.
- Drink liquids between meals.
- Avoid spicy or greasy foods.
- Sit up while eating.
- Wait an hour after eating before lying down.
- Wait 2 hours after eating before exercising.

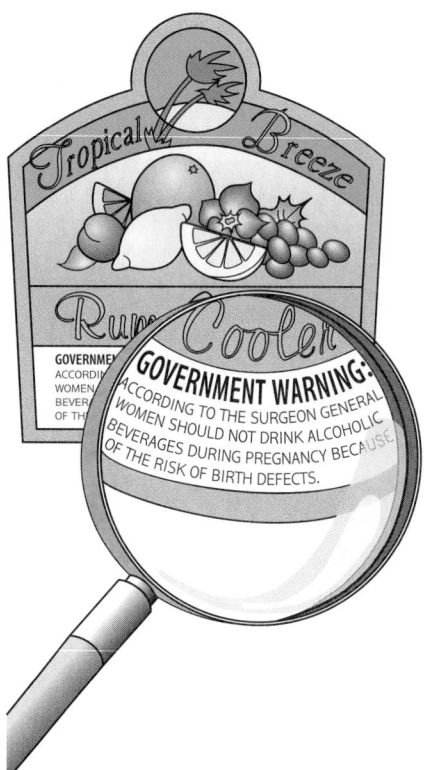

Fetal Effects of Abused Drugs:

Amphetamines: Suspected nervous system damage; behavioral abnormalities.

Barbiturates: Drug withdrawal symptoms in the newborn, lasting up to six months.

Cocaine: Uncontrolled jerking motions; paralysis; permanent mental and physical damage.

Marijuana: Short-term irritability at birth.

Opiates (including heroin): Drug withdrawal symptoms in the newborn, permanent learning disability (attention deficit disorder).

removal of wastes. It slows growth, thus retarding physical development in the uterus; and it may cause behavioral or intellectual problems later on.[19] Constituents of cigarette smoke such as nicotine, cyanide, and others pose a danger to the fetus. Growing evidence links a woman's smoking during pregnancy and exposure of her newborn to second-hand smoke with sudden infant death syndrome (SIDS), the unexplained deaths that sometimes occur in otherwise healthy infants.[20] The Surgeon General has warned that parental smoking can kill an otherwise normal fetus or newborn.

Other drugs taken during pregnancy can cause serious birth defects. The use of drugs not prescribed by a physician, even over-the-counter drugs or high-dose vitamin supplements, is inadvisable. Research shows that mothers who abuse drugs such as marijuana and cocaine during pregnancy inflict serious health consequences, including nervous system disorders, on their future infants.[21] Crack and other forms of cocaine pose hazards to infants who may face low-birthweight complications, heartbeat abnormalities, the pain of withdrawal, and even death as they first experience life outside the womb.[22] Some effects of other drugs of abuse on the fetus are listed in the margin.

Among vitamins, a single massive dose of vitamin A (100 times the RDA) has caused birth defects. Chronic lower-dose vitamin A supplement use (three to four times the RDA) also causes birth defects.[23] Women taking supplements should take heed—experts urge pregnant women not to exceed daily intakes of three times the RDA of vitamin A. Fetuses can also be injured by other poisons, including household insecticides and solvents, lead or other heavy metals from any source, and many other toxins.

Dieting, even for short periods, is also hazardous during pregnancy. Low-carbohydrate diets or fasts that cause ketosis deprive the growing brain of needed glucose and may impair its development. Such diets are also likely to be deficient in other nutrients vital to fetal growth. Energy restriction during pregnancy is dangerous, regardless of the woman's prepregnancy weight or the amount of weight gained in the previous month.

Caffeine crosses the placenta, and the fetus has only a limited ability to metabolize it. No firm limit for caffeine intake is yet available. Intakes of up to the amount in three or four cups of coffee or tea spaced throughout a day are generally thought to be safe.[24] (Caffeine amounts in food and beverages are listed in this chapter's Controversy.)

✓ **KEY POINT** **Abstinence from smoking and other drugs, avoiding dieting, and limited caffeine use are recommended during pregnancy.**

DRINKING DURING PREGNANCY

Alcohol is arguably the most hazardous drug to future generations because it is legally available, heavily promoted, and widely abused. Society often sends mixed messages concerning alcohol. Companies promote an image of drinkers as wealthy, healthy, young, and active while health authorities warn that alcohol may have adverse effects, especially during pregnancy (see Figure 12-5). Every container of beer, wine, or liquor for sale in the United States is now required to warn pregnant women of the danger of drinking during pregnancy. In the past, many women who would have ceased drinking during pregnancy, had they known the danger, unwittingly damaged their infants. Women of childbearing age need to know about alcohol's effects.

Alcohol's Effects

Oxygen is indispensable on a minute-to-minute basis to the development of the fetus's central nervous system. A sudden dose of alcohol can halt the delivery of oxygen through the umbilical cord. Alcohol also slows cell division, reducing the number of cells produced and inflicting abnormalities on those that are produced.[25] During the first month of pregnancy, even a few minutes of alcohol exposure can exert a major effect on the fetal brain, which at that time is growing at the rate of 100,000 new brain cells a minute. Alcohol also interferes with placental transport of nutrients to the fetus and can cause malnutrition in the mother; then all of malnutrition's harmful effects compound the effects of the alcohol.

✔ **KEY POINT** Alcohol limits oxygen delivery to the fetus, slows cell division, and reduces the number of cells organs produce. Alcoholic beverages must bear warnings to pregnant women.

Apgar score a system of scoring an infant's physical condition right after birth. Heart rate, respiration, muscle tone, response to stimuli, and color are ranked 0, 1, or 2. A low score indicates that medical attention is required to facilitate survival.

fetal alcohol syndrome (FAS) the cluster of symptoms seen in an infant or child whose mother consumed excess alcohol during her pregnancy. FAS includes, but is not limited to, brain damage, growth retardation, mental retardation, and facial abnormalities.

Fetal Alcohol Syndrome

Drinking alcohol during pregnancy threatens the fetus with irreversible brain damage, growth retardation, mental retardation, facial abnormalities, vision abnormalities, low **Apgar scores,** and more than 40 identifiable health problems, a cluster of symptoms known as **fetal alcohol syndrome** or **FAS.**[26] The fetal brain is extremely vulnerable to a glucose or oxygen deficit, and alcohol causes both by disrupting placental functioning. In addition, alcohol itself crosses the placenta freely and is directly toxic to the defenseless fetal brain and nervous system. The result is permanent brain damage and lifelong mental retardation. FAS is preventable by limiting alcohol intake during pregnancy, but once present, it is incurable.

Over the past 15 years, incidence of FAS has increased sixfold.[27] About a fifth of women continue drinking alcohol after they learn that they are pregnant. For women who want to drink during their pregnancies, then, the important question is how much alcohol is too much.

Clearly, 3 ounces of alcohol (about 6 drinks) a day is too much early in pregnancy, even if the woman stops drinking immediately after she learns that she is pregnant. Birth defects have been observed in the children of some women who drank 2 ounces (4 drinks) of alcohol daily during pregnancy. Low birthweight has been observed in infants born to some women who drank 1 ounce (2 drinks) per day during pregnancy. At that level of alcohol intake, a sizable and significant increase in the rate of spontaneous abortions occurs; the reason is unclear, but perhaps the alcohol poisons the fetus or causes the placenta to detach. FAS is also known to occur with as few as 2 drinks a day.

All studies of alcohol doses and fetal damage report that the pattern of drinking, even more than the average alcohol intake, may play an important role. For example, a woman whose average intake was only 1 ounce of alcohol a day might not drink at all during the week, but then might have 14 drinks each weekend. Thus the fetus might be intermittently exposed to high alcohol doses. No matter what the intake or pattern, the most severe impact is likely to occur in the first month, before the woman may be aware that she is pregnant.

Controversy 11 defined "a drink" as:
- ✔ 3 to 4 ounces wine.
- ✔ 10 ounces wine cooler.
- ✔ 12 ounces beer.
- ✔ 1 ounce hard liquor.

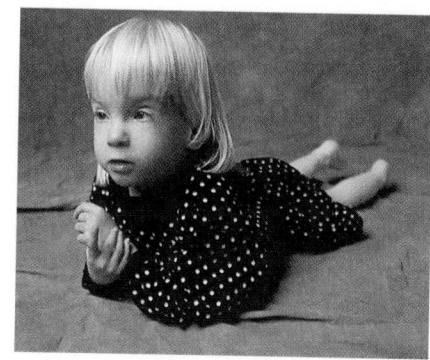

A child with FAS.

fetal alcohol effect (FAE) partial abnormalities from prenatal alcohol exposure, not sufficient for diagnosis with FAS, but impairing to the child. Also called *alcohol-related birth defects (ARBD)* or *subclinical FAS*.

Research using animals shows that one-fifth of the amount of alcohol needed to produce major, outwardly visible defects will surely produce learning impairment in the offspring, a condition known as **fetal alcohol effect (FAE).** Some children show no outward sign of the impairment, but the damage is there on the inside. Others may be short in stature or display subtle facial abnormalities. Most perform poorly in school and in social interactions and suffer a subtle form of brain damage. Anyone exposed to alcohol before birth may always respond differently to it, and also to certain drugs, than if no exposure had occurred. Even before fertilization, alcohol may damage the ovum or sperm in the mother or father-to-be, and so lead to abnormalities in children.

Although the syndrome was named for damage evident at birth, it has been shown that children born with it remain damaged. They may live, but they never fully recover. Figure 12-6 shows the facial abnormalities of FAS, because they are easy to depict. A visual picture of the internal harm is impossible, but it is that damage that virtually seals the fate of the child for life. About 3 in every 1,000 children are victims of this preventable damage, making FAS the leading known cause of mental retardation in the world. Moreover, for every baby diagnosed with FAS, 3 or 4 with FAE may go undiagnosed until problems

FIGURE 12-6

TYPICAL FACIAL CHARACTERISTICS OF FAS

The severe facial abnormalities shown here are just outward signs of severe mental impairments and internal organ damage. These defects, though hidden, may create major health problems later.

SOURCE: Adapted from J. O. Beattie, Alcohol exposure and the fetus, *European Journal of Clinical Nutrition* 46 (1992): S7–S17.

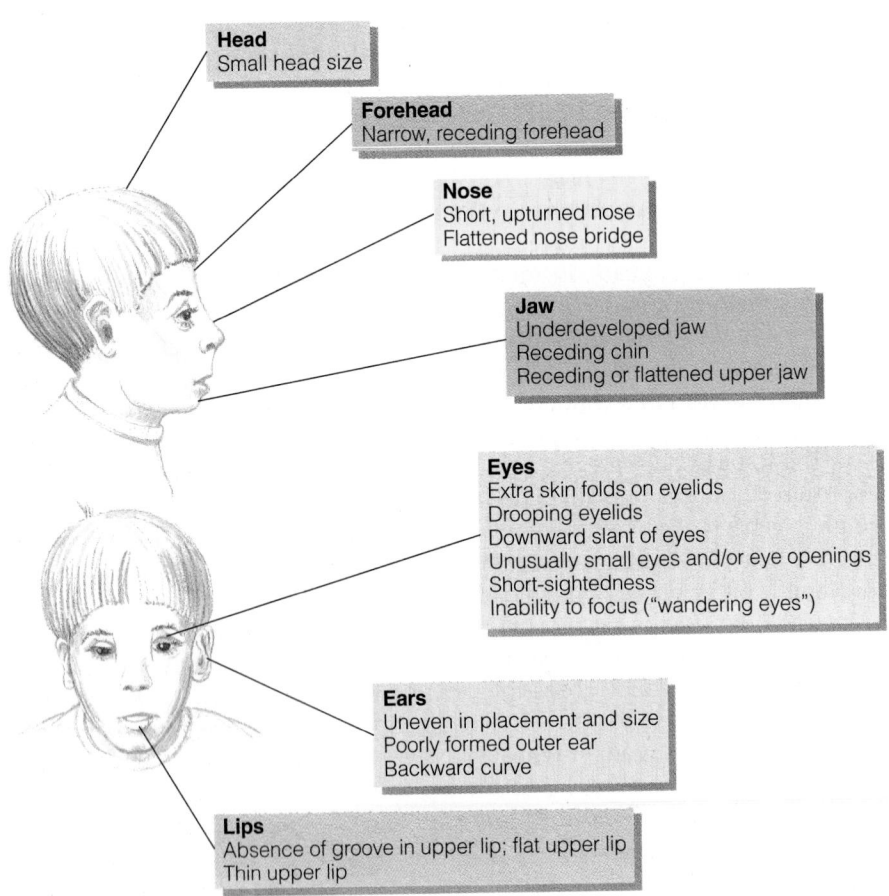

Head
Small head size

Forehead
Narrow, receding forehead

Nose
Short, upturned nose
Flattened nose bridge

Jaw
Underdeveloped jaw
Receding chin
Receding or flattened upper jaw

Eyes
Extra skin folds on eyelids
Drooping eyelids
Downward slant of eyes
Unusually small eyes and/or eye openings
Short-sightedness
Inability to focus ("wandering eyes")

Ears
Uneven in placement and size
Poorly formed outer ear
Backward curve

Lips
Absence of groove in upper lip; flat upper lip
Thin upper lip

develop later in the preschool years. Upon reaching adulthood, such children are ill equipped for employment, relationships, and the other facets of life most adults take for granted.

✔ KEY POINT **The birth defects of fetal alcohol syndrome arise from severe damage to the fetus caused by alcohol. A lesser condition, fetal alcohol effect, may be harder to diagnose but also robs the child of a normal life.**

Experts' Advice

The American Academy of Pediatrics takes the position that women should stop drinking as soon as they *plan* to become pregnant.[28] As mentioned, this step is important for fathers-to-be as well. It is important to know, though, that a woman who has drunk heavily during the first two-thirds of her pregnancy, can still prevent some organ damage by stopping heavy drinking during the third trimester.

Experts have not always agreed that women need to abstain totally from using alcohol during pregnancy. Researchers looking for a "safe" intake limit have come full circle to concede that abstinence from alcohol is the best policy for pregnant women. The authors of this book do, too. It is a personal choice, but if we had it to make, we would give up even the pleasure of wine with meals "for the duration." After the birth of our healthy baby, we would celebrate, if at all, with one glass of the finest champagne.

✔ KEY POINT **Abstinence from or strict restriction of alcohol is critical to prevent irreversible damage to the fetus.**

TROUBLESHOOTING

Some additional measures can help women to avoid the most common problems encountered during pregnancy. Pregnancy precipitates **gestational diabetes** in some women. Without proper management, diabetes can lead to fetal or infant sickness and death. Properly managed, it will cause no harm at all except that surgical birth may be necessary.[29] It is therefore standard procedure that all pregnant women be screened for diabetes at about the sixth month. Thereafter, at every checkup, urine testing for ketone bodies is in order.

A certain degree of **edema** is to be expected in late pregnancy, and some women also develop hypertension during that time. If a rise in blood pressure is mild, it may subside after childbirth and cause no harm.[30] If it is the **pregnancy-induced hypertension (PIH)** that is part of a condition known as **preeclampsia,** however, the effects can be serious.

Preeclampsia causes severe edema; threatens the pregnant woman's circulatory system, liver, kidneys, and brain; and endangers the lives of both mother and fetus. Three key elements help to identify women with preeclampsia: edema, hypertension, and protein in the urine. It is important to keep track of maternal indicators throughout pregnancy and to initiate medical treatment promptly if preeclampsia is diagnosed.

Pregnancy is a time of adjustment to major changes, physical, social, emotional, and financial. The couple who are expecting a baby will have to change their lifestyles as they take on the responsibility of caring for a child. Ideally,

gestational diabetes abnormal glucose tolerance appearing during pregnancy, with subsequent return to normal after the end of pregnancy.

edema accumulation of fluid in the tissues (also defined in Chapter 6).

pregnancy-induced hypertension (PIH) a form of high blood pressure that can develop in later pregnancy.

preeclampsia a potentially dangerous condition during pregnancy characterized by edema, hypertension, and protein in the urine.

Warning Signs of PIH:
✔ Headaches.
✔ Swelling, especially facial swelling.
✔ Dizziness.
✔ Blurred vision.
✔ Sudden weight gain.

The normal edema of pregnancy is a response to gravity: fluid from blood pools in the ankles. The edema of PIH causes swelling of the face and hands as well as of the feet and ankles.

colostrum (co-LAHS-trum) a milklike secretion from the breast during the first day or so after delivery before milk appears; rich in protective factors.

the mother will start developing this sense of responsibility by caring for herself during pregnancy. The expectant parents need support in thinking of themselves as important people with a new and challenging task that they can and will perform well.

✔ **KEY POINT** **Common medical problems associated with pregnancy are gestational diabetes and pregnancy-induced hypertension (PIH). These should be managed to minimize associated risks.**

BREASTFEEDING

As the time of childbirth nears, a woman must decide whether she will feed her baby breast milk or formula. Before she makes this choice, she should be aware of some things about breastfeeding. Both the American Academy of Pediatrics (AAP) and the Canadian Pediatric Society stand behind the statement, "Breastfeeding is strongly recommended for full term infants, except in the few instances where specific contraindications exist." The American Dietetic Association advocates breastfeeding for the nutritional health it confers on the infant as well as for the physiological, social, economic, and other benefits it gives to the mother.[31] All other legitimate nutrition authorities share this view, but some makers of baby formula try to convince women otherwise, as the Consumer Corner that follows the next section points out.

Breast Milk

Breast milk is tailor-made to meet the nutrient needs of the human infant.[32] Its carbohydrate is lactose, and its fat provides a generous portion of the essential omega-6 fatty acid linoleic acid and its products. In addition, a mother who consumes food rich in omega-3 fatty acids will pass these beneficial nutrients on to her child through her milk. Breast milk contains fat-digesting enzymes that help ensure efficient fat absorption by the infant.[33] Breast milk also conveys information to the infant's body about its environment by way of antibodies, whole proteins, and other constituents.

Breast milk also offers the infant unsurpassed protection against infection. This protection includes antiviral and antibacterial agents and infection inhibitors. Some of these immune molecules are proteins that the infant absorbs whole, but greatest protection may occur in the milk itself. These immune factors interfere with growth of bacteria that could otherwise attack the infant's vulnerable digestive tract linings.[34]

During the first two or three days of lactation, the breasts produce **colostrum,** a premilk substance containing antibodies and white cells from the mother's blood. Colostrum is relatively free of bacteria as it leaves the breast, and the baby cannot contract a bacterial infection from it even if the mother has one. Because it contains immunity factors, colostrum helps protect the newborn infant from those infections against which the mother has developed immunity, precisely those in the environment likely to infect the infant. Maternal antibodies from colostrum inactivate harmful bacteria within the infant's digestive tract. Later, breast milk also delivers antibodies, although not as many as colostrum. The degree to which antibodies are delivered in milk depends partly on how well nourished the woman is herself.[35] Malnourished

The effects of malnutrition on immunity were presented in Chapter 11.

women often have abnormal immune responses, so they do not have enough antibodies to share.

Certain factors in colostrum and breast milk favor the growth of "friendly" bacteria in the infant's digestive tract, so that other, harmful bacteria cannot grow there.* Another factor present in colostrum and breast milk stimulates the development of the infant's digestive tract. Worn cells in the infant's digestive tract are promptly replaced, facilitating the tract's functioning.

Breast milk changes in composition throughout lactation. Milk from the mother of a premature infant meets the developmental needs of a preterm infant in ways that full-term mother's milk cannot match. For example, the milk for a premature infant provides more protein in less volume, just the right mix to support the rapid growth required to help a premature infant survive its first critical weeks. Some preliminary research even suggests that preterm infants who are breastfed may have an intellectual advantage over formula-fed preterm infants.[36] More research is needed to support or refute this idea, however. Breast milk composition keeps on changing from early to late infancy, to meet the infant's changing energy and nutrient needs.

The protein in breast milk is largely **alpha-lactalbumin,** a protein the human infant can easily digest. Another breast milk protein, **lactoferrin,** indirectly benefits the baby's iron nutrition and also acts as an antibacterial agent. Lactoferrin is an iron-gathering compound that helps absorb iron into the infant's bloodstream, keeps intestinal bacteria from getting enough iron to grow out of control, and also works directly to kill some bacteria.

The vitamin content of the breast milk of a well-nourished mother is ample. Even vitamin C, for which cow's milk is a poor source, is supplied generously by the breast milk of such a mother. The concentration of vitamin D in breast milk is low, but this is not a threat to light-skinned infants who are taken out into the sunshine regularly. The dark-skinned infant, or one who has little exposure to sunlight, however, may not make enough vitamin D to prevent rickets. Because so many variables exist regarding vitamin D and sunlight exposure, the AAP recommends vitamin D supplementation (400 IU per day) beginning at birth for many breastfed babies.

As for minerals, the 2-to-1 calcium-to-phosphorus ratio of breast milk is ideal for calcium absorption, and both of these minerals, along with magnesium, support the rate of growth expected in a human infant. Breast milk is also low in sodium. The limited amount of iron in breast milk is highly absorbable, and its zinc, too, is absorbed better than from cow's milk, thanks to the presence of a zinc-binding protein.

Supplements are not necessary for a breast-fed baby, except possibly for vitamin D and, after six months, fluoride and iron. Fluoride is not an essential nutrient, but it does help to prevent dental caries. Breast milk provides little fluoride, regardless of the mother's intake. Before four months, supplemental iron is unnecessary. Babies are born with enough iron in their livers to last about half a year, and iron deficiency is rarely seen in very young infants. By about six months, it seems desirable to begin feeding the breastfed infant iron-fortified cereals.

Other factors in breast milk include several enzymes, several hormones, and lipids, all of which protect the infant against infection. Prolonged breastfeeding (six months or more) may reduce the incidence of allergic or autoimmune

alpha-lactalbumin (lact-AL-byoo-min) the chief protein in human breast milk. The chief protein in cow's milk is *casein* (CAY-seen).

lactoferrin (lack-toe-FERR-in) a factor in breast milk that binds iron and keeps it from supporting the growth of the infant's intestinal bacteria.

---

*The "friendly" bacteria are the *Lactobacillus bifidus* type.

certified lactation consultant a health-care provider, often a registered nurse, with specialized training in breast and infant anatomy and physiology who teaches the mechanics of breastfeeding to new mothers. Certification is granted after passing a standardized post-training examination.

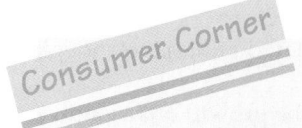

FORMULA'S ADVERTISING ADVANTAGE

Scientific consensus is strong that breastfeeding is preferable for most infants, yet a third more women chose bottle feeding in 1990 than in 1980.[37] When every legitimate nutrition authority strongly recommends breast-feeding, why do so many women who could breastfeed choose formula?

Certainly, most women are free to choose whatever feeding method best suits their needs. For only a few is breastfeeding either prohibited for medical reasons or medically indicated for special needs of the infant. For many women, though, the decision to forgo breastfeeding is influenced not only by social and personal concerns but also by aggressive advertising of formulas.[38] The ads can lead women to believe that formula is just as good for infants as human milk.

Advertisers of infant formulas often strive to create the illusion that formula is identical to human milk. In reality, no formula can match the nutrients, agents of immunity, and environmental information conveyed to infants through human milk. The ads are convincing, though: "Like mother's milk, our formula provides complete nutrition" or "Why trust anything but our brand? It's scientifically formulated to meet your baby's needs." These ads imply, falsely, that breast milk is "unscientific," unknown, and therefore untrustworthy.

To augment their market share, formula sellers give coupons and samples of free formula to pregnant women who are deciding whether to breastfeed. After childbirth, women in the hospital receive "goodie bags" with more coupons to tempt them to go and receive their "gifts." Later, drugstores dispense still more coupons whenever computerized cash registers ring up items related to breastfeeding, such as pads that protect clothing from milk. And still more coupons arrive by mail three months later, at a time when some women give up breastfeeding, even though authorities urge continued breastfeeding for several more months.[39]

An unwelcome trend of earlier and earlier dismissal of new mothers and newborns from hospitals has had a negative impact on breastfeeding. In an attempt to cut costs, some insurance companies limit payments for hospital stays after childbirth to as short a time as possible. Two physicians in New Jersey expressed concern about the impact of early release upon breastfeeding:

> With early discharge, the mother's milk secretion has not started and she will be lucky to meet the lactation expert at the door as she leaves.[40]

The physicians go on to cite a reduced incidence of breastfeeding with early release, even in hospitals that employ **certified lactation consultants** who specialize in helping new mothers to establish a healthy breast-feeding relationship with their newborns. Counseling can have considerable influence on a woman's decision to breastfeed.[41]

The U.S. Surgeon General set a goal that 75 percent of new mothers should be breastfeeding on discharge from the hospital in 1990. In 1990, the actual number of women breastfeeding at the time of leaving the hos-

Healthy People 2000 goal: Increase to at least 75% the proportion of mothers who breastfeed their babies in the early weeks and to at least 50% the proportion who continue breastfeeding until their babies are five to six months old.

pital was barely above 50 percent, and the government-sponsored WIC program was providing almost $500 million in free formula each year to impoverished new mothers.[42]

Contrary to appearances, the WIC program is not passing off baby formula on new mothers. The registered dietitians who advise WIC mothers promote breastfeeding at every opportunity. Many mothers who seek help from WIC, however, have already begun to feed formula but cannot afford its price. Once a mother starts feeding her infant formula, her own milk dries up. Then she must continue feeding formula. At this point WIC has no choice but to supply her baby with the formula it needs.

Formula-fed infants in developed nations are generally healthy, and they usually grow normally on formula, but they miss out on the breastfeeding advantages pointed out in the text.[43] In developing nations, however, the consequence of not choosing to breastfeed can be tragic. Feeding formula is often fatal to the infant where poverty limits access to formula mixes, where clean water is unavailable for safe formula preparation, and where medical help is limited. The World Health Organization strongly supports breastfeeding for the world's infants and actively opposes the marketing of infant formulas to new mothers. Table 12-9 lists important provisions of WHO's code of ethics for formula makers worldwide.

Women should, of course, be free to choose between breast and bottle, but the decision is important and should be made by carefully weighing valid factual information. The choice should not be influenced by sophisticated advertising ploys created by an industry that profits from formula sales.

TABLE 12-9

Ten Provisions of the International Code for Marketing Breastmilk Substitutes

- NO advertising of any of these products to the public.
- NO free samples to mothers.
- NO promotion of products, including the distribution of free or low-cost supplies, in health care facilities.
- NO company sales representatives to advise mothers.
- NO gifts or personal samples to health workers.
- NO words or pictures idealizing artificial feeding, or pictures of infants on labels of infant milk containers.
- Information to health workers should be scientific and factual.
- ALL information on artificial infant feeding, including that on labels, should explain the benefits of breastfeeding and the costs and hazards associated with artificial feeding.
- Unsuitable products, such as sweetened condensed milk, should not be promoted for babies.
- Manufacturers and distributors should comply with the *Code's* provisions even if countries have not adopted laws or other measures.

SOURCE: World Health Organization International Code of Marketing of Breast-milk Substitutes, World Health Organization, Geneva, 1981 as summarized by INFACT Canada.

disease in babies with family histories of such diseases. Much remains to be learned about the composition and characteristics of human milk. Clearly, it is a very special substance.

✓ **KEY POINT**   **Breast milk is normally the ideal food for infants. It contains not only the needed nutrients in the right proportions but also protective factors. It is especially valuable for premature infants.**

Concerns for the Breastfeeding Mother

Toward the end of her pregnancy, a woman who plans to breastfeed her baby should begin to prepare. No elaborate or expensive preparations are needed, but the expectant mother might want to read at least one of the many handbooks available on breastfeeding.* Among the preparations is to learn what

---

*An international organization that helps women with breastfeeding concerns is the LaLeche League. See Appendix E for the address.

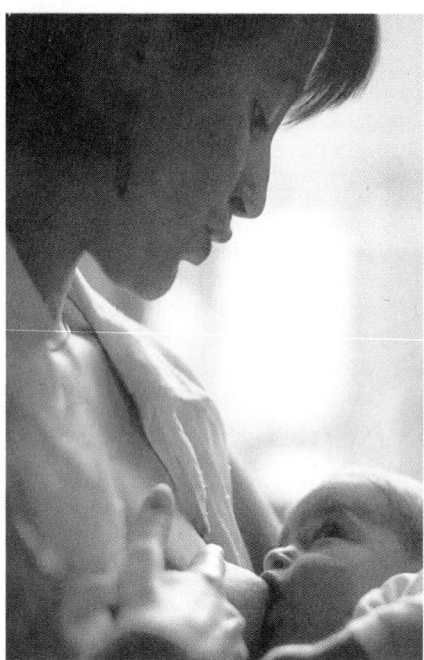

Breastfeeding goes most smoothly for the woman who prepares.

dietary changes are needed. Adequate nutrition is essential to successful lactation; without it, lactation may falter.

A nursing mother produces about 25 ounces of milk a day (more in early lactation, less later on when the baby begins eating other foods). Producing this milk costs a woman almost 650 calories per day. About 500 calories of this energy should be provided by the diet. The other 150 calories may be drawn from the fat stores the woman accumulated during pregnancy.

The food energy consumed by the nursing mother should carry with it abundant nutrients, especially those needed to make milk, such as calcium, protein, magnesium, zinc, and enough fluid to prevent dehydration. Figure 12-3 showed the differences between a lactating woman's nutrient needs and those of a nonpregnant woman, and Table 12-6 suggested a food pattern that meets them.

The volume of breast milk produced depends not on how much fluid the mother drinks but on how much milk the baby demands.[44] The nursing mother is nevertheless advised to drink at least 2 quarts of liquids each day to protect herself from dehydration. To help themselves remember to drink enough liquid, many women make a habit of drinking a glass of milk, juice, or water each time the baby nurses as well as at mealtimes.

People often ask about the old adage "beer makes good milk." Beer does seem to stimulate prolactin, a hormone important to lactation. However, the alcohol in beer enters breast milk and can easily overwhelm an infant's immature alcohol-degrading system. A woman's hormones need no external assistance to perform perfectly, and even beer should be strictly limited to an occasional 12-ounce serving. Even this amount may alter the taste of the milk to the disapproval of the nursing infant, who may, in protest, drink less milk than normal.[45] Similarly, excess caffeine can make a baby jittery and wakeful. Other drugs have worse effects.

Some infants may be sensitive to foods such as cow's milk, onions, or garlic in the mother's diet and become uncomfortable when she eats them. Nursing mothers should not automatically avoid such foods, however. A mother who is nursing her baby is advised to eat whatever nutritious foods she chooses. Then, if a particular food seems to cause the infant discomfort, she can try eliminating that food from her diet for a few days and see if the problem goes away.

Another question often raised is whether a mother's milk may lack a nutrient if she fails to get enough in her diet. The answer differs from one nutrient to the next, but in general, the effect of nutritional deprivation of the mother is to reduce the *quantity*, not the *quality*, of her milk. For protein, carbohydrate, and most minerals, the milk of a healthy mother has a fairly constant composition. Any excess water-soluble vitamins the mother takes in are excreted in the urine; the body does not release them into the milk. The amounts of fat-soluble vitamins in human milk are affected, however, by the mother's excessive or deficient intakes. For example, large doses of vitamin A correspondingly raise the concentration of this vitamin in breast milk. Vitamin supplementation of undernourished women appears to help normalize the vitamin concentrations in their milk and may be beneficial.

If a mother does not breastfeed, she may find it hard to lose the fat she gained during pregnancy.[46] This does not mean that a breastfeeding woman can eat unlimited food and still effortlessly return to prepregnancy weight. Breastfeeding costs energy, true, but carefully chosen programs of diet and exercise are still the cornerstones of weight control. Exercise in particular helps to reduce body fatness and improve fitness without much affecting a woman's milk production or her infant's weight gain.[47] A gradual weight loss (1 pound per week) is safe and does not reduce milk output. Too large an energy deficit, however, especially soon after birth, will inhibit lactation.

✓ KEY POINT **The lactating woman needs extra fluid and enough energy and nutrients to make sufficient milk each day. Malnutrition most often diminishes the quantity of the milk produced without altering quality. Lactation facilitates loss of the extra fat gained during pregnancy.**

When Not to Breastfeed

If a woman has an ordinary cold, she can go on nursing without worry. The infant will probably catch it from her anyway, and thanks to immunological protection, a breastfed baby may be less susceptible than a formula-fed baby would be. If a woman has a serious communicable disease such as tuberculosis or hepatitis, then mother and baby have to be separated. Breastfeeding may be continued by pumping the mother's breasts several times a day and letting the baby drink the milk from a bottle (see margin).

The virus responsible for causing AIDS (HIV) can be passed from an infected mother to her infant during pregnancy, at birth, or through breastfeeding, so women in developed countries who have tested positive for HIV should not breastfeed. They should choose a safe alternative feeding method, such as breast milk from a milk bank.[48] In developing countries, an infant who is not breastfed faces hazards even more dire than the risk of HIV transmission. Milk banks in the United States pasteurize donated human milk and make it available to infants who lack access to milk from their own mothers. Pasteurization destroys harmful organisms, such as HIV, but leaves intact the beneficial constituents of the milk.

Similarly, if a nursing mother must take medication that is secreted in breast milk and is known to affect the infant, then breastfeeding must be put off for the duration of treatment. Meanwhile, the flow of milk can be sustained by pumping the breasts and discarding the milk. Many prescription drugs do not reach nursing infants in sufficient quantities to affect them adversely. Other drugs are not compatible with breastfeeding either because they are secreted into the milk and can harm the infant or because they suppress lactation.[49] A nursing mother should consult with the prescribing physician prior to taking any drug.

Many women wonder about using oral contraceptives during lactation. One type that combines the hormones estrogen and progestin seems to suppress milk output, lower the nitrogen content of the milk, and shorten the duration of breastfeeding. In contrast, progestin-only pills have no effect on breast milk or breastfeeding and are considered appropriate for lactating women.

Drug addicts, including alcohol abusers, are capable of taking such high doses that their infants can become addicts by way of breast milk. In these cases, too, breastfeeding is contraindicated.

A few women, about 5 of every 100, produce too little milk to nourish their infants adequately. Severe consequences, including infant dehydration, malnutrition, and brain damage, can occur should the condition go undetected for long. Early warning signs of insufficient milk are dry diapers (a well-fed infant

For Safe Breast Milk Storage:
- Wash hands thoroughly before pumping.
- Clean pumping equipment according to manufacturer's directions.
- Sterilize bottles, nipples, and rings before using.
- Refrigerate milk to be fed within 48 hours.
- Freeze milk to be stored longer than 48 hours.
- Thaw milk gently on defrost cycle of microwave or in refrigerator.
- Do not refreeze thawed milk.

wets about six diapers a day) and infrequent bowel movements. In such cases, formula feeding is essential.

A woman sometimes hesitates to breastfeed because she has heard that environmental contaminants may enter breast milk and harm her infant. While some contaminants do enter breast milk, others may be filtered out of the milk. Formula-fed infants consume a great deal of tap water because formula is made with water, and so they receive directly any contaminants that may be in the water supply. The decision whether to breastfeed on this basis might best be made after consultation with a physician or dietitian familiar with the local circumstances.

For more about contaminants and nutrition, turn to Chapter 14.

✓ **KEY POINT**   **Most ordinary infections such as colds have no effect on breastfeeding. Breastfeeding may be inadvisable if milk is contaminated with drugs or environmental pollutants.**

FEEDING THE INFANT

For a while the infant drinks only breast milk or formula, but later becomes able to handle other foods. Early nutrition affects later development, and early feedings establish eating habits that influence nutrition throughout life.

Trends change and experts argue the fine points, but nourishing a baby is relatively simple. Common sense in the selection of infant foods and a nurturing, relaxed environment go far to promote the infant's well-being.

Nutrient Needs

A baby grows faster during the first year of life than ever again, as Figure 12-7 shows. Pediatricians carefully monitor the growth of infants and children, since growth is an important reflection of nutrition status. The birthweight doubles around four months of age and triples by the age of one year. (If a 150-pound adult were to grow like this, the person's weight would increase to 450 pounds in a single year.) By the end of the first year, the growth rate slows considerably, so that the weight gained between the first and second birthdays amounts to less than 10 pounds.

The rapid growth and metabolism of the infant demand an ample supply of all the nutrients. Of special importance during infancy are the energy nutrients and those vitamins and minerals critical to the growth process, such as vitamin A, vitamin D, calcium, and iron.

Because they are small, babies need smaller total amounts of these nutrients than adults do; but as a percentage of body weight, babies need over twice as much of most nutrients. Figure 12-8 compares a five-month-old baby's needs (per unit of body weight) with those of an adult man. As you can see, some of the differences are extraordinary. Sometime around six months of age, energy needs increase less rapidly as the growth rate begins to slow down, but some of the energy saved by slower growth is spent in increased activity. When their growth slows, infants spontaneously reduce their energy intakes. Thus parents should expect their babies to adjust their food intakes downward when appropriate and should not force or coax them to eat more.

Vitamin K nutrition for newborns presents a unique case. A newborn's digestive tract is sterile, and vitamin K–producing bacteria take weeks to establish

FIGURE 12-7

WEIGHT GAIN OF HUMAN INFANTS IN THE FIRST FIVE YEARS OF LIFE

The colored vertical bars show how the yearly increase in weight gain slows its pace over the years.

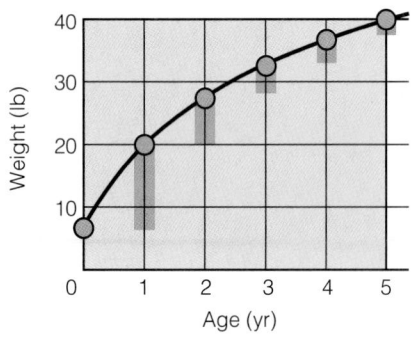

FIGURE 12-8

NUTRIENT RDA OF A FIVE-MONTH-OLD INFANT AND AN ADULT MALE COMPARED ON THE BASIS OF BODY WEIGHT

Infants may be relatively small and inactive, but they use large amounts of energy and nutrients in proportion to their body size to keep all their metabolic processes going.

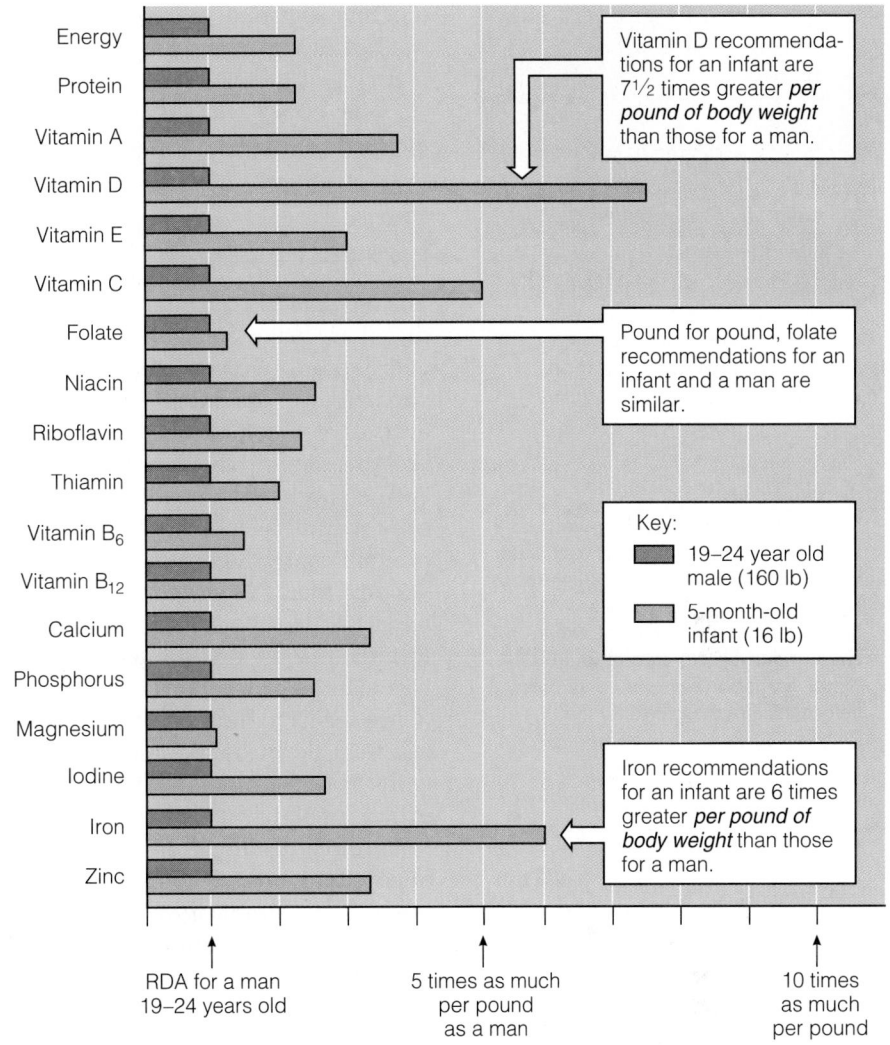

Vitamin D recommendations for an infant are 7½ times greater *per pound of body weight* than those for a man.

Pound for pound, folate recommendations for an infant and a man are similar.

Key:
- 19–24 year old male (160 lb)
- 5-month-old infant (16 lb)

Iron recommendations for an infant are 6 times greater *per pound of body weight* than those for a man.

RDA for a man 19–24 years old

5 times as much per pound as a man

10 times as much per pound

themselves in the baby's intestines. To prevent uncontrolled bleeding in the newborn, a single dose of vitamin K is given at birth, usually by injection.

The most important nutrient of all, for infants as for everyone, is the one easiest to forget: water. The younger a child is, the more of its body weight is water and the faster the water is lost and replaced. Proportionately more of an infant's body water than an adult's is between the cells and in the vascular space, and this water is easy to lose. Conditions that cause fluid loss, such as hot weather, vomiting, diarrhea, or sweating, can rapidly propel an infant into life-threatening dehydration.

In early infancy, breast milk or infant formula normally provides enough water for a healthy infant to replace water losses from the skin, lungs, feces, and urine. When the infant starts eating solid foods, additional water is required. If the weather is hot and the mother is thirsty, her infant probably is,

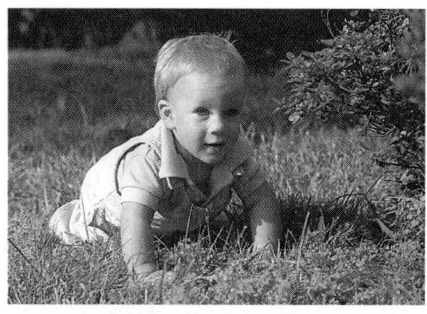

After age six months, energy saved by the slowing of growth is spent on increasing activity.

Formula Options:

- ✓ Liquid concentrate (inexpensive, relatively easy)—mix with equal part water.
- ✓ Powdered formula (cheapest, lightest for travel)—read label directions.
- ✓ Ready-to-feed (easiest, most expensive)—pour directly into clean bottles.
- ✓ Never an option—whole cow's milk before 12 months of age.

too. Infants cannot tell you what they are crying for; remember that they may need plain water, and let them drink it until they quench their thirst.

✓ **KEY POINT** **Infants' rapid growth and development depend heavily on adequate nutrient supplies. Adequate water is also crucial.**

Formula Feeding and Weaning to Milk

The type of milk the infant receives and the age at which solid foods are introduced are major areas of concern in infant nutrition research. Under most circumstances a woman can freely choose to feed breast milk or formula; either one will meet the infant's nutrient needs. If the family has a low income, however, or if other factors threaten the baby's health, then the advantages of breastfeeding tip the balance in its favor.

The substitution of formula feeding for breastfeeding involves striving to copy nature as closely as possible. Human and cow's milks differ; cow's milk is significantly higher in protein, calcium, and phosphorus, for example, to support the calf's faster growth rate. A formula can be prepared from cow's milk that does not differ significantly from human milk in these respects; the formula makers first dilute the milk and then add carbohydrate and nutrients to make the proportions comparable to those of human milk. Still, some evidence seems to indicate that formula-fed infants attain larger size at an earlier age than do breastfed infants. It is unknown what, if any, long-term effects early feeding choices may have on children's later growth, or whether this extra growth harms or benefits health or is just neutral.

Formula feeding offers a reasonable alternative to the mother whose attempts at breastfeeding have met with frustration. Nourishment for the infant from formula is adequate, and a mother can choose this course with confidence. Other advantages are that parents can see that the baby is getting enough milk during feedings. Also, other family members can participate in feeding sessions, giving them a chance to develop the special closeness that feeding fosters and freeing the mother to devote time to her other children or to herself. Mothers who resume employment early after giving birth may choose formula for their infants, but they have another option. Breast milk can be pumped into bottles and given to the baby in day care. At home, mothers may breastfeed as usual. Many mothers use both methods—they breastfeed at first but wean to formula within the first six months.

Table 12-10 compares the composition of human milk with typical formulas. For infants with special problems, formulas can be adapted to meet their special needs (adjusted protein ratio, lower linoleic acid, lower minerals). For premature babies, special premature formulas are available. For infants of strict vegetarians or for those allergic to milk protein, special formulas based on soy protein are available. For infants with lactose intolerance, formulas with the lactose replaced can be used. For infants with other special needs, many other variations are available.

For as long as formula or breast milk is the baby's major food, ordinary milk is an inappropriate replacement, primarily because milk provides less iron and vitamin C.[50] Plain, unmodified cow's milk (including whole, skim, low-fat, or evaporated milk) is not recommended before the baby's first birthday. The

TABLE 12-10

Human Milk Compared with Infant Formula for Selected Nutrients

Content	Mature Human Milk	Fortified Infant Formula
Energy (cal/100 ml)	64	67
Protein (% of cal)	6	9
Fat (% of cal)	40–50	50
Carbohydrate (% of cal)	41	42
Iron (mg/L)	0.5	1.5–12
Vitamin A (µg/L)	675	660
Niacin (mg/L)	1.5	7.5
Vitamin D (µg/L)	2.2	41
Inositol (mg/L)	149	32

SOURCE: L. A. Barness, ed., Committee on Nutrition, American Academy of Pediatrics, *Pediatric Nutrition Handbook* (Elk Grove, Ill.: American Academy of Pediatrics, 1993), Appendix E.

infant's digestive tract may be sensitive to the protein content and, if so, may bleed and worsen iron deficiency. A lasting allergy to cow's milk may develop. Also, the infant's immature kidneys are stressed by plain cow's milk. Some evidence suggests that exposure to cow's milk in early infancy may bear some relation to the development of insulin-dependent diabetes later on; researchers are working to establish what, if any, relationship may exist in this regard.[51] In the meanwhile, breastfeeding circumvents the issue.

Once the baby is obtaining at least two-thirds of total daily food energy from a balanced mixture of cereals, vegetables, fruits, and other foods (usually after 12 months of age), then whole cow's milk, fortified with vitamins A and D, is an acceptable accompanying beverage. Low-fat milk is not recommended before age two years. Table 12-11 defines some terms applied to types of milk.

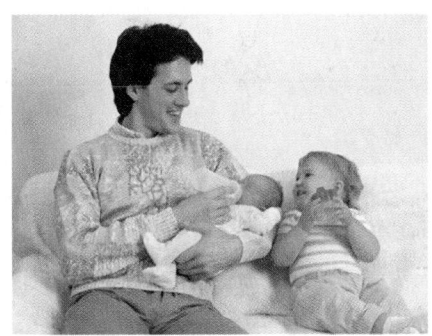

Feeding expressed breast milk, formula, or water from a bottle lets other family members in on the fun.

✓ **KEY POINT** **Infant formulas are designed to resemble breast milk and must meet an AAP standard for nutrient composition. Special formulas are available for premature babies, allergic babies, and others. Formula should be replaced with milk only after the baby is eating a balanced assortment of foods, no earlier than at six months; a year is preferred.**

First Foods

Foods can be introduced into a baby's diet as the baby becomes physically ready to handle them. This readiness develops in stages. A newborn baby can swallow only liquids that are well back in the throat. Later (at four months or so), the baby's tongue can move against the palate to swallow semisolid food such as cooked cereal. Still later, the first teeth erupt, but not until sometime during the second year can a baby begin to handle chewy food. The stomach and intestines are immature at first; they can digest milk sugar (lactose) but not starch. At about four months, most babies can begin to digest starchy foods.

The baby's kidneys are unable to concentrate waste efficiently, so a baby must excrete relatively more water than an adult to carry off a comparable amount of waste. This means that the risk of dehydration is higher for infants

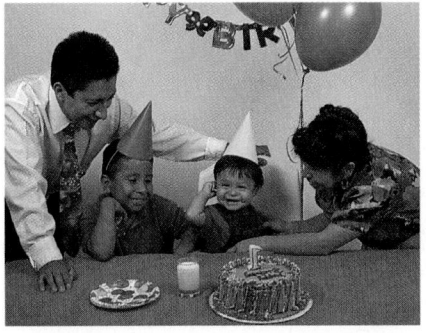

A day of firsts: the first birthday party and the first taste of whole, unmodified cow's milk.

milk anemia iron-deficiency anemia caused by drinking so much milk that iron-rich foods are displaced from the diet.

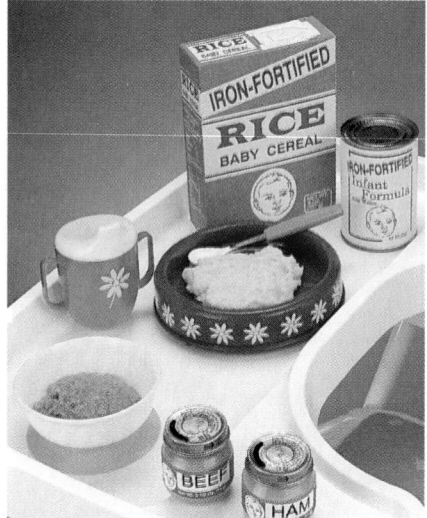

Foods such as iron-fortified cereals and formulas, mashed legumes, and strained meats provide iron.

than for adults, and it becomes even greater once solid foods are introduced. Water and other fluids take on added importance to prevent dehydration.

Iron deficiency is prevalent in children between the ages of six months and three years due to their rapid growth rate and the significant place that milk has in their diets. This can lead to iron-deficiency anemia, popularly called **milk anemia.**

Iron ranks highest on the list of nutrients most needing attention in infant nutrition. A baby's stored iron supply from before birth runs out after the birthweight doubles, so formula with iron for formula-fed babies, then iron-fortified cereals, and then meat or meat alternates are recommended. By the end of the first year, half or more of all infants are receiving less than the RDA for iron, and one-fourth are receiving less than two-thirds of the RDA. Six-month-old infants who are weaned to cow's milk have lower blood iron measures than those who remain on formula.[52] While iron is of primary importance, vitamin C is also important.

The timing for adding solid foods to a baby's diet depends on several factors. Formula or breast milk alone is sufficient until age four to six months. Babies who are ready for solid foods thrive on receiving them and develop new skills through handling the foods. Any of the following indicates readiness:

- When the infant can sit with support and can control its head movements.
- When the birthweight has doubled.
- When the infant is about six months old.

TABLE 12-11

Milk Terms

- **casein** or **sodium caseinate** the principal protein of cow's milk. Another milk protein found in human milk's whey is **lactalbumin.**
- **condensed milk** evaporated milk to which a large amount of sugar (sucrose) is added during processing; intended for making desserts, not for feeding babies. Accidental use of condensed milk in preparation of infant formula can cause dehydration.
- **evaporated milk** milk concentrated to half volume by evaporation. Adding water reconstitutes the milk; the taste is altered by the processing, however.
- **evaporated milk formula** formula made at home from evaporated milk, sugar, and water, seldom used today and not recommended.
- **fortified** (with respect to milk) milk to which vitamins A and D have been added.
- **homogenized milk** milk treated to mix the fat evenly with the watery part (fat ordinarily floats to the top as cream). Heated milk is forced under high pressure through small openings to emulsify the fat.
- **lactalbumin** see *casein.*
- **pasteurized milk** milk that is heat treated to eliminate disease-causing microbes and to reduce its total bacterial count to an acceptable level.
- **powdered milk** dehydrated milk solids. Some powdered milks rehydrate easily (instant milk); others require extensive blending. Both whole and nonfat milk can be powdered.
- **whey** the liquid that remains after milk has coagulated (see also *casein*).
- **whole milk** full-fat cow's milk.

TABLE 12-12

First Foods for the Infant

Age (Months)	Addition
0–4	Breast milk or formula only—no advantage gained from supplemental foods
4–6	Iron-fortified rice cereal, followed by other cereals (for iron; baby can swallow and can digest starch now)[a]
5–7	Strained vegetables and/or fruits and their juices,[b] one by one (perhaps vegetables before fruits, so the baby will learn to like their less-sweet flavors)
6–8	Soft or strained protein foods (cheese, yogurt, and tofu; cooked beans, meat, fish, chicken, and egg yolk)
8–10	Finely chopped meat (baby can chew now), toast, teething crackers (for emerging teeth) and soft table foods (start slowly)
10–12	Whole cooked egg (allergies are less likely now), whole milk (at 12 months), more table foods[c]

[a]Later you can change cereals, but don't forget to keep on using the iron-fortified varieties.

[b]All baby juices are fortified with vitamin C, but they are more expensive than adult varieties. Orange juice causes allergies in some babies; apple juice is often recommended.

[c]Avoid sweetened baby food desserts and other desserts that contribute much food energy but few nutrients.

All babies develop according to their own schedules, and while Table 12-12 presents a suggested sequence, individuality is important. Three considerations are relevant: the baby's nutrient needs, the baby's physical readiness to handle different forms of foods, and the need to detect and control allergic reactions.

Foods introduced at the right times contribute to an infant's physical development. For example, experience with solid food at four to six months, when swallowing ability is developing, helps to desensitize the gag reflex. When the baby can sit up, can handle finger foods, and is teething, then hard crackers and other hard finger foods may be introduced under the watchful eye of an adult. These foods promote the development of manual dexterity and control of the jaw muscles, but the caretaker must make sure that the infant does not choke on them at first. Hard crackers that melt slowly to a mush that is easy to swallow are best. Babies and even young children can easily choke on popcorn, nuts, hot dogs, raw carrots, whole grapes, and hard candy; these foods are not worth the risk.

Some parents want to feed solids as early as possible on the theory that "stuffing the baby" at bedtime will promote sleeping through the night. There is no proof for this theory. Babies start to sleep through the night whenever they are ready, no matter when solid foods are introduced. By three months, most are sleeping adequately regardless.

New foods should be introduced one at a time, so that allergies or other sensitivities can be detected. For example, when fortified baby cereals are introduced, try rice cereal first for several days; it causes allergy least often. Try wheat-containing cereal last; it is a common offender. Egg whites, soy products, peanut products, cow's milk, and citrus fruits are introduced still later for the same reason. If a food causes an allergic reaction (irritability due to skin rash, digestive upset, or respiratory discomfort), discontinue its use before

Chapter 13 offers more information on allergies.

Children love to eat what their families eat.

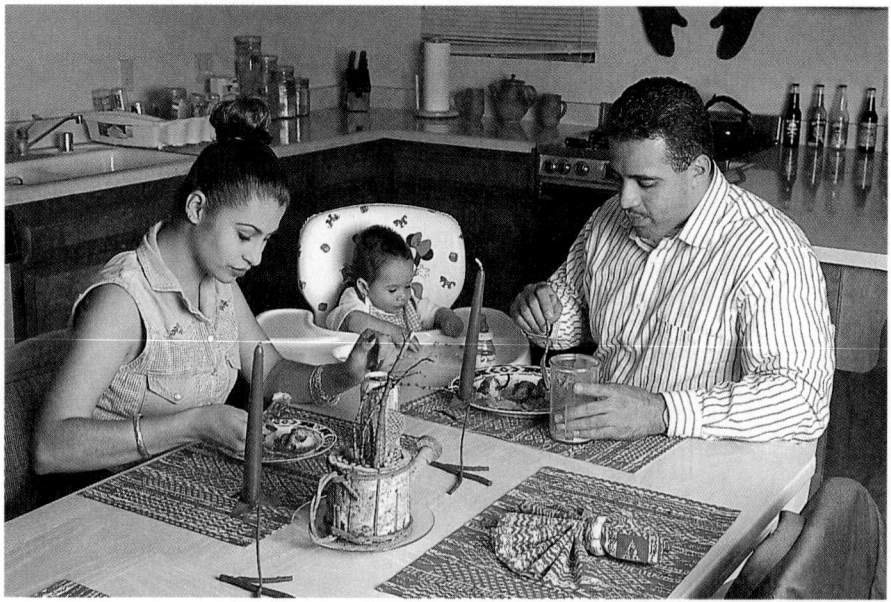

going on to the next food. About nine times out of ten, the allergy won't be evident immediately but will manifest itself in vague symptoms occurring up to five days after the offending food is eaten. Wait a month or two to try the food again; many sensitivities disappear with maturity. If the family history indicates allergies, apply extra caution in introducing new foods. Parents who detect allergies early in an infant's life can spare the whole family much grief.

As for the choice of foods, baby foods commercially prepared in the United States and Canada are safe, nutritious, and of high quality. In response to consumer demand, baby food companies have removed much of the added salt and sugar their products contained in the past, and baby foods also contain few or no additives. Nutrient density is generally high with the exception of mixed dinners with added starch fillers and heavily sweetened desserts. Brands vary in their use of starch and sugar—the ingredient lists distinguish one from another. Parents should not feed directly from the jar but should remove portions to a dish for feeding so as not to contaminate the unused food that will be stored in the jar.

Appendix A includes the nutrient composition of many commercial baby foods.

An alternative to commercial baby food for the parent who wants the baby to have family foods is to process a small portion of the table food in a blender, food processor, or baby food grinder. This necessitates cooking without salt or sugar, though, as the best baby food manufacturers do. The adults can season their own food after taking out the baby's portion. After a meal, leftover baby food can be frozen in an ice cube tray to yield a dozen or so servings that can be quickly thawed, heated, and served on a busy day.

Chapter 14 provides details about botulism.

Canned vegetables are not appropriate for babies. Often the salt content is too high, and some nutrient value is lost in the canning process. Also, awareness of food poisoning and precautions against it are imperative. Honey should never be fed to infants because of the risk of botulism.

Liquids remain important and should deliver nutrients. It is unfortunate, but not uncommon to see infants' bottles filled with soft drinks, sports drinks, sugary juice drinks, or punches. Infants and children thrive best on water, milk, or juice. They have high nutrient needs but can extract only water and sugar from colored, sweetened, fruit-flavored water.

Ideally, the one-year-old sits at the table, eats many of the same foods everyone else eats, and drinks liquids from a cup, not a bottle. A meal plan that meets the requirements for the one-year-old is shown in Table 12-13.

✔ KEY POINT   **Solid food additions to a baby's diet should begin at about six months and should be governed by the baby's nutrient needs and readiness to eat. By one year, the baby should be receiving foods from all food groups.**

Looking Ahead

The first year of a baby's life is the time to lay the foundation for future health. From the nutrition standpoint, the problems most common in later years are obesity and dental disease. Prevention of obesity can also help prevent the obesity-related diseases: atherosclerosis, diabetes, and cancer.

The idea that obese babies grow into obese adults is popular, although questions still surround it. A researcher who wants to determine whether the relationship holds up must spend up to 50 years following people's health histories. From what is known, though, it seems that an obese child in an obese family is more likely to remain obese than an obese child in a normal-weight family.[53]

To discourage development of the behaviors and attitudes that are associated with obesity, parents should not teach babies to seek food as a reward, to expect food as comfort for unhappiness, or to associate food deprivation with punishment. If they cry for thirst, give them water, not milk or juice. If they cry

TABLE 12-13

Meal Plan for a One-Year-Old

Breakfast	**Afternoon snack**
½ c whole milk	½ c whole milk
3 tbs cereal	Teething crackers
1 to 2 tbs fruit[a]	1 tbs peanut butter
Teething crackers	
Morning snack	**Dinner**
½ c whole milk	1 c whole milk
1 to 2 tbs fruit[a]	1 egg
Teething crackers	2 tbs cereal or potato
	2 to 3 tbs vegetables[b]
Lunch	2 to 3 tbs fruit[a]
1 c whole milk	
2 to 3 tbs vegetables[b]	
2 tbs chopped meat or well-cooked, mashed legumes	

[a]Include citrus fruits, melons, and berries.
[b]Include dark green, leafy and deep yellow vegetables.

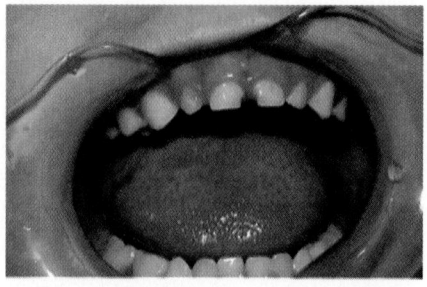

Nursing bottle syndrome in an early stage.

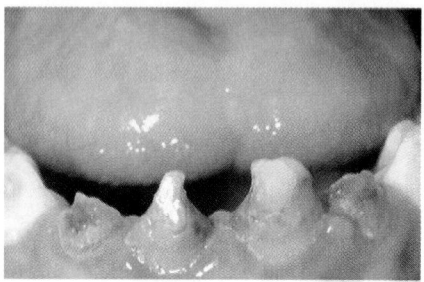

Nursing bottle syndrome, an extreme example. The lower teeth have decayed all the way to the gum line.

for companionship, pick them up, don't feed them. If they are hungry, by all means, feed them appropriately.

An irrational fear of obesity leads some parents to underfeed their infants, depriving them of the energy and nutrients they need to grow. Some people wonder if they should feed their infants a very low-fat diet to reduce heart disease risk, but the AAP recommends a normal fat intake for infants. As mentioned, dietary lipids are used to build a normal central nervous system. Furthermore, growth failure is common in children on fat-restricted diets, even when energy from other sources is ample. With rare exceptions, to be identified by physicians, babies need the food energy and fat of whole milk until two years of age. The only precaution parents should take is not to feed high-calorie baby foods such as sugar-sweetened desserts in overly large quantities.

The same strategies promote normal dental development: supplying nutritious foods, avoiding sweets, and discouraging the association of food with reward or comfort. In addition the practice of giving a baby a bottle as a pacifier is strongly discouraged by dentists. Sucking for long periods of time pushes the normal jawline out of shape and causes a bucktoothed profile: protruding upper and receding lower teeth. Furthermore, prolonged sucking on a bottle of milk or juice bathes the upper teeth in a carbohydrate-rich fluid that favors the growth of decay-producing bacteria. The bacteria produce acid that dissolves tooth material. Babies regularly put to bed with a bottle are sometimes seen with their upper teeth decayed all the way to the gum line, a condition known as nursing bottle syndrome, shown in the margin.

✔ **KEY POINT** **The early feeding of the infant lays the foundation for life-long eating habits. It is desirable to foster preferences that will support normal development throughout life and ward off common lifestyle diseases.**

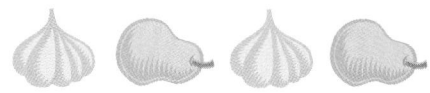

FOOD FEATURE

MEALTIMES WITH INFANTS

The wise parent of a one-year-old offers nutrition and affection together. It is literally true that "feeding with love" produces better growth in both weight and height of children than feeding the same food in an emotionally negative climate.[54] It also promotes better brain development because the formation of nerve-to-nerve connections in the brain depends both on nutrients and on environmental stimulation.

The person feeding a one-year-old has to be aware that the child's exploring and experimenting are normal and desirable behaviors. The child is developing a sense of autonomy that, if allowed to flower, will provide the foundation for later assertiveness in choosing when and how much to eat and when to stop eating. The child's self-direction, if consistently overridden, can later turn into shame and self-doubt. In light of the developmental and nutrient needs of one-year-olds and in the face of their often contrary and willful behavior, a few feeding guidelines may be helpful. Following are several problem situations with suggestions for handling them:

■ *He stands and plays at the table instead of eating.* Don't let him. To discourage him, put him down, and let him eat later. Be consistent and firm, not punitive. If he is really hungry, he will soon learn to sit still while eating.

■ *She wants to poke her fingers into her food.* Let her. She has much to learn from feeling the texture of her food. When she knows all about it, she'll naturally graduate to the use of a spoon.

■ *He wants to manage the spoon himself, but can't handle it.* Let him try. As he masters it, withdraw your help gradually until he is feeding himself competently. At this age a baby can learn to feed himself and intensely wants to do so. He will spill, of course, but he'll outgrow that soon.

■ *She refuses food that her mother knows is good for her.* This way of demonstrating autonomy, one of the few available to the one-year-old, is most satisfying. Don't force. Poor eating habits that develop in the one- to two-year-old stage can last throughout life. As long as she is getting enough milk and is given a variety of nutritious foods to choose from, she will gradually learn to like different foods, provided that she feels she is making the choice.

If a baby refuses milk, though, do provide an alternative source of the bone- and muscle-building nutrients that milk supplies. Milk-based puddings, custards, and cheeses are often successful substitutes. For the baby who is allergic to milk, use calcium-fortified soy milk formulas.

■ *He prefers sweets such as candy and sugary confections to foods containing more nutrients.* All human beings love sweets, but limit them strictly and in the house, and keep them out of sight. There is no room in a baby's daily 1,000 calories for nutrient-poor sweets. The meal plan shown earlier in Table 12-11 provides more than 500 calories from milk; one or two servings of each of the other types of food provide the other 500. A candy bar, substituted for any of these foods, displaces valuable nutrients.

These recommendations reflect a spirit of tolerance that serves the best interest of the infant emotionally as well as physically. This attitude, carried throughout childhood, helps the child to develop a healthy relationship with food. The next chapter finishes the story of growth and nutrition.

SELF-CHECK

Answers to these Self-Check questions are in Appendix G.

1. A deficiency of which nutrient appears to be related to an increased risk of neural tube defects in the newborn?
   a. vitamin B_6
   b. folate
   c. calcium
   d. niacin

2. Which of the following may be hazardous during pregnancy?
   a. vitamin A supplementation
   b. dieting for weight loss
   c. drinking alcohol
   d. all of the above

3. Breastfed infants may need supplements of:
a. fluoride, iron, and vitamin D
b. zinc, iron, and vitamin C
c. vitamin E, calcium, and fluoride
d. vitamin K, magnesium, and potassium

4. Breastfeeding is contraindicated if a woman has:
a. AIDS
b. hepatitis
c. tuberculosis
d. all of the above

5. Only a slightly increased intake is recommended during pregnancy for:
a. folate
b. iron
c. energy
d. protein

6. A major reason why a woman's nutrition before pregnancy is crucial is that it determines whether her uterus will support the growth of a normal placenta.   T   F

7. Fetal alcohol syndrome (FAS) is the leading known cause of mental retardation in the world.   T   F

8. A sure way to get a baby to sleep through the night is to feed solid foods as soon as the baby can swallow them.   T   F

9. In general, the effect of nutritional deprivation on a breastfeeding mother is to reduce the quality of her milk.   T   F

10. Caffeine seems relatively harmless to normal adults when used in moderation (the equivalent of, say, two average-sized cups of coffee a day). (Read about this in the upcoming Controversy.)   T   F

NOTES

Notes are in Appendix F.

Medicines, Other Drugs, and Nutrition

A 45-year-old Chicago business executive attempts to give up smoking with the help of nicotine gum. At the same time she decides to replace smoking breaks with beverage breaks and begins drinking frequent servings of tomato juice, coffee, and colas. She is discouraged when her craving for tobacco continues unabated after chewing the prescription gum and her stomach becomes upset. Problem: nutrient-drug interaction.

A 14-year-old girl begins to develop frequent and prolonged respiratory infections. In the last six months, she has complained of constant fatigue despite adequate sleep; she has had trouble completing school assignments; and she has quit the volleyball team because she runs out of energy on the court. During the same six months, she has tried a new weight-loss fad that requires taking three times the recommended dosage of antacid pills each day. Her pediatrician has diagnosed iron-deficiency anemia. Problem: nutrient-drug interaction.

A 30-year-old schoolteacher who takes antidepressant medication enjoys an after-school faculty wine and cheese party. After sampling the cheese with a glass or two of red wine, his face becomes flushed. His behavior prompts others to drive him home. In the early morning hours, he awakens with severe dizziness, a migraine headache, vomiting, and trembling. An ambulance delivers him to an emergency room where a physician takes swift action to save his life. Problem: nutrient-drug interaction.

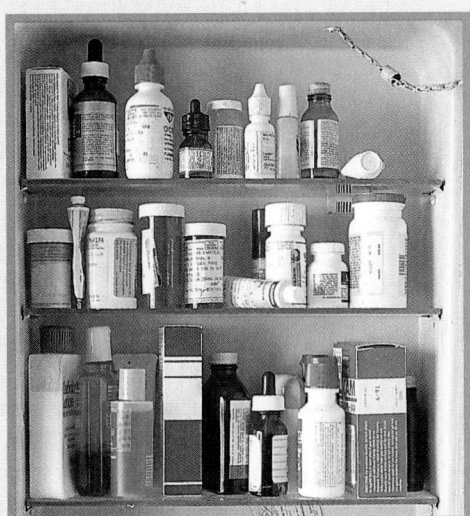

- Drugs can delay or prevent nutrient absorption.
- Drugs can modify taste, appetite, or food intake.
- Nutrients can interfere with drug action, metabolism, or excretion.
- Drugs can interfere with nutrient action or excretion.

Absorption of Drugs and Nutrients   The business executive described earlier felt the effects of a variation of the type of interaction mentioned first in the list above. Acid from the tomato juice, coffee, and colas she drank before chewing nicotine gum kept the nicotine from being absorbed through the lining of her mouth.[1] With this route blocked, the nicotine traveled to her stomach, remained unabsorbed, and caused nausea. Other foods and beverages can have similar effects (Table C12-1). Once identified, the problem is easy to prevent by waiting to eat or drink until after chewing the gum.

Drugs can also interfere with the small intestine's absorption of nutrients, particularly minerals. This is what the tired 14-year-old experienced. Her overuse of antacids abolished the stomach's normal acidity, on which iron absorption depends. The medicine bound tightly to the iron molecules, forming an insoluble, unabsorbable complex. Her iron stores already bordered on deficiency, as is typical of young girls, so her misuse of antacids pushed her over the edge into frank deficiency.

MEDICINES AND NUTRITION

People sometimes think that medical drugs do only good, not harm. The opening stories illustrate that both "prescription" and "over-the-counter (OTC)" medicines can and do cause harm when they interact with the body's normal use of nutrients. Just as alcohol and nutrition interact, so do drugs and nutrition:

- Foods can delay or prevent drug absorption.

Metabolic Interactions   As for the teacher who landed in the emergency room, he was taking an antidepressant medicine, one of the monoamine oxidase inhibitors (MAOI). At the party, he suffered a dangerous chemical interaction between the medicine and the compound tyramine in his cheese and wine. Tyramine is produced during the fermenting process in cheese and wine manufacturing.

505

TABLE C12-1

Foods and Beverages that Limit the Effectiveness of Nicotine Gum

- Apple juice.
- Beer.
- Coffee.
- Colas.
- Grape juice.
- Ketchup.
- Lemon-lime soda.
- Mustard.
- Orange juice.
- Pineapple juice.
- Soy sauce.
- Tomato juice.

The MAOI medication works by depressing the activity of enzymes that destroy the brain neurotransmitter dopamine. With less enzyme activity, more dopamine is left, and depression lifts. At the same time, the drug also depresses enzymes in the liver that destroy tyramine. Ordinarily, the man's liver would have quickly destroyed the tyramine from the cheese and wine. Tyramine built up too high in the man's body and caused the potentially fatal reaction. Table C12-2 (page 508) lists some examples of other possible drug-nutrient interactions, including both prescription and OTC medications.

Over-the-Counter (OTC) Medications OTC drugs are readily available and widely used in the United States and can harm people's nutrition status, especially when they are misused. For example, people who use laxatives daily for weeks or months may find that their intestines can no longer function without them. Laxative dependence and chronic use can lead to malnutrition by carrying nutrients so rapidly through the intestines that many vitamins have no time to be absorbed. The laxative mineral oil, which the body cannot absorb, can rob a person of fat-soluble vitamins. Vitamin D deficiencies can occur this way; calcium, too, may be excreted with the oil, accelerating adult bone loss.

Advertisers promote antacids as a panacea for those who overindulge in rich food and drink. In such cases, the drugs may do no harm, but people with recurrent stomach pain should be checked by a physician. Such pain can indicate a serious condition such as an ulcer. Antacids containing calcium are also promoted as min-

eral supplements, but taking antacids every day can cause an iron deficiency, and those with aluminum hydroxide can inhibit phosphorus absorption.[2] Phosphorus is necessary for bone mineralization, and chronic use of some antacids can eventually impair bone health. One elderly woman had to be admitted to the hospital because of the bone pain in her legs; she could barely stand up or walk unassisted. Not long before, she had more than doubled her antacid dose. Once she stopped taking the antacids, the pain in her legs subsided.

Many people take large quantities of aspirin, easily 10 to 12 tablets each day, to relieve the pain of arthritis, backaches, and headaches. This much aspirin can speed up blood loss from the stomach by as much as ten times, enough to cause iron-deficiency anemia in some people.[3] People who take aspirin regularly should make sure they eat iron-rich foods regularly as well.

Oral Contraceptives and Estrogen Millions of women use oral contraceptives, daily doses of hormones that prevent pregnancy by creating hormonal climate similar to that of pregnancy itself. For 30 years, these have been the most studied drugs in the United States. Research has uncovered several risks of taking these drugs, and now, new doses and formulas produce effective contraceptives with wide safety margins. The case of the oral contraceptives illustrates that interactions between just one drug and nutrients can be complex.

Oral contraceptives clearly do alter blood nutrient levels. Significantly, they also alter blood lipids, possibly raising the risk of cardiovascular disease in menstruating women.[4] This effect poses very little risk for young healthy women who do not smoke.[5] Beyond

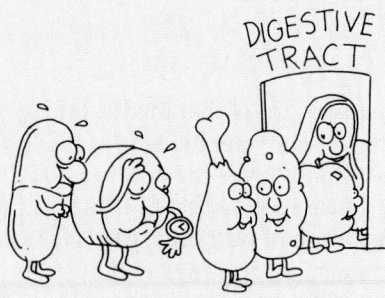

Foods can slow down the absorption of drugs in the digestive tract.

about age 35, however, most oral contraceptives raise total cholesterol and triglyceride concentrations and lower HDL, amplifying the risk of stroke and heart disease. A few women using oral contraceptives also experience mild hypertension. A leading expert in contraceptive technology compares these risks with risks from other activities in the life of a woman who both smokes and uses oral contraceptives. For example, a ride in a car is more than twice as risky to life, and a motorcycle ride carries 16 times the risk.[6]

Each nutrient responds differently to oral contraceptive use (see Table C12-2). At first glance this might seem to indicate that women using oral contraceptives are on their way to suffering deficiencies of some nutrients and have somehow enlarged their body stores of others. The research in the area has yielded conflicting results, however, so any such assumptions would be premature. Take vitamin A, for example. Researchers were concerned that the high blood vitamin A in oral contraceptive users might be due to release of the liver's stored vitamin A and indicate impending deficiency.[7] They found otherwise. Oral contraceptives do not appear to deplete liver vitamin A or cause deficiency. Similarly, research shows that iron in the blood of oral contraceptive users stays well within the normal range.

The vitamin B_6 status of oral contraceptive users has been extensively studied. Research shows that some oral contraceptive users have low blood vitamin B_6. Since vitamin B_6 assists in the body's handling of the amino acid tryptophan, this pathway is impaired, but other vitamin B_6-dependent functions remain normal. Excessive vitamin B_6 can be toxic (see Chapter 7), so oral contraceptive users are generally advised to rely on vitamin-rich, nutrient-dense foods and to avoid supplements.

Some women lose, and some gain, weight when taking oral contraceptives. Some may gain 20 pounds or more, from fat deposited in the hips, thighs, and breasts, or because they retain fluid.[8] Some lean tissue is also deposited in response to an androgenic (steroid) effect of the pills. Sometimes a switch to another form of pill can normalize body weight.

As with oral contraceptives, women's responses to estrogen replacement drugs must be assessed individually. Some women may suffer edema because estrogen promotes sodium conservation by the kidneys. Sodium restriction can correct this condition.[9] Others may develop abnormally low blood folate or vitamin B_6, indicating a need to include more vitamin-rich, nutrient-

dense foods in the diet. All women taking estrogen should be aware that vitamin C doses of a gram or more may elevate serum estrogen and falsely suggest that a lower dose is needed.

If a woman who uses oral contraceptives or estrogen replacement therapy thinks she may have a nutrient deficiency, she should refrain from taking individual supplements and seek testing and a diagnosis from a health-care professional to rule out other causes of her symptoms. For most women a nutritious diet is all that is needed. If a woman feels compelled to take a supplement, however, a multivitamin-mineral supplement that does not exceed the RDA is probably harmless, as long as it accompanies a well-balanced diet. Chapter 7 showed how to select a supplement.

CAFFEINE

The well-known "wake-up" effect of caffeine is the primary reason why people in every society use it in some form. Compared with the drugs discussed so far, though, caffeine's interactions with foods and nutrients are subtle. And yet in one important way caffeine's relationship to nutrition is more notable. Caffeine comes in many foods and beverages, and people may be unaware that it is there. Many OTC cold and headache remedies also contain caffeine because it perks up even sick people and relieves the headache caused by caffeine withdrawal that no other pain reliever can touch.[10] Table C12-3 lists the caffeine contents of beverages and foods.

Caffeine is a true stimulant drug. Like all stimulants, it increases the respiration rate, heart rate, blood pressure, and secretion of stress and other hormones. It stimulates the digestive tract, promoting efficient elimination, and promotes water loss from the body as well.

Caffeine is the most popular and widely consumed drug in the United States. One in three U.S. citizens consumes about 200 milligrams of caffeine per day (as in 2 small cups of coffee), but many others consume much more. Some people's intake patterns fulfill all the accepted criteria for a diagnosis of drug dependence.[11] High caffeine intakes seem to accompany advanced age, high body weight, and cigarette and alcohol use.[12]

Children are especially sensitive to caffeine's effects because they are small and, at first, not adapted to its use. Parents should be aware that caffeine is present in chocolate bars, colas, and other soft drinks.

Despite caffeine's tremendous popularity, many people today are using less because they fear that it harms

TABLE C12-2

Nutrition Effects of a Few Commonly Used Drugs

Medicines and Caffeine	Effects on Absorption	Effects on Excretion	Effects on Metabolism
Antacids (aluminum containing)	Reduce iron absorption	Increase calcium and phosphorus excretion	May accelerate destruction of thiamin
Antibiotics (long-term usage)	Reduce absorption of fats, amino acids, folate, fat-soluble vitamins, vitamin B_{12}, calcium, copper, iron, magnesium, potassium, phosphate, zinc	Increase excretion of folate, niacin, potassium, riboflavin, vitamin C	Destroy vitamin K–producing bacteria and reduce vitamin K production
Aspirin (large doses, long-term usage)	Lowers blood concentration of folate	Increases excretion of thiamin, vitamin C, vitamin K; causes iron and potassium losses through blood loss	
Caffeine		Increases excretion of small amounts of calcium and magnesium	Stimulates release of fatty acids into the blood
Diuretics		Raise blood calcium and zinc; lower blood folate, chloride, magnesium, phosphorus, potassium, vitamin B_{12}; increase excretion of calcium, sodium, thiamin, potassium, chloride, magnesium	Interfere with storage of zinc
Laxatives (effects vary with type)	Reduce absorption of glucose, fat, carotene, vitamin D, other fat-soluble vitamins, calcium, phosphate, potassium	Increase excretion of all unabsorbed nutrients	
Oral contraceptives	Reduce absorption of folate, may improve absorption of calcium	Cause sodium retention	Raise blood vitamin A, copper, iron; may lower blood folate, riboflavin, vitamin B_6, vitamin B_{12}, vitamin C; may elevate requirements for riboflavin and vitamin B_6
Estrogen replacement therapy	May reduce absorption of folate	Causes sodium retention	May raise blood glucose, triglycerides, vitamin A, vitamin E, copper, and iron; may lower blood vitamin C, folate, vitamin B_6, riboflavin, calcium, magnesium, and zinc

SOURCE: Data from Z. M. Pronsky, *Food Medication Interactions*, 9th ed. (Pottstown, Pa.: Food-Medication Interactions, 1995).

health. Research in the last decade has yielded sporadic reports linking caffeine to health problems such as cancer, birth defects, and hypertension. However, much other research refutes any links between caffeine and cancer or birth defects and finds only weak links between caffeine and hypertension.[13]

Moderate caffeine intakes may speed up metabolic energy expenditures.[14] In one study, only 100 milligrams of caffeine (about what is in a cup of coffee) noticeably raised the metabolic rates of both lean and previously obese people for several hours.

Caffeine seems relatively harmless when used in moderation (again, as in 2 cups of coffee a day). In higher doses, caffeine can cause symptoms associated with anxiety: sweating, tenseness, and inability to concentrate. High doses may also accelerate bone loss in women past midlife.[15] Caffeine may also contribute to painful but benign fibrocystic breast disease.

If you like caffeine-containing foods or beverages, the most reasonable approach may be to limit your intake to the equivalent of about 2 small cups of coffee per day. For most people this is enough to produce reduced drowsiness and keen awareness of tasks at hand without paying too high a price. Pregnant women, especially, should exercise moderation in using caffeine, and parents should monitor and control their children's intakes.

TOBACCO

Cigarette and other tobacco use causes thousands of people to suffer from cancer and other diseases of the cardiovascular, digestive, and respiratory systems. These effects are beyond nutrition's scope, but smoking does depress hunger and body fatness and change nutrient status, and the nutrition effects are also linked to lung cancer. Chapter 9 provided details on smoking and body fatness.

Nutrient intakes of smokers and nonsmokers differ.[16] Smokers have lower intakes of dietary fiber, vitamins, and minerals, even when their energy intakes are quite similar to those of nonsmokers. The association between smoking and low vitamin intake may be noteworthy, considering the altered metabolism of vitamin C in smokers and their lower blood values for a number of nutrients. The research has just begun on many nutrients, but much is known about vitamin C.[17]

Research shows that the vitamin C requirement of smokers exceeds that of nonsmokers.[18] Smokers break down vitamin C faster and so must take in more vita-

TABLE C12-3

Caffeine Content of Beverages and Foods

Drinks and Foods	Average (mg)	Range (mg)
Coffee (5 oz cup)		
Brewed, drip method	130	110–150
Brewed, percolator	94	64–124
Instant	74	40–108
Instant "lite"	30	no data
Decaffeinated, brewed or instant	3	1–5
Tea (5 oz cup)		
Brewed, major U.S. brands	40	20–90
Brewed, imported brands	60	25–110
Instant	30	25–50
Iced (12 oz glass)	70	67–76
Herb teas (caffeine-free)	0	0
Soft drinks (12 oz can)		
Dr. Pepper		40
Colas and cherry colas:		
Regular		30–46
Diet		2–58
Clear and caffeine-free		0–trace
Extra caffeine (Jolt)		75–100
Mountain Dew, Mello Yello		52
Big Red		38
Fresca, 7-Up, Sprite, Squirt, Sunkist Orange, seltzers, root beers		0
Cocoa beverage (5 oz cup)	4	2–20
Chocolate milk beverage (8 oz)	5	2–7
Milk chocolate candy (1 oz)	6	1–15
Dark chocolate, semisweet (1 oz)	20	5–35
Baker's chocolate (1 oz)	26	26
Chocolate-flavored syrup (1 oz)	4	4
Carob	0	0

NOTE: Many over-the-counter medications such as pain relievers and cold medicines also contain caffeine. Their labels must list the milligram amounts of caffeine per dose of medicine. Read medicine labels carefully.

min C–containing foods to achieve steady body pools comparable to those of nonsmokers. It is estimated that the vitamin C requirement of smokers may be twice as high as that of nonsmokers. The evidence for this is so strong that the vitamin C RDA is set at 100 milligrams per day for smokers compared to 60 for nonsmokers.[19]

ILLICIT DRUGS

People know that illicit drugs are harmful, but many choose to abuse them anyway in spite of the risks. Like

OTC and prescription drugs, illegal drugs modify body functions. They are unlike medicines, however, in that no watchdog agency such as the Food and Drug Administration (FDA) monitors them for safety, effectiveness, or even purity. Drugs purchased on the street are likely to contain impurities or to be mixed with cheaper drugs to maximize profits for the pushers. No two batches are alike. The risks of using illicit drugs are many and diverse, ranging from health risks to imprisonment to death. Marijuana and cocaine are the most extensively studied of the illicit drugs.

Smoking a marijuana cigarette affects several senses including the sense of taste. It produces an enhanced enjoyment of eating, especially of sweets, commonly known as "the munchies." Why or how this effect occurs is not known. Despite higher food intakes, marijuana abusers often consume fewer nutrients than do nonabusers, because the extra foods they choose tend to be high-calorie, low-nutrient snack foods. Besides the nutrition effects, regular marijuana users face the same risk of lung cancer as people who smoke a pack of cigarettes a day.

Cocaine elicits effects such as intense euphoria, restlessness, heightened self-confidence, irritability, insomnia, and loss of appetite. Weight loss is a common side effect, and cocaine abusers often develop eating disorders. Repeated use can cause a rapid heart rate, irregular heartbeats, heart attacks, and even death. Cocaine use continues to escalate as cheaper and more dangerous forms of the drug become available. Cocaine in its smokable form, crack, has greater addictive power than any other drug; it is overwhelming and terrifying. One former crack addict tells of holding a gun to his brother's head to demand money for his next crack purchase.

Unlike marijuana use, cocaine use causes serious malnutrition. The craving for the drug replaces hunger; the stronger the craving for cocaine, the less a drug abuser wants nutritious food. Rats given unlimited access to cocaine will choose the drug over food until they die of starvation. The effects of the other addictive drugs vary in degree but are similar in kind to those of cocaine. A few are listed in Table C12-4. Drug abusers face multiple nutrition problems:

- They spend their food money on drugs.
- They lose interest in food during "high" times.
- Their days often lack the regularity and routine that promote good eating habits.

TABLE C12-4

Nutrition Effects of Four Nonmedical Drugs

Drug of Abuse	Possible Effects on Nutrition Status
Cocaine	Reduces intakes of nutritious foods; increases intakes of alcohol, coffee, and fat; may induce or aggravate eating disorders
Heroin	Heightens and delays insulin response to glucose; reduces intakes of nutritious foods
Marijuana	Increases intakes of foods, especially sweets; may cause weight gain
Nicotine	Reduces intake of sweet foods and water; increases intakes of fat; reduces fetal weight; lowers blood concentration of beta-carotene.

SOURCES: Data from M. E. Mohs, R. R. Watson, and T. Leonard-Green, Nutritional effects of marijuana, heroin, cocaine, and nicotine, *Journal of the American Dietetic Association* 90 (1990): 1261–1267; G. van Poppel, S. Spanhaak, and T. Ockhuizen, Effects of beta carotene on immunological indexes in healthy male smokers, *American Journal of Clinical Nutrition* 57 (1993): 402–407.

- They may contract hepatitis, a viral liver disease spread via infected needles, which causes taste changes, loss of appetite, and loss of weight. (They risk contracting AIDS in the same way.)
- Treatments and medicines may alter their nutrition status.
- Those who become ill with infectious diseases develop increased needs for nutrients.

During withdrawal from drugs, an important aspect of treatment is the identification and correction of nutrition problems.

Not all the interactions discussed here occur every time a person takes a drug. Some people are more vulnerable than others to drug-nutrient interactions. The potential for undesirable drug-nutrient interactions is greatest for those who:

- Take drugs (or medicines) for long times.
- Take two or more drugs at the same time.
- Are poorly nourished to begin with or are not eating well.

PERSONAL STRATEGY

In conclusion, when you need to take a medicine, do so wisely. Ask your physician, pharmacist, or other health-care provider for specific instructions about the doses, times, and how to take them—for example, with meals or on an empty stomach. If you notice new symptoms or if a drug seems not to be working well, consult your physician. The only instruction people need about illicit drugs is to avoid them altogether for countless reasons. As for smoking and chewing tobacco, the same advice applies: don't take these habits up, or if you already have, take steps to quit. For drugs with lesser conse-quences to health, such as caffeine, use moderation.

Try to live life in a way that requires less chemical assistance. If sleepy, try a 15-minute nap or meditation instead of a 15-minute coffee break. The coffee will stimulate your nerves for an hour, but the alternatives will refresh your attitude for the rest of the day. If you suffer constipation, try getting enough exercise, fiber, and water for a few days. Chances are that a laxative will be unnecessary. The strategy being suggested here is to take control of your body, allowing your reliable, self-healing nature to make fine adjustments that you need not force with chemicals. Bodies have few requests: adequate nutrition, rest, exercise, and hygiene. Give yours what it asks for, and let it function naturally, day-to-day, without interference from drugs.

NOTES

Notes are in Appendix F.

CHILD, TEEN, AND OLDER ADULT

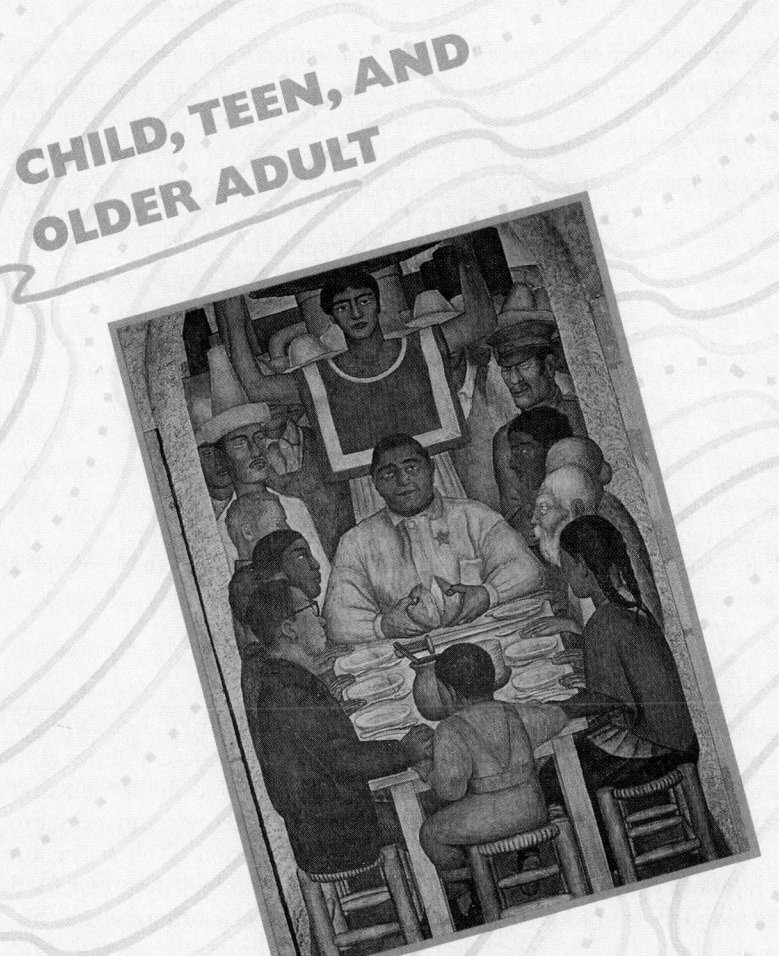

13

CONTENTS

Diego Rivera 1886–1957, *El Pan Nuestro*, Education Secretariat, Mexico, © SuperStock.

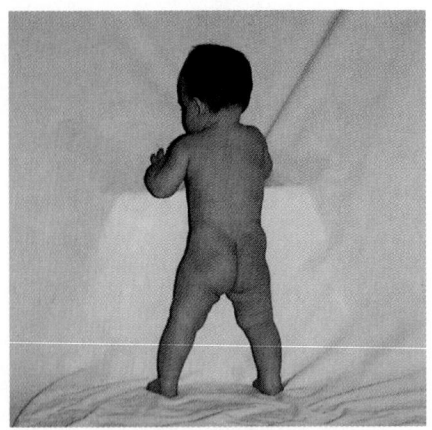

The body shape of a one-year-old (above) changes dramatically by age two (below). The two-year-old has lost much baby fat; the muscles (especially in the back, buttocks, and legs) have firmed and strengthened; and the leg bones have lengthened.

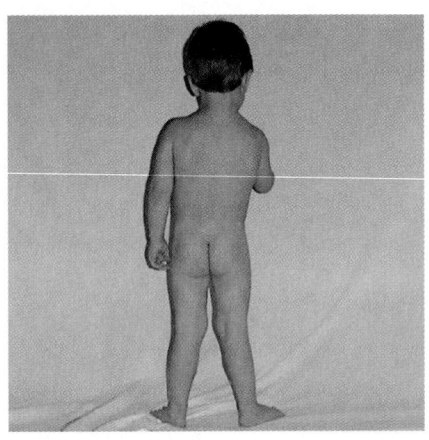

Example: A 174-pound adult male needs 1,000 RE of vitamin A. That is 5.75 RE per pound. A 44-pound five-year-old needs 500 RE of vitamin A. That is 11.4 RE per pound.

13 To grow and to function well in the adult world, children need a solid background of sound eating habits. These habits begin at babyhood with the introduction of solid foods, as shown in the last chapter. But at that point nutrition has just begun; the plot thickens. Nutrient needs change steadily throughout life into old age, depending on the rate of growth, gender, activities, and many other factors. Nutrient needs also vary from individual to individual, but generalizations are possible and useful.

EARLY AND MIDDLE CHILDHOOD

After the age of one year, a child's growth rate slows, but the body continues to change dramatically. At age one, infants have just learned to stand and toddle; by two years, they can take long strides with solid confidence and are learning to run, jump, and climb. These new accomplishments are possible thanks to the accumulation of a larger mass and greater density of bone and muscle tissue. Thereafter, the same trends, a lengthening of the long bones and an increase in musculature, continue until adolescence, though unevenly and more slowly.

Growth and Nutrient Needs of Young Children

An infant's appetite decreases markedly near the first birthday, in line with the great reduction in growth rate. Thereafter the appetite fluctuates. At times children seem to be insatiable, and at other times they seem to live on air and water. Parents need not worry about this: a child will need and demand more food during periods of rapid growth than during slow periods. The perfection of appetite regulation in children of normal weight guarantees that their food energy intakes will be right for each stage of growth.[1] One caution: some children may overeat in response to external cues, disregarding satiety signals and thereby inviting the onset of obesity.

A one-year-old child needs perhaps 1,000 calories a day; a three-year-old needs 300 calories more. The next seven years add 700 more calories for a total of about 2,000 calories a day. Thus, even though total energy needs have doubled by age ten, the child's energy need per pound of body weight has steadily declined. More active children of any age need more energy because they spend more, and an inactive child can become obese even when eating less than average.

Growth enlarges the demand for all the nutrients per pound of body weight. On this basis, a five-year-old's need for, say, vitamin A is about double the need of an adult man (see margin). Before the adolescent growth spurt, children accumulate stores of nutrients that they will need in the years ahead. Then, when they take off on that growth spurt and their nutrient intakes cannot meet the demands of rapid growth, they draw on the nutrients they stored earlier. This is especially true of calcium; the denser the bones are in childhood, the better prepared they will be to support teen growth and still withstand the inevitable bone losses of later life. A tried and true means of providing these nutrients is to follow the Daily Food Guide. The recommendations for children are shown in Table 13-1.

Careful food selection is essential to ensure that a child receives the right amounts of nutrients. When a child consistently skips breakfast or is allowed to choose sugary foods (candy or marshmallows) in place of nourishing ones

TABLE 13-1

Daily Food Guide for Children

FOOD GROUP	SERVINGS PER DAY	SERVING SIZES BY AGE GROUP		
		2 to 3 Years	4 to 6 Years	7 to 12 Years
Bread and cereals (whole grain or enriched)	6 or more	½ slice	1 slice	1 slice
Vegetables	3 or more	2–3 tbs or 3–4 oz juice	3–4 tbs or ½ c juice	¼–½ c or ½ c juice
Fruits	2 or more	2–3 tbs or 3–4 oz juice	3–4 tbs or ½ c juice	¼–½ c or ½ c juice
Meat and meat alternates	2–3	1–2 oz	1–2 oz	2–3 oz
Milk and milk products	3 to 4	½ c	½–¾ c	½–1 c

SOURCE: Serving sizes from P. M. Queen and C. E. Lang, *Handbook of Pediatric Nutrition* (Gaithersburg, Md.: Aspen Publishers, 1993), p. 152.

(whole-grain cereals), it is virtually certain that the child will fail to get enough of several nutrients. The nutrients missed from a skipped breakfast won't be "made up" at lunch and dinner but will be completely left out that day. A child can't be trusted to choose nutritious foods on the basis of taste alone; the preference for sweets is inborn, as Figure 3-7 of Chapter 3 made clear.

Active, normal-weight children may enjoy occasional treats of high-calorie but nutritious foods. From the milk group, ice cream or pudding is good now and then; from the bread group, whole-grain or enriched cakes, cookies, or even doughnuts are an acceptable addition to a balanced diet. These foods are made from milk and grain, they carry valuable nutrients, and they encourage a child to learn, appropriately, that eating is fun. However, should a child regularly eat large quantities of these treats, the only possible outcomes are nutrient deficiencies, obesity, or both. Parents of wandering elementary school children should be aware that they may be spending pocket money at nearby stores and filling up on sweets.[2]

While it is important to teach children nutrition principles that can help to avoid obesity, it is also important to use sensitivity in teaching. Children are impressionable and can easily get the idea that their worthiness or lovability is somehow tied to body weight. Some parents fail to realize that society's ideal of slimness can be perilously close to starvation. A child encouraged to "diet" cannot obtain the nutrients required for normal growth and development. Even healthy children without diagnosable eating disorders have been observed to stunt their own growth through "dieting."[3] Weight gain in truly overweight children can be controlled safely without compromising growth, but should be overseen by a registered dietitian.

Desirable weight-control behaviors to instill in children are to relax while eating, to pause and enjoy their table companions, and to stop eating when they are full. Parents can assist further by not exceeding recommended serving sizes of food unless needed. Healthy snacks such as milk, crackers, and fruit, rather than colas and chips, set a pattern for healthy choices later on. The next section presents more tips for feeding children.

✔ **KEY POINT** **Children's nutrient needs reflect their stage of growth. Positive parental guidance can help establish food patterns that provide adequate nourishment for growth without obesity.**

Mealtimes and Snacking

The childhood years are a parent's last chance to influence food choices. Appropriate eating habits and attitudes toward food ensure positive development during growth and help future adults maintain healthy weights and reduce risks of degenerative diseases in later life.

Children's Preferences Children naturally like nutritious foods in all the food groups, with one exception—vegetables, which some young children frequently refuse. Here presentation may be the key.

Many children prefer vegetables that are mild flavored, slightly undercooked and crunchy, bright in color, and easy to eat. Cooked foods should be served warm, not hot, because a child's mouth is much more sensitive than an adult's. The mild flavors of carrots, peas, and corn are preferred because a child has more taste buds. Smooth foods such as grits, oatmeal, mashed potatoes, and pea soup should have no lumps in them. Children prefer familiar foods; fear of new foods is practically universal among children. Suggesting, rather than commanding, that a child try small amounts of new foods at the beginning of a meal, when the child is hungry, seems to work best.[4]

Choking A child may make no sound when choking, so an adult should keep an eye on children when they are eating. Encouraging the child to sit when eating is a good practice; choking is more likely when children are running or reclining.[5] Round foods such as grapes, nuts, hard candies, and pieces of hot dog can easily become lodged in a child's small windpipe. Other potentially dangerous foods include tough meat, popcorn, chips, and peanut butter eaten by the spoon.

Little children like to eat small portions of food at little tables.

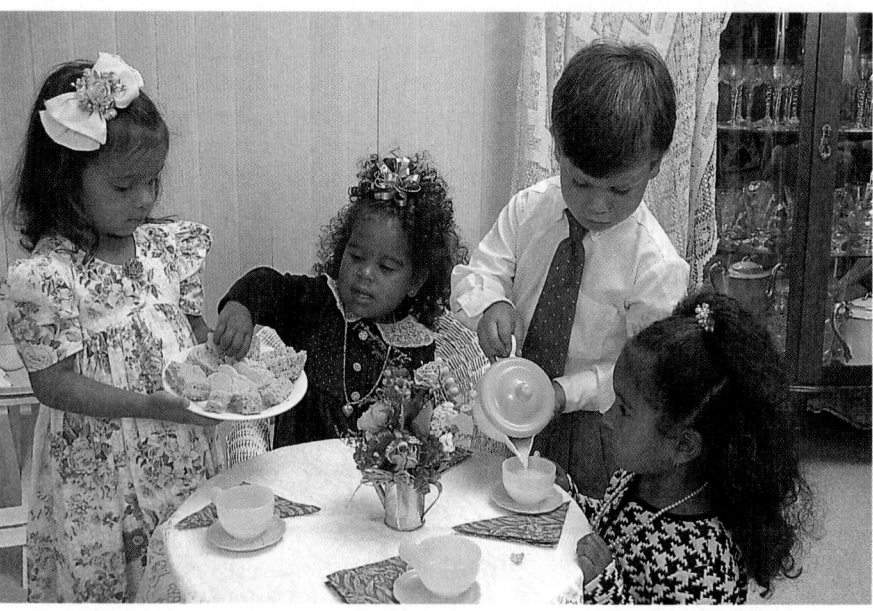

Portion Sizes   Little children like to eat small portions of food at little tables. If offered large portions, children may well fill up on favorite foods, ignoring others. Toddlers often go on food jags eating only one or two favored foods. The best way to handle food jags lasting a week or so is to make no response, since two-year-olds regard any form of attention as a reward. After two weeks of indulging the jag, try serving tiny portions of many foods, including the favored items. Distract the child with friends at meals, and make other foods as attractive as possible.

Remember, too, that just as parents are entitled to their likes and dislikes, a child who genuinely and consistently rejects a food should be allowed the same privilege. Also, children should be believed when they say they are full: the "clean-your-plate" dictum should be stamped out for all time. Children who are forced to override their own satiety signals are essentially in training for obesity. Encourage children to listen to their bodies, and do not make an issue of food acceptance. The parent is responsible for *what* the child is offered to eat, but the child is responsible for *how much* and even *whether* to eat.

Snacking and Other Healthy Habits   Parents may find that their children often snack so much that they are not very hungry at mealtimes. This need not be a problem as long as children know how to snack. Snacks that are nutritious can meet the same needs as nutritious small meals do. Keep snack foods simple and readily available. Milk, cheese, fruit, yogurt, peanut butter sandwiches, and cereal can all satisfy children and help meet nutrient needs.

A bright, unhurried atmosphere free of conflict is conducive to good appetite. Parents who serve meals in a relaxed and casual manner, without anxiety, provide a climate in which a child can learn to enjoy eating. Parents who beg, cajole, and demand that their children eat set up power struggles. A child may find mealtimes unbearable if they are accompanied by a barrage of accusations—"Susie, your hands are filthy . . . your report card . . . and clean your plate!" The child's stomach recoil as both body and mind react to stress of this kind.

Children love to be included in meal preparation. Children as young as age two can develop new skills by helping out (see Table 13-2 in the margin). A positive experience is most likely when tasks match children's developmental abilities, and when enthusiasm and enjoyment, not criticism or drudgery, surrounds them. Praise for a job well done (or at least well attempted) expands a child's sense of pride and helps to develop skills and positive feelings toward healthy foods. Children also like to eat foods they help to prepare.

Many parents may overlook perhaps the single most important influence on their child's food habits—their own habits. Parents who don't prepare, serve, and eat carrots shouldn't be surprised when their child refuses to eat carrots. A child learns much through imitation. Parents set an irresistible example by enjoying nutritious foods at meals and snacks.

While preparing, serving, and enjoying food, caretakers can promote not only physical but also emotional growth at every stage of a child's life. It is important for parents to help Joey and Susie to remember that they are good kids. What they do may sometimes be unacceptable, but they are still normal, healthy, growing, fine human beings.

KEY POINTS   Healthy eating habits and positive relationships with food are learned in childhood. Parents teach children best by example.

TABLE 13-2

Food Skills of Preschoolers[a]

Age 1–2 years, when large muscles develop, the child:
- uses short-shanked spoon.
- helps feed self.
- lifts and drinks from cup.
- helps scrub, tear, break, or dip foods.

Age 3 years, when medium hand muscles develop, the child:
- spears food with fork.
- feeds self independently.
- helps wrap, pour, mix, shake, spread, and crack nuts with supervision.

Age 4 years, when small finger muscles develop, the child:
- uses all utensils and napkin.
- helps roll, juice, mash, peel, and crack egg shells.

Age 5 years, when fine coordination of fingers and hands, the child:
- helps measure, grind, cut, and grate.
- uses hand-cranked egg beater with supervision.

[a]These ages are approximate. Healthy, normal children develop at their own pace.

SOURCES: Adapted from M. Sigman-Grant, Feeding Preschoolers: Balancing nutrition and developmental needs, *Nutrition Today,* July/August 1992, pp. 13–17; A. A. Hertzler, Preschoolers' food handling skills—motor development, *Journal of Nutrition Education* 21 (1989): 100B–100C.

TABLE 13-3

Iron-Rich Foods Kids Like[a]

Breads, Cereals, and Grains
Canned macaroni (½ c)
Canned spaghetti (½ c)
Cream of wheat (¼ c)
Fortified dry cereals (1 oz)[b]
Noodles, rice, or barley (½ c)
Tortillas (1 flour, 2 corn)
Whole-wheat, enriched, or
    fortified bread (1 slice)

Vegetables
Baked flavored potato skins
    (½ skin)
Cooked mushrooms (½ c)
Cooked mung bean sprouts or
    snow peas (½ c)
Green peas (½ c)
Mixed vegetable juice (1 c)

Fruits
Apple juice (1 c)
Canned plums (3 plums)
Cooked dried apricots (¼ c)
Dried peaches (4 halves)
Raisins (1 tbs)

Meats and Legumes
Bean dip (¼ c)
Canned pork and beans (⅓ c)
Mild chili or other bean/meat
    dishes (¼ c)
Liverwurst (½ oz)
Meat casseroles (½ c)
Peanut butter and jelly sandwich
    (½ sandwich)
Lean roast beef or cooked ground
    beef (1 oz)
Sloppy joes (½ sandwich)

[a]Each serving provides at least 1 milligram iron, or one-tenth of a child's iron RDA. Vitamin C–rich foods included with these snacks increase iron absorption.

[b]Some fortified breakfast cereals contain more than 10 milligrams iron per half-cup serving (read the labels).

SOURCE: Many of these ideas reflect data in A. A. Hertzler, Children's food patterns—A review: I. Food preferences and feeding problems, *Journal of the American Dietetic Association* 83 (1983): 551–554.

Controversy 13 details the mental symptoms of anemia.

Nutrient Deficiencies and Behavior

A child who suffers from nutrient deficiencies exhibits physical and behavioral symptoms: the child is sick and out of sorts. Diet-behavior connections are of keen interest to caretakers who both feed children and live with them.

Deficiencies of protein, energy, vitamin A, iron, and zinc plague children the world over. In developing nations, such deficiencies cause or contribute to nearly half the deaths of children under four and inflict blindness, stunted growth, and vulnerability to infections on millions more.

In developed countries such as the United States and Canada, most deficiencies have subtle, even unnoticeable, effects. A study of British children, found about 40 percent of them to have intakes of less than half the RDA of folate, vitamin D, calcium, iron, magnesium, selenium, zinc, and many other minerals. The researchers gave multinutrient supplements to some of the children and later administered intelligence tests to all of them. Those who had received the supplements scored significantly higher on the tests than the others did. The researchers took the findings to mean that although children may be well-nourished in terms of protein and some vitamins, as they are in the United States, brain function may be sensitive to borderline deficiencies of many other nutrients, a conclusion supported by many previous findings.[6]

Iron deficiency is the most common nutrient deficiency in children and adolescents, and reducing its incidence should be a top priority according to U.S. nutritionists.[7] Besides carrying oxygen in the blood, iron works within cells as part of large molecules to release energy. A lack of iron not only causes an energy crisis but also directly affects behavior, mood, attention span, and learning ability. Iron also plays key roles in many molecules of the brain and nervous system. Deficiencies of iron produced experimentally in animals have caused abnormal metabolism in neurotransmitters, notably those that regulate the ability to pay attention, which is crucial to learning.

Iron deficiency is usually diagnosed by a deficit of iron in the *blood*, after anemia has developed. A child's *brain*, however, is sensitive to slightly lowered iron concentrations long before the blood effects appear. It is difficult to distinguish the effects of iron deficiency from those of other factors in children's lives, but studies have found connections between iron deficiency and behavior. Iron deficiency seems to manifest itself in a lowering of the motivation to persist in intellectually challenging tasks, a shortening of the attention span, and a reduction of overall intellectual performance.[8] A child with such symptoms may be irritable, aggressive, and disagreeable or sad and withdrawn. One might label such a child "hyperactive," "depressed," or "unlikable," but these traits may not be purely psychological; they may arise from malnutrition. Inspection of a disruptive or apathetic child's diet by a qualified health-care professional can identify these reversible problems, and additions to the diet can correct them. Table 13-3 lists some iron-rich foods kids like to eat. Only a health-care provider should make the decision to give iron supplements, of course, and if used, supplements should be kept out of children's reach.

✔ **KEY POINT**   **The detrimental effects of nutrient deficiencies in children of developed nations can be subtle. Iron deficiency is the most widespread nutrition problem of children and causes abnormalities in both physical health and behavior.**

The Problem of Lead

Malnutrition is often a complex condition involving multiple nutrients and non-nutritional factors. One such factor is lead poisoning, which can cause iron-deficiency anemia. Conversely, iron deficiency impairs the body's defenses against lead. A child with iron-deficiency anemia is three times as likely to have elevated blood lead as a child with normal iron status. Calcium may slow lead's absorption or interfere with its toxic effects in the body.[9]

Babies like to explore, and they put everything into their mouths, including things that may harm them, such as chips of old paint, pieces of metal, and other unlikely substances. These are normal baby activities, but they may be silently raising blood lead until toxic concentrations have built up. Not until much later, after lead toxicity has set in, do caretakers notice unusual symptoms.

Joey was such a child. This normal-appearing baby grew up in an inner city, where dust from heavily traveled streets settled on his playthings, sprinkling lead from old gasoline deposits into his environment. He loved to taste everything: table legs, toys, the spindles of flaky paint railings—whatever was within his reach. And his mother often mixed his morning formula with the first water from the tap, water that had spent the night absorbing lead from the old building's lead pipes. Figure 13-1 shows the origins of lead in children's environments.

Joey grew to become a cautious, quiet preschooler who clung to stair railings with both hands as he slowly climbed up and down. He was late in walking, small for his age, seldom played as vigorously as other children, and was prone to small health disturbances, such as diarrhea, irritability, and lethargy. While his health quietly deteriorated, his parents shrugged off subtle symptoms as normal variations in children. They explained away his small size, awkward stair climbing, lack of fine motor coordination, hearing difficulties, and slow learning. Finally, a pediatrician detected lead toxicity in Joey's blood and started treating him with lead-scavenging drugs.[10] Except for persistent, minor learning disabilities, Joey is now growing normally and playing vigorously.

For kids like Joey, the truth can easily come too late, since even one year of lead exposure can permanently impair the brain, nervous system, and psychological functioning.[11] Older children with high blood lead, as compared with their peers, have more physical complaints and are more delinquent, aggressive, and distractable.[12] The effects occur with lower doses than those originally defined as toxic, so the Centers for Disease Control have lowered the official poisoning threshold and have called for universal screening of children's blood.[13] The Public Health Service says lead poisoning is the most serious environmental threat children face today.

Lead is an indestructible metal element; the body cannot alter it. Because it is similar chemically to nutrient minerals like iron, calcium, and zinc, lead displaces these minerals from their sites of action, but then is unable to perform their biological functions. Consequently, lead interferes with many of the body's systems, particularly the vulnerable tissues of the nervous system, kidneys, blood, and bone marrow.

The body absorbs lead greedily during times of rapid growth and then hoards it possessively. During pregnancy, lead crosses the placenta, invades the developing fetus, and inflicts severe damage on the fetal nervous system.

The Environmental Protection Agency (EPA) provides this toll-free hotline for lead information: 1-800-LEAD-FYI (1-800-532-3394).

FIGURE 13-1

OUR CHILDREN'S DAILY LEAD
Lead finds its way into the bodies of children when they ingest lead-containing foods, water, dust, or paint chips, or when they breathe lead-laden air.

TITLE SOURCE: Title borrowed from M. A. Wessel and A. Dominski. Our children's daily lead, *American Scientist* 6 (1977): 294–298.

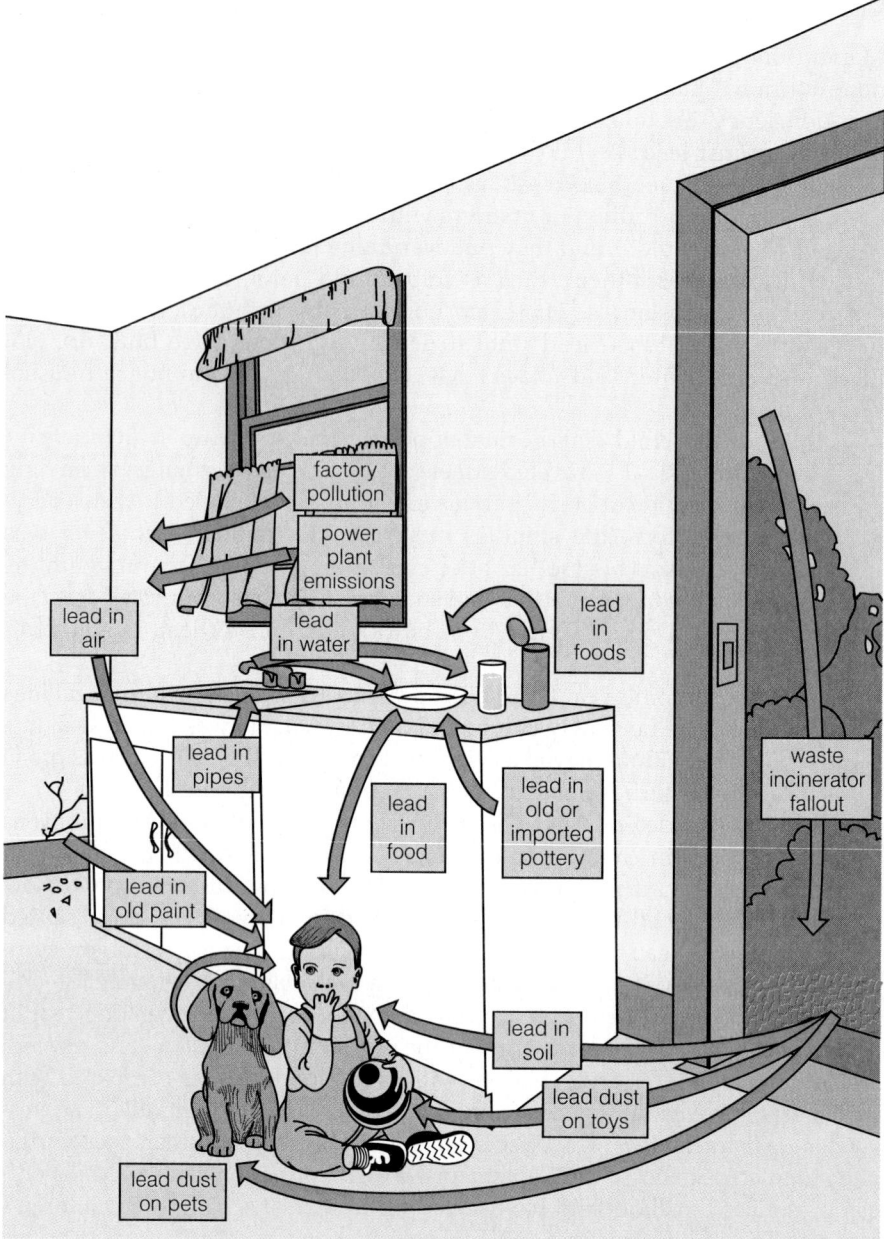

Infants and young children absorb five to ten times as much lead as do adults. One of every six children between the ages of six months and five years and one of every nine fetuses are exposed to threatening levels of lead.[14]

As toddlers, children expand their ranges for exploring, and they still taste and chew everything. Thus the toddler years see a marked rise in blood lead concentrations.[15] While the neuromuscular system is maturing, high blood lead interferes with balance, motor development,[16] and the relay of nerve messages to and from the brain. Children with the highest blood lead at ages two and three years suffer the greatest developmental delays at age four.

Researchers studying young children's development must keep in mind that lead intoxication may affect their results.[17]

Reductions in the use of leaded gasolines and other products mandated by federal law in past years have helped to limit the amounts of lead in the environment—and in children's blood. The decline in blood lead concentrations in children during the late 1970s paralleled exactly the decline in the nation's use of leaded gasoline, leaded house paint, and lead-soldered food cans. Even so, many children's blood lead concentrations remain unacceptably high because some lead is still discharged into the environment. Legislation is now in place that requires warnings to prospective home buyers if lead paint is present in houses before purchase. It also increases state budgets to pay for aggressive programs of testing and treating children for lead poisoning. Additionally, a federal tracking system is attempting to gather data so that areas of greatest concern can be identified and the problems corrected.

As mentioned earlier, lead competes in the body with iron, calcium, and zinc.[18] Deficiencies of these minerals are common in young children and enhance lead absorption and retention. Prevention of lead toxicity rests primarily on reduced exposure, but parents can protect their children to some degree by making sure that they receive adequate calcium and other minerals.

Once diagnosed, nutrient deficiencies and even lead toxicity are easy to treat. The trick is to identify these conditions before too much damage has set in. Sometimes abnormal behavior is the only observable sign of poor nutrition.

✓ **KEY POINT**   **Lead poisoning remains a serious environmental threat to children. It can inflict severe, irreparable damage on growing children. Environmental lead levels have declined in recent years but not enough to safeguard children's health.**

Food Allergy, Intolerance, and Aversion

Food **allergy** is frequently blamed for physical and behavioral abnormalities in children. In truth, the prevalence of food allergy among children is far less (up to 8 percent) than many grown-ups believe.[19] Among adults, allergies are even less common, occurring in 2 percent of the population.

A true food allergy occurs when a whole food protein or other large molecule enters the body tissues. Recall that most large molecules of food are normally dismantled to smaller ones in the digestive tract before absorption. Some, however, are not digested but enter the bloodstream whole. Once they are inside, the body's immune system reacts to undigested food proteins or other large molecules as it does to any other **antigen:** it releases **antibodies, histamine,** or other defensive agents. A problem not involving the immune system that results from exposure to food substances is known as a **food intolerance.**

Allergies may have one or two components. They always involve antibodies; they may or may not involve symptoms. A person may produce antibodies *without* exhibiting any symptoms or may produce antibodies *and* exhibit symptoms. Symptoms without antibody production are not due to allergy. This means that allergies cannot be diagnosed from symptoms alone; they have to be diagnosed by testing for antibodies.

A food allergy can produce many different symptoms. In the digestive tract, it may cause cramping, bloating, nausea, diarrhea, or vomiting; in the skin, it

allergy an immune reaction to a foreign substance, such as a component of food. Also called *hypersensitivity* by researchers.

antigen a substance foreign to the body that elicits the formation of antibodies or an inflammation reaction from immune system cells. Food antigens are usually glycoproteins (large proteins with glucose molecules attached). Inflammation consists of local swelling and irritation and attracts white blood cells to the site.

antibodies as defined in Chapter 6, large protein molecules that are produced in response to the presence of antigens and then inactivate the antigens.

histamine a substance that participates in causing inflammation; produced by cells of the immune system as part of a local immune reaction to an antigen.

food intolerance an adverse effect of a food or food additive not involving the immune response.

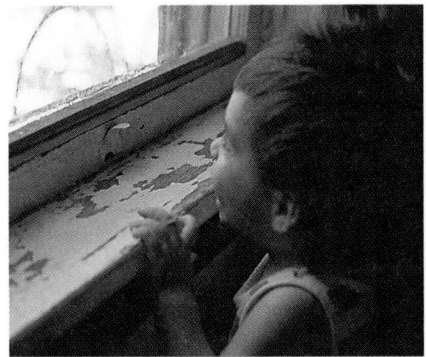

Paint is the main source of lead in most children's lives.

Alternative agricultural and industrial processes that can help to reduce environmental lead and other contaminants are discussed in Chapter 15.

anaphylactic (an-AFF-ill-LAC-tic) **shock** a life-threatening whole-body allergic reaction to an offending substance.

food aversion an intense dislike of a food, possibly biological in nature, resulting from an illness or other negative experience associated with that food.

A concern exists about allergic reactions to new genetically engineered foods. See Controversy 14.

Warning signs of allergic anaphylactic shock: itching tongue and tightness in the throat, abdominal pain, itchy and blotchy skin, nausea, vomiting, diarrhea, inflamed nasal membranes, chest pain, swelling, low blood pressure, shock, and respiratory arrest.

These normally wholesome foods are most likely to induce symptoms in people with allergies.

may cause hives, swelling, and rashes; in the lungs, it can cause asthma; it can also cause a runny nose or irritated, reddened eyes. A severe, dangerous, generalized reaction is **anaphylactic shock.**

Allergic reactions to food can occur with different timings; symptoms may appear within minutes or up to 24 hours later. Identifying a food that causes an immediate allergic reaction is easy because symptoms correlate closely with the time of eating the food. If the reaction is delayed, though, identifying the offending food is more difficult because many other foods will have been eaten by the time the symptoms have appeared. Many people are allergic to just one food, but some are allergic to many.

Almost 75 percent of allergic reactions are caused by just three foods: eggs, peanuts, and milk.[20] The other 25 percent are caused by a variety of foods from almonds to yeast breads. The life-threatening reaction of anaphylactic shock is most often caused by peanuts, nuts, fish, or shellfish.[21]

A skin prick test and a double-blind food challenge can confirm a true food allergy. These tests are time-consuming and often expensive, however, so people—and even physicians—often try to guess the cause of an adverse reaction and use the term *food allergy* loosely. A parent whose child has any kind of discomfort after eating, such as stomachache, headache, pain, rapid pulse rate, nausea, wheezing, hives, bronchial irritation, or cough, may decide that an allergy is responsible, when in fact the cause is something else entirely. Only careful, skilled testing by a physician can distinguish the many possibilities, and such testing is seldom done.

Because reliable tests for food allergy are inconvenient and expensive, people are tempted to believe quacks offering quick and easy but sophisticated-sounding laboratory work. For example, "cytotoxic testing" involves mixing blood with foods to see what blood cells "react" to. As you might guess, this test is invalid for detecting allergy because isolated blood cells are cut off from the body's immune system, which produces the allergic response. Other terms relating to allergy quackery are *brain allergy, metabolic rejectivity syndrome,* and the term *ecology* when applied to body functions.

A **food aversion,** an intense dislike of a food, may be a biological response to a food that once caused trouble. Children's food aversions may be the result of nature's efforts to protect them from allergic or other adverse reactions. Parents are advised to watch for signs of food dislikes and to take them seriously. Such a dislike may turn out to be a whim or fancy, but it should be respected. Although many cases of suspected allergies turn out to be something else, real allergies do exist, as do other valid reasons to avoid certain foods. In any case, don't prejudge. Test. Then, if an important staple food must be excluded from the diet, find other foods to provide the omitted nutrients and ensure the child's continued good nutrition.

Allergies are often blamed when behavior problems arise, but children who are sick from any cause are likely to be cranky. Evidence does not support the hypothesis that allergy can cause misbehavior without other symptoms. The next section singles out a type of misbehavior that is not caused by foods.

✔ KEY POINT **Food allergies cause illness, but diagnosis is difficult. Tests are imperative to determine whether allergy exists. Food aversions can be related to food allergies or to adverse reactions to foods.**

Hyperactivity, "Hyper" Behavior, and Diet

Hyperactivity, one kind of **learning disability,** occurs in 5 to 10 percent of young, school-aged children, that is, in 2 or 3 in every classroom of 30 children. It can lead to academic failure and major behavioral problems. Parents and teachers need to deal effectively with it wherever it appears to avert the grief that can otherwise result.

Food allergies have been blamed for hyperactivity. Research to date does not support the idea that food allergies or intolerances cause hyperactivity in children, but studies continue. Research has also all but dismissed the idea that sugar makes children hyperactive (see Controversy 4 for details). One study did find an association between doses of the food colorant tartrazine and increased irritability, restlessness, and sleep disturbances in a small percentage of hyperactive children.[22] Parents who wish to avoid tartrazine can find it listed with the ingredients on labels of the processed foods that contain it.

Physicians often diagnose hyperactivity by conducting trials with stimulant drugs. Stimulants normally speed up people's activity, but they calm down children with hyperactivity. The reason is unclear, but the drugs may stimulate centers in the brain that control behavior. *In children who are responsive,* prescription medication should at least be considered as the treatment of choice for hyperactivity.

Many parents, resistant to the idea of drugs for hyperactive children, hope that altering children's diets might improve their behavior. While optimal nutrition is critical to mental and physical health, appealing-sounding but unfounded dietary "treatments" may serve only to delay effective medical help. Such treatments may seem to help for a while due to the placebo effect, but they fail to provide lasting cures.

Hyperactivity is not the same as "hyper" behavior, or excitability and anxiety in children. This kind of behavior is sometimes linked to diet through excess caffeine, which can overstimulate children. A 12-ounce cola or a 8-ounce glass of iced tea, for example, contains up to 50 milligrams of caffeine. Two or more such beverages in the body of a 60-pound child are equivalent to the caffeine in 8 cups of coffee for a 175-pound man. High caffeine intakes bring on sleeplessness, restlessness, irregular heartbeats, and general misery. The great majority of U.S. children consume caffeine. Children cannot be expected to resist tempting colas and candy bars. It is the task of concerned adults to limit children's access to such foods. Eventually, children develop self-control, but only within the limits that were provided for them when they were young.

Without any magic answers, parents still may have to deal with excitable, rambunctious, and unruly children. Common sense says that all children at times get wild and "hyper." There are many normal, everyday causes of such behavior:

- Desire for attention.
- Lack of sleep.
- Overstimulation.
- Too much television.
- Lack of exercise.

hyperactivity (in children) a syndrome characterized by inattention, impulsiveness, and excess motor activity. Usually occurs before age seven, lasts six months or more, and does not entail mental illness or mental retardation. Also called *attention deficit disorder* or *hyperkinesis* and may be associated with minimal brain damage.

learning disability an altered ability to learn basic cognitive skills such as reading, writing, and mathematics.

The placebo effect was defined earlier. It is the healing effect produced by faith in a treatment, rather than by the treatment itself.

Controversy 12 presented a table of the caffeine in some foods and beverages.

A child who often fills up on cookies, misses lunch, becomes too cranky to nap, misses out on outdoor play, and spends hours in front of a television suffers stresses that trigger chronic patterns of crankiness. This self-perpetuating cycle of tension and fatigue resolves itself when the caretakers begin giving more consistent care to the child's welfare. It especially helps to insist on regular hours of sleep, regular mealtimes, and regular outdoor exercise.

KEY POINT   Hyperactivity is not caused by poor nutrition, but "hyper" behavior may reflect excess caffeine consumption or inconsistent care. A wise parent will limit children's caffeine intakes and meet their needs for structure to prevent tension and fatigue.

Television and Children's Nutrition

Television has adverse effects on children's nutrition. On the average, children in the United States spend as much time watching television as they do attending school; over 20 percent of children seldom play outside; and 80 percent watch television every schoolday afternoon and on Saturdays.[23] Television exerts four major kinds of impacts on children's nutrition. First, television viewing requires no energy. It seems to reduce the metabolic rate to a level below that of rest, requiring even less energy than daydreaming. The effect may be most pronounced in obese children.[24] Second, it consumes time that could be spent in energetic play. Third, watching television correlates with between-meal snacking and with buying and eating the calorically dense foods most heavily advertised on children's programs. Fourth, it encourages food behaviors that damage dental health.

Many research teams have found that obesity in children correlates strongly with television viewing. The best accepted research strongly supports the opinion that " . . . 29 percent of the cases of [childhood] obesity could be prevented by reducing television viewing to 0 to 1 hours per week."[25]

Children who watch more than two hours of television per day may also have higher serum cholesterol than do more active children.[26] In most cases the high cholesterol accompanies obesity, and in many it predicts an elevated risk of heart disease in adult life. While some experts recommend regular cholesterol screening for all children, others find such measures unjustified and favor testing only those whose parents or grandparents developed cardiovascular disease.[27] No harm can come to children over the age of two who are encouraged to eat a variety of foods, to reach or maintain a desirable weight, and, within reason, to obtain enough fiber and limit fat and cholesterol intakes.[28]

Children who watch hours of television a day are also prone to frequent snacking on high-sugar foods, a major factor in dental caries development. Sticky, high-carbohydrate snack foods cling to the teeth and provide an ideal environment for the growth of mouth bacteria that cause caries. What child can resist the delicious-looking, sugar-filled fun foods that dance across their television screens? Television commercials only prompt children to buy and eat sugary foods—they have no stake in promoting dental health. Parents must combat this influence by teaching children to do the following:

TABLE 13-4

Dietary Recommendations for Controlling Dental Caries

Food Group	Low Caries Potential	High Caries Potential[a]
Dairy	Milk, cheese, plain yogurt	Chocolate milk, ice cream, ice milk, milkshakes, fruited yogurt
Meat/meat alternates	Lean meat, fish, poultry; eggs; legumes	Peanut butter with added sugar, lunch meats with added sugar, meats with sugared glazes
Fruits	Fresh or packed in water	Dried (raisins, figs, dates), packed in syrup or juice, jams, jellies, preserves, fruit juices or drinks
Vegetables	Salad greens, cauliflower, cucumbers, radishes, carrots, celery	Candied sweet potatoes, glazed carrots
Bread/cereal	Popcorn, toast, hard rolls, pretzels, pizza, bagels	Cookies, sweet rolls, pies, doughnuts, muffins, cakes, potato chips, oatmeal,[b] oatmeal cookies,[b] puffed oat cereal,[b] dry ready-to-eat sugared cereals, snack crackers, granola bars, sandwich cookies, peanut butter crackers
Other	Sugarless gum, sugarless soft drinks, sugarless candy	Sugared gum, soft drinks, candy, fudge, caramels, honey, creme-filled cakes, sugars, syrups, jelly beans

[a]Brush and rinse the teeth especially well and quickly after eating these foods.
[b]The soluble fiber in oats makes this grain particularly sticky and therefore cariogenic.

- Limit between-meal snacking.
- Brush and floss daily, and brush or rinse after eating snacks.
- Choose foods that don't stick to teeth and are swallowed quickly.
- Snack on crisp or fibrous foods to stimulate the release and rinsing action of saliva.

Table 13-4 lists foods that promote dental health and those that require speedy removal from the teeth.

Evidence from these many points of view suggests that television's effects on children's nutritional health are negative. It seems prudent, therefore, to advise parents to limit children's television viewing time to one or two hours a day or less.

✓ **KEY POINT**   **Television viewing can contribute to obesity through lack of exercise and overconsumption of snacks. Television advertising of sugary foods promotes sugar consumption and tooth decay.**

Breakfast Ideas for Rushed Mornings:

✔ Make ahead and freeze 5 sandwiches to thaw and serve with juice. Fillings may include peanut butter, low-fat cream cheese, other cheeses, jams, fruit slices, or meats. Or use flour tortillas with cheese, roll up, wrap, and freeze for later heating in a toaster oven or microwave oven.

✔ Teach school-aged children to help themselves to dry cereals, milk, and juice. Keep unbreakable bowls, spoons, and cups in low cupboards, and keep milk and juice in small unbreakable pitchers on a low refrigerator shelf.

✔ Keep a bowl of fresh fruit and small containers of shelled nuts, trail mix (the kind without candy), or roasted peanuts for grabbing. Granola or other grain cereal poured into an 8-ounce yogurt tub is easy to eat on the run. So are plain toasted whole-grain frozen waffles—no syrup needed.

✔ Untraditional choices are often acceptable. Purchase or make ahead enough carrot sticks to divide among several containers; serve with yogurt or bean dip. Leftover casseroles, stews, or pasta dishes are nutritious choices that children can eat hot or cold.

The Importance of Breakfast

While parents are doing what they can to establish nutrition-promoting eating behaviors in their children, grade school exposes children to foods prepared and served by outsiders. The U.S. government funds several programs to provide nutritious, high-quality meals, including breakfast, to children at school. Meeting the nutrition and education needs of children is critical to supporting their healthy growth and development.[29]

Children who eat no breakfast perform poorly in tasks requiring concentration, their attention spans are shorter, they achieve lower test scores, and they are tardy or absent more often than their well-fed peers. Common sense tells us that it is unreasonable to expect anyone to study and learn when no fuel has been provided. Even children who have eaten breakfast suffer from distracting hunger by late morning. Unfed children suffer all the more.

Schools that begin to participate in the federal school breakfast program observe higher achievement test scores and lower tardiness and absence rates.[30] Being fed at the day's start may account for these improvements, but evidence suggests that nutrients consumed at breakfast also affect a child's overall nutrition profile.[31] In other words, kids who eat breakfast are better nourished overall than those who miss out. A Canadian study found that an astonishing 15 to 20 percent of children attended school once or more each week without eating breakfast, and just 30 percent consumed adequate daily servings from all food groups.[32]

✔ **KEY POINT** **Breakfast is critical to school performance. Not all children start the day with an adequate breakfast, but school breakfast programs help to fill the need for some.**

Lunches at School

For the past 50 years, lunches served at school have been meeting many of the nutrient needs of the nation's children. Today's lunches must include specified servings of milk, protein-rich foods (meat, poultry, fish, cheese, eggs, legumes, or peanut butter), vegetables, fruits, and breads or other grain foods. The design is intended to provide at least a third of the RDA for each of the nutrients. Table 13-5 shows school lunch patterns for different ages.

Parents often rely on school lunches to meet a significant part of their children's nutrient needs on school days. Indeed, students who regularly eat school lunches have higher intakes of energy and nutrients than students who do not. Children don't always like what they are served, though, and school lunch programs must strike a balance between what children want to eat and what will nourish them and guard their health.

Many schoolchildren in the United States have significant risk factors for developing cardiovascular disease.[33] In an effort to help reduce their risk, the U.S. Department of Agriculture (USDA) ruled that, by 1998, all government-supported meals served at schools must follow the *Dietary Guidelines for Americans*.[34] Many schools already serve such meals, but cannot prevent private vendors from offering other, unregulated meals, even fast foods, side-by-side with the school lunches in school cafeterias. U.S. children develop a taste for fat and salt early in life and thus may reject foods that are low in fat and high in nutrient density.[35] Children receive a mixed message when they are left on

TABLE 13-5

School Lunch Patterns for Different Ages

FOOD GROUP	PRESCHOOL (AGE)		GRADE SCHOOL THROUGH HIGH SCHOOL (GRADE)ᵃ		
	1 to 2	3 to 4	K to 3	4 to 6	7 to 12
Milk					
1 serving of fluid milkᵇ	¾ c	¾ c	1 c	1 c	1 c
Meat or Meat Alternate					
1 serving:					
Lean meat, poultry, or fish	1 oz	1½ oz	1½ oz	2 oz	2 oz
Cheese	1 oz	1½ oz	1½ oz	2 oz	2 oz
Large egg(s)	½	¾	¾	1	1
Cooked dry beans or peas	¼ c	⅜ c	⅜ c	½ c	½ c
Peanut butter	2 tbs	2 tbs	3 tbs	3 tbs	4 tbs
Peanuts, soynuts, tree nuts, or seedsᶜ	½ oz	¾ oz	¾ oz	1 oz	1 oz
Vegetable and/or Fruit					
2 or more servings, both to total	½ c	½ c	¾ c	¾ c (plus ½ c extra over a week)	1 c
Bread or Bread Alternate					
Servingsᵈ	5 per week (minimum ½ per day)	8 per week (minimum 1 per day)	10 per week (minimum 1 per day)	12 per week (minimum 1 per day)	15 per week (minimum 1 per day)

ᵃThese patterns may be used so long as the meals served meet the *Dietary Guidelines for Americans* and provide one-third of the child's RDA for nutrients.

ᵇWhole milk and unflavored low-fat milk must be offered; flavored milks or nonfat milk may also be offered.

ᶜThese foods may meet no more than one-half a serving of meat and must be accompanied by other meat or alternate in the meal.

ᵈA serving is 1 slice of whole-grain or enriched bread; a whole-grain or enriched biscuit, roll, muffin, or the like; or ½ c cooked rice, pasta, or other grain.

SOURCE: U.S. Department of Agriculture.

their own to choose between the health-supporting school lunch and high-fat, high-salt, low–nutrient density foods that their taste buds may prefer.[36]

School officials trying to lower the fat in school lunches often run into problems. When schools make an effort to meet the *Dietary Guidelines* for fat intakes, the meals may fall short of the RDA goals for iron and other nutrients. The American Dietetic Association urges the development of a special set of guidelines especially for children to ensure that school lunches will both provide the needed nutrients and protect health.[37]

Some children in high schools also face the option of choosing soft drinks, frozen confections, candies, and other low-nutrient treats from school snack bars, vending machines, or school stores.[38] No federal laws exist to restrict sales of these items to schoolchildren. The administrators of the school lunch program have tried to outlaw such sales on school grounds, but have been defeated by the powerful lobbying efforts of industries that reap profits from children's pocket money. Given a choice, though, many children still select nutritious snacks, such as yogurt, milk, or fruit, when these foods are also made available.

✓ KEY POINT   School lunches are designed to meet at least a third of the daily nutrients needed by growing children. Schools are challenged to appeal to children's food preferences while providing meals that meet the

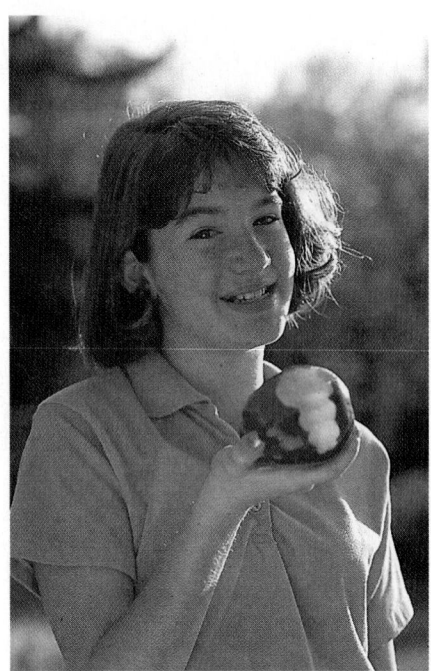

Nutritious snacks play an important role in an active teen's diet.

Food sources of iron and calcium are listed in Chapter 8.

Dietary Guidelines. **Vending machines, school stores, and snack bars tempt children with sweet treats.**

Nutrition Education

Coincident with the school lunch program is a program of nutrition education and training (NET program) in all public schools. Although minimally funded, the program remains in effect. Children are indeed learning basic nutrition facts at school.[39] As children grow, they will need this knowledge of nutrition to enable them to make healthy food choices as the choices become theirs to make.

✓ KEY POINT **Schools share with families the responsibility of offering nutrition education to children.**

THE TEEN YEARS

Teenagers are not fed; they eat. Self-directed food choices play a natural part in the search for an identity, which is acquired largely by trial and error, apart from the guidance of adult advice. Teens face tremendous pressures from peers and the media, especially regarding body image. Many teens readily adopt fads and scams offering promises of slenderness, good-looking muscles, freedom from acne, or control over symptoms that may accompany menstruation. At the same time, nutrient needs are high. Choices made during the teen years profoundly affect health, both now and in the future.

Growth and Nutrient Needs of Teenagers

With the onset of adolescence, needs for all nutrients become greater than at any other time of life except during pregnancy and lactation. The need for iron is especially great to support menstruation in girls and to develop lean body mass in boys.

Adolescence is a crucial time for bone development. The requirement for calcium reaches its peak during these years.[40] At the same time, low calcium intakes are all too common. Especially when paired with physical inactivity, these low intakes may compromise the development of peak bone mass.[41] The attainment of maximal bone mass during the young years is considered the best protection against age-related bone loss and fractures in later life.[42] Teenagers who choose soft drinks instead of milk at most meals do no favor for their future bone health.

As they grow to adults, girls develop a somewhat higher percentage of body fat than boys do. This intensive growth period brings hormonal changes that profoundly affect every organ of the body, including the brain.

Teenagers' rates and patterns of growth vary tremendously. Girls' growth spurts begin at 10 or 11 years of age and peak at about 12 years. Boys' growth spurts begin at 12 or 13 years and peak at about 14 years, slowing down at about 19. Growth charts used for children don't fit teens very well, but height and weight charts meant for adults fit even less well. Two boys of the same age may vary in height by a foot, but if both have been growing steadily, each is fulfilling his genetic destiny according to an inborn schedule of events. Parents should watch only for reasonably smooth progress; to apply external standards that a child cannot "live up to" is to invite a lasting diminished self-image. The only way to be sure that a teenager is growing satisfactorily is to compare each new height and weight measure with his or her own measures taken earlier. Health-care providers also compare measures of the changes of **puberty** with standard rating scales.[43]

The energy needs of adolescents vary tremendously. An active, rapidly growing boy of 15 may need 4,000 calories or more a day just to maintain his weight, but an inactive girl of the same age who is growing slowly may need less than 2,000 calories to keep from becoming obese. The insidious problem of obesity may first become apparent in adolescence, mostly in girls, and may last a lifetime. Teen athletes especially need energy and nutrients, and the nutrition advice to athletes in Chapter 10 is especially important for them.

One of the many changes girls face as they become women is the onset of menstruation. The hormones that regulate the menstrual cycle powerfully affect not just the uterus and the ovaries but metabolic rate, glucose tolerance, appetite, food intake, mood, and behavior. Most women live easily with the cyclic rhythm of the menstrual cycle, but some are afflicted with physical and emotional pain prior to menstruation, a condition called **premenstrual syndrome,** or **PMS.** This chapter's Consumer Corner offers more on PMS.

✔ KEY POINT **Nutrient and energy needs of teens vary with gender, body size, and activity level. Growth patterns vary widely.**

Eating Patterns and Food Choices

Teenagers come and go as they choose. They are no longer fed; they eat. With a multitude of afterschool, social, and job activities, they almost inevitably fall into irregular eating habits. The adult becomes a **gatekeeper,** controlling availability but not intakes of food in the teenager's environment. Teens typically turn a deaf ear to adults' attempts at coercion or persuasion to eat particular foods. Wise gatekeepers will set examples to follow and will provide access to nutritious foods that are low in sugar and fat. They welcome their teenage sons and daughters and their friends into the kitchen with the invitation, "Help yourselves! There's plenty of food in the refrigerator" (meats and peanut butter for sandwiches, raw vegetables, milk, fruit juices) "and more on the table" (breads, fruits, nuts, popcorn, cereals).

On the average, about a fourth of a teenager's total daily energy intake comes from snacks. This is one way that teens with irregular schedules can gain all the protein, thiamin, riboflavin, vitamin B_6, magnesium, and zinc that they need. Their calcium intakes may fall short unless they snack on dairy products, and they often fail to obtain enough iron and vitamin A. For iron, a teen might snack on iron-containing hard-cooked eggs, low-fat bran muffins, or tortillas with spicy bean spread along with a glass of orange juice to help maximize the iron's absorption. For vitamin A, why not carrot sticks, mixed vegetable juice, cantaloupe, or some dried apricots?

Inevitably, teenagers do a lot of eating away from home. They love fast food, and fortunately, more and more fast-food establishments are offering nutritious choices alongside their standard fat-laden fare. This is a positive trend,

puberty the period in life when a person develops sexual maturity and the ability to reproduce.

premenstrual syndrome (PMS) a cluster of symptoms that some women experience prior to and during menstruation. They include, among others, abdominal cramps, back pain, swelling, headache, painful breasts, and mood changes.

gatekeeper with respect to nutrition, a key person who controls other people's access to foods and thereby affects their nutrition profoundly. Examples are the spouse who buys and cooks the food, the parent who feeds the children, and the caretaker in a day-care center.

The nutritive values of selected fast foods are presented in the Table of Food Composition, Appendix A.

prostaglandins hormonelike compounds (eicosanoids) related to and derived from polyunsaturated fatty acids (*prostagland* because the first such compound discovered was from the prostate gland).

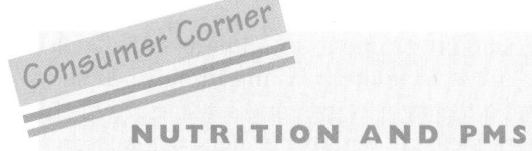

NUTRITION AND PMS

A woman suffering from PMS may complain of any or all of the following symptoms: cramps and aches in the abdomen, back pain, headaches, acne, swelling of the face and limbs associated with water retention, food cravings (especially for chocolate and other sweets), abnormal thirst, pain and lumps in the breasts, diarrhea, and mood changes, including both nervousness and depression. Some researchers are attempting to define clusters of these symptoms in hopes of assigning each cluster to a different cause.

Two things are believed to happen during the two weeks prior to menstruation that may affect a woman's nutrition:

- The basal metabolic rate during sleep speeds up, although the daytime rate may not change.[44]
- Appetite and calorie intakes may increase.[45]

Most studies seem to indicate that women take in an average of 300 calories a day more during the ten days prior to menstruation than during the ten days after. This may mean that women who wish to control their weight may find it relatively easy to restrict calories during the two weeks following menstruation. During the two weeks before the next menstruation, they may find it harder to limit calories because they are fighting a natural, hormone-governed increase in appetite.

Among candidates for causes of PMS are: abnormal secretion of **prostaglandins,** and altered secretion of the two major regulatory hormones of the menstrual cycle, estrogen and progesterone. One possible *nutrition*-related cause of PMS is sodium retention, with the water retention that accompanies it. Some doctors prescribe diuretics to get rid of the excess sodium and water, with mixed results. The placebo effect is extraordinarily powerful in PMS, so much so that even an agent that appears to relieve symptoms for several months may not prove to be a cure in the long run.[46] Diuretic therapy causes loss of minerals such as potassium, possibly making PMS symptoms worse. Also, if women do retain sodium and water just before menstruation, this may be normal and desirable.

One nutrient heavily researched with regard to PMS is vitamin B_6. The logic of ascribing PMS to a vitamin B_6 deficiency is that women with PMS may have abnormal levels of hormones that require vitamin B_6 for their action. One of the symptoms of PMS is depression, a mood disorder that many people, both male and female, experience under a wide variety of conditions, including vitamin B_6 deficiency. Trials of vitamin B_6 in PMS have not proved conclusive, however. A few subjects may respond favorably to treatment with vitamin B_6, but the improvement is not statistically meaningful. For some women, a relative or absolute vitamin B_6 deficiency may aggravate or even cause PMS, whereas for others it may have no effect on the syndrome. No need exists for megadoses of vitamin B_6, and the hazards associated with such doses are well documented (see Table 7-6 of Chapter 7).

Vitamin E deficiency is another possible contributor to PMS. One research study, a double-blind, placebo-controlled study of 75 women, suggested that supplemental vitamin E brought relief from sore breasts associated with PMS, while the placebo did not. However, some women *without* PMS also have sore breasts, and they, too, can sometimes be relieved by vitamin E. In another study of 41 women, vitamin E improved many other symptoms of PMS, such as nervousness, breast pain, edema, headaches, cravings, and others. Possibly, the correct logic is that vitamin E deficiency does not cause PMS, but can worsen symptoms associated with the menstrual period.

Tea consumption has been strongly linked with PMS. Women who drink the most tea seem to have the worst symptoms. Which component of tea is responsible, the caffeine, the pigments, or other substances, is not known, but evidence indicates a role for caffeine. Data from questionnaires administered to more than 800 women correlated caffeine intakes with PMS in a linear fashion: the more caffeine-containing beverages the women reported drinking, up to 10 cups per day, the more symptoms of PMS they reported suffering.[47] Even one cup of caffeinated beverage a day accompanied slight increases in PMS symptoms. So any woman who finds menstrual symptoms troublesome may want to try a caffeine-free lifestyle for a while and see if her symptoms improve.

One thing seems clear: the woman with PMS should look to her total lifestyle, diet being only a part of it. Adequate sleep and physical activity help, and she should be moderate in her intakes of sugar, caffeine, salt, alcohol, and any other abusable substances. Finally, she should watch out for snake-oil salespeople selling PMS "cures," for they are everywhere.

but teenagers must choose the foods they need from among those offered. The gatekeeper can take action to arm the teen with the needed nutrition information presented in a meaningful way to the individual teen. Often teens who are prone to gain weight will open their ears to news about the fat and calorie contents of some fast foods. Others attend best to information about the negative effects of a high-fat diet on sport performance.

Teenagers are intensely involved in day-to-day life with their peers and in preparation for their future lives as adults. The gatekeeper can set an example, provide an environment with plenty of nutritious foods, and stand by with reliable nutrition information and advice, but the rest is up to the teens themselves. Ultimately, they make the choices.

✓ KEY POINT **With planning, the gatekeeper can encourage teens to meet nutrient requirements by providing nutritious snacks.**

acne chronic inflammation of the skin's follicles and oil-producing glands, which leads to an accumulation of oils inside the ducts that surround hairs; usually associated with the maturation of young adults.

Acne

No one knows why some people get **acne** while others do not, but heredity plays a role—acne runs in families.[48] The hormones of adolescence also play a role by stimulating the glands in the skin. The skin's natural oil is made in deep glands and is supposed to flow out through tiny ducts to the skin's surface. In acne, the ducts become clogged, and oily secretions build up in the ducts.

One medical treatment for acne is to apply a vitamin A relative, retinoic acid or Retin A, directly to the skin. This loosens the plugs that form in the ducts, allowing the oil to flow normally, but the acid may burn the skin and may cause pimples to form, making the acne look worse at first. The Food and Drug Administration (FDA) has also recently approved Retin A* as a prescription topical wrinkle treatment for older skin.

Prescribed antibiotic pills and ointments work for some, and antibiotic ointments do not burn the skin. The oral prescription medicine Accutane is synthesized from vitamin A, but it is much more powerful than the vitamin itself and is effective against the deep lesions of cystic acne. Accutane is highly toxic and causes serious birth defects in the infants of women who have taken it during their pregnancies. Women with acne who wish to use Accutane should use contraception diligently before beginning treatment and for a time after treatment has ceased.

Although medicines made from vitamin A are successful in treating acne, vitamin A itself has no effect, and supplements of the vitamin can be toxic. Quacks remain undaunted by these facts, though, and market vitamin A supplements to people hoping to cure acne. Of course a certain amount of vitamin A is essential for healthy skin, but too much can damage the body.

Among foods charged with aggravating acne are chocolate, cola beverages, fatty or greasy foods, milk, nuts, sugar, and foods or salt containing iodine. None of these factors has been proved to worsen acne, and two, chocolate and sugar, have been shown not to worsen it. Psychological stress, though, clearly worsens acne. Vacations from school often bring acne relief. Sun and swimming also help, perhaps because they are relaxing and also because the sun's rays kill bacteria and water cleanses the skin. Too much sun exposure in a teen may make skin cancer likely in later life, however.

One remedy always works: time. While waiting, attend to basic needs. Petal-smooth, healthy skin reflects a tended, cared-for body whose owner provides it with nutrients and fluids to sustain it, exercise to stimulate it, and rest to restore its cells.

✔ KEY POINT **Although no foods have been proven to aggravate acne, stress can worsen it. Supplements are useless against acne, but stress relief, sunlight, and proved medications can help.**

SPECIAL CONCERNS OF WOMEN

Being female in our society raises a person's risks of suffering from disabling diseases.[49] Some such diseases are unrelated to nutrition, cancers of the ovaries or uterus, for example. Others, such as osteoporosis and breast can-

---

*The trade name of retinoic acid sold as a wrinkle cream is Renova.

cer, correlate with a woman's nutrition status. Importantly, women often erroneously discount some other diseases that take a severe toll on their health. For example, cardiovascular disease, the number one killer of women over 50, is often wrongly believed to be primarily of concern to men. Messages concerning diet and exercise to prevent CVD, therefore, often escape women, even the many who will develop and die from the disease.

Many more women than men live in poverty, which greatly raises their risks of illnesses. Given that a woman's physical health plays many pivotal roles in bringing forth future generations, and that women contribute vastly to society economically, socially, and politically, it is no exaggeration to say that "good health for women means good health for society as a whole."[50]

One of the largest disease prevention studies ever undertaken is the Women's Health Initiative, a 15-year study of more than 164,000 women over age 50 from across the nation. By 2005, the study will yield sorely needed data on the effects on women's health of diet modification, hormone replacement, and vitamin and mineral supplementation. The researchers hope it will also provide some answers about ways in which diet relates to breast and other cancers.

Campaigns are underway to advance such research and to educate professionals and consumers about women's health and nutrition. The American Dietetic Association's Nutrition and Health Campaigns for Women represents a major national effort to deliver accurate nutrition information to women as the food providers and gatekeepers of the nation. The Dietitians of Canada have launched similar efforts, and their benefits will be felt for generations to come.

> ✔ **KEY POINT** **Women suffer from more illnesses than do men, yet less is known about the links between diet and women's health. Many efforts are under way to fill the gaps in research on and services to women.**

THE LATER YEARS

This looks like a section about older people, but it is relevant even if the reader is only 20 years old. How you live and think at 20 years of age can profoundly affect the quality of your life at 60 or 80 years. Without realizing it, most people hold a stereotype, largely negative, of what it is like to be old—and then, later, they become that way. An old saying has it that "as the twig is bent, so grows the tree." Unlike a tree, however, you can bend your own twig.

Before you will adopt nutrition behaviors that will enhance your health in old age, you must accept on a personal level that you yourself are aging. People who fear age may make the mistake of equating age with disease. Aging affects everyone, given time; but disease can strike anyone at any stage of the life cycle. To learn what negative and positive views you hold about aging, try answering the questions in the margin. Your answers reveal not only what you think of older people now but also what will probably become of you. You may wish to review some of the reasons for your answers and, if they are not supported by science, to change your beliefs.

The majority of the U.S. population is now middle-aged. As that group ages, the ratio of old people to young people is growing larger. The fastest-growing age group is people over 85 years old.[51]

In the United States, the **life expectancy** at birth is 79 years for women and 72 years for men, up from about 50 years in 1900.[52] Once a person survives the

life expectancy the average number of years lived by people in a given society.

How Will You Age?
- ✔ In what ways do you expect your appearance to change as you age?
- ✔ What physical activities do you see yourself engaging in at age 70?
- ✔ What will be your financial status? Will you be independent?
- ✔ What will your sex life be like? Will others see you as sexy?
- ✔ How many friends will you have? What will you do together?
- ✔ Will you be happy? Cheerful? Curious? Depressed? Uninterested in life or new things?

life span the maximum number of years of life attainable by a member of a species.

longevity long duration of life.

TABLE 13-6

Changes with Age You Probably Must Accept

These changes are probably beyond your control:

✔ Graying of hair

✔ Balding

✔ Some drying and wrinkling of skin

✔ Impairment of near vision

✔ Some loss of hearing

✔ Reduced taste and smell sensitivity

✔ Reduced touch sensitivity

✔ Slowed reactions (reflexes)

✔ Slowed mental function

✔ Diminished visual memory

✔ Menopause (women)

✔ Loss of fertility (men)

✔ Loss of joint elasticity

Differences in maximum life-span between animals eating normally and those that are energy restricted:

Rats
     normal diet, 33 months
     restricted diet, 47 months

Spiders
     normal diet, 100 days
     restricted diet, 139 days

Single-celled animals (protozoans)
     normal diet, 13 days
     restricted diet, 25 days

SOURCE: R. Weindruch, Caloric restriction and aging, *Scientific American*, January 1996, pp. 46–52.

perils of youth and reaches age 65, the average person's life expectancy jumps to 83 years. Advances in medical science, including antibiotics and other treatments, are largely responsible for almost doubling the life expectancy in this century. Still, the biological schedule that we call aging cuts off life at a genetically fixed point in time. The **life span** (the maximum length of life possible for a species) of human beings, 115 years, has not changed over the years and is probably the upper limit of human **longevity.**

Nutrition and other lifestyle habits work together in the aging of the body. In a classic study, researchers in California observed nearly 7,000 adults and noticed that some were young for their ages, others old for their ages.[53] To find out what made the difference, the researchers focused on health habits and identified six factors that affect physiological age. Three of the six factors were related to nutrition: abstinence from, or moderation in, alcohol use; regularity of meals; and weight control. (The others were regular adequate sleep, abstinence from smoking, and regular physical activity.) The physical health of those who reported all six positive health practices was comparable to that of people 30 years younger who reported few or none. Numerous studies have since confirmed the benefits of these six factors. The findings suggest that even though people cannot alter the years of their births, they can alter the probable lengths and quality of their lives. The pair of tables in the margin, Tables 13-6 and 13-7, list some changes of aging that are unpreventable and also some that may yield to lifestyle influences.

✔ **KEY POINT** **Life expectancy for U.S. adults has increased in the last century. The lifestyle factors that can make a difference in aging are limited or no alcohol use, regular balanced meals, weight control, adequate sleep, abstinence from smoking, and regular physical activity.**

NUTRITION AND LONGEVITY

Throughout history, human beings have sought ways to prolong youth and life. The search is as relentless today as it has ever been. Scientists who study the aging process have found no specific diet or nutrient supplement that will prolong life, despite hundreds of unproven claims to the contrary, but they have discovered several links to nutrition.

The first evidence that diet might extend life came more than half a century ago from experiments on rats. Researchers fed young rats diets adequate in all nutrients but short in energy. The rats stopped growing. Then the researchers increased the energy, and growth resumed. Meanwhile, control rats were allowed to eat and grow normally. Many of the rats in the energy-deficient group died young from the effects of malnutrition. A few survivors, however, lived an extraordinarily long time, and they developed the diseases of old age later in life, even though they had suffered malformations and stunting that did not improve with normal feed. These rats remained alive far beyond the normal life span for such animals.

In the study just described, food restriction was begun as soon as the animals were weaned (at three weeks). More moderate energy restriction with adequate nutrient intake later in life also seems to prolong survival without incurring such severe physical malformations. In fact, restricted rats seem to retain youthfulness longer and develop fewer of the factors associated with chronic diseases. Energy restriction in adult animals has been reported to lower blood pressure and blood glucose and to improve the insulin response to glucose.[54] Similar work on primates is in an early stage, so whether restricting these animals' diets will prolong their lives is not yet known. Evidence from other species (see the margin) suggests that it may.

Several mechanisms to explain how energy restriction prolongs life in rats have been proposed, but none has been proved. Research suggests that food restriction may delay age-related diseases, reduce body fat, slow the metabolic rate, control blood glucose, prevent lipid oxidation, and minimize the damage from free radicals.[55] Researchers hope that by discovering how food restriction slows aging in animals, they may better understand how aging occurs in people and how best to slow its effects. From what is known now, nutrition in the later years plays a key role in maintaining health into old age.[56]

✔ **KEY POINT**   **In rats, food energy deprivation may lengthen the lives of individuals who survive the treatment.**

NUTRITION IN THE LATER YEARS

Knowledge of nutrition in older adults has grown considerably in the last decade. The current RDA tables, however, still combine everyone over 50 into one group, even though needs change as aging progresses. The next edition is likely to provide more specific recommendations for an aging population.

Nutrient needs become more individual with age, depending on genetics and individual medical history. For example, one person's stomach acid secretion, which helps in iron absorption, may decline, so that person may need more iron. Another person may excrete more folate due to past liver disease and thus need a higher dose. Despite their shortcomings, the RDA still present a standard with which nutrient intakes may be compared, and despite physical changes, health-promoting lifestyle choices may avert some of the problems facing the elderly. Table 13-8 lists some changes that can affect nutrition.

✔ **KEY POINT**   **No special RDA exist for groups past 50 years old, even though nutrient needs change. Individual histories strongly influence older people's nutrient needs.**

Energy and Activity

Energy needs often decrease with advancing age. For one thing, the number of active cells in each organ decreases, reducing the body's overall metabolic rate (although much of this loss may not be inevitable). For another, older people usually reduce their physical activity, and so their lean tissue diminishes. After about the age of 50 years, the RDA for energy assumes about a 5 percent reduction in energy output per decade (see the inside front cover). For those who must limit energy, there is little leeway for foods of low nutrient density such as sugars, fats, and, of course, alcohol.[57] Current thinking, however, seems to refute the idea that declining energy needs are unavoidable. Physical activity, along with proper nutrition, probably holds part of the key not only to maintaining energy needs but to upholding many other functions as well.[58] It also seems an effective preventer of a destructive spiral of sedentary

TABLE 13-7

Changes with Age You Probably Can Slow or Prevent

By exercising, eating an adequate diet, reducing stress, and planning ahead, you may be able to slow or prevent:

✔ Wrinkling of skin due to sun damage
✔ Some forms of mental confusion
✔ Raised blood pressure
✔ Speeded-up resting heart rate
✔ Reduced breathing capacity and oxygen uptake
✔ Increased body fatness
✔ Raised blood cholesterol
✔ Slowed energy metabolism
✔ Decreased maximum work rate
✔ Loss of sexual functioning
✔ Loss of joint flexibility
✔ Oral health: loss of teeth, gum disease
✔ Bone loss
✔ Digestive problems, constipation

The Canadian RNI provide separate recommendations for those 50 to 74 years and for those 75 and older. See the Canadiana Appendix.

TABLE 13-8

Examples of Physical Changes of Aging That Affect Nutrition

Digestive Tract	Intestines lose muscle strength resulting in sluggish motility that leads to constipation. Stomach inflammation, abnormal bacterial growth, and greatly reduced acid output impair digestion and absorption. Pain may cause food avoidance or reduced intake.
Hormones	For example, the pancreas secretes less insulin and cells become less responsive, causing abnormal glucose metabolism.
Mouth	Tooth loss, gum disease, and reduced salivary output impede chewing and swallowing. Choking may become likely; pain may cause avoidance of hard-to-chew foods.
Sensory Organs	Diminished senses of smell and taste can reduce appetite; diminished sight can make food shopping and preparation difficult.
Body Composition	Weight loss and decline in lean body mass lead to lowered energy requirements. May be preventable or reversible through physical activity.

The "dwindles" refers to a complex of interacting failures in the elderly including:

✔ Weight loss.
✔ Diminished mental function.
✔ Decreased physical ability to function.
✔ Social withdrawal.
✔ Malnutrition.

SOURCE: A. M. Egbert, The dwindles: Failure to thrive in older patients, *Nutrition Reviews* 54 (1996): S25–S30.

behavior and mental and physical losses in the elderly that one expert has called "the dwindles."[59]

A nutrition expert stresses the importance of exercise to the elderly:

> We now know that physically active elders can build and rebuild muscle mass. Even the frail elderly can improve function by a remarkable 200 percent on a short, focused exercise regimen. No single feature of aging can more dramatically affect basal metabolism, insulin sensitivity, calorie intake, appetite, breathing, ambulation, mobility, and independence than muscle mass.[60]

Even institutionalized people in their nineties have been able to gain muscle bulk and strength and to regain some pep in their walking steps after just eight weeks of weight training.[61] Training not only improves muscles but also increases the blood flow to the brain. Besides, a person spending energy in physical activity can afford to eat more food, and with it come more nutrients. Any exercise, even a ten-minute walk a day, provides a benefit. Older people should feel free to exercise in their own way, at their own pace. They should not hold themselves to standards set in younger days because aging necessarily brings a lessened capacity to perform exercise.[62]

✔ KEY POINT **Energy needs decrease with age, but exercise burns off excess fuel and brings health benefits.**

Carbohydrates and Fiber

The recommendation to obtain 6 to 11 servings of breads, grains, or pasta is appropriate for older people. It is especially wise to choose the majority of those servings from whole grains. With age, fiber takes on extra importance for its role against constipation, a common complaint among older adults and especially among nursing home residents. Older adults generally do not obtain the recommended daily 27 to 40 grams of fiber.[63] When low fiber intakes are combined with low fluid intakes, inadequate exercise, and constipating medications, constipation becomes almost inevitable.

✔ KEY POINT   **Generous carbohydrate intakes are recommended for older adults. Including fiber in the diet is important to avoid constipation.**

Fats and Arthritis

Fats should be limited in the diet of older adults for many reasons. Foods low in fat are often rich in vitamins and minerals. Diets constructed from such foods may help retard the onset of cancer, atherosclerosis, obesity, and other diseases.

Fat in the diet is under surveillance for a possible role in causing **arthritis,** the painful deterioration and swelling of the joints that troubles many older people. During movement, the ends of normal bones are protected by small sacs of fluid that act as lubricants. With arthritis, the sacs erode, cartilage and bone ends disintegrate, and joints become malformed and painful to move.

Dietary fat may affect the pain of rheumatoid arthritis, a severe form of arthritis that is seen to improve in many people when they adopt a low-fat diet. When these people resume eating fats and oils (except fish oils), their symptoms recur. One explanation is that the active products of both omega-6 and omega-3 fatty acids are involved in regulating pain-producing inflammation and may be responsible for the effect. According to this theory, omega-6 fatty acids worsen the pain while omega-3 acids relieve it. Another theory links free-radical damage to arthritis.[64]

Another fat-arthritis connection may be that low-fat diets help people to lose weight and that the weight loss produces the improvements. Sufficient lean body mass may be important to reduce arthritis symptoms as well.[65] More research is needed to clarify these connections.

One form of arthritis known as **gout** worsens when sufferers consume foods that are high in purines, compounds that cause crystals of uric acid to form in the joints. Some of the best sources of omega-3 fatty acids, unfortunately, are also the highest in purines—among them, sardines, herring, anchovies, mackerel, and other fish and shellfish. This makes attempts at self-diagnosis and treatment of arthritis especially unwise. While some with arthritis may benefit from increased fish intakes, others may make themselves worse.

Other dietary changes that may affect arthritis include fasting, vegetarianism, increased intakes of vitamin E[66] or other antioxidant nutrients, and elimination diets. No one universally effective diet for arthritis relief is known. Many *ineffective* "cures" are sold, however, as the margin list shows. The safest bet for those with arthritis is to obtain a medical diagnosis and treatment.

✔ KEY POINT   **A low-fat diet may improve some symptoms of arthritis. Omega-3 fatty acids may also have a positive effect. Foods high in purines can worsen the arthritis of gout.**

arthritis a usually painful inflammation of joints caused by many conditions, including infections, metabolic disturbances, or injury; usually results in altered joint structure and loss of function.

gout a painful form of arthritis resulting from a metabolic abnormality in which excessive amounts of the waste product uric acid collect in the blood and uric acid salt is deposited as crystals in the joints. Also defined in Controversy 11.

Not Effective as Cures for Arthritis:
- Alfalfa tea.
- Aloe vera liquid.
- Any of the amino acids.
- Burdock root.
- Calcium.
- Celery juice.
- Copper or copper complexes.
- Dimethyl sulfoxide (DMSO).
- Fasting.
- Fresh fruit.
- Honey.
- Inositol.
- Kelp.
- Lecithin.
- Melatonin.
- Para-aminobenzoic acid (PABA).
- Raw liver.
- Selenium.
- Superoxide dismutase (SOD).
- Vitamins D, E, C, or any B vitamin supplements.
- Watercress.
- Yeast.
- Zinc.
- 100 other substances.

cataracts (CAT-uh-racts) thickening of the lens of the eye that can lead to blindness. Cataracts can be caused by injury, viral infection, toxic substances, genetic disorders, and possibly by some nutrient deficiencies or imbalances.

Protein

Protein needs of older people seem to remain about the same as for the young adult years. The choice of which protein-containing foods to eat takes on extra importance, however. Some older people have lost their teeth, and this makes chewing tough meats next to impossible. They need soft or chopped foods. Individuals with chronic constipation, heart disease, or diabetes may receive benefits from fiber-rich low-fat vegetables rich in proteins, such as legumes and grains. Such foods are easy to chew and can help stretch limited food budgets as well.

✔ **KEY POINT** **Protein needs remain about the same through adult life, but choosing low-fat fiber-rich protein foods may help control other health problems.**

Controversy 13 discusses the importance of some vitamins and minerals to the brain.

Macular degeneration is another cause of sight loss in the elderly that is believed to be related to diets low in fruits and vegetables; see Controversy 7.

Vitamins

Vitamin A stands alone among the vitamins, in that its absorption appears to increase with aging.[67] For this reason researchers have proposed lowering the vitamin A RDA for aged populations. Some resist such a change, though, because vitamin A and its precursor beta-carotene are active in prevention of oxidative damage to body tissues, an effect described in Chapter 7.

Older adults face a greater risk of vitamin D deficiency than younger people do. Many older adults drink little or no vitamin D–fortified milk, and many go day after day with no exposure to sunlight, especially if they reside in nursing homes. Additionally, as people age, vitamin D synthesis declines, setting the stage for deficiency. These age-related changes have inspired the suggestion that a higher RDA for vitamin D for the elderly is needed, but a better solution would be to ensure that every elderly person obtains the RDA of vitamin D and gets outside more often or even just sits by an open window some of the time.

Many elderly people consume far less than the RDA for vitamin D, vitamin B_6, folate, and many minerals.[68] In fact, one study indicated that many elderly people, while not frankly deficient, may need more vitamin B_{12}, vitamin B_6, and folate than they are consuming.[69]

Of particular interests are two theories linking low intakes of antioxidant vitamins and other antioxidants with age-related changes in the eyes. One theory concerns eye changes that lead to the permanent blindness of macular degeneration, already described in Controversy 7. People with lifelong high intakes of vegetables rarely suffer from macular degeneration.

The other theory concerns **cataracts**. A cataract is a thickening of the lens that impairs vision and ultimately leads to blindness. Cataracts can occur even in well-nourished individuals due to injury or other trauma, but most cataracts are vaguely called senile cataracts, meaning "caused by aging." Only 5 percent of people younger than 50 years have cataracts; by age 75, the percentage jumps by nine times that number to over 45 percent.[70] People who eat few fruits and vegetables obtain too few antioxidants, both nutrients and phytochemicals, and this puts them at risk of developing cataracts. The lens of the eye is easily oxidized, and such damage is believed to lead to cataracts. The

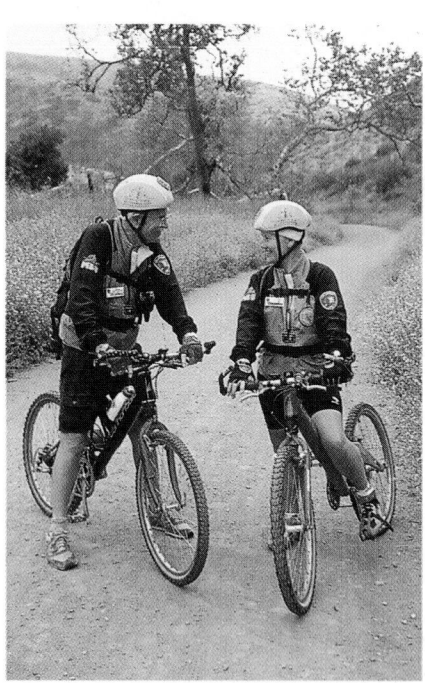

Energy like this requires continued physical activities and all the nutrients to support it.

amounts of nutrients that seem to be protective against both macular degeneration and cataracts are easily provided by several servings a day of the vegetables, fruits, and other foods that contain them.

✔ KEY POINT   **Vitamin A absorption increases with aging. Older people suffer more from vitamin D deficiency than do young people. Cataracts may be most likely in those with low fruit and vegetable intakes.**

Water and the Minerals

Dehydration is a major risk for older adults, who may not notice or pay attention to their thirst. With age, the thirst mechanism may become imprecise, and older people may go for long periods without drinking fluids.[71] The kidneys also gradually lose the ability to efficiently recapture water before it is lost as urine.[72] This causes some problems and worsens others, such as dehydration, constipation, and other intestinal problems. In a person with asthma, dehydration thickens mucus in the lungs which may block airways. Even muscle weakness and mental confusion can result. Regardless of age, adults need to drink 6 to 8 glasses of water each day. A person we know uses this trick to ensure getting enough water: he keeps six inexpensive 8-ounce cups in the cupboard. Through the day he uses each one to drink water only once and then collects them in the dish drain. In the afternoon he checks the cupboard and makes sure to drink from any remaining cups. For him, drinking water has become a habit, and seldom are any cups left in the cupboard after supper.

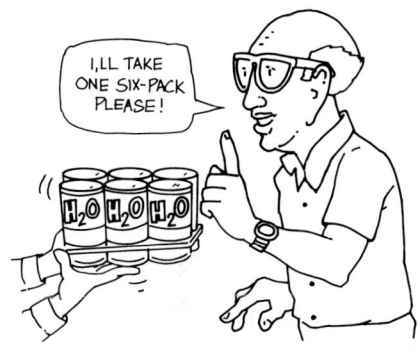

Adults of all ages need 6 to 8 glasses of water each day.

Iron   Among the minerals, iron deserves mention. Iron-deficiency anemia is less common in older adults than in younger people, and in fact, iron status generally improves in later life, especially for women when menstruation ceases.[73] Iron deficiency still occurs in some elderly people, however, especially in those with low food energy intakes. Aside from diet, other factors in many older people's lives make iron deficiency likely:

- Chronic blood loss from ulcers, hemorrhoids, or the like.
- Poor iron absorption due to reduced stomach acid secretion.
- Antacid use, which interferes with iron absorption.
- Use of medicines that cause blood loss, including anticoagulants, aspirin, and arthritis medicines.

Older people take more medicines than others, and nutrition effects are common.

Zinc   Zinc deficiencies are common in older people. As many as 95 percent of older adults may not get the zinc they need, and many miss the mark by more than half. Zinc deficiency, in turn, may depress appetite and blunt the sense of taste, thereby leading to low food intakes and poor zinc status.

Some research suggests that older adults absorb zinc less efficiently than younger people do.[74] Many medications interfere with the body's absorption or use of zinc, and elderly people often take many medicines.[75] The bright side of the zinc story is that some healthy older adults may need less than they did when they were younger.

These foods provide iron and zinc together: meat, poultry, liver, oysters, whole grains, fortified breakfast cereals,* and legumes.

*Cereals fortified with iron and zinc may not be available in Canada.

These foods provide calcium and zinc together: milk, yogurt, canned fish with bones, and oysters. A few dry cereals available in the United States are fortified with both calcium and zinc (read the labels).

Calcium-rich foods are listed in Chapter 8, and Controversy 8 discusses osteoporosis.

Calcium   Abundant dietary calcium throughout life is important to protect against osteoporosis, which can set in during later life. The calcium intakes of many people, especially women, in the United States are well below the RDA. If fresh milk causes stomach discomfort, as the majority of older people report, then lactose-modified milk or other calcium-rich foods should take its place.

A summary of the effects of aging on nutrient needs appears in Table 13-9. As people live longer lives, attention to nutrition concerns can help to ensure the best possible quality of life.

✓ KEY POINT   **Aging alters vitamin and mineral needs. Some needs rise, some decline.**

Senile Dementia—Alzheimer's Disease

Alzheimer's disease is now the third costliest health problem in the United States, following heart disease and cancer.[76] In Alzheimer's disease, the brain deteriorates abnormally with brain cell death occurring in areas of the brain that coordinate memory and cognition. Alzheimer's may rob as many as 5 percent of U.S. adults of productive life by age 65 and 20 percent of those over 80.[77] A cluster of symptoms justify diagnosis: losses of memory and reasoning power, loss of the ability to communicate, and loss of physical capabilities, finally causing death. More research is needed, and quickly, to find solutions.

A newly established connection to a human gene that makes part of a lipoprotein* has sparked new hope for prevention of Alzheimer's.[78] Ultimately, researchers hope to use this genetic finding to develop an early test to identify people who are prone to Alzheimer's.

The brain of a person with Alzheimer's has an abnormally small amount of an enzyme that synthesizes acetylcholine from choline. Acetylcholine is essential to memory. Experimental administration of acetylcholine-blocking drugs leads normal people to perform poorly on memory tests. Conversely, when subjects are given drugs that enhance concentrations of acetylcholine in the brain, they perform well on the same tests.[79] To date, oral supplements of choline or lecithin (which contains choline, first mentioned in this regard in Chapter 7) have had no effect on memory, mental functioning, or the progression of Alzheimer's, but researchers are still collecting data that may reveal a connection.[80] Recent trials of lecithin given in combination with certain drugs do report improvement in a few cognitive deficiencies.[81]

"Smart" drugs, drinks, and supplements, sold with promises of brainpower enhancement, are discussed in this chapter's Controversy.

A new drug† seems to slow Alzheimer's advance in about 20 percent of users, but cannot reverse the damage already done.[82] Meanwhile, other drugs, such as the nicotine of tobacco and estrogen hormone therapy, seem to favorably influence older people's ability to remember.

Nutrition bears only weak links to Alzheimer's. Most people have heard of an association between the mineral aluminum and Alzheimer's disease. A causal connection, however, seems unlikely. Brain aluminum in people with

---

*The gene associated with Alzheimer's is apo E4, one of three apolipoprotein E varieties. A report on the genetic and other aspects of Alzheimer's is available from Alzheimer's Disease Education and Referral Center, P.O. Box 8250, Silver Springs, MD 20907-8250.
†The trade name of this drug for Alzheimer's disease is Cognex.

TABLE 13-9

Summary of Nutrient Concerns in Aging

Nutrient	Effect of Aging	Comments
Energy	Need decreases.	Physical activity moderates the decline.
Fiber	Low intakes make constipation likely.	Inadequate water intakes and physical activity, along with some medications, compound the problem.
Protein	Needs stay the same.	Choices of low-fat, high-fiber legumes and grains meet both protein and other needs.
Vitamin A	Absorption increases.	Supplements not normally needed.
Vitamin D	Increased likelihood of inadequate intake; skin synthesis declines.	Daily moderate exposure to sunlight may be of benefit.
Water	Lack of thirst and increased urine output make dehydration likely.	Mild dehydration is a common cause of confusion.
Iron	In women, status improves after menopause; deficiencies linked to chronic blood losses and low stomach acid output.	Stomach acid required for absorption; antacid or other medicine use may aggravate iron deficiency; vitamin C and meat enhance absorption.
Zinc	Intakes are often inadequate and absorption may be poor, but needs may also decrease.	Medications interfere with absorption; deficiency may depress appetite and sense of taste.
Calcium	Intakes may be low; osteoporosis becomes common.	Lactose intolerance commonly prevents milk intake; substitutes are needed.

Alzheimer's exceeds normal brain aluminum by some 10 to 30 times. Still, blood and hair aluminum remains normal, indicating that the accumulation is caused by something in the brain itself, not by high aluminum in the diet. Thus the high brain aluminum must be more a result, than a cause, of the disease.

Finally, nutrient deficiencies, and especially those that continue over many years, may contribute to losses of memory and thinking ability that some older adults experience. Subtle vitamin deficits also impair cognition and are currently under study.[83] Such deficiencies are not believed to cause Alzheimer's disease, and they can be largely reversed with diet.

✓ KEY POINT   **Alzheimer's disease causes brain deterioration in one-fifth of people past age 80. A genetic link to Alzheimer's may open the way to prevention. Current treatment helps only marginally; dietary aluminum is probably unrelated.**

Food Choices of Older Adults

Results of national surveys help indicate what older adults are eating. Many older people seem to have heard and heeded nutrition messages. They have cut down on saturated fats in dairy foods and meats and are eating slightly more vegetables and whole-grain breads.[84] Smart marketers appeal to this growing group, many of whom are willing and able to spend more money on food than are people of other ages. Store shelves now prominently display good-tasting, low-fat, nutritious foods in easy-to-open, single-serving packages with labels that are easy to read. Many nutrient supplements are marketed for older adults. Whether to take a supplement is a personal choice, but

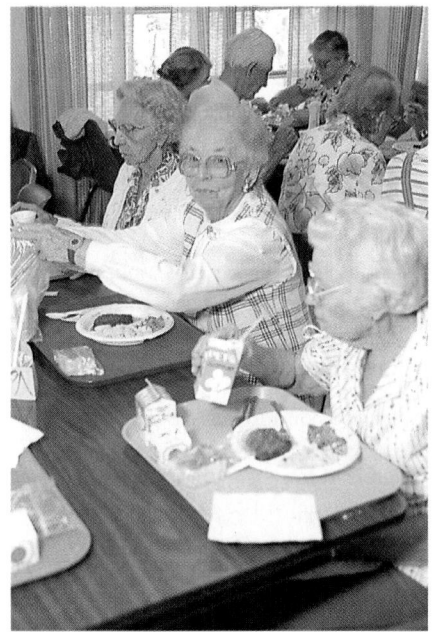

Shared meals can be the high point of the day.

Healthy People 2000: Increase to at least 80% the receipt of home foodservices by people aged 65 and older who have difficulty in preparing their own meals or are otherwise in need of home-delivered meals.

evidence supports the idea that a single low-dose multivitamin and mineral tablet a day can improve resistance to disease in the elderly.[85]

Obstacles to Adequacy   The food choices and eating habits of older adults are affected not just by preference but by the changes that accompany the experience of aging in our society. Those who live alone, with others and in institutions all eat differently.[86]

Some life circumstances seem to make older people vulnerable to malnutrition. Two factors stand out: use of multiple medications and abuse of alcohol. People over age 65 take about a fourth of all the medications, both prescription and over-the-counter, sold in the United States. Typically, an older person receives prescriptions from several physicians, usually specialists, who are not aware that other drugs have been prescribed. While medications may enable a person with health problems to live longer and more comfortably, they may also pose a threat to nutrition status because they interact with nutrients, depress the appetite, or alter the perception of taste (see Controversy 12).

The incidence of alcoholism, alcohol abuse, or problem drinking among the elderly in the United States is estimated at between 2 and 10 percent.[87] Evidence is also mounting that loneliness, isolation, and depression in the elderly accompany the overuse of alcohol. It isn't possible to say whether the depression or the alcohol abuse comes first, for each worsens the other, and both detract from nutrient intakes. Table 13-10 and the margin list provide means of identifying who might be at risk for malnutrition.

Men living alone are likely to consume poorer-quality diets than those living with spouses.[88] Some older people suffer medical conditions that affect nutrition. They may have difficulty chewing, or because of reduced taste sensitivity, they may have lost a form of taste-induced satiety so that they no longer seek a wide variety of foods.[89]

Programs That Help   For older people who lack funds to buy nutritious foods, federal programs can be of at least some help. One is the Supplemental Security Income program, intended to assist the very poor by increasing their income to the defined poverty level. Another is the Title IIIC Older Americans Act of 1965, still in effect today, that provides for nutrition for the elderly. The program provides nutritious meals, social interaction, education and shopping assistance, counseling and referral to other needed services, and transportation. Many people say that the shared midday meals this program provides are the high point of their day. They enjoy gathering with friends to share both conversation and nutritious meals. For the homebound, Meals on Wheels volunteers deliver meals to the door, a benefit even though the recipients miss out on the social atmosphere of the congregate program.

Many of these programs are now threatened by efforts to cut government spending. The Assistant Secretary for Aging sees these cuts as shortsighted:

> At this critical time, the basic right to adequate food and nutrition, which is a basic safety net for those in need and at risk, is under attack.[90]

Besides, proper nutrition plays a critical role in preventing avoidable illnesses later on, and thereby averts medical costs much higher than the cost of the meals.

TABLE 13-10

Nutrition Screening Initiative Checklist

Circle the number to the right if the statement applies to you.

Statement	Yes	Score:
I have an illness or condition that makes me eat different kinds and/or amounts of food.	2	**0-2: Good.** Recheck your score in 6 months.
I eat fewer than 2 meals per day.	3	
I eat few fruits or vegetables and use few milk products.	2	**3-5: Moderate nutritional risk.** Visit your local office on aging, senior nutrition program, senior citizens center, or health department for tips on improving eating habits.
I have 3 or more drinks of beer, liquor, or wine almost every day.	2	
I have tooth or mouth problems that make it hard for me to eat.	2	
I don't always have enough money to buy the food I need.	4	
I eat alone most of the time.	1	
I take 3 or more different prescribed or over-the-counter drugs a day.	1	**6 or more: High nutritional risk.** See your doctor, dietitian, or other health-care professional for help in improving your nutrition status.
Without wanting to, I have lost or gained 10 pounds in the last 6 months.	2	
I am not always physically able to shop, cook, and/or feed myself.	2	
Total		

NOTE: The Nutrition Screening Initiative is part of a national effort to identify and treat nutrition problems in older Americans.

Nutritionists are wise not to focus solely on nutrient and food intakes of the elderly, because social interactions may be as important. A professor of psychiatry wrote perceptively of many elderly people, using the pronoun "he" to mean a typical elderly person:

> It is not what the older person eats but with whom that will be the deciding factor in proper care for him. The oft-repeated complaint of the older patient that he has little incentive to prepare food only for himself is not merely a statement of fact but also a rebuke to the questioner for failing to perceive his isolation and aloneness and to realize that food . . . for one's self lacks the condiment of another's presence which can transform the simplest fare to the ceremonial act with all its shared meaning.[91]

The need for companionship surrounding meals is as great today as it was when these words were written.

Nutrition knowledge meets health in the real world of cooking, cleaning, and shopping, but many older people, even able-bodied ones with financial resources, find themselves unable to perform these tasks. For anyone living alone and for those of advanced age especially, it is important to work through the problems that food preparation presents.[92] This chapter's Food Feature presents some ideas.

Sources of Support for the Elderly:
✓ Social Security.
✓ Food Stamps.
✓ Supplemental Security Income program.
✓ Title IIIC of the Older Americans Act.
✓ Meals on Wheels.

✓ **KEY POINT** **Food choices of the elderly are affected by aging, altered health status, and changed life circumstances. Assistance programs can help both by providing nutritious meals and by easing financial problems. Social stimulation also helps people eat well by relieving loneliness.**

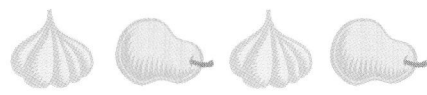

FOOD FEATURE

SINGLE SURVIVAL

Singles of all ages face problems concerning the purchasing, storing, and preparing of food. Whether a single person is a student in a college dormitory, an elderly person in a retirement apartment, or a professional in an efficiency apartment, the problems of preparing nourishing meals are the same. Many college students live in dormitories, most without kitchens and freezers, and for them, purchasing and storage problems are compounded. Following is a collection of ideas gathered from single people who have devised answers to some of these problems.

Large packages of meat and vegetables are often suitable for a family of four or more, and even a head of lettuce can spoil before one person can use it all. Buy only what you will use. Don't be timid about asking the grocer to break open a family-sized package of wrapped meat or fresh vegetables. Look for bags of prepared salad greens to take the place of lettuce in both salads and sandwiches. Small-sized containers of food may be expensive, but it is also expensive to let the unused portion of a large-sized container spoil. Buy only three pieces of each kind of fresh fruit: a ripe one, a medium-ripe one, and a green one. Eat the first right away and the second soon, and let the last one ripen to eat days later.

Think up a variety of ways to use a vegetable that you must buy in large quantity. For example, you can divide a head of cauliflower into thirds. Cook one-third and eat it as a hot vegetable. Toss another third into a salad dressing marinade for use as an appetizer. Save the rest to use raw in salad.

Make mixtures using what you have on hand. A thick stew prepared from any leftover vegetables and bits of meat, with some added onion, pepper, cel-

Buy only what you will use.

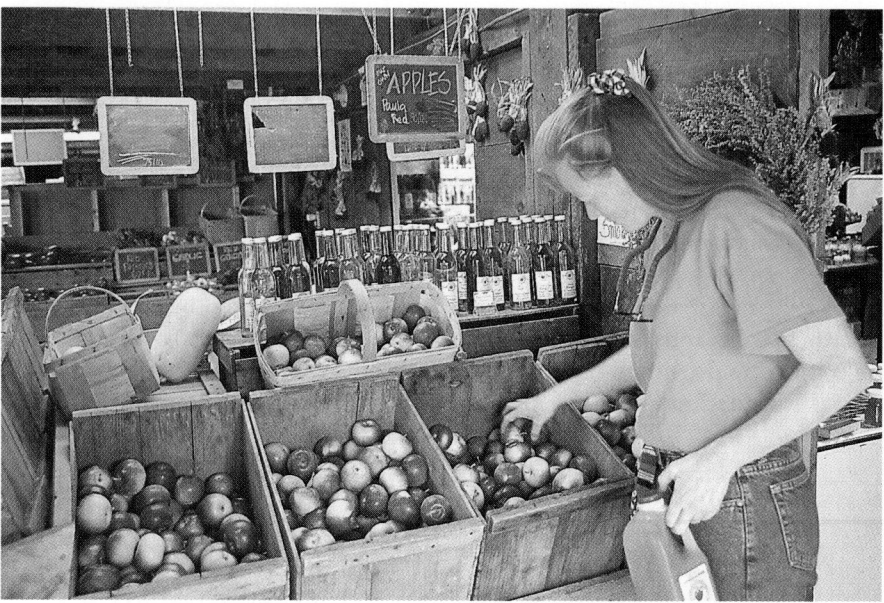

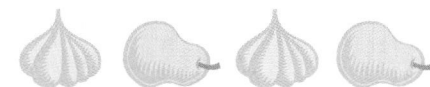

ery, and potatoes, makes a complete and balanced meal, except for milk. If you like creamed gravy, add nonfat dry milk to your stew.

Buy fresh milk in the sizes you can best use. If your grocer doesn't carry pints or quarts of milk, try a convenience store. If you eat lunch in a cafeteria, buy two pints of milk—one to drink and one to take home and store.

For shelf-stable items that you can't buy in single-serving quantities, prepare a space for rows of glass jars. Use the jars to store rice, tapioca, lentils, other dry beans, flour, cornmeal, dry nonfat milk, and cereal, to name only a few possibilities. Cut the directions-for-use label from the package of each item and store it in the jar. Place each jar, tightly sealed, in a freezer for a few days to kill any eggs or organisms before storing it on the shelf. Then the jars will keep bugs out of the foods indefinitely. The jars make an attractive display and will remind you of possibilities for variety in your menus.

Experiment with stir-fried foods. A large fry pan often works as well or better than a wok on modern ranges. A variety of vegetables and meats can be enjoyed this way; inexpensive vegetables such as cabbage and celery are delicious when crisp cooked in a little oil with soy sauce or lemon juice added. Interesting frozen vegetable mixtures are available in larger grocery stores. Cooked, leftover vegetables can be dropped in at the last minute. A bonus of a stir-fried meal is that you'll have only one pan to wash.

If you can afford a microwave oven, buy one. You'll use fewer pots and pans and you can freeze or refrigerate meals in microwavable containers to reheat whenever you like.

Depending on your freezer space, make a regular-sized recipe of a dish that takes time to prepare: a casserole, vegetable pie, or meat loaf. Freeze individual portions in containers that can be microwaved or heated later. Be sure to date these so you will use the oldest first.

Buy a loaf of bread and immediately store half, well wrapped, in the freezer (not the refrigerator, which will make it stale). Buy frozen vegetables in a bag, toss in a variety of herbs, and divide among single-serving containers. Vary your choices to prevent boredom.

For nutrition's sake, it is important to attend to loneliness at mealtimes. The person who is living alone must learn to connect food with socializing. Cook for yourself with the idea that you will invite guests, and make enough food so that you can enjoy the leftovers later on. If you know an older person who eats alone, you can bet that person would love to join you for a meal now and then. Invite the person often.

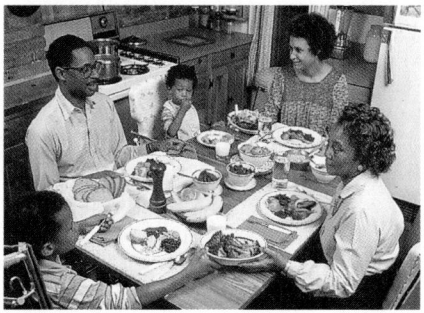

Invite guests to share a meal.

Light destroys riboflavin, so use opaque jars for enriched pasta and dry milk.

✔ **SELF-CHECK**

Answers to these Self-Check questions are in Appendix G.

1. Which of the following can contribute to choking in children?
   a. peanut butter eaten by itself
   b. reclining while eating
   c. popcorn and nuts
   d. all of the above

2. Which of the following is most commonly deficient in children and adolescents?
   a. folate
   b. zinc
   c. iron
   d. vitamin D

3. An allergic reaction to a food always involves:
   a. anaphylactic shock
   b. dislike of a particular food
   c. antibodies
   d. all of the above

4. Which of the following may alleviate symptoms of PMS?
   a. adequate vitamin E and vitamin B_6
   b. exercise
   c. omitting caffeine from the diet
   d. all of the above

5. Which of the following have been shown to improve acne?
   a. avoiding chocolate and fatty foods
   b. retinoic acid or Retin A
   c. vitamin A supplements
   d. all of the above

6. Research to date supports the idea that food allergies or intolerances are common causes of hyperactivity in children. T F

7. Dietary fat may play a role in causing arthritis. T F

8. Vitamin A absorption decreases with age. T F

9. Children who watch more than two hours of television per day may be prone to develop elevated serum cholesterol and dental caries. T F

10. Some severe nutrient deficiencies can cause mental symptoms. (Read about this in the upcoming Controversy.) T F

NOTES

Notes are in Appendix F.

Food, Mind, and Memory

Why do you feel like eating a steak at one meal and a doughnut at another? Why do you feel sleepy after lunch and not after dinner? Do some foods help you to think or to remember? Human behavior and the brain are still largely mysterious territory, and research is uncovering layer below layer of complexity. Researchers no longer doubt that intakes of food and nutrients affect the mind and memory, and they are beginning to understand how and why. The neurosciences are sure to be the focus of many future nutrition investigations.[1]

THE BRAIN AND ITS NEUROTRANSMITTERS

The brain has special needs. Encased in its protective skull, a hard, bony, inelastic helmet, the brain cannot expand and contract as can, say, the liver or adipose tissue. It cannot store its own reserve supply of glycogen or fat because those fuels take up space. It cannot store oxygen to oxidize those fuels, or nutrients to help it do so. Therefore the brain must depend on the passing blood supply for both its fuels and its oxygen. Furthermore, its needs for those substances are extraordinary. It comprises only 2 percent of the adult's body weight, but at any given time the brain contains 15 percent of the body's blood, and it devours 20 to 30 percent of the fuels that support the basal metabolism. Should the blood deliver too little oxygen or glucose, the brain's cells would cease communicating with each other (see Figure C13-1), and coma would occur within minutes. Should the blood supply be interrupted altogether, coma would ensue within 10 seconds.

Nutrients of all kinds are crucial to brain function, and the blood supply must deliver these, too. For example, the brain requires amino acids to make its messenger molecules, some 30 to 40 **neurotransmitters** and related compounds. The brain also needs electrically charged minerals to help transmit its electrical

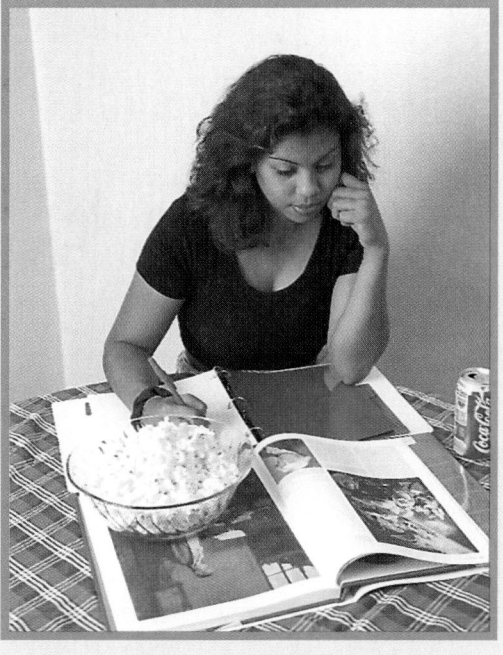

impulses, vitamins and other minerals to facilitate these processes, lipids to repair its cell membranes, and water to maintain the fluids in which many of the chemical processes take place. Table C13-1 defines some terms relating to brain function.

The brain is extremely sensitive to fluctuations in its own internal chemical composition. To keep its internal environment constant, it has its own molecular sieve to filter from the blood, the fluid and chemicals it needs: see the **blood-brain barrier** in Table C13-1. No matter how widely blood fluctuates in chemical composition, the brain's internal milieu hardly changes at all.

Because of its dependence on blood borne fuels, oxygen, and nutrients, the brain monitors the blood closely and sends messages to other organs to signal its needs for these substances. At one time the brain may need glucose; at another, amino acids. Animals regulate their intakes of protein and carbohydrate, each proportional to the other, in response to promptings from the brain. People probably do this, too, unconsciously.[2]

A day's intake of lipids, vitamins, and minerals are unlikely to affect the brain's functioning immediately, although they probably do affect it over time. Amino acids, in contrast, are used to form neurotransmitters within the day they are eaten, and their effects are seen within minutes or hours of ingestion. Scientists exploring the effects of nutrients on the brain are especially interested in these associations:

- Some amino acids serve as the starting material from which some neurotransmitters are built.

- Vitamins and minerals assist enzymes in the syntheses of neurotransmitters.

If the quantity of a nutrient eaten is to affect the brain directly, the nutrient must be free to come and go as it pleases; its brain concentration must fluctuate in

FIGURE C13-1

COMMUNICATION WITHIN THE BRAIN

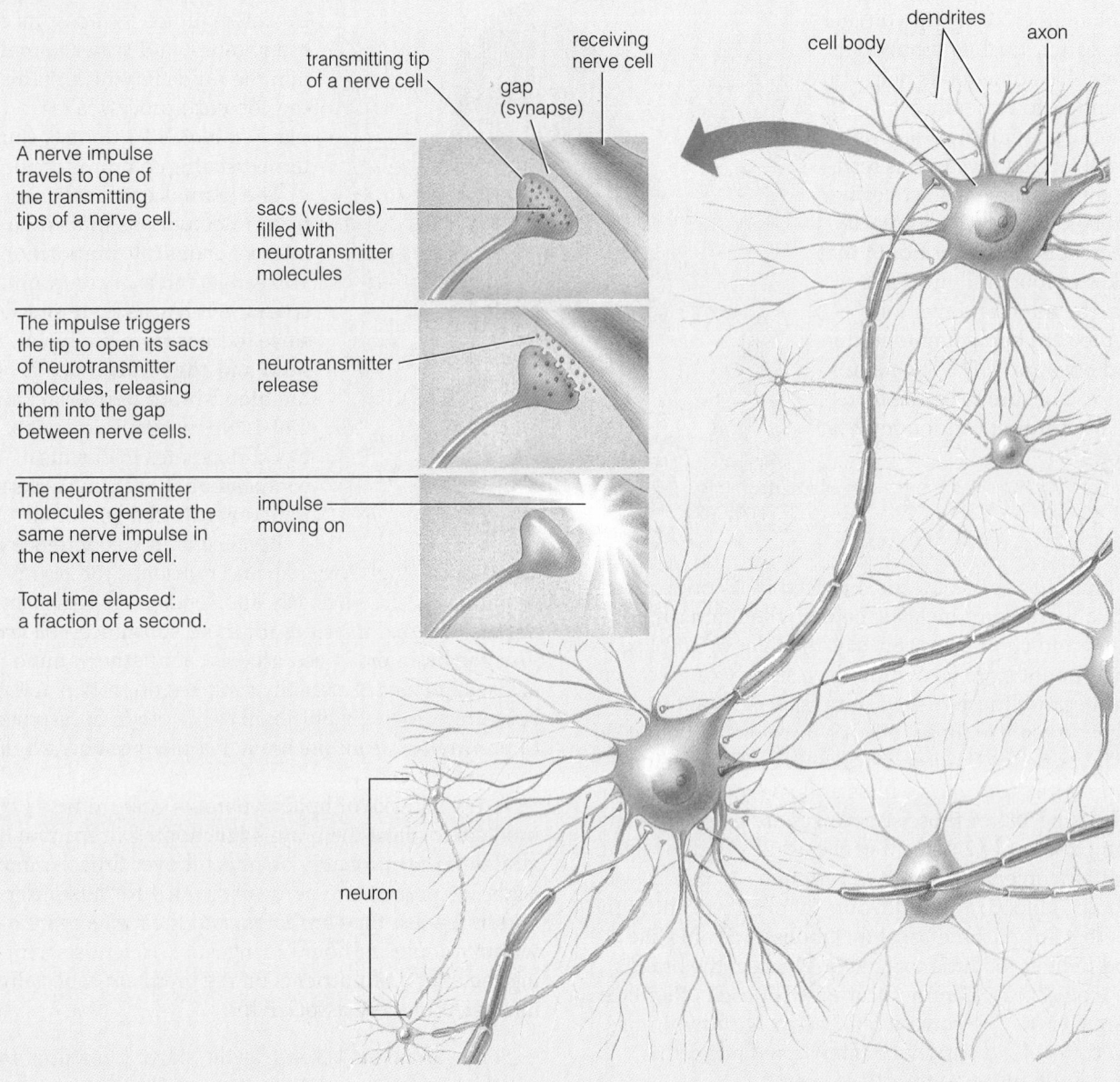

transmitting tip of a nerve cell

receiving nerve cell

gap (synapse)

cell body

dendrites

axon

A nerve impulse travels to one of the transmitting tips of a nerve cell.

sacs (vesicles) filled with neurotransmitter molecules

The impulse triggers the tip to open its sacs of neurotransmitter molecules, releasing them into the gap between nerve cells.

neurotransmitter release

The neurotransmitter molecules generate the same nerve impulse in the next nerve cell.

impulse moving on

Total time elapsed: a fraction of a second.

neuron

response to diet. Most amino acids never exceed a given level in the brain no matter how much of them is consumed, but the brain's regulatory amino acids cross the blood-brain barrier freely. Furthermore, once in the brain, these precursor nutrients exert **precursor control**; that is, the brain responds to larger or smaller amounts of them by making larger or smaller amounts of neurotransmitters from them. Thus the food a person eats can influence brain chemistry by changing the rates at which the brain makes its neurotransmitters. These facts link eating directly to brain chemistry, and thereby, as you will see in a moment, the eater's mood and other sensations.

One neurotransmitter whose brain concentration is especially sensitive to changes in precursor supply has been studied in depth: **serotonin**, whose precursor is

TABLE C13-1
Brain Terms

- **blood-brain barrier** a barrier composed of the cells lining the blood vessels in the brain. These cells are so tightly glued to each other that blood-borne substances cannot get into the brain between the cells, but only by crossing the cell bodies themselves. Thus the cells, using all their sophisticated equipment, can screen substances for entry.
- **catecholamines** neurotransmitters made from the amino acid tyrosine: dopamine, epinephrine, and norepinephrine.
- **neurotransmitter** a chemical messenger released by a nerve cell when that cell is firing (conducting a nerve impulse). The neurotransmitter diffuses to the next nerve cell and alters the membrane of that cell, making it either less or more likely to fire. Exposed to enough neurotransmitter molecules, the next nerve cell will fire.
- **precursor control** control of a compound's synthesis by the availability of that compound's precursor. The more precursor there is, the more of the compound is made.
- **serotonin** a compound related in structure to (and made from) the amino acid tryptophan. It serves as one of the brain's principal neurotransmitters.

the amino acid tryptophan. Similarly, a set of neurotransmitters, the **catecholamines**, depend on the availability of their precursor amino acid, tyrosine. The discussion that follows centers on serotonin because more details about it are known.

Tryptophan to Serotonin Ordinary meals of the kind people eat every day raise or lower the concentration of serotonin in the brain, depending on the meal's protein and carbohydrate content.[3] Serotonin release, in turn, affects sensations and mood, so the ingredients of meals may have real effects on how people feel afterward.[4] Many people report feeling relaxed, peaceful, or sleepy after eating certain foods; these sensations are sometimes attributed to serotonin's effects on the brain. Research shows that a lack of tryptophan flowing into the brain can manifest itself in wakefulness, depresses mood, a tendency to startle, and an enhanced sensitivity to pain. Animals that have been made tryptophan-deficient exhibit these symptoms, and when given tryptophan, they return to normal as their brain serotonin is restored. Tests show that tryptophan reduces sensitivity to pain in people, too.[5]

The amount of tryptophan that enters the brain depends not only on the amount of tryptophan the person eats but also on the total protein and carbohydrate eaten with it. If tryptophan is taken as a single amino acid, then brain serotonin increases proportionately. Normally, however, whole proteins, not just tryptophan, are eaten. In this case some of the other large amino acids in the proteins compete with tryptophan for entry into the brain because they use the same transport mechanism to get across the blood-brain barrier. In this situation tryptophan fails to enter the brain in increased quantities and so does not effectively enhance brain serotonin synthesis.

If carbohydrate is fed instead of protein, however, the carbohydrate can "help" to deliver tryptophan, already in the bloodstream, to the brain because it elicits the secretion of the hormone insulin. Insulin drives the *other* amino acids, but not tryptophan, into *body* cells, leaving the tryptophan free to enter the brain without competition. Thus, paradoxically, food high in carbohydrate—*not* food high in protein—eases tryptophan's transport into the brain and so promotes serotonin synthesis.

Choosing a meal to raise brain serotonin presents a problem, though. The amount of protein in most mixed meals, even those high in carbohydrate, is generally more than sufficient to block the tryptophan-delivering effect of carbohydrate.[6]

Researchers speculate that people's food choices may be partly governed by the brain's reactions to prior foods eaten. This idea is that, when a meal elicits top mental performance, the brain of the eater may be "trained" to prefer those foods and so to choose them often.[7] That could partly explain why, in the great majority of societies of the world, people seem naturally to prefer mixed meals over single foods. It may be that meals with mixed protein and carbohydrate sources provide just the right balance to support brain function.

Serotonin and Appetite An understanding of the absorption of tryptophan by the brain may help explain how animals and human beings, depending on what kinds of foods they have eaten last, seem to know what foods to choose next time to ensure balance. According to one theory, since a high-carbohydrate meal raises brain serotonin, this satisfies a need and so reduces the urge to eat more carbohydrate. A person or animal who has eaten plenty of carbohydrate therefore will seek out more protein at the next meal. A high-protein meal creates a serotonin deficit, awakens the carbohydrate craving, and once again leads to the consumption of carbohydrate-containing foods.

Though not everyone agrees, a chief appeal of this theory is that it seems to account for what is often observed to happen with low-carbohydrate diets. The more dieters try to restrict carbohydrate, the more they seem to crave it. The effect is accentuated if they are insulin resistant, as is likely if they are obese. When an insulin-resistant person eats carbohydrate, insulin's normal actions do not follow, and the cells continue to hunger for glucose. Furthermore, brain serotonin does not rise, and so the carbohydrate craving is intensified.

Another theory links serotonin to obesity. The theory gains support from the finding that serotonin is often below average in the brains of obese people and of people of normal weight who report craving carbohydrate-rich food.[8] While direct cause-and-effect conclusions are not yet possible, the authors of the study suggest that high-carbohydrate weight-loss diets may be most successful because they work *with* many people's brain chemistry rather than against it.

Dieting in general seems to disrupt mental functioning somewhat.[9] During dieting, people are easily distracted from tasks requiring vigilance and have slower reaction times. They also score lower on memory tests than at times of normal eating. Whether these effects are related to neurotransmitter synthesis or are equally likely to result from any sort of change in regular eating habits remains a mystery.

Some evidence weakens the theory that links serotonin to the appetite for carbohydrate. When animals were injected with tryptophan, which should stimulate protein intake according to the theory, no preference for protein or carbohydrate was observed.[10] Ongoing research should ultimately help to untangle this problem, but it may well first become more knotty.

Serotonin, Mood, and Sleep Some people describe themselves as anxious, tense, and somewhat depressed before eating carbohydrate, and say they experience reversal of these symptoms afterward. The amino acid tryptophan given by itself often has similar effects, consistent with the notion that it is the indirect agent of carbohydrate's effect. When tryptophan is restricted in the diet, some people report depressed feelings.[11] When tryptophan is restored, depressed feelings lift, but in their place come drowsiness, clumsiness, and mental slowing.[12]

Reports exist of disturbed serotonin metabolism in people with major depression. Researchers interested in studying the effects of food on people's emotions fed tryptophan-deficient diets to two groups of young men: one with long family histories of depression and a matched (control) group with no reported depression in the family.[13] As blood tryptophan concentrations dropped, the men with family histories of depression scored significantly lower on a mood scale, indicating depression. None of the controls scored lower on the test—their moods hadn't changed. Major depression is a serious condition that is not reversible through diet alone. Still, those who tend to be depressed may be more sensitive to the effects of serotonin than are others. Such people would do well to eat balanced meals at regular intervals to supply the brain with the materials needed to make serotonin.

Carbohydrate or tryptophan may also induce fatigue or sleepiness. The tryptophan effect is particularly well known; from at least 50 studies in people and animals. Carbohydrate or tryptophan can also increase the error rate in performance tests. Elevated brain serotonin is known to reduce aggression in rats, and it may have that effect on people, too.[14]

Studies demonstrate clearly that single amino acids, when administered alone, act like drugs in the body. These effects are interesting, but they are not well characterized, and people should not dose themselves with amino acids seeking mental effects. The Consumer Corner of Chapter 6 warned that to do so is to imperil health.

EFFECTS OF OTHER NUTRIENTS AND FOODS ON THE BRAIN

Nutrients other than amino acids are also involved in the synthesis of neurotransmitters. Iron is needed in one of the first steps of neurotransmitter synthesis. Vitamin B_6 and riboflavin are needed in later steps. These nutrients are but three among many; deficiencies of them are reflected in depressed or otherwise disturbed mood.[15] Deficiencies of many nutrients also cause anemia, which produces mental symptoms of its own (see Table C13-2). Some mental effects of nutrient deficiencies become apparent only in severe deficiency states, but others such as fatigue or depressed mood can be among the first symptoms of a developing deficiency. Administration of the missing nutrient rapidly reverses these effects.

An interesting idea currently under study concerns the possibility that lipids may affect human emotions, too.[16] Several years ago, a research team examined mortality data from subjects participating in ongoing

TABLE C13-2

The Mental Symptoms of Anemia

Apathy, listlessness
Behavior disturbances
Clumsiness
Hyperactivity
Irritability
Lack of appetite
Learning disorders (vocabulary, perception)
Low scores on latency and associative reactions
Lowered IQ
Reduced physical work capacity
Repetitive hand and foot movements
Shortened attention span

NOTE: These symptoms are not caused by anemia itself but by iron deficiency in the brain. Children with much more severe anemias from other
causes, such as sickle-cell anemia and thalassemia, show no reduction in
IQ when compared with children without anemia.

cholesterol-lowering studies.[17] People receiving cholesterol-lowering drugs or dietary treatments were twice as
likely as controls to die from suicide or violence. The
possibility that lowering blood cholesterol might cause
negative emotion gained strength with the report of a
study of monkeys fed diets either high or low in fat and
cholesterol. Monkeys fed the low-fat, low-cholesterol
diet were rated as significantly more aggressive and less
social and had lower brain serotonin than controls.[18]
Low serum cholesterol in human beings has been linked
with both suicide and aggression.[19] In contrast, fish oil
was shown to reduce aggression in college students
under the stress of final exams.[20]

A number of plausible mechanisms exist for the
associations just described, but none has yet been
proved. Heart disease brought on by high blood cholesterol is a proven threat to health and life; people
receiving treatments for high blood cholesterol should
make no changes until more studies make clear the
implications of these early findings.

CAN EXTRA NUTRIENTS OR "SMART" SUPPLEMENTS ENHANCE BRAIN FUNCTION?

If deficiencies of nutrients can cause mental disturbances, can extra amounts of some nutrients make
brain function excel? The idea has appeal, especially to
business people, students, textbook authors, medical
workers, and others who must remain alert despite
long hours, little sleep, or international travel.

Purveyors of "smart" drugs, supplements, and
drinks say they can speed thinking and learning, jump-
start a failing memory, and reverse aging processes.
Some drugs sold with these claims are just now being
tested for reversal of the mental deterioration of
Alzheimer's disease common in old age. Some are
available by prescription in this country, but people
have to order others from foreign countries because
they are not approved for use in the United States. The
idea seems to be that if a drug can reverse or slow deterioration in a diseased brain, then perhaps it can boost
the thinking power of a normal brain. An expert in the
field of the neurobiology of learning and memory com-
mented concisely on smart drugs: "I think they are
silly."[21]

Experts at the FDA have warned that many of the
smart drugs produce well-known side effects such as
gastrointestinal distress, headaches, ulcers of the nasal
cavity, and insomnia. They warn that long-term effects
of other drugs are not known.[22]

Among herbs, an extract of the evergreen *Gingko
biloba* is sold as a "brain-power" enhancer. Some studies support a theory that the herb's antioxidant effects
may improve the mental functioning of the impaired
aging brain.[23] Unknown is whether the herb can boost
functioning in a healthy brain and whether long-term
use is safe. Until more is known, it cannot be recommended.

The supplements and drinks, which may also be
promoted as a legal high (euphoria) to people too
young to buy alcohol, are made mostly of amino acids,
vitamins, choline, and lecithin. In reality, no known
nutrient supplement produces euphoria, but the
placebo effect can do so.

Users tell convincing stories about the effects of
these drinks, but none of the products has been shown
to improve intelligence in clinical trials. Researchers
who attempt to measure people's feelings of being
smart, witty, energetic, and able to remember run into
problems. Measurements of this sort are always
clouded by the placebo effect and wishful thinking.
Also a person with slight nutrient deficiencies may well
respond favorably to a potion that provides the missing
nutrients.

Other mental effects of nutrients may exist as well.
Some inquiries have suggested a role for ingestion of
carbohydrate on the formation of memory.[24] It may be
that blood glucose somehow sparks the formation of
memory or improves recall. The very act of eating also
enhances memory, although the details of how it does
so are not known. People given a snack during a learning task exhibit better recall later than when no snack is
given. Hungry mice, fed immediately after learning a

task, later remember how to perform that task better than do mice fed before the learning session. This effect may be a survival adaptation; in the wild, individuals who learn something new and obtain food as a result benefit from remembering the new behavior.

A curious response to food is the almost universal love for the taste of chocolate, which some claim is a craving akin to an addiction. Most chocolate lovers say that eating chocolate lifts their spirits.[25] Chocolate contains phytochemicals, such as caffeine (a central nervous system stimulant), theobromine (another stimulant), and phenylethylamine (a biologically active amine), all of which could conceivably affect mood. One group of researchers suggested that one amine in chocolate may activate some of the same brain areas that marijuana targets.[26] Of course, chocolate has none of the mind-altering effects of marijuana, but if it stimulates the brain in ways that enhance the sensory qualities of food, as marijuana is known to do, this effect might make chocolate seem extra delicious. The vast majority of studies of chocolate's effects have not found chocolate to affect the brain's functioning, however, doubtless a disappointment to chocoholics everywhere.[27]

APPLICATIONS

Can a person choose foods to maximize the brain's performance? With some qualifications, the answer seems to be that choices surrounding mealtimes probably can minimize diet-induced sluggishness, clumsiness, or poorer-than-normal memory capacity. The opposite food choices may also bring on those effects in some people who want to go to sleep.

A student who wishes to perform optimally on an examination, for example, may be wise to consider carefully the foods chosen for breakfast or lunch before the exam. Right away it should be said that normal variations in meals presenting mixtures of carbohydrate, fat, and protein are unlikely to produce any noticeable effects on mental functioning. That is, mixed meals generally support mental functioning well. When the eater strays far from normal eating, however, brain functioning can change.[28]

Our exam-taking student might best avoid foods extremely high in carbohydrate and low in protein (5% of calories or lower) in the hours before the test. Otherwise, the carbohydrate might speed up the brain's production of serotonin, producing mental grogginess. As already mentioned, carbohydrate stimulates insulin

TABLE C13-3

High-Carbohydrate, Low-Protein Foods

These foods present enough carbohydrate, without too much protein, to induce sleep:

- Plain white rice
- Spaghetti noodles with tomato sauce (no meat or cheese)
- Plain baked potato
- Muffin
- Pancakes or waffles with syrup
- White bread
- Cooked cream of wheat cereal, plain, no milk
- Fruits
- Fruit juices
- Peanut butter and jelly sandwich
- Whole-wheat bread
- Oatmeal, plain, no milk

release and triggers the synthesis of serotonin. Serotonin's calming, sleep-inducing effect is exactly the wrong effect for the test taker who needs alertness. Foods that provide protein along with carbohydrate do not induce serotonin synthesis, so regular, mixed meals seem best in this regard.

Research, as well as common sense, tells us that breakfast is of prime importance to a person taking an exam in the morning hours, while lunch is linked to mental performance in the afternoon. While any effects from food on the neurotransmitters of the brain take at least an hour to become manifest, food in the digestive tract seems to have an immediate, unexplained effect on performance. No one knows why, but a common finding is the "post-lunch dip"—an early afternoon period of less-than-optimal mental performance. Paying attention to mental tasks can seem harder after lunch, especially after a large meal, but the effect is by no means universally observed. A prudent action for those taking tests in the early afternoon would be to eat lightly at the lunch hour and save heavier eating for after the test.

If the student is accustomed to taking caffeine in beverages, then it may be especially important to do so on exam day. Persons missing their normal caffeine intakes experience headaches, drowsiness, and fatigue that interfere with mental tasks. For people not accustomed to caffeine, its addition will not improve performance. Alcohol, of course, worsens mental performance.

An interesting finding is that mental performance seems most adversely affected by food that is different in composition from that ordinarily eaten.[29] Among people who eat breakfasts, those eating foods that differ more from the norm perform worse than those eating foods of more typical composition. The advice to be gleaned from this finding is, simply, don't rock the boat on examination day. Stick to normal mealtime choices to sidestep adverse effects on mental functioning.

For those seeking the calming effect of serotonin, for example, to induce sleep, the opposite advice holds. Foods that provide less than 1 gram of protein per 100 calories are the best choices for this purpose.[30] Table C13-3 lists some foods with the right carbohydrate-to-protein ratio to induce sleep, but note that these foods carry a lot of calories. A person who eats an extra meal before bedtime must reduce intakes at other meals or risk gaining body fat. Ample daily exercise can both burn off calories and help induce healthy sleep.

Finally, it goes without saying that the diet should be adequate to supply all the precursor and supporting nutrients needed for mental functioning. No manipulation of energy nutrients will correct less-than-optimal brain functioning if needed nutrients are missing. Fluid is also important. Even slight dehydration can cause confusion.

With all of its unsolved mysteries, the human brain remains fascinating to researchers. The ideas presented here, and others like them, offer plenty of grist for the mills of researchers for many years to come.

NOTES

Notes are in Appendix F.

FOOD SAFETY AND FOOD TECHNOLOGY

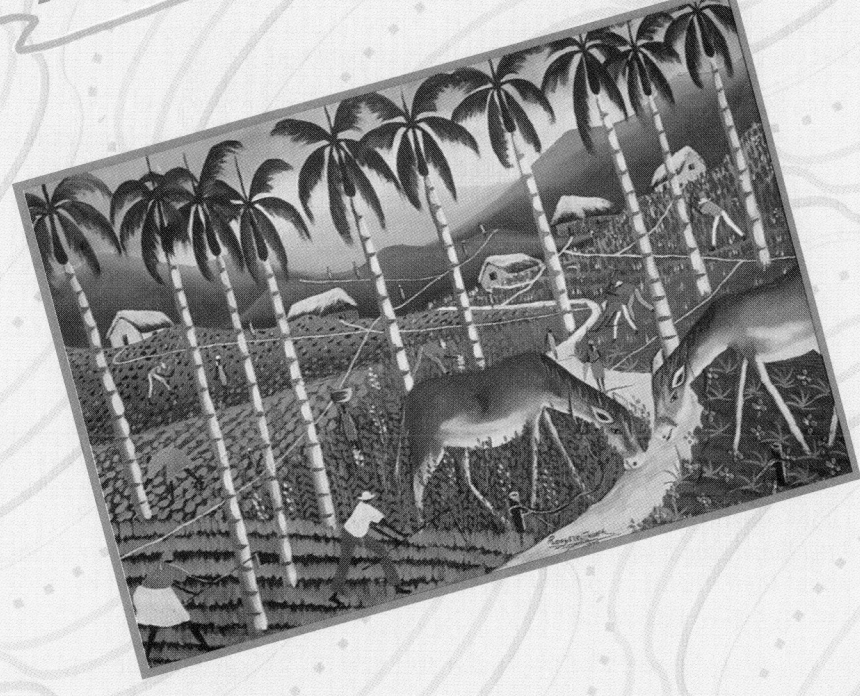

CONTENTS

Roosevelt, 1952, *Landscape with Royal Palms*, Haitian Private Collection, © SuperStock.

food poisoning illness transmitted to human beings through food; caused by a poisonous substance (*food intoxication*) or an infectious agent (*food-borne infection*). Also called *food-borne illness.*

hazard a state of danger; used to refer to any circumstance in which harm is possible under normal conditions of use.

14 Consumers have questions about their food. Are today's food products nutritious? Are they pure and free from contamination? Are the additives in them safe? And who is looking out for these consumer concerns?

The Food and Drug Administration (FDA) is the major agency charged with monitoring the food supply. Other agencies are listed in Table 14-1. The areas of concern the FDA has identified in our food supply are listed below. The one listed first, microbial **food poisoning,** also called *food-borne illness,* constitutes a true **hazard,** and so is of most concern. The one listed last, food additives, is of least concern. The others fall somewhere in between.

1. *Microbial food poisoning.* This affects the most people every year.
2. *Natural toxins in foods.* These constitute a hazard whenever people consume single foods either by choice (fad diets) or by necessity (poverty).
3. *Residues in food.*
   a. Environmental contaminants (other than pesticides) such as household and industrial chemicals. These are increasing yearly in number and concentration, and their impacts are hard to foresee and to forestall.
   b. Pesticides. These are a subclass of environmental contaminants, but are listed separately because they are applied intentionally to foods and so, in theory, can be controlled.
   c. Animal drugs. These include metabolically active proteins that increase growth or milk production in food animals and dairy cows.
4. *Nutrients in foods.* These require close attention as more and more artificially constituted foods appear on the market.
5. *Intentional food additives.* These are listed last because so much is known about them that they pose virtually no hazard to consumers, and because their use is well regulated.[1]

These concerns are remarkably similar to those of other nations around the world.[2]

TABLE 14-1

Agencies That Monitor the U.S. Food Supply

- **CDC (Centers for Disease Control and Prevention)** a branch of the Department of Health and Human Services that is responsible, among other things, for monitoring food-borne diseases.
- **EPA (Environmental Protection Agency)** a federal agency that is responsible, among other things, for regulating pesticides and establishing water quality standards.
- **FDA (Food and Drug Administration)** a part of the Department of Health and Human Services' Public Health Service that is responsible for ensuring the safety and wholesomeness of all foods sold in interstate commerce except meat, poultry, and eggs (which are under the jurisdiction of the USDA); inspecting food plants and imported foods; and setting standards for food consumption.
- **USDA (U.S. Department of Agriculture)** the federal agency responsible for enforcing standards for the wholesomeness and quality of meat, poultry, and eggs produced in the United States; conducting nutrition research; and educating the public about nutrition.
- **WHO (World Health Organization)** an international agency that, among other responsibilities, develops standards to regulate pesticide use. A related organization is the FAO (Food and Agricultural Organization).

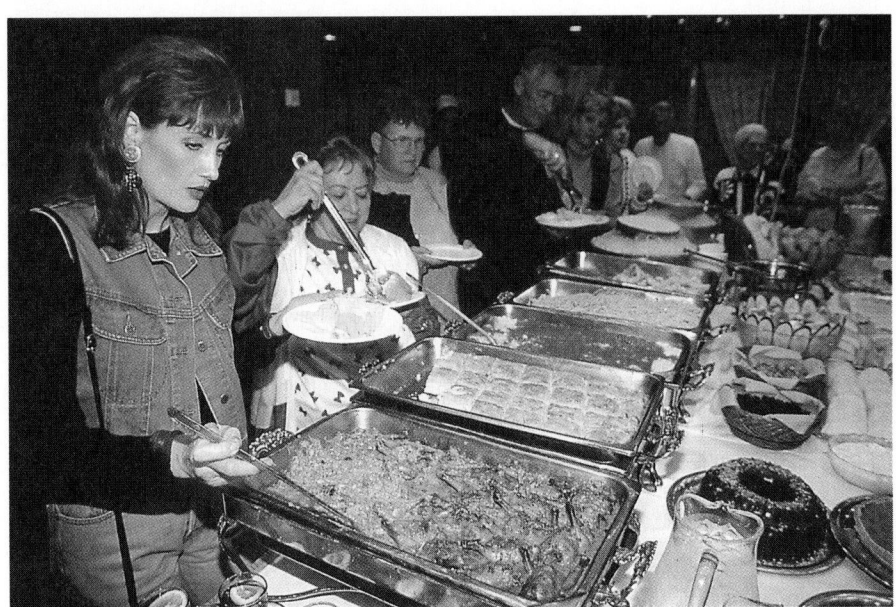

With the privilege of abundance comes the responsibility to choose wisely.

In our free market, where food companies compete for sales, the consumer enjoys the safest, most pleasing, and most abundant food supply in the world. With this benefit comes the consumer's responsibility of distinguishing between foods with a good **safety** record and foods that may pose a hazard. Often foods are safe until they are mishandled or misused.

This chapter provides the information consumers need to purchase, handle, and use foods with confidence. It begins with the most pressing concern of the FDA, food producers, and food consumers alike: food poisoning.[3]

safety the practical certainty that injury will not result from the use of a substance.

entertoxins poisons that act upon mucous membranes, such as those of the digestive tract.

neurotoxins poisons that act upon the cells of the nervous system.

MICROBES AND FOOD SAFETY

Episodes of food poisoning cause illness in at least one-third of the U.S. population each year, and their number is steadily increasing. Between 21 million and 81 million cases of diarrhea that are treated in the United States each year are from food-borne illnesses. Some 9,000 people a year die of food poisoning.[4] Nearly everyone else experiences illness from food poisoning every year, but may mistakenly pass it off as "flu."

The Threat from Microbial Contamination

Food-borne illness can be caused either by infection or by intoxication. Microorganisms such as *Salmonella* varieties that occur in foods commonly infect the human body themselves. Other microorganisms in foods produce **enterotoxins** or **neurotoxins** in foods or in the human digestive tract. Bacteria may multiply or act in food during improper preparation or storage, or within the digestive tract after a person eats contaminated food. If you experience the digestive tract disturbances listed in Table 14-2 as the major or only symptoms of your next bout of "flu," chances are excellent that what you really have is food poisoning. For people who are otherwise ill or malnourished or for the very old or young, even these relatively mild disturbances can be fatal.

TABLE 14-2
Food-Borne Illnesses

Disease and Organism That Causes It	Most Frequent Food Source	Onset and General Symptoms	Prevention Methods
Food-Borne Infections			
Campylobacteriosis *Campylobacter jejuni* bacterium	Raw poultry, beef, lamb, unpasteurized milk (foods of animal origin eaten raw or undercooked or recontaminated after cooking).	Onset: 2 to 5 days. Diarrhea, nausea, vomiting, abdominal cramps, fever; sometimes bloody stools; lasts 7 to 10 days.	Cook foods thoroughly; use pasteurized milk; use sanitary food-handling methods.
Giardiasis *Giardia lamblia* protozoa	Contaminated water; uncooked foods.	Onset: 5 to 25 days. Diarrhea (but occasionally constipation), abdominal pain, gas, abdominal distension, digestive disturbances, anorexia, nausea, and vomiting.	Use sanitary food-handling methods; avoid raw fruits and vegetables where protozoa are endemic; dispose of sewage properly.
Hepatitis Hepatitis A virus	Undercooked or raw shellfish.	Onset: 15 to 20 days (28 to 30 days average). Inflammation of the liver with tiredness; nausea, vomiting, or indigestion; jaundice (yellowed skin and eyes from buildup of wastes); muscle pain.	Cook foods thoroughly.
Listeriosis *Listeria monocytogenes* bacterium	Raw meat and seafood, raw milk, and soft cheeses.	Onset: 7 to 30 days. Mimics flu; blood poisoning, complications in pregnancy, and meningitis (stiff neck, severe headache, and fever).	Use sanitary food-handling methods; cook foods thoroughly; use pasteurized milk.
Perfringens food poisoning *Clostridium perfringens* bacterium	Meats and meat products stored at between 120 and 130°F.	Onset: 8 to 12 hr (usually 12). Abdominal pain, diarrhea, nausea, and vomiting; symptoms last a day or less and are usually mild; can be serious in old or weak people.	Use sanitary food-handling methods; cook foods thoroughly; refrigerate foods promptly and properly.
Salmonellosis *Salmonella* bacteria	Raw or undercooked eggs, meats, poultry, milk and other dairy products, shrimp, frog legs, yeast, coconut, pasta, and chocolate.	Onset: 6 to 48 hr. Nausea, fever, chills, vomiting, abdominal cramps, diarrhea, and headache; can be fatal.	Use sanitary food-handling methods; use pasteurized milk; cook foods thoroughly; refrigerate foods promptly and properly.
Traveler's diarrhea *Escherichia coli* (usually)	Contaminated water, undercooked ground beef, raw foods, imported unpasteurized soft cheeses.	Onset: 12 to 18 hr. Loose and watery stools, nausea, bloating, and abdominal cramps.	Cook foods thoroughly; use safe, treated water and pasteurized milk; wash fruits and vegetables.

(continued on next page)

TABLE 14-2

Food-Borne Illnesses continued

Disease and Organism That Causes It	Most Frequent Food Source	Onset and General Symptoms	Prevention Methods
Food-Borne Infections continued			
Trichinosis *Trichinella spiralis* parasite	Raw or undercooked pork or wild game (bear). Worms burrow through the body tissues to reach muscle tissue where they remain alive.	Onset: 24 hr. Abdominal pain, nausea, vomiting, diarrhea, and fever. One to two weeks later, muscle pain, low-grade fever, pain on breathing, edema (swelling), skin eruptions, loss of appetite, and weight loss. Drug therapy kills the worms and deaths are rare.	Cook foods thoroughly.
Food Intoxications			
Botulism Botulinum toxin (produced by the *Clostridium botulinum* bacterium)	Anaerobic environment of low acidity (canned corn, peppers, green beans, soups, beets, asparagus, mushrooms, ripe olives, spinach, tuna, chicken, chicken liver, liver paté, luncheon meats, ham, sausage, stuffed eggplant, herb-flavored oils, lobster, and smoked and salted fish).	Onset: 4 to 36 hr. Nervous system symptoms, including double vision, inability to swallow, speech difficulty, and progressive paralysis of the respiratory system; often fatal; leaves prolonged symptoms in survivors.	Use proper canning methods for low-acid foods; avoid commercially prepared foods with leaky seals or with bent, bulging, or broken cans.
Staphylococcal food poisoning Staphylococcal toxin (produced by the *Staphylococcus aureus* bacterium)	Toxin produced in meats, poultry, egg products, tuna, potato and macaroni salads, and cream-filled pastries.	Onset: ½ to 8 hr. Diarrhea, nausea, vomiting, abdominal cramps, and fatigue; mimics flu; lasts 24 to 48 hr; rarely fatal.	Use sanitary food-handling methods; cook food thoroughly; refrigerate foods promptly and properly.

The symptoms of one neurotoxin stand out as severe and commonly fatal—those of **botulism,** caused by the toxin of the *Clostridium botulinum* bacterium that grows inside improperly canned (and especially home-canned) foods, improperly prepared vacuum-packed foods, or in oils flavored with herbs, garlic, vegetables, or other edible agents and stored at room temperature. The microbe grows only in the absence of oxygen, in low-acid conditions, and at temperatures that support growth of most bacteria—40° to 120° Fahrenheit.[5]

Botulism danger signs constitute a true medical emergency (see the next page's margin). Even with medical assistance, survivors can suffer symptoms for months, years, or a lifetime. So potent is the botulinum toxin that an amount as tiny as a single grain of salt can kill several people within an hour. The

botulism an often-fatal food poisoning caused by botulinum toxin, a toxin produced by the *Clostridium botulinum* bacterium that grows without oxygen in nonacidic canned foods.

pasteurization the treatment of milk with heat sufficient to kill certain pathogens (disease-causing microbes) commonly transmitted through milk; not a sterilization process. Pasteurized milk retains bacteria that cause milk spoilage. Raw milk, even if labeled "certified," transmits many food-borne diseases to people each year and should be avoided.

Hazard Analysis Critical Control Point (HACCP) a systematic plan to identify and correct potential microbial hazards in the manufacturing, distribution, and commercial use of food products.

Warning Signs of Botulism:
- Double vision.
- Weak muscles.
- Difficulty swallowing.
- Difficulty breathing.

For other forms of food poisoning, get medical help when these symptoms occur:
- bloody stools.
- headache accompanied by muscle stiffness and fever.
- rapid heart rate, fainting, dizziness.
- fever of longer than 24 hours duration.
- diarrhea of more than 3 days' duration.
- numbness, muscle weakness, tingling sensations in the skin.

botulinum toxin is destroyed by heat, so canned foods that contain the toxin can be rendered harmless by boiling them for ten minutes. Home-canned food can be prepared safely ony if proper canning techniques are followed to the letter.*

✔ KEY POINT **Each year in the United States, many millions of people suffer from mild to life-threatening symptoms caused by food poisoning.**

Safety in the Marketplace

Overwhelmingly, most food poisoning results from errors consumers make in handling foods *after* purchase. While commercially prepared food is usually safe, rare accidents do occur, however, and they can affect many people at once. This makes news reporters take notice. Milk producers, for example, rely on **pasteurization,** a process of heating milk to kill many disease-causing organisms and make milk safe for consumption. When, on occasion, a major dairy develops flaws in its pasteurization system, tens of thousands of cases of food-borne illness may result.

In 1994, a fast-food restaurant chain in the Northwest served undercooked hamburgers tainted with a particularly dangerous strain of *E. coli* bacteria. As a result, three lives were lost and hundreds of other patrons were stricken with serious illness.[6] This incident focused the national spotlight on two important food safety issues; that live, disease-causing organisms of many types are routinely found in raw meats, and that thorough cooking is necessary to make animal-derived foods safe. These revelations have led to a much needed overhaul of the country's mechanisms for ensuring food safety.

One outcome of the concern about food-borne illness is a law requiring that producers of meat, poultry, and seafood employ an effective prevention method, the **Hazard Analysis Critical Control Point (HACCP)** plan.[7] The method requires identification of "critical control points" in food production where the risk of food contamination is high. A plan must then be developed and implemented to prevent loss of control at those critical points. For many years, meat and seafood inspectors relied on their senses of sight, smell, and touch to detect bad meat and seafood. Unfortunately, human senses cannot detect dangerous organisms until after the food has begun to decay. Newer, more accurate tests for microbial contamination must be used to verify that each HACCP plan for a food-producing company is effective. The FDA estimates that these safety regulations should prevent up to 60,000 to 80,000 cases of food-borne illness each year from seafood poisoning alone.[8]

Luckily, large-scale commercial incidents, while dramatic, make up only a fraction of the nation's total food-poisoning cases each year. Most cases arise from one person's error in a small setting and affect just a few victims. Some people have come to accept a yearly bout or two of intestinal illness as inevitable, but in truth, these illnesses can and should be prevented. To protect themselves, consumers need to learn how to select, prepare, and store food safely.

Canned and packaged foods sold in grocery stores are easily controlled, but rare accidents do happen. Batch numbering makes it possible to recall conta-

*Complete, up-to-date, safe home-canning instructions are included in the USDA's 172-page *Complete Guide to Home Canning,* available for $11.00 from the Superintendent of Documents, Government Printing Office, Washington, DC 20402.

minated foods through public announcements via newspapers, television, and radio, and the FDA monitors large suppliers. You can help protect yourself, too. Carefully inspect the seals and wrappers of packages. Reject leaking or bulging cans. Many jars have safety "buttons," areas of the lid designed to pop up once opened; make sure that they are firmly sealed. If a package on the shelf looks ragged, soiled, or punctured, do not buy the product; turn it in to the store manager. A badly dented can or a mangled package is useless in protecting food from microorganisms, insects, spoilage, or even vandals. Frozen foods should be solidly frozen, and those in a chest-type freezer case should be stored below the frost line.

Raw foods from the grocery store, especially meats, poultry, eggs, and seafood, contain microbes, as all things do. Whether or not the microbes from these sources will multiply and cause illness can be largely a matter of what you do or fail to do in your own kitchen.

✔ KEY POINT   **Industry employs sound practices to safeguard the commercial food supply from microbial threats. Still, incidents of commercial food poisoning have incurred widespread harm to health.**

Food Safety in the Kitchen

Food can provide ideal conditions for bacteria to thrive and produce their toxins. Disease-causing bacteria require three things: (1) warmth (40°F to 140°F), (2) moisture, and (3) nutrients. To defeat bacteria, people who prepare food should keep in mind that food poisoning is always possible. Do these three things: keep hot food hot, keep cold food cold, and keep the kitchen clean. Keeping hot food hot includes cooking foods for long enough to reach an internal temperature that will kill microbes as described in the next section. Cooked foods must be held at 140° or higher until served. Refrigerate foods immediately after serving a meal, and definitely before two hours have passed (one hour if room temperature approaches 90°F).

Keeping cold food cold starts when you leave the grocery store. If you are running errands, shop last, so that the groceries will not stay in the car too long. (If ice cream begins to melt, it has been too long.) Upon arrival home, load foods into the refrigerator or freezer immediately. Keeping foods cold applies to defrosting foods, too. Thaw meats or poultry in the refrigerator, not at room temperature. Table 14-3 lists some safe keeping times for foods kept at or below 40° F.

Keeping the kitchen clean requires using freshly washed utensils and laundered towels, and washing your hands with soap before and during food handling. If you are ill or have open sores, stay away from food. Clean equipment frequently. Microbes love to nestle down in small, damp spaces such as the inner cells of sponges or the pores between the fibers of wooden cutting boards. It isn't true that wooden boards do not support microbial growth; they support microbial growth as much as other boards do. You can ensure safety of cutting boards and sponges by washing them in a dishwasher or by treating them as suggested below. Alternatively, sponges can be saved for car washing and other heavy cleaning chores, while the kitchen is cleaned with washable dishcloths that can be laundered often. Sponges with special antibacterial characteristics are also becoming available for purchase.

TABLE 14-3

Safe Refrigerator Storage Times (40°F)

1 to 2 days
Raw ground meats, breakfast or other raw sausages, raw fish or poultry; gravies

3 to 5 days
Raw steaks, roasts, or chops; cooked meats, vegetables, and mixed dishes; ham slices; mayonnaise salads (chicken, egg, pasta, tuna)

1 week
Hard-cooked eggs, bacon or hot dogs (opened packages); smoked sausages.

2 to 4 weeks
Raw eggs (in shells); bacon or hot dogs (packages unopened); dry sausages (pepperoni, hard salami); most aged and processed cheeses (Swiss, brick)

2 months
Mayonnaise (opened jar); most dry cheeses (parmesan, romano)

SOURCE: A. Hecht, Preventing food-borne illnesses, *FDA Consumer*, January/February 1991, p. 21; Refrigerator storage times for selected foods, *Consumer Reports on Health*, December 1991, p. 93.

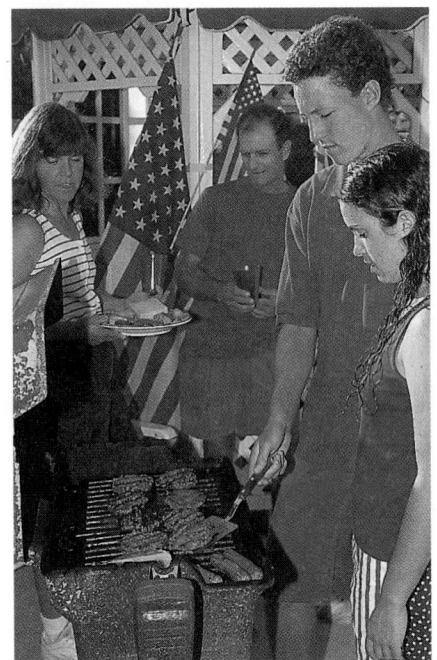

A safe hamburger is cooked well-done, appears brown (not pink) throughout, and is steaming hot. Place it on a clean plate when it's done.

mad cow disease formally, bovine spongiform encephalopathy (BSE); a fatal disease of cattle affecting the nerves and brain. Research has not yet determined whether the bovine disease is related to an extremely rare form of a fatal brain disease of people. BSE has plagued cattle herds of Great Britain and in 1996 some ten people there died from the human disease, leading researchers to suspect a link. In the United States, USDA's ongoing surveillance of herds has found them consistently free of BSE. In Great Britain, diseased cattle and their products are promptly destroyed, and no British beef or milk are imported into the United States.

To eliminate microbes you have three choices, each with benefits and drawbacks. One is to poison the microbes on boards, sponges, and other equipment with toxic chemicals such as bleach (one capful per gallon of water). The benefit is that chlorine can kill even the hardiest organism. The drawback is that chlorine that washes down household drains into the water supply forms chemicals that can harm waterways and fish.

A second option is to treat kitchen equipment with heat. Soapy water heated to 140°F kills most harmful organisms and washes most others away. This takes effort, though, since you have to use truly scalding water heated well beyond the temperature of the tap. An automatic dishwasher accomplishes both of the above: it washes in water hotter than hands can tolerate. Also, dishwasher detergents may contain chlorine. Whichever strategy you use, for a small initial investment, you can use truly safe implements to prepare your food.

✓ KEY POINT **To prevent food poisoning, always remember that it can happen. Keep hot foods hot, keep cold foods cold, and keep the kitchen clean.**

Troublesome Foods

Some foods are more hospitable to microbial growth than others. In general, foods that are high in moisture and nutrients and those that are chopped or ground are especially favorable hosts.

Meats and Poultry Meats and poultry require special handling. Raw meats and poultry bear labels to instruct consumers on meat safety (see Figure 14-1). Meats often contain all sorts of bacteria, and they provide a moist, nutritious environment that is just right for microbial growth. If you take burgers out to the grill on a plate, wash that plate in hot, soapy water before using it to hold the cooked burgers. Ground meat or poultry is handled more than other kinds and exposes much more surface area for bacteria to land on, so experts advise cooking to at least medium well done. For meat loaf, use a thermometer to test the internal temperature. Don't waste energy being alarmed by the media's latest sensation, such as **mad cow disease.** Pay attention, instead, to real threats from undercooked or improperly stored meats. Figure 14-2 lists safe internal temperatures of cooked meats, and other important temperatures.[*]

It goes without saying that any food with an "off" appearance or odor should not be used or even tasted. However, you cannot rely on your senses of smell and sight alone to warn you, because most hazards are not detectable by odor, taste, or appearance. Also, cooking does not destroy all bacterial toxins. Even hot cooked food, if handled improperly prior to serving, can cause illness.

To protect yourself as far as you can, always keep the possibility of food poisoning in mind. Delicious looking meatballs on a buffet should be steaming hot. Food at 140°F feels hot, not just warm.

Eggs Over the past 10 years, surveillance of food safety has revealed a threatening trend. Increasingly, when blood samples from food poisoning victims or samples of illness-causing foods are studied, *Salmonella* of a most virulent type

---

[*]The USDA's meat and poultry hotline answers questions about meat and poultry safety: 1-800-535-4555.

FIGURE 14-1

SAFE HANDLING INSTRUCTIONS FOR MEAT AND POULTRY

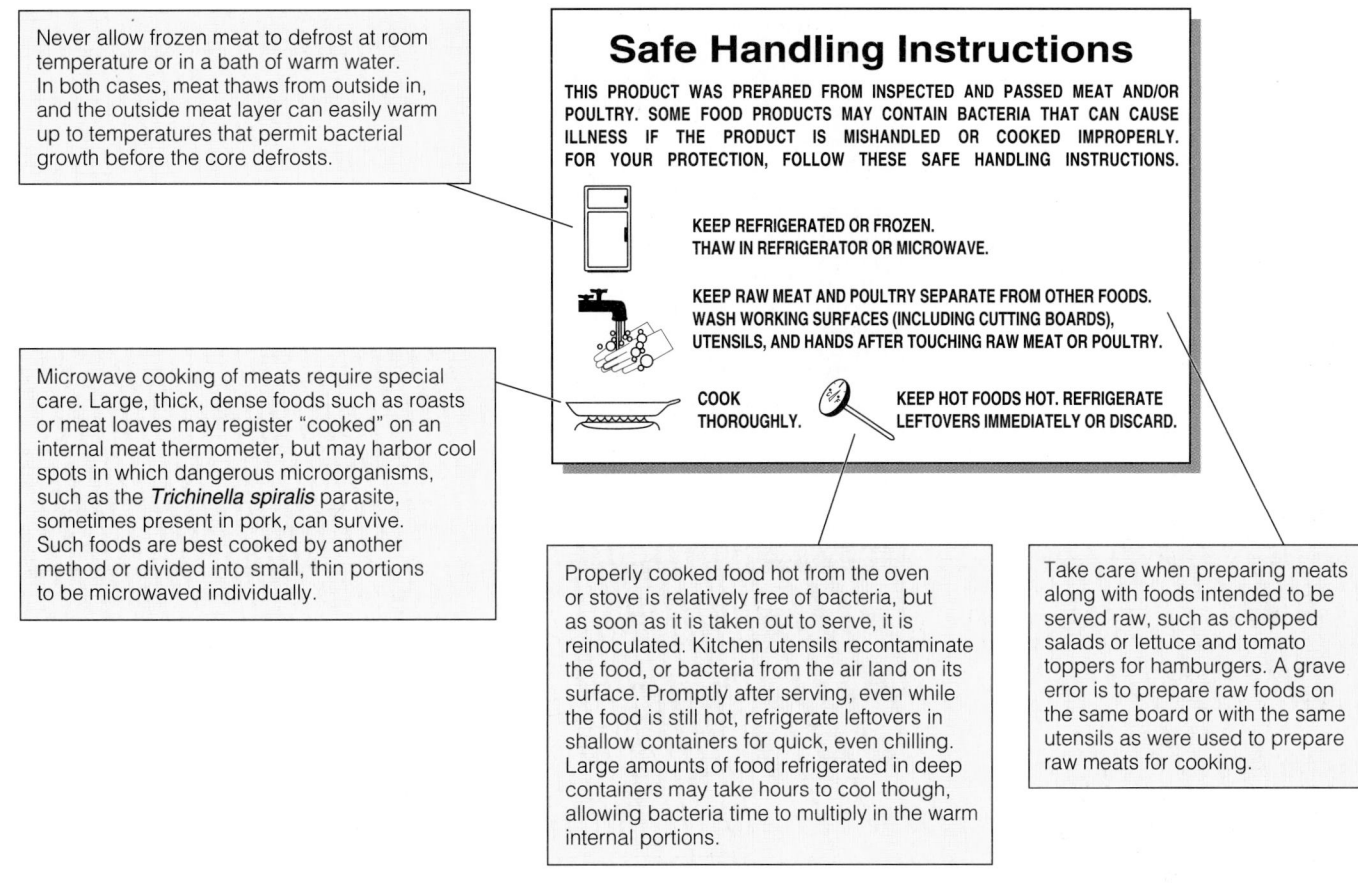

Never allow frozen meat to defrost at room temperature or in a bath of warm water. In both cases, meat thaws from outside in, and the outside meat layer can easily warm up to temperatures that permit bacterial growth before the core defrosts.

Microwave cooking of meats require special care. Large, thick, dense foods such as roasts or meat loaves may register "cooked" on an internal meat thermometer, but may harbor cool spots in which dangerous microorganisms, such as the *Trichinella spiralis* parasite, sometimes present in pork, can survive. Such foods are best cooked by another method or divided into small, thin portions to be microwaved individually.

Safe Handling Instructions

THIS PRODUCT WAS PREPARED FROM INSPECTED AND PASSED MEAT AND/OR POULTRY. SOME FOOD PRODUCTS MAY CONTAIN BACTERIA THAT CAN CAUSE ILLNESS IF THE PRODUCT IS MISHANDLED OR COOKED IMPROPERLY. FOR YOUR PROTECTION, FOLLOW THESE SAFE HANDLING INSTRUCTIONS.

KEEP REFRIGERATED OR FROZEN. THAW IN REFRIGERATOR OR MICROWAVE.

KEEP RAW MEAT AND POULTRY SEPARATE FROM OTHER FOODS. WASH WORKING SURFACES (INCLUDING CUTTING BOARDS), UTENSILS, AND HANDS AFTER TOUCHING RAW MEAT OR POULTRY.

COOK THOROUGHLY.

KEEP HOT FOODS HOT. REFRIGERATE LEFTOVERS IMMEDIATELY OR DISCARD.

Properly cooked food hot from the oven or stove is relatively free of bacteria, but as soon as it is taken out to serve, it is reinoculated. Kitchen utensils recontaminate the food, or bacteria from the air land on its surface. Promptly after serving, even while the food is still hot, refrigerate leftovers in shallow containers for quick, even chilling. Large amounts of food refrigerated in deep containers may take hours to cool though, allowing bacteria time to multiply in the warm internal portions.

Take care when preparing meats along with foods intended to be served raw, such as chopped salads or lettuce and tomato toppers for hamburgers. A grave error is to prepare raw foods on the same board or with the same utensils as were used to prepare raw meats for cooking.

is detected in the samples.[9] Raw, unpasteurized eggs seem especially likely to be contaminated. The Centers for Disease Control and Prevention warn that consumers should cooks eggs until the whites are set firmly, and the yolks begin to thicken, before eating them. No longer is it safe to drop a raw egg into a food or beverage that will not be cooked before consumption. You can still safely enjoy classic foods that call for raw eggs, such as Caesar salad dressing and hollandaise sauce, by preparing them with pasteurized egg replacers, sold in cartons in the dairy case, instead of raw eggs.

Seafood   For adults and children alike, eating raw or lightly steamed seafood is a risky proposition even if it is prepared by a master chef. The microorganisms that lurk there are undetectable, even to an expert.

People who like **sushi** know that not all varieties are made from raw fish. Many types are made with cooked crab meat and vegetables, avocado, or other delicacies and are perfectly safe to enjoy. Also, the rumor that freezing fish will make it safe to eat raw is only partly true. Freezing fish will kill mature parasitic worms, but only cooking can kill all worm eggs and other microorganisms that can cause illness.

sushi a Japanese dish that consists of vinegar-flavored rice, seafood, and colorful vegetables, typically wrapped in seaweed. Some sushi is wrapped in raw fish; other sushi contains only cooked ingredients.

FIGURE 14-2

FOOD SAFETY TEMPERATURES (FAHRENHEIT)

SOURCE: U.S. Department of Agriculture, 1993.

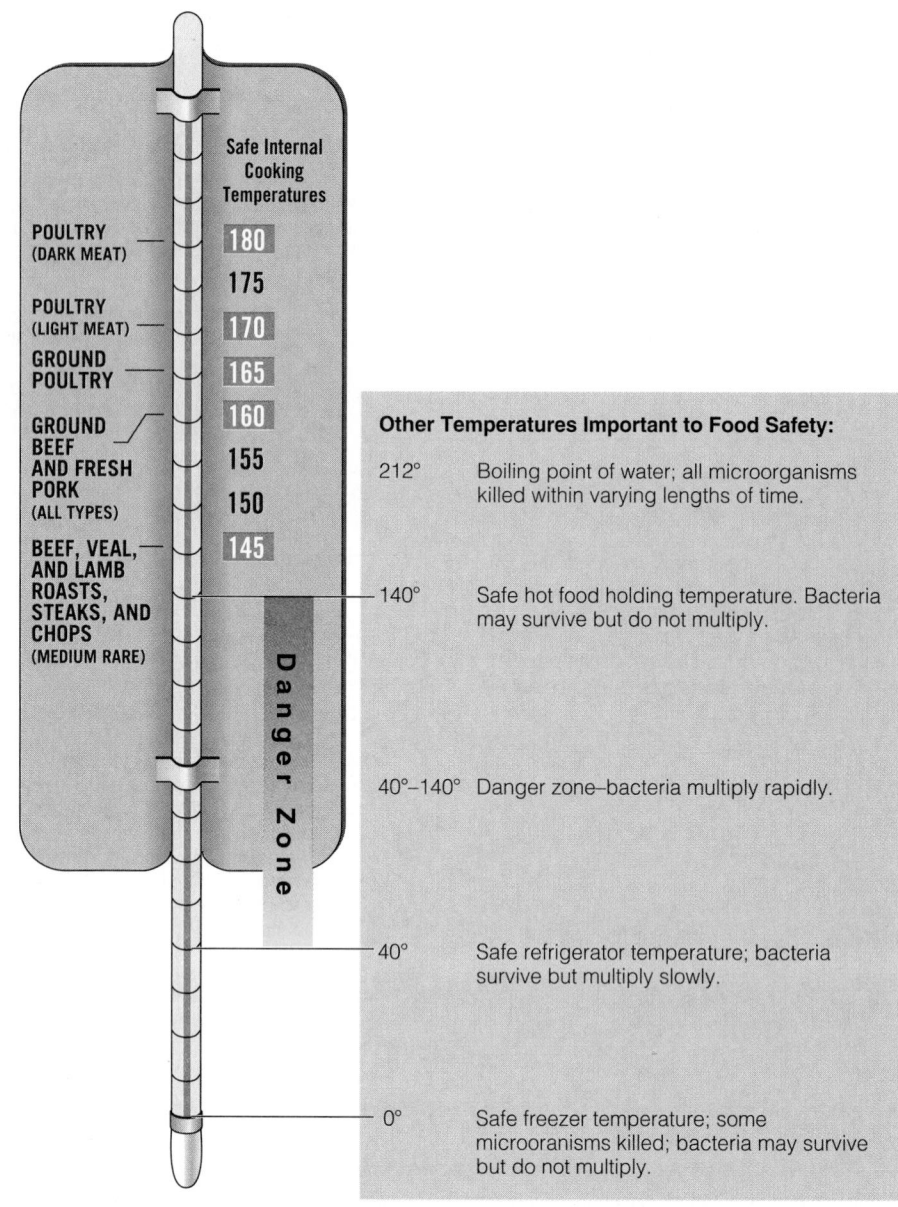

As population density increases along the shores of seafood-harvesting waters, pollution of those waters inevitably invades the seafood living there.* Watchdog agencies monitor commercial fishing waters and try to keep harvesters out of the worst areas. They eventually do catch cheaters, but meanwhile, unwholesome food can reach the market. In one season alone, black-market dealers may sell millions of dollars worth of clams and oysters taken illegally from closed harvesting areas.[10]

*To speak with an expert on seafood safety, call the FDA seafood hotline: 1-800-FDA-4010.

The food-borne infections that lurk in normal-appearing seafood can be even worse than those of spoilage: hepatitis; worms, flukes, and other parasites; severe viral intestinal disorders; poisoning by naturally occurring toxins; and other diseases.[11] Hepatitis infection causes prolonged illness that persists for months or years, severely damages the liver, greatly increases the risk of developing liver cancer, and, once in the body, is transmissible to others. Many types of worms depend on the blood of their host for food and reproduction; they attack digestive membranes, sometimes causing life-threatening perforations. Flukes attack the liver, damaging it.

People who have loved and eaten raw oysters and other seafood for years may try to brush off these threats because they have never experienced serious illness. Some have heard that alcoholic beverages taken with raw seafood eliminate risks or that hot sauce kills the bacteria, but these assertions are not true. A study did find a correlation between taking one drink of whiskey or wine and a reduced risk of disease after eating contaminated seafood, but this evidence is no guarantee of protection.[12] Hot sauce is useless against the bacteria that contaminate oysters.[13] Experts agree unanimously that the risks of eating raw or lightly cooked seafood today are unacceptably high due to environmental contamination.[14]

Hope for the future purity of foods, and especially of poultry, meats, and seafoods, comes on the crest of new advances in **biotechnology.** Geneticists are now able to tailor the DNA inside a living bacterial cell to yield a **biosensor** organism. The biosensor can detect chemicals that disease-causing microorganisms create in foods.[15] Such tests promise to be superior to today's methods of detecting harmful organisms in food products.[16] Their use may soon dramatically improve the safety of raw seafoods and other foods for sale in the market.

Picnics and Lunch Bags   For picnics that are fun and safe, and for safe packed lunches, keep these precautions in mind. Choose foods that last without refrigeration, such as fresh fruits and vegetables, breads and crackers, and canned spreads and cheeses that you can open and use on the spot. Aged cheeses, such as cheddar and Swiss, do well at environmental temperatures for an hour or two, but for longer periods, carry them in a cooler or thermal lunch bag. To keep lunch bag foods chilled, choose a thermal lunch bag and freeze beverages to pack in them with the foods. The beverages keep foods cold as they thaw in the hours before lunch. Keep mayonnaise cold. Mayonnaise is resistant to spoilage because of its acid content, but when it is mixed with chopped ingredients in pasta, meat, or vegetable salads, the mixtures spoil easily. The chopped ingredients have extensive surface areas for bacteria to invade, and foods that have been in contact with cutting boards, hands, and kitchen utensils have picked up at least a few bacteria earlier. Chill chopped salads well in shallow containers before, during, and after a picnic, and keep salad sandwiches cold until eaten.

Honey   Another danger lurks in honey. Honey can contain dormant spores of *Clostridium botulinum* that can awaken (germinate) in the human body to produce the deadly botulinum toxin mentioned earlier. Mature adults are usually protected against this threat, but infants under one year of age should never be fed honey, which can also be contaminated with environmental pollutants picked up by the bees. Honey has been implicated in several cases of sudden infant death.

Because food poisoning so common, the following Consumer Corner is devoted to it. Much grief can be averted by applying its advice.

biotechnology the science that manipulates biological systems or organisms to modify their products or components or create new products (see the Controversy).

biosensor a genetically altered microbe that provides a rapid, low-cost, and accurate test for toxic products of microbial agents in foods.

In many states, containers of raw oysters must bear this warning: "There is a risk associated with consuming raw oysters or any raw animal protein. If you have chronic illness of the liver, stomach or blood or have immune disorders, you are at greater risk of serious illness from raw oysters and should eat oysters fully cooked. If unsure of your risk, consult a physician."

More on biotechnology in this chapter's Controversy.

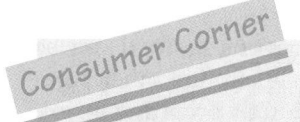

FOOD SAFETY WHILE TRAVELING

About half of the people who travel to places where cleanliness standards are lacking suffer from food-borne illnesses. Commonly known as traveler's diarrhea, these illnesses can ruin a trip. To avoid illness while traveling:

■ Before you travel, ask your physician which medicines to take with you in case you get sick.

■ Wash your hands often with soap and water, especially before handling food or eating.

■ Eat only cooked and canned foods. Eat raw fruits or vegetables only if you have washed them with your own clean hands in boiled water and peeled them yourself. Skip salads.

■ Be aware that water, and ice made from it, may be unsafe, too. Take along disinfecting tablets or an element that boils water in a cup. Drink only treated, boiled, canned, or bottled beverages, and drink them without ice, even if they are not chilled to your liking.

■ Avoid using the local water supply, even if you are just brushing your teeth, unless you boil or disinfect it first.

One journalist succinctly sums up these recommendations: "Boil it, cook it, peel it, or forget it."[17] If you follow these rules, chances are excellent that you will remain well.

✔ **KEY POINT**   **Some foods pose special microbial threats and so require special handling. Seafood is especially likely to be contaminated. Almost all types of food poisoning can be prevented by safe food preparation, storage, and cleanliness. Biosensors may one day ensure safety of raw foods.**

NATURAL TOXINS IN FOODS

Consumers may naively think they can eliminate all poisons from their diets by eating only "natural" foods. On the contrary, nature has provided natural foods with the natural poisons they need to fend off diseases, insects, and other predators. Humans rarely suffer actual harm from such poisons, but the *potential* for harm does exist.

A table in Chapter 11 names belladonna and hemlock as deadly poisons in the form of natural herbs. Few people know, however, that the herb sassafras contains a cancer-causing agent and is banned from use in commercially produced foods and beverages. Equally surprising is that cabbage, turnips, mustard greens, and radishes all contain small quantities of harmful goitrogens, compounds that can enlarge the thyroid gland and aggravate thyroid problems.

Cabbages and their relatives are celebrated for the nonnutrients they contain, compounds associated with low cancer rates. The protection seems to result when the mild toxins these foods contain force the body to build up its arsenal of carcinogen-destroying equipment.[18] Then, when a potent carcinogen arrives, the prepared body deals with it swiftly.

Other natural poisons in *raw* lima beans, and, in fruit seeds such as apricot pits, are members of a group called cyanogens, precursors to the deadly poison cyanide. Many countries restrict commercially grown lima beans to those varieties with the lowest cyanogen contents. As for fruit seeds, they are seldom deliberately eaten. An occasional swallowed seed or two presents no danger, but a couple of dozen seeds could be fatal to a small child. Perhaps the most infamous cyanogen is laetrile, a compound erroneously represented as a cancer cure. True, the poison laetrile kills cancer cells, but only at doses that kill the person, too. Research over the past 100 years has proven laetrile to be an ineffective cancer treatment and dangerous to the taker.

Potatoes contain many natural poisons, including solanine, a bitter, powerful, narcotic-like substance. The small amounts of solanine normally found in potatoes are harmless, but solanine can build up to toxic levels when potatoes are exposed to light during storage. Cooking does not destroy solanine, but because most of a potato's solanine is in the green layer that develops just beneath the skin, it can be peeled off, making the potato safe to eat. If the potato tastes bitter, however, throw it out.

At some times of the year, seafood may become contaminated with the so-called red tide toxin that occurs during algae blooms. Eating seafood contaminated with red tide causes a form of food poisoning that paralyzes the eater. The FDA monitors fishing waters for red tide algae and closes waters to fishing whenever it appears.

These examples of naturally occurring toxins should serve as a reminder of three principles. First, any substance can be toxic when consumed in excess. Practice moderation in the use of all foods. Second, poisons are poisons, whether made by people or by nature. It is not the source of a chemical that makes it hazardous, but its chemical structure. Third, by including a variety of foods in the diet, consumers ensure that toxins in foods are diluted by the volume of the other foods eaten.

✔ **KEY POINT** **Natural foods contain natural toxins that can be hazardous if consumed in excess. To avoid poisoning by toxins, eat all foods in moderation, treat chemicals from all sources with respect, and choose a variety of foods.**

ENVIRONMENTAL CONTAMINANTS

A justifiably high-ranking concern about the food supply everywhere is environmental contamination of foods. As populations increase worldwide and nations become more industrialized, the problem looms ever larger. A food **contaminant** is anything that does not belong there.

The potential harmfulness of a contaminant depends in part on the extent to which it lingers in the environment or in the human body—that is, on how **persistent** it is. Some contaminants are short-lived because microorganisms or agents such as sunlight or oxygen can break them down. Some contaminants linger in the body only for a short time because the body can rapidly excrete them or metabolize them to harmless compounds. These contaminants present little cause for concern. Some contaminants resist breakdown, however, and interact with the body's systems without being metabolized or excreted. These

contaminant any substance occurring in food by accident; any food constituent that is not normally present.

persistent of a stubborn or enduring nature; with respect to food contaminants, the quality of remaining unaltered and unexcreted in plant foods or in the bodies of animals and human beings.

FIGURE 14-3

BIOACCUMULATION OF TOXINS IN THE FOOD CHAIN

If none of the chemicals are lost along the way, one person ultimately receives all of the toxic chemicals that were present in the original several tons of producer organisms.

❹ A person whose principal animal-protein source is fish may consume about 100 pounds of fish in a year.

❸ Larger fish consume a few tons of plankton-eating fish in the course of their lifetimes—and the toxic chemicals from the small fish become more concentrated in the flesh of the larger species.

❷ The toxic chemicals become more concentrated in the plankton-eating fish that consume several tons of producer organisms in their lifetimes.

❶ Producer organisms may become contaminated with toxic chemicals.

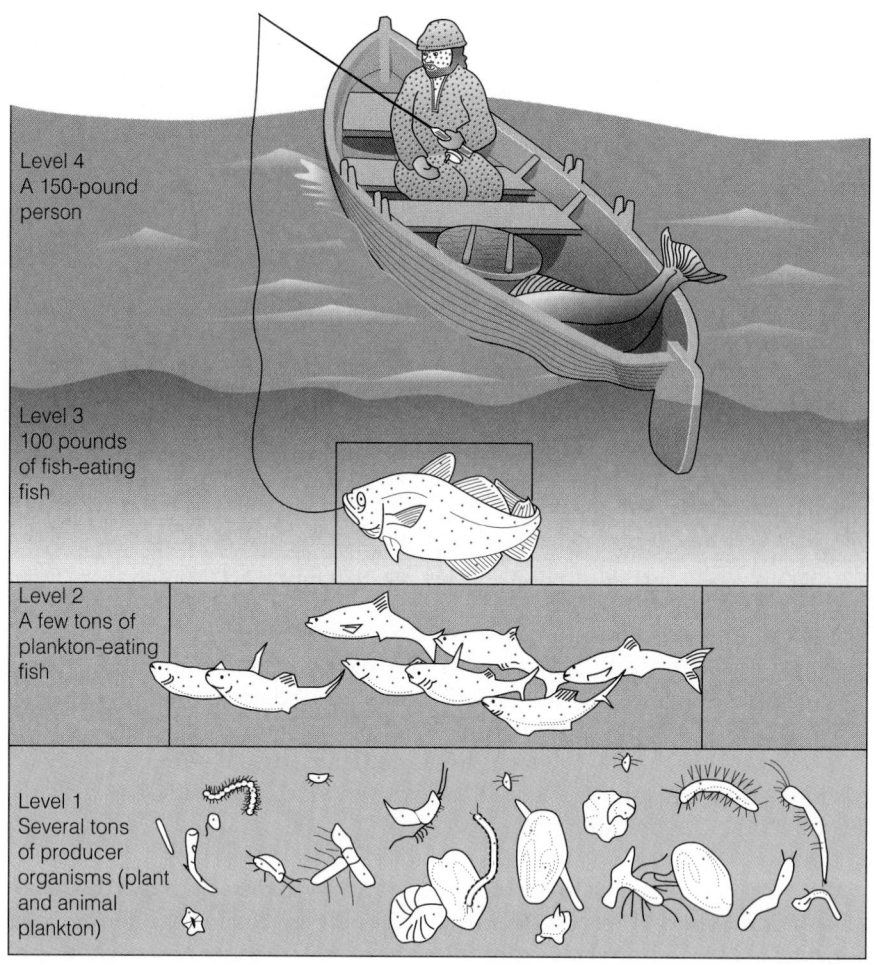

Level 4
A 150-pound person

Level 3
100 pounds of fish-eating fish

Level 2
A few tons of plankton-eating fish

Level 1
Several tons of producer organisms (plant and animal plankton)

Toxic chemicals :·

bioaccumulation the accumulation of a contaminant in the tissues of living things at higher and higher concentrations along the food chain.

heavy metal any of a number of mineral ions such as mercury and lead; so called because they are of relatively high atomic weight. Many heavy metals are poisonous.

organic halogen an organic compound containing one or more atoms of a halogen—fluorine, chlorine, iodine, or bromine.

can pass from one species to the next and accumulate at higher concentrations in each level of the food chain, a process called **bioaccumulation.** Figure 14-3 shows how toxic chemicals accumulate in the food chain.

How much of a threat do environmental contaminants pose to the food supply? For the most part, the hazards appear to be small because the FDA monitors the presence of contaminants in foods and requires that contaminated foods be removed from the market. In the event of an accidental industrial spill or one caused by a natural event, such as a volcano, however, the hazard can suddenly become great. The following paragraphs describe how two different types of contaminants have found their way into the food supply in the past. One is a **heavy metal** (mercury) that was released into waterways by industry and accumulated in fish that people ate. The other is an **organic halogen** (polybrominated biphenyl or PBB) that was accidentally spilled into livestock feed and eaten by animals whose meat people eventually ate in turn.

A classic example of acute contamination occurred in 1953 when a number of people in Minamata, Japan, became ill with a disease no one had seen before. By 1960, 121 cases had been reported, including 23 in infants. Mortality was high; 46 died, and the survivors suffered progressive blindness, deafness, loss of coordination, and impaired mental function. The cause of this misery was ultimately revealed: Manufacturing plants in the region were discharging mercury into the waters of the bay, the mercury was turning to methylmercury on leaving the factories, and the fish in the bay were accumulating this poison in their bodies. Some of the people who were poisoned had been eating fish from the bay every day. The infants who contracted the disease had not eaten any fish, but their mothers had, and even though the mothers exhibited no symptoms during their pregnancies, the poison had been affecting their unborn babies.

As for PBB, in 1973, half a ton of the toxic compound was accidentally mixed into some livestock feed that was distributed throughout the state of Michigan. The chemical found its way into millions of animals and then into people who ate their meat. The seriousness of the accident began to come to light when dairy farmers reported that their cows were going dry, aborting their calves, and developing abnormal growths on their hooves. More than 30,000 cattle, sheep, and swine and more than a million chickens were destroyed, but the effects on people were not prevented. An estimated 97 percent of Michigan's residents had been exposed to PBB. Some of the exposed farm residents suffered nervous system aberrations and liver disorders.

Mercury is a heavy metal and PBB is an organic halogen. These two classes of chemicals are among the most toxic and are still being liberated into our environment daily. The number of contaminants we could discuss here, and the amount of information available about them, is far beyond our scope. Table 14-4 selects a few contaminants of great concern in foods to show how pervasively a contaminant can affect the body.

✔ KEY POINT **Persistent environmental contaminants pose a small but significant threat to the safety of food. An accidental spill can create an extreme hazard.**

PESTICIDES

The use of **pesticides** helps to ensure the survival of some crops, but the damage pesticides do to the environment is considerable and increasing. Moreover, there is some question about whether the widespread use of pesticides has really improved the overall yield of food. Even with extensive pesticide use, U.S. agriculture loses about one-fifth of its crops to pests, and worldwide, pests destroy about one-third of food crops every year.[19]

No doubt, pesticides do help preserve some crops, but at a considerable cost in other respects. Many pesticides are broad-spectrum poisons that damage all living cells, not just those of pests. Their use, therefore, can pose hazards to the plants and animals in natural systems, and especially to workers involved with pesticide production and transport. High doses of pesticides applied to laboratory animals cause birth defects, sterility, tumors, organ damage, and central nervous system impairment. At one time, a legal requirement stated that no traces of pesticides found to cause cancer in animals would be allowed in

pesticides chemicals used to control insects, diseases, weeds, fungi, and other pests on crops and around animals. Used broadly, the term includes *herbicides* (to kill weeds), *insecticides* (to kill insects), and *fungicides* (to kill fungi).

Chemical Contaminants of Concern in Foods:

Heavy metals:
  Lead
  Mercury
  Cadmium
  Selenium
  Arsenic
Halogens and organic halogens:
  Chlorine
  Iodine
  Vinyl chloride
  Ethylene dichloride
  Trichloroethylene (TCE)
  Polybrominated biphenyl (PBB)
  Polychlorinated biphenyls (PCBs)
Others:
  Asbestos
  Dioxins
  Acrylonitrile
  Lysinoalanine
  Diethylstilbestrol (DES)
  Heat-induced mutagens
  Antibiotics (in animal feed)

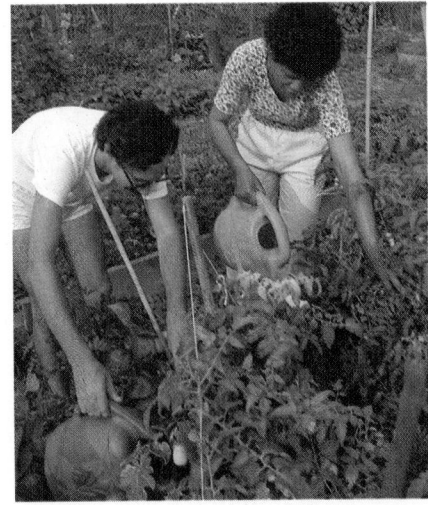

In some small gardens, handwork can take the place of pesticides.

TABLE 14-4

Examples of Contaminants in Foods

Name and Description	Sources	Toxic Effects	Typical Route to Food Chain
Cadmium (heavy metal)	Used in industrial processes including electroplating, plastics, batteries, alloys, pigments, smelters, and burning fuels. Present in cigarette smoke and in smoke and ash from volcanic eruptions.	No immediately detectable symptoms; slowly and irreversibly damages kidneys and liver.	Enters air in smokestack emissions, settles on ground, absorbed into food plants, consumed by farm animals, and eaten in vegetables and meat by people. Sewage sludge and fertilizers leave large amounts in soil; runoff contaminates shellfish.
Lead[a] (heavy metal)	Lead crystal decanters and glassware, painted china, old house paint, batteries, pesticides, old plumbing, and some food-processing chemicals.	Displaces calcium, iron, zinc, and other minerals from their sites of action in the nervous system, bone marrow, kidneys, and liver, causing failure to function.	Originates from industrial plants and pollutes air, water, and soil. Still present in soil from many years of leaded gasoline use.
Mercury (heavy metal)	Widely dispersed in gases from earth's crust; local high concentrations from industry, electrical equipment, paints, and agriculture.	Poisons the nervous system, especially in fetuses.	Inorganic mercury released into waterways by industry and acid rain is converted to methylmercury by bacteria and ingested by food species of fish (tuna, swordfish, and others).
Polychlorinated biphenyls (PCBs) (organic compounds)	No natural source; produced for use in electrical equipment (transformers, capacitors).	Long-lasting skin eruptions, eye irritations, growth retardation in children of exposed mothers, anorexia, fatigue, others.	Discarded electrical equipment; accidental industrial leakage, or reuse of PCB containers for food.

[a]For answers to questions concerning lead, call the National Lead Information Center at 1-800-424-LEAD.

Pesticides:

✔ Kill pests' natural predators.
✔ Accumulate in the food chain.
✔ Pollute the water, soil, and air.

foods. In 1996, this provision of the law was eliminated, but the law still applies to food additives, as a later section explains.

Ironically, pesticides also promote the survival of the very pests they are intended to wipe out. Consider a pesticide aimed at some insects that are attacking a crop. The pesticide may kill *almost* 100 percent of them, but thanks to the genetic variability of large populations, some insects are likely to survive exposure. The resistant insects can then multiply free of competition and soon will produce many offspring—offspring that have inherited resistance to the pesticide. This new strain of insects can attack the crop with enhanced vigor. To control these resistant insects requires application of a new and more powerful pesticide—and this leads to the emergence of a population of still more resistant insects. The same effects arise from use of herbicides and fungicides. One alternative to this destructive series of events is to manage pests using a combination of natural and biological controls, as discussed in Controversy 15.

Pesticides are not produced only in laboratories; they also occur in nature. The nicotine in tobacco and psoralens in celery are examples. Natural pesticides, however, are less damaging to other living things and less persistent in the environment than most human-made ones.

If an ideal pesticide could be made, it would be one that would destroy only the pest, not accumulate in the food chain, and quickly degrade to nontoxic products so that by the time consumers ate the food, no harmful **residues** would remain. Unfortunately, no such perfect pesticide exists, although biological controls substituted for them may qualify (see Controversy 15). Developing new pesticides and monitoring their use are ongoing activities that require continued vigilance on the part of government agencies.

As Figure 14-4 demonstrates, pesticide residues on agricultural products can sometimes survive processing and may be present in and on foods served to people.[20] Risks to health from pesticide exposure are probably small for healthy adults, but children, because of their lower body weights and immature detoxifying systems, may be more at risk for some types of pesticide poisoning.[21] When asked, most people in the United States say they are very concerned about pesticide residues in and on their foods.

The legal **tolerance limits** for pesticide residues in foods are low, generally 1/100 to 1/1,000 the level found to cause no effect in laboratory animals. Over 10,000 tolerance regulations state maximum levels for over 300 pesticide chemicals used on various specific crops in the United States. If a pesticide is misused, growers risk fines, lawsuits, and destruction of their crops. In 25 years of testing, the FDA has seldom found residues above tolerance levels, so it appears that pesticides are generally used according to regulations. This makes sense, because growers are not anxious to spend extra capital on unneeded chemicals.[22]

residues whatever remains. In the case of pesticides, those amounts that remain on or in foods when people buy and use them.

tolerance limit the maximum amount of a residue permitted in a food when a pesticide is used according to label directions.

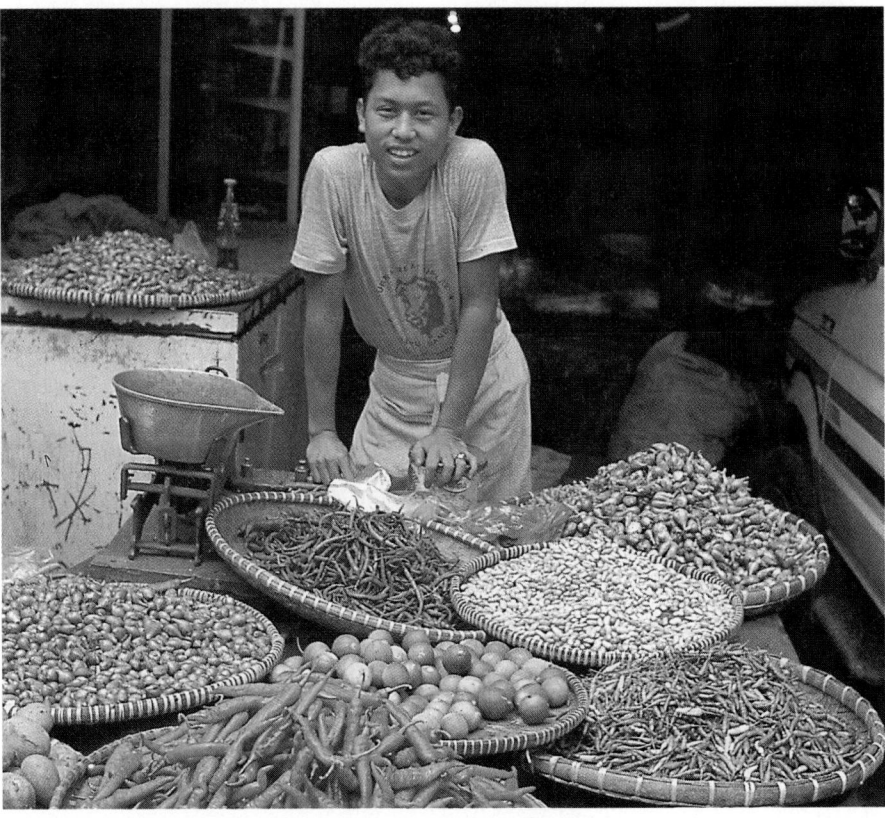

Foods imported from other countries may contain residues of pesticides that are banned from use here.

FIGURE 14-4

POSSIBLE PATHWAYS OF PESTICIDE RESIDUES TO A FAST-FOOD MEAL
The red dots in the figure represent pesticide residues left on foods from field spraying or postharvest application. Notice that most pesticides follow fats in foods, and that some processing methods, such as washing and peeling vegetables, reduce pesticide concentrations while others tend to concentrate them.

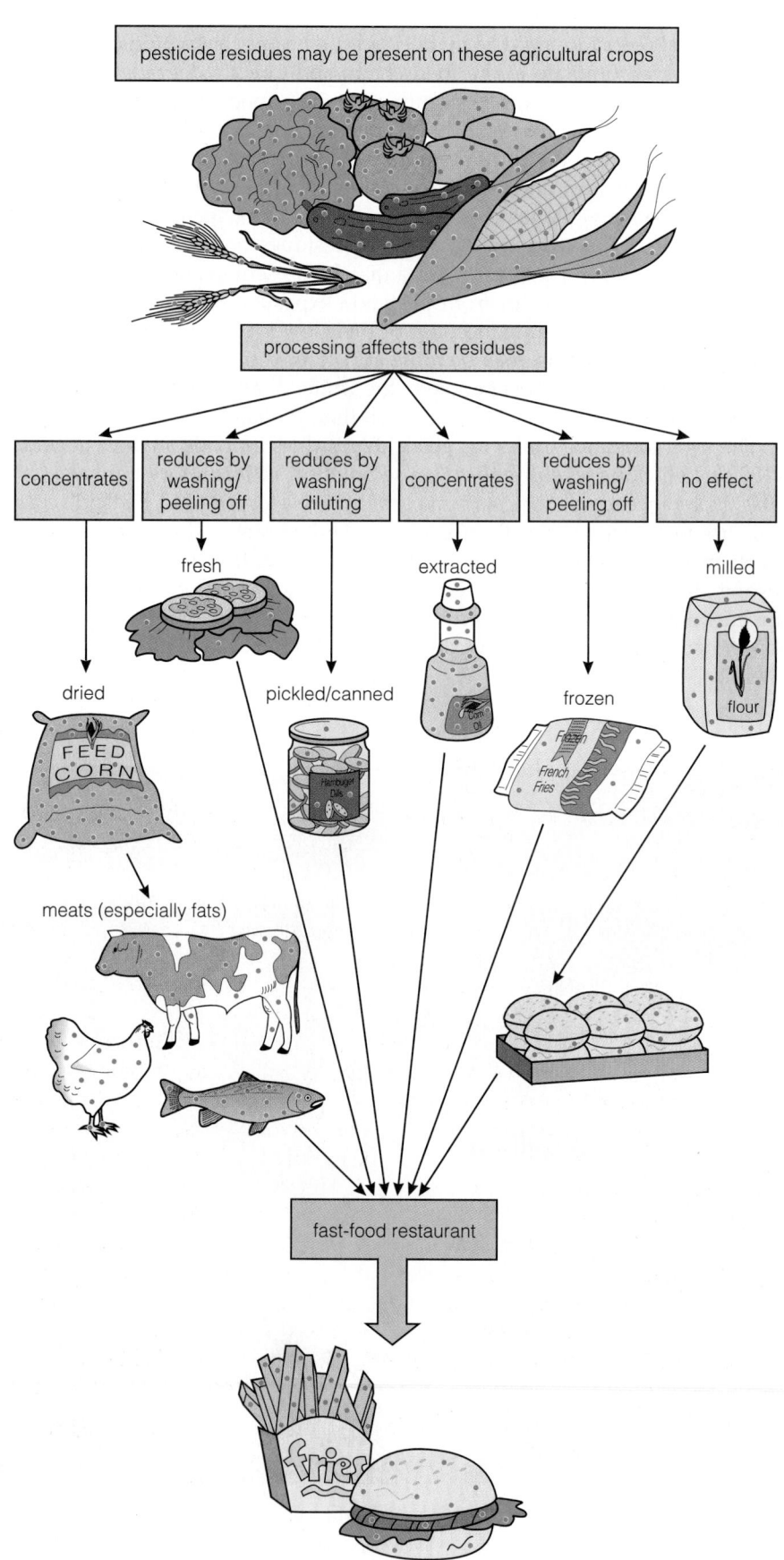

TABLE 14-5

Ways to Reduce Pesticide Residue Intake

- Trim fat from meat and remove skin from poultry and fish; discard fats and oils in broths and pan drippings. (Pesticide residues concentrate in the animal's fat.)
- Vary meat, poultry, and fish choices from day to day and do not take fish oil capsules.
- Wash fresh produce in water. Use a scrub brush, and rinse thoroughly.
- Use a knife to peel an orange or grapefruit, do not bite into the peel.
- Discard the outer leaves of leafy vegetables such as cabbage and lettuce.
- Peel waxed fruit and vegetables. (Waxes don't wash off and can seal in pesticide residues.)
- Peel vegetables such as carrots and fruits such as apples when appropriate. (Peeling removes pesticides that remain in or on the peel, but also removes fibers, vitamins, and minerals.)

A loophole in federal regulations allows companies in the United States to make banned pesticides and export them to other countries. The banned pesticides then return to the United States on imported foods, a circuitous route that has been called the "circle of poison." When imported foods are found to contain illegal residues, they may be refused entry. The FDA collects some samples of both domestic and imported foods and analyzes them using methods that can detect residues well below tolerances. If the FDA finds products that exceed permitted limits, it can seize the products or order them destroyed. The overwhelming majority of the foods tested by the FDA are found to contain either no residues or residues within federally permitted limits.[23] A problem is that budget restraints limit the FDA's testing capacity.

In addition to monitoring pesticides in the marketplace, the FDA also monitors people's pesticide intakes, along with their intakes of essential minerals, industrial chemicals, heavy metals, and radioactive materials. Four times a year FDA surveyors buy more than 200 foods in U.S. grocery stores in several cities, prepare them ready to serve, and then analyze them. Food preparation often destroys or removes contaminants, so the FDA tests for levels at least five times lower than permitted limits. FDA's findings confirm that the bulk of the U.S. food supply contains no excessive pesticide residues.[24]

The FDA does not sample *all* food shipments or test for *all* pesticides. Fewer than 700 inspectors and scientists test food samples from the multitude of farms, groves, docks, airports, warehouses, and processing plants the agency oversees. The FDA cannot (nor can it be expected to) guarantee 100 percent safety in the food supply. Instead, it sets conditions so that substances do not become a hazard and acts promptly when problems or suspicions arise.

Consumers also bear some responsibility for their own health and safety with respect to pesticides. They can learn about the potential benefits and dangers of pesticide use, discuss regulations and alternatives with others, advise their government representatives about their findings, and apply pressure wherever it will help change inappropriate procedures. Meanwhile, people can minimize their risks by following the guidelines offered in Table 14-5.*

---

*For answers to any questions about any sort of pesticides, call the EPA's 24-hour National Pesticide Hotline: 1-800-858-PEST.

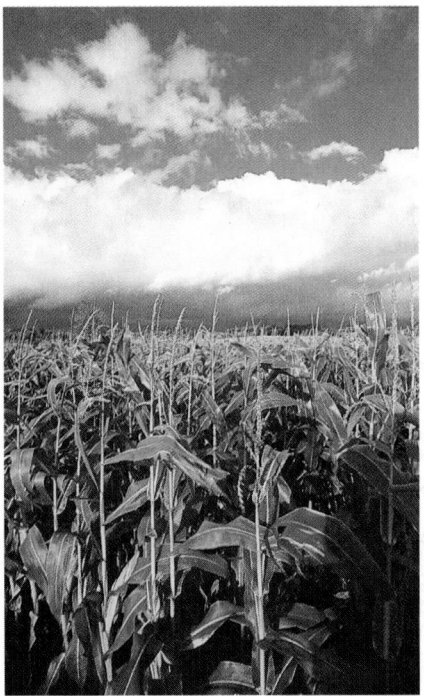

Crops like these can be kept safe from pests through a combination of natural and biological controls.

ultrahigh temperature (UHT) short-time exposure of a food to temperatures above those normally used, to sterilize it.

modified atmosphere packaging (MAP) preservation of a perishable food by packaging it in a gas-impermeable container from which air has been removed, or to which another gas mixture has been added.

canning preservation by killing all microorganisms present in food and by then sealing out air. The food, container, and lid are heated until sterile; as the food cools, the lid makes an airtight seal, preventing contamination.

freezing preservation by lowering food temperature to a point that halts life processes. Microorganisms do not die but remain dormant until the food is thawed.

drying preservation by removing sufficient water from food to inhibit microbial growth.

extrusion a process by which the form of food is changed, such as changing corn to corn chips; not a preservation measure.

In addition to the suggestions in the table, consumers who buy fresh foods grown locally can confirm that the growers have used responsible methods. Consumers who want pesticide-free produce shouldn't look for "perfect" fruits and vegetables. Pesticide-free produce may have a few minor blemishes, but these are not a hazard.

People who want quick meals may often rely on convenience foods and fast foods, and prepare few foods at home from farm-fresh produce. The gains in convenience and speed in food preparation must be weighed against a loss of control over how, exactly, foods are processed and what, exactly, they contain. The next sections describe a much debated issue concerning the safety of some foods.

✓ KEY POINT   **Pesticides can be part of a safe food protection program, but can also be hazardous when handled or used inappropriately. The FDA tests for pesticide residues in both domestic and imported foods. Consumers can take steps to minimize their ingestion of pesticide residues in foods.**

FOOD PROCESSING AND THE NUTRIENTS IN FOODS

Much of the total food eaten today, whether in restaurants or at home, has been prepared in some way by industry. People often ask what processing does to foods and to their nutritional value.

Many forms of processing aim to extend the usable life of a food—that is, to preserve it. To preserve food, a process must prevent three processes: (1) microbial growth, (2) oxidative changes, and (3) enzymatic destruction of food molecules. The first two of these were mentioned in earlier sections. Enzymatic destruction occurs as active enzymes in food cells break down their internal molecular structures and cell membranes and walls. Processes involving heat denature the enzymes, and those applying cold slow enzyme activity.

In general, food processing involves trade-offs. It makes food safer, or it gives food a longer usable lifetime, or it cuts preparation time—but at the cost of some vitamin and mineral losses. A process such as pasteurization, which makes milk safe to drink, is clearly worth that cost. Incidentally, those boxes of milk on the shelves of the grocery store that can be kept at room temperature at home have been treated with a process called **ultrahigh temperature (UHT)**. The milk is exposed to temperatures above those of pasteurization for just long enough to sterilize it.

Other processed foods may even gain a nutritional edge over their unprocessed counterparts, such as when fat is removed by processing from milk or other foods. The next sections explain each of these preservation or processing techniques—**modified atmosphere packaging (MAP), canning, freezing, drying, extrusion**—and their effects on nutrients.

✓ KEY POINT   **Processing aims to protect food from microbial, oxidative, and enzymatic spoilage. Some nutrients are lost in processing.**

Modified Atmosphere Packaging

Today, in most produce departments, shoppers choose bags of washed, trimmed, fresh, chilled salads and chopped vegetables. These products are convenient for busy cooks who have little time for preparation. True, they are more expensive to purchase than comparable loose vegetables, but, unopened, they last much longer and so save on waste. The secret to these vegetables' long shelf life is a technique called modified atmosphere packaging (MAP). The method also preserves freshness in soft pasta noodles, baked goods, prepared foods, fresh and cured meats, seafoods, dry beans and other dry products, ground and whole-bean coffee, and other foods.

Food manufacturers using MAP first package foods in plastic film or other wraps that oxygen cannot penetrate. Then, they remove the air inside the package, creating a vacuum, or they replace the air with a mixture of oxygen-free gases, such as carbon dioxide and nitrogen. By excluding oxygen MAP:

- slows ripening of fruits and vegetables.
- reduces spoilage by mold and bacterial growth.
- prevents discoloration of cut vegetables and fruits.
- prevents spoilage by rancidity of fats.
- slows development of "off" flavors from accelerated enzyme action that breaks down flavor and aroma molecules.
- slows enzyme-induced breakdown of vitamins.

Chilling of all foods packaged this way is imperative to keep them fresh and safe.

MAP foods retain their vitamins much longer than the same foods when exposed to the air. MAP foods also taste fresh, making them especially popular with consumers. One concern about the MAP method is that it may permit growth of the *Clostridium botulinum* bacterium in moist, low acid foods, such as lunch meats or cooked dishes, when they are kept for long periods at too-warm temperatures. Properly stored, however, the foods are as safe and nutritious as fresh foods.

✔ KEY POINT **Modified atmosphere packaging makes many fresh packaged foods available to consumers. MAP foods compare well to fresh foods in terms of nutrient quality.**

Canning

Canning is one of the more effective methods of protecting food against the growth of microbes (bacteria, fungi, and yeasts) that might otherwise spoil it, but canned foods, unfortunately, do have fewer nutrients. Like other heat treatments, the canning process is based on time and temperature. Each small increase in temperature has a major killing effect on microbes and only a minor effect on nutrients. In contrast, long heating times are costly in terms of nutrient losses. Therefore industry chooses treatments that employ the **high-temperature–short-time (HTST) principle** for canning.

Which nutrients does canning affect, and how? To answer these questions, food scientists have performed many experiments. They have paid particular attention to three vulnerable water-soluble vitamins: thiamin, riboflavin, and vitamin C.

high-temperature–short-time (HTST) principle the rule that every 10°C (18°F) rise in processing temperature brings about an approximately tenfold increase in microbial destruction, while only doubling nutrient losses.

The Food Feature later in this chapter gives tips on preserving nutrients during cooking.

Acid stabilizes thiamin, but heat rapidly destroys it; therefore the foods that lose the most thiamin during canning are the low-acid foods such as lima beans, corn, and meat. Up to half, or even more, of the thiamin in these foods can be lost during canning. Unlike thiamin, riboflavin is stable to heat but sensitive to light, so glass-packed, not canned, foods are most likely to lose riboflavin. Vitamin C's special enemy is an enzyme (ascorbic acid oxidase) present in fruits and vegetables as well as in microorganisms. By destroying this enzyme, HTST processes such as canning actually help to preserve at least some of the product's vitamin C. Some will be destroyed by the heat of the process, though. As for the fat-soluble vitamins, they are relatively stable and are not affected much by canning.

Minerals are unaffected by heat, so they cannot be destroyed as vitamins can be. Both minerals and water-soluble vitamins can be lost, however, when they leak into canning or cooking water that the preparer then throws away. Losses are closely related to the extent to which a food's tissues have been broken, cut, or chopped and to the length of time the food is in the water.

Some minerals are added when foods are canned. Important in this respect is sodium chloride, table salt, which is added for flavoring. Many food companies have begun making low-salt versions of their products. Unfortunately, because the low-salt batches are smaller, these products may cost more than the higher-salt versions.

✔ **KEY POINT** **Some water-soluble vitamins are destroyed by canning, but many more diffuse into the canning liquid. Fat-soluble vitamins and minerals are not affected by canning, but minerals also leach into canning liquid.**

Freezing

Freezing is an alternative to canning as a means of preserving food. People often ask how frozen foods compare with canned. In general, frozen foods' nutrient contents are similar to those of fresh foods; losses are minimal. The freezing process itself does not destroy any nutrients, but some losses may occur during the steps taken before freezing, such as the quick dunking into boiling water (blanching), washing, trimming, or grinding. Vitamin C losses are especially likely because they occur whenever tissues are broken and exposed to air (oxygen destroys vitamin C). Uncut fruits, especially if they are acidic, do not lose their vitamin C; strawberries, for example, may be kept frozen for over a year without losing any vitamin C. Mineral contents of frozen foods are much the same as for fresh.[25]

Frozen foods may even be more nutritious than fresh. Fresh foods are often shipped long distances, and to ensure that they make the trip without bruising or spoiling, they are often harvested unripe. Frozen foods are shipped frozen, so that produce is allowed to ripen in the field and to develop nutrients to their fullest potential. If foods are frozen and stored under proper conditions, they will often contain more nutrients when served at the table than fresh fruits and vegetables that have stayed in the produce department of the grocery store even for a day.

Frozen foods have to be kept solidly frozen at below 32°F or 0°C, if they are to retain their nutrients. Vitamin C converts to its inactive forms rapidly at warmer temperatures. Food may seem frozen at 36°F or 2°C, but much of it is actually unfrozen, and enzyme-mediated changes can occur fast enough to completely destroy the vitamin C in only two months. If you want to maximize the nutritive value of the foods you store at home, invest in a freezer thermometer, monitor your frozen-food storage place, and keep it at below freezing temperature (0°F).

✓ KEY POINT   Foods frozen promptly and kept frozen lose few nutrients.

Drying

Consumers wonder how dried or dehydrated foods compare with canned and frozen foods. Dried or dehydrated foods have their own special characteristics. Drying offers several advantages. It eliminates microbial spoilage (because microbes need water to grow), and it greatly reduces the weight and volume of foods (because foods are mostly water). Furthermore, commercial drying does not cause major nutrient losses. Foods dried in heated ovens at home, however, may sustain dramatic nutrient losses. Vacuum puff drying and freeze drying, which take place in cold temperatures, conserve nutrients especially well.

Sulfite additives are added during the drying of fruits such as peaches, grapes (raisins), and plums (prunes) to prevent browning. Some people suffer allergic reactions when they consume sulfites. Sulfur dioxide helps to preserve vitamin C as well, but it is highly destructive to thiamin. This is of small concern, however, because most dehydrated products with added sulfur dioxide were not major sources of thiamin before processing.

✓ KEY POINT   Commercially dried foods retain most of their nutrients, but home-dried foods often sustain dramatic losses.

Extrusion

Some food products, particularly cereals and snack foods, have undergone a process known as extrusion. In this process the food is heated, ground, and pushed through various kinds of screens to yield different shapes, such as breakfast "puffs," some fast-food potato products, the "bits" you sprinkle on salad, and so-called food novelties. Considerable nutrient losses occur during extrusion, and nutrients are usually added to compensate. But foods this far removed from the original fresh state are still lacking significant nutrients (notably, vitamin E), and consumers should not rely on them as staple foods. Enjoy them, but only as occasional snacks and as additions to enhance the appearance, taste, and variety of meals.

✓ KEY POINT   Extrusion involves heat and destroys nutrients.

FOOD ADDITIVES

People ask valid questions about **additives.** What are they, why are they there, and are they dangerous in any way? In FDA's list of concerns presented at the start of this chapter, food additives were not a high priority. Compared with the FDA's other concerns, additives pose little danger to consumers, and the FDA has confidence in the ability of regulations already in place to control additive use in the food industry.

additives substances that are added to foods, but are not normally consumed by themselves as foods.

GRAS (generally recognized as safe) list a list established by the FDA, of food additives long in use and believed safe.

Manufacturers use food additives to give foods desirable characteristics: color, flavor, texture, stability, enhanced nutrient composition, or resistance to spoilage. Additives, classed by their functions, are listed with their definitions in Table 14-6, and some are discussed further in the section that follows.

Regulations Governing Additives

The FDA is charged with the responsibility for deciding what additives shall be in foods. The FDA's judgments on additives hinge primarily on their safety and effectiveness for the stated purpose. To obtain permission to use a new additive in food products, a manufacturer must test the additive and then satisfy the FDA that:

- It is effective (it does what it is supposed to do).
- It can be detected and measured in the final food product.

Then the manufacturer must study the effects of the additive when fed in large doses to animals under strictly controlled conditions to prove that:

- It is safe (it causes no cancer, birth defects, or other injury).

Finally, the manufacturer must submit all test results to the FDA. The whole process may take many years.

The FDA then schedules a public hearing and announces the date and location in its official publication, *FDA Consumer.* Consumers are invited to participate at these hearings, where experts present testimony for and against granting permission to use the additive. Thus the consumer's rights and responsibilities are written into the provisions for deeming additives safe.

FDA's approval of an additive does not give manufacturers free license to add it to foods with abandon. On the contrary, the FDA writes a regulation stating in what amounts, for what purposes, and in what foods the additive may be used. No additives are permanently approved; all are periodically reviewed.

The GRAS List Many substances were exempted from complying with this procedure at the time it was first instituted because they had been used for a long time and their use entailed no known hazards. Some 700 substances in all were put on the **generally recognized as safe (GRAS) list.** When substantial scientific evidence or public outcry has questioned the safety of a GRAS list additive, however, its safety has been reevaluated. All substances about which any legitimate question was raised have been removed or reclassified.

To remain on the GRAS list, an additive must not have been found to cause cancer in any test on animals or human beings. The Delaney clause (the part of the law that states this criterion) is uncompromising in addressing carcinogens in food and drugs; in fact, this policy has been challenged in court.[26] One congressional report called the Delaney clause "scientifically unmanageable" and noted that it does not allow food safety to keep up with science.[27] For now the Delaney clause remains in effect with regard to food additives.

The Problem with Delaney The Delaney clause states that "no additive shall be deemed to be safe if it is found to induce cancer when ingested by man or animal." That sounds simple and clear enough, yet you may be aware of

TABLE 14-6

Food Additives by Function

- **antimicrobial agents** preservatives that prevent spoilage by mold or bacterial growth. Familiar examples are acetic acid (vinegar) and sodium chloride (salt). Others are benzoic, propionic, and sorbic acids; nitrites and nitrates; and sulfur dioxide.
- **antioxidants** preservatives that prevent rancidity of fats in foods and other damage to food caused by oxygen. Examples are vitamins E and C, BHA, BHT, propyl gallate, and sulfites.
- **artificial colors** certified food colors, added to enhance appearance. (*Certified* means approved by the FDA). Vegetable dyes are extracted from vegetables such as beta-carotene from carrots. Food colors are a mix of vegetable dyes and synthetic dyes approved by the FDA for use in food.
- **artificial flavors, flavor enhancers** chemicals that mimic natural flavors and those that enhance flavor.
- **bleaching agents** substances used to whiten foods such as flour and cheese. Peroxides are examples.
- **chelating agents** defined in Chapter 4 as molecules that bind other molecules. As additives, they prevent discoloration, flavor changes, and rancidity that might occur because of processing. Examples are citric acid, malic acid, and tartaric acid (cream of tartar).
- **nutrient additives** vitamins and minerals added to improve nutritive value.
- **preservatives** antimicrobial agents, antioxidants, chelating agents, radiation, and other additives that retard spoilage or preserve desired qualities, such as softness in baked goods.
- **radiation** ionizing rays that act as a preservative by disrupting chemical structures within cells, including the cell bodies of microorganisms. Irradiation is a process, but it causes new substances to form in the food; therefore radiation is considered to be an additive. Controversy 14 discusses food irradiation.
- **thickening and stabilizing agents** ingredients that maintain emulsions, foams, or suspensions or lend a desirable thick consistency to foods. Dextrins (short chains of glucose formed as a breakdown product of starch), starch, and pectin are examples. (Gums such as carrageenan, guar, locust bean, agar, and gum arabic are others.

exceptions made for additives in some products. Saccharin was the first of these. In the 1970s, the FDA tried to ban saccharin because tests had failed to prove that saccharin did not cause cancer in animals, but Congress voted to allow saccharin to remain in products and carry a warning. This move was an attempt to balance the Delaney clause with current food safety and cancer knowledge. A little historical background may provide some insight.

The Delaney clause was adopted over 30 years ago at a time when scientists' awareness of cancer causes was limited to radiation, tobacco smoke, a chemical used to make dyes, and soot. Since then researchers have identified more than three dozen human carcinogens and several hundred animal carcinogens. In addition, technology has advanced so that substances once detectable only in parts per thousand can now be measured in parts per billion or even per trillion. (One part per trillion is equivalent to about one grain of sugar in an Olympic-sized swimming pool.) We cannot provide absolute protection from all carcinogens in foods, as Congressman Delaney once thought we could. Current laws that mandate such protection are asking the impossible.

toxicity the ability of a substance to harm living organisms. All substances are toxic if high enough concentrations are used.

margin of safety in reference to food additives, a zone between the concentration normally used and that at which a hazard exists. For common table salt, for example, the margin of safety is 1/5 (five times the concentration normally used would be hazardous).

The Margin-of-Safety Concept An important distinction governs decisions about an additive's safety—the distinction between **toxicity** and hazard associated with substances. Toxicity is a general property of all substances; hazard is the capacity of a substance to produce injury *under conditions of its use.* All substances can be toxic at some level of consumption, but they are called hazardous only if they are actually consumed in sufficiently large quantities. An additive is not a hazard if it proves toxic only in an immense amount that people never consume. The additive is a hazard only if it is toxic as actually used.

A food additive is supposed to have a wide **margin of safety.** Most additives that involve risk are allowed in foods only at levels 100 times below those at which the risk is still known to be zero. Experiments to determine the extent of risk involve feeding test animals the substance at different concentrations throughout their lifetimes. The additive is then permitted in foods at 1/100 the level that causes no harmful effect whatever in the animals. In many foods, *naturally* occurring toxins appear at levels that bring their margins of safety closer to 1/10. Even nutrients, as you have seen, involve risks at high dosage levels. The margin of safety for vitamins A and D is 1/25 to 1/40; it may be less than 1/10 in infants. For some trace elements, it is about 1/5. People consume common table salt daily in amounts only three to five times less than those that cause serious toxicity.

The margin-of-safety concept also applies to nutrients used to fortify foods. Iodine has been added to salt to prevent iodine deficiency, but it has to be added with care because it is a deadly poison in excess. Similarly, iron added to grain products has doubtless helped prevent many cases of iron-deficiency anemia in women and children but iron in excess can cause iron overload in men. The upper limit has to be remembered.

Most additives used in foods are there because they offer benefits that outweigh their risks or that make the risks worth taking. In the case of color additives that only enhance the appearance of foods but do not improve their health value or safety, no amount of risk may be deemed worth taking. Only 10 of an original 80 synthetic color additives are still approved by the FDA for use in foods, and screening of these substances continues.[28]

Manufacturers must comply with other regulations as well. Additives must not be used:

- In quantities larger than those necessary to achieve the needed effects.
- To disguise faulty or inferior products.
- To deceive the consumer.
- Where they significantly destroy nutrients.
- Where their effects can be achieved by economical, sound manufacturing processes.

The regulations in force governing the management of intentional additives are well conceived, and on the whole, they have been effective. Funding shortages limit the capabilities of watchdog agencies such as the FDA, however, and some mistakes and false reports do slip by.

✔ KEY POINT **The FDA regulates the use of intentional additives. Additives must be safe, effective, and measurable in the final product. Additives on the GRAS list are assumed to be safe because they have long been used. No additive may be used that has been found to cause cancer in animals or people. Additives used must have wide margins of safety.**

A Closer Look at Selected Food Additives

The following sections focus on those few individual food additives that receive the most negative publicity because people ask questions about them most often. The order is alphabetical; it is not an order of importance.

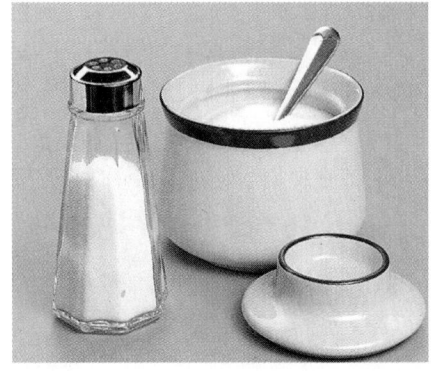

Two long-used preservatives.

Antimicrobial Agents   Foods can go bad in two ways: one dangerous, one not. The dangerous way is by becoming hazardous to health; the other way is by losing their flavor and attractiveness. An example of the dangerous way is the growth of microbes that can cause food poisoning. Preservatives known as *antimicrobial agents* protect food from these microbes.

The best-known, most widely used antimicrobial agents are two common substances—salt and sugar. Salt has been used since before recorded history to preserve meat and fish; sugar serves the same purpose in jams, jellies, and canned and frozen fruits. (Any jam or jelly that toots its "no preservatives" horn is exaggerating. There is no need to add extra preservatives, so most makers do not.) Both salt and sugar work by withdrawing water from the food; microbes cannot grow without water. Today, other additives such as potassium sorbate and sodium propionate are also used to extend the shelf life of baked goods, cheese, beverages, mayonnaise, margarine, and many other products.

The *nitrites*, another group of antimicrobial agents, are added to meats and meat products for three main purposes: to preserve their color (especially the pink color of hot dogs and other cured meats); to enhance their flavor by inhibiting rancidity (in cured meats); and to protect against bacterial growth. In particular, in amounts much smaller than needed to confer color, nitrites prevent the growth of the bacterium that produces the deadly botulinum toxin described earlier in the chapter.

Nitrites clearly perform important jobs, but they have been the object of controversy because they can be converted in the human body to nitrosamines, which cause cancer in animals. Some cured meats are available without nitrites. However, reducing nitrites consumed in meats would hardly make a difference in a person's overall exposure to nitrosamine-related compounds. For example, an average cigarette smoker inhales 100 times the nitrosamines that the average bacon eater ingests. Likewise, a beer drinker imbibes up to roughly five times the amount that the bacon eater receives, and cosmetics release into the skin about twice as much as is delivered from bacon. Even the air inside automobiles delivers measurable nitrites.[29]

✔ **KEY POINT**   **Microbial food spoilage can be prevented by antimicrobial additives. Of these, sugar and salt have a long history of use. Nitrites added to meats have been associated with cancer in laboratory animals.**

Antioxidants   The other way food can go bad is by undergoing changes in color and flavor caused by exposure to oxygen in the air (oxidation). Often these changes involve little hazard to health, but they damage the food's appearance, taste, and nutritional quality. Familiar examples of these changes are sliced apples or potatoes turning brown and oil going rancid. Antioxidant preservatives protect food from this kind of spoilage. Some 27 antioxidants are approved for use in foods, vitamin C (ascorbate) and vitamin E (tocopherol) among them.

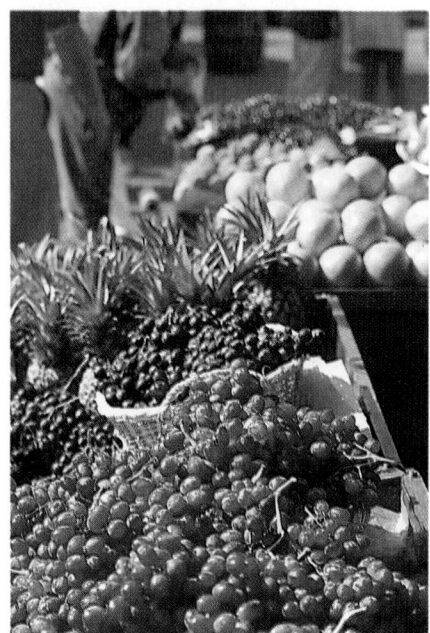

Raw grapes may legally be treated with sulfites. Wash them thoroughly before eating them.

Another group of antioxidants is the sulfites. They are used to prevent oxidation in many processed foods, in alcoholic beverages (especially wine), and in drugs. They used to be popular with restaurant owners for use on salad bars because they kept raw fruits and vegetables looking fresh, but this use was banned after a few people experienced dangerous allergic reactions to the sulfites. The FDA now prohibits sulfite use on food meant to be eaten raw, with the exception of grapes, and it requires foods and drugs to list on their labels any sulfites that are present. For most people, sulfites do not pose a hazard in the amounts used in products, but they have one other drawback. As mentioned earlier, sulfites can destroy a lot of thiamin in foods. A person choosing a food that contains sulfites should not count on that food to provide a share of the daily need for thiamin.

The ban on sulfites has stimulated a search for alternatives, with pleasing results. Some producers now use honey to clarify browned apple juice. Agriculturists have also created a hybrid apple that doesn't brown.[30] The combination of four GRAS additives can also perform the tasks of substitute sulfites.[31*]

Two other antioxidants in wide use are the well-known BHA and BHT, which prevent rancidity in baked goods and snack foods. BHT provides a refreshing change from the many tales of woe and cancer scares associated with other additives. Among the many tests performed on BHT were several showing that animals fed large amounts of this substance developed *less* cancer when exposed to carcinogens and lived longer than controls. BHT apparently protects against cancer through an antioxidant effect similar to that of vitamin E. To obtain this effect, though, a much larger amount of BHT must be present in the diet than the U.S. average. A caution: used experimentally at levels of intake even higher than this, the substance has *produced* cancer.

This discussion provides the opportunity to mention an important point about additives. No two additives are alike. Generalizations about them are meaningless. No single valid statement can apply to all of the 3,000-odd different substances commonly added to foods. Questions about which additives are safe and under what conditions of use have to be asked and answered item by item.

✓ **KEY POINT** **Antioxidants prevent oxidative changes in foods that would lead to unacceptable discoloration and texture changes in the food. Ingestion of the antioxidants sulfites can cause problems for some people; BHT may offer antioxidant effects in the body.**

Artificial Colors   As mentioned, only about 10 synthetic artificial colors are still on the GRAS list, a highly select group that has survived considerable screening. They are among the most intensively investigated of all additives. In fact, they are much better known than the *natural* pigments of plants, and the limits on the safety of their use can be stated with greater certainty.

Still, the food colors, because they are dispensable have been more heavily criticized than almost any other group of additives. Simply stated, they only make foods pretty, whereas other additives, such as preservatives, make foods

---

*The four GRAS additives are citric acid, ascorbic acid, sodium acid pyrophosphate, and calcium chloride.

safe. Hence with food colors we can afford to require that their use entail no risk, whereas with other additives we may have to compromise between the risks of using them and the risks of *not* using them.

The food color tartrazine (yellow number 5) causes an allergic reaction in susceptible people. Symptoms include hives, itching, and nasal congestion, sometimes severe enough to require medical treatment. It is not a common problem; only 1 or 2 in 10,000 individuals may have the reaction. Still, that is over 20,000 individuals in the nation as a whole. In addition, some hyperactive children may be sensitive to tartrazine, as Chapter 12 explained. People with allergy and parents of children who react to tartrazine rightly demand to know where the dye is in foods so that they can avoid it. They cannot just avoid yellow-colored foods, because tartrazine is used to confer turquoise, green, and maroon colors on foods and drugs as well. Legislation is now in force requiring that tartrazine be listed on all labels of foods that contain it so that consumers can avoid it if they wish.

✔ KEY POINT **The addition of artificial colors is tightly controlled. Some people react adversely to the colorant tartarzine.**

Artificial Flavors and Flavor Enhancers While only a few artificial colors are currently permitted in foods, close to 2,000 artificial flavors and flavor enhancers are approved, making them the largest single group of food additives. One of the best-known members of this group is monosodium glutamate, or MSG (trade name, Accent), the monosodium salt of the amino acid glutamic acid. MSG is used widely in restaurants, especially Asian restaurants, as a flavor enhancer. In addition to enhancing other flavors, research indicates that MSG may itself possess a basic taste independent of the well-known sweet, salty, bitter, and sour tastes.[32]*

MSG has received publicity because it can produce a cluster of adverse reactions, recently named the **MSG symptom complex** by FDA, in many individuals. Symptoms include burning sensations, chest and facial flushing or pain, throbbing headaches, and the others listed in the margin. MSG has been investigated extensively enough to be deemed safe for adults to use (except people who react adversely to it, of course), but it is kept out of foods for infants because very large doses have been shown to destroy brain cells in developing mice. Infants have not yet developed the capacity to fully exclude such substances from their brains and so are more sensitive to them. No one really knows how common this reaction to MSG is or why it might occur. A probable link may lie in elevated blood levels of the MSG component glutamate, a compound known to stimulate the release of some types of pituitary hormones in experimental animals.[33] FDA is currently considering banning the words "no MSG" from labels of foods that contain other sources of glutamate. Meals containing carbohydrate seem less likely to induce adverse effects from MSG than meals of broth, so when dining on Asian-style foods, potentially sensitive people should perhaps order dishes such as soups that contain noodles, and eat plenty of plain rice with main dishes to provide carbohydrate, as do Asians themselves.

---

*The taste produced by MSG is termed *umami.*

MSG symptom complex the acute, temporary, and self-limiting reactions experienced by many people upon ingesting a large dose of MSG. The name MSG symptom complex, given by FDA, replaces the former *Chinese restaurant syndrome.*

Foods Containing Tartrazine:
Orange drinks (Tang, Daybreak, Awake).
Gatorade (lime flavored).
Gelatin desserts (Jell-O, Royal).
Golden Blend Italian dressing (Kraft).
Some cake mixes and icings (Duncan Hines, Pillsbury, Cake Mate).
Imitation banana or pineapple extract (McCormick).
Seasoning salt (French's).
Macaroni and cheese dinner (Kraft).
'Cheez' curls and balls (Planter's).
Fruit chews (Skittles).
Butterscotch squares and candy corn (Brach's).

MSG Symptom Complex:
✔ Breathing problems in people with asthma.
✔ Burning sensations on forearms, chest, and back of neck.
✔ Chest pain.
✔ Drowsiness.
✔ Facial pressure or tightness of skin.
✔ Headache.
✔ Nausea.
✔ Numbness of the neck that spreads to arms and back.
✔ Palpitations.
✔ Tingling, warmth, weakness in face, upper back, neck, and arms.
✔ Weakness.

SOURCE: D. J. Raiten, J. M. Talbot, and K. D. Fisher, Executive summary from the report: Analysis of adverse reactions to monosodium glutamate (MSG), *Journal of Nutrition* 125 (1995): 2892S–2906S.

incidental additives substances that can get into food not through intentional introduction but as a result of contact with the food during growing, processing, packaging, storing, or some other stage before the food is consumed. The terms *accidental* and *indirect additives* mean the same thing.

✓ **KEY POINT**   **Among flavorings added to foods, the flavor enhancer MSG has been determined to cause reactions in people with sensitivities to it.**

Nutrient Additives   Nutrients added to improve or to maintain the nutritional value of foods make up another class of additives. Among them are the enrichment nutrients added to refined grains, the iodine added to salt, vitamins A and D added to dairy products, and the nutrients used to fortify breakfast cereals. When nutrients are added to a nutrient-poor food, it may appear from its label to be nutrient-rich. It is, but only in those nutrients chosen for addition. Nutrients are sometimes also added for other purposes. Vitamins C and E used as antioxidants are examples already mentioned.

✓ **KEY POINT**   **Nutrients are added to foods to enrich or to fortify them. These additives do not necessarily make the foods nutritious, only rich in the vitamins and minerals that have been added.**

Incidental Food Additives

Indirect or **incidental additives** are called *additives,* but are really contaminants that find their way into food as the result of some phase of production, processing, storage, or packaging. For example, among incidental additives are tiny bits of plastic, glass, paper, tin, and the like from packages, and chemicals from processing, such as the solvent used to decaffeinate some coffees.

Some microwave products are sold in "active packaging" that participates in cooking the food. Pizza, for example, may rest on a cardboard pan coated with a thin film of metal that absorbs microwave energy and may heat up to 500°F. During the intense heat, some particles of the packaging components migrate into the food.[34] Regular microwave packages heat up less, but particles still migrate. Materials from both kinds of packaging are under study to determine their safety for consumption. Until more is known, a wise choice is to use only glass or ceramic containers and to avoid reusing disposable containers, such as margarine tubs, for microwaving.

Coffee filters, milk cartons, paper plates, and frozen food packages can all be made of bleached paper and so can contaminate foods with trace amounts of compounds known as dioxins. Dioxins form during the chlorination step in making bleached paper. Dioxins can migrate into foods that come in contact with bleached paper, but the amounts entering food are infinitesimally small—one part per trillion, or the equivalent of one second in 32,000 years. Such amounts do not appear to present a health risk to people, and drinking milk from bleached cartons appears to be safe.[35] Dioxins are persistent, however, and they leach into the environment by way of both paper mill effluent and discarded paper products in landfills. Dioxins accumulate as do heavy metals and organic halogens, becoming more and more concentrated in land, water, and animals until they build up to hazardous levels.

Incidental additives sometimes find their way into foods, but adverse effects are rare. These additives are well regulated, just as intentional additives are. All food packagers are required to perform specific tests to discover whether materials from packages are migrating into foods. If they are, their safety must be confirmed by strict procedures like those governing intentional additives.

A topic of interest to many consumers, but of small concern to the FDA are the hormones administered to livestock that produce food. FDA has deemed the practice safe, and does not require testing of food products for traces of the drugs. The next section provides the details about the hormones that prompted FDA's decision.

✓ **KEY POINT**   **Incidental additives are substances that get into food during processing. They are well regulated, and most present no hazard.**

GROWTH HORMONE IN MEAT AND MILK

"Hormone milk" is what opponents call the milk of dairy cattle treated with the cattle form of **growth hormone, bovine somatotropin (BST).** The hormone is produced by genetically engineered bacteria, and livestock growers administer it to cattle as a drug.[36] Many people fear the introduction of this "artificial" drug into meat animals or dairy herds. In truth, synthetic growth hormone is virtually identical to growth hormone made naturally in the pituitary gland of the animal's brain.[37]

Many ranchers and farmers advocate the use of growth hormone because it makes meat animals develop more meat and less pure fat and dairy cows produce up to 25 percent more milk.[38] At the same time, they eat only three-quarters the normal allotment of feed. To the farmers, these changes mean higher profits from more market-ready product without the high costs of more cattle, more farmhands, or more equipment. The environment may profit as well. Smaller herds can live on smaller plots of cleared land, and less feed means less feed production, less fuel transportation, and less overall environmental impact (Chapter 15 gives details).

As for the safety of BST, in a report from its Technology Assessment Conference, the National Institutes of Health concludes, "As currently used in the United States, meat and milk from [hormone-] treated cows are as safe as those from untreated cows."[39] The FDA has approved BST for agricultural use.[40]

Any claims of danger from BST fall apart under scientific scrutiny.[41] Most fears of BST stem from failure to distinguish steroid hormones, which can be taken orally because they survive digestion, from peptide hormones, which are destroyed by digestive enzymes. Estrogen, found in many oral contraceptives, is a steroid hormone; BST, however, is a peptide hormone. Also, the amount of hormone found in the milk of BST-treated cows is within the range that can occur naturally.[42] Besides, about 90 percent of all BST, regardless of its source, is destroyed by pasteurization.

Even if some BST were to survive digestion and processing to enter the bloodstream, it would have no effect on the body. This is because the chemical structures of growth hormones from animals differ widely from the structure of **human somatotropin (HST),** the hormone active in human beings. When BST was first discovered, scientists hoped to use it to treat growth hormone–deficient children. Tests proved disappointing, for BST failed to stimulate receptors for human growth hormone and thus had no effect on the children's growth.

Cows treated with BST suffer more udder infections (mastitis) and so are given more antibiotics—and these drugs then show up in the cows' milk and meat.[43] Eating the meat could thus pose a hazard to those allergic to the drugs but all milk and meat are tested for drug residues and contaminated

growth hormone a hormone (somatotropin) that promotes growth and that is produced naturally in the pituitary gland of the brain.

bovine somatotropin (BST) growth hormone of cattle, which can be produced for agricultural use by genetic engineering. Also called *bovine growth hormone (BGH).*

human somatotropin (HST) human growth hormone.

products not sold. Whether consumers will reject milk or meat from hormone-treated cattle will be the final word on BST. Other such issues are raised in this chapter's Controversy.

✓ **KEY POINT**   **Bovine somatotropin causes cattle to produce more meat and milk on less feed than untreated cattle. Opponents raise ethical issues concerning this practice, but the FDA has deemed it safe.**

To sum up the messages of this chapter, U.S. foods are safe and hazards are rare. Precautions against food poisoning are the most important measures people can take to protect themselves from illness caused by foods. For optimal nutrition, though, which lies beyond safety, people can do more. The Food Feature that follows offers pointers on the selection and cooking of foods for the healthiest possible diet.

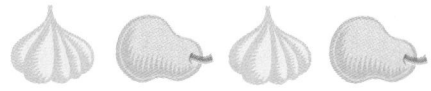

FOOD FEATURE

MAKING WISE FOOD CHOICES AND COOKING TO PRESERVE NUTRIENTS

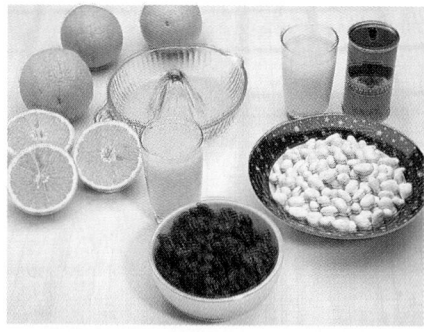

In terms of nutrient density, canned juice is almost as nutritious as fresh, but yogurt-covered raisins are *not* as nutritious as plain raisins.

In general, the more heavily processed foods are, the less nutritious they become. Does that mean, then, that everyone should avoid all processed food? The answer is not simple: in each case it depends on the food and on the process. Consider the case of orange juice and vitamin C. Orange juice is available in several forms, each processed a different way. Fresh juice is simply squeezed from the orange, a process that extracts the fluid juice from the fibrous structures that contain it. Each 100 calories of the fresh-squeezed juice contains 111 milligrams of vitamin C. When this juice is condensed by heat, frozen, and then reconstituted, as is the juice from the freezer case of the grocery store, 100 calories of the reconstituted juice contain just 88 milligrams of vitamin C, because vitamin C is destroyed in the condensing process. Canning is even harder on vitamin C: 100 calories of canned orange juice has 82 milligrams of vitamin C.

These figures may seem to indicate that fresh juice is the superior food, and so it may be. But consider this: most people's RDA of vitamin C (60 milligrams) is covered by a single serving of any of the above choices. In this case, at least for vitamin C, the losses due to processing are not a problem. Besides, processing confers enormous convenience and distribution advantages. Fresh orange juice spoils. Shipping fresh juice to distant places in refrigerated trucks costs much more than shipping frozen juice (which takes up less space) or canned juice (which requires no refrigeration). The fresh product still contains active enzymes that continue to degrade its compounds (including vitamin C) and so cannot be stored indefinitely without compromising nutrient quality. Frozen and canned juices remain virtually unchanged for long periods. The savings gained from shipping and storing canned and frozen juices are passed on to consumers. Without canned or frozen juice, people with limited incomes or those with no access to fresh juice would be deprived of this excellent food.

Some processing stories are not so rosy. In Chapter 8, for instance, you saw how processed foods are often loaded with sodium as their potassium is leached away, exactly the wrong effect for people with hypertension. A related mischief of processing is the addition of sugar and fat—palatable, high-calorie additives that reduce nutrient density. For example, consider nuts and raisins covered with "natural yogurt." This may sound like one healthy food being added to another, but a look at the ingredient panel warns that generous amounts of sugar and fat accompany the yogurt. About 75 percent of the weight of the product is sugar and fat; only 8 percent is yogurt. To pick just one nutrient for an example, here is what happens to the iron density of the raisins: 100 calories of raisins = 0.71 milligrams of iron; 100 calories of "yogurt" raisins = 0.26 milligrams of iron. These foods taste so good that wishful thinking can easily take hold, but the reality is that sugar- and fat-coated food is candy. The word *yogurt* on the label means only that one of the ingredients of the candy coating is some small amount of yogurt.

Names, even whole-food names, written on labels do not prove that foods so named provide any nutritional benefit to consumers. The foods themselves have to be nutritious. Incidentally, do not conclude from this example that raisins are a good source of iron. Compared with other food sources of iron on a per-calorie basis, raisins fall short. The iron Snapshot in Chapter 8 showed some iron-rich foods.

A good general rule for making food choices is to choose whole foods to the greatest extent possible and to seek out among processed foods only the ones that processing has improved nutritionally. (When processing removes fat, as in skim milk, it is often a benefit to the consumer.) Being realistic, few people have the time to bake all their own bread from scratch, to shop every few days for fresh meats, or to wash, peel, chop, and cook fresh fruits and vegetables at every meal. This is where food processing comes in. Commercially prepared whole-grain breads, frozen cuts of meats, bags of frozen vegetables, and canned or frozen fruit juices do little disservice to nutrition and enable the consumer to eat a wide variety of foods at great savings in time and human energy. The nutrient contents of processed foods exist on a continuum:

Whole-grain bread > refined white bread > sugared doughnuts.

Milk > fruit-flavored yogurt > canned chocolate pudding.

Corn on the cob > canned creamed corn > caramel popcorn.

Oranges > orange juice > orange-flavored drink.

Baked ham > deviled ham > fried bacon.

The nutrient continuum is paralleled by another continuum—the nutrition status of the consumer. The closer to the farm the foods you eat, the better nourished you are, but that doesn't mean you have to live in the fields.

Wise food choices are half the story of smart nutrition self-care; skillful food preparation is the other half. In modern commercial processing, losses of vitamins seldom exceed 25 percent. In contrast, losses in food preparation at home can be close to 100 percent, and it is not unusual to see losses in the 60 to 75 percent range. These facts put the matter of food processing into perspective. The kinds of foods you buy certainly make a difference, but what you do with them in your kitchen can make an even greater difference.

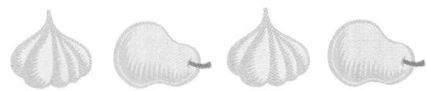

1. Purchase mostly fresh foods or those that processing has benefitted nutritionally.

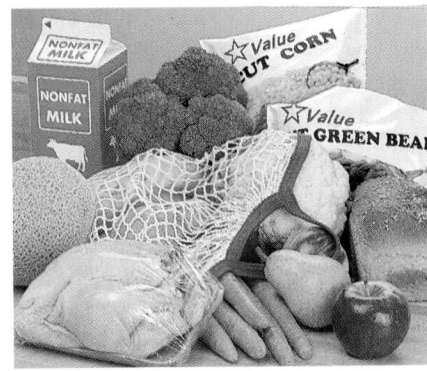

2. Steam vegetables or cook them in a microwave oven.

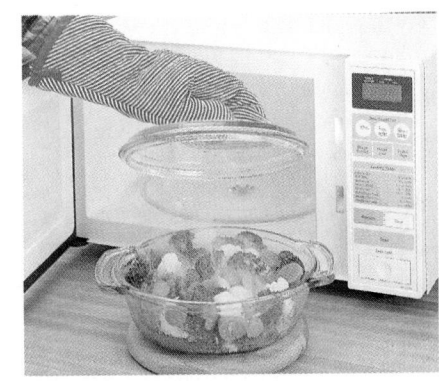

3. Wrap foods tightly and refrigerate them. Space foods to allow chilled air to circulate around them.

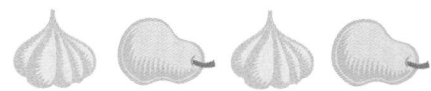

To develop skill in preparing foods requires some understanding of the effects of cooking and storing foods on nutrients. Vitamins are organic compounds synthesized and broken down by enzymes found in the foods that contain them. The enzymes that break down nutrients in fruits and vegetables, like all enzymes, have a temperature optimum. They work best at the temperatures at which the plants grow, normally about 70°F (25°C), which is also the room temperature in most homes. Chilling fresh produce slows down enzymatic destruction of nutrients. To protect the vitamin content, most fruits and vegetables should be vine ripened (if possible), chilled immediately after picking, and kept cold until use.

Besides being vulnerable to enzyme-mediated spoilage, the vitamin riboflavin is light sensitive. It can be destroyed by the ultraviolet rays of the sun or by fluorescent light. For this reason milk is not sold (and should not be stored) in transparent glass containers. Cardboard or opaque plastic containers screen out light, protecting the riboflavin. Since grain products such as macaroni and rice are also important sources of riboflavin, cooks who store them in glass jars should stow the jars in closed cupboards.

Some vitamins are acids or antioxidants and so are most stable in an acid solution away from air. Citrus fruits, tomatoes, and many juices are acid. As long as the skin is uncut or the can is unopened, their vitamins are protected from air. If you store a cut vegetable or fruit or an opened carton of juice, cover it with an airtight wrapper, or close it tightly and store it in the refrigerator.

Labels on frozen foods tell you "Do not refreeze." As food freezes, the cellular water expands into long, spiky ice crystals that puncture cell membranes and disrupt tissue structures, changing the texture of the food. There is usually no danger in eating a twice-frozen food although some nutrients are lost upon thawing and refreezing. Provided that it hasn't spoiled while it was thawed or wasn't thawed at warm temperature, the main problem with a twice-frozen food is that it may be unappealing.

Minerals and water-soluble vitamins in fresh-cut vegetables readily dissolve into the water in which they are washed, boiled, or canned. If the water is discarded, as much as half of the vitamins and minerals in foods go down the drain with it. A bit of Southern folk wisdom is to serve the cooking liquid with the vegetable rather than throwing it away; this liquid is known as the "pot liquor" and may be used to moisten cornbread or to make gravies or soups. Other ways to minimize cooking losses: steam vegetables over water rather than in it, stir-fry them in small amounts of oil, or microwave them. Wash the intact food vigorously and briefly, don't soak it. Cut vegetables after washing except for those such as broccoli that you have to cut to wash adequately. For peeled vegetables, such as potatoes, add them to water that is vigorously boiling, not to cold water, to minimize the length of time the vegetables are exposed to nutrient-leaching water. Microwave ovens are excellent for conserving nutrients. They cook fast without requiring the addition of fats or excess liquid. Some special microwaving concerns appear in the margin.

Take care when cooking in a microwave oven. Food can become extraordinarily hot or build up steam that may scald unprotected hands or face. Before cooking eggs, sausages, or any food encased in a membrane, pierce the membrane to prevent explosion of the food. Never warm baby formula or food in a microwave oven.

Here's a way to tell if glass or other containers are made of microwave-safe materials. Microwave the empty container for one minute and carefully touch it.

Warm = unsafe for microwave.

Lukewarm = safe for short reheating use.

Cool = safe for long microwave cooking times.

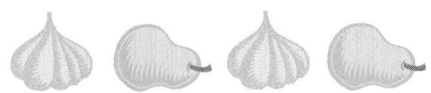

During other types of cooking, minimize the destruction of vitamins by avoiding high temperatures and long cooking times. Iron destroys vitamin C by catalyzing its oxidation, but perhaps the benefit of increasing the iron content of foods by cooking in iron utensils outweighs this disadvantage. Each of these tactics is small by itself, but saving a small percentage of the vitamins in foods each day can mean saving significant amounts in a year's time.

Meanwhile, however, a law of diminishing returns operates. Most vitamin losses under reasonable conditions are not catastrophic. You need not fret over small vitamin losses that occur in your kitchen; you may waste energy or time that is valuable to you in other ways. Be assured that if you start with fresh, whole foods containing ample amounts of vitamins and are reasonably careful in their preparation, you will receive a bounty of the nutrients that they contain.

✓ SELF-CHECK

Answers to these Self-Check questions are in Appendix G.

1. Which of the following food hazards has the FDA identified as its number one concern?
   a. pesticides in food
   b. microbial food poisoning
   c. intentional food additives
   d. environmental contaminants

2. To prevent food-borne illnesses, cooked foods should be held at temperatures higher than:
   a. 85°F
   b. 100°F
   c. 140°F
   d. 212°F

3. Which diseases may be contracted from normal-appearing seafood?
   a. hepatitis
   b. worms and flukes
   c. viral intestinal disorders
   d. all of the above

4. Which of the following heavy metals is *not* among those considered to be chemical contaminants of concern?
   a. zinc
   b. cadmium
   c. lead
   d. mercury

5. Which of the following are likely sources of nitrates?
   a. cosmetics
   b. cigarette smoke
   c. bacon and hot dogs
   d. all of the above

6. Foods that smell good, look good, and taste good are always safe to eat.   T   F

7. Vitamins are unaffected by heat processing because they cannot be destroyed, as minerals can be.   T   F

8. The artificial flavors and flavor enhancers are the largest single group of food additives.   T   F

9. The canning industry chooses treatments that employ the low-temperature–long-time (LTLT) principles for canning.   T   F

10. Foods produced through biotechnology, if not substantially different from foods already in use, require no special safety testing or labeling. (Read about this in the upcoming Controversy.)   T   F

NOTES

Notes are in Appendix F.

Future Foods: Are the New Food Technologies Safe?

Food futurists who gaze ahead to the 21st century see a world with many more people, greater food demands, and less available farmland on which to grow food. Foods will have to be easy to grow in abundance. Furthermore, people in developed countries will have little or no time for cooking or sitting down to meals.[1] Foods will have to be easy and quick to prepare. Already today, consumers need nutritious, affordable, easy-to-prepare foods that are low in fat and taste good. And, of course, the foods must be safe to eat—free from microbial and other contamination. Also, the production of foods must economically support food growers and producers, and must have as little environmental impact as possible. These diverse needs may seem to oppose each other, and yet all are promised by advocates of new technologies. Should we believe these promises?

The developing world has an even greater need for foods with all these qualities than do developed nations. An unrelenting population explosion within the borders of less developed nations foretells of widespread famine to come unless, as many scientists hope, new food technologies can stave off disastrous famines by increasing crop yields and food safety and reducing food waste.

Today the world is witnessing the beginning of a revolution of applied technology in food science and agriculture. Upon surveying government, business, and university experts about technologies now under development, the FDA concluded, "the floodgates of innovation are opening. Nearly 800 different developments [are] reported as technically feasible." Many of those developments are nearing reality.[2]

While new technologies promise immense benefits in solving food problems, some consumers feel uneasy about possible risks. They question whether the processors of foods or the consumers stand to benefit. This Controversy focuses on both sides of two major food technology issues that hold vast potential for changing

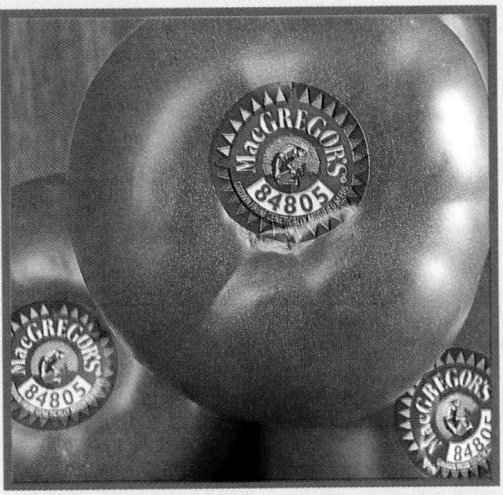

the food supply. The first is **genetic engineering,** a form of biotechnology, and the second is **irradiation** of foods.

GENETIC ENGINEERING

For centuries farmers have been changing the genetic makeup of their crop plants and farm animals. Season after season they have selectively bred plants or animals possessing desirable traits, hoping to obtain offspring that reliably display those traits. Today's lush, hefty, healthy agricultural crops and animals, from cabbage and squash to pigs and cattle, all are the results of those efforts.

Among the successes of selective breeding is corn. Its large, full, sweet cobs and high yields bear little resemblance to the original wild, native corn with its sparse two or three kernels to a stalk. Some new strains of corn lack the enzyme that normally turns sugar to starch within days, so the new corn retains the sweet taste that people prefer instead of turning starchy. Selective breeding, called by some the "old biotechnology," works, but slowly and imprecisely.

Recently, scientists have discovered a way of speeding up and refining the process of genetic change through biotechnology. The changes in corn just mentioned required centuries, but today's genetic engineering methods could have accomplished the same things in about a year or two of work. Genetic engineering is more than just an improved means of selective breeding. The technique wields awesome power—the power to change the most basic patterns of life in ways never before possible.[3] Figure C14-1 compares the genetic results of selective breeding and genetic engineering.

The Products of Genetic Engineering The products of genetic engineering are currently of three main types. First, new strains of agricultural crops offer new desired traits, such as improved resistance to diseases or insect pests. Second, strains of microorganisms have been engineered to produce

Traditional Breeding

DNA is a strand of genes, much like a strand of pearls. Traditional plant breeding combines many genes at once.

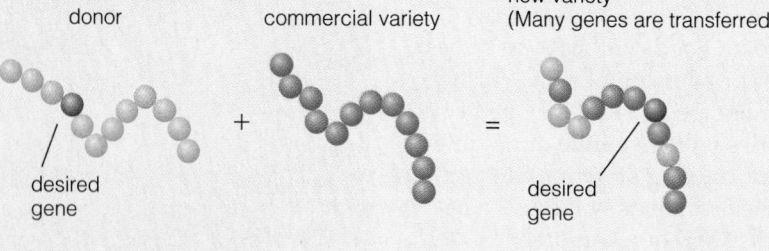

donor   commercial variety   new variety (Many genes are transferred.)

desired gene   desired gene

Genetic Engineering

Through genetic engineering, a single gene may be transferred from one strand of DNA to another.

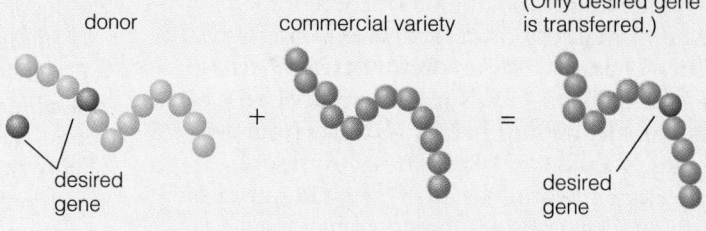

donor   commercial variety   new variety (Only desired gene is transferred.)

desired gene   desired gene

substances that occur in only small amounts or not at all in nature (such as bovine somatotropin, the cattle growth hormone mentioned in the preceding chapter). Third, agricultural crops have been developed that resist destruction by herbicides.

Plant cells make likely candidates for genetic engineering because a single plant cell can often be coaxed to reproduce an entire new plant. Cells with this talent include fertilized ova, stem or germ cells, and some embryonic cells. Each cell contains an exact replica of the genetic information contained in the original cell. If any DNA fragments have been introduced by scientists, the cells will faithfully reproduce these, too.

For example, scientists can start with an undifferentiated cell, known as a stem cell, from the "eye" of a potato plant. Into that cell they can implant some DNA with genes for the protein coat (but not the infective part) of a virus that attacks potato plants. Then they can stimulate the stem cell to begin growing a whole new **transgenic** potato plant that replicates the piece of viral protein coat in each of its cells. The presence of the protein stimulates the plant to develop immunity to an attack from the real virus.

Products from transgenic bacteria often assist food manufacturers. One bacterium, for example, was given the ability to make the enzyme renin, a substance necessary to produce cheese. Before this innovation, renin was traditionally harvested from the stomachs of calves, an expensive process. Through recombinant DNA technology, the gene responsible for making renin was snipped from some calf DNA and transferred to a single bacterial cell. That cell divided many times, producing a whole colony of transgenic bacteria. With each bacterial cell contributing just a minute amount of renin, a large colony becomes a factory of mass production. By the same process, human hormones, such as the once-scarce human growth hormone, can be produced abundantly. Today, many children with growth

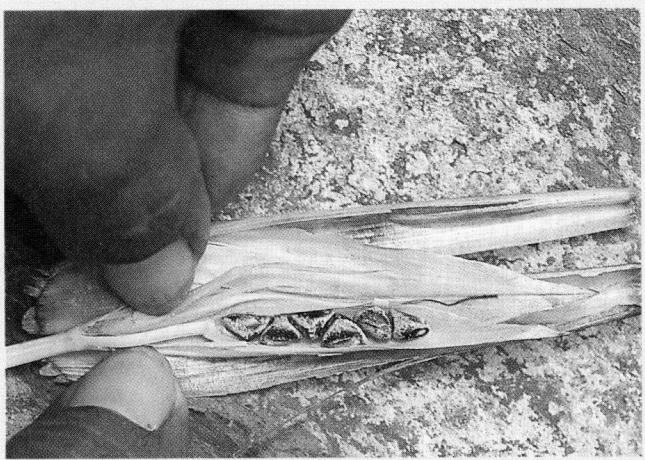

The original wild corn from which today's corn was developed over centuries of selective breeding.

hormone deficiency can grow normally thanks to a reliable supply of human growth hormone harvested from transgenic bacteria.

The technique just described allows an organism to make proteins native to some other living thing. Another option is to block or suppress production of unwanted cell products, as in the corn with the long-lasting sweet taste, mentioned earlier. Lately, this procedure has brought to market an especially long-lasting tomato.[4] Normally, tomatoes produce a protein that softens them after they have been picked. Scientists introduced into a tomato plant an **antisense gene,** a mirror image of the native gene that coded for the "softening" enzyme. The new antisense gene blocked the softening enzyme (see Figure C14-2). A vine-ripe tomato with the antisense gene can be harvested at its most flavorful and nutritious red-ripe stage and still last long enough to go to market.

Another group of crops are intended to benefit farmers by easing the task of controlling weeds. These plants are genetically engineered to withstand potent herbicides. As a result, farmers can spray whole fields with the herbicides and kill every other plant growing there, leaving only the desired crop.

Other possibilities for the near future are tomatoes and cotton that produce their own insecticides, which may render pesticide sprays unnecessary. Shrimp may soon fight diseases with genetic ammunition borrowed from sea urchins. Some plants may even be given special molecules to help them grow food in soil so polluted that all other plants wither and die.

These projects are already in progress. Close on their heels are many more ingenious ideas. What if salt tolerance could be transplanted from a coastal marsh plant into crop plants? Could crops then be irrigated with seawater, thus conserving dwindling freshwater supplies? Would the world food supply increase if rice farmers were able to grow plants that were immune to disease? What if consumers could dictate which traits scientists insert into food plants? Would they choose to add extra cancer-fighting phytochemicals or hard-to-get nutrients? These ideas may sound fantastic, but many such organisms are already on laboratory shelves, awaiting FDA approval for use in agriculture.

Safety and Regulation   While both scientists and food industrialists hail biotechnology with confidence, some consumers fear what they call "Frankenfoods." They question the safety of direct genetic tampering that produces effects not yet fully understood, even by the scientists who developed the techniques. Some feel uncomfortable when the power of direct control over the genes lies in the hands of human beings who may not act in everyone's best interest. They feel genetic

TABLE C14-1

Food Technology Terms

- **antisense gene** the chemical opposite of a gene, which adheres to the native working gene and keeps it from producing proteins.
- **genetic engineering** a field within biotechnology that involves the direct, intentional manipulation of the genetic material of living things in order to obtain some desirable trait not present in the original organism; also called *recombinant DNA technology.*
- **irradiation** application of ionizing radiation to foods to reduce insect infestation or microbial contamination, or slow the ripening or sprouting process.
- **outcrossing** the unintented breeding of a domestic crop with a related wild species.
- **radiolytic products** chemicals formed during irradiation of food.
- **transgenic organism** an organism that grows from an embryonic, stem, or germ cell into which a new gene has been inserted. The organism carries the new gene in all of its cells.
- **plant-pesticides** substances produced within plant tissues that kill or repel attacking organisms.

FIGURE C14-2

HOW BIOTECHNOLOGY TECHNIQUES CAN BLOCK FORMATION OF SPECIFIC PROTEINS

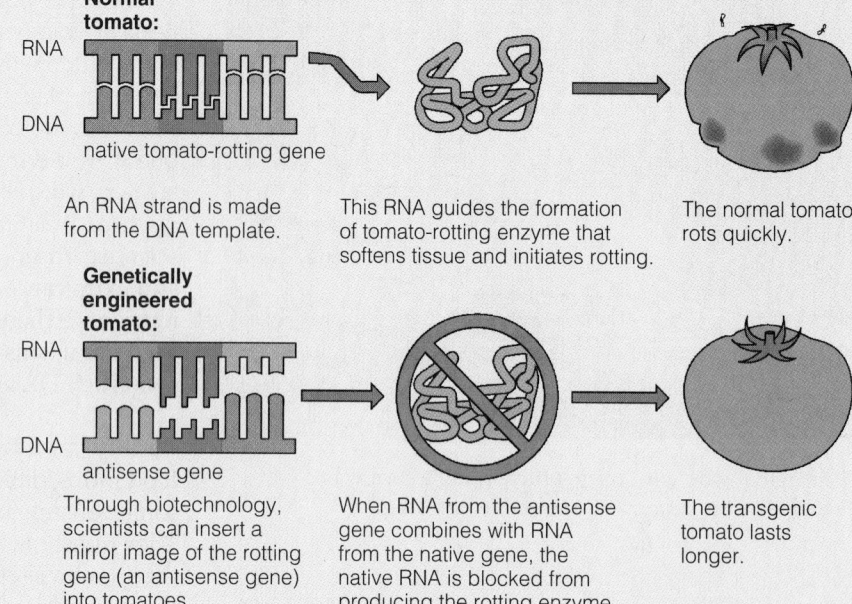

Normal tomato:

RNA

DNA

native tomato-rotting gene

An RNA strand is made from the DNA template.

This RNA guides the formation of tomato-rotting enzyme that softens tissue and initiates rotting.

The normal tomato rots quickly.

Genetically engineered tomato:

RNA

DNA

antisense gene

Through biotechnology, scientists can insert a mirror image of the rotting gene (an antisense gene) into tomatoes.

When RNA from the antisense gene combines with RNA from the native gene, the native RNA is blocked from producing the rotting enzyme.

The transgenic tomato lasts longer.

CD ROM   Outline > Food Safety > Intro > Technology > produce photograph

---

decisions are best left to the powers of nature. Those given to flights of imagination envision a biotechnology run amok, used for frivolous, greedy purposes such as cloning dinosaurs for entertainment.*

Many legitimate safety questions exist, however. Many focus on the "foreign" proteins produced by organisms that receive new genes. Students of nutrition know that DNA governs the synthesis of protein and that, in the human body, proteins are degraded by digestive enzymes and rendered nontoxic. Several dangerous exceptions exist, though, including the botulinum toxin and certain other peptide toxins. Some scientists worry that such peptides may accidentally form and not be detected promptly enough to prevent harm to those who eat the foods.

Among the newest transgenic foods are yellow squash with two viral genes that confer resistance to the most common viral diseases and a potato that produces a beetle-killing toxin. These two new plants, which are currently being grown around the United States, produce what the Environmental Protection Agency (EPA) calls **plant-pesticides,** a group of pesticides made by the plants themselves. Plant-pesticides require regulation under an EPA proposal.[5] A concern of scientists about disease-resistant crops is the possibility of **outcrossing,** accidental cross-pollination with related wild weeds that would give the weeds an enormous survival advantage over other wild species and crowd them out. Questions are also raised about the environmental impacts of spraying large areas with lethal herbicides and, leaving only one genetically engineered plant species alive. Others dismiss these concerns.

The case for requiring rigorous testing is strong.[6] For example, when a new gene has been introduced into a food, tests should make sure that other, unwanted genes have not accompanied it. If a disease-producing microorganism has donated genetic material to make the recombinant DNA, scientists must prove that no dangerous characteristic from the microorganism has also entered the food. If the inserted genetic material comes from a source to which some people develop allergies, such as nuts, then the new product may produce allergies in those people, and labeling may be necessary.[7] Furthermore, the newly altered genetic material may create proteins never before encountered by the human body—unique proteins. Their effects should be studied and their presence regulated to ensure that people can eat them safely.[8]

---

*Michael Crichton's novel *Jurassic Park* (New York: Ballantine Books, 1990) and the film that followed paint a frightening but unrealistic picture of rampaging dinosaurs let loose on an unsuspecting world. Biotechnology cannot create living things from DNA samples.

The FDA's Position   The FDA has taken the position that whole foods produced through biotechnology require no special safety testing or labeling, if they are not substantially different from foods already in use.[9] The FDA holds developers of new foods responsible for testing those that differ significantly from traditional foods. Any product with an antisense gene, including the tomato described earlier, is assumed to be safe, since the antisense gene prevents synthesis of a protein and adds nothing but a tiny fragment of genetic material. On the other hand, any extra substances introduced, such as new enzymes, hormones, or resistance traits, must meet the same safety standards applied to all additives.[10] A tomato with a gene that produces an insecticide, for example, could not be marketed unless the insecticide "additive" was proved safe to eat at the levels people would normally encounter.[11]

Speaking in defense of the FDA's decision are the FDA itself, recognized as the nation's leading expert and advocate for food safety, and the American Dietetic Association, which represents current scientific thinking in nutrition.[12] Many other scientific organizations agree, contending that biotechnology can deliver on promises for an improved food supply if we give it a fair chance to do so.[13]

To help determine the safety of the products of biotechnology, the FDA has established a new National Center for Food Safety and Technology (NCFST) in Illinois. Studies performed at the NCFST guide the FDA in setting regulations governing food processes and products.

A lack of scientific understanding underlies many fears of biotechnology. The same lack of understanding breeds fear in consumers who adamantly oppose another food technology—irradiation.

IRRADIATED FOODS

Proponents claim that ionizing radiation applied to foods can solve some of our food safety and supply problems.[14] But do the potential hazards inherent in the technology outweigh theoretical benefits?

Today, consumers bear the responsibility for safety from food-borne illnesses. They must cook meats and eggs to the well-done stage to kill dangerous microorganisms lurking in the raw products. They must scrub vegetables and fruits to remove pesticide residues applied to kill molds and insects that attack food during storage. Even then they cannot be certain that foods

such as grains are free of sprays. Could food irradiation relieve consumers of these burdens?

The Irradiation Process   Irradiation easily kills many disease-producing microorganisms and so could save many of the millions of children worldwide who die each year from food-borne illnesses. Radiation also sexually sterilizes the parasite *Trichinella* and interrupts its destructive life cycle.[15] Irradiation might replace some types of postharvest pesticides because it can kill mold spores and insect pests and their eggs. Supporters argue that between a quarter and half of the food produced annually is lost to pests and decay after harvest, and that irradiation could eliminate most of this waste. While some scientists agree with these assessments, critics counter that food irradiation also may pose some serious and unnecessary threats.

Irradiation works by exposing foods to controlled doses of gamma rays from the radioactive compound cobalt 60 or from X rays generated by machines. As radiation passes through a living cell, it disrupts the internal structures and so kills or deactivates the cell. Low doses can kill the growth cells in the "eyes" of potatoes and ends of onions, preventing them from sprouting. They can also delay ripening of bananas, avocados, and other fruits. High doses can penetrate tough insect exoskeletons and mold or bacterial cell walls to destroy their life-maintaining DNA, proteins, and other molecules and thereby reduce microorganism and insect threats.* Doses high enough to sterilize food completely cannot be used, because they would also destroy the food. They can, however, sterilize spices. Technicians expose spices to the highest doses of radiation allowed by law.

A perspective on the doses used is gained by comparing them to the lethal human dose. The lowest doses of radiation needed to treat fragile fruits and vegetables are 10 to 20 times the doses that would kill human beings. The doses required to sterilize foods are still higher. Needless to say, irradiation technology requires extremely cautious handling.

Irradiated foods must now bear a label stating that the foods have been treated with radiation or must display the irradiation symbol shown here. Exceptions are

---

*The spores of one dangerous bacterium are naturally beyond the reach of even the highest legal doses of irradiation—those of *Clostridium botulinum*, the bacterium responsible for the lethal food-poisoning agent, botulinum toxin.

The symbol for foods treated with radiation.

permitted for spices that are mixed with processed foods, and for irradiated foods served in restaurants.

Many consumers indicate they are willing to purchase irradiated foods, but some vigorously challenge the whole idea of food irradiation. A few in the latter group mistakenly believe that irradiated foods themselves become radioactive. This is not true. Properly irradiated food does not become radioactive any more than teeth become radioactive after dental X-ray procedures. The use of radioactivity demands great care, though. Foods exposed to extremely high doses of the wrong sort of radiation can indeed become radioactive. A point of reassurance is that such abuses would also render them inedible.[16]

A fear not easily put to rest concerns chemicals called **radiolytic products,** which are produced in foods as they undergo irradiation. A very few radiolytic products are unique, appearing only in irradiated foods; others are commonly found in many foods after all sorts of processing, including cooking. Their effects on human health and nutrition, if any, are unknown, but many studies on animals indicate no effect on the animals' health. Among radiolytic products are highly reactive free radicals, which, as described in Controversy 7, attack other molecules, setting up chain reactions. The attacked molecules go on to attack others that, in turn, become attackers, causing chaos within cell structures. Irradiation changes some of the molecules in living tissue of foods into free radicals. Whether the extra free radicals formed during food irradiation are absorbed into the body or are linked to any diseases in human beings is not known.

Irradiation's Effects on Nutrients Nutrients in foods are known to be attacked by free radicals from irradiation. Many amino acids withstand attack by irradiation and free radicals, but the side chains of certain individual amino acids are open to destruction by these influences. When those amino acids are part of a protein chain, it, too, is destroyed. Irradiation also destroys some vitamins such as vitamin E, whose primary function is to scavenge reactive free radicals and thus to protect cell membranes. Other vitamins, including beta-carotene, vitamin B_6, vitamin C, and especially thiamin, are also vulnerable to free radicals. Theoretically, if marginally nourished people were to consume a steady diet of nothing but irradiated foods, they might well develop frank nutrient deficiencies.[17] Dr. David Murray, a powerful critic of irradiation, uses these words to describe the nutrient losses sustained through irradiation:

> If irradiation were to be applied to the meats, fruits and vegetables that form the bulk of most human diets, the nutritional impoverishment of those diets would be so extensive that sufficiency thresholds for many essential nutrients would no longer be met. The phrase 'empty calories' would take on a new dimension.

Countering this opinion is one from the American Council on Science and Health (ACSH), a group that advocates irradiation. While acknowledging that doses of radiation high enough to sterilize food do cause vitamin losses, the ACSH describes the losses sustained during low-dose irradiation to be similar to those caused by other processing techniques such as canning. The ACSH therefore concludes that irradiation is not a health hazard.

The FDA concurs that irradiation of chicken to reduce *Salmonella* contamination produces thiamin losses, but of less than 2 percent of total thiamin, losses not considered significant. Any food that suffers greater than a 2 percent loss of any nutrient during irradiation is required by the FDA to be labeled as an "imitation food."

Murray responds that the studies showing minimal vitamin losses were performed immediately after irradiation, before the free radicals and "weeping" (fluid losses) resulting from irradiation had finished destroying the vitamin contents of the foods. The longer a food is stored, the greater the losses of nutrients, and losses from irradiated foods far exceed those incurred by any other type of processing.

If the purpose of irradiation is to preserve food and increase its shelf life, then nutrient destruction and loss during storage warrants further investigation. If losses are significant, then a label alerting consumers to that fact should probably be mandatory.[18] After all, a person who buys and eats a food from the grocery store trusts the food to provide vitamins. If the food has been irradiated, the buyer should be warned to obtain vitamins from another source. Even if consumers were willing to compensate for nutrient losses sustained through radiation, one question above all others still remains: Are irradiated foods safe to eat?

Safety Concerns   Radiation changes foods in ways whose health effects are still not completely understood. For example, when irradiated food is heated in a laboratory within three months after treatment, it emits light detectable by instruments.[19] (People fearful of this phenomenon say, "It glows.")[20] This light energy, called thermoluminescence, arises from overexcited electrons, stimulated by radiation.

Another poorly understood phenomenon occurs in laboratory experiments in which freshly irradiated food is fed to rats. The rats develop chromosomal abnormalities, impaired fertility, and depressed immune responses.[21] Evidence that freshly irradiated food may also adversely affect people comes from one study performed on malnourished children. In the days before current ethics would have prevented such a study, researchers fed freshly irradiated wheat to malnourished children to study its effects. The results showed increased chromosomal abnormalities in all but one of the children.[22] Children fed irradiated wheat that had been held in storage for longer than three months or fed nonirradiated wheat showed no increased chromosomal abnormalities.

Animal experiments could perhaps prove or disprove the existence of some of the feared effects, but testing irradiated foods is difficult. The safety of other additives is tested by feeding animals hundreds of times the amount of a substance that a person might consume in a day, but researchers cannot feed animals hundreds of times more irradiated food than people would consume.[23] In its publication *Priorities*, the ACSH attacks the validity of studies showing ill effects:

> Arguments against food irradiation are largely based on poorly planned, rejected experiments, pseudo science, and emotion, which are fronts for an antinuclear political agenda.[24]

Some people oppose food irradiation on other safety grounds. The method necessitates transporting radioactive materials, exposing workers to them, and then disposing of the spent wastes, which remain radioactive for many years. They claim that these processes pose an unacceptable and unnecessary risk to human health and reproduction. Birth defects are common in children who were exposed to nonlethal low doses of radiation dur-

ing their fetal development and even in children whose parents were exposed to radiation before the children were conceived. These concerns are echoed by food industrialists and others who hope to gain acceptance for the process, but are unwilling to risk human health. They hope to safeguard both workers and future generations through strict operating standards and enforcement of regulations limiting radiation exposure.

Finally, some consumers worry that food manufacturers might use the technology unethically. It could allow the sale of old or tainted food that would otherwise be condemned by FDA because of high bacterial counts. For example, food stored in unsanitary conditions might be contaminated with rodent or insect feces. If fecal bacteria are killed by irradiating the food, FDA inspectors might judge the food to be wholesome and allow its sale to unwitting consumers.

In the end, the objectives of irradiation technology may be achievable by less expensive methods such as higher cleanliness standards for food-animal facilities to prevent microbial contamination, selective breeding of produce to permit safe storage for longer times, and application of gases and pesticides that dissipate before product use to ensure destruction of pests and infestations. These methods pose none of the hazards associated with transport and handling of radioactive materials, and they have been proved safe for the human food supply.

Will our impressive new technologies provide foods to meet the needs of the future? Optimists would say yes. Biotechnology holds a world of promise, and with proper safeguards and controls, it may yield products that meet the needs of consumers almost perfectly.[25] Even irradiation, with its potential for hazard, may, with proper safety controls in place, prove useful in helping to provide safe, abundant food for the world's growing population.[26] All products of technology must pass a final examination, though—the test of consumer acceptance. If the products meet people's needs, are attractive, economical, and tasty, and have been proven safe, consumers will buy them. If they fail to meet these standards, consumers will bypass them, and the technologies themselves will fade into history.

NOTES

Notes are in Appendix F.

HUNGER AND THE GLOBAL ENVIRONMENT

15

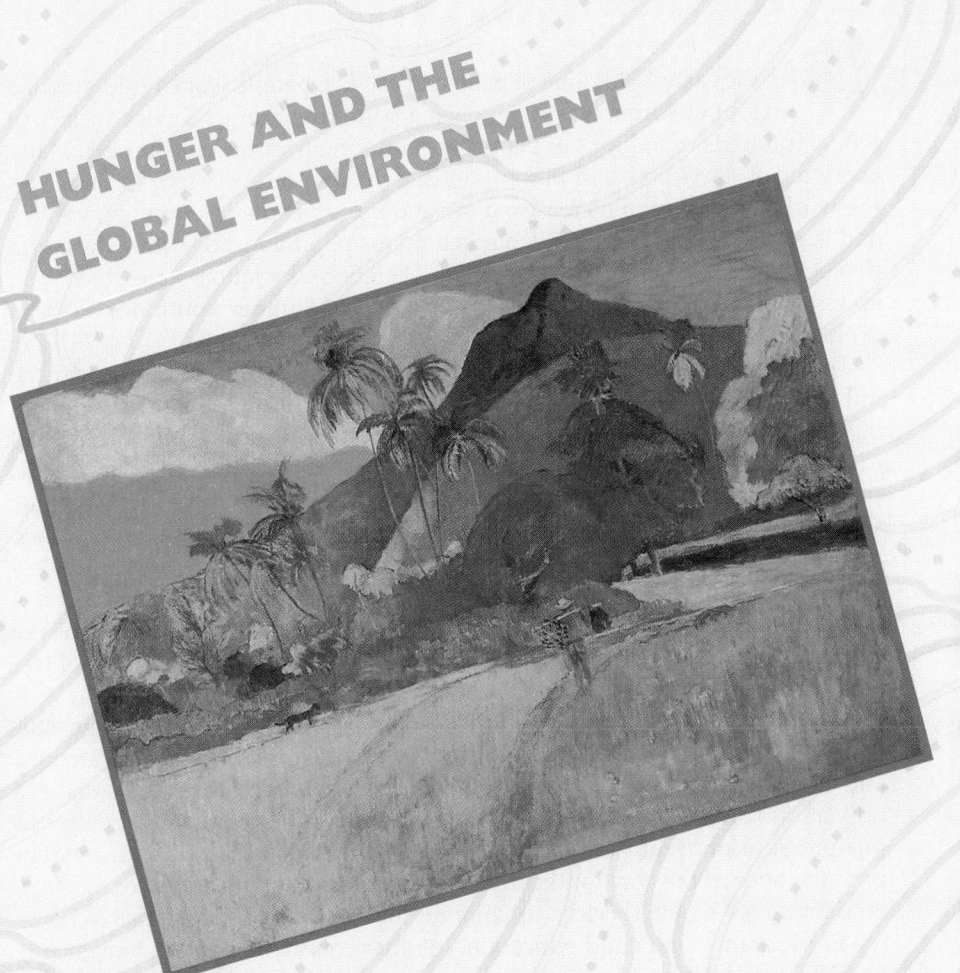

CONTENTS

Paul Gauguin 1848–1903, *Tahitian Landscape with a Mountain*, Minneapolis Institute of Art, Minnesota,
© SuperStock.

fossil fuel coal, oil, and natural gas. These are nonrenewable fuels that pollute. Renewable or alternative fuels, such as solar and wind energy, pollute less or not at all.

15 In the early 1990s, one person in every five people worldwide, and one in four children, was experiencing pain from hunger caused by lack of food. Hundreds of millions of people are suffering from chronic hunger. Many are dying of starvation: tens of thousands each day, one every two seconds.[1] As the world's population increases, more and more people face hunger; yet less and less food is becoming available as humans populate and pollute the earth, depleting its resources.[2] The American Dietetic Association states that ". . . access to food is a fundamental human right. Hunger continues to be a problem of staggering proportions."[3]

The tragedy described on these pages may seem at first to be beyond the influence of the ordinary person. What possible difference can one person make? Can one person's choice to recycle a bottle or to eat a vegetarian meal or to join a hunger-relief organization make a difference? In truth, such choices produce several benefits. For one, a single person's awareness and example, shared with others, may influence many other people over time. For another, an action repeated becomes a habit. For still another, a person who makes choices with awareness of their impacts has a sense of having some control over those impacts. That sense of personal control, in turn, helps people to take effective action in many areas. People without a sense of personal control feel hopeless and become ineffective.

Students, especially, can play a powerful role in bringing about change. Students everywhere are helping to change governments, human predicaments, and environmental problems for the better. Student movements persuaded 127 universities and many institutions, corporations, and government agencies to put pressure on South Africa, and succeeded in ending apartheid. Student pressure opened the way for the first deaf president at a university for the deaf. Students offer major services to communities through soup kitchens, home repair programs, and child education. In other countries, student movements have hastened the coming of cultural and political autonomy, the reform of universities, and advances in peace and human rights causes. Students have launched significant protests against totalitarianism in China and have mounted successful environmental cleanups and defense efforts.[4]

"Never doubt that a small group of thoughtful, committed people can change the world. Indeed, it is the only thing that ever has."

—Margaret Mead

THE NEED FOR CHANGE

In the mid-1990s, the earth's total food supply is sufficient to feed all of its people adequately, but uneven distribution of resources leaves some without enough food. In the near future, however, we may face more global food insecurity as many forces compound to threaten world food production and distribution. During the 1990s, all of the following trends are taking place:

■ *Hunger, poverty, and population growth.* Millions of people are starving. Fifteen children die of malnutrition every 30 seconds, but 75 children are born during that same 30 seconds.

■ *Loss of food-producing land.* Food-producing land is becoming saltier, is eroding, and is being paved over. Each year, the world's farmers try to feed some 90 million more people with 24 billion fewer tons of topsoil. Overall food security is threatened.[5]

■ *Accelerating* **fossil fuel** *use.* Fuel use is accelerating, with attendant pollution of air, soil, and water; ozone depletion; and global warming.

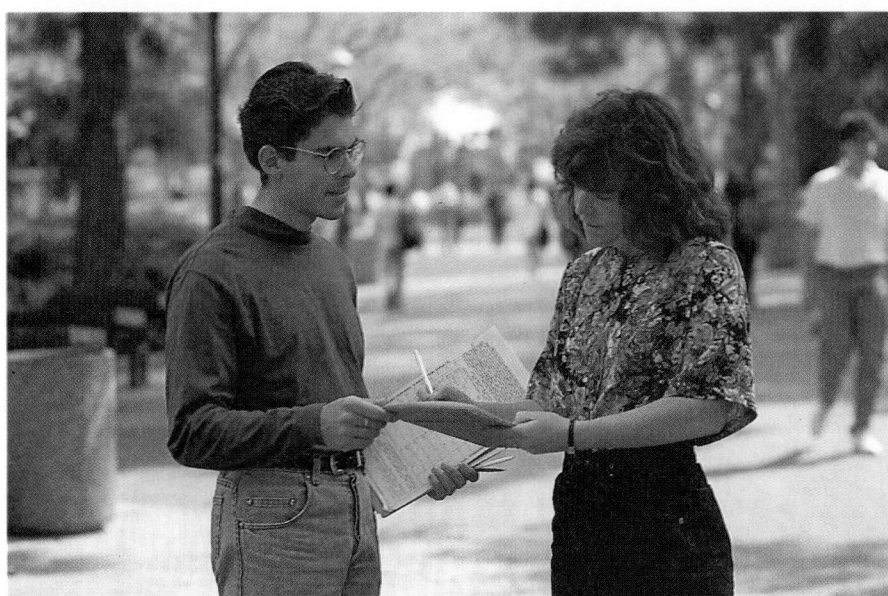

Personal choices, made by many people, can have large impacts.

- *Increasing air pollution.* Air quality is diminishing all over the globe.*
- *Global warming, droughts, and floods.* Climbing atmospheric levels of heat-trapping carbon dioxide are a concern. The concentration of carbon dioxide is now 26 percent higher than 200 years ago. As a result, a massive warming trend seems to be taking place.[6] Climate change causes both droughts and floods, which destroy crops and people's homelands.[7]
- *Ozone loss from the outer atmosphere.* The outer atmosphere's protective ozone layer is growing thinner, permitting harmful radiation from the sun to damage crops and ecosystems and to cause cancers and cataracts in people and animals.[8]
- *Water shortages.* The world's supplies of fresh water are dwindling and becoming polluted.[9]
- *Deforestation and desertification.* Forests are shrinking and deserts are growing.
- *Ocean pollution.* Ocean pollution is killing fish; overfishing is depleting the numbers of those that remain.[10]
- *Extinctions of species.* More than 140 species of animals and plants are going extinct each day. Another 20 percent of all species are expected to die out in the next ten years. Many kinds of whales, birds, giant mammals, colorful butterflies, and thousands of other animals and plants will never again be seen in the universe.[11]

These global problems are all related. The causes overlap, and so do the solutions. To think positively, this means that any initiative a person takes to help solve one problem will help solve many others. Figure 15-1 shows how all of today's global environmental problems tend to worsen each other, with human population growth linked to all of them. A later section spells out the

---

* Many older references have been removed to save space, but they are available in older editions of this book.

FIGURE 15-1

THE GIANT WEB OF GLOBAL PROBLEMS

Follow the arrows to see how each problem intensifies others.

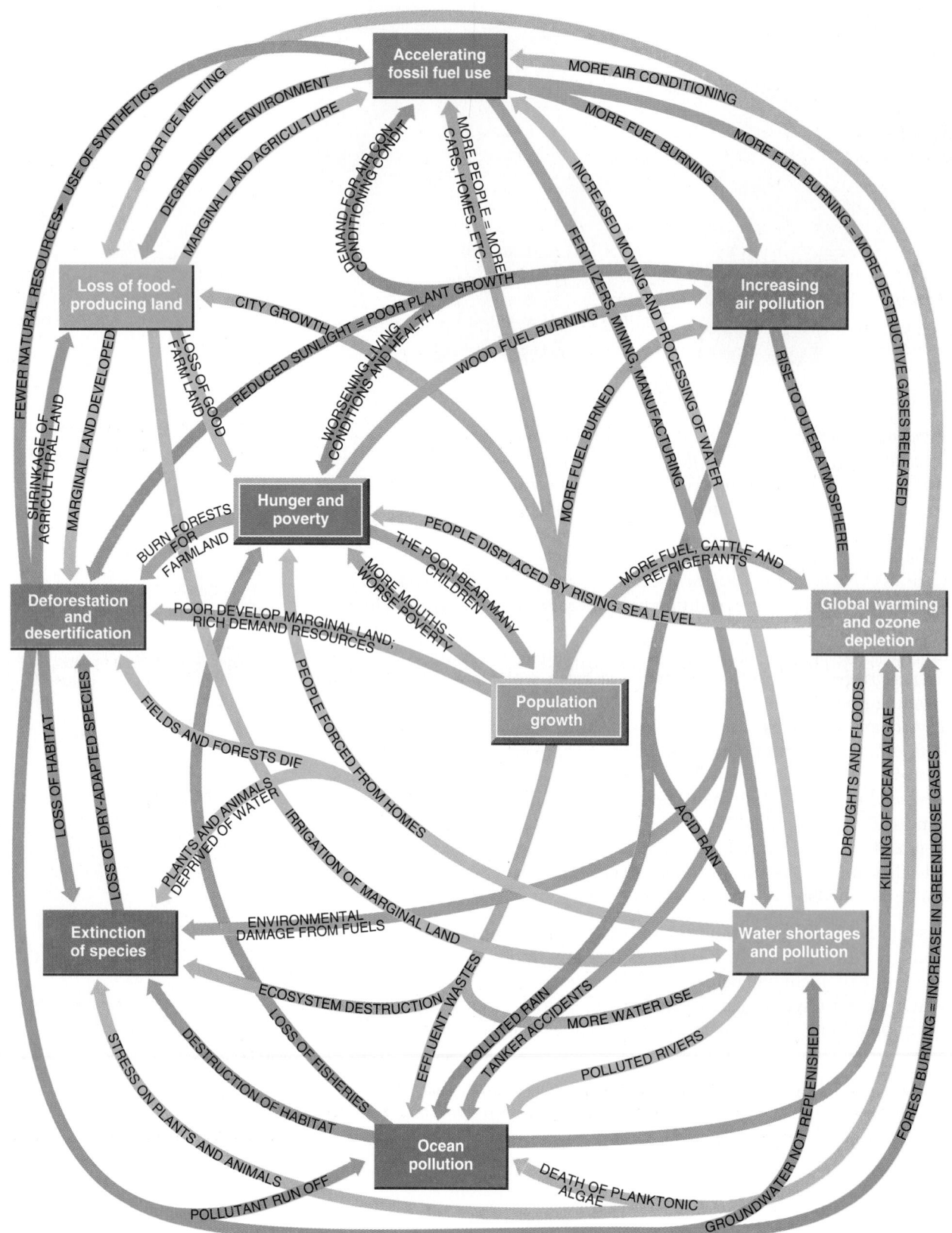

urgency of effective controls on overpopulation. The Controversy section shows how U.S. consumers fit in, by highlighting some of our current food-production choices and showing how they contribute to global food problems.

HUNGER

The hunger of concern here is not the healthy appetite we all feel, which leads us to sit down and eat a hearty meal, but the chronic, painful hunger people feel when no food is available.[12] Severe deficiencies of vitamin A and the minerals iodine and iron accompany this hunger, afflicting more than 40 percent of the world's people. The terms of Table 15-1 help to define concepts relating to hunger.

Worldwide, many children are hungry and children comprise three-fourths of those who die each year from starvation and related illnesses.[14] In the United States, one of every five children is hungry at least some of the time; these children live in families who do not know where their next meal is coming from, or when it will come.[15] In developed countries, food poverty causes hunger; people are hungry not because there is no food nearby to purchase, but because they lack money with which to buy the food.[16]

In the United States, food poverty reaches into all segments of society, affecting not only the chronic poor (migrant workers, ethnic minorities, the unskilled and unemployed, the homeless, and some elderly) but also the so-called new poor. Some are displaced farm families. Some are former blue-collar and white-collar workers forced out of their trades and professions into minimum-wage jobs. These people outnumber the chronic poor, and they are not on welfare; they have jobs, but the pay is too low to meet their needs. Families with incomes below a certain level are simply unable to buy sufficient amounts of nourishing foods, even if they are skilled in food shopping.

Hunger is not always easy to recognize. Table 15-2 shows how national surveys identify it in the United States. A family that would answer "Yes" to the questions in the table is a family that suffers from this type of hunger. Such hunger affects not just individual families but the whole nation:

> Hunger, particularly childhood hunger, [is] not only a moral issue [but] a competitiveness issue. . . . Hunger compromises the ability to learn. Hungry children have more school absence rates, and when they are in school, their powers of concentration are greatly reduced. The malnutrition that results from chronic hunger can even slow or permanently inhibit the physical development of the brain. So hunger is . . . an issue of failed beginnings for millions of American children—the future of our country.[17]

The causes of hunger in developed nations are many, but the primary causes are poverty and lack of employment. Other causes that contribute to hunger are abuse of alcohol and other drugs; mental or physical illness; depression; lack of awareness of or access to available food programs; and the reluctance of people, particularly the elderly, to accept what they perceive as "welfare" or "charity."[18] Still, poverty remains the major cause of hunger, and solving the poverty problem would do a lot to relieve hunger.[19]

✔ **KEY POINT** **Chronic hunger causes many deaths worldwide, especially among children. Intermittent hunger is frequently seen in U.S. children. The immediate cause of hunger is poverty.**

TABLE 15-1

Hunger Terms

- **hunger** lack or shortage of basic foods needed to provide the energy and nutrients that support health.
- **food insecurity** the condition of uncertain access to food of sufficient quality or quantity.
- **food poverty** hunger occurring when enough food exists in an area but some of the people cannot obtain it because they lack money, they are being deprived for political reasons, they live in a country at war, or because of other problems such as lack of transportation.[13]
- **food shortage** hunger occurring when an area of the world lacks enough total food to feed its people.

Food poverty is the prevailing form of hunger in the United States.

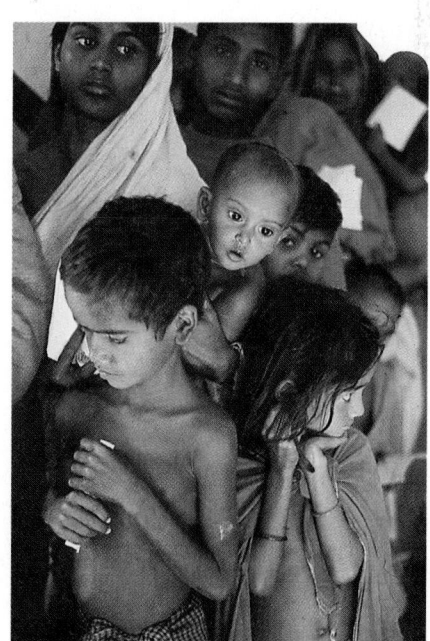

A primary cause of hunger is poverty.

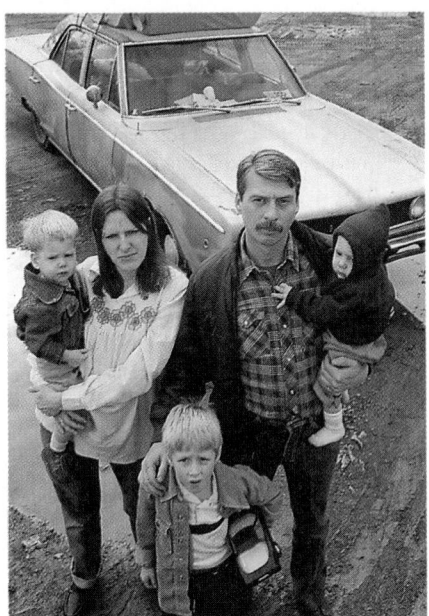

These people and many others like them in the United States face food insecurity daily.

U.S. federal food programs include:

✔ Special Supplemental Food Program for Women, Infants, and Children (WIC, see Chapter 12).

✔ WIC Farmers' Market Nutrition Program.

✔ Food Stamp Program.

✔ National School Lunch and Breakfast Programs (see Chapter 13).

✔ Emergency Food Assistance Program.

✔ Commodity Supplemental Food Program.

✔ Commodity Distribution to Charitable Institutions.

✔ Nutrition Program for Older Americans (see Chapter 13).

✔ Food Distribution Program on Indian Reservations.

✔ Nutrition Assistance to Puerto Rico.

TABLE 15-2

How to Diagnose Food Insecurity in a U.S. Household

Questions like these are asked on surveys to determine the extent of food insecurity in a household. The more questions that receive a "Yes" answer, the more intense the hunger the household is experiencing.

Do you often go hungry?

Do you often have too little food to eat because you have no money, transportation, or kitchen appliances that work?

Do you ever rely on nutritionally inferior foods to feed yourself or your children because you lack any of these resources?

Do you ever eat less than you feel you should because you lack any of these resources?

Do you ever skip meals or cut the size of meals because you lack any of these resources?

Do you ever rely on neighbors, friends, relatives, or schools to feed any of your children because there is not enough food in the house?

Do your children ever say they are hungry because there is not enough food in the house?

Do you or any of your children ever go to bed hungry because there is not enough food in the house?

SOURCES: Adapted from C. A. Wehler, R. I. Scott, and J. J. Anderson, The Community Childhood Hunger Identification Project: A model of domestic hunger—demonstration project in Seattle, Washington, *Journal of Nutrition Education* (1 Supplement), January/February 1992, pp. 29S–35S; and R. R. Briefel and C. E. Woteki, Development of food sufficiency questions for the Third National Health and Nutrition Examination Survey, *Journal of Nutrition Education* (1 Supplement), January/February 1992, pp. 24S–28S.

U.S. Food Programs

For the moment, many U.S. programs take aim at preventing or relieving domestic malnutrition and hunger. Several such programs have been described in earlier chapters: children's school lunch and school breakfast programs; and child care food programs; programs to supply low-income pregnant women and mothers with nourishing food (WIC); and food assistance programs for older adults such as congregate meals and Meals on Wheels.

Another program for low-income people is the Food Stamp program, administered by the U.S. Department of Agriculture (USDA). The USDA issues food stamp coupons through state social services or welfare agencies to households (defined as people who buy and prepare food together). Recipients may use the coupons like cash to purchase food and food-bearing plants and seeds, but not to buy tobacco, cleaning items, alcohol, or other nonfood items. More than 27 million people in the United States receive food stamps at a cost of over $22 billion per year; over 20 million more who have not applied for food stamps are thought to have incomes low enough to qualify for them.[20]

By delivering life-giving foods to millions of U.S. citizens daily, these federal programs and others support both health and well-being. For example, children in Project Head Start, an educational program that includes breakfast, are twice as likely to graduate from high school and to become employed as their peers in the same circumstances who do not participate.[21]

Despite the government's efforts, federal programs intended to remedy hunger are not fully successful. Many more people now need welfare and food assistance than in the 1980s.[22] For example, of the estimated 2 million home-less people in the United States who are eligible for food assistance, only 15 percent of single adults and 50 percent of families receive food stamps.

In an effort to assist the hungry where federal programs fall short, private efforts have sprung up in many communities. Concerned citizens work through local agencies and churches to help deliver food to hungry people. Community-based soup kitchens and shelters generally provide good-quality meals. The meals average only 1,000 calories each, though, and most homeless people receive fewer than one and a half meals a day, so many are inade-quately nourished.[23] Food pantries and community gardens contribute gro-ceries to families in need. Table 15-3 shows how individuals can directly assist in local hunger-relief efforts; it presents a 14-step program for developing a hunger-free community. Although these efforts provide emergency relief to

TABLE 15-3

Fourteen Ways Communities Can Address Their Local Hunger Problems

1. Establish a community-based emergency food-delivery network.
2. Assess food-insecurity problems and evaluate community services. Create strategies for responding to unmet needs.
3. Establish a group of individuals, including low-income participants, to develop and to implement policies and programs to combat food insecurity; monitor responsiveness of existing services; and address underlying causes of hunger.
4. Participate in federally assisted nutrition programs that are easily assessible to targeted populations.
5. Integrate public and private resources, including local businesses, to relieve food insecurity.
6. Establish an education program that addresses the food needs of the com-munity and the need for increased local citizen participation in activities to alleviate food insecurity.
7. Provide information and referral services for accessing both public and pri-vate programs and services.
8. Support programs to provide transportation and assistance in food shop-ping, where needed.
9. Identify high-risk populations, and target services to meet their needs.
10. Provide adequate transportation and distribution of food from all resources.
11. Coordinate food services with parks and recreation programs and other community-based outlets to which area residents have easy access.
12. Improve public transportation to human service agencies and food resources.
13. Establish nutrition education programs for low-income citizens to enhance their food purchasing and preparation skills and to make them aware of the connections between diet and health.
14. Establish a program for collecting and distributing nutritious foods, either agricultural commodities in farmers' fields or prepared foods that would have been wasted.

SOURCE: House Select Committee on Hunger, legislation introduced by Tony P. Hall, excerpted in *Seeds*, Sprouts edition, January 1992, p. 3 with permission (SEEDS Magazine; P.O. Box 6170; Waco, TX 76706). For more on developing a hunger-free community, write: Hunger Free, House Select Committee on Hunger, 505 Ford House Office Building, Washington, DC 20515.

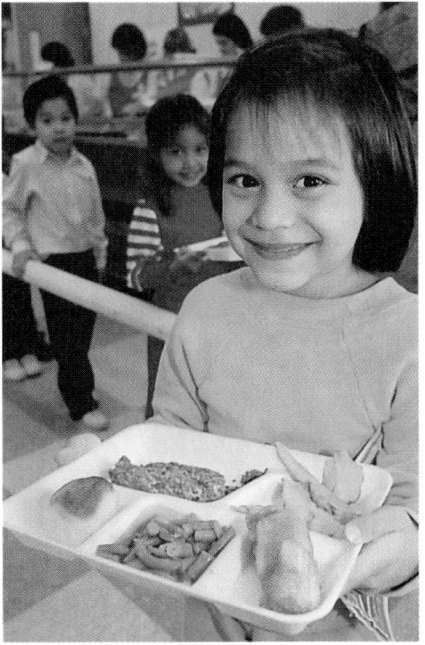

School lunches provide low-income children with nourishment for little or no cost.

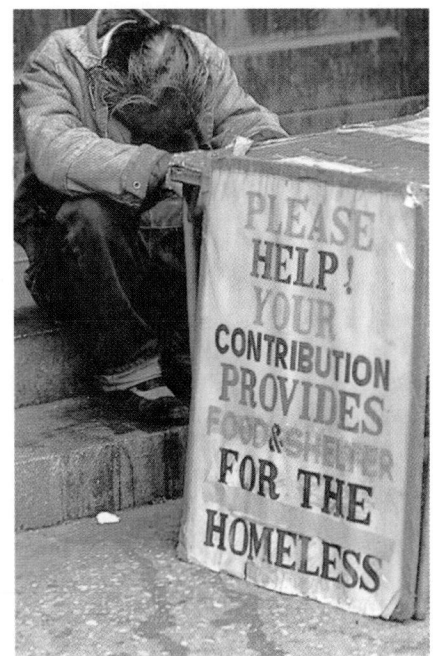

In the United States, at least 20 million people are hungry for at least part of every month.

famine widespread scarcity of food in an area that causes starvation and death in a large portion of the population.

hungry people, they leave unsolved the greater problems of low wages and too few jobs for people who lack higher education or training.

✔ **KEY POINT** **Poverty and hunger are widespread in the United States, not only among the unemployed, but also among working people. Government programs to relieve poverty and hunger are not fully successful.**

World Hunger

In the developing world, hunger and poverty are even more intense. People face more extreme hunger problems than the United States, and the causes are more diverse. The primary form of hunger is still food poverty, but the poverty is more extreme. Most people absolutely cannot grasp the severity of poverty in the developing world. One-fifth of the world's 5 billion people have no land and no possessions *at all*. They survive on less than one dollar a day each, they lack water that is safe to drink, and they cannot read or write.[24] Many spend about 80 percent of all they earn on food, but still cannot meet their needs. The average U.S. housecat eats twice as much protein every day as one of these people, and the cost of keeping that cat is greater than such a person's annual income.[25]

Food Shortage   The most visible form of hunger is **famine,** a true food shortage in an area that causes multitudes of people to starve and die. The natural causes of famine—drought, flood, and pests—have, in recent years, taken second place behind the social causes. Between 15 and 30 million people died during the Chinese famine of 1959 through 1961, the worst famine of this century. The main cause was government policies associated with the "great leap forward," which devastated the Chinese agricultural system.[26]

In the 1990s, the violence of war has become a dominant cause of famine worldwide. In all of the countries that have reported famine so far in this decade—Angola, Ethiopia, Liberia, Mozambique, Somalia, and Sudan—armed conflict has been a major cause. Farmers become warriors, their agricultural fields become battlegrounds, the citizens go hungry, and the warring factions often get in the way of famine relief. The world continues to struggle to find a middle ground between respecting the sovereignty of nations and insisting that all nations allow humanitarian assistance to reach their people.

Since the 1950s, food aid from other countries has provided a safety net for countries whose crops fail. But food aid now does more than just offset poor harvests; it also delivers food relief to countries, such as Ethiopia, that are chronically short of food and without resources to buy it. Some people are concerned that as many countries cut their support of foreign aid, this food aid backup may become insufficient. It has been called a "band-aid" approach when radical surgery is needed.

Chronic Hunger   While famine is the image we usually associate with world hunger, the numbers affected by famine are relatively small compared with those suffering from less severe but chronic hunger. Nearly 800 million people, mostly women and children, in developing countries suffer from chronic malnutrition.[27] In addition, one child in six in the world is born underweight, and

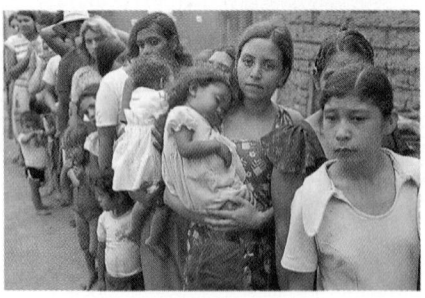

Staving off starvation—emergency food relief in Nicaragua.

almost two in five children are underweight by age five. Around 2 billion people, mostly women and children, are deficient in iron, iodine, or vitamin A.[28] The ravages to the body of such deficiencies were spelled out in earlier chapters of this book.

Tens of thousands die of malnutrition every day. Many are afflicted by the diseases of poverty: parasitic and infectious diseases such as dysentery, whooping cough, measles, tuberculosis, cholera, and malaria—which interact with poor nutrition in a fatal cycle. Most children who die of malnutrition do not starve to death—they die because their health has been compromised by dehydration from infections that cause diarrhea. Currently, **oral rehydration therapy (ORT)** is saving an estimated 1 million lives each year by helping to stop the infection-diarrhea cycle. The ORT solution increases a body's ability to absorb fluids 25-fold. Clean or boiled drinking water is essential, however, for contaminated water will reinfect the child.

Malnourished women in poverty bear sickly infants who cannot fend off the diseases of poverty, and many succumb within the first years of life. Breastfeeding helps prolong an infant's life, but eventually the child must be weaned. Weaning foods may consist of thin gruels made with unclean water, and even these foods are scanty in quantity. All too often, children sicken and die soon after weaning. Because of poverty, infection, and malnutrition, the life expectancy in some African countries averages 50 years; in Uganda it is only 38 years, half of the U.S. life expectancy.[29]

Diminishing World Food Supply   Until 1988, the world's reserves of stored grain, an index of the sufficiency of the world food supply, increased nearly every year. The often-repeated statement that "We have enough food to feed everyone" was true. Efforts at relieving hunger focused on transporting food to where it was needed and on improving storage. Also, because in many developing countries most of the men were involved in producing **cash crops** for export, hunger-relief efforts focused on educating and empowering women to grow and use nutritious food to feed their families. These efforts, thought to be aiming at the right targets, were expected to solve the world's hunger problem.

Since 1988, however, the situation has changed. The world's population is growing at the rate of about 90 million persons each year, and food production is no longer keeping pace. In recent years, grain reserves have fallen dangerously low (see Figure 15-2). Grain reserves in 1995 were enough to feed the world for only about 50 days.[30] Shortfalls of U.S. corn and wheat harvests in the early part of 1996 have been labeled "extreme."[31] Further growth in the world's food output is being blocked by environmental degradation and drought in many agricultural areas. People in developed nations may feel safely insulated against food shortages, but this is a false feeling of security. Developed countries may be last to feel the effects, but they do finally go as the world goes.

✔ **KEY POINT**   **Natural causes such as drought, flood, and pests and social causes such as armed conflicts and overpopulation all contribute to hunger and poverty of developing countries. International food production is falling behind demand and world food surpluses are diminishing.**

oral rehydration therapy (ORT) oral fluid replacement for children with severe diarrhea caused by infectious disease. ORT enables a mother to mix a simple solution for her child from substances that she has at home.

cash crops crops grown for sale or export, as opposed to food crops grown for local consumption.

The symptoms of malnutrition vary according to the nutrients lacking and the individual's stage of life. See Chapter 6 for effects of protein and energy deficiency; Chapters 7 and 8 for vitamin and mineral deficiencies; Chapter 11 for effects on immunity; Chapter 12 for effects on newborns and pregnant women; and Chapter 13 for effects on children, teens, and the elderly.

FIGURE 15-2

WORLD GRAIN CARRYOVER STOCKS EXPRESSED AS DAYS OF CONSUMPTION, 1963–1996

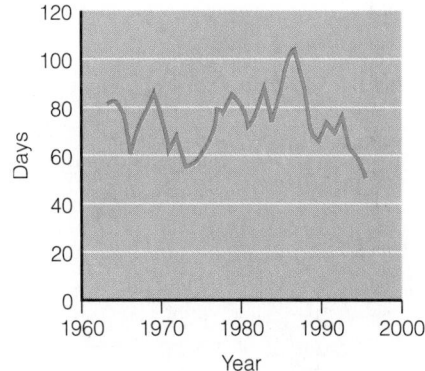

SOURCE: L. R. Brown, Facing food scarcity, *World Watch*, November/December 1995, pp. 10–20.

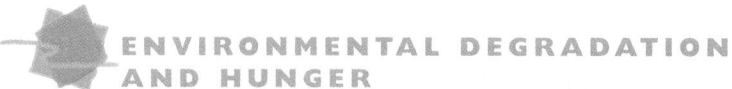

ENVIRONMENTAL DEGRADATION AND HUNGER

Hunger and poverty interact with a third force: environmental degradation. Poor people often destroy the very resources they need for survival. In desperation, they sell everything they own to obtain money for food, even the seeds that would have provided next year's crops. They cut their trees for firewood or timber to sell, then lose the soil to erosion. Without these resources, they become still poorer. Thus poverty causes environmental ruin, and the ruin leads to hunger.[32]

Soil Erosion Worldwide crop yields are declining by an estimated 6 percent per year due to soil erosion in every nation.[33] Deforestation of the world's rainforests dramatically adds to land loss. In Sierra Leone, where 60 percent of the land was primary rainforest in 1961, only 6 percent is now.[34] Without the forest covering to hold the land in place, mud and silt wash off the rocks beneath, drastically reducing the land's productivity.[35]

Around the world, irrigation can no longer compensate by improving crop yields, because all the land that can benefit from irrigation is already receiving it. In fact, continuous irrigation leaves deposits of salt in the soil, and rising salt concentrations are lowering yields on close to a quarter of the world's irrigated cropland. Nor can fertilizer enhance agricultural production much more; it is already being used to maximum effect in major agricultural areas. Genetic improvements in crops are also already in use. During the middle of this century, major genetic improvements led to rapid advances in agricultural outputs. Now, despite the exciting technological advances reported in Controversy 14, not many more such ways of improving the world's total output are forthcoming.[36]

More about overgrazing appears in Controversy 15.

Grazing Lands and Fisheries Meat and fish outputs are also falling. Grasslands for growing beef are already being fully used or overused on every continent. The yield of fish from the oceans is declining for the first time in history due to overfishing and pollution. Big fish, such as tuna, swordfish, and shark, are being overfished. Atlantic stocks of the heavily fished bluefin tuna have dropped by 94 percent.[37] Cod are rapidly disappearing off the New England coast and are almost gone farther north.

Inland fisheries have also suffered tremendous drops in yield as a result of environmental damage. The Aral Sea, located between Kazakhstan and Uzbekistan, yielded 40,000 tons of fish per year in 1960 and today is biologically dead. As water was diverted for irrigation over the last 30 years, the sea became increasingly salty until finally no fish could live in it.[38] Acidification has also taken a toll on inland fisheries. In Canada, 14,000 lakes are considered biologically dead as a result of acid rain.[39]

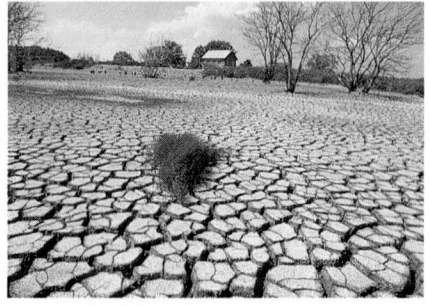

As groundwater is used up, deserts spread.

Climate and Water Other forms of environmental degradation that reduce food outputs include both air pollution and climate change. An unusually hot and dry summer in 1988 pushed the U.S. grain harvest below consumption for the first time in history. In 1994, new heat records were set throughout the western United States, northern Europe, the Baltic, and Japan.[40] A rise of only a degree or so in average global temperature may reduce soil moisture, impair pollination of major food crops such as rice and corn, slow growth, weaken disease resistance, and disrupt many other factors affecting crop yields.

Supplies of fresh water, too, have shrunk to the point where they are limiting the numbers of people who can survive in some areas. In fact, water availability may limit human population growth even before food availability does.[41]

carrying capacity the total number of living organisms that a given environment can support without deteriorating in quality.

Overpopulation   The extent to which the world grain harvest can be amplified by means of improved technology is now estimated at no better than 1 percent a year. Meanwhile, the world's population is rising at the rate of at least 2 percent per year.[42] The earth's population is expected to double by the year 2033, but will exceed the world's estimated **carrying capacity** before this time. Many authorities in many fields—and more every year—are calling for a reduction in the rate at which the world's population is allowed to increase; Figure 15-3 provides historical perspective on current trends in population growth. Overpopulation may well be the most serious threat that humankind faces today.

FIGURE 15-3

WORLD POPULATION GROWTH

The earth's human population has experienced by far its greatest expansion during the last 200 years of history.

Years needed for the human population to reach . . .

Its 1st billion	. . . . .2,000,000 years
2nd billion	. . . . .105 years
3rd billion	. . . . .30 years
4th billion	. . . . .15 years
5th billion	. . . . .12 years
6th billion	. . . . .11 years

Is it any wonder that, despite modern agricultural technology, food supplies are falling behind?

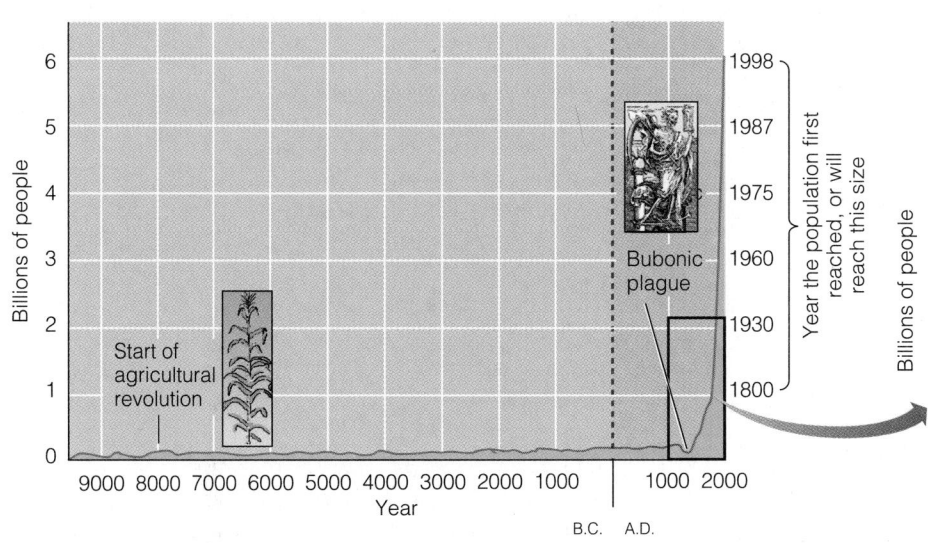

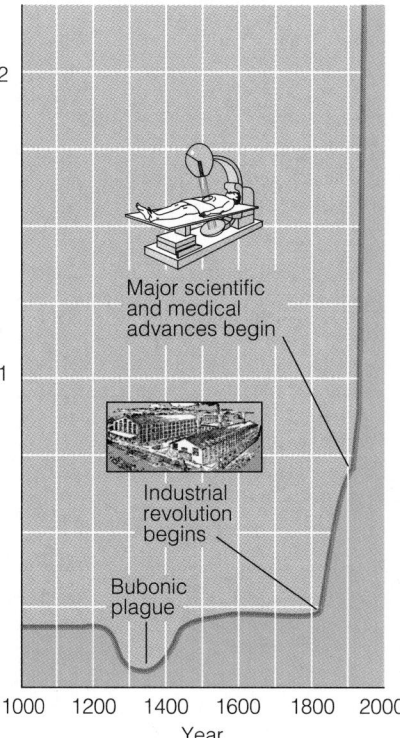

The sheer magnitude of our annual population increase is difficult to comprehend. Each month the world adds the equivalent of another New York City.[43] During six months of the terrible 1992 famine in Somalia, an estimated 300,000 people starved to death. Yet it took the world only 29 *hours* to replace their numbers! Ninety million people born a year, spread over 365 days, comes to a quarter-million people a day—or just over 10,000 people born every hour.[44]

Population stabilization has become one of the most pressing needs of this time in history: it appears to be the only way to enable the world's food output to keep up with the world's overwhelming numbers of people with people's growing numbers. Without population stabilization, the nations of the world can neither support the lives of people already born nor remedy or halt global environmental deterioration. And before the population problem can be resolved, it may be necessary to remedy the poverty problem. In countries around the world, economic growth has been accompanied by slowed population growth.[45] Of the 90-odd million people being added to the population each year, 88 million are born in the most poverty-stricken areas of the world.[46]

Thus, together, overpopulation and environmental problems are reducing the world's ability to produce enough food for its people. Today there is barely enough food to feed everyone, so the present hunger remains largely a problem of unequal distribution of resources and is not yet a worldwide food shortage. If present trends continue, however, the time is rapidly approaching when the world will experience an absolute deficit of food.[47] This conclusion seems inescapable. Skyrocketing human numbers threaten the earth's capacity to produce adequate food and imperil health in innumerable other ways. To resolve the population problem, a necessary first step is to remedy poverty problems, for reasons discussed next.

✓ **KEY POINT** **Environmental degradation caused by the impacts of growing numbers of people is reducing the world's food output per person.**

FIGURE 15-4

INCOME AND FERTILITY
Greater wealth means lower rates of birth.

SOURCE: H. R. Pulliam and N. M. Haddad, Human population growth and the carrying capacity concept, *Bulletin of the Ecological Society of America*, September 1994, pp. 141–157.

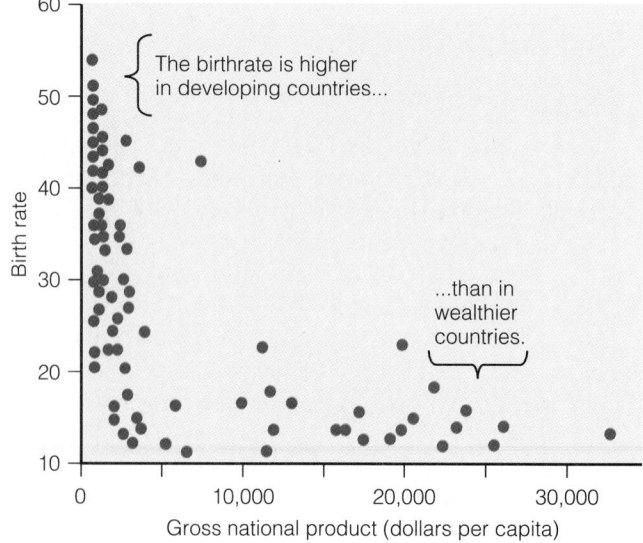

Improvements in agriculture can no longer keep up with people's growing numbers. Solving the population problem is an urgent necessity.

POVERTY AND OVERPOPULATION

The giant web of global problems, shown in Figure 15-1, centered population growth among the many factors contributing to poverty and hunger. The figure also showed the reverse: poverty and hunger contribute to population growth (see Figure 15-4).

The first of these cause-effect relationships is easy to understand. As a population grows larger, more mouths must be fed, and the worse poverty and hunger become. How does poverty lead to overpopulation? Poverty and hunger exert an ironic effect on people, driving them to bear more children. Poverty and hunger typically go hand in hand with ignorance, including ignorance of how to control family size. Also, a family in poverty depends on its children to farm the land, haul water, and care for the adults in their old age. Poverty claims many of a family's young children, who are among the most likely to die from disease and other causes. If a family faces ongoing poverty, the parents will choose to have many children as a form of "insurance" that some will survive to adulthood. People are willing to risk having fewer children only if they are sure that their children will live. The environment also suffers, for the more people must share meager resources, the more heavily they draw on trees for fuel and on water supplies. This sets up the damaging cycle shown in Figure 15-5: more resources are needed, more hands are needed to help gather them, so more children are produced.[48]

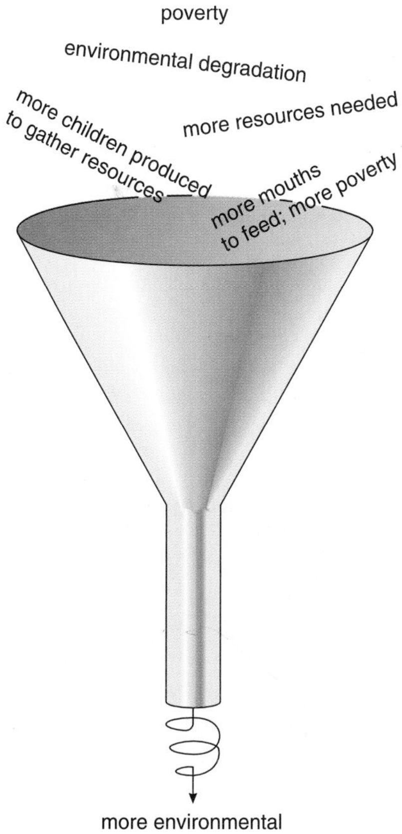

Population growth also contributes to hunger indirectly by preempting good agricultural land for growing cities and industry and forcing people onto marginal land, where they cannot produce sufficient food for themselves. The world's poorest people live in the world's most damaged and inhospitable environments. There they experience, daily, tens of thousands of early deaths from malnutrition and disease.

Relieving poverty and hunger, then, may be a necessary first step in curbing population growth. When people attain better access to health care, education, and family planning, the death rate falls. At first there is a "bulge" in the population, because births outnumber deaths, but as the standard of living continues to improve, families become willing to risk having smaller numbers of children. Then the birth rate falls. Thus, after a short but necessary lag time, improvements in living standards help stabilize the population.

The link between improved economic status and slowed population growth has been demonstrated in country after country.[49] Central to this success is **sustainable** development that includes not only economic growth, but also a sharing of resources among all groups. Where this has happened, population growth has slowed the most. Examples are parts of Sri Lanka, Taiwan, Malaysia, and Costa Rica. Where economic growth has occurred but only the rich have grown richer, population growth has remained high. Examples include Brazil, Mexico, the Philippines, and Thailand, where large families continue to be a major economic asset for the poor.

As a society gains economic footing, education also becomes a greater priority. A society that educates its children, both male and female, sees fertility

sustainable able to continue indefinitely. Here the term refers to the use of resources at such a rate that the earth can keep on replacing them, for example, cutting trees no faster than new ones grow and producing pollutants at a rate with which the environment and human cleanup efforts can keep pace. In a sustainable economy, resources do not become depleted, and pollution does not accumulate.

FIGURE 15-5

THE WORSENING OF POVERTY, OVERPOPULATION, AND ENVIRONMENTAL DEGRADATION
Population growth, poverty, and environmental degradation combine to worsen each other.

poverty

environmental degradation

more children produced to gather resources

more resources needed

more mouths to feed; more poverty

more environmental degradation and povery

FIGURE 15-6

EDUCATION AND FERTILITY
Higher education means lower rates of birth.

SOURCE: H. R. Pulliam and N. M. Haddad, Human population growth and the carrying capacity concept, *Bulletin of the Ecological Society of America,* September 1994, pp. 141–157.

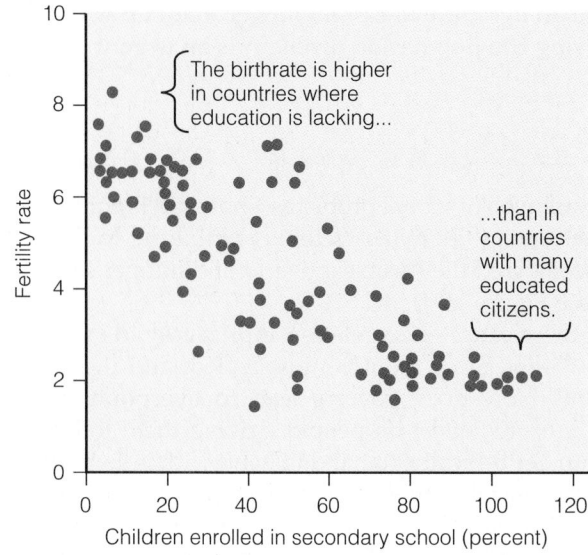

rates decline (see Figure 15-6). Education for girls and women yields improvements in family life, including improved nutrition, better sanitation, effective birth control, and elevated status for women. Educated women also take more control of family planning and can earn esteem through employment, and not solely through fertility.

✔ **KEY POINT** **More people means more mouths to feed, which worsens poverty, hunger, and environmental problems. Poverty, hunger, and a degraded environment, in turn, prompt parents to have more children. Breaking this cycle requires improving the economic status of the people and providing them with health care, education, and family planning.**

Solutions

The keys to solving the world's environmental, poverty, and hunger problems are in the hands of both the poor and the rich nations, but require different efforts from them. The poor nations need to make contraceptive technology and information more widely available, educate their citizens (particularly women), develop better programs to assist the poor, and slow and reverse the destruction of their environmental resources, such as forests, waterways, and soil. The rich nations need to stem their wasteful and polluting uses of resources and energy, which are contributing to global environmental degradation. They also must become willing to ease the debt burden that many poor nations face. One way is to offer debt forgiveness in return for the poor nations' taking recommended steps to help their own people and conserve their resources.

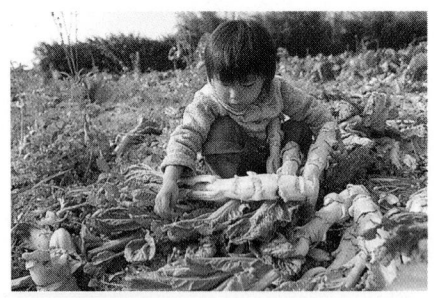

In some countries, every pair of little hands is needed to help feed the family.

Sustainable Development Worldwide

Many nations now agree that improvement of all nations' economies is a prerequisite to meeting the world's other urgent needs: population stabilization, arrest of environmental degradation, sustainable treatment of resources, and relief of hunger. An important step was taken when a United Nations convention on the Rights of the Child was ratified by over 100 nations. Significantly, for the first time in world history, the document mentioned nutrition as an internationally recognized human right.[50] Another first step was taken in 1992, when over 100 nations met for the Earth Summit in Rio de Janeiro, Brazil, and discussed the relationships of the environment to poverty and hunger.

The formal name of the summit was the United Nations Conference on Environment and Development, or UNCED for short. At this meeting, many nations agreed for the first time to 27 principles of sustainable development, which the conferees defined as development that would equitably meet both the economic and the environmental needs of present and future generations.

The participants at UNCED discussed climate change and the possibility of setting legally binding targets and timetables for every nation to cut its emissions of global-warming gases. They also signed agreements to protect the earth's remaining species of plants and animals and to preserve the world's forests. The participating nations also began to discuss ways of alleviating the problems of poverty in the developing world. Since then, a third international conference on climate change has taken place, and some 200 nations including the United States have made firmer commitments to reduce their releases of gases that warm the globe. In 1996, the United States began passing legislation to accomplish these objectives.

Such discussions have opened vistas of hope. Much remains to be done, though, and all nations have major parts to play. For our part, in the United States, the challenges are many. For one, we are being urged to reduce our consumption of fossil fuel and thereby our disproportionate contribution to global environmental degradation. For another, it has been suggested that the United States can help directly by supporting international moves to relieve poverty and environmental degradation worldwide. The steps identified in the next paragraphs are recommended.

Relieve Interest Payments First, a plan is needed to relieve the developing countries of the gigantic interest payments they have been making to U.S. and international banks. In the early 1980s, those countries received $50 billion more a year from the developed world than they paid out, and they were able to make some progress toward solving their internal poverty and environmental problems. Today, however, they pay out $50 billion more than they take in, so they are becoming poorer every year.[51] They sell a bounty of cash crops to the developed world, such as cotton, tobacco, coffee, sugar, and palm oil, but they cannot put the proceeds back into their economies. All the money they make goes to pay the interest on their loans, and they even have to borrow more. It has been called "one of the great ironies of the world" that some of the world's richest farmland is being used to produce nonnutritious crops for U.S. dollars, only to pour the money down the interest-payment drain while the producing nations' people starve.[52] The debtor nations could use that same land to grow food crops to feed their own people.

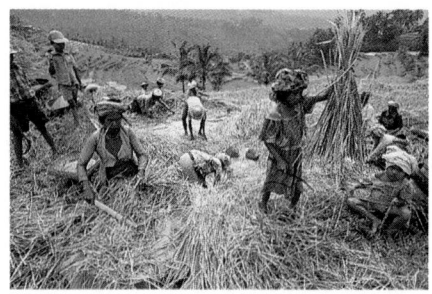

Labor-intensive agriculture that is low in technical inputs is most often the appropriate technology in developing countries.

Support Land Reform Second, the debt relief must reach those within the countries who need it, and not just the wealthy. In some poor countries, astronomically wealthy upper classes control all the good crop land and use it to produce luxury cash crops for export while the landless poor starve and multiply. Relieving hunger requires land reform—returning sufficient land to the dispossessed so that they can live and grow food on it. Simultaneous community development is needed to ensure that the people become able to support themselves permanently.

Encourage Labor-Intensive Methods Third, rather than emphasizing *technology*-intensive methods of harvesting resources, developing countries could shift toward *labor*-intensive means of *maintaining* their resources. That way, succeeding generations can also benefit from those resources.[53]

Account for Environmental Costs Fourth, to account correctly for the great value of environmental resources such as soil, water, and trees, a new system of economic accounting must come into use. Soil, water, and trees should be counted in economic balance sheets. Systems of national accounting must recognize that depletion of natural resources is a step backward economically. Government accounting systems must subtract lost resources from the gross national product. This would promote the making of decisions that would more accurately take into account future environmental costs and benefits and encourage the use of investment criteria that would stem the loss of natural capital.[54]

The United States can exert international leadership along these lines. It can encourage other developed nations to support the same measures.

The idea behind all these measures is that relieving poverty will help relieve environmental degradation and hunger. To rephrase a well-known adage, If you give a man a fish, he will eat for a day. If you teach him to fish, so that he can buy and maintain his own gear and bait, he will eat for a lifetime and help to feed you. In comparison with food giveaways and money doles, which are only stop-gap measures, social reforms that permanently better the lot of the poor can permanently solve the hunger problem.[55]

Activism and Simpler Lifestyles at Home

Every segment of our society can play a role in the fight against poverty, hunger, and environmental degradation. The federal government, the states, local communities, big business and small companies, educators, and all individuals, including dietitians and foodservice managers, have many opportunities to forward the effort.

Government policies can change to promote sustainability. For example, the government can stop using tax money to pay for the wasteful use of fossil fuels and of fertilizers and pesticides made from them. Instead, it can pay for energy-conservation services and crop protection.[56]

Businesses can take initiatives to help; some already have. Several, such as AT&T, Prudential, and Kraft General Foods, are major supporters of anti-hunger programs.[57]

Educators, including nutrition educators, have a crucial role to play. They can teach others about the underlying social and political causes of poverty, the root cause of hunger. At the college level, they can teach the relationships between hunger and population, hunger and environmental degradation, hunger and the status of women, hunger and the global debt crisis.[58] They can advocate legislation to address poverty problems. They can teach the poor to develop and run their own nutrition programs in their own communities and to fight on their own behalf for antipoverty, antihunger legislation.[59]

Dietitians and foodservice managers have a special role to play. They are being urged by their professional organization, the American Dietetic Association (ADA), to promote the saving of resources by reuse, recycling (including composting), energy conservation, and water conservation in both their professional and their personal lives.[60] In addition, the ADA urges its members to work for policy changes in private and government food assistance programs, to intensify education about hunger, and to be advocates on the local, state, and national levels to help end hunger in the United States.[61]

All individuals can also become involved in these large trends. Many small decisions each day add up to large impacts on the environment, and Figure 15-7 shows that consumers can choose to minimize their negative impacts in many ways. Consider this list:

- Shop "carless" and plan to make fewer shopping trips. Motor vehicles constitute the largest single source of air pollution. Air pollution harms children and adults with lung problems, reduces crop yields, causes acid rain, and damages forests.
- Choose foods that are low on the food chain (see the Controversy section). Growing animals for their meat and dairy products by feeding them grain uses much more land and other resources than growing grain and other crops for direct use by people.
- Avoid canned beef products of any kind, including stews, chili, corned beef, and pet foods. Many of these foods come at the expense of cleared rainforest land: 200 square feet of rainforest are lost *permanently* for every pound of beef produced.
- Choose chicken and small fish more often. Chickens are often grown locally and use fewer resources to produce; small fish eat low on the food chain. Avoid large species endangered by overfishing, such as some varieties of tuna, swordfish, and shark.
- Buy foods grown close to home. Locally grown foods require less transportation, packaging, and refrigeration.
- Avoid overly packaged items; buy bulk items with minimal packages or reusable or recyclable ones. Each can, foam tray, waxed or clay-coated cardboard container, plastic bottle, or glass jar requires land and many other resources to produce, and its disposal pollutes and costs more land.
- Avoid disposable pans, dishes, and other items that are used once and thrown away. Avoid spray cans—they are hard to recycle because they are made of many materials.
- Carry reusable string or cloth grocery sacks. Production of paper and plastic grocery bags represents a huge drain on resources. Paper factories use chemicals such as toxic forms of chlorine bleach, which they release into waterways in quantities so large that the chemicals can destroy whole bays and fisheries.[62]
- Use fast cooking methods. Stir-frying, pressure cooking, and microwaving all use less energy than conventional stovetop or oven cooking methods.

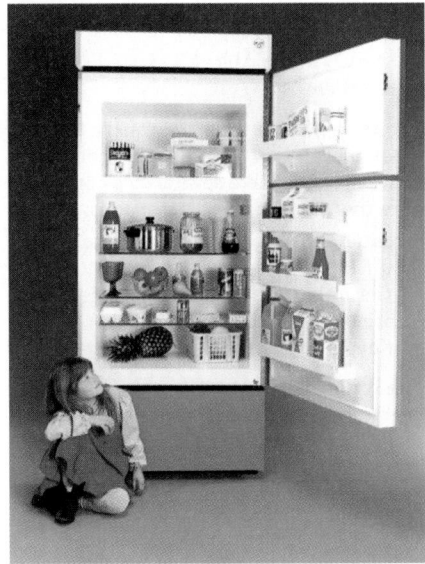

This energy-saving refrigerator requires less than a twentieth of the energy used by a regular refrigerator, but chills and freezes food just as well. The motor is small, releases little heat, and is on top. In contrast, with a "regular" refrigerator's inefficient design, the large motor is below the unit, so it heats the very unit it is trying to cool.

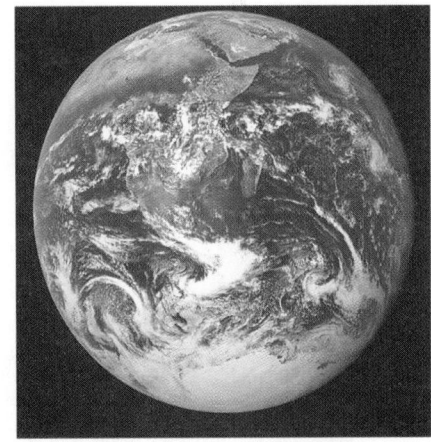

"We do not inherit the earth from our ancestors, we borrow it from our children."

Often ascribed to Chief Seattle, Native American Indian Chief, 1854, but author unknown.

FIGURE 15-7

DOMESTIC FOODWAYS THAT RESPECT THE ENVIRONMENT

The refrigerator uses more energy than any other appliance in most people's homes. Consumers can take several steps to minimize the energy a refrigerator uses:

✔ Set it at 37° to 40°F; set the freezer at 0°F.

✔ Clean the coils and the insulating gaskets around the doors regularly.

✔ Keep it in good repair.

The water heater can also waste a lot of energy. Keep the water heater set at 120° to 130°F (no hotter) to save energy. For safe household dishes, sterilization is not necessary. Water of 120° to 130°F enhances the action of dishwashing detergents, making microorganisms slippery and removing them from the dishes. These measures will keep food fresh and dishes clean while keeping energy use low.

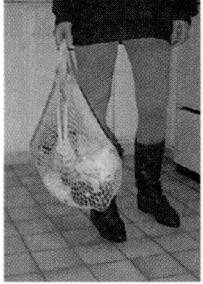

Shop carless. It can be a pleasure and a great source of exercise.

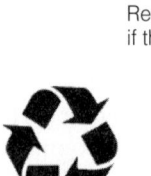

Recycle throwaways if they must be used.

Use reusable bags instead of throwaway bags.

Use items that don't use energy . . .

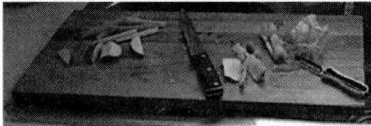

. . . instead of those that do use energy (even small appliances).

Use reusable items . . .

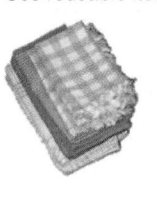 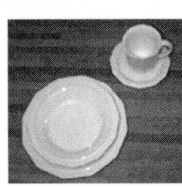

. . . instead of nonreusable items.

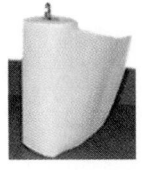 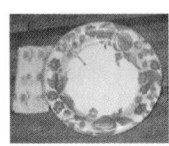

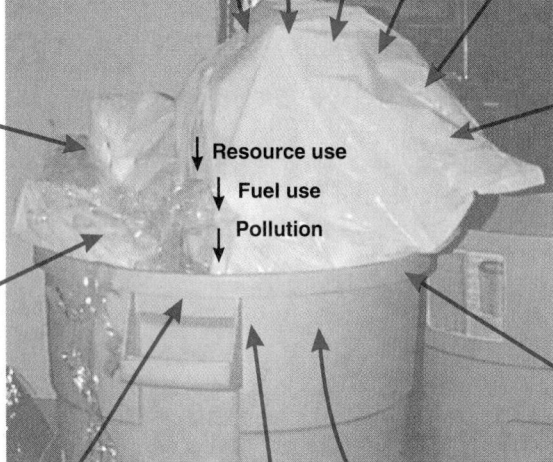

↓ **Resource use**
↓ **Fuel use**
↓ **Pollution**

Buy recycled goods to close the loop.

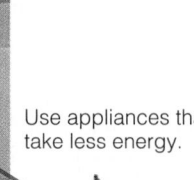

Use appliances that take less energy.

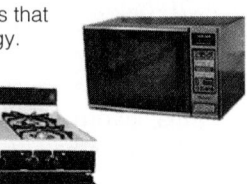

Make a switch from a meat-centered diet to a plant-centered diet. [a]

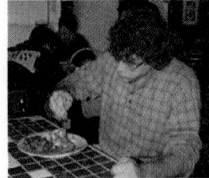 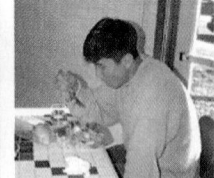

Buy fruits of differing ripeness.

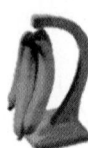

Eat most perishable foods first.

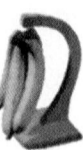

Run your refrigerator efficiently. [b]

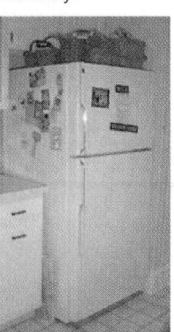

[a] Plant-centered diets are healthier and more environmentally responsible.
[b] Refer to the caption to learn how to run your refrigerator efficiently.

- Reduce use of aluminum foil, paper towels, plastic wraps, plastic storage bags, sponges, and other disposable items. Find permanent reusable replacements for each, such as pans with lids, reusable storage containers, and washable cloths and towels.
- Use fewer electric gadgets. Mix batters, chop vegetables, and open cans by hand.
- Purchase the most efficient large appliances possible.
- Insulate the home.
- Consider using solar power, especially to heat water.
- Reduce, reuse, recycle.

The personal rewards of all these behaviors are many, from saving money to the satisfaction of knowing that you are treading lightly on the earth. But do they really help? They do, if enough people join in. Perhaps most importantly, each person can support organizations that lobby for the needed changes in economic policies toward developing countries. According to one nutrition educator, "This [lobbying] is probably the most effective single thing that Joe or Jane Average Citizen can do [to help solve the world's hunger and environment problems]."[63]

Another way people can assist the global community in solving its poverty and hunger problems is to join and work for international hunger-relief organizations. Table 15-4 lists some of the major ones.

Then, in their own homes, schools, and workplaces, all people can take many small steps to help. All aspects of our lifestyles relate to global problems. Consider the personal actions just mentioned: reduce, reuse, recycle, and cut energy use for cars and homes. Admittedly, these approaches to solving today's global problems seem simple, but because we number 5 billion plus, such actions taken by many people can exert an immense impact. If each of the world's 5 billion people takes one five-billionth share of the responsibility for improving things, the job can get done. Just to be sure, though, those who can do more are encouraged to do so to compensate for those who are, as yet, too poor, ignorant, powerless, or inflexible to join in.

Finally, it makes sense for everyone in this world, rich or poor, in the United States or any other country, to plan on bearing no more than one or two children. For those who want large families, there are plenty of children to adopt. And for those who love children and want to help them in other ways, there are numerous opportunities to play with, teach, and nurture the world's children, from the community center downtown to the remotest primitive village on the globe.

"Be part of the solution, not part of the problem," an adage says. In other words, don't waste time or energy moaning and groaning about how tough things are; do something to improve them. This adage is as applicable to today's global environmental problems as it is to an unwashed dish in the kitchen sink. They are our problems: human beings created them, and human beings must solve them.

✔ KEY POINT **Government, business, educators, and all individuals have many opportunities to promote sustainability worldwide and wise resource use at home.**

TABLE 15-4

Hunger-Relief Organizations People Can Join

Bread for the World Institute
1100 Wayne Ave., Suite 1000
Silver Spring, MD 20910
(301) 608-2400

International Labour Organization
1828 L St. NW, Suite 801
Washington, DC 20036
(202) 653-7652

OXFAM America
26 West St.
Boston, MA 02111-1206
(617) 482-1211

Seeds
P.O. Box 6170
Waco, TX 76706

United Nations International Children's Emergency Fund (UNICEF)
3 United Nations Plaza
New York, NY 10017-4414
(212) 326-7035

United Nations Food and Agriculture Organization (FAO)
1001 22nd St. NW, Suite 300
Washington, DC 20437
(202) 653-2400

World Health Organization (WHO)
525 23rd St. NW
Washington, DC 20037
(202) 861-3200

World Hunger Program
Brown University
Box 1831
Providence, RI 02912
(401) 863-2700

SELF-CHECK

Answers to these Self-Check questions are in Appendix G.

1. Which of the following is an example of environmental degradation?
   a. soil erosion
   b. damaged grazing lands
   c. air pollution
   d. all of the above

2. Which of the following activities is recommended due to the small negative impact it has on the environment?
   a. Use the oven whenever possible.
   b. Line pans with aluminum foil to reduce cleanup time.
   c. Use a pressure cooker or microwave to cook foods.
   d. Carry groceries home in paper bags rather than plastic bags.

3. What is the primary cause of famine in the world?
   a. poverty
   b. drought
   c. social causes such as war
   d. flood

4. Which of the following is a symptom of food insecurity?
   a. You worry about gaining weight.
   b. You sometimes rely on neighbors to feed your children because there is not enough food in the house.
   c. You shop daily to get the best prices.
   d. You buy organic foods to avoid harm from chemicals.

5. Which of the following is a sustainable agricultural practice? (Read about this in the upcoming Controversy.)
   a. Plant legumes between grain crops.
   b. Use fertilizers generously.
   c. Irrigate on a large scale.
   d. Grow the same crop repeatedly on the same land.

6. At least 140 species of animals and plants are going extinct every day in the world.   T   F

7. More people in the world suffer from famine than from chronic hunger.   T   F

8. The higher a nation's economic status, the faster its population grows over the long run.   T   F

9. In the United States, fewer people need welfare and food assistance in the 1990s than in the 1980s due to the success of government programs.   T   F

10. An example of "eating lower on the food chain" would be to eat more fruits and grains and less beef. (A topic of this chapter's Controversy.)   T   F

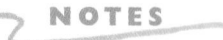 NOTES

Notes are in Appendix F.

Agribusiness and Food Production: How to Go Forward?

While some individuals are attempting to make their own personal lifestyles more environmentally benign, as suggested in the chapter, others are seeking ways to improve whole sectors of human enterprise, such as agriculture. To date, large agricultural enterprises have been among the world's biggest polluters and resource users. Is it possible for agriculture to become sustainable? And if so, will the change hurt farmers? These questions are addressed in this Controversy.

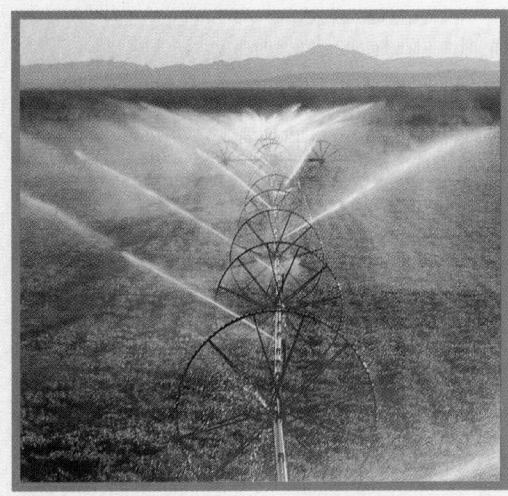

COSTS OF PRODUCING FOOD UNSUSTAINABLY

The environmental and social costs of agriculture and the food industry take many forms. Among them are resource waste and pollution, energy overuse, and tolls on life in farm communities. Table C15-1 offers some terms important to these concepts.

Resources and Pollution Producing food has always cost the earth dearly. First of all, to grow food, we clear land—prairie, wetland, or forest. This always causes losses of native ecosystems and wildlife.

Then we plant crops or graze animals on the land. Negative impacts on soil and water follow. The soil loses nutrients as each crop is taken from it, so fertilizer is applied. Some fertilizer runs off and pollutes the waterways. Some plowed soil runs off, clouds the water, and interferes with the growth of aquatic plants and animals.

Then, to protect crops against weeds and pests, we apply herbicides and pesticides. These chemicals also pollute the water and, wherever the wind carries them, the air. Most herbicides and pesticides kill not only weeds and pests, but also native plants, native insects, and animals that eat those plants and insects.

Finally, we irrigate, a practice that adds salts to the soil in many areas. The water evaporates, but the salts do not, so the soil becomes more and more salty, hindering plant growth. Irrigation can also deplete the water supply over time because it pulls water from surface waters or from underground, and then evaporates or runs off. This process, carried to an extreme, can dry up rivers and lakes and lower the water table of whole regions. This sets a vicious cycle in motion, for the lower the water table, the more farmers must irrigate; and the more they irrigate, the more groundwater they use up.

Agricultural pesticides and herbicides, if not used conservatively, also pollute rivers, lakes, and groundwater. In 1989, the nation's most prestigious national scientific research body, the National Research Council of the National Academy of Sciences, produced a report that said, in part, that agriculture is the largest single source of **nonpoint pollution** of surface water in the nation. Pollution from "point sources," such as sewage plants or factories, is relatively easy to control, but runoff from fields and pastures enters waterways from all over broad regions and is nearly impossible to control.

Widespread use of pesticides and herbicides also causes resistant pests and weeds to evolve. This makes necessary the use of still more pesticides and herbicides. Some farmers have been buying so many pesticides, herbicides, fertilizers, and soil boosters that their costs for these items have risen too high to bear. Pesticide residues are even becoming a problem for *people* who eat foods produced this way, not to mention the hazard the pesticides pose to farm workers who handle and apply them. In short, our ways of producing foods are, for the most part, not sustainable.[1]

Some agricultural practices also deplete the soil—particularly indiscriminate land clearing (deforestation) and overuse by cattle (overgrazing). In 1992, the World Resources Institute presented the results of a massive study of human impacts on the soil, showing that agriculture is destroying its own foundation. In just the past 40 years, the study said, human agricultural activities have ruined more than 10 percent of the earth's most fertile land, an area the size of China and India combined. Over 20 million acres have been so damaged that they will be impossible to reclaim, the study said. Soil erosion, if unchecked, is predicted to result in a 20 percent decline in global food production by the end of this century, and by 2025 the amount of food-producing land per person may shrink by nearly 40 percent.[2]

Agriculture is also weakening its own underpinnings by failing to conserve species diversity. By the year 2050, some 40,000 more plant species, existing in 1990, may go extinct.[3] The United Nations' Food and Agriculture Organization attributes many of the losses, which are already occurring daily, to modern farming practices, as well as to population growth. Global eating habits, too, have become uniform. People everywhere are eating the same limited array of foods, so that local regions' native, genetically diverse plants are not enough in demand to make them seem worth preserving. Yet in the future, as the climate warms and the earth changes, those may be the very plants that people will need as food sources.[4] A wild species of corn that grows in a dry climate, for example, might contain just the genetic information necessary to help make the domestic corn crop resistant to drought. Controversy 14

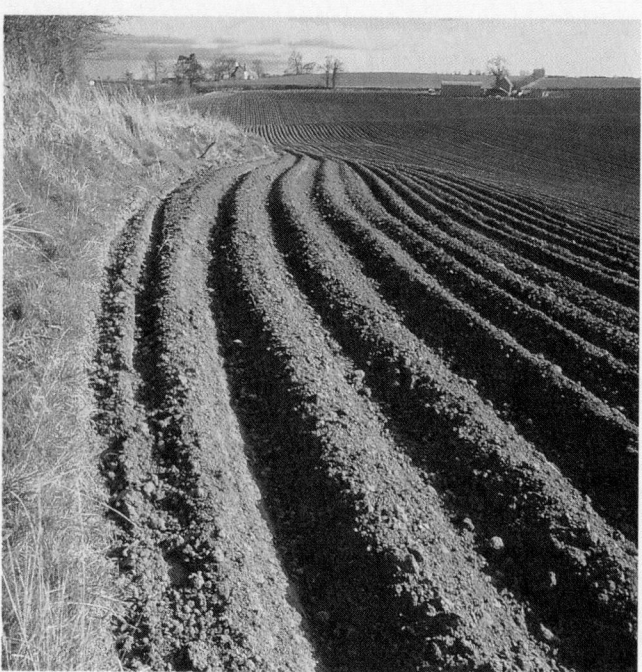

Vast areas are under plow, and those that must be irrigated can, over time, become salty and unusable.

TABLE C15-1

Agricultural and Environmental Terms

- **agribusiness** agriculture practiced on a massive scale by large corporations owning vast acreages and employing intensive technological, fuel, and chemical inputs.
- **alternative (low-input,** or **sustainable) agriculture** agriculture practiced on a small scale using individualized approaches that vary with local conditions so as to minimize technological, fuel, and chemical inputs.
- **externalities** hidden costs that are not reflected in the prices of things, such as the costs of subsidies that permit agribusiness foods to be sold at artificially low prices.
- **integrated past management (IPM)** management of pests using a combination of natural and biological controls and minimal or no application of pesticides.
- **nonpoint pollution** water pollution caused by runoff from all over an area, rather than from discrete "point" sources. An example is the pollution in runoff from farm fields.
- **subsidies** government money, derived from taxes, used to support (subsidize) practices that otherwise would force producers to set their prices too high to compete successfully.

offered other examples of genes that might be needed to improve food crops.

The culprits that attend the growing of crops—land clearing, irrigation, fertilizer overuse, pesticide overuse, herbicide overuse, and loss of genetic diversity—have always taken a tremendous toll on the earth. Agriculture has already destroyed many once-fertile regions, where high civilizations formerly flourished. The deserts of North Africa were once wheat fields, the breadbasket of the Roman Empire. Plowing and irrigation reduced them to dry, salty dust. Today, such damage is accelerating as the population grows faster and agriculturalists use more technology every year. Mistreatment of soil and water is now causing destruction on a scale never known before.[5]

Raising livestock also takes a toll. Like plant crops, herds of livestock occupy land that once maintained itself in a natural state. The land pays a price in losses of native plants and animals, soil erosion, water depletion, and desert formation. Alternatively, if animals are raised in concentrated areas (such as cattle feedlots or giant hog farms), a high price is paid when animal wastes cause water pollution.[6] And animals in feedlots still have to be fed; grain is grown for them on other land. That grain may require fertilizers, herbicides, pesticides, and irrigation, too. More cropland is used in the United States, one-fifth of the total, to produce grain for livestock than to produce grain for people.

Other environmental costs attend fishing. Fishing easily becomes overfishing and depletes stocks of the very food fish that people need to eat. Some kinds of fishing involve methods that kill aquatic animals other than those sought and deplete large populations of ecologically important nonfood animals, such as dolphins.

Energy The entire food industry, whether based on crop growing, cattle ranching, or fishing, requires energy, which entails burning fossil fuel. Massive fossil fuel use is threatening our planet by causing global warming, ozone depletion, water pollution, ocean pollution, and other ills.

In the United States, the food industry consumes about 20 percent of all the energy the nation uses. Each year we spend 1,500 liters (over 350 gallons) of oil per person to produce, process, distribute, and prepare our food. Energy is used to run farm machinery and to produce fertilizers and pesticides. Energy is also used to prepare, package, transport, refrigerate, and otherwise store, cook, and wash our foods.

Losses of Family Farms During the early and mid-1980s, U.S. agriculture encountered serious economic problems: declining markets for U.S. farm produce abroad as other countries increased their agricultural production and exports, a long recession at home, and an increase in the cost of federal loans. Many U.S. farmers, particularly those who specialized in export crops, suffered heavy financial losses. Some were unable to pay their debts and had to leave farming. At the dawn of the 1990s, tens of thousands of farms were still struggling, especially medium-sized family farms.[7] Between 1980 and 1993, more than 350,000 farms, representing 15 percent of the farms in the United States, disappeared.[8]

Most U.S. farmers today have little or no control over what products they produce, the costs of their supplies, or the prices they receive for their goods. Just prior to 1980, the USDA urged farmers to increase corn and soybean production for export. To expand their production capabilities, farmers borrowed heavily. Since that time, the costs of seed, fertilizer, equipment, and loans have risen. Thousands of U.S. farmers are frustrated, in debt, and threatened with poverty. Incidentally, we might note that the crop prices farmers receive are only a small part of the cost of the foods we eat. In 1985, for example, consumers paid $29 million just for the packages on their foods. In the same year, farmers received less than $29 million for the food itself.[9]

Farmers and ranchers can theoretically obtain financial support from the government in the form of **subsidies** and tax write-offs. Subsidies support practices such as the use of irrigation, pesticides, fertilizers, and fuels that farmers could not otherwise afford. Farmers and ranchers who receive subsidies can charge lower prices for their crops and meats, which helps them compete for buyers. Tax write-offs permit farmers and ranchers to pay lower taxes than other citizens, in effect making their enterprises more profitable.

Unfortunately, huge corporation-owned farms find it much easier to obtain and use subsidies than do small

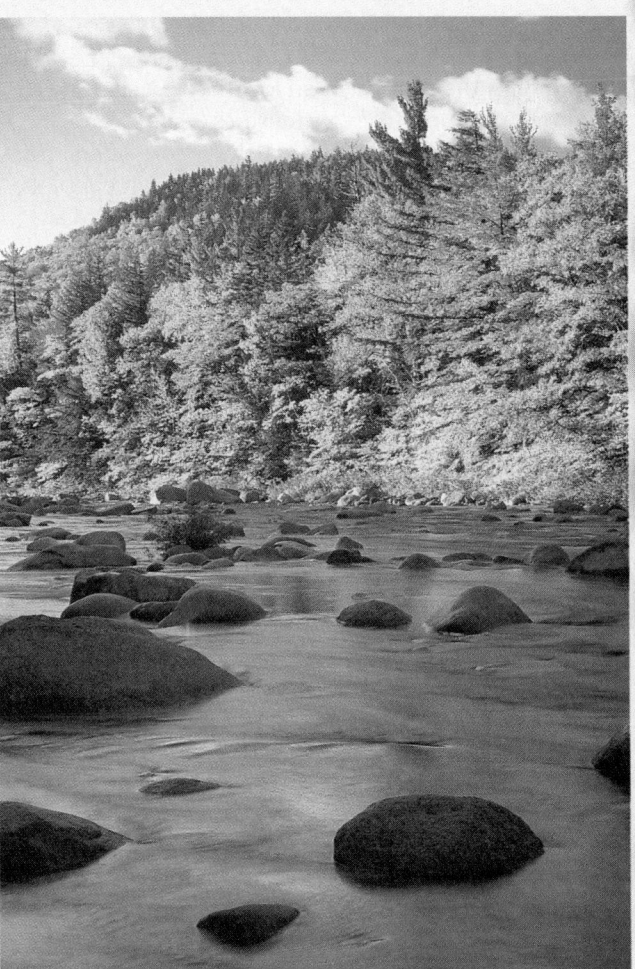

Pure rivers represent irreplaceable water resources.

family farms. Subsidies accomplish the most for the money when they support technology-intensive practices using large machines over large land areas. Huge farms and ranches, collectively part of the massive food-producing enterprise called **agribusiness,** tend to use little local labor, and the profits they make tend not to stay in local communities. In fact, subsidies to agribusiness may actually be helping to drive families out of farming.

Farm subsidies also tend to promote unsustainable practices. Subsidies encourage farmers to place a higher priority on producing abundant food than on protecting soil, water, and local biodiversity. Subsidies make it easy to overuse fertilizers and pesticides, to overuse land at the cost of soil erosion, and to use irrigation water wastefully.[10] For ranchers, billions of dollars in subsidies promote intensive forms of livestock production.[11] Evidence suggests that subsidies are unsound both economically and environmentally.[12]

A third problem is that subsidies permit sellers to set the prices of their products so low that buyers tend to buy more products from agribusiness than from smaller, local farms. The local grocery store offers broccoli from Mexico, carrots from California, pineapples from Hawaii, and bananas from Central America at prices no local operators could beat, even if they could grow those products. Roadside stands offer bundles of greens and baskets of local fruits and vegetables, but less conveniently and sometimes at higher prices than many shoppers are willing to pay.

Environmental and social costs, such as pollution and hardship to farmers, are not reflected in the *prices* of products. These costs are therefore called *external* costs, or **externalities.** People don't pay for these when they buy the products; they pay in tax money used to defray these costs. Sometimes people do not pay in money at all, but in health and social stresses; and the environment pays in resource losses and environmental deterioration. If these costs were included in prices, the prices of unsustainably produced products would be much higher. People then buy more products produced by smaller farms and ranches with less technology, less pollution, and more labor.

Agribusiness is usually the kind of agricultural system that produces the most food on the smallest land area. With the help of subsidies, agribusiness also produces the cheapest food.[13] If subsidies and other price supports were removed, many food prices would be higher. And if the prices had to include a "tax" to pay for pollution cleanup, water protection, and land

restoration, they would be higher still. It has been suggested that the dollar prices of foods produced with so much irrigation, pesticides, fertilizers, and fossil fuel should even be high enough to pay for "the costs of unemployment when farms fail, . . . national security to protect our supply of imported petroleum [for tractor fuel], . . . medical care for thousands of workers injured each year by pesticides, . . . ground water contamination," and other such external costs.[14] Still other needs include education and benefits for the nation's silent slave labor force—the migrant farm workers.

PROPOSED SOLUTIONS

For each of the problems described above, solutions have been devised. To put them into practice will require some new learning.

After reviewing problems associated with U.S agriculture, the members of the National Research Council expressed the intent to develop an alternative mode of producing food. The goals were to conserve land, water, and energy, to exert minimal environmental impacts, and to produce abundant food profitably. They named this solution **alternative agriculture.**[15]

Alternative agriculture is not one system but a set of practices that can be matched to particular needs in local areas. It emphasizes careful use of natural processes, wherever possible, rather than chemically intensive methods.[16] For example, a farmer using **integrated pest management** employs many techniques, such as crop rotation and natural predators, to control pests rather than depending on heavy use of pesticides alone. Table C15-2 contrasts alternative agriculture methods with unsustainable methods. Many sustainable techniques are not really new, incidentally; they would be familiar to our great grandparents. Many farmers today are rediscovering the benefits of old techniques as they adapt and experiment with them in the search for sustainable methods.

Farming by these methods produces crops reliably and lowers farmers' financial risks by reducing the impacts of changing prices of pesticides, fertilizers, and the like. Both large and small farms can use these practices, and many different machineries are compatible with them. Each technique has a different value for farmers of different crops in different regions. For example, corn and soybean farmers in the Midwest can eliminate routine insecticide use relatively easily, whereas fruit and vegetable growers in the hot and humid Southeast would find this harder to do.[17] Not

TABLE C15-2

Alternative Agricultural Techniques

Nonsustainable Practice	Sustainable Practice
- Growing the same crop repeatedly on the same patch of land. This takes more and more nutrients out of the soil, makes fertilizer use necessary; favors soil erosion; and invites weeds and pests to become established, making pesticide use necessary.	- Rotate crops. This increases nitrogen in the soil so there is less need to buy fertilizers. If used with appropriate plowing methods, crop rotation reduces soil erosion. An acre of land planted one year in corn, the next in wheat, and the next in clover loses 2.7 tons of topsoil each year, but if it is planted only in corn three years in a row, it will lose 19.7 tons a year. Crop rotation also reduces problems caused by weeds and pests.
- Using fertilizers generously. Excess fertilizer pollutes ground and surface water and costs both farmers' household money and consumers' tax money.	- Reduce the use of fertilizers and use livestock manure more effectively. Store manure during the nongrowing season and apply it during the growing season.
	- Alternate nutrient-devouring crops with nutrient-restoring crops.
	- Plant legumes between grain crops (because legumes' roots leave nitrogen in the soil).
	- Compost on a large scale, including all plant residues not harvested. Plow the compost into the soil to improve its water-holding capacity.
- Feeding livestock in feedlots where their manure produces a major water pollutant problem. Piled in heaps, manure also releases methane, a global-warming gas.	- Feed livestock or buffalo on the open range where their manure will fertilize the ground on which plants grow and will release no methane. Alternatively, at least collect feedlot animals' manure and use it as fertilizer, or, at the very least, treat it before release.
- Spraying herbicides and pesticides over large areas to wipe out weeds and pests.	- Apply ingenuity in weed and pest control. Use rotary hoes twice instead of herbicides once. Treat when and where necessary only. Spot treat weeds by hand.
	- Rotate crops to foil pests that lay their eggs in the soil where last year's crop was grown.
	- Use resistant crops. Genetically improve crops so that they resist pests and diseases.
	- Time the planting of crops so that pests that hatch at other times cannot gain access to them.
	- Use biological controls such as predators that destroy the pests.
- Plowing the same way everywhere, allowing unsustainable water runoff and erosion.	- Plow in ways tailored to different areas. Conserve both soil and water by using cover crops, crop rotation, no-till planting, and contour plowing.
- Injecting animals with antibiotics to prevent disease in livestock.	- Maintain animals' health so that they can resist disease by way of their own vigor.
- Irrigating on a large scale.	- Irrigate only during dry spells and apply only spot irrigation.

all crops can grow reliably without pesticides, but many can.

Alternative agriculture has some apparent disadvantages, but advantages offset them. For example, as chemical use falls, yields per acre also fall somewhat, but costs per acre also fall, so that the return per acre may be the same as or greater than before. More money goes to farmers and less to the fuels, fertilizers, pesticides, and irrigation that subsidies would help pay for. Prices for farm products may rise, but taxes can fall, because subsidies can be reduced or eliminated. The end result is to make both farmers and consumers better off financially.

Some economists and scientists have suggested that rather than subsidizing pesticide and fertilizer use, we should be taxing it. Some states are trying that strategy with success.[18] Some are proposing to tax products such as sugar at the grocery store level to raise money to repair the environmental damage they cause.[19] Mentioned in the Chapter 14 Controversy, plant biotechnology can offer economic, environmental, and agricultural benefits by shrinking the acreage needed for crops, reducing soil losses, minimizing use of chemical insecticides, and bettering crop protection.

Low-input agriculture works. More than 30,000 of the nation's farmers are successfully using sustainable techniques such as those described in Table C15-2. Notable among them are farmers in seven states who began pioneering these methods on a large scale in the 1980s and before. Low-input agriculture has been called "an idea whose time has come."[20] It is seen as "a food production system that can indefinitely sustain a healthy food supply, restore our soil and water resources, and revitalize individual farms and rural communities, all with little reliance on fossil fuels."[21]

Energy Efficiency   Fuel used in agriculture can amount to some 6,560 calories to produce a can of corn or 7,980 calories to produce a package of frozen corn. Much of this energy input could be reduced, as Table C15-3 shows. The last suggestion in the table implies that consumers should center their diets on foods that require low energy inputs, a choice that is described next. Often that means choosing plants over meats.

Eating Lower on the Food Chain   Studies of energy use in the U.S. food system have revealed which foods require the most and least energy to produce. The least energy is needed for grain: about one-third calorie of fuel is burned to produce each calorie of grain. Fruits and vegetables are intermediate, and most animal protein requires from 10 to 90 calories of fossil energy per calorie of usable food. Thus most animal-protein products require much more energy, as well as more land and water, than do plant-protein products. An exception is livestock raised on the open range; these animals require low energy inputs as do most plant foods. We grow so much more grain-fed, than range-fed, beef, however, that the average energy requirement for beef production is high. Figure C15-1 shows how much less fuel vegetarian diets require than meat diets and shows that vegan diets require the least fuel of all.

To support our meat intake we maintain several billion livestock, about four times our own weight in animals. Livestock consume ten times as much grain each day as we do. We could use much of that grain to make grain products for ourselves and share them. The shift

TABLE C15-3

Sustainable Energy-Saving Agricultural Techniques

- Use machinery scaled to the job at hand and operate it at efficient speeds.
- Combine operations. Harrow, plant, and fertilize in the same operation.
- Use diesel fuel. Use solar and wind energy on farms. Use methane from manure. Be open-minded to alternative energy sources.
- Use new disease- and pest-resistant plant varieties developed through genetic engineering.
- Save on technological and chemical inputs and spend some of the savings paying people to do manual jobs. Increasing labor inputs has been considered inefficient. Reverse this thinking: creating more jobs is preferable to using more machinery and fuel.
- Partially return to the techniques of using animal manure and crop rotation. This would save energy because chemical fertilizers require large energy inputs to produce.
- Eliminate subsidies to truckers. Change highway funding so that the tax burden falls more heavily on truckers than on other highway users. Transport foods by rail or water (building and maintaining rail lines can add more jobs than are lost in trucking). To move lettuce by truck from California to New York requires 36 calories for each calorie in the lettuce. Railways are five times more efficient than trucks.
- Choose crops that require low energy inputs (fertilizer, pesticides, irrigation).
- Educate people to cook food efficiently.

FIGURE C15-1

AVERAGE AMOUNTS OF FUEL REQUIRED TO FEED PEOPLE EATING AT DIFFERENT LEVELS ON THE FOOD CHAIN

Three people who eat differently are compared here. Each has the same energy intake: 3,300 calories a day. The fossil fuel amounts necessary to produce these different diets are calculated based on U.S. conditions.

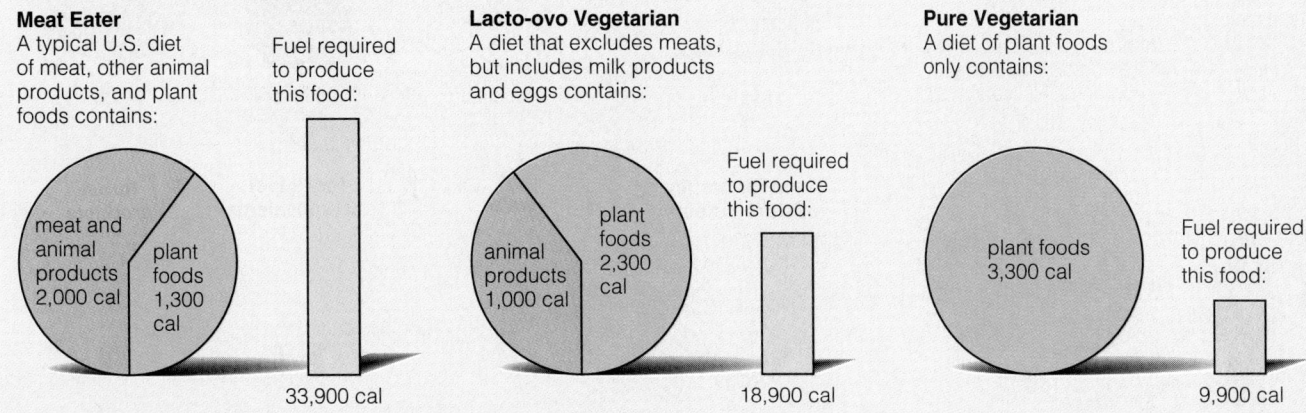

Meat Eater
A typical U.S. diet of meat, other animal products, and plant foods contains:

Fuel required to produce this food:

meat and animal products 2,000 cal

plant foods 1,300 cal

33,900 cal

Lacto-ovo Vegetarian
A diet that excludes meats, but includes milk products and eggs contains:

Fuel required to produce this food:

animal products 1,000 cal

plant foods 2,300 cal

18,900 cal

Pure Vegetarian
A diet of plant foods only contains:

plant foods 3,300 cal

Fuel required to produce this food:

9,900 cal

SOURCE: Adapted from D. Pimentel, *Food, Energy and the Future of Society* (Boulder, Colo.: Associated University Press, 1980), Figure 5, p. 27.

could free up enough grain to feed 400 million people and would necessitate burning less fuel and using less water. It could also free up much more land. The contrast between resource use in the United States and in China, a society that does live largely on plant foods, is startling (see Figure C15-2).

Part of the solution to the livestock problem may be to cease feeding grain to livestock and return to grazing animals on the open range, which can be a sustainable practice. Ranchers have to manage the grazing carefully to hold the cattle's numbers to what the land can support without degradation. To accomplish this, the economic favoritism shown to livestock and feed-growing operations would have to end. If producers were to pay the true costs of the irrigation water, fertilizers, pesticides, fuels, and lands they use rather than paying artificially lowered prices, the prices of meats might rise to two or three times what they are now. According to classic economic theory, people would then buy less meat (reducing demand), and producers would respond by producing less meat (reducing supply). Meat production would then fall to a sustainable level.

Some individuals are taking action without waiting for prices to change. Some meat eaters are choosing to

cut down on their meat portions or to eat range-fed beef or buffalo only. Livestock on the range eat grass, which people cannot eat.[22] "Rangeburger" buffalo also offers nutrition advantages over grain-fed beef. It is lower in fat, and the fat has more polyunsaturated fatty acids, including the omega-3 type.[23] Some people are switching to nonmeat, and even pure vegan, diets.[24] Shifting to a fish diet appears not to be a practical alternative at present, although fish farming shows promise of becoming practical in the future and could help greatly to provide nutritious meat at a price people and the environment could afford.[25] For the last quarter of the 20th century, overfishing so drastically reduced so many ocean fish species that ocean fishing cannot meet the need. Also, much fish production is energy intensive, requiring large inputs of fuel for boats, refrigeration, processing, packing, and transport. Moreover, bioaccumulation of toxins in fish is becoming a serious problem in some areas; in others it rules out fish use altogether.

Chapter 15 and its Controversy have suggested that, while many problems are global in scope, the actions of individual people lie at the heart of their solutions. On learning this, concerned people may take a perfectionist

FIGURE C15-2

RESOURCE USE IN THE UNITED STATES AND CHINA COMPARED

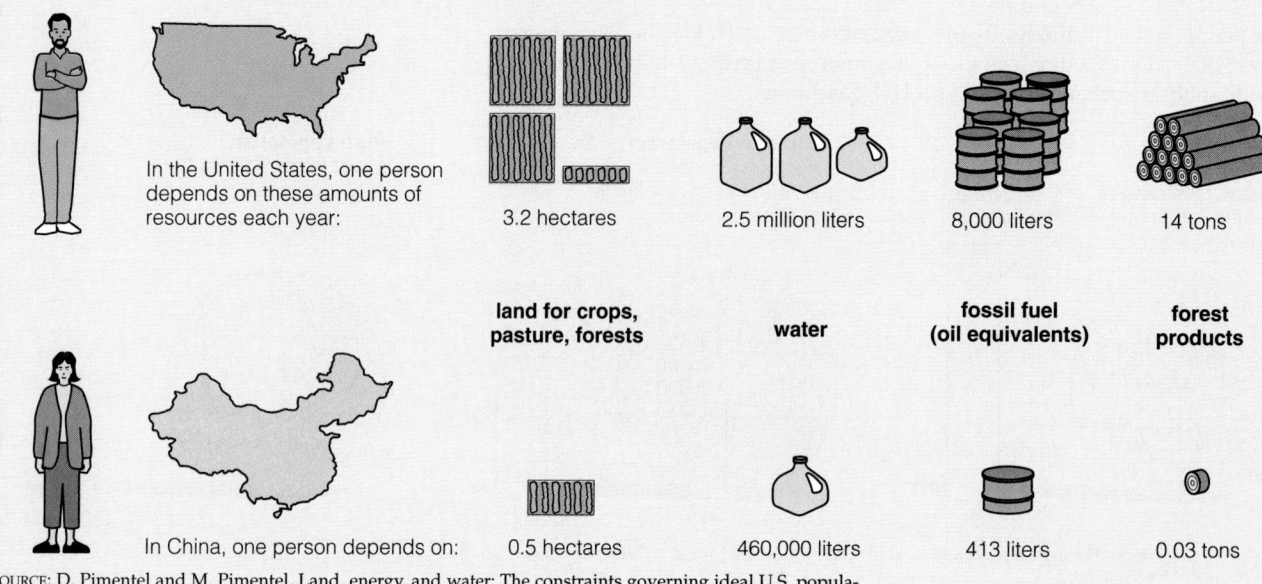

SOURCE: D. Pimentel and M. Pimentel, Land, energy, and water: The constraints governing ideal U.S. population size. *The NPG* (Negative Population Growth) *Forum*, January 1990, Table 2, p. 2.

attitude, believing that they "should" be doing more than they realistically can, and so feel defeated. Yet, striving for perfection, even while falling short, is a way to achieve progress well worth celebrating. A positive attitude can bring about improvement, and improvement is enough to be proud of. Celebrate the changes that are possible today by making them a permanent part of your life; do the same with changes that become possible tomorrow and every day thereafter. The results may add up to more than you dared to hope for.

NOTES

Notes are in Appendix F.

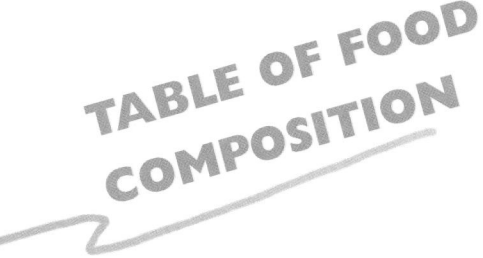

TABLE OF FOOD COMPOSITION

A

This table of food composition is specifically designed for this textbook. It contains more complete values for dietary fiber; saturated, monounsaturated, and polyunsaturated fat; vitamin B$_6$; folate; magnesium; and zinc than any comparable table. Also, a wide variety of foods from all food groups are included, and updated yearly to reflect current food patterns. For example, this edition includes about 300 more foods than are in the table in the previous edition.

To achieve a complete and reliable listing of nutrients for all the foods, over 1,000 sources of information are researched. Government sources of information are the primary base for all the data: the USDA *Handbook* series and its current supplemental data, as well as current data on baked goods, snacks, and sweets. In addition, provisional USDA information—both published and unpublished—is included. Many conversations with the staff members at the USDA Human Nutrition Information Service in Hyattsville, Maryland, provided additional professional information to refine the data.

Even with all the government sources available, there are still missing nutrient values; and as the various government data are updated, conflicting values are reported from the USDA for the same items. To fill in the missing values and resolve discrepancies, other sources of information are used. These reliable sources include refereed journal articles, food composition tables from Canada and England, information from other nutrient data banks and publications, unpublished scientific data, and manufacturers' data.

Estimates of nutrient amounts for foods and nutrients include all possible adjustments, in the interest of accuracy. When multiple values are reported for a nutrient, the numbers are averaged and weighted with consideration given to the original number of samples from the separate sources. Whenever water percentages are available, estimates of nutrient amounts are adjusted for water content. When no water is given, water percentage is assumed to be that shown in the table. Whenever a reported weight appeared inconsistent (cooked eggplant, for example), many kitchen tests were made, and the average weight of the typical product was given as tested.

When estimates of nutrient amounts in cooked foods are derived from reported amounts in raw foods, published retention factors are applied. Some reported data for combination foods are modified in this table to include the newer data available for major ingredients. For example, since the "pies" were analyzed and reported, newer data on fruits have been published. Bakery items reflect the most current data with the new enrichment levels for certain nutrients. And, new information on some snacks and sweets is reflected in this edition.

Considerable effort has been made to report the most accurate data available and to eliminate missing values. The table is updated annually, and the authors welcome any suggestions or comments for future editions.

IT IS IMPORTANT TO KNOW

There can be many different nutrient values reported for foods, even by reliable sources. Many factors influence the amounts of nutrients in foods, including the mineral content of the soil, the method of processing, genetics, the diet of the animal or the fertilizer of the plant, the season of the year, methods of analysis, the difference in moisture content of the samples analyzed, the length and method of storage, and methods of cooking the food.

Although each nutrient from USDA government data is presented as a single number in some USDA publications, each number is actually an average of a range of data. In the more detailed reports (Handbook 8 series), the number of samples is identified, and the standard deviation of the data is also noted. USDA data will have different reported values for foods as well, as older information is replaced with newer data in the more recent publications. Therefore, nutrient data should be viewed and used only as a guide, a close approximation of nutrient content.

Dietary fiber deserves a special word. Estimates of dietary fiber are included for all the foods in this table. The sources of this information are primarily extensive published and unpublished information from the USDA Human Nutrition Information Service in Hyattsville, Maryland; *Composition of Foods by Southgate* (England); and many journal articles.

It is important to know that data for dietary fiber is still undergoing review in the scientific community. No doubt, there will be changes in the data as analytical techniques are refined and interpretations clarified.

Vitamin A is reported in retinol equivalents. The amount of this vitamin can vary by the season of the year and the maturity of the plant. (Note the difference between collard greens from fresh and from frozen, items 843 and 844.) Reported values in both dairy products and plants are higher in summer and early fall than in winter. The values reported here represent year-round averages. In the organ meats of all animal products (liver especially), there are large amounts of vitamin A, and these amounts vary widely, depending on the background of the animal. The vitamin is present in very small amounts in regular meat and is often reported as a trace.

Vitamin E values have been added to this edition of the table, expressed as alpha tocopherol equivalent milligrams. These units adjust for the differing degrees of activity among various forms of vitamin E found in foods. Vitamin E activity also varies with such conditions as high-temperature cooking and rancidity, which destroy it, or air-tight packaging and the presence of other antioxidants, which preserve it.

The energy and nutrients in recipes and combination foods vary widely, depending on the ingredients. The various fatty acids and cholesterol are influenced by the type of fat used (the specific type of oil, vegetable shortening, butter, margarine, etc.).

Total fats, as well as the breakdown of total fats to saturated, monounsaturated, and polyunsaturated fats, are listed in the table. The fatty acids seldom add up to the total. This is due to rounding and to the existence of small amounts of other fatty acid components that are not included in the three basic categories, including trans fatty acids and glycerol.

Niacin values are for preformed niacin and do not include additional niacin that may form in the body from the conversion of tryptophan.

The items in this table have been organized into several categories, which are listed at the head of each right-hand page. As the key shows, each group has been color-coded to ease paging through this table.

In an effort to conserve space, abbreviations have been used in some food descriptions. The following abbreviations have been used in the food descriptions and nutrient breakdowns:

- diam = diameter
- enr = enriched
- f/ = from
- g = grams
- liq = liquid
- pce = piece

- w/ = with
- w/o = without
- t = trace
- 0 = zero (no nutrient value)
- — = information not available

This table has been prepared for West Publishing Company and is copyrighted by ESHA Research in Salem, Oregon—the developer and publisher of the Food Processor®, Nutrition Pro®, and Genesis® nutrition software systems. The major sources for the data from the U.S. Department of Agriculture are supplemented by over 1000 additional sources of information. Because the list of references is so extensive, it is not provided in this textbook, but it is available from the publisher.

Table A–1
Food Composition

Computer Code Number	Food Description	Measure	Wt (g)	H$_2$O (%)	Ener (cal)	Prot (g)	Carb (g)	Dietary Fiber (g)	Fat (g)	Fat Breakdown (g)		
										Sat	Mono	Poly
BEVERAGES												
	Alcoholic:											
	Beer:											
1	Regular (12 fl oz)	1½ c	356	92	146	1	13	3	0	0	0	0
2	Light (12 fl oz)	1½ c	354	95	99[1]	1	5	1	0	0	0	0
1506	Nonalcoholic (12 fl oz)	1 ea	360	98	32	1	5	0	0	0	0	0
	Gin, rum, vodka, whiskey:											
3	80 proof	1½ fl oz	42	67	97	0	0	0	0	0	0	0
4	86 proof	1½ fl oz	42	64	105	0	<1	0	0	0	0	0
5	90 proof	1½ fl oz	42	62	110	0	0	0	0	0	0	0
	Liqueur:											
1359	Coffee liqueur, 53 proof	1½ fl oz	52	31	175	<1	24	0	<1	.1	t	.1
1360	Coffee & cream liqueur, 34 proof	1½ fl oz	47	46	154	1	10	0	7	4.5	2.1	.3
1361	Crème de menthe, 72 proof	1½ fl oz	50	28	186	0	21	0	<1	t	t	.1
	Wine:											
6	Dessert (4 fl oz)	½ c	118	72	181[2]	<1	14	0	0	0	0	0
7	Red	3½ fl oz	103	88	74	<1	2	0	0	0	0	0
8	Rosé	3½ fl oz	103	89	73	<1	1	0	0	0	0	0
9	White medium	3½ fl oz	103	90	70	<1	1	0	0	0	0	0
1592	Nonalcoholic	1 c	232	98	14	1	3	0	0	0	0	0
1593	Nonalcoholic light	1 c	251	98	15	1	3	0	0	0	0	0
1409	Wine cooler, bottle (12 fl oz)	1½ c	340	90	169	<1	20	<1	<1	0	0	t
1595	Wine cooler, cup	1 c	227	90	113	<1	13	<1	<1	0	0	t
	Carbonated:[3]											
10	Club soda (12 fl oz)	1½ c	355	100	0	0	0	0	0	0	0	0
11	Cola beverage (12 fl oz)	1½ c	370	89	152	0	38	0	<1	0	0	.1
12	Diet cola w/aspartame (12 fl oz)	1½ c	355	100	4	<1	<1	0	0	0	0	0
13	Diet cola w/saccharin (12 fl oz)	1½ c	355	100	0	0	<1	0	0	0	0	0
14	Ginger ale (12 fl oz)	1½ c	366	91	124	0	32	0	0	0	0	0
15	Grape soda (12 fl oz)	1½ c	372	89	160	0	42	0	0	0	0	0
16	Lemon-lime (12 fl oz)	1½ c	368	90	147	0	38	0	0	0	0	0
17	Orange (12 fl oz)	1½ c	372	88	179	0	46	0	0	0	0	0
18	Pepper-type soda (12 fl oz)	1½ c	368	89	151	0	38	0	<1	.3	0	0
19	Root beer (12 fl oz)	1½ c	370	89	152	0	39	0	0	0	0	0
20	Coffee,[3] brewed	1 c	240	99	5[4]	<1	1	0	<1	0	0	0
21	Coffee,[3] prepared from instant	1 c	240	99	5[4]	<1	1	0	<1	0	0	0
	Fruit drinks, noncarbonated:[5]											
22	Fruit punch drink, canned	½ c	126	88	59	0	15	0	<1	0	0	0
1358	Gatorade	1 c	240	94	60	0	15	0	0	0	0	0
23	Grape drink, canned	½ c	125	87	63	<1	16	<1	0	0	0	0
1304	Kool-Aid, with sugar	1 c	240	90	89	0	23	0	<1	0	0	0
1356	Kool-Aid, with NutraSweet	1 c	240	95	43	0	11	0	0	0	0	0

[1]Calories can vary from 78 to 131 for 12 fl. oz.

[2]Values are for sweet dessert wine. Dry dessert wines contain 149 cal and 5 g of carbohydrate.

[3]Mineral content varies depending on water source.

[4]Calorie values from USDA vary from 1 to 5 cal per cup.

[5]Usually less than 10% fruit juice.

(Computer code number is for West Diet Analysis program)

PAGE KEY: A–4 = BEV   A–6 = DAIRY   A–12 = EGGS   A–14 = FAT/OIL   A–18 = FRUIT   A–26 = BAKERY   A–36 = GRAIN   A–44 = FISH
A–48 = MEATS   A–50 = POULTRY   A–54 = SAUSAGE   A–56 = MIXED/FAST   A–64 = NUTS/SEEDS   A–68 = SWEETS   A–70 = VEG/LEG
A–84 = MISC   A–88 = SOUPS/SAUCES   A–90 = FAST   A–106 = FRZN ENTREE   A–112 = BABY FOODS

Chol (mg)	Calc (mg)	Iron (mg)	Magn (mg)	Pota (mg)	Sodi (mg)	Zinc (mg)	VT-A (RE)	Thia (mg)	Ribo (mg)	Niac (mg)	V-B6 (mg)	Fola (μg)	VT-C (mg)	VT-E α-TE (mg)
0	18	.11	21	89	18	.07	0	.04	.11	1.60	.18	21	0	0
0	18	.14	18	64	11	.11	0	.04	.11	1.38	.11	15	0	0
0	25	.04	32	90	18	.04	0	.02	.09	1.63	.18	22	0	0
0	0	.02	0	1	<1	.02	0	<.01	0	0	0	0	0	0
0	0	.02	0	1	<1	.02	0	<.01	0	0	0	0	0	0
0	0	.02	0	1	<1	.02	0	<.01	0	0	0	0	0	0
0	1	.03	2	16	4	.02	0	0	.01	.07	0	0	0	0
7	8	.06	1	15	43	.08	20	0	.03	.04	.01	0	0	0
0	0	.04	0	0	2	.02	0	0	0	0	0	0	0	0
0	9	.28	11	108	11	.08	0	.02	.02	.25	0	<1	0	0
0	8	.44	13	116	5	.09	0	.01	.03	.08	.03	2	0	0
0	8	.39	10	102	5	.06	0	0	.02	.07	.02	1	0	0
0	9	.33	10	83	5	.07	0	0	.01	.07	.01	<1	0	0
0	21	.93	23	204	16	.19	0	0	.02	.23	.05	2	0	0
0	23	1	25	221	18	.2	0	0	.03	.25	.05	3	0	0
0	19	.92	18	152	29	.2	1	.02	.02	.16	.04	4	6	.02
0	13	.61	12	101	19	.13	<1	.01	.02	.10	.03	3	4	.02
0	18	.04	4	7	75	.36	0	0	0	0	0	0	0	0
0	11	.11	4	4	15	.04	0	0	0	0	0	0	0	0
0	14	.11	4	0	21[6]	.28	0	.02	.08	0	0	0	0	0
0	14	.14	4	7	57	.18	0	0	0	0	0	0	0	0
0	11	.66	4	4	26	.18	0	0	0	0	0	0	0	0
0	11	.3	4	4	56	.26	0	0	0	0	0	0	0	0
0	7	.26	4	4	40	.18	0	0	0	.06	0	0	0	0
0	19	.22	4	7	45	.37	0	0	0	0	0	0	0	0
0	11	.15	0	4	37	.15	0	0	0	0	0	0	0	0
0	19	.19	4	4	48	.26	0	0	0	0	0	0	0	0
0	5	.12	12	130	5	.05	0	0	0	.53	0	<1	0	0
0	7	.12	10	86	7	.07	0	0	<.01	.68	0	0	0	0
0	10	.26	3	32	28	.15	2	.03	.03	.03	0	2	37	0
0	0	.12	2	26	96	.05	0	.01	0	0	0	0	0	0
0	4	.13	5	44	1	.04	0	.01	.01	.13	.03	1	20	0
0	38	.12	2	2	34	.07	0	0	<.01	<.01	0	<1	28	0
0	17	.65	5	50	50	.26	2	.02	.05	.05	0	5	77	0

[6] Value for product sweetened with aspartame only; sodium is 32 mg if a blend of aspartame and sodium saccharin is used.

(For purposes of calculations, use "0" for t, <1, <.1, <.01, etc.)

Table A–1
Food Composition

Computer Code Number	Food Description	Measure	Wt (g)	H$_2$O (%)	Ener (cal)	Prot (g)	Carb (g)	Dietary Fiber (g)	Fat (g)	Fat Breakdown (g)		
										Sat	Mono	Poly
	BEVERAGES—Cont.											
	Fruit drinks, noncarbonated—Cont.											
26	Lemonade, frozen concentrate (6-oz can)	¾ c	219	52	396	1	103	1	<1	.1	t	.1
27	Lemonade, from concentrate	1 c	248	89	99	<1	26	<1	<1	t	t	t
28	Limeade, frozen concentrate (6-oz can)	¾ c	218	50	408	<1	107	1	<1	t	t	.1
29	Limeade, from concentrate	1 c	247	89	101	0	27	<1	<1	0	0	t
24	Pineapple grapefruit, canned	1 c	250	88	118	<1	29	<1	<1	t	t	.1
25	Pineapple orange, canned	1 c	250	87	125	3	30	<1	0	0	0	0
	Fruit and vegetable juices: see Fruit and Vegetable sections											
	Slim Fast:[1]											
1612	Chocolate malt with nonfat milk	1 c	273	82	190	14	32	2	1	.3	.1	t
1613	Strawberry with nonfat milk	1 c	273	82	190	14	32	2	1	.3	.1	t
1611	Vanilla with nonfat milk	1 c	273	82	190	14	32	2	1	.3	.1	t
	Ultra Slim Fast:[1]											
1616	Chocolate with nonfat milk	1 c	278	81	200	14	36	5	1	.3	.1	t
1614	French vanilla with nonfat milk	1 c	278	81	190	14	36	4	1	.3	.1	t
1615	Strawberry Supreme with nonfat milk	1 c	278	81	190	14	36	4	1	.3	.1	t
1357	Water, bottled: Perrier (6½ fl oz)	1 ea	192	100	0	0	0	0	0	0	0	0
1594	Water, bottled: Tonic water	1½ c	366	91	124	0	32	0	0	0	0	0
	Tea:[2]											
30	Brewed, regular	1 c	240	100	2	0	1	0	<1	0	0	t
1662	Brewed, herbal	¾ c	178	100	2	0	<1	0	t	0	0	t
32	From instant, sweetened	1 c	262	91	89	<1	22	0	<1	t	0	t
31	From instant, unsweetened	1 c	237	100	2	0	<1	0	0	0	0	0
	DAIRY											
	Butter: see Fats and Oils, #158,159,160											
	Cheese, natural:											
33	Blue	1 oz	28	42	100	6	1	0	8	5.3	2.2	.2
34	Brick	1 oz	28	41	105	7	1	0	8	5.3	2.4	.2
35	Brie	1 oz	28	48	95	6	<1	0	8	4.9	2.3	.2
36	Camembert	1 oz	28	52	85	6	<1	0	7	4.3	2	.2
37	Cheddar:	1 oz	28	37	114	7	<1	0	9	6	2.7	.3
38	1" cube	1 ea	17	37	69	4	<1	0	6	3.6	1.6	.2
39	Shredded	1 c	113	37	455	28	1	0	37	23.8	10.6	1.1
1406	Low fat, low sodium	1 oz	28	65	49	7	1	0	2	1.3	0.6	.1
	Cottage:											
984	Low sodium, low fat	1 c	225	84	162	28	6	0	2	1.4	.6	.1
40	Creamed, large curd	1 c	225	79	232	28	6	0	10	6.4	2.9	.3
41	Creamed, small curd	1 c	210	79	216	26	6	0	9	6	2.7	.3
42	With fruit	1 c	226	72	280	22	30	0	8	4.9	2.2	.2
43	Low fat 2%	1 c	226	79	203	31	8	0	4	2.8	1.2	.1
44	Low fat 1%	1 c	226	82	164	28	6	0	2	1.5	.7	.1
46	Cream	1 oz	28	54	99	2	1	0	10	6.2	2.8	.4
983	Low fat	1 oz	28	64	65	3	2	0	5	3.1	1.4	.2
47	Edam	1 oz	28	42	101	7	<1	0	8	5	2.3	.2
48	Feta	1 oz	28	55	75	4	1	0	6	4.2	1.3	.2

[1]See Chapter 9 for healthy weight loss strategies. The formulas for these products change periodically; these data reflect nutrient values as of our publication date.

[2]Mineral content varies depending on water source.

(Computer code number is for West Diet Analysis program)

PAGE KEY: A–4 = BEV   A–6 = DAIRY   A–12 = EGGS   A–14 = FAT/OIL   A–18 = FRUIT   A–26 = BAKERY   A–36 = GRAIN   A–44 = FISH   A–48 = MEATS   A–50 = POULTRY   A–54 = SAUSAGE   A–56 = MIXED/FAST   A–64 = NUTS/SEEDS   A–68 = SWEETS   A–70 = VEG/LEG   A–84 = MISC   A–88 = SOUPS/SAUCES   A–90 = FAST   A–106 = FRZN ENTREE   A–112 = BABY FOODS

Chol (mg)	Calc (mg)	Iron (mg)	Magn (mg)	Pota (mg)	Sodi (mg)	Zinc (mg)	VT-A (RE)	Thia (mg)	Ribo (mg)	Niac (mg)	V-B6 (mg)	Fola (µg)	VT-C (mg)	VT-E α-TE (mg)
0	15	1.58	11	146	9	.18	21	.06	.21	.16	.05	22	39[3]	0
0	7	.4	5	37	7	.1	5	.01	.05	.04	.01	5	10[3]	0
0	11	.22	9	128	0	.09	0	.02	.02	.22	0	9	26	0
0	7	.07	2	32	5	.05	0	0	0	.05	0	2	7	0
0	18	.78	15	152	35	.15	9	.08	.04	.67	.1	26	115	0
0	13	.68	15	115	7	.15	133	.08	.05	.52	.12	27	56	0
4	450	6.3	140	690	230	5.25	350	.53	.59	7	.7	120	21	5
4	450	6.3	140	720	220	5.25	350	.53	.59	7	.7	120	21	5
4	450	6.31	140	721	220	5.24	350	.53	.59	7	.7	120	21	5
<1	450	6.3	140	800	230	5.25	350	.52	.59	7	.7	120	21	10
<1	450	6.3	140	730	250	5.25	350	.52	.59	7	.7	120	21	10
<1	450	6.3	140	710	250	5.25	350	.52	.59	7	.7	120	21	10
0	27	0	0	0	2	0	0	0	0	0	0	0	0	0
0	4	.04	0	0	15	.37	0	0	0	0	0	0	0	0
0	0	.05	7	89	7	.05	0	0	.03	0	0	12	0	0
0	4	.14	2	16	2	.07	0	.02	.01	0	0	1	0	0
0	5	.05	5	50	8	.08	0	0	.05	.09	.01	10	0	0
0	5	.05	5	47	7	.07	0	0	<.01	.09	0	1	0	0
21	150	.09	6	73	395	.75	65	.01	.11	.29	.05	10	0	.18
27	191	.12	7	39	159	.74	86	0	.1	.03	.02	6	0	.14
28	52	.14	6	43	178	.67	52	.02	.15	.11	.07	18	0	.18
20	110	.09	6	53	239	.67	71	.01	.14	.18	.06	18	0	.18
30	204	.19	8	28	176	.88	86	.01	.11	.02	.02	5	0	.1
18	123	.12	5	17	106	.53	51	0	.06	.01	.01	3	0	.06
119	815	.77	31	111	702	3.53	342	.03	.43	.09	.08	21	0	.41
6	199	.2	8	32	6	.88	18	.01	.01	.03	.02	5	0	.25
9	137	.32	11	193	29	.86	25	.05	.36	.3	.15	27	0	.23
33	135	.32	12	190	911	.83	108	.05	.37	.28	.15	27	0	.28
31	126	.29	11	177	851	.78	101	.04	.34	.26	.14	26	0	.26
25	108	.25	9	151	915	.65	81	.04	.29	.23	.12	22	0	.21
19	155	.36	14	217	918	.95	45	.05	.42	.33	.17	30	0	.13
10	138	.32	12	193	918	.86	25	.05	.37	.29	.15	28	0	.25
31	23	.34	2	34	84	.15	124	0	.06	.03	.01	4	0	.26
16	32	.48	2	47	84	.22	63	.01	.08	.04	.02	5	0	.14
25	207	.12	8	53	274	1.07	72	.01	.11	.02	.02	5	0	.21
25	140	.18	5	18	316	.82	36	.04	.24	.28	.12	9	0	.01

[3] Vitamin C can range from 5 to 72 mg in a small can of frozen concentrate, and from 1 to 18 mg in 1 c of prepared lemonade.

(For purposes of calculations, use "0" for t, <1, <.1, <.01, etc.)

Table A–1
Food Composition

Computer Code Number	Food Description	Measure	Wt (g)	H$_2$O (%)	Ener (cal)	Prot (g)	Carb (g)	Dietary Fiber (g)	Fat (g)	Fat Breakdown (g)		
										Sat	Mono	Poly
	DAIRY—Cont.											
	Cheese—Cont.											
49	Gouda	1 oz	28	42	101	7	1	0	8	5	2.2	.2
50	Gruyère	1 oz	28	33	117	8	<1	0	9	5.4	2.8	.5
51	Gorgonzola	1 oz	28	39	111	7	0	0	9	5.5	2.4	.5
52	Liederkranz	1 oz	28	53	87	5	<1	0	8	5.3	2.2	.2
1676	Limburger	1 oz	28	48	93	6	<1	0	8	4.7	2.4	.1
53	Monterey Jack	1 oz	28	41	106	7	<1	0	9	5.4	2.5	.3
54	Mozzarella, whole milk	1 oz	28	54	80	5	1	0	6	3.7	1.9	.2
55	Mozzarella, part-skim milk, low moisture	1 oz	28	49	79	8	1	0	5	3.1	1.4	.1
56	Muenster	1 oz	28	42	104	7	<1	0	9	5.4	2.5	.2
1399	Nonfat (Kraft Singles)	1 oz	28	60	45	6	4	0	0	0	0	0
	Parmesan, grated:											
57	Cup, not pressed down	1 c	100	18	456	42	4	0	30	19	8.7	.7
58	Tablespoon	1 tbs	5	18	23	2	<1	0	2	1	.4	t
59	Ounce	1 oz	28	18	129	12	1	0	9	5.4	2.5	.2
60	Provolone	1 oz	28	41	100	7	1	0	8	4.8	2.1	.2
61	Ricotta, whole milk	1 c	246	72	428	28	8	0	32	20.4	8.9	1
62	Ricotta, part-skim milk	1 c	246	74	339	28	13	0	19	12.1	5.7	.6
63	Romano	1 oz	28	31	109	9	1	0	8	4.8	2.2	.2
64	Swiss	1 oz	28	37	106	8	1	0	8	5	2.1	.3
976	Low fat	1 oz	28	60	51	8	1	0	1	.9	.4	<.1
	Pasteurized processed cheese products:											
65	American	1 oz	28	39	106	6	<1	0	9	5.6	2.5	.3
66	Swiss	1 oz	28	42	94	7	1	0	7	4.6	2	.2
67	American cheese food, jar	1 oz	28	43	93	6	2	0	7	4.4	2	.2
68	American cheese spread	1 oz	28	48	82	5	2	0	6	3.8	1.8	.2
982	Velveeta cheese spread, low fat, low sodium	1 oz	28	63	51	7	1	0	2	1.3	0.6	.1
69	Cream, sweet:	1 c	242	81	315	7	10	0	28	17.3	8	1
	Half & half (cream & milk):											
70	Tablespoon	1 tbs	15	81	19	<1	1	0	2	1.1	.5	.1
71	Light, coffee or table:	1 c	240	74	468	6	9	0	46	28.8	13.4	1.7
72	Tablespoon	1 tbs	15	74	29	<1	1	0	3	1.8	.8	.1
73	Light whipping cream, liquid:[1]	1 c	239	64	698	5	7	0	74	46.1	21.7	2.1
74	Tablespoon	1 tbs	15	64	44	<1	<1	0	5	2.9	1.4	.1
75	Heavy whipping cream, liquid:[1]	1 c	238	58	821	5	7	0	88	54.7	25.5	3.3
76	Tablespoon	1 tbs	15	58	52	<1	<1	0	6	3.4	1.6	.2
77	Whipped cream, pressurized:	1 c	60	61	154	2	8	0	13	8.3	3.8	.5
78	Tablespoon	1 tbs	4	61	10	<1	<1	0	1	.6	.3	t
79	Cream, sour, cultured:	1 c	230	71	492	7	10	0	48	29.9	13.9	1.8
80	Tablespoon	1 tbs	14	71	30	<1	1	0	3	1.8	.8	.1
	Cream products—imitation and part dairy:											
81	Coffee whitener, frozen or liquid	1 tbs	15	77	20	<1	2	0	2	1.4	t	0
82	Coffee whitener, powdered	1 tsp	2	2	11	<1	1	0	1	.6	t	t
83	Dessert topping, frozen, nondairy:	1 c	75	50	239	1	17	0	19	16.4	1.2	.4
84	Tablespoon	1 tbs	5	50	16	<1	1	0	1	1.1	.1	t
85	Dessert topping, mix with whole milk:	1 c	80	67	151	3	13	0	10	8.6	.7	.2
86	Tablespoon	1 tbs	5	67	9	<1	1	0	1	.5	t	t

[1]For whipped cream, (non-pressurized), double the liquid cream volume of codes 73, 74 or 75, 76. One tablespoon liquid cream becomes 2 tablespoons when "whipped."

(Computer code number is for West Diet Analysis program)

Chol (mg)	Calc (mg)	Iron (mg)	Magn (mg)	Pota (mg)	Sodi (mg)	Zinc (mg)	VT-A (RE)	Thia (mg)	Ribo (mg)	Niac (mg)	V-B6 (mg)	Fola (µg)	VT-C (mg)	VT-E α-TE (mg)
32	198	.07	8	34	232	1.11	49	.01	.09	.02	.02	6	0	.1
31	286	.05	10	23	95	1.11	85	.02	.08	.03	.02	3	0	.1
25	149	.12	8	26	512	.57	103	.01	.09	.2	.04	9	0	.22
21	110	.12	7	68	389	.7	91	.01	.18	.1	.04	34	0	.21
26	141	.04	6	36	227	.6	90	.02	.14	.04	.02	16	0	.18
25	211	.2	8	23	152	.85	72	0	.11	.03	.02	5	0	.1
22	146	.05	5	19	105	.63	68	0	.07	.02	.02	2	0	.1
15	207	.07	7	27	149	.89	54	.01	.1	.03	.02	3	0	.13
27	203	.12	8	38	178	.8	90	0	.09	.03	.02	3	0	.13
5	224	0	–	81	438	–	128	–	.10	–	–	–	0	0
79	1375	.95	51	107	1861	3.19	173	.04	.39	.31	.1	8	0	.8
4	69	.05	3	5	93	.16	9	0	.02	.02	.01	<1	0	.04
22	390	.27	14	30	528	.9	49	.01	.11	.09	.03	2	0	.22
20	214	.15	8	39	247	.92	75	0	.09	.04	.02	3	0	.1
124	509	.93	28	258	206	2.88	330	.03	.48	.26	.11	30	0	.86
76	669	1.08	36	308	308	3.3	278	.05	.45	.19	.05	32	0	.53
29	300	.22	12	24	340	.73	40	.01	.1	.02	.02	2	0	.2
26	272	.05	10	31	74	1.11	72	.01	.1	.03	.02	2	0	.14
10	272	.05	10	31	74	1.11	18	.01	.1	.03	.02	2	0	.06
27	174	.11	6	46	405	.85	82	.01	.1	.02	.02	2	0	.13
24	219	.17	8	61	388	1.03	65	0	.08	.01	.01	2	0	.19
18	163	.24	9	79	336	.85	62	.01	.13	.04	.04	2	0	.2
16	159	.09	8	69	380	.73	54	.01	.12	.04	.03	2	0	.2
10	194	.12	7	51	2	.94	18	.01	.11	.02	.02	3	0	.14
89	254	.17	25	315	98	1.23	259	.08	.36	.19	.09	6	2	.27
6	16	.01	2	19	6	.08	16	.01	.02	.01	.01	<1	<1	.02
158	230	.1	21	293	95	.65	437	.08	.35	.14	.08	6	2	.36
10	14	.01	1	18	6	.04	27	.01	.02	.01	0	<1	<1	.02
265	165	.07	17	231	82	.6	705	.06	.3	.1	.07	9	1	1.43
17	10	0	1	14	5	.04	44	.01	.02	.01	0	1	<1	.09
326	153	.07	17	179	89	.55	1001	.05	.26	.09	.06	9	1	1.5
21	10	0	1	11	6	.03	63	0	.02	.01	0	1	<1	.1
46	61	.03	6	88	78	.22	124	.02	.04	.04	.02	2	0	.36
3	4	0	<1	6	5	.01	8	0	0	0	0	<1	0	.02
102	267	.14	26	331	122	.62	449	.08	.34	.15	.04	25	2	1.3
6	16	.01	2	20	7	.04	27	0	.02	.01	0	2	<1	.08
0	1	<.01	<1	29	12	0	1	0	0	0	0	0	0	.24
0	<1	.02	<1	16	4	.01	<1	0	0	0	0	0	0	.01
0	5	.09	1	14	19	.02	64[2]	0	0	0	0	0	0	.14
0	<1	.01	<1	1	1	0	4[2]	0	0	0	0	0	0	.01
8	72	.03	8	120	53	.22	39[2]	.02	.09	.05	.02	3	1	.11
<1	5	0	<1	8	3	.01	2[2]	0	.01	0	0	<1	<1	.01

[2]Vitamin A value is from beta-carotene used for coloring.

(For purposes of calculations, use "0" for t, <1, <.1, <.01, etc.)

Table A–1
Food Composition

Computer Code Number	Food Description	Measure	Wt (g)	H$_2$O (%)	Ener (cal)	Prot (g)	Carb (g)	Dietary Fiber (g)	Fat (g)	Fat Breakdown (g)		
										Sat	Mono	Poly
DAIRY—Cont.												
88	Dessert topping, pressurized:	1 c	70	60	185	1	11	0	16	13.2	1.3	.2
87	Tablespoon	1 tbs	4	60	11	<1	1	0	1	.8	.1	t
91	Sour cream, imitation:	1 c	230	71	478	6	15	<1	45	40.9	1.3	.1
92	Tablespoon	1 tbs	14	71	29	<1	1	0	3	2.5	.1	t
89	Sour dressing, part dairy:	1 c	235	75	418	8	11	0	39	31.3	4.6	1.1
90	Tablespoon	1 tbs	15	75	27	<1	1	0	2	2	.3	.1
	Milk, fluid:											
93	Whole milk	1 c	244	88	150	8	11	0	8	5.1	2.3	.3
94	2% low-fat milk	1 c	244	89	121	8	12	0	5	2.9	1.3	.2
95	2% milk solids added[1]	1 c	245	89	124	9	12	0	5	2.9	1.4	.2
96	1% low-fat milk	1 c	244	90	102	8	12	–	3	1.6	.8	.1
97	1% milk solids added[1]	1 c	245	90	104	9	12	0	2	1.5	.7	.1
98	Nonfat milk, vitamin A added	1 c	245	91	86	8	12	0	<1	.3	.1	t
99	Nonfat milk solids added[1]	1 c	245	90	90	9	12	0	1	.4	.2	t
100	Buttermilk, nonfat	1 c	245	90	99	8	12	0	2	1.3	.6	.1
	Milk, canned:											
101	Sweetened condensed	1 c	306	27	982	24	166	0	27	16.8	7.4	1
102	Evaporated, whole	1 c	252	74	338	17	25	0	19	11.6	5.9	.6
103	Evaporated, nonfat	1 c	255	79	199	19	29	0	1	.3	.2	t
	Milk, dried:											
104	Buttermilk, sweet	1 c	120	3	464	41	59	0	7	4.3	2	.3
105	Instant, nonfat, envelope[2]	1 ea	91	4	325	32	47	0	1	.4	.2	t
106	Instant nonfat, cup	1 c	68	4	243	24	35	0	<1	.3	.1	t
107	Goat milk	1 c	244	87	167	9	11	0	10	6.5	2.7	.4
108	Kefir, 2% milkfat[3]	1 c	233	82	122	9	9	0	5	2.9	1.2	.1
	Milk beverages and powdered mixes:											
	Chocolate:											
109	Whole	1 c	250	82	208	8	26	3	9	5.2	2.5	.3
110	2% fat	1 c	250	83	178	8	26	3	5	3.1	1.5	.2
111	1% fat	1 c	250	85	157	8	26	3	3	1.5	.7	.1
	Chocolate-flavored beverages:											
112	Powder containing nonfat dry milk:	1 oz	28	2	102	3	22	<1	1	.7	.4	t
113	Prepared with water	¾ c	206	86	103	4	22	<1	1	.7	.4	t
114	Powder without nonfat dry milk:	¾ oz	22	1	77	1	20	1	1	.4	.2	t
115	Prepared with whole milk	1 c	266	81	226	9	31	<1	9	5.5	2.6	.3
116	Eggnog, commercial	1 c	254	74	343	10	34	0	19	11.3	5.7	.9
974	2% low-fat eggnog	1 c	254	85	189	12	17	0	8	3.8	2.7	.7
1027	Instant Breakfast, envelope, powder only:	1 ea	37	7	131	7	24	<1	1	.3	.1	t
1028	Prepared with whole milk	1 c	281	77	280	15	36	<1	9	5.4	2.5	.3
1029	Prepared with 2% milk	1 c	281	78	252	15	36	<1	5	3.3	1.5	.2
1283	Prepared with 1% milk	1 c	281	79	233	16	36	<1	3	2	.9	t
1284	Prepared with nonfat milk	1 c	281	80	215	16	36	<1	1	.6	.3	t
117	Malted milk, chocolate, powder:[4]	¾ oz	21	1	79	1	18	<1	1	.5	.2	.1
118	Prepared with whole milk	1 c	265	81	228	9	30	1	9	5.5	2.6	.4
1661	Ovaltine with whole milk	1 c	265	81	225	9	29	1	9	5.5	2.6	.4
119	Malted milk, regular, powder:[4]	¾ oz	21	2	87	2	16	<1	2	.9	.4	.3
120	Prepared with whole milk	1 c	265	81	236	10	27	<1	10	5.9	2.8	.6

[1]Milk solids added, label claims less than 10 g protein per cup.

[2]Yields 1 qt fluid milk when reconstituted according to package directions.

[3]Most values provided by product labeling.

[4]The latest USDA data from *Handbook 8–14* on beverages updates previous USDA data.

(Computer code number is for West Diet Analysis program)

PAGE KEY: A–4 = BEV   A–6 = DAIRY   A–12 = EGGS   A–14 = FAT/OIL   A–18 = FRUIT   A–26 = BAKERY   A–36 = GRAIN   A–44 = FISH   A–48 = MEATS   A–50 = POULTRY   A–54 = SAUSAGE   A–56 = MIXED/FAST   A–64 = NUTS/SEEDS   A–68 = SWEETS   A–70 = VEG/LEG   A–84 = MISC   A–88 = SOUPS/SAUCES   A–90 = FAST   A–106 = FRZN ENTREE   A–112 = BABY FOODS

Chol (mg)	Calc (mg)	Iron (mg)	Magn (mg)	Pota (mg)	Sodi (mg)	Zinc (mg)	VT-A (RE)	Thia (mg)	Ribo (mg)	Niac (mg)	V-B6 (mg)	Fola (μg)	VT-C (mg)	VT-E α-TE (mg)
0	4	.01	1	13	43	.01	33[5]	.0	0	0	0	0	0	.12
0	<1	0	<1	1	2	0	2[5]	0	0	0	0	0	0	.01
0	6	.9	15	370	235	2.74	0	0	0	0	0	0	0	.34
0	<1	.05	1	23	14	.16	0	0	0	0	0	0	0	.02
13	266	.07	23	381	113	.87	5[5]	.09	.38	.17	.04	28	2	.29
1	17	0	1	24	7	.06	<1[5]	.01	.02	.01	0	2	<1	.02
33	290	.12	33	371	120	.93	76	.09	.39	.2	.1	12	2	.24
18	298	.12	33	376	122	.95	139	.09	.4	.21	.1	12	2	.17
18	311	.12	35	397	128	.98	140	.1	.42	.22	.11	13	2	.17
10	300	.12	34	381	123	.95	144	.09	.41	.21	.1	12	2	.1
10	311	.12	35	397	128	.98	145	.1	.42	.22	.11	13	2	.1
4	301	.1	28	407	126	.98	149	.09	.34	.22	.1	13	2	.1
5	316	.12	35	419	129	1	149	.1	.43	.22	.11	13	2	.1
9	284	.12	27	370	257	1.03	20	.08	.38	.14	.08	12	2	.15
104	869	.58	79	1135	389	2.88	248	.27	1.27	.64	.16	34	8	.66
74	658	.48	61	764	267	1.94	136	.12	.8	.49	.13	20	5	.45
9	740	.74	69	847	293	2.29	298	.11	.79	.44	.14	22	3	.01
83	1421	.36	132	1910	620	4.84	65	.47	1.9	1.05	.41	57	7	.48
17	1119	.28	106	1552	500	4.01	646[6]	.38	1.58	.81	.31	45	5	.02
12	836	.21	80	1159	373	3	483[6]	.28	1.18	.61	.23	34	4	.01
28	327	.12	34	498	122	.73	137	.12	.34	.68	.11	1	3	.22
10	350	.5	28	205	50	.9	155	.45	.44	.3	.09	23	<1	.12
30	280	.6	33	418	149	1.03	73	.09	.41	.31	.1	12	2	.23
17	285	.6	33	423	151	1.03	143	.09	.41	.32	.1	12	2	.13
7	288	.6	33	425	152	1.03	148	.09	.42	.32	.1	12	2	.07
1	92	.34	24	202	143	.41	1	.03	.16	.17	.03	0	1	.04
2	97	.35	25	202	148	.45	1	.03	.17	.18	.04	3	1	.08
0	8	.69	22	129	46	.34	<1	.01	.03	.11	<.01	1	<1	.09
32	301	.8	53	497	164	1.28	77	.1	.43	.32	.1	12	2	.27
149	330	.51	47	419	138	1.17	203	.09	.48	.27	.13	2	4	.58
194	269	.71	32	367	155	1.26	197	.11	.55	.21	.15	30	2	1.02
4	105	4.74	84	350	142	3.16	554	.31	.07	5.25	.42	105	28	5.31
38	396	4.86	117	721	262	4.09	630	.41	.47	5.46	.52	118	31	5.51
23	403	4.87	118	726	264	4.12	693	.41	.48	5.46	.53	118	31	5.41
14	406	4.87	118	731	266	4.12	698	.41	.48	5.45	.52	118	31	5.28
9	406	4.84	112	755	268	4.14	703	.4	.42	5.47	.52	118	31	5.28
1	13	.48	15	129	53	.17	4	.04	.04	.42	.03	4	<1	.08
34	305	.61	48	498	172	1.09	80	.13	.44	.62	.13	16	3	.27
34	385	4	53	620	244	1.17	901	.74	1.26	10.9	1.02	32	34	.45
4	63	.15	20	159	104	.21	18	.11	.19	1.1	.09	10	1	.08
37	355	.26	53	530	223	1.14	95	.2	.59	1.31	.19	22	3	1.06

[5]Vitamin A value is from beta-carotene used for coloring.

[6]With added vitamin A.

(For purposes of calculations, use "0" for t, <1, <.1, <.01, etc.)

Table A–1
Food Composition

Computer Code Number	Food Description	Measure	Wt (g)	H₂O (%)	Ener (cal)	Prot (g)	Carb (g)	Dietary Fiber (g)	Fat (g)	Fat Breakdown (g)		
										Sat	Mono	Poly
DAIRY—Cont.												
121	Milk shakes, chocolate (10 fl oz)	1¼ c	283	72	359	10	58	<1	10	6.5	3	.4
122	Milk shakes, vanilla (10 fl oz)	1¼ c	283	75	314	10	51	<1	8	5.3	2.4	.3
	Milk desserts:											
134	Custard, baked	1 c	265	79	278	13	28	0	12	6.2	4	1
1548	Low-fat frozen dessert bars	1 ea	81	72	90	2	18	0	1	.2	.1	.4
	Ice cream, vanilla (about 10% fat):											
123	Hardened: ½ gallon	1 ea	1064	61	2138	37	251	1	117	72.4	33.8	4.4
124	Cup	1 c	133	61	267	5	31	<1	15	9	4.2	.6
125	Fluid ounces	3 oz	50	61	101	2	12	<1	6	3.4	1.6	.2
126	Soft serve	1 c	173	60	372	7	38	<1	22	12.9	6	.8
	Ice cream, rich vanilla (16% fat):											
127	Hardened: ½ gallon	1 ea	1188	60	2554	49	264	1	154	88.9	41.5	5.5
128	Cup	1 c	148	57	357	5	33	<1	24	14.8	6.9	.9
1724	Ben & Jerry's	½ c	106	64	230	4	21	0	17	10	–	–
	Ice milk, vanilla (about 4% fat):											
129	Hardened: ½ gallon	1 ea	1048	68	1456	40	238	1	45	27.7	12.9	1.7
130	Cup	1 c	131	68	182	5	30	<1	6	3.5	1.6	.2
131	Soft serve (about 3% fat)	1 c	175	70	221	9	38	<1	5	2.8	1.3	.2
	Pudding, canned (5-oz can = .55 cup):											
135	Chocolate	1 ea	142	69	189	4	32	1	6	1	2.4	2
136	Tapioca	1 ea	142	74	169	3	27	<1	5	.9	2.2	1.9
137	Vanilla	1 ea	142	71	185	3	31	<1	5	.8	2.2	1.9
	Puddings, dry mix with whole milk:											
138	Chocolate, instant	1 c	260	75	289	8	49	3	8	4.8	2.4	.5
139	Chocolate, regular, cooked	½ c	130	74	144	4	23	1	4	2.7	1.3	.2
140	Rice, cooked	½ c	132	72	161	4	27	1	4	2.3	1.1	.2
141	Tapioca, cooked	½ c	130	74	148	4	25	<1	4	2.3	1.1	.1
142	Vanilla, instant	½ c	130	74	148	4	26	<1	4	2.3	1.1	.2
143	Vanilla, regular, cooked	½ c	130	75	144	4	24	<1	4	2.4	1.1	.2
132	Sherbet (2% fat): ½ gallon	1 ea	1542	66	2127	17	469	0	31	17.9	8.3	1.2
133	Cup	1 c	193	66	266	2	59	0	4	2.2	1	.2
144	Soy milk	1 c	240	93	79	7	4	3	5	.5	.8	2
1584	Yogurt, frozen, low-fat[1]	½ c	87	65	138	3	21	0	5	3	1.4	.2
1512	Scoop	1 ea	79	74	78	4	16	0	<1	.1	t	0
	Yogurt, low-fat:											
1172	Fruit added with low-calorie sweetener	1 c	241	86	122	11	19	1	<1	.2	.1	t
145	Fruit added[2]	1 c	227	75	232	10	43	<1	2	1.6	.7	.1
146	Plain	1 c	227	85	144	12	16	0	4	2.3	1	.1
147	Vanilla or coffee flavor	1 c	227	79	194	11	31	0	3	1.8	.8	.1
148	Yogurt, made with nonfat milk	1 c	227	85	127	13	17	0	<1	.3	.1	t
149	Yogurt, made with whole milk	1 c	227	88	139	8	11	0	7	4.8	2	.2
EGGS[3]												
	Raw, large:											
150	Whole, without shell	1 ea	50	75	74	6	1	0	5	1.5	1.9	.7
151	White	1 ea	33	88	17	4	<1	0	0	0	0	0
152	Yolk	1 ea	17	49	59	3	<1	0	5	1.6	1.9	.7

[1]Data is from 1992 USDA data on snacks and sweets.

[2]Carbohydrate and calories vary widely—consult label if more precise values are needed.

[3]This data is newest revised information from the USDA with 24% less cholesterol.

(Computer code number is for West Diet Analysis program)

PAGE KEY: A–4 = BEV   A–6 = DAIRY   A–12 = EGGS   A–14 = FAT/OIL   A–18 = FRUIT   A–26 = BAKERY   A–36 = GRAIN   A–44 = FISH
A–48 = MEATS   A–50 = POULTRY   A–54 = SAUSAGE   A–56 = MIXED/FAST   A–64 = NUTS/SEEDS   A–68 = SWEETS   A–70 = VEG/LEG
A–84 = MISC   A–88 = SOUPS/SAUCES   A–90 = FAST   A–106 = FRZN ENTREE   A–112 = BABY FOODS

Chol (mg)	Calc (mg)	Iron (mg)	Magn (mg)	Pota (mg)	Sodi (mg)	Zinc (mg)	VT-A (RE)	Thia (mg)	Ribo (mg)	Niac (mg)	V-B6 (mg)	Fola (μg)	VT-C (mg)	VT-E α-TE (mg)
37	320	.88	48	566	275	1.16	65	.16	.69	.46	.14	10	1	.19
31	345	.25	34	492	232	1.02	91	.13	.52	.52	.15	9	2	.17
231	297	.79	37	405	204	1.4	159	.09	.6	.22	.13	27	1	.64
1	82	.07	10	111	47	.26	38	.03	.11	.06	.03	3	1	.07
468	1362	.96	149	2117	851	7.34	1245	.44	2.55	1.23	.51	53	6	0
59	170	.12	19	265	106	.92	156	.05	.32	.15	.06	7	1	0
22	64	.04	7	100	40	.34	59	.02	.12	.06	.02	3	<1	0
157	227	.36	21	306	106	.9	266	.08	.31	.16	.08	16	1	.64
1081	1556	2.49	143	2102	725	6.18	1829	.58	2.16	1.13	.57	107	10	4.4
90	173	.07	16	235	83	.59	272	.06	.24	.12	.06	7	1	0
95	150	.36	–	–	55	–	225	–	–	–	–	–	0	0
147	1456	1.05	157	2211	891	4.61	493	.61	2.78	.94	.68	63	8	0
18	182	.13	20	276	111	.58	62	.08	.35	.12	.08	8	1	0
21	275	.1	25	387	123	.93	51	.09	.35	.21	.08	11	2	0
4	128	.72	30	256	183	.6	16	.04	.22	.49	.04	4	3	.18
1	119	.33	11	148	168	.38	0	.03	.14	.44	.14	6	1	.13
10	125	.18	11	160	192	.35	9	.03	.2	.36	.02	0	0	.18
29	265	.75	47	432	738	1.09	55	.09	.37	.25	.1	10	2	.16
16	144	.47	20	212	134	.58	34	.04	.23	.13	.05	5	1	.08
15	133	.5	17	165	140	.6	26	.1	.18	.6	.04	5	1	.13
16	135	.08	16	172	157	.44	35	.04	.18	.09	.05	5	1	.1
14	131	.09	16	166	372	.43	33	.04	.18	.1	.05	5	1	.08
16	139	.06	17	177	208	.45	35	.04	.18	.1	.04	5	1	.08
77	833	2.16	123	1480	709	7.4	216	.39	1.05	1.48	.52	62	66	.88
10	104	.27	15	185	89	.93	27	.05	.13	.18	.07	8	8	.11
0	10	1.39	46	338	29	.55	7	.39	.17	.35	.1	4	0	.02
2	124	.26	12	184	76	.36	50	.03	.19	.25	.07	5	1	.04
1	137	.07	13	175	53	.67	1	.03	.16	.09	.04	8	1	<.01
3	369	.61	41	550	139	1.83	6	.1	.45	.5	.11	32	26	.17
10	345	.16	33	440	133	1.68	25	.08	.4	.22	.09	21	2	.07
14	415	.18	40	529	159	2.02	36	.1	.49	.26	.11	25	2	.1
11	388	.16	37	497	149	1.88	30	.09	.46	.24	.1	24	2	.08
4	452	.2	43	579	174	2.2	5	.11	.53	.28	.12	28	2	.01
29	275	.11	26	350	105	1.34	68	.07	.32	.17	.07	17	1	.2
213	25	.72	5	61	63	.55	96	.03	.25	.04	.07	24	0	.525
0	2	.01	4	47	54	0	0	<.01	.15	.03	0	1	0	0
218	23	.59	2	16	7	.52	99	.03	.11	0	.06	25	0	.537

(For purposes of calculations, use "0" for t, <1, <.1, <.01, etc.)

Table A–1
Food Composition

Computer Code Number	Food Description	Measure	Wt (g)	H₂O (%)	Ener (cal)	Prot (g)	Carb (g)	Dietary Fiber (g)	Fat (g)	Fat Breakdown (g) Sat	Mono	Poly
	EGGS—Cont.											
	Cooked:											
153	Fried in margarine	1 ea	46	69	92	6	1	0	7	1.9	2.8	1.3
154	Hard-cooked, shell removed	1 ea	50	75	78	6	1	0	5	1.6	2	.7
155	Hard-cooked, chopped	1 c	136	75	211	17	2	0	14	4.5	5.6	1.9
156	Poached, no added salt	1 ea	50	75	75	6	1	0	5	1.6	1.9	.7
157	Scrambled with milk & margarine	1 ea	61	73	101	7	1	0	7	2.2	2.9	1.3
1681	Egg substitute, liquid	½ c	126	83	106	15	1	0	4	.8	1.1	2
1254	Egg Beaters, Fleischmann's	¼ c	61	–	30	6	1	0	0	0	0	0
1262	Egg substitute, liquid, prepared	⅓ c	69	81	66	9	1	0	3	.5	.7	1.3
	FATS and OILS											
158	Butter: Stick	½ c	113	16	810	1	<1	0	92	57.1	27.6	3.4
159	Tablespoon	1 tbs	14	16	100	<1	<1	0	11	7.1	3.4	.4
160	Pat (about 1 tsp)[1]	1 ea	5	16	36	<1	<1	0	4	2.5	1.2	.2
1682	Whipped	1 tsp	3	16	22	<1	<1	0	3	1.5	.7	.1
	Fats, cooking:											
1363	Bacon fat	1 tbs	14	0	125	0	0	0	14	6.4	5.9	1.1
1362	Beef fat/tallow	1 c	205	0	1849	0	0	0	205	103	85.7	8.2
1364	Chicken fat	1 c	205	<1	1845	0	0	0	205	61.1	91.6	42.8
161	Vegetable shortening:	1 c	205	0	1812	0	0	0	205	51.5	91.2	53.5
162	Tablespoon	1 tbs	13	0	115	0	0	0	13	3.3	5.8	3.4
163	Lard:	1 c	205	0	1849	0	0	0	205	80.4	92.5	23
164	Tablespoon	1 tbs	13	0	117	0	0	0	13	5.1	5.9	1.5
	Margarine:											
165	Imitation (about 40% fat), soft:	1 c	227	58	783	1	1	0	88	14.5	33	37
166	Tablespoon	1 tbs	14	58	48	<1	<1	0	5	.9	2	2.3
167	Regular, hard (about 80% fat):	½ c	113	16	812	1	1	0	91	14.8	42	29.6
168	Tablespoon	1 tbs	14	16	101	<1	<1	0	11	1.8	5	3.6
169	Pat	1 ea	5	16	36	<1	<1	0	4	.8	1.8	1.3
170	Regular, soft (about 80% fat):	1 c	227	16	1625	2	1	0	183	30.7	83	61
171	Tablespoon	1 tbs	14	16	100	<1	<1	0	11	1.9	5.1	3.8
2056	Saffola, unsalted	1 tbs	14	20	101	0	0	0	11	1.9	4.8	4.7
2057	Saffola, reduced fat	1 tbs	14	37	71	0	0	0	9	1.3	2.7	4.5
172	Spread (about 60% fat), hard:	½ c	113	37	610	1	0	0	69	15.9	29.4	20.5
173	Tablespoon	1 tbs	14	37	76	<1	0	0	9	2	3.6	2.5
174	Pat[1]	1 ea	5	37	27	<1	0	0	3	.7	1.2	1
175	Spread (about 60% fat), soft:	1 c	227	37	1226	1	0	0	138	29.1	71.5	31.3
176	Tablespoon	1 tbs	14	37	76	<1	0	0	9	1.8	4.4	1.9
2160	Touch of Butter (47% fat)	1 tbs	14	36	77	<1	0	0	9	2	4.4	1.9
	Oils:											
1585	Canola:	1 c	218	0	1927	0	0	0	218	15.5	128	64.5
1586	Tablespoon	1 tbs	14	0	124	0	0	0	14	1	8.2	4.1
177	Corn:	1 c	218	0	1927	0	0	0	218	29.4	52.8	127
178	Tablespoon	1 tbs	14	0	124	0	0	0	14	1.8	3.4	8.2

[1]Pat is 1" square, ⅓" thick; about 1 tsp; 90 per lb.

(Computer code number is for West Diet Analysis program)

PAGE KEY: A–4 = BEV   A–6 = DAIRY   A–12 = EGGS   A–14 = FAT/OIL   A–18 = FRUIT   A–26 = BAKERY   A–36 = GRAIN   A–44 = FISH   A–48 = MEATS   A–50 = POULTRY   A–54 = SAUSAGE   A–56 = MIXED/FAST   A–64 = NUTS/SEEDS   A–68 = SWEETS   A–70 = VEG/LEG   A–84 = MISC   A–88 = SOUPS/SAUCES   A–90 = FAST   A–106 = FRZN ENTREE   A–112 = BABY FOODS

Chol (mg)	Calc (mg)	Iron (mg)	Magn (mg)	Pota (mg)	Sodi (mg)	Zinc (mg)	VT-A (RE)	Thia (mg)	Ribo (mg)	Niac (mg)	V-B6 (mg)	Fola (μg)	VT-C (mg)	VT-E α-TE (mg)
211	25	.72	5	61	162	.55	114	.03	.24	.04	.07	17	0	.75
212	25	.59	5	63	62	.53	84	.03	.26	.03	.06	22	0	.53
577	68	1.62	14	171	169	1.44	228	.09	.7	.09	.17	60	0	1.43
212	25	.72	5	60	61	.56	95	.02	.22	.03	.06	18	0	.53
215	43	.73	7	84	171	.62	119	.03	.27	.05	.07	18	<1	.8
1	67	2.65	11	416	223	1.65	272	.14	.38	.14	<.01	19	0	.61
0	40	1.08	–	85	100	–	–	–	–	–	–	–	–	.3
1	42	1.65	7	260	139	1.02	170	.07	.22	.08	0	9	0	.38
247	27	.18	2	29	935[2]	.06	852[3]	.01	.04	.05	<.01	3	0	1.79
31	3	.02	<1	4	117[2]	.01	107[3]	<.01	<.01	.01	0	<1	0	.22
11	1	.01	<1	1	41[2]	<.01	38[3]	0	<.01	<.01	0	<1	0	.08
7	1	0	<1	1	26[2]	<.01	24[3]	0	<.01	<.01	0	<1	0	.05
14	<1	0	<1	<1	76	<.01	0	0	0	0	0	0	0	.31
223	0	0	0	<1	<1	0	0	0	0	0	0	0	0	5.54
174	0	0	0	0	0	0	351	0	0	0	0	0	0	5.54
0	0	0	0	0	0	0	0	0	0	0	0	0	0	17
0	0	0	0	0	0	0	0	0	0	0	0	0	0	1.08
195	<1	0	<1	<1	<1	.23	0	0	0	0	0	0	0	2.46
12	<1	0	<1	<1	<1	.01	0	0	0	0	0	0	0	.16
0	40	0	4	57	800[4]	0	2254[5]	.01	.05	.03	.01	2	<1	5.29
0	2	0	<1	4	49[4]	0	139[5]	<.01	<.01	<.01	<.01	<1	<1	.33
0	34	0	3	48	1065[4]	.23	1122[5]	.01	.04	.03	.01	1	<1	14.5
0	4	0	<1	6	132[4]	.03	139[5]	<.01	<.01	<.01	<.01	<1	<1	1.8
0	2	0	<1	2	47[4]	.01	50[5]	<.01	<.01	<.01	0	<1	<1	.64
0	60	0	5	86	1678[4]	0	2254[5]	.02	.07	.04	.02	2	<1	27.2
0	4	0	<1	5	103[4]	0	139[5]	<.01	<.01	<.01	<.01	<1	<1	1.68
–	0	0	–	–	0	–	52	–	–	–	–	–	0	–
–	0	0	–	–	116	–	52	–	–	–	–	–	0	.14
0	24	0	2	34	1122[4]	.17	1122[5]	.01	.03	.02	.01	1	<1	5.65
0	3	0	<1	4	139[4]	0	139[5]	<.01	<.01	<.01	<.01	<1	<1	.7
0	1	0	<1	1	50[4]	0	50[5]	0	<.01	<.01	0	<1	<1	.25
0	47	0	4	68	2256[4]	0	2254[5]	.02	.06	.04	.01	2	<1	20.5
0	3	0	<1	4	139[4]	0	139[5]	<.01	<.01	<.01	<.01	<1	<1	1.26
1	3	0	<1	4	140	0	152	<.01	<.01	<.01	<.01	<1	0	1.27
0	0	0	0	0	0	0	0	0	0	0	0	0	0	45.8
0	0	0	0	0	0	0	0	0	0	0	0	0	0	2.94
0	0	0	0	0	0	0	0	0	0	0	0	0	0	46
0	0	0	0	0	0	0	0	0	0	0	0	0	0	2.95

[2] For salted butter, unsalted butter contains 12 mg sodium per stick or ½ c, 1.5 mg/tbs, or .5 mg/pat.

[3] Values for vitamin A are a year-round average.

[4] For salted margarine.

[5] Based on average vitamin A content of fortified margarine. Federal specifications require a minimum of 15,000 IU/lb.

(For purposes of calculations, use "0" for t, <1, <.1, <.01, etc.)

Table A–1
Food Composition

Computer Code Number	Food Description	Measure	Wt (g)	H₂O (%)	Ener (cal)	Prot (g)	Carb (g)	Dietary Fiber (g)	Fat (g)	Fat Breakdown (g)		
										Sat	Mono	Poly
	FATS and OILS—Cont.											
	Oils—Cont.											
179	Olive:	1 c	216	0	1909	0	0	0	216	29.2	159	18.4
180	Tablespoon	1 tbs	14	0	124	0	0	0	14	1.9	10.3	1.2
1683	Olive, extra virgin	1 tbs	14	<1	126	0	0	0	14	1.96	10.8	1.3
181	Peanut:	1 c	216	0	1909	0	0	0	216	35.6	113	56.8
182	Tablespoon	1 tbs	14	0	124	0	0	0	14	2.4	7.3	3.7
183	Safflower:	1 c	218	0	1927	0	0	0	218	19.8	26.4	162
184	Tablespoon	1 tbs	14	0	124	0	0	0	14	1.3	1.7	10.4
185	Soybean:	1 c	218	0	1927	0	0	0	218	31.4	50.8	126
186	Tablespoon	1 tbs	14	0	124	0	0	0	14	2	3.3	8.1
187	Soybean/cottonseed:	1 c	218	0	1927	0	0	0	218	40	64.3	105
188	Tablespoon	1 tbs	14	0	124	0	0	0	14	2.5	4.1	6.7
189	Sunflower:	1 c	218	0	1927	0	0	0	218	25	45	144
190	Tablespoon	1 tbs	14	0	124	0	0	0	14	1.5	2.9	9.2
	Salad dressings/sandwich spreads:											
191	Blue cheese, regular	1 tbs	15	32	76	1	1	<1	8	1.5	1.9	4.4
1040	Low calorie	1 tbs	15	80	15	1	<1	<1	1	.2	.5	.4
1684	Caesar's	1 tbs	12	36	55	1	<1	<1	5	.9	3.5	.5
192	French, regular	1 tbs	16	38	69	<1	3	<1	9	1.5	1.2	3.4
193	Low calorie	1 tbs	16	69	21	<1	3	<1	1	.1	.2	.5
194	Italian, regular	1 tbs	15	38	70	<1	1	<1	9	1	1.6	4.1
195	Low calorie	1 tbs	15	82	16	<1	1	<1	1	.2	.3	.9
	Kraft, Deliciously Right											
2150	1000 Island	2 tbs	32	–	70	0	8	0	4	1	–	–
2153	Bacon & tomato	2 tbs	31	–	60	1	3	0	5	1	–	–
2154	Cucumber ranch	2 tbs	31	–	60	0	2	0	5	1	–	–
2151	French	2 tbs	32	–	50	0	6	0	3	.5	–	–
2152	Ranch	2 tbs	31	–	100	0	5	0	9	1.5	–	–
199	Mayo type, regular	1 tbs	15	40	58	<1	3	0	5	.7	1.4	2.7
1030	Low calorie	1 tbs	15	54	39	<1	1	0	3	.4	.8	1.4
	Mayonnaise:											
197	Imitation, low calorie	1 tbs	15	63	35	<1	2	0	3	.5	.7	1.6
196	Regular (soybean)	1 tbs	14	15	100	<1	<1	0	11	1.6	3.1	5.7
1488	Regular, low calorie, low sodium	1 tbs	14	63	32	<1	2	0	3	.5	.6	1.4
1493	Regular, low calorie	1 tbs	16	63	37	<1	3	0	3	.5	.7	1.6
2058	Saffola, light	1 tbs	15	–	44	0	1	0	4	.5	1	2.9
198	Ranch, regular	½ c	119	35	436	4	6	0	45	6.7	19.4	17
2251	Low calorie	2 tbs	28	70	60	0	2	0	5	1	–	–
1685	Russian	1 tbs	15	35	74	<1	2	0	8	1.1	1.8	4.5
1502	Salad dressing, low calorie, oil free	1 tbs	15	88	4	<1	1	<1	<1	0	0	0
	Salad dressing, no cholesterol											
1605	(Miracle Whip)	1 tbs	15	57	48	0	2	0	4	1.1	1.1	2.1
203	Salad dressing, from recipe, cooked[1]	1 tbs	16	69	25	1	2	<1	2	.5	.6	.3
200	Tartar sauce, regular	1 tbs	14	34	74	<1	1	<1	8	1.5	2.6	4.1
1503	Low calorie	1 tbs	14	63	31	<1	2	<1	2	.4	.6	1.3
201	Thousand island, regular	1 tbs	16	46	60	<1	2	<1	6	1	1.3	3.2
202	Low calorie	1 tbs	15	69	24	<1	2	<1	2	.2	.4	.9
204	Vinegar & oil	1 tbs	16	47	72	0	<1	0	8	1.5	2.4	3.9

[1]Fatty acid values apply to product made with regular margarine.

(Computer code number is for West Diet Analysis program)

PAGE KEY: A–4 = BEV   A–6 = DAIRY   A–12 = EGGS   A–14 = FAT/OIL   A–18 = FRUIT   A–26 = BAKERY   A–36 = GRAIN   A–44 = FISH   A–48 = MEATS   A–50 = POULTRY   A–54 = SAUSAGE   A–56 = MIXED/FAST   A–64 = NUTS/SEEDS   A–68 = SWEETS   A–70 = VEG/LEG   A–84 = MISC   A–88 = SOUPS/SAUCES   A–90 = FAST   A–106 = FRZN ENTREE   A–112 = BABY FOODS

Chol (mg)	Calc (mg)	Iron (mg)	Magn (mg)	Pota (mg)	Sodi (mg)	Zinc (mg)	VT-A (RE)	Thia (mg)	Ribo (mg)	Niac (mg)	V-B6 (mg)	Fola (μg)	VT-C (mg)	VT-E α-TE (mg)
0	<1	.82	<1	0	<1	.13	0	0	0	0	0	0	0	26.8
0	<1	.05	<1	0	<1	.01	0	0	0	0	0	0	0	1.74
0	–	–	–	–	–	–	0	0	0	0	0	0	0	1.74
0	<1	.06	<1	<1	<1	.02	0	0	0	0	0	0	0	27.9
0	<1	0	<1	0	<1	0	0	0	0	0	0	0	0	1.81
0	0	0	0	0	0	0	0	0	0	0	0	0	0	94
0	0	0	0	0	0	0	0	0	0	0	0	0	0	6.03
0	<1	.04	<1	0	0	0	0	0	0	0	0	0	0	39.7
0	<1	0	<1	0	0	0	0	0	0	0	0	0	0	2.55
0	0	0	0	0	0	0	0	0	0	0	0	0	0	61.5
0	0	0	0	0	0	0	0	0	0	0	0	0	0	3.95
0	0	0	0	0	0	0	0	0	0	0	0	0	0	110
0	0	0	0	0	0	0	0	0	0	0	0	0	0	7.08
3	12	.03	0	6	164	0	10	<.01	.02	.02	.01	1	<1	1.4
<1	13	.08	1	1	180	.04	<1	<.01	.02	.01	<.01	<1	<1	.14
12	22	.19	3	20	202	.12	6	<.01	.02	.49	.01	2	1	.7
9	2	.06	0	13	219	.01	3	<.01	<.01	<.01	<.01	1	0	1.63
1	2	.06	0	13	126	.03	0	0	0	0	0	0	0	.19
0	2	.03	<1	2	118	.02	4	<.01	<.01	0	<.01	1	0	1.53
1	<1	.03	0	2	118	.02	0	0	0	0	0	0	0	.68
5	0	0	–	55	320	–	0	–	–	–	–	–	0	.38
3	0	0	–	40	300	–	0	–	–	–	–	–	0	1.45
0	0	0	–	20	450	–	0	–	–	–	–	–	0	1.41
0	0	0	–	15	260	–	100	–	–	–	–	–	0	.85
0	0	0	–	0	320	–	0	–	–	–	–	–	0	2.54
4	2	.03	<1	1	107	.03	13	<.01	<.01	<.01	<.01	1	0	.6
4	2	.03	<1	1	107	.03	10	<.01	<.01	0	0	1	0	.65
4	<1	0	<1	2	75	.02	0	0	0	0	0	0	0	.97
8	3	.07	<1	5	80	.02	12	0	0	<.01	.08	1	0	1.7
3	0	0	0	1	15	.02	1	0	<.01	0	0	<1	0	.53
4	<1	0	<1	2	80	02	0	0	0	0	0	0	0	1.03
–	0	0	–	–	103	–	0	–	–	–	–	–	0	4.79
47	119	.31	12	158	522	.44	86	.04	.17	.08	.05	6	1	4.76
10	20	0	–	–	240	–	0	–	–	–	–	–	0	1.41
3	3	.1	.23	24	130	.06	31	.01	.01	.1	<.01	1.59	1	1.53
0	1	.04	2	7	256	<.01	<1	0	0	<.01	<.01	<1	<1	0
0	0	0	0	0	102	0	2	0	0	0	0	0	0	.65
9	13	.08	0	19	117	0	20	.01	.02	.04	0	0	<1	.3
7	3	.13	<1	11	99	.02	9	<.01	<.01	0	.01	1	<1	2.24
3	2	.09	<1	5	83	.02	2	<.01	<.01	.01	<.01	<1	<1	.83
4	2	.09	<1	18	112	.02	15	<.01	<.01	<.01	<.01	1	0	1.14
2	2	.09	<1	17	150	.02	14	<.01	<.01	<.01	<.01	1	0	1.19
0	0	0	0	1	<1	0	0	0	0	0	0	0	0	1.41

(For purposes of calculations, use "0" for t, <1, <.1, <.01, etc.)

Table A–1
Food Composition

Computer Code Number	Food Description	Measure	Wt (g)	H₂O (%)	Ener (cal)	Prot (g)	Carb (g)	Dietary Fiber (g)	Fat (g)	Fat Breakdown (g) Sat	Mono	Poly
	FATS and OILS—Cont.											
	Salad dressings/sandwich spreads—Cont.											
	Wishbone											
2179	French, fat-free	1 tbs	16	–	6	0	1	–	0	0	–	.1
2180	Creamy Italian, lite	1 tbs	15	–	26	<1	2	–	2	.4	–	.7
2166	Italian, lite	1 tbs	16	77	6	0	1	–	–	0	–	.1
2167	Ranch, lite	1 tbs	15	–	42	<1	3	0	4	.7	–	2.3
	FRUITS and FRUIT JUICES											
	Apples:											
	Fresh, raw, with peel:											
205	2 ¾" diam (about 3 per lb w/cores)	1 ea	138	84	81	<1	21	3	<1	.1	t	.1
206	3 ¼" diam (about 2 per lb w/cores)	1 ea	212	84	125	<1	32	4	1	.1	t	.2
207	Raw, peeled slices	1 c	110	85	63	<1	16	2	<1	.1	t	.1
208	Dried, sulfured	10 ea	64	32	155	1	42	6	<1	t	t	.1
209	Apple juice, bottled or canned	1 c	248	88	116	<1	29	<1	<1	<1	t	<.1
210	Applesauce, sweetened	1 c	255	80	193	<1	51	3	<1	.1	t	.1
211	Applesauce, unsweetened	1 c	244	88	104	<1	28	3	<1	<1	t	t
	Apricots:											
212	Raw, w/o pits (about 12 per lb w/ pits)	3 ea	106	86	51	1	12	2	<1	t	.2	.1
	Canned (fruit and liquid):											
213	Heavy syrup	1 c	258	78	214	1	55	3	<1	t	.1	t
214	Halves	3 ea	85	78	70	<1	18	1	<1	t	t	t
215	Juice pack	1 c	248	87	119	2	30	3	<1	t	t	t
216	Halves	3 ea	84	87	40	1	10	1	<1	t	t	t
217	Dried, halves	10 ea	35	31	83	1	22	3	<1	t	.1	t
218	Dried, cooked, unsweetened, w/liquid	1 c	250	76	212	3	55	9	<1	t	.2	.1
219	Apricot nectar, canned	1 c	251	85	140	1	36	2	<1	t	.1	t
	Avocados, raw, edible part only:											
220	California (2 lb with refuse)	1 ea	173	73	306	4	12	6	30	4.5	19.4	3.5
221	Florida (1 lb with refuse)	1 ea	304	80	340	5	27	8	27	5.3	14.8	4.5
222	Mashed, fresh, average	1 c	230	74	370	5	17	9	35	5.6	22.1	4.5
	Bananas, raw, without peel:											
223	Whole, 8¾" long (175 g w/peel)	1 ea	114	74	104	1	27	2	1	.2	t	.1
224	Slices	1 c	150	74	137	2	35	3	1	.3	.1	.1
1285	Bananas, dehydrated slices	1 oz	28	3	98	1	25	2	1	.2	t	.1
225	Blackberries, raw	1 c	144	86	75	1	18	6	1	.3	.1	.1
	Blueberries:											
226	Fresh	1 c	145	85	81	1	20	4	1	t	.2	.3
227	Frozen, sweetened	10 oz	284	77	230	1	62	6	<1	.1	.1	.2
228	Frozen, thawed	1 c	230	77	186	1	50	5	<1	.1	.1	.2
	Cherries:											
229	Sour, red pitted, canned water pack	1 c	244	90	88	2	22	2	<1	.1	.1	.1
230	Sweet, red pitted, raw	10 ea	68	81	49	1	11	<1	1	.1	.2	.2
231	Cranberry juice cocktail[1]	1 c	253	85	144	0[2]	36	<1	<1	.1	t	.1
1411	Cranberry juice, low calorie	¾ c	178	95	34	0	8	1	0	0	0	0
232	Cranberry-apple juice	1 c	253	83	169	<1	43	<1	<1[3]	t	t	.1

[1]Data here are from the newest USDA *Handbook 8–14* on beverages. These data are somewhat different from that presented in *Handbook 8–9* on fruits and fruit juices.

[2]The newest USDA *Handbook 8–14* data on beverages indicates "0" for protein.

[3]The newest USDA *Handbook 8–14* data on beverages indicates "0" for fat.

(Computer code number is for West Diet Analysis program)

PAGE KEY: A–4 = BEV   A–6 = DAIRY   A–12 = EGGS   A–14 = FAT/OIL   A–18 = FRUIT   A–26 = BAKERY   A–36 = GRAIN   A–44 = FISH
A–48 = MEATS   A–50 = POULTRY   A–54 = SAUSAGE   A–56 = MIXED/FAST   A–64 = NUTS/SEEDS   A–68 = SWEETS   A–70 = VEG/LEG
A–84 = MISC   A–88 = SOUPS/SAUCES   A–90 = FAST   A–106 = FRZN ENTREE   A–112 = BABY FOODS

Chol (mg)	Calc (mg)	Iron (mg)	Magn (mg)	Pota (mg)	Sodi (mg)	Zinc (mg)	VT-A (RE)	Thia (mg)	Ribo (mg)	Niac (mg)	V-B6 (mg)	Fola (µg)	VT-C (mg)	VT-E α-TE (mg)
0	–	–	–	–	249	–	–	–	–	–	–	–	–	–
<1	0	0	–	–	148	–	–	0	0	0	–	–	0	.56
0	1	0	–	–	249	–	–	0	0	0	–	–	–	.24
5	0	0	0	0	148	0	–	0	0	0	–	–	0	–
0	10	.25	7	159	0	.05	7	.02	.02	.11	.07	4	8	.442
0	15	.38	11	244	0	.08	11	.04	.03	.16	.1	6	12	.68
0	4	.08	3	124	0	.04	5	.02	.01	.1	.05	<1	4	.09
0	9	.9	10	288	56[2]	.13	6	0	.1	.59	.08	0	2	.35
0	17	.92	7	295	7	.07	<1	.05	.04	.25	.07	<1	2	.03
0	10	.89	8	155	8	.1	3	.03	.07	.48	.07	2	4[4]	.03
0	7	.29	7	183	5	.07	7	.03	.06	.46	.06	1	3[4]	.02
0	15	.57	8	313	1	.28	277	.03	.04	.64	.06	9	11	.94
0	23	.77	18	361	10	.28	317	.05	.06	.97	.14	4	8	2.3
0	8	.25	6	119	3	.09	105	.02	.02	.32	.05	1	3	.76
0	30	.74	25	409	10	.27	419	.04	.05	.85	.13	4	12	2.21
0	10	.25	8	139	3	.09	142	.01	.02	.29	.04	1	4	.75
0	16	1.65	16	482	4	.26	253	<.01	.05	1.05	.05	4	1	.53
0	40	4.18	42	1222	8	.66	590	.01	.07	2.36	.28	0	4	1.25
0	18	.95	13	286	8	.23	331	.02	.03	.65	.05	3	2[5]	.201
0	19	2.04	71	1096	21	.73	106	.19	.21	3.32	.48	113	14	2.32
0	33	1.61	103	1483	15	1.28	185	.33	.37	5.84	.85	162	24	2.37
0	25	2.37	90	1377	23	.97	140	.25	.28	4.42	.64	142	18	3.08
0	7	.35	33	451	1	.18	9	.05	.11	.62	.66	22	10	.31
0	9	.46	43	594	2	.24	12	.07	.15	.81	.87	29	14	.41
0	6	.33	31	417	1	.17	9	.05	.07	.79	.15	11	2	.29
0	46	.82	29	282	0	.39	24	.04	.06	.58	.08	49	30	1.02
0	9	.25	7	129	9	.16	15	.07	.07	.52	.05	9	19	1.45
0	17	1.11	6	170	3	.17	13	.06	.15	.72	.17	19	3	2.02
0	14	.9	5	138	2	.14	10	.05	.12	.58	.14	15	2	1.63
0	27	3.37	15	239	17	.17	183	.04	.1	.43	.11	19	5	.32
0	10	.26	7	152	0	.04	14	.03	.04	.27	.02	3	5	.09
0	8	.38	5	45	5	.18	1	.02	.02	.09	.05	1	90[6]	0
0	16	.07	4	39	5	.04	1	.02	.02	.06	.03	<1	57	0
0	18	.15	5	68	5	.1	1	.01	.05	.15	.05	1	81[6]	0

[4]Value based on products without added vitamin C. Bottled apple juice with added vitamin C usually contains 41.6 mg/100 g, or 103 mg per cup. Check label for specific vitamin C values.

[5]Without added vitamin C. Products with added vitamin C contain 136 mg per cup. Check label.

[6]Nutrient added.

(For purposes of calculations, use "0" for t, <1, <.1, <.01, etc.)

Table A–1
Food Composition

Computer Code Number	Food Description	Measure	Wt (g)	H$_2$O (%)	Ener (cal)	Prot (g)	Carb (g)	Dietary Fiber (g)	Fat (g)	Fat Breakdown (g) Sat	Mono	Poly
	FRUITS and FRUIT JUICES—Cont.											
233	Cranberry sauce, canned, strained	1 c	277	61	418	1	107	3	<1	t	.1	.2
234	Dates, whole, without pits	10 ea	83	22	228	2	61	6	<1	.2	.1	t
235	Dates, chopped	1 c	178	22	490	4	130	13	1	.3	.2	t
236	Figs, dried	10 ea	187	28	477	6	122	17	2	.4	.5	1
	Fruit cocktail, canned, fruit and liq:											
237	Heavy syrup pack	1 c	255	80	186	1	48	3	<1	t	t	.1
238	Juice pack	1 c	248	87	114	1	29	3	<1	t	t	t
	Grapefruit:											
	Raw 3¾" diam (half w/rind = 241 g)											
239	Pink/red, half fruit, edible part	1 ea	123	91	37	1	9	2	<1	t	t	t
240	White, half fruit, edible part	1 ea	118	90	39	1	10	2	<1	t	t	t
241	Canned sections with light syrup	1 c	254	84	152	1	39	1	<1	t	t	.1
	Grapefruit juice:											
242	Fresh, raw	1 c	247	90	96	1	23	<1	<1	t	t	.1
243	Canned, unsweetened	1 c	247	90	94	1	22	<1	<1	t	t	.1
244	Sweetened	1 c	250	87	115	1	28	<1	<1	t	t	.1
	Frozen concentrate, unsweetened:											
245	Undiluted, 6-fl-oz can	¾ c	207	62	302	4	71	1	1	.1	.1	.2
246	Diluted with 3 cans water	1 c	247	89	101	1	24	<1	<1	.1	t	.1
	Grapes, raw European (adherent skin):											
247	Thompson seedless	10 ea	50	81	35	<1	9	<1	<1	.1	t	.1
248	Tokay/Emperor, seeded types	10 ea	57	81	40	<1	10	<1	<1	.1	t	.1
	Grape juice:											
249	Bottled or canned	1 c	253	84	154	1	38	2	<1	.1	t	.1
	Frozen concentrate, sweetened:											
250	Undiluted, 6-fl-oz can	¾ c	216	54	387	1	96	<1	1	.2	t	.2
251	Diluted with 3 cans water	1 c	250	87	127	<1	32	<1	<1	.1	t	.1
1410	Low calorie	1 c	250	84	153	1	37	<1	<1	.1	t	.1
252	Kiwi fruit, raw, peeled (88 g with peel)	1 ea	76	83	46	1	11	1	<1	t	.1	.1
253	Lemons, raw, without peel and seeds (about 4 per lb whole)	1 ea	58	89	17	1	5	2	<1	t	t	.1
	Lemon juice:											
254	Fresh:	1 c	244	91	61	1	21	1	<1	.1	t	.2
255	Tablespoon	1 tbs	15	91	4	<1	1	<1	<1	t	t	t
256	Canned or bottled, unsweetened:	1 c	244	93	51	1	16	1	1	.1	t	.2
257	Tablespoon	1 tbs	15	93	3	<1	1	<1	<1	t	t	t
258	Frozen, single strength, unsweetened:	1 c	244	92	54	1	16	1	1	.1	t	.2
2298	Tablespoon	1 tbs	15	92	3	<1	1	<1	<1	t	t	t
	Lime juice:											
260	Fresh:	1 c	246	90	66	1	22	1	<1	t	t	.1
261	Tablespoon	1 tbs	15	90	4	<1	1	<1	<1	t	t	t
262	Canned or bottled, unsweetened	1 c	246	93	52	1	16	1	1	.1	.1	.2
263	Mangoes, raw, edible part (300 g w/skin & seeds)	1 ea	207	82	134	1	35	6	1	.1	.2	.1

(Computer code number is for West Diet Analysis program)

PAGE KEY: A–4 = BEV   A–6 = DAIRY   A–12 = EGGS   A–14 = FAT/OIL   A–18 = FRUIT   A–26 = BAKERY   A–36 = GRAIN   A–44 = FISH   A–48 = MEATS   A–50 = POULTRY   A–54 = SAUSAGE   A–56 = MIXED/FAST   A–64 = NUTS/SEEDS   A–68 = SWEETS   A–70 = VEG/LEG   A–84 = MISC   A–88 = SOUPS/SAUCES   A–90 = FAST   A–106 = FRZN ENTREE   A–112 = BABY FOODS

Chol (mg)	Calc (mg)	Iron (mg)	Magn (mg)	Pota (mg)	Sodi (mg)	Zinc (mg)	VT-A (RE)	Thia (mg)	Ribo (mg)	Niac (mg)	V-B6 (mg)	Fola (µg)	VT-C (mg)	VT-E α-TE (mg)
0	11	.61	8	72	80	.14	6	.04	.06	.28	.04	2	6	.28
0	27	.95	29	541	2	.24	4	.07	.08	1.83	.16	10	0	.08
0	57	2.05	62	1160	5	.52	9	.16	.18	3.92	.34	22	0	.18
0	269	4.19	110	1331	21	.95	24	.13	.16	1.3	.42	14	2	0
0	15	.74	13	224	15	.2	51	.05	.05	.95	.13	7	5	.74
0	20	.52	17	235	10	.22	77	.03	.04	1	.13	6	7	.5
0	13	.15	10	159	0	.09	32[1]	.04	.02	.23	.05	15	47	.31
0	14	.07	11	175	0	.08	1	.04	.02	.32	.05	12	39	.3
0	36	1.02	25	328	5	.2	2	.1	.05	.62	.05	22	54	.64
0	22	.49	30	400	2	.12	2[2]	.1	.05	.49	.11	25	94	.12
0	17	.49	25	378	2	.22	2	.1	.05	.57	.05	26	72	.12
0	20	.9	25	405	5	.15	2	.1	.06	.8	.05	26	67	.13
0	56	1.01	79	1001	6	.37	6	.3	.16	1.6	.32	26	248	.37
0	20	.35	27	336	2	.12	2	.1	.05	.54	.11	9	83	.12
0	6	.13	3	92	1	.03	3	.05	.03	.15	.05	2	5	.35
0	6	.15	3	105	1	.03	4	.05	.03	.17	.06	2	6	.4
0	23	.61	25	334	8	.13	3	.07	.09	.66	.16	7	<1	0
0	28	.78	32	159	15	.28	6	.11	.2	.93	.32	9	179[3]	.38
0	10	.25	10	52	5	.1	2	.04	.06	.31	.1	3	60[3]	.13
0	22	.6	25	330	8	.12	2	.06	.09	.65	.16	6	<1	0
0	20	.31	23	252	4	.08[4]	13	.01	.04	.38	.04	17	74	.85
0	15	.35	5	80	1	.03	2	.02	.01	.06	.05	6	31	.14
0	17	.07	15	303	2	.12	5	.07	.02	.24	.12	31	112	.22
0	1	0	1	19	<1	.01	<1	0	0	.01	.01	2	7	.01
0	27	.32	19	249	51	.15	4	.1	.02	.48	.1	25	60	.22
0	2	.02	1	15	3	.01	<1	.01	0	.03	.01	2	4	.01
0	19	.29	19	217	2	.12	3	.14	.03	.33	.15	23	77	.22
0	1	.02	1	13	<1	.01	<1	.01	0	.02	.01	1	5	.01
0	22	.07	15	268	2	.15	2	.05	.02	.25	.11	20	72	.22
0	1	0	1	16	2	.01	<1	0	0	.01	.01	1	4	.01
0	29	.57	17	184	39[5]	.15	4	.08	.01	.4	.07	19	16	.17
0	21	.27	19	323	4	.08	805	.12	.12	1.21	.28	39	57	2.32

[1]Vitamin A in Texas red grapefruit would be 74 RE.

[2]This is vitamin A for white grapefruit juice; pink or red grapefruit juice = 109 RE per cup.

[3]With added vitamin C (ascorbic acid).

[4]Data are estimated from other fruit data.

[5]Sodium benzoate and sodium bisulfite added as preservatives.

(For purposes of calculations, use "0" for t, <1, <.1, <.01, etc.)

Table A–1
Food Composition

Computer Code Number	Food Description	Measure	Wt (g)	H$_2$O (%)	Ener (cal)	Prot (g)	Carb (g)	Dietary Fiber (g)	Fat (g)	Fat Breakdown (g)		
										Sat	Mono	Poly
	FRUITS and FRUIT JUICES—Cont.											
	Melons, raw, without rind and contents:											
264	Cantaloupe, 5" diam (2 ⅓ lb whole with refuse), orange flesh	½ ea	267	90	93	2	22	2	1	.1	.1	.2
265	Honeydew, 6½" diam (5¼ lb whole with refuse), slice = ⅒ melon	1 pce	129	90	45	1	12	1	<1	t	t	t
266	Nectarines, raw, w/o pits, 2½" diam	1 ea	136	86	67	1	16	2	1	.1	.2	.3
	Oranges, raw:											
267	Whole w/o peel and seeds, 2 ⅝" diam (180 g with peel and seeds)	1 ea	131	87	62	1	15	3	<1	t	t	t
268	Sections, without membranes	1 c	180	87	85	2	21	4	<1	t	t	t
	Orange juice:											
269	Fresh, all varieties	1 c	248	88	112	2	26	<1	<1	.1	.1	.1
270	Canned, unsweetened	1 c	249	89	105	1	24	<1	<1	t	.1	.1
271	Chilled	1 c	249	88	110	2	25	<1	1	.1	.1	.2
	Frozen concentrate:											
272	Undiluted (6-oz can)	¾ c	213	58	339	5	81	2	<1	.1	.1	.1
273	Diluted w/3 parts water by volume	1 c	249	88	112	2	27	<1	<1	t	t	t
1345	Orange juice, from dry crystals	1 c	248	88	114	0	29	0	<1	t	t	t
274	Orange and grapefruit juice, canned	1 c	247	89	106	1	25	<1	<1	t	t	t
	Papayas, raw:											
275	½" slices	1 c	140	89	54	1	14	3	<1	.1	.1	t
276	Whole, 3½" diam by 5⅛" w/o seeds and skin (1 lb w/refuse)	1 ea	304	89	118	2	30	5	<1	.1	.1	.1
1031	Papaya nectar, canned	1 c	250	85	142	<1	36	2	<1	.1	.1	.1
	Peaches:											
277	Raw, whole, 2½" diam, peeled, pitted (about 4 per lb whole)	1 ea	87	88	37	1	10	2	<1	t	t	t
278	Raw, sliced	1 c	170	88	73	1	19	3	<1	t	.1	.1
	Canned, fruit and liquid:											
279	Heavy syrup pack:	1 c	256	79	189	1	51	3	<1	t	.1	.1
280	Half	1 ea	81	79	60	<1	16	1	<1	t	t	t
281	Juice pack:	1 c	248	88	109	2	29	4	<1	t	t	t
282	Half	1 ea	77	88	34	<1	9	1	<1	t	t	t
283	Dried, uncooked	10 ea	130	32	311	5	80	12	1	.1	.4	.5
284	Dried, cooked, fruit and liquid	1 c	258	78	198	3	51	7	1	.1	.2	.3
	Frozen, slice, sweetened:											
285	10-oz package	1 ea	284	75	266	2	68	4	<1	t	.1	.2
286	Cup, thawed measure	1 c	250	75	235	2	60	4	<1	t	.1	.2
1032	Peach nectar, canned	1 c	249	86	134	1	35	1	<1	t	t	t
	Pears:											
	Fresh, with skin, cored:											
287	Bartlett, 2½" diam (about 2½ per lb)	1 ea	166	84	98	1	25	4[1]	1	t	.1	.2
288	Bosc, 2 1/5" diam (about 3 per lb)	1 ea	141	84	83	1	21	3[1]	1	t	.1	.1
289	D'Anjou, 3" diam (about 2 per lb)	1 ea	200	84	118	1	30	5[1]	1	t	.2	.2
	Canned, fruit and liquid:											
290	Heavy syrup pack:	1 c	255	80	188	1	49	5[1]	<1	t	.1	.1
291	Half	1 ea	79	80	58	<1	15	2[1]	<1	t	t	t
292	Juice pack:	1 c	248	86	124	1	32	5[1]	<1	t	t	t
293	Half	1 ea	77	86	38	<1	10	2[1]	<1	t	t	t

[1]Dietary fiber data vary 2.4 to 3.4 g/100 g for fresh pears; 1.6 to 2.6 g/100 g for canned pears.

(Computer code number is for West Diet Analysis program)

PAGE KEY: A–4 = BEV   A–6 = DAIRY   A–12 = EGGS   A–14 = FAT/OIL   A–18 = FRUIT   A–26 = BAKERY   A–36 = GRAIN   A–44 = FISH   A–48 = MEATS   A–50 = POULTRY   A–54 = SAUSAGE   A–56 = MIXED/FAST   A–64 = NUTS/SEEDS   A–68 = SWEETS   A–70 = VEG/LEG   A–84 = MISC   A–88 = SOUPS/SAUCES   A–90 = FAST   A–106 = FRZN ENTREE   A–112 = BABY FOODS

Chol (mg)	Calc (mg)	Iron (mg)	Magn (mg)	Pota (mg)	Sodi (mg)	Zinc (mg)	VT-A (RE)	Thia (mg)	Ribo (mg)	Niac (mg)	V-B6 (mg)	Fola (μg)	VT-C (mg)	VT-E α-TE (mg)
0	29	.56	29	825	24	.43	860	.1	.06	1.53	.31	45	113	.4
0	8	.09	9	350	13	.11	5	.1	.02	.77	.08	39	32	.19
0	7	.2	11	288	0	.12	101	.02	.06	1.35	.03	5	7	1.21
0	52	.13	13	237	0	.09	27	.11	.05	.37	.08	40	70	.31
0	72	.18	18	326	0	.13	38	.16	.07	.51	.11	54	96	.43
0	27	.5	27	496	2	.12	50	.22	.07	.99	.1	75	124	.22
0	20	1.1	27	436	5	.17	45	.15	.07	.78	.22	45	86	.22
0	25	.42	27	473	3	.1	20²	.19	.28	.05	.7	45²	82²	.47
0	68	.75	72	1435	6	.38	59	.6	.14	1.53	.33	330	294	.68
0	22	.25	25	473	3	.12	20	.2	.04	.5	.11	109	97	.47
0	62	.2	2	50	12	.1	551	0	.04	0	0	142	121	0
0	20	1.14	25	390	7	.17	30	.14	.07	.83	.06	35	72	.17
0	34	.14	14	360	4	.1	39	.04	.04	.47	.03	53	86	1.6
0	73	.3	30	781	9	.21	85	.08	.1	1.03	.06	115	187	3.4
0	25	.85	7	77	13	.37	27	.01	.01	.37	.02	5	8	.05
0	4	.1	6	171	0	.12	47	.01	.04	.86	.02	3	6	.61
0	8	.19	12	335	0	.24	92	.03	.07	1.68	.03	6	11	1.2
0	8	.69	13	235	15	.23	84	.03	.06	1.57	.05	8	7	2.28
0	2	.22	4	74	5	.07	27	.01	.02	.5	.01	3	2	.72
0	15	.67	17	317	10	.27	94	.02	.04	1.44	.05	8	9	3.72
0	5	.21	5	99	3	.08	29	.01	.01	.45	.01	3	3	1.2
0	36	5.28	55	1293	9	.74	281	<.01	.28	5.69	.09	<1	6	0
0	23	3.38	33	826	5	.46	52	.01	.05	3.92	.1	<1	10	0
0	9	1.05	14	369	17	.14	81	.04	.1	1.85	.05	9	267³	2.53
0	8	.92	12	325	15	.12	71	.03	.09	1.63	.04	8	236³	2.23
0	12	.47	10	100	17	.2	64	.01	.03	.72	.02	3	13	.03
0	18	.41	10	208	0	.2	3	.03	.07	.17	.03	12	7	.83
0	16	.35	8	176	0	.17	3	.03	.06	.14	.02	10	6	.71
0	22	.5	12	250	0	.24	4	.04	.08	.2	.04	15	8	1
0	13	.56	10	165	13	.2	1	.03	.06	.62	.04	3	3	1.28
0	4	.17	3	51	4	.06	<1	.01	.02	.19	.01	1	1	.4
0	22	.72	17	238	10	.22	2	.03	.03	.5	.03	3	4	1.24
0	7	.22	5	74	3	.07	1	.01	.01	.15	.01	1	1	.39

(2)Values for juice from California oranges indicate the following values for 1 c: 36 RE of vitamin A, 72 μg of folate, and 106 mg of vitamin C.

(3)With added vitamin C (ascorbic acid).

(For purposes of calculations, use "0" for t, <1, <.1, <.01, etc.)

Table A–1
Food Composition

Computer Code Number	Food Description	Measure	Wt (g)	H₂O (%)	Ener (cal)	Prot (g)	Carb (g)	Dietary Fiber (g)	Fat (g)	Fat Breakdown (g)		
										Sat	Mono	Poly
	FRUITS and FRUIT JUICES—Cont.											
294	Dried halves	10 ea	175	27	459	3	121	13	1	.1	.2	.3
1033	Pear nectar, canned	1 c	250	84	150	<1	39	2	<1	t	t	t
	Pineapple:											
295	Fresh chunks, diced	1 c	155	87	76	1	19	2	1	t	.1	.2
	Canned, fruit and liquid:											
	Heavy syrup pack:											
296	Crushed, chunks, tidbits	⅓ c	84	79	65	<1	17	1	<1	t	t	t
297	Slices	1 ea	58	79	45	<1	12	<1	<1	t	t	t
298	Juice pack, crushed, chunks, tidbits	1 c	250	84	150	1	39	2	<1	t	t	.1
299	Juice pack, slices	1 ea	58	84	35	<1	9	<1	<1	t	t	t
300	Pineapple juice, canned, unsweetened	1 c	250	86	140	1	35	<1	<1	t	t	.1
	Plantains, without peel:											
301	Raw slices (whole = 179 g w/o peel)	1 c	148	65	181	2	47	3[1]	1	.3	.1	.1
302	Cooked, boiled, sliced	1 c	154	67	179	1	48	4	<1	.1	t	.1
	Plums:											
303	Fresh, medium, 2⅛" diam	1 ea	66	85	36	1	9	1	<1	t	.3	.1
304	Fresh, small, 1½" diam	1 ea	28	85	15	<1	4	<1	<1	t	.1	t
	Canned, purple, with liquid:											
305	Heavy syrup pack:	1 c	258	76	229	1	60	3	<1	t	.2	.1
306	Plums	3 ea	110	76	98	<1	26	1	<1	t	.1	t
307	Juice pack:	1 c	252	84	146	1	38	3	<1	t	t	t
308	Plums	3 ea	95	84	55	<1	14	1	<1	t	t	t
1698	Pomegranate, fresh	1 ea	154	81	105	1	27	5	<1	–	–	–
	Prunes, dried, pitted:											
309	Uncooked (10 = 97 g w/pits, 84 g w/o pits)	10 ea	84	32	200	2	53	8[2]	<1	t	.3	.1
310	Cooked, unsweetened, fruit & liq (250 g w/pits)	1c	212	70	227	3	60	14	<1	t	.3	.1
311	Prune juice, bottled or canned	1c	256	81	182	2	45	3	1	t	.5	t
	Raisins, seedless:											
312	Cup, not pressed down	1 c	145	15	435	5	115	5	1	.2	t	.2
313	One packet, ½ oz	½ oz	14	15	42	<1	11	1	<1	t	t	t
	Raspberries:											
314	Fresh	1 c	123	87	60	1	14	5	1	t	.1	.4
315	Frozen, sweetened:	10 oz	284	73	293	2	74	13	<1	t	t	.3
316	Cup, thawed measure	1 c	250	73	258	2	66	11	<1	t	t	.2
317	Rhubarb, cooked, added sugar	1 c	240	68	278	1	75	5	<1	t	t	.1
	Strawberries:											
318	Fresh, whole, capped	1 c	149	92	45	1	10	2	1	t	.1	.3
	Frozen, sliced, sweetened:											
319	10-oz container	10 oz	284	73	272	2	74	5	<1	t	.1	.2
320	Cup, thawed measure	1 c	255	73	244	1	66	5	<1	t	t	.2
	Tangerines, without peel and seeds:											
321	Fresh (2⅜" whole) 116 g w/refuse	1 ea	84	88	37	1	9	1	<1	t	t	t
322	Canned, light syrup, fruit and liquid	1 c	252	83	153	1	41	2	<1	t	t	t
323	Tangerine juice, canned, sweetened	1 c	249	87	124	1	30	<1	<1	t	t	.1

[1]Dietary fiber value partially derived from data for bananas.

[2]Dietary fiber data can vary between 6 and 13 g for 10 prunes.

(Computer code number is for West Diet Analysis program)

PAGE KEY: A–4 = BEV   A–6 = DAIRY   A–12 = EGGS   A–14 = FAT/OIL   A–18 = FRUIT   A–26 = BAKERY   A–36 = GRAIN   A–44 = FISH
A–48 = MEATS   A–50 = POULTRY   A–54 = SAUSAGE   A–56 = MIXED/FAST   A–64 = NUTS/SEEDS   A–68 = SWEETS   A–70 = VEG/LEG
A–84 = MISC   A–88 = SOUPS/SAUCES   A–90 = FAST   A–106 = FRZN ENTREE   A–112 = BABY FOODS

Chol (mg)	Calc (mg)	Iron (mg)	Magn (mg)	Pota (mg)	Sodi (mg)	Zinc (mg)	VT-A (RE)	Thia (mg)	Ribo (mg)	Niac (mg)	V-B6 (mg)	Fola (μg)	VT-C (mg)	VT-E α-TE (mg)
0	59	3.68	58	933	10	.68	1	.01	.25	2.4	.13	0	12	0
0	12	.65	7	32	10	.17	<1	<.01	.03	.32	.03	3	3	.25
0	11	.57	22	175	2	.12	4	.14	.06	.65	.13	16	24	.16
0	12	.32	13	87	1	.1	1	.08	.02	.24	.06	4	6	.08
0	8	.22	9	60	1	.07	1	.05	.01	.17	.04	3	4	.06
0	35	.7	35	305	3	.25	10	.24	.05	.71	.18	12	24	.25
0	8	.16	8	71	1	.06	2	.05	.01	.16	.04	3	6	.06
0	42	.65	32	335	3	.27	1	.14	.05	.64	.24	58	27[3]	.05
0	4	.89	55	739	6	.21	167[4]	.08	.08	1.02	.44	33	27	.4
0	3	.89	49	716	8	.2	140	.07	.08	1.16	.37	40	17	.22
0	3	.07	5	113	0	.07	21	.03	.06	.33	.05	1	6	.4
0	1	.03	2	48	0	.03	9	.01	.03	.14	.02	1	3	.17
0	23	2.17	13	234	49	.18	67	.04	.1	.75	.07	6	1	1.81
0	10	.92	5	100	21	.08	29	.02	.04	.32	.03	3	<1	.77
0	25	.86	20	388	3	.28	255	.06	.15	1.19	.07	7	7	1.76
0	10	.32	8	146	1	.1	96	.02	.06	.45	.03	2	3	.67
0	5	.46	5	399	5	–	0	.05	.05	.46	.16	–	9	.85
0	43	2.08	38	625	3	.44	167	.07	.14	1.65	.22	3	3	1.22
0	49	2.35	42	708	4	.51	65	.05	.21	1.53	.46	<1	6	<.01
0	31	3	36	707	10	.54	1	.04	.18	2	.56	1	11	.03
0	71	3.02	48	1088	17	.39	1	.23	.13	1.19	.36	5	5	1.02
0	7	.29	5	105	2	.04	<1	.02	.01	.11	.03	<1	<1	.1
0	27	.7	22	186	0	.57	16	.04	.11	1.11	.07	32	31	.55
0	43	1.85	37	324	3	.51	17	.05	.13	.65	.1	74	47	1.28
0	37	1.63	32	285	3	.45	15	.05	.11	.57	.08	65	41	1.13
0	348	.5	29	230	2	.19	17	.04	.05	.48	.05	13	8	.48
0	21	.57	15	247	1	.19	4	.03	.1	.34	.09	26	84	.21
0	31	1.68	20	278	9	.17	7	.04	.14	1.14	.08	42	117	.4
0	28	1.51	18	250	8	.15	6	.04	.13	1.02	.08	38	105	.4
0	12	.08	10	131	1	.2	77	.09	.02	.13	.06	17	26	.2
0	18	.93	20	196	15	.6	212	.13	.11	1.12	.11	12	50	.9
0	45	.5	20	443	3	.07	105	.15	.05	.25	.08	11	55	.22

[3] If vitamin C is added, it contains 96 mg per cup.
[4] Vitamin A values range from 1.5 RE for white-fleshed varieties to 178 RE for yellow-fleshed varieties.

(For purposes of calculations, use "0" for t, <1, <.1, <.01, etc.)

Table A–1
Food Composition

Computer Code Number	Food Description	Measure	Wt (g)	H₂O (%)	Ener (cal)	Prot (g)	Carb (g)	Dietary Fiber (g)	Fat (g)	Fat Breakdown (g)		
										Sat	Mono	Poly
	FRUITS and FRUIT JUICES—Cont.											
	Watermelon, raw, without rind & seeds:											
324	Piece, 1" by 10" diam (2 lb w/refuse or 926 g)	1 pce	482	91	154	3	35	1	2	.6	.4	1.1
325	Diced	1 c	160	91	51	1	11	1	1	.2	.1	.4
	BAKED GOODS: BREADS, CAKES, COOKIES, CRACKERS, PIES											
326	Bagels, plain, enriched, 3½" diam	1 ea	68	33	187	7	36	2	1	.1	.1	.5
1663	Bagel, oat bran	1 ea	71	33	181	8	38	8	1	.1	.2	.4
	Biscuits:											
327	From home recipe	1 ea	28	29	100	2	13	<1	5	1.2	2	1.2
328	From mix	1 ea	28	29	94	2	14	1	3	.8	1.2	1.2
329	From refrigerated dough	1 ea	20	27	75	1	9	<1	4	2	1	.1
330	Bread crumbs, dry, grated (see #364, 365 for soft crumbs)	1 c	100	6	395	12	72	4	5	1.3	2.1	2
2087	Bread sticks, brown & serve	1 ea	57	34	150	7	28	1	2	.5	.5	.5
	Breads:											
331	Boston brown, canned, 3¼" slice	1 pce	45	47	88	2	19	2	1	.1	.1	.3
332	Cracked wheat (¼ cracked-wheat & ¾ enr wheat flour): 1-lb loaf	1 ea	454	36	1180	39	225	27	18	4.2	8.6	3.1
333	Slice (18 per loaf)	1 pce	25	36	65	2	12	2	1	.2	.5	.2
334	Slice, toasted	1 pce	21	30	59	2	11	1	1	.2	.4	.2
335	French/Vienna, enriched: 1-lb loaf	1 ea	454	34	1243	40	236	13	14	2.9	5.5	3.1
337	Slice, 4¾ x 4 x ½"	1 pce	25	34	68	2	13	1	1	.2	.3	.2
336	French, slice, 5 x 2½"	1 pce	35	34	96	3	18	1	1	.2	.4	.2
	French toast: see Mixed Dishes, and											
	Fast Foods, #691											
2083	Honey wheatberry	1 pce	38	3	100	3	18	2	2	0	.5	0
338	Italian, enriched: 1-lb loaf	1 ea	454	36	1230	40	227	14	16	3.9	3.7	6.3
339	Slice, 4½ x 3¼ x ¾"	1 pce	30	36	81	3	15	1	1	.3	.2	.4
340	Mixed grain, enriched: 1-lb loaf	1 ea	454	38	1135	45	211	32	17	3.7	6.9	4.2
341	Slice (18 per loaf)	1 pce	25	38	62	3	12	2	1	.2	.4	.2
342	Slice, toasted	1 pce	23	32	63	3	12	2	1	.2	.4	.2
343	Oatmeal, enriched: 1-lb loaf	1 ea	454	37	1221	38	220	18	20	3.2	7.2	7.7
344	Slice (18 per loaf)	1 pce	25	37	67	2	12	1	1	.2	.4	.4
345	Slice, toasted	1 pce	23	31	67	2	12	1	1	.2	.4	.4
346	Pita pocket bread, enr, 6½" round	1 ea	60	32	165	5	33	1	1	.1	.1	.3
347	Pumpernickel (⅔ rye & ⅓ enr wheat flour): 1-lb loaf	1 ea	454	38	1135	39	216	33	14	2	4.2	5.6
348	Slice, 5 x 4 x ⅜"	1 pce	32	38	80	3	15	2	1	.1	.3	.4
349	Slice, toasted	1 pce	29	32	80	3	15	2	1	.1	.3	.4
350	Raisin, enriched: 1-lb loaf	1 ea	454	34	1243	36	237	20	20	4.9	10.4	3.1
351	Slice (18 per loaf)	1 pce	25	34	68	2	13	1	1	.3	.6	.2
352	Slice, toasted	1 pce	21	28	62	2	12	1	1	.2	.5	.2
353	Rye, light (⅓ rye & ⅔ enr wheat flour): 1-lb loaf	1 ea	454	37	1177	39	219	28	15	2.8	6	3.6
354	Slice, 4¾ x 3¾ x ⁷⁄₁₆"	1 pce	25	37	65	2	12	2	1	.2	.3	.2
355	Slice, toasted	1 pce	22	31	62	2	12	2	1	.2	.3	.2

PAGE KEY: A–4 = BEV   A–6 = DAIRY   A–12 = EGGS   A–14 = FAT/OIL   A–18 = FRUIT   A–26 = BAKERY   A–36 = GRAIN   A–44 = FISH   A–48 = MEATS   A–50 = POULTRY   A–54 = SAUSAGE   A–56 = MIXED/FAST   A–64 = NUTS/SEEDS   A–68 = SWEETS   A–70 = VEG/LEG   A–84 = MISC   A–88 = SOUPS/SAUCES   A–90 = FAST   A–106 = FRZN ENTREE   A–112 = BABY FOODS

Chol (mg)	Calc (mg)	Iron (mg)	Magn (mg)	Pota (mg)	Sodi (mg)	Zinc (mg)	VT-A (RE)	Thia (mg)	Ribo (mg)	Niac (mg)	V-B6 (mg)	Fola (μg)	VT-C (mg)	VT-E α-TE (mg)
0	39	.82	53	559	10	.34	178	.39	.1	.96	.69	11	46	.72
0	13	.27	18	186	3	.11	59	.13	.03	.32	.23	4	15	.24
0	50	2.43	20	69	363	.6	0	.37	.21	3.1	.03	15	0	.02
0	9	2.2	39	139	360	1.42	3	.24	.23	2.1	.14	31	<1	.17
1	67	.81	5	34	163	.15	6	.1	.09	.84	.01	3	<1	.68
1	52	.58	7	53	267	.17	7	.1	.1	.86	.02	2	<1	.11
1	24	.44	2	23	158	.08	7	.07	.05	.44	.01	2	0	.12
0	227	6.13	46	221	862	1.23	<1	.76	.43	6.85	.1	25	0	.88
0	60	2.7	–	–	290	–	0	.225	.102	1.6	–	–	0	–
<1	31	.95	28	143	284	.22	5	.01	.05	.5	.04	3	0	.14
0	195	12.8	236	804	2452	5.68	0	1.63	1.09	16.7	1.38	177	0	2.6
0	11	.7	13	44	135	.31	0	.09	.06	.92	.08	10	0	.14
0	10	.64	12	40	123	.29	0	.07	.05	.75	.06	6	0	.13
0	341	11.5	123	513	2764	3.95	0	2.36	1.49	21.6	.19	141	0	1.07
0	19	.63	7	28	152	.22	0	.13	.08	1.19	.01	8	0	.06
0	26	.89	9	40	213	.3	0	.18	.11	1.66	.01	11	0	.08
0	20	.72	–	–	200	–	0	.12	.07	.8	–	–	0	.24
0	354	13.4	123	499	2648	3.9	0	2.15	1.33	19.9	.22	136	0	1.26
0	23	.88	8	33	175	.26	0	.14	.09	1.31	.01	9	0	.08
0	413	15.8	241	926	2216	5.81	0	1.85	1.55	19.8	1.51	218	1	2.79
0	23	.87	13	51	122	.32	0	.1	.09	1.09	.08	12	<1	.15
0	23	.87	13	51	122	.32	0	.08	.08	.98	.07	9	<1	.15
0	300	12.3	168	645	2724	4.68	9	1.81	1.09	14.3	.31	123	2	1.56
0	16	.68	9	36	150	.26	<1	.1	.06	.78	.02	7	<1	.09
0	17	.68	9	35	150	.26	<1	.08	.05	.71	.01	5	<1	.09
0	52	1.58	16	72	322	.5	0	.36	.2	2.78	.02	14	0	.02
0	309	13.1	245	944	3050	6.76	0	1.48	1.38	14	.57	155	0	2.3
0	22	.92	17	67	215	.48	0	.1	.1	.99	.04	11	0	.16
0	22	.92	17	66	214	.47	0	.08	.09	.89	.04	8	0	.17
0	300	13.2	118	1030	1770	3.27	<1	1.54	1.81	15.8	.31	154	2	3.44
0	17	.73	7	57	97	.18	0	.08	.1	.87	.02	9	<1	.19
0	15	.66	6	52	89	.16	<1	.06	.08	.71	.01	5	<1	.173
0	331	12.9	182	754	2996	5.22	0	1.97	1.52	17.3	.34	232	0	2.51
0	18	.71	10	42	165	.29	0	.11	.08	.95	.02	13	0	.14
0	18	.68	9	40	160	.28	0	.08	.07	.83	.02	9	<1	.13

(For purposes of calculations, use "0" for t, <1, <.1, <.01, etc.)

Table A–1
Food Composition

Computer Code Number	Food Description	Measure	Wt (g)	H_2O (%)	Ener (cal)	Prot (g)	Carb (g)	Dietary Fiber (g)	Fat (g)	Fat Breakdown (g) Sat	Mono	Poly
	BAKED GOODS: BREADS, CAKES, COOKIES, CRACKERS, PIES—Cont.											
356	Wheat (enr wheat & whole-wheat flour):[1] 1-lb loaf	1 ea	454	37	1180	41	213	25	19	3.9	7.3	4.5
357	Slice (18 per loaf)	1 pce	25	37	64	2	12	1	1	.2	.4	.2
358	Slice, toasted	1 pce	23	32	65	2	12	1	1	.2	.4	.2
359	White, enriched: 1-lb loaf	1 ea	454	37	1213	38	225	12	16	3.7	7.3	3.4
360	Slice (18 per loaf)	1 pce	25	37	67	2	12	1	1	.2	.4	.2
361	Slice, toasted	1 pce	22	30	64	2	12	1	1	.2	.4	.2
362	Slice (22 per loaf)	1 pce	20	37	53	2	10	1	1	.2	.3	.2
363	Slice, toasted	1 pce	17	30	50	2	9	<1	1	.2	.3	.1
364	White bread cubes, soft	1 c	30	36	81	3	15	1	1	.2	.5	.2
365	White bread crumbs, soft	1 c	45	36	120	4	23	1	1	.3	.6	.4
366	Whole-wheat: 1-lb loaf	1 ea	454	38	1116	44	209	28	19	4.2	7.6	4.5
367	Slice (16 per loaf)	1 pce	28	38	69	3	13	2	1	.3	.5	.3
368	Slice, toasted	1 pce	25	30	69	3	13	2	1	.3	.5	.3
	Bread stuffing, prepared from mix:											
369	Dry type	1 c	140	65	249	4	30	4	12	2.4	5.3	3.6
370	Moist type, with egg and margarine	1 c	203	65	341	8	45	4	15	3	6.5	4.3
	Cakes, prepared from mixes:[1]											
	Angel food:											
371	Whole cake, 9¾" diam tube	1 ea	635	33	1641	38	367	10	5	.8	.5	2.3
372	Piece, 1/12 of cake	1 pce	53	33	137	3	31	1	<1	.1	t	.2
373	Boston cream pie, 1/8 of cake	1 pce	120	45	302	3	52	2	10	3	5.3	1.2
	Coffee cake:											
374	Whole cake, 7¾ x 5⅝ x 1¼"	1 ea	430	31	1368	24	227	7	41	8	16.6	13.6
375	Piece, 1/6 of cake	1 pce	72	31	229	4	38	1	7	1.3	2.8	2.3
	Devil's food, chocolate frosting:											
376	Whole cake, 2 layer, 8 or 9" diam	1 ea	1107	23	4059	45	605	31	182	51.4	99.6	21.1
377	Piece, 1/16 of cake	1 pce	69	23	253	3	38	2	11	3.2	6.2	1.3
378	Cupcake, 2½" diam	1 ea	42	23	154	2	23	1	7	1.9	3.8	.8
	Gingerbread:											
379	Whole cake, 8" square	1 ea	570	33	1764	23	289	18	58	14.8	21.9	7.6
380	Piece, 1/9 of cake	1 pce	63	33	195	3	32	2	6	1.6	3.5	.8
	Yellow, chocolate frosting, 2 layer:											
381	Whole cake, 8 or 9" diam	1 ea	1108	22	4207	42	613	20	193	52.4	107	23.2
382	Piece, 1/16 of cake	1 pce	69	22	262	3	38	1	12	3.3	6.7	1.4
	Cakes from recipes w/enr flour:											
	Carrot cake, cream cheese frosting:[2]											
383	Whole, 9 x 13" cake	1 ea	1536	21	6693	71	725	20	406	75.1	100	208
384	Piece, 1/16 of cake, 2¼ x 3¼" slice	1 pce	112	23	488	5	53	1	30	5.5	7.3	15.2
	Fruitcake, dark:											
385	Whole cake, 7½" diam tube, 2¼" high	1 ea	1361	25	4409	39	838	48	124	15.2	56.8	44.1
386	Piece, 1/32 of cake, ⅔" arc	1 pce	43	25	139	1	26	2	4	.5	1.8	1.4
	Sheet, plain, no frosting:[3]											
387	Whole cake, 9" square	1 ea	777	23	2773	42	444	6	96	25	41.3	24.5
388	Piece, 1/9 of cake	1 pce	86	23	307	5	48	<1	11	3.3	5	2.8

(1)Excepting angel food cake, cakes were made from mixes containing vegetable shortening, and frostings were made with margarine. All mixes use enriched flour.

(2)Made with vegetable oil.

(3)Cake made with vegetable shortening.

(4)Made with margarine.

(Computer code number is for West Diet Analysis program)

PAGE KEY: A–4 = BEV   A–6 = DAIRY   A–12 = EGGS   A–14 = FAT/OIL   A–18 = FRUIT   A–26 = BAKERY   A–36 = GRAIN   A–44 = FISH
A–48 = MEATS   A–50 = POULTRY   A–54 = SAUSAGE   A–56 = MIXED/FAST   A–64 = NUTS/SEEDS   A–68 = SWEETS   A–70 = VEG/LEG
A–84 = MISC   A–88 = SOUPS/SAUCES   A–90 = FAST   A–106 = FRZN ENTREE   A–112 = BABY FOODS

Chol (mg)	Calc (mg)	Iron (mg)	Magn (mg)	Pota (mg)	Sodi (mg)	Zinc (mg)	VT-A (RE)	Thia (mg)	Ribo (mg)	Niac (mg)	V-B6 (mg)	Fola (µg)	VT-C (mg)	VT-E α-TE (mg)
0	476	15	209	913	2414	4.77	0	2	1.28	18.7	.49	185	0	3
0	26	.83	12	50	133	.26	0	.11	.08	1.13	.03	11	0	.17
0	26	.83	12	50	132	.26	0	.08	.06	.93	.02	7	0	.14
5	490	12.9	109	541	2452	2.81	0	2.13	1.5	17	.29	154	0	1.3
<1	27	.71	6	30	135	.15	0	.12	.09	.99	.01	9	0	.07
<1	26	.73	6	29	130	.15	0	.09	.08	.86	.01	6	0	.04
<1	22	.57	5	24	108	.12	0	.09	.07	.75	.01	7	0	.06
<1	20	.57	4	22	101	.12	0	.07	.06	.67	.01	4	0	.03
<1	25	.84	6	32	151	.19	0	.14	.1	1.19	.02	10	0	.05
<1	38	1.3	9	48	227	.28	0	.18	.11	1.5	.15	16	0	.08
0	327	15	390	1144	2382	8.85	0	1.59	.93	17.4	.81	227	0	4.72
0	20	.94	24	72	147	.55	0	.1	.06	1.09	.05	14	0	.29
0	20	.93	24	71	148	.55	0	.08	.05	.97	.05	10	0	.23
0	45	1.54	17	104	760	.39	113	.19	.15	2.07	.06	24	0	1.96
0	130	3.35	30	266	936	.65	140	.34	.29	3.23	.11	35	3	2.44
0	889	3.3	76	591	4756	.44	0	.65	3.12	5.61	.2	19	0	.64
0	74	.28	6	49	397	.04	0	.05	.26	.47	.02	2	0	.05
44	28	.46	7	47	173	.19	28	.49	.32	.23	.03	10	<1	1.27
211	585	6.19	77	482	1810	1.94	172	.72	.75	6.54	.21	52	1	7.14
35	98	1.04	13	81	303	.32	29	.12	.13	1.09	.04	9	<1	1.2
509	476	24.5	376	2214	3690	7.64	310	.3	1.47	6.39	.41	89	1	18.7
32	30	1.52	23	138	230	.48	19	.02	.09	.4	.03	6	<1	1.17
19	18	.93	14	84	140	.29	12	.01	.06	.24	.02	3	<1	.71
200	393	18.9	91	1375	2615	2.34	91	1.08	1.06	8.89	.22	57	1	7.81
22	43	2.09	10	152	289	.26	10	.12	.12	.98	.02	6	<1	.86
609	410	23.2	332	1975	3742	6.87	299	1.33	1.74	13.9	.32	89	1	29.9
38	25	1.44	21	123	233	.43	19	.08	.11	.86	.02	6	<1	1.86
829	384	19.4	276	1714	3	7.53	5897	2.09	2.4	15.5	1.17	184	17	64.8
60	28	1.41	20	125	276	.55	480	.15	.17	1.13	.08	13	1	4.73
68	449	28.3	218	2082	3674	3.67	475	.68	1.35	10.8	.63	41	5	–
2	14	.89	7	66	116	.12	15	.02	.04	.34	.02	1	<1	1.34
505	497	11.7	108	613	2331	2.75	130	1.24	1.4	10.1	.26	54	2	11.03
56	55	1.3	12	68	258	.3	14	.14	.15	1.12	.03	6	<1	1.22

(For purposes of calculations, use "0" for t, <1, <.1, <.01, etc.)

Table A–1
Food Composition

Computer Code Number	Food Description	Measure	Wt (g)	H_2O (%)	Ener (cal)	Prot (g)	Carb (g)	Dietary Fiber (g)	Fat (g)	Fat Breakdown (g) Sat	Mono	Poly
	BAKED GOODS: BREADS, CAKES, COOKIES, CRACKERS, PIES—Cont.											
	Sheet, plain, uncooked white frosting:[4]											
389	Whole cake, 9" square	1 ea	1096	22	4085	38	644	10	159	26.1	67	56.1
390	Piece, ⅙ of cake	1 pce	121	22	451	4	71	1	18	2.9	7.4	6.2
	Pound cake:											
2299	Loaf, 8½ x 3½ x 3¼"	1 ea	478	25	1863	26	234	4	95	53	26.7	5.21
392	Piece, 1/17 of loaf, ½" slice	1 pce	28	25	109	2	14	<1	6	3	1.5	.31
	Cakes, commercial:											
	Cheesecake:											
401	Whole cake, 9" diam	1 ea	1110	46	3559	61	283	23	250	128	86	15.3
402	Piece, 1/12 of cake	1 pce	92	46	295	5	23	2	21	10.6	7.1	1.3
	Pound cake:											
393	Loaf, 8½ x 3½ x 3"	1 ea	500	25	1948	27	244	3	99	55.5	27.9	5.4
394	Slice, 1/17 of loaf, 2" slice	1 pce	29	25	113	2	14	<1	6	3.2	1.6	.3
	Snack: 2 small cakes per package											
395	Chocolate w/creme filling (Ding Dong)	1 ea	28	20	105	1	17	<1	4	.9	1.5	1.2
396	Sponge w/creme filling (Twinkie)	1 ea	42	20	153	1	27	<1	5	1.1	1.9	1.5
1677	Sponge cake, 1/12 of 12" cake	1 pce	65	30	188	4	40	<1	2	.5	.6	.3
1678	Strawberry shortcake, fresh	1 ea	254	74	327	5	40	4	17	10.1	4.9	1
	White, white frosting, 2 layer:											
397	Whole cake, 8 or 9" diam	1 ea	1140	20	4271	38	718	11	154	45.7	68.1	39.8
398	Piece, 1/16 of cake	1 pce	71	20	266	2	45	1	10	2.8	4.2	2.5
	Yellow, chocolate frosting, 2 layer:											
399	Whole cake, 8 or 9" diam	1 ea	1108	22	4207	42	614	20	193	52.4	107	23.2
400	Piece, 1/16 of cake	1 pce	69	22	262	3	38	1	12	3.3	6.7	1.4
1332	Bagel chips	5 pce	70	4	298	6	52	6	7	1.2	1.9	3.3
2225	Bagel chips, onion garlic, toasted	½ oz	14	–	70	2	9	–	2	0	2	0
1035	Cheese puffs/Cheetos	1 oz	28	1	155	2	15	<1	10	1.9	5.8	1.3
	Cookies made with enriched flour:											
	Brownies with nuts:											
403	Commercial w/frosting, 1½ x 1¾ x ⅞"	1 ea	25	14	101	1	16	1	4	1.1	2.1	.6
404	Home recipe, 1¾ x 1¾ x ⅞"[1]	1 ea	20	13	93	1	10	<1	6	1.5	2.2	1.9
1902	Fat free fudge, Entenmann's	1 pce	40	24	110	2	27	1	0	0	0	0
	Chocolate chip:											
405	Commercial, 2¼" diam	4 ea	42	12	192	1	25	1	10	3.1	5.5	1.1
406	Home recipe, 2¼" diam	4 ea	40	6	195	2	23	1	11	3.2	4.2	3.4
407	From refrigerated dough, 2¼" diam	4 ea	48	13	213	2	29	1	10	3.3	4.8	1
408	Fig bars	4 ea	56	16	195	2	40	3	4	.7	2.2	.7
2052	Fruit bar, no fat	1 ea	28	–	90	2	21	0	0	0	0	0
2162	Fudge, fat free, Snackwell	1 ea	16	14	53	1	12	<1	<1	.1	.1	<.1
2002	Granola cookie, fat free	3 ea	28	17	85	2	19	2	0	0	0	0
409	Oatmeal raisin, 2⅝" diam	4 ea	52	6	226	3	36	2	8	1.7	3.6	2.6
410	Peanut butter, home recipe, 2⅝" diam[2]	4 ea	48	6	228	4	28	1	11	2.1	5.2	3.5
411	Sandwich-type, all	4 ea	40	2	189	2	28	1	8	1.7	4.7	1.1
412	Shortbread, commercial, small	4 ea	32	4	161	2	21	1	8	2	4.3	1
413	Shortbread, home recipe, large[3]	2 ea	28	3	153	2	16	1	9	5.8	2.7	.4

(1)Made with vegetable oil.
(2)Made with vegetable shortening.
(3)Made with butter.
(4)Made with margarine.

(Computer code number is for West Diet Analysis program)

PAGE KEY: A–4 = BEV   A–6 = DAIRY   A–12 = EGGS   A–14 = FAT/OIL   A–18 = FRUIT   A–26 = BAKERY   A–36 = GRAIN   A–44 = FISH   A–48 = MEATS   A–50 = POULTRY   A–54 = SAUSAGE   A–56 = MIXED/FAST   A–64 = NUTS/SEEDS   A–68 = SWEETS   A–70 = VEG/LEG   A–84 = MISC   A–88 = SOUPS/SAUCES   A–90 = FAST   A–106 = FRZN ENTREE   A–112 = BABY FOODS

Chol (mg)	Calc (mg)	Iron (mg)	Magn (mg)	Pota (mg)	Sodi (mg)	Zinc (mg)	VT-A (RE)	Thia (mg)	Ribo (mg)	Niac (mg)	V-B6 (mg)	Fola (μg)	VT-C (mg)	VT-E α-TE (mg)
614	680	11.8	66	581	3770	2.74	208	1.1	.77	5.48	.38	99	2	20.8
68	75	1.31	7	64	416	.3	23	.12	.08	.6	.04	11	<1	2.3
0	85	1.71	–	324	1502	–	745	0	.51	6.26	.07	53	0	–
0	5	.1	–	19	88	–	44	0	.03	.4	<.01	3	0	–
611	566	6.99	122	999	2297	5.66	1787	.31	2.14	2.16	.58	167	7	11.7
51	47	.58	10	83	190	.47	148	.03	.18	.18	.05	14	1	.97
1105	175	6.95	55	595	1983	2.3	779	.68	1.15	6.55	.17	55	1	3.29
64	10	.4	3	34	115	.13	45	.04	.07	.38	.01	3	<1	.19
5	21	.94	12	35	119	.16	1	.06	.08	.69	.01	2	<1	.56
7	19	.55	3	38	153	.13	2	.06	.06	.51	.01	2	<1	.82
66	46	1.77	7	64	158	.33	30	.16	.18	1.25	.03	8	0	.29
53	209	2.33	29	359	510	.57	172	.29	.33	2.26	.13	40	95	.73
91	547	9.12	60	661	2665	1.77	369	1.14	1.48	10.3	.16	64	1	20.5
6	34	.57	4	41	166	.11	23	.07	.09	.64	.01	4	<1	1.28
609	410	23.2	332	1975	3742	6.87	299	1.33	1.74	13.9	.32	89	1	29.9
38	25	1.44	21	123	233	.43	19	.08	.11	.86	.02	6	<1	1.86
0	9	1.38	41	137	418	.88	0	.1	.12	1.57	.1	58	0	.47
0	–	–	–	–	80	–	–	.09	.03	1.20	–	–	–	<.01
1	16	.67	5	47	294	.11	10	.07	.1	.92	.04	34	<1	1.43
4	7	.56	8	37	78	.18	5	.06	.05	.43	.01	3	<1	.53
15	11	.37	11	35	69	.19	40	.03	.04	.2	.02	3	<1	.58
0	0	1.08	–	90	140	–	0	–	–	–	–	–	0	<.01
0	6	1.02	15	39	137	.19	21	.05	.08	.68	.07	2	0	1.22
13	16	.99	22	90	144	.37	66	.07	.07	.54	.03	5	<1	1.16
11	12	1.08	11	86	100	.24	8	.09	.09	.95	.02	4	0	.98
0	36	1.63	15	116	196	.22	2	.09	.12	1.05	.04	6	<1	.39
0	0	.36	–	–	95	–	0	–	–	–	–	–	0	.01
0	3	.29	5	26	71	.08	–	.02	.02	.26	0	–	0	<.01
0	–	.72	–	85	80	–	–	.09	.03	.40	–	–	4	–
17	52	1.38	22	124	280	.45	85	.13	.09	.65	.04	6	<1	1.3
15	19	1.08	19	111	249	.39	75	.11	.1	1.68	.04	9	<1	1.82
0	10	1.56	18	70	242	.32	0	.03	.07	.83	.01	2	0	1.21
6	11	.88	5	32	146	.17	4	.11	.1	1.07	.01	3	0	.98
25	5	.75	4	20	132	.12	85	.1	.07	.83	.01	3	0	.22

(For purposes of calculations, use "0" for t, <1, <.1, <.01, etc.)

Table A–1
Food Composition

Computer Code Number	Food Description	Measure	Wt (g)	H₂O (%)	Ener (cal)	Prot (g)	Carb (g)	Dietary Fiber (g)	Fat (g)	Fat Breakdown (g)		
										Sat	Mono	Poly
	BAKED GOODS: BREADS, CAKES, COOKIES, CRACKERS, PIES—Cont.											
414	Sugar, from refrigerated dough, 2" diam	4 ea	48	5	232	2	31	<1	11	2.8	6.2	1.4
1874	Vanilla sandwich, Snackwell's	2 ea	26	4	109	1	21	1	2	.5	.8	.2
415	Vanilla wafers	10 ea	40	5	176	2	29	8	6	1.4	2.4	1.5
416	Corn chips	1 oz	28	1	151	2	16	1	9	1.3	2.7	4.7
	Crackers:[1]											
1034	Armenian cracker bread	4 pce	28	4	110	3	23	1	.3	<.1	<.1	<.1
417	Cheese	10 ea	10	3	50	1	6	<1	3	.9	.9	.5
418	Cheese with peanut butter	4 ea	30	4	145	4	17	<1	7	1.5	3.6	1.3
	Fat Free:											
2161	Cracked pepper, Snackwell	1 ea	15	2	60	2	13	<1	<1	.1	.1	.2
2159	Wheat, Snackwell	7 ea	15	1	60	2	12	1	<1	.1	.1	.1
2075	Whole wheat, herb seasoned	½ oz	14	5	45	2	9	2	0	0	0	0
2077	Whole wheat, onion	½ oz	14	5	45	2	9	2	0	0	0	0
419	Graham	2 ea	14	4	59	1	11	<1	1	.4	.7	.2
420	Melba toast, plain	1 pce	5	5	19	1	4	<1	<1	<.1	<.1	<.1
1514	Rice cakes, unsalted	2 ea	18	6	69	1	14	<1	1	.2	.2	.2
421	Rye wafer, whole grain	2 ea	14	5	47	1	11	2	<1	<.1	<.1	<.1
422	Saltine®[2]	4 ea	12	4	52	1	9	<1	1	.3	.8	.2
1971	Saltine®, unsalted tops	2 ea	6	–	25	1	4	0	1	0	0	0
423	Snack-type, round like Ritz	3 ea	9	3	45	1	5	<1	2	.4	1	.8
424	Wheat, thin	4 ea	8	3	38	1	5	1	2	.7	.8	.2
425	Whole-wheat wafers	2 ea	8	3	35	1	5	1	1	.2	.8	.2
426	Croissants, 4½ x 4 x 1¾"	1 ea	57	23	231	5	26	1	12	6.7	3.2	.7
1699	Croutons, seasoned	½ c	15	4	70	2	10	<1	3	.8	1.4	.4
	Danish pastry:											
427	Packaged ring, plain, 12 oz	1 ea	340	21	1349	19	181	1	65	13.5	40.8	6.4
428	Round piece, plain, 4¼" diam, 1" high	1 ea	57	21	226	3	30	<1	11	2.3	6.8	1.1
429	Ounce, plain	1 oz	28	21	111	2	15	<1	5	1.1	3.4	.5
430	Round piece with fruit	1 ea	65	29	231	3	31	–	11	2.3	7	1.1
	Desserts, 3 x 3" piece:											
1348	Apple crisp	1 pce	78	61	127	1	25	–	3	.6	1.2	.8
1353	Apple cobbler	1 pce	104	57	199	2	35	1	6	1.3	2.7	1.9
1349	Cherry crisp	1 pce	138	75	158	2	27	1	5	1	2.4	1.7
1352	Cherry cobbler	1 pce	129	66	198	2	34	1	6	1.3	2.7	1.9
1350	Peach crisp	1 pce	139	73	166	1	30	1	5	1	2.3	1.6
1351	Peach cobbler	1 pce	130	65	204	2	36	1	6	1.3	2.7	1.9
	Doughnuts:											
431	Cake type, plain, 3¼" diam	1 ea	50	21	211	3	25	1	11	1.9	4.8	4.1
432	Yeast-leavened, glazed, 3¾" diam	1 ea	60	25	242	4	27	1	14	3.5	7.7	1.7
	English muffins:											
433	Plain, enriched	1 ea	57	42	134	4	26	2	1	.1	.2	.5
434	Toasted	1 ea	50	37	128	4	25	2	1	.1	.2	5
1504	Whole wheat	1 ea	50	46	102	4	20	5	1	.2	.3	.4
2010	Fruit & fitness bar, fat free	1 ea	38	20	110	2	27	1	0	0	0	0
1414	Granola bar, soft	1 ea	42	6	188	3	29	2	7	3.1	1.6	2.3
1415	Granola bar, hard	1 ea	28	4	132	3	18	2	6	.7	1.2	3.4

[1]Crackers made with enriched white (wheat) flour except for rye wafers and whole-wheat wafers.

[2]Made with lard.

(Computer code number is for West Diet Analysis program)

PAGE KEY: A–4 = BEV   A–6 = DAIRY   A–12 = EGGS   A–14 = FAT/OIL   A–18 = FRUIT   A–26 = BAKERY   A–36 = GRAIN   A–44 = FISH   A–48 = MEATS   A–50 = POULTRY   A–54 = SAUSAGE   A–56 = MIXED/FAST   A–64 = NUTS/SEEDS   A–68 = SWEETS   A–70 = VEG/LEG   A–84 = MISC   A–88 = SOUPS/SAUCES   A–90 = FAST   A–106 = FRZN ENTREE   A–112 = BABY FOODS

Chol (mg)	Calc (mg)	Iron (mg)	Magn (mg)	Pota (mg)	Sodi (mg)	Zinc (mg)	VT-A (RE)	Thia (mg)	Ribo (mg)	Niac (mg)	V-B6 (mg)	Fola (µg)	VT-C (mg)	VT-E α-TE (mg)
15	43	.89	4	78	225	.13	5	.09	.06	1.16	.01	3	0	1.54
<1	17	.61	5	28	95	.16	–	.05	.07	.69	.01	–	0	–
23	19	.96	6	39	125	.14	7	.11	.13	1.24	.03	4	0	.54
0	36	.37	21	40	179	.36	3	.01	.04	.33	.07[3]	6[4]	<1	.38
0	5	1.4	7	32	140	.2	0	.19	.13	1.6	.01	5	0	1.11
1	15	.48	4	14	99	.11	9	.06	.04	.47	.05	3	0	.1
2	24	.88	17	73	298	.33	3	.12	.1	1.96	.45	8	0	1.33
<1	26	.73	4	19	148	.14	–	.05	.06	.78	.01	–	<1	–
<1	28	.58	7	43	169	.21	–	.04	.07	.73	.02	–	0	–
0	–	.36	–	70	80	–	–	.06	–	.4	–	–	–	–
0	–	.36	–	70	80	–	–	.06	–	.4	–	–	–	–
0	3	.52	4	19	85	.11	0	.03	.04	.58	.01	2	0	.27
0	5	.19	3	10	41	.1	0	.02	.01	.21	<.01	1	0	.01
0	2	.37	25	52	5	.54	1	0	.03	1.4	.02	4	0	.02
0	6	.83	17	69	111	.39	<1	.06	.04	.22	.04	6	<1	.28
0	14	.65	3	15	156	.09	0	.07	.05	.63	<.01	4	0	.2
0	–	.36	–	5	50	–	–	–	–	–	–	–	–	.1
0	11	.32	2	12	76	.06	0	.03	.03	.36	<.01	1	0	.4
2	3	.25	6[5]	17	69	.24[5]	0	.04	.03	.4	.01	1	0	.31
0	4	.25	8[5]	24	53	.17	0	.02	.01	.36	.01	2	0	.31
43	21	1.16	9	67	424	.43	78	.22	.14	1.25	.03	16	<1	.25
<1	14	.42	6	27	186	.14	1	.08	.06	.7	.01	6	0	.24
105	143	6.94	54	371	1261	1.87	20	.99	.75	8.5	.2	54	10	3.06
18	24	1.16	9	62	211	.31	3	.16	.12	1.43	.03	9	2	.51
9	12	.58	4	31	105	.16	2	.08	.06	.71	.02	5	1	.25
13	15	.97	10	76	230	.33	17	.2	.14	1.24	.04	10	1	.59
0	22	.58	5	76	142	.12	24	.07	.06	.6	.03	4	2	–
1	31	.78	6	87	304	.16	76	.1	.09	.74	.04	3	<1	.99
0	29	2.15	12	164	73	.15	145	.07	.08	.59	.06	10	3	.98
1	37	1.81	10	114	311	.2	135	.1	.11	.85	.05	9	2	1.07
0	23	.95	13	198	69	.2	104	.05	.05	1.03	.03	6	5	2.48
1	33	.91	10	140	308	.23	105	.09	.09	1.18	.03	6	3	2.2
18	22	.98	10	63	273	.27	9	.11	.12	.92	.03	4	<1	1.73
4	26	1.23	13	65	205	.46	6	.22	.13	1.71	.03	13	0	1.75
0	99	1.43	12	75	264	.4	0	.25	.16	2.21	.02	21	<1	.07
0	94	1.37	11	71	252	.38	0	.19	.14	1.9	.02	14	<1	.06
0	133	1.23	35	105	319	.8	0	.15	.07	1.71	.08	24	0	.35
0	–	1.08	–	120	35	–	–	.12	.07	.8	–	–	6	–
<1	45	1.09	31	136	118	.64	0	.12	.07	.22	.04	10	0	3.22
0	17	.84	27	95	83	.58	4	.07	.03	.45	.02	7	<1	2.15

[3]Vitamin B₆ values vary between brands. Check the label.

[4]Values from 1992 USDA data for snacks and sweets.

[5]Values derived from whole-wheat recipes and retention values.

(For purposes of calculations, use "0" for t, <1, <.1, <.01, etc.)

Table A–1
Food Composition

Computer Code Number	Food Description	Measure	Wt (g)	H₂O (%)	Ener (cal)	Prot (g)	Carb (g)	Dietary Fiber (g)	Fat (g)	Fat Breakdown (g)		
										Sat	Mono	Poly
	BAKED GOODS: BREADS, CAKES, COOKIES, CRACKERS, PIES—Cont.											
	Granola bar, fat free:											
1985	Blueberry	1 ea	43	7	140	3	33	3	0	0	0	0
2012	Chocolate chip	1 ea	43	7	140	3	33	3	0	0	0	0
1983	Date almond	1 ea	43	7	140	3	33	3	0	0	0	0
1984	Raisin	1 ea	43	7	140	3	33	3	0	0	0	0
2011	Strawberry	1 ea	43	7	140	3	33	3	0	0	0	0
	Muffins, 2½" diam, 1½" high:											
	From home recipe											
435	Blueberry[1]	1 ea	45	39	131	3	18	7	5	1.1	1.2	2.4
436	Bran, wheat[2]	1 ea	45	35	130	3	19	3	6	1.2	1.4	2.8
437	Cornmeal	1 ea	45	32	144	3	20	2	6	1.2	1.4	2.8
	From commercial mix:											
438	Blueberry	1 ea	45	36	135	2	22	1	4	.7	1.6	1.4
439	Bran, wheat	1 ea	45	35	124	3	21	4	4	1.1	2.1	.6
440	Cornmeal	1 ea	45	30	144	3	22	2	5	1.3	2.4	.6
	Nabisco Newtons, fat free:											
1864	Cranberry	1 ea	23	–	68	1	16	–	0	0	0	0
1867	Fig	1 ea	23	–	68	1	16	–	0	0	0	0
1865	Raspberry	1 ea	23	–	68	1	16	–	0	0	0	0
1868	Strawberry	1 ea	23	–	68	1	16	–	0	0	0	0
	Pancakes, 4" diam:											
441	Buckwheat, from mix w/ egg and milk	1 ea	27	54	56	2	8	1	2	.5	.5	.8
442	Plain, from home recipe	1 ea	27	53	61	2	8	<1	3	.6	.7	1.2
443	Plain, from mix; egg, milk, oil added	1 ea	27	53	52	1	10	<1	1	.1	.2	.2
1468	Pan dulce, sweet roll w/topping	1 ea	79	21	291	5	48	1	9	2	3.9	2.7
	Piecrust, with enriched flour, vegetable shortening, baked:											
444	Home recipe, 9" shell	1 ea	180	10	949	11	85	3	62	15.5	27.4	16.4
	From mix:											
445	For 2-crust pie	1 ea	320	10	1686	20	152	6	111	27.6	48.6	29.2
446	1 pie shell	1 ea	180	11	902	12	91	3	55	13.9	31.1	6.9
	Pies, 9" diam; crust made with vegetable shortening, enriched flour:											
447	Apple:[3] Whole pie	1 ea	945	52	2239	18	321	16	104	19.9	56.1	19.8
448	Piece, ⅙ of pie	1 pce	158	52	374	3	54	3	17	3.3	9.4	3.3
449	Banana cream: Whole pie	1 ea	1188	48	3195	52	391	–	162	44.7	68	39.2
450	Piece, ⅙ of pie	1 pce	198	48	533	9	65	–	27	7.4	11.3	6.5
451	Blueberry:[3] Whole pie	1 ea	945	51	2315	25	317	13	112	27.6	48.4	29.1
452	Piece, ⅙ of pie	1 pce	158	51	387	4	53	2	19	4.6	8.1	4.9
453	Cherry:[3] Whole pie	1 ea	945	46	2551	26	364	14	115	28.3	50.2	30.7
454	Piece, ⅙ of pie	1 pce	158	46	427	4	61	2	19	4.7	8.4	5.1
455	Chocolate cream:[4] Whole pie	1 ea	1194	46	3367	57	372	6	192	62	78	40
456	Piece, ⅙ of pie	1 pce	199	46	561	10	62	1	32	10	13	6.7
457	Custard:[3] Whole pie	1 ea	910	61	1911	50	189	11	106	25.3	52.4	17.5
458	Piece, ⅙ of pie	1 pce	152	61	319	8	32	2	18	4.2	8.8	2.9
459	Lemon meringue:[3] Whole pie	1 ea	840	42	2251	13	396	10	73	13.1	30.5	24.3
460	Piece, ⅙ of pie	1 pce	140	42	375	2	66	2	12	2.2	5.1	4
461	Peach: Whole pie	1 ea	945	45	2603	22	377	13	108	26.4	49	31.8

[1]Made with vegetable shortening.
[2]Made with vegetable oil.
[3]Values from latest USDA data for Baked Goods.
[4]Values based on recipe: pie crust, cooked chocolate pudding, whipped cream topping.

(Computer code number is for West Diet Analysis program)

PAGE KEY: A–4 = BEV   A–6 = DAIRY   A–12 = EGGS   A–14 = FAT/OIL   A–18 = FRUIT   A–26 = BAKERY   A–36 = GRAIN   A–44 = FISH   A–48 = MEATS   A–50 = POULTRY   A–54 = SAUSAGE   A–56 = MIXED/FAST   A–64 = NUTS/SEEDS   A–68 = SWEETS   A–70 = VEG/LEG   A–84 = MISC   A–88 = SOUPS/SAUCES   A–90 = FAST   A–106 = FRZN ENTREE   A–112 = BABY FOODS

Chol (mg)	Calc (mg)	Iron (mg)	Magn (mg)	Pota (mg)	Sodi (mg)	Zinc (mg)	VT-A (RE)	Thia (mg)	Ribo (mg)	Niac (mg)	V-B6 (mg)	Fola (μg)	VT-C (mg)	VT-E α-TE (mg)
0	20	3.6	–	120	10	–	–	.03	.07	.4	–	–	–	–
0	20	3.6	–	120	10	–	–	.03	.07	.4	–	–	–	–
0	20	3.6	–	120	10	–	–	.03	.07	.4	–	–	–	–
0	20	3.6	–	120	10	–	–	.03	.07	.4	–	–	–	–
0	20	3.6	–	120	10	–	–	.03	.07	.4	–	–	–	–
18	85	1.03	7	55	198	.24	13	.12	.13	.99	.02	5	1	.81
16	84	1.89	35	143	265	1.24	108	.15	.2	1.81	.14	23	4	1.04
20	116	1.18	10	65	263	.27	18	.14	.14	1.07	.04	8	<1	.86
21	11	.51	5	35	197	.17	10	.07	.14	1.01	.03	5	<1	.63
31	14	1.14	26	66	210	.52	14	.09	.11	1.29	.08	7	0	.68
28	34	.88	9	59	358	.29	20	.11	.12	.94	.05	5	<1	.68
–	–	–	–	–	76	–	–	–	–	–	–	–	–	–
–	–	–	–	–	76	–	–	–	–	–	–	–	–	–
–	–	–	–	–	76	–	–	–	–	–	–	–	–	–
–	–	–	–	–	76	–	–	–	–	–	–	–	–	–
18	69	.51	15	63	144	.32	18	.05	.07	.36	.04	5	<1	.27
16	59	.49	4	36	119	.15	15	.05	.08	.42	.01	3	<1	.38
3	34	.42	5	47	170	.1	2	.06	.06	.46	.03	2	<1	.11
26	13	1.82	10	57	140	.35	88	.23	.21	1.98	.04	22	<1	1.35
0	18	5.22	25	121	976	.79	0	.7	.5	5.96	.04	20	0	9.94
0	32	9.28	45	214	1734	1.41	0	1.25	.89	10.6	.08	35	0	17.7
0	108	3.89	27	112	1312	.7	0	.54	.33	4.27	.1	22	0	9.94
0	104	4.25	66	614	2513	1.51	284	.26	.25	2.49	.36	38	30	15.6
0	17	.71	11	103	420	.25	47	.04	.04	.42	.06	6	5	2.61
606	891	12.5	190	1960	2851	5.7	832	1.65	2.46	12.5	1.58	131	19	17.5
101	149	2.08	32	327	475	.95	139	.27	.41	2.08	.26	22	3	2.91
0	66	11.7	76	473	1748	1.89	38	1.45	1.25	11.2	.32	47	7	19.8
0	11	1.96	13	79	292	.32	6	.24	.21	1.88	.05	8	1	3.32
0	94	17.6	85	728	1804	1.89	454	1.4	1.18	12.1	.32	66	9	18
0	16	2.94	14	122	302	.32	76	.23	.2	2.02	.05	11	2	3
632	967	15.3	311	1755	2924	7.6	872	1.6	2.4	12	.56	119	6	18.6
105	161	2.04	52	292	487	1.3	145	.27	.4	2	.09	20	1	3.1
300	728	5.28	100	965	2184	4.73	456	.35	1.89	2.66	.44	182	3	10.8
50	122	.88	17	161	365	.79	76	.06	.32	.44	.07	30	<1	1.81
378	470	5.12	126	748	1226	4.12	437	.52	1.76	5.45	.25	67	27	12
63	78	.85	21	125	204	.69	73	.09	.29	.91	.04	11	4	2
17	79	3	68	1132	2660	1.59	187	.28	.5	1	.42	49	11	22.3

(For purposes of calculations, use "0" for t, <1, <.1, <.01, etc.)

Table A–1
Food Composition

Computer Code Number	Food Description	Measure	Wt (g)	H_2O (%)	Ener (cal)	Prot (g)	Carb (g)	Dietary Fiber (g)	Fat (g)	Fat Breakdown (g) Sat	Mono	Poly
	BAKED GOODS: BREADS, CAKES, COOKIES, CRACKERS, PIES—Cont.											
462	Piece, ⅙ of pie	1 pce	158	45	435	4	63	2	18	4.4	8.2	5.3
463	Pecan:[1] Whole pie	1 ea	825	19	3300	33	472	29	153	31	88	24.5
464	Piece, ⅙ of pie	1 pce	138	19	552	6	79	5	25	5.2	14.9	4.1
465	Pumpkin:[1] Whole pie	1 ea	1240	58	2604	48	339	33	118	25	62.1	19.8
466	Piece, ⅙ of pie	1 pce	206	58	433	8	56	6	20	4.2	10.3	3.3
467	Pies, fried, commercial: Apple	1 ea	85	40	266	2	33	2	14	6.5	5.8	1.2
468	Pies, fried, commercial: Cherry	1 ea	85	40	269	3	36	2	14	2	6	4.6
	Pretzels, made with enriched flour:											
469	Thin sticks, 2¼" long	10 ea	3	3	11	<1	2	<1	<1	t	t	t
470	Dutch twists, 2¾ x 2⅝"	1 ea	16	3	61	1	13	<1	1	.1	.2	.2
471	Thin twists, 3¼ x 2¼ x ¼"	10 ea	60	3	229	5	47	2	2	.4	.8	.7
	Rolls & buns, enriched, commercial:											
472	Cloverleaf rolls, 2½" diam, 2" high	1 ea	28	32	85	2	14	1	2	.5	1.1	.3
473	Hot dog buns	1 ea	40	34	114	3	20	1	2	.5	1	.4
474	Hamburger buns	1 ea	45	34	129	4	23	1	2	.5	1.1	.4
475	Hard roll, white, 3¾" diam, 2" high	1 ea	50	31	147	5	26	1	2	.3	.6	.9
476	Submarine rolls/hoagies, 11½ x 3 x 2½"	1 ea	135	31	392	12	75	4	4	.9	1.3	1.4
	Rolls & buns, enriched, home recipe:											
477	Dinner rolls 2½" diam, 2" high	1 ea	35	29	112	3	19	1	3	.7	1.1	.7
	Sports/fitness bar:											
2043	Forza energy bar	1 ea	70	18	231	11	45	4	1	–	–	–
2042	Power bar	1 ea	65	21	225	10	40	3	1	–	–	–
2041	Tiger sports bar	1 ea	65	17	230	11	40	4	2	–	–	–
478	Toaster pastries, fortified (Poptarts)	1 ea	54	12	212	3	38	1	6	.8	2.2	2.1
2132	Toaster strudel pastry—cream cheese	1 ea	53	32	184	3	28	<1	9	2.8	–	–
2134	Toaster strudel pastry—french toast	1 ea	53	31	177	3	27	1	7	2.8	–	–
	Tortilla chips:											
1271	Plain	1 oz	28	7	140	2	18	2	6	2	4.4	1
1036	Nacho flavor	1 oz	28	2	139	2	18	1	7	1.4	4.3	1
1037	Taco flavor	1 oz	28	2	134	2	18	2	7	1.3	4	1
	Tortillas:											
479	Corn, enriched, 6" diam	1 ea	30	44	67	2	14	2	1	.1	.2	.3
480	Flour, 8" diam	1 ea	35	27	115	3	20	1	2	.4	1	1
1301	Flour, 10" diam	1 ea	57	27	185	5	32	1	4	.6	1.6	1.6
481	Taco shells	1 ea	14	4	66	1	9	1	3	.4	1.5	.6
	Waffles, 7" diam:											
482	From home recipe	1 ea	75	42	218	6	25	1	11	2.1	2.6	5.1
483	From mix, egg/milk added	1 ea	75	42	218	5	26	1	10	1.7	2.7	5.2
1510	Whole grain, prepared from frozen	1 ea	39	44	106	4	12	1	5	1.6	1.9	1
	GRAIN PRODUCTS: CEREAL, FLOUR, GRAIN, PASTA and NOODLES, POPCORN											
484	Barley, pearled, dry, uncooked	1 c	200	10	704	20	155	27	2	.5	.3	1.1
485	Barley, pearled, cooked	1 c	157	69	193	4	44	8	1	.1	.1	.3
	Breakfast bars, fat free:											
2009	Apple	1 ea	38	21	110	2	24	3	0	0	0	0
2005	Chocolate	1 ea	38	21	110	2	24	3	0	0	0	0
2003	Strawberry	1 ea	38	21	110	2	24	3	0	0	0	0

(1)Values from latest USDA data for Baked Goods.

(Computer code number is for West Diet Analysis program)

PAGE KEY: A–4 = BEV   A–6 = DAIRY   A–12 = EGGS   A–14 = FAT/OIL   A–18 = FRUIT   A–26 = BAKERY   A–36 = GRAIN   A–44 = FISH
A–48 = MEATS   A–50 = POULTRY   A–54 = SAUSAGE   A–56 = MIXED/FAST   A–64 = NUTS/SEEDS   A–68 = SWEETS   A–70 = VEG/LEG
A–84 = MISC   A–88 = SOUPS/SAUCES   A–90 = FAST   A–106 = FRZN ENTREE   A–112 = BABY FOODS

Chol (mg)	Calc (mg)	Iron (mg)	Magn (mg)	Pota (mg)	Sodi (mg)	Zinc (mg)	VT-A (RE)	Thia (mg)	Ribo (mg)	Niac (mg)	V-B6 (mg)	Fola (μg)	VT-C (mg)	VT-E α-TE (mg)
3	13	.57	11	789	445	.27	31	.05	.09	.2	.07	8	2	3.73
264	140	8.66	149	611	3498	4.7	388	.75	1.01	2.05	.17	49	9	20.9
44	23	1.45	25	102	585	.79	65	.13	.17	.34	.03	8	2	3.49
248	744	9.8	186	1909	3496	5.58	5951[2]	.68	1.9	2.32	.71	186	19	20
41	124	1.63	31	317	581	.93	989[2]	.11	.31	.38	.12	31	3	3.32
13	13	.88	8	51	325	.17	8	.1	.08	.98	.03	4	2	.37
13	19	.88	9	55	318	.17	15	.1	.08	.98	.03	3	1	.37
0	1	.13	1	4	51	.03	0	.01	.02	.16	<.01	2	0	.01
0	6	.69	6	23	274	.14	0	.07	.1	.84	.02	13	0	.03
0	22	2.59	21	88	1029	.51	0	.28	.37	3.15	.07	50	0	.13
<1	34	.89	6	38	148	.22	0	.14	.09	1.14	.01	8	<1	.22
0	56	1.27	8	56	224	.25	0	.19	.12	1.57	.02	11	0	.19
0	63	1.43	9	63	252	.28	0	.22	.14	1.77	.02	12	0	.21
0	47	1.65	14	54	272	.47	0	.24	.17	2.12	.03	8	0	.09
0	122	3.78	27	122	783	.85	0	.54	.33	4.47	.05	41	0	.1
13	21	1.04	7	53	145	.24	28	.14	.14	1.21	.02	15	<1	.35
0	300	6.3	160	220	65	5.25	–	1.5	1.7	20	2	400	60	20
–	300	5.4	140	120	20	5.25	–	1.5	1.7	20	2	400	60	–
–	350	4.5	140	280	100	–	50	1.5	1.7	20	2	400	60	20
0	14	1.89	10	60	226	.36	57[3]	.16	.2	2.13	.21	43	<1	1
12	12	.95	–	–	–	–	17	–	–	–	–	–	0	.99
6	6	.84	–	–	191	–	2	–	–	–	–	–	0	.99
0	0	0	25	65	135	.43	0	.02	.05	.36	.08	3	0	.38
1	42	.4	23	61	198	.34	12	.04	.05	.4	.08	4	1	.38
1	44	.57	25	61	221	.36	25	.07	.06	.57	.08	6	<1	.38
0	52	.42	19	46	48	.28	8	.03	.02	.45	.07	5	0	.05
0	44	1.17	9	46	169	.25	0	.19	.1	1.26	.02	4	0	.45
0	71	1.88	15	74	272	.4	0	.3	.17	2.03	.03	7	0	.72
0	22	.35	15	25	51	.18	5	.04	.02	.23	.04	1	0	.59
52	191	1.74	14	119	383	.51	49	.2	.26	1.55	.04	11	<1	1.73
52	91	1.23	14	119	383	.5	49	.15	.3	1.55	.04	11	<1	1.5
39	84	.7	15	91	150	.41	25	.08	.12	.75	.05	7	<1	.53
0	58	5	158	560	18	4.26	4	.38	.23	9.22	.52	46	0	.26
0	17	2.09	34	146	5	1.29	2	.13	.1	3.23	.18	25	0	.08
0	20	.72	–	160	65	–	–	.09	.03	.4	–	–	2	–
0	20	.72	–	160	65	–	–	.09	.03	.4	–	–	2	–
0	20	.72	–	160	65	–	–	.09	.03	.4	–	–	2	–

[2] Latest USDA values of vitamin A for canned pumpkin are almost 3.5 times greater than previously published values. Canned pumpkin is usually a blend of pumpkin and winter squash.
[3] Vitamin A values from label declarations vary.

(For purposes of calculations, use "0" for t, <1, <.1, <.01, etc.)

Table A–1
Food Composition

Computer Code Number	Food Description	Measure	Wt (g)	H$_2$O (%)	Ener (cal)	Prot (g)	Carb (g)	Dietary Fiber (g)	Fat (g)	Fat Breakdown (g)		
										Sat	Mono	Poly
	GRAIN PRODUCTS: CEREAL, FLOUR, GRAIN, PASTA and NOODLES, POPCORN—Cont.											
	Breakfast bar, Snackwell											
2165	Apple-cinnamon	1 ea	37	16	119	1	29	1	0	0.1	<.1	.1
2164	Blueberry	1 ea	37	16	121	1	29	1	0	0.1	<.1	.1
2163	Strawberry	1 ea	37	16	120	1	29	1	0	<.1	<.1	.1
	Breakfast cereals, hot, cooked:											
	Corn grits (hominy) enriched:											
486	Regular and quick, prepared, yellow	1 c	242	85	145	3	31	5	<1	.1	.1	.2
487	Instant, prepared from packet, white	1 ea	137	85	82	2	18	<1	<1	t	t	<.1
	Cream of wheat:											
488	Regular, quick, instant	1 c	244	87	131	4	27	1	<1	.1	.1	.2
489	Mix and eat, plain, packet	1 ea	142	82	102	3	21	<1	<1	t	t	.1
1664	Farina cereal, cooked	½ c	117	87	58	2	12	2	<1	t	t	t
490	Malt-O-Meal	1 c	240	88	122	4	26	1	<1	t	t	.1
494	Maypo	1 c	242	83	172	6	32	6	2	.4	.8	.1
	Oatmeal or rolled oats:											
491	Regular, quick, instant, nonfort	1 c	234	85	145	6	25	4	2	.4	.7	.9
	Instant, fortified:											
492	Plain, from packet	¾ c	177	85	104	4	18	3	2	.3	.6	.7
493	Flavored, from packet	¾ c	164	76	167	4	33	2	2	.3	.6	.7
	Breakfast cereals, ready to eat:											
495	All-Bran	⅓ c	28	3	70	4	21	10	1	.1	.1	.3
1306	Alpha Bits	1 c	28	1	109	2	24	1	1	.1	.2	.3
1307	Apple Jacks	1 c	28	2	109	2	25	1	<1	t	t	t
1308	Bran Buds	1 c	84	3	217	12	64	31	2	.4	.3	1.1
1305	Bran Chex	1 c	49	2	156	5	39	8	1	.2	.2	.8
1309	Honey BucWheat Crisp	¾ c	28	5	109	3	23	2	1	.2	.2	.4
1310	C. W. Post, plain	1 c	97	2	432	9	70	7	15	11.3	1.7	1.4
1311	C. W. Post, with raisins	1 c	103	4	446	9	74	14	15	11	1.7	1.4
496	Cap'n Crunch	1 c	37	2	156	2	30	1	3	2.2	.4	.5
1312	Cap'n Crunchberries	1 c	38	3	160	2	31	1	3	2.1	.4	.5
1313	Cap'n Crunch, peanut butter	1 c	38	2	167	3	29	<1	5	2.1	1.5	1.1
497	Cheerios	1 c	23	5	90	3	16	2	1	.3	.5	.6
1314	Cocoa Krispies	1 c	36	2	139	2	32	<1	1	.1	.1	.2
1316	Cocoa Pebbles	1 c	31	2	127	1	27	<1	2	t	t	t
1315	Corn Bran	1 c	36	2	125	2	30	7	1	.2	.3	.7
1317	Corn Chex	1 c	28	2	110	2	25	<1	1	.1	.2	.6
498	Corn Flakes, Kellogg's	1¼ c	28	3	109	2	24	1	<1	t	t	t
499	Corn Flakes, Post Toasties	1¼ c	28	3	108	2	24	1	<1	t	t	t
1340	Corn Pops	1 c	28	3	107	1	25	<1	<1	t	t	.1
1318	Cracklin' Oat Bran	1 c	60	4	229	6	41	10	9	2.1	2.3	3.5
1038	Crispy Wheat `N Raisins	1 c	43	7	150	3	35	3	1	.1	.1	.4
1319	Fortified Oat Flakes	1 c	48	3	177	9	35	1	1	.1	.3	.3
500	40% Bran Flakes, Kellogg's	1 c	39	3	127	5	31	6	1	.1	.1	.4
501	40% Bran Flakes, Post	1 c	47	3	152	5	37	9	1	.2	.2	.3
502	Froot Loops	1 c	28	3	111	2	25	1	1	.2	.1	.1
518	Frosted Flakes	1 c	35	3	133	2	32	1	<1	t	t	t
1320	Frosted Mini-Wheats	4 ea	31	5	111	3	26	2	<1	.1	t	.2
1321	Frosted Rice Krispies	1 c	28	3	108	1	26	<1	<1	t	t	t
1324	Fruit & Fibre w/dates	½ c	28	9	95	2	21	4	1	.2	.6	.5
1325	Fruitful Bran	¾ c	34	1	144	3	37	6	<1	.1	.1	.2

(Computer code number is for West Diet Analysis program)

PAGE KEY: A–4 = BEV   A–6 = DAIRY   A–12 = EGGS   A–14 = FAT/OIL   A–18 = FRUIT   A–26 = BAKERY   A–36 = GRAIN   A–44 = FISH   A–48 = MEATS   A–50 = POULTRY   A–54 = SAUSAGE   A–56 = MIXED/FAST   A–64 = NUTS/SEEDS   A–68 = SWEETS   A–70 = VEG/LEG   A–84 = MISC   A–88 = SOUPS/SAUCES   A–90 = FAST   A–106 = FRZN ENTREE   A–112 = BABY FOODS

Chol (mg)	Calc (mg)	Iron (mg)	Magn (mg)	Pota (mg)	Sodi (mg)	Zinc (mg)	VT-A (RE)	Thia (mg)	Ribo (mg)	Niac (mg)	V-B6 (mg)	Fola (µg)	VT-C (mg)	VT-E α-TE (mg)
<1	17	5	6	68	103	3.88	–	.39	.44	5.2	.52	–	<1	–
<1	14	4.83	5	44	107	3.85	–	.39	.44	5.2	.52	–	<1	–
<1	14	4.82	6	47	102	3.83	–	.39	.44	5.2	.52	–	2	–
0	0	1.55[1]	10	53	0[2]	.17	14[3]	.24[1]	.14[1]	1.96[1]	.06	2	0	.12
0	7	1.01[1]	5	29	343	.08	0	.18[1]	.08[1]	1.3[1]	.03	1	0	.03
0	51[1]	10.5[1]	12	46	141[4]	.34	0	.24[1]	0[1]	1.46[1]	.03	10	0	.03
0	20[1]	8.09[1]	7	38	241	.24	376[1]	.43[1]	.28[1]	4.97[1]	.57	101	0	.02
0	2	.58	2	15	0[5]	.08	0	.09	.06	.64	.01	2	0	.02
0	5	9.6[1]	5	31	2[5]	.17	0	.48[1]	.24[1]	5.76[1]	.02	5	0	.03
0	126	8.47	51	213	9.7	1.5	709	.73	.73	9.44	.97	10	29	.24
0	19	1.59	56	131	2[5]	1.15	4	.26	.05	.3	.05	9	0	.23
0	162[1]	6.3[1]	42	99	283[1]	.87	453[1]	.53[1]	.28[1]	5.47[1]	.74	150	0	.21
0	172[1]	7[1]	38	156	235[1]	1	458[1]	.53[1]	.38[1]	5.9[1]	.76	156	0	.21
0	23	4.52[1]	105	345	315	3.75	371[1]	.37[1]	.43[1]	5[1]	.51	100	15[1]	.52
0	8	2.7	17	108	177	1.51	371	.37	.43	5	.51	100	0	.02
0	3	4.52	6	23	124	3.75	370	.37	.43	5	.51	100	15	.05
0	56	13.4	267	1403	515	11.1	1111	1.09	1.26	14.8	1.51	296	44	1.33
0	29	7.79	125	393	454	2.14	11	.64	.26	8.62	.88	172	26	.56
0	40	8.12	32	106	266	.51	673	.68	.77	9	1.4	9	27	6.62
<1	47	15.4	67	197	166	1.64	1283	1.26	1.46	17.1	1.75	342	0	.68
<1	50	16.4	74	260	160	1.64	1362	1.34	1.55	18.1	1.85	363	0	.72
0	6	9.81[1]	15	48	278	4	5[1]	.66[1]	.71[1]	8.62[1]	1	238	0	.18
<1	12	9.8	15	54	265	3.88	5	.65	.74	8.92	1.02	140	0	.27
0	8	10	20	62	291	4.15	6	.66	.77	9.73	1.14	265	0	.21
0	39	3.66[1]	32	82	249	.64	304[1]	.3[1]	.34[1]	4.05[1]	.41	5	12[1]	.16
<1	6	2.27	12	53	275	1.91	476	.47	.54	6.34	.65	127	19	.17
0	5	1.97	13	52	148	1.66	411	.41	.47	5.52	.56	109	0	.04
0	41	12.2	18	70	310	4	8	.37	.7	10.9	.86	232	0	.19
0	3	1.8	4	23	268	.1	14	.37	.07	5	.51	100	15	.07
0	1	1.8[1]	3	26	286	.08	370[1]	.36[1]	.42[1]	4.93[1]	.5	99	15[1]	.04
0	1	.74[1]	4	32	293	.08	370[1]	.36[1]	.42[1]	4.93[1]	.5	99	0	.07
0	1	1.8	2	17	103	1.51	370	.37	.43	5	.51	100	15	.03
0	40	3.78	116	355	487	3.18	794	.78	.9	10.6	1.08	212	32	.4
0	71	6.84	34	173	204	.51	569	.56	.64	7.57	.77	15	0	.45
0	68	13.7	58	343	429	1.5	635	.62	.72	8.45	.86	169	0	.34
0	19	24.8[1]	71	247	302	5.15	516[1]	.51[1]	.58[1]	6.86[1]	.7	137	0	7.22
0	21	7.47[1]	101	250	430	2.49	622[1]	.61[1]	.7[1]	8.27[1]	.85	165	0	.54
0	3	4.52[1]	7	26	144	3.75	370[1]	.37[1]	.43[1]	5[1]	.51	100	15[1]	.1
0	1	2.21[1]	3	22	283	.05	463[1]	.45[1]	.52[1]	6.16[1]	.63	123	19[1]	.05
0	10	1.95	25	105	9	1.64	410	.4	.46	5.46	.56	109	16	.28
0	1	1.79	5	21	237	.31	370	.37	.43	5	.51	100	15	.03
0	15	5	40	167	132	1.51	356	.37	.43	5	.5	100	0	.65
0	23	5	67	276	264	1.3	270	.46	.43	6	.5	100	<1	.79

(1)Nutrient added (values sometimes based on label declaration).
(2)Cooked without salt. If salt is added according to label recommendation, sodium content is 540 mg.
(3)Value for yellow corn grits; cooked white corn grits contain 0 RE of vitamin A.
(4)Values for quick cereal.
(5)Cooked without salt. If added according to label recommendations, sodium content is 390 mg for Cream of Wheat; 324 mg for Malt-O-Meal; 374 mg for oatmeal; 385 mg for Farina.

(For purposes of calculations, use "0" for t, <1, <.1, <.01, etc.)

Table A–1
Food Composition

Computer Code Number	Food Description	Measure	Wt (g)	H₂O (%)	Ener (cal)	Prot (g)	Carb (g)	Dietary Fiber (g)	Fat (g)	Fat Breakdown (g)		
										Sat	Mono	Poly
	GRAIN PRODUCTS: CEREAL, FLOUR, GRAIN, PASTA and NOODLES, POPCORN—Cont.											
	Breakfast cereals, ready to eat—Cont.											
1322	Fruity Pebbles	1 c	32	3	131	1	28	1	2	.4	.3	.4
503	Golden Grahams	1 c	39	2	150	2	33	1	1	1	.1	.2
504	Granola, homemade	½ c	61	3	297	8	34	6	17	2.9	4.7	8.6
1670	Granola, low fat, commercial	½ c	47	3	179	4	36	3	3	0	–	–
505	Grape Nuts	½ c	57	3	203	7	47	6	<1	t	t	.2
1326	Grape Nuts Flakes	1 c	32	3	116	3	26	3	<1	.1	t	.1
1665	Heartland Natural with raisins	1 c	101	5	430	10	70	6	14	–	–	–
1327	Honey & Nut Corn Flakes	1 c	38	4	151	2	31	1	2	.3	.7	1
506	Honey Nut Cheerios	1 c	33	3	126	4	27	1	1	.1	.3	.3
1328	HoneyBran	1 c	35	2	119	3	29	4	1	.1	.1	.4
1329	HoneyComb	1 c	22	1	86	1	20	<1	<1	.1	.1	.2
1330	King Vitaman	1 c	19	2	77	1	16	1	1	.7	.1	.2
1039	Kix	1 c	19	3	74	2	16	<1	<1	.1	.1	.2
1331	Life	1 c	43	5	158	8	31	3	1	.1	.2	.4
507	Lucky Charms	1 c	32	3	125	3	26	1	1	.2	.4	.5
1323	Mueslix Five Grain	1 c	82	5	279	7	63	7	3	.5	1	1.2
1416	Granola, low-fat	⅓ c	31	3	119	3	25	2	2	0	–	–
	Health Valley Granola, fat-free:											
2081	Date & almond	1 oz	28	7	90	2	21	3	0	0	0	0
2080	Raisin cinnamon	1 oz	28	7	90	2	21	3	0	0	0	0
2082	Tropical fruit	1 oz	28	7	90	2	21	3	0	0	0	0
508	Nature Valley Granola	1 c	113	4	502	12	75	6	20	13	2.9	2.8
1666	Nutri Grain Almond Raisin	⅔ c	40	9	140	3	31	3	2	0	–	–
1333	Nutri-Grain—corn	1 c	42	3	160	3	35	3	1	.1	.2	.6
1335	Nutri-Grain—wheat	1 c	44	3	158	4	37	3	<1	.1	.1	.3
1336	100% Bran	1 c	66	3	177	8	48	20	3	.6	.6	1.9
509	100% Natural cereal, plain	½ c	57	2	267	7	36	5	12	8.2	2.3	1.1
1337	100% Natural with apples & cinnamon	1 c	104	2	478	11	70	7	20	15.4	1.8	1.3
1338	100% Natural with raisins & dates	1 c	110	3	496	11	72	7	20	13.6	3.7	1.7
510	Product 19	1 c	33	3	125	3	27	1	<1	t	t	.1
1339	Quisp	1 c	30	2	124	2	25	<1	2	1.5	.3	.3
511	Raisin Bran, Kellogg's	1 c	49	8	152	5	37	5	1	.2	.1	.4
512	Raisin Bran, Post	1 c	56	9	171	5	42	8	1	.2	.2	.4
1667	Raisin Squares	½ c	28	8	90	2	23	2	0	0	0	0
1041	Rice Chex	¾ c	19	3	75	1	17	<1	1	.2	.2	.3
513	Rice Krispies, Kellogg's	1 c	29	2	114	2	25	<1	<1	t	t	.1
514	Rice, puffed	1 c	14	3	56	1	13	<1	<1	t	t	t
515	Shredded Wheat	1 c	43	5	155	5	34	4	1	.2	.2	.5
516	Special K	1 c	21	2	83	4	16	1	<1	t	t	t
517	Super Golden Crisp	1 c	33	1	123	2	30	1	<1	t	t	.1
519	Honey Smacks	1 c	38	3	142	3	33	<1	1	.1	.1	.3
1341	Tasteeos	1 c	24	2	94	3	19	3	1	.2	.2	.3
1342	Team	1 c	42	4	164	3	36	<1	1	.2	.2	.3
520	Total, wheat, with added calcium	1 c	33	4	116	3	26	4	1	.1	.1	.3
521	Trix	1 c	28	2	109	2	25	<1	<1	.2	.1	.1
1344	Wheat Chex	1 c	46	2	168	5	38	4	1	.2	.2	.6

(Computer code number is for West Diet Analysis program)

Chol (mg)	Calc (mg)	Iron (mg)	Magn (mg)	Pota (mg)	Sodi (mg)	Zinc (mg)	VT-A (RE)	Thia (mg)	Ribo (mg)	Niac (mg)	V-B6 (mg)	Fola (μg)	VT-C (mg)	VT-E α-TE (mg)
0	4	2.04	9	25	178	1.73	424	.42	.49	5.6	.58	114	0	.03
<1	24	6.21[1]	16	86	386	.34	517[1]	.51[1]	.59[1]	6.87[1]	.7	6	21[1]	.29
0	38	2.42	71	306	6	2.23	2	.37	.15	1.07	.21	49	1	7.87
0	19	7	38	136	47	5.66	329	.55	.64	7.55	.76	146	–	7.26
0	5	2.47[1]	38	190	396	1.25	755[1]	.74[1]	.85[1]	9.98[1]	1.03	201	0	.14
0	13	9.28	36	113	181	.65	423	.42	.49	5.71	.58	114	0	.08
0	61	3.7	130	382	207	2.61	6	.29	.13	1.43	.18	41	1	.71
0	5	2.39	8	48	302	.14	503	.49	.57	6.67	.68	133	20	.1
0	23	5.3[1]	39	116	299	.87	437[1]	.43[1]	.5[1]	5.87[1]	.6	22	18[1]	.34
0	16	5.57	46	150	202	.9	463	.45	.52	6.16	.63	23	19	.81
0	4	2.09	7	70	123	1.17	291	.29	.33	3.87	.4	78	0	.09
0	2	11.4	6	23	145	.15	644	.83	.95	11.6	1.06	259	30	1.29
0	24	5.44	8	30	194	.16	252	.25	.28	3.35	.34	67	10	.05
0	150	11.3	14	192	224	1.42	9	.93	.97	11.3	.08	36	0	.22
0	36	5.09[1]	27	66	227	.56	424[1]	.42[1]	.48[1]	5.63[1]	.58	6	17[1]	.14
0	38	8.94	82	369	107	7.46	747	.75	.84	9.84	.99	197	1	8.94
0	–	1.8	24	95	60	3.74	150	.37	.42	4.99	.5	100	–	4.99
0	–	.36	–	85	35	–	–	.06	–	.4	–	–	–	–
0	–	.36	–	85	35	–	–	.06	–	.4	–	–	–	–
0	–	.36	–	85	35	–	–	.06	–	.4	–	–	–	–
0	71	3.77	115	388	232	2.19	7	.4	.19	.82	.09	85	0	7.97
0	16	.8	11	130	220	3.75	–	.38	.43	5	.5	100	–	–
0	1	.89	27	98	276	5.54	556	.55	.63	7.39	.76	148	22	11.1
0	12	1.24	34	119	299	5.81	583	.57	.66	7.74	.79	155	23	11.6
0	46	8.12	312	824	457	5.74	0	1.58	1.78	20.9	2.11	47	63	1.53
<1	99	1.68	68	281	24	1.28	3	.17	.31	1.3	.1	17	0	.65
1	157	2.9	72	515	52	2	6	.33	.57	1.88	.11	17	1	.73
1	159	3.12	124	537	47	2.11	6	.31	.65	2.09	.16	45	0	.77
0	4	21[1]	12	51	378	.49	1746[1]	1.75[1]	1.98[1]	23.3[1]	2.34	465	70[1]	24.4
0	9	6.33	12	45	240	.18	5	.54	.76	5.79	.91	8	0	.16
0	17	22.2[1]	63	254	271	5	498[1]	.49[1]	.59[1]	6.66[1]	.69	132	0	.45
0	26	8.9[1]	95	344	365	2.97	741[1]	.73[1]	.84[1]	9.86[1]	1.01	197	0	1.3
0	10	8.1	26	110	0	1.5	0	.38	.43	5	.5	100	–	.61
0	3	1.2	5	22	158	.26	1	.25	.01	3.34	.34	67	10	.03
0	5	1.83[1]	12	28	213	.49	0[1]	.12[1]	.03[1]	.2[1]	.05	3	15[1]	.03
0	1	.15[1]	4	16	<1	.14	0	.01[1]	.01[1]	.42[1]	.01	3	0	.01
0	16	1.8	57	156	4	1.41	0	.11	.12	2.24	.11	21	0	.23
<1	6	3.39[1]	12	37	196	2.82	275[1]	.28[1]	.32[1]	3.75[1]	.38	75	11[1]	.05
0	7	2.08[1]	20	123	29	1.75	437[1]	.43[1]	.49[1]	5.81[1]	.59	116	0	.12
0	4	2.39[1]	18	56	100	.38	503[1]	.49[1]	.57[1]	6.67[1]	.68	133	20[1]	.2
0	11	3.82	26	71	182	.69	318	.31	.36	4.22	.43	9	13	.17
0	6	2.57	19	71	259	.58	556	.55	.63	7.39	.76	7	22	.1
0	282	21[1]	37	123	326	.78	1746[1]	1.75[1]	1.98[1]	23.3[1]	2.34	465	70[1]	25.8
0	6	4.52[1]	6	27	179	.13	371[1]	.37[1]	.43[1]	5[1]	.51	3	15[1]	.56
0	18	7.31	58	173	308	1.23	0	.6	.17	8.1	.83	162	24	.17

[1]Nutrient added (values sometimes based on label declaration).

(For purposes of calculations, use "0" for t, <1, <.1, <.01, etc.)

Table A–1
Food Composition

Computer Code Number	Food Description	Measure	Wt (g)	H$_2$O (%)	Ener (cal)	Prot (g)	Carb (g)	Dietary Fiber (g)	Fat (g)	Fat Breakdown (g)		
										Sat	Mono	Poly
	GRAIN PRODUCTS: CEREAL, FLOUR, GRAIN, PASTA and NOODLES, POPCORN—Cont.											
1043	Wheat cereal, puffed, fortified	1 c	12	3	44	2	10	1	<1	t	t	.1
522	Wheaties	1 c	29	5	101	3	23	3	<1	.1	t	.2
	Buckwheat flour:											
523	Dark	1 c	98	11	328	12	69	8	3	.7	.9	.9
524	Light	1 c	98	12	340	6	78	6	1	.2	.4	.4
525	Buckwheat, whole grain, dry	1 c	175	10	600	23	125	18	6	1.3	1.8	1.8
526	Bulgar, dry, uncooked	1 c	140	9	479	17	106	26	2	.3	.2	.8
527	Bulgar, cooked	1 c	182	78	151	6	34	8	<1	<.1	<.1	.2
	Cornmeal:											
528	Whole-ground, unbolted, dry	1 c	122	10	442	10	94	9	4	.6	1.2	2
529	Bolted, nearly whole, dry	1 c	122	10	441	10	94	12	4	.6	1.2	2
530	Degermed, enriched, dry	1 c	138	12	505	12	107	10	2	.3	.6	1
531	Degermed, enriched, cooked	1 c	240	78	209	5	44	4	1	.1	.2	.4
	Macaroni, cooked:											
532	Enriched	1 c	140	66	197	7	40	2	1	.1	.1	.4
533	Whole wheat	1 c	140	67	174	7	37	5	1	.1	.1	.3
534	Vegetable, enriched	1 c	134	68	172	6	36	6	<1	t	t	.1
535	Millet, cooked	½ c	120	71	143	4	28	2	1	.2	.2	.6
	Noodles (see also Pasta and Spaghetti)											
1507	Cellophane noodles, cooked	1 c	190	79	160	<1	39	<1	<1	t	t	t
1995	Cellophane noodles, dry	½ c	70	13	246	<1	60	<1	<1	<.1	<.1	<.1
537	Chow mein, dry	1 c	45	1	237	4	26	2	14	2	3.5	7.8
536	Egg noodles, cooked, enriched	1 c	160	69	213	8	40	2	2	.5	.7	.7
538	Spinach noodles, dry	3½ oz	100	8	372	13	75	11	2	.2	.2	.6
1343	Oat bran, dry	¼ c	23	7	57	4	16	4	2	.3	.6	.7
	Pasta, cooked:											
1418	Fresh	2 oz	57	69	74	3	14	1	1	.1	.1	.2
1417	Linguini	1 c	140	66	197	7	40	2	1	.1	.1	.4
1598	Rotini	1 c	140	66	197	7	40	2	1	.1	.1	.4
	Popcorn:											
539	Air popped, plain	1 c	8	4	31	1	6	1	<1	<.1	.1	.2
1042	Microwaved, low fat, low sodium	1 c	6	3	24	1	4	1	1	.1	.2	.3
540	Popped in vegetable oil/salted	1 c	11	2	55	1	6	1	3	.5	.9	1.5
541	Sugar-syrup coated	1 c	35	2	151	1	28	2	4	1.3	1	1.6
	Rice:											
542	Brown rice, cooked	1 c	195	73	216	5	45	4	2	.4	.6	.6
2215	Mexican rice, cooked	½ c	113	–	410	8	90	3	15	2	.1	.1
2216	Spanish rice, cooked	½ c	123	85	65	2	14	1	1	–	–	–
	White, enriched, all types:											
543	Regular/long grain, dry	1 c	185	11	675	13	148	2	1	.3	.4	.3
544	Regular/long grain, cooked	1 c	205	68	267	6	58	1	<1	.2	.2	.2
545	Instant, prepared without salt	1 c	165	76	161	3	35	1	<1	.1	.1	.1

(Computer code number is for West Diet Analysis program)

PAGE KEY: A–4 = BEV   A–6 = DAIRY   A–12 = EGGS   A–14 = FAT/OIL   A–18 = FRUIT   A–26 = BAKERY   A–36 = GRAIN   A–44 = FISH   A–48 = MEATS   A–50 = POULTRY   A–54 = SAUSAGE   A–56 = MIXED/FAST   A–64 = NUTS/SEEDS   A–68 = SWEETS   A–70 = VEG/LEG   A–84 = MISC   A–88 = SOUPS/SAUCES   A–90 = FAST   A–106 = FRZN ENTREE   A–112 = BABY FOODS

Chol (mg)	Calc (mg)	Iron (mg)	Magn (mg)	Pota (mg)	Sodi (mg)	Zinc (mg)	VT-A (RE)	Thia (mg)	Ribo (mg)	Niac (mg)	V-B6 (mg)	Fola (μg)	VT-C (mg)	VT-E α-TE (mg)
0	3	.57	17	42	<1	.28	0	.02	.03	1.3	.02	4	0	.08
0	44	4.61[1]	32	108	276	.65	384[1]	.38[1]	.43[1]	5.1[1]	.52	102	15[1]	.36
0	40	3.98	246	565	11	3.06	0	.41	.19	6.03	.57	53	0	1.01
0	11	1	47	314	1	2.56	0	.09	.05	.47	.09	100	0	.5
0	32	3.85	405	805	2	4.2	0	.18	.74	12.3	.37	52	0	1.8
0	49	3.44	230	574	24	2.7	0	.32	.16	7.15	.48	38	0	.224
0	18	1.75	58	123	9	1.04	0	.1	.05	1.82	.15	33	0	.053
0	7	4.21	155	350	43	2.22	57	.47	.24	4.43	.37	31	0	.82
0	7	4.21	154	350	43	2.22	57	.37	.1	2.3	.37	31	0	.96
0	7	5.7	55	224	4	.99	57	.99	.56	6.96	.35	66	0	.46
0	3	2.35	22	91	1	.41	23	.3	.21	2.42	.12	22	0	.21
0	10	1.96	25	43	1	.74	0	.29	.14	2.34	.05	10	0	.04
0	21	1.48	42	62	4	1.13	0	.15	.06	.99	.11	7	0	.14
0	15	.66	26	41	8	.59	7	.15	.08	1.43	.03	8	0	.05
0	4	.76	53	74	2	1.09	0	.13	.1	1.6	.13	23	0	.22
0	14	1	3	5	9	.23	0	.07	0	.09	.02	1	0	.06
0	18	1.53	2	7	7	.29	0	.11	0	.14	.04	1	0	.09
0	18	1.53	2	7	7	.29	0	.11	0	.14	.04	1	0	.07
53	19	2.54	30	45	11	.99	10	.3	.13	2.38	.06	11	0	.08
0	58	2.13	174	376	36	2.76	46	.37	.2	4.55	.32	48	0	.04
0	13	1.27	55	130	1	.73	0	.27	.05	.22	.04	12	0	.39
19	3	.65	10	14	3	.32	3	.12	.09	.56	.02	4	0	.06
0	10	1.96	25	43	1	.74	0	.29	.14	2.34	.05	10	0	.08
0	10	1.96	25	43	1	.74	0	.29	.14	2.34	.05	10	0	.04
0	1	.21	11	24	<1	.27	2	.02	.02	.15	.02	2	0	.01
0	1	.13	9	14	28	.22	1	.02	.01	.12	.01	1	0	.06
0	1	.31	12	25	97	.29	2	.01	.01	.17	.02	2	<1	.01
2	15	.61	12	38	72	.2	4	.02	.02	.77	.01	1	0	.42
0	19	.82	84	84	10	1.23	0	.19	.05	2.98	.28	8	0	1.4
0	150	4.5	–	–	1350	–	–	–	–	–	–	–	48	–
0	–	.36	–	–	670	–	–	–	–	–	–	–	–	–
0	52	8	46	213	9	2.02	0	1.07	.09	7.75	.3	15	0	.24
0	20	2.48	25	72	2	1	0	.33	.03	3.03	.19	6	0	.1
0	13	1.04	8	7	5[2]	.4	0	.12	.08	1.45	.02	7	0	.08

[1]Nutrient added (values sometimes based on label declaration).

[2]If prepared with salt according to label recommendation, sodium would be 608 mg.

(Computer code number is for West Diet Analysis program)

Table A–1
Food Composition

Computer Code Number	Food Description	Measure	Wt (g)	H$_2$O (%)	Ener (cal)	Prot (g)	Carb (g)	Dietary Fiber (g)	Fat (g)	Fat Breakdown (g)		
										Sat	Mono	Poly
	GRAIN PRODUCTS: CEREAL, FLOUR, GRAIN, PASTA and NOODLES, POPCORN—Cont.											
	Parboiled/converted rice:											
546	Raw, dry	1 c	185	10	686	13	151	3	1	.3	.3	.3
547	Cooked	1 c	175	73	200	4	43	1	<1	.1	.1	.1
1486	Sticky rice (glutinous), cooked	1 c	241	76	234	5	51	2	<1	.1	.2	.2
548	Wild rice, cooked	1 c	164	73	166	7	35	2	1	.1	.1	.4
1700	Rice and pasta (Rice-a-Roni), cooked	½ c	109	71	133	3	23	4	3	.6	1.2	1
549	Rye flour, medium	1 c	102	10	361	10	79	15	2	.2	.2	.8
1044	Soy flour, low-fat	1 c	88	2	324	45	30	1	6	.9	1.3	3.3
	Spaghetti pasta:											
550	Without salt, enriched	1 c	140	66	197	7	40	2	1	.1	.1	.4
551	With salt, enriched	1 c	140	66	197	7	40	2	1	.1	.1	.4
552	Whole-wheat spaghetti, cooked	1 c	140	67	174	7	37	6	1	.1	.1	.3
1302	Tapioca, pearl, dry	1 c	152	11	518	<1	134	2	<1	.01	.01	.01
553	Wheat bran, crude	½ c	30	10	65	5	19	13	1	.2	.2	.7
554	Wheat germ, raw	1 c	100	11	360	23	52	15	10	1.7	1.4	6
555	Wheat germ, toasted	1 c	113	5	432	33	56	16	12	2.1	1.7	7.5
1669	Wheat germ, with brown sugar & honey	½ c	57	5	215	12	35	3	5	.8	.7	2.8
556	Rolled wheat, cooked	1 c	240	83	149	5	33	4	1	.2	.2	.4
557	Whole-grain wheat, cooked	⅓ c	50	86	28	1	7	1	<1	t	t	.1
	Wheat flour (unbleached):											
	All-purpose white, enriched:											
558	Sifted	1 c	115	11	419	12	88	3	1	.2	.1	.5
559	Unsifted	1 c	125	11	455	13	95	3	1	.2	.1	.5
560	Cake or pastry, enriched, sifted	1 c	96	12	348	8	75	2	1	.1	.1	.4
561	Self-rising, enriched, unsifted	1 c	125	11	443	12	93	3	1	.2	.1	.5
562	Whole wheat, from hard wheats	1 c	120	10	406	16	87	15	2	.4	.3	.9
	MEATS: FISH and SHELLFISH											
1045	Bass, baked or broiled	4 oz	113	68	166	27	0	0	5	1.1	2.1	1.5
1046	Bluefish, baked or broiled	4 oz	113	62	180	29	0	0	6	1.3	2.6	1.5
1047	Bluefish, fried in bread crumbs	4 oz	113	61	232	26	5	<1	11	2.4	4.9	2.8
1686	Catfish, breaded/flour fried	4 oz	113	48	325	21	14	1	20	5	9	5
	Clams:											
563	Raw meat only	4 oz	113	81	84	14	3	0	1	.1	.1	.3
564	Canned, drained	4 oz	113	72	168	29	6	0	2	.2	.2	.6
1290	Steamed, meat only	20 ea	90	71	133	23	5	0	2	.2	.2	.5
	Cod:											
565	Baked with butter	4 oz	113	75	150	26	0	0	4	.4	.3	.6
566	Batter fried	4 oz	113	76	196	20	8	<1	9	2.2	3.6	2.6
567	Poached, no added fat	4 oz	113	77	116	25	0	0	1	.2	.1	.3
	Crab, meat only:											
1048	Blue crab, cooked	4 oz	113	77	115	23	0	0	2	.3	.3	.8
1049	Dungeness crab, cooked	4 oz	113	73	124	25	1	0	1	.2	.2	.5
568	Blue crab, canned	4 oz	113	76	112	23	0	0	1	.3	.2	.5
1587	Crab, imitation, from surimi	4 oz	113	74	115	14	12	0	1	.3	.2	.8
569	Fish sticks, breaded pollock	2 ea	57	46	155	9	14	<1	7	1.8	2.9	1.8
	Flounder/sole, baked w/lemon juice:											
570	With butter	4 oz	113	73	160	21	<1	0	8	4.3	2	.7
571	With margarine	4 oz	113	73	160	21	<1	0	8	1.6	3.1	2.5

(Computer code number is for West Diet Analysis program)

PAGE KEY: A–4 = BEV   A–6 = DAIRY   A–12 = EGGS   A–14 = FAT/OIL   A–18 = FRUIT   A–26 = BAKERY   A–36 = GRAIN   A–44 = FISH
A–48 = MEATS   A–50 = POULTRY   A–54 = SAUSAGE   A–56 = MIXED/FAST   A–64 = NUTS/SEEDS   A–68 = SWEETS   A–70 = VEG/LEG
A–84 = MISC   A–88 = SOUPS/SAUCES   A–90 = FAST   A–106 = FRZN ENTREE   A–112 = BABY FOODS

Chol (mg)	Calc (mg)	Iron (mg)	Magn (mg)	Pota (mg)	Sodi (mg)	Zinc (mg)	VT-A (RE)	Thia (mg)	Ribo (mg)	Niac (mg)	V-B6 (mg)	Fola (µg)	VT-C (mg)	VT-E α-TE (mg)
0	111	6.6	57	222	9	1.78	0	1.1	.13	6.72	.65	31	0	.241
0	33	1.98	21	65	5	.54	0	.44	.03	2.45	.03	7	0	.09
0	5	.34	12	24	12	.99	0	.05	.03	.7	.06	2	0	.07
0	5	.98	52	166	5	2.2	0	.08	.14	2.12	.22	43	0	.38
1	9	1.02	13	46	619	.31	0	.13	.08	1.94	.11	8	<1	–
0	24	2.16	76	347	3	2.03	0	.29	.12	1.76	.27	19	0	1.36
0	165	5.27	201	2260	16	1.04	4	.33	.25	1.9	.46	360	0	.2
0	10	1.96	25	43	1	.74	0	.29	.14	2.34	.05	10	0	.084
0	10	1.96	25	43	140	.74	0	.29	.14	2.34	.05	10	0	.38
0	21	1.48	42	62	4	1.13	0	.15	.06	.99	.11	7	0	.07
0	30	2.4	2	17	2	.18	0	.01	0	0	.01	6	0	0
0	22	3.18	183	355	1	2.18	0	.16	.17	4.08	.39	24	0	.7
0	39	6.26	239	892	12	12.3	0	1.88	.5	6.81	1.3	281	0	18
0	51	10.3	362	1070	5	18.8	0	1.89	.93	6.32	1.11	398	7	20.5
0	19	3.86	136	405	2	7.06	0	.71	.35	2.37	.42	150	7	12.54
0	17	1.49	53	170	0	1.15	0	.17	.12	2.14	.17	26	0	.48
0	3	.29	12	33	<1	.24	0	.04	.01	.5	.03	4	0	.1
0	17	5.34	25	122	2	.8	0	.9	.57	6.79	.05	30	0	.07
0	19	5.8	27	133	2	.87	0	.98	.62	7.38	.05	32	0	.08
0	13	7	15	101	2	.6	15	.36	.4	6.5	.03	18	0	.06
0	423	5.84	24	155	1586	.77	0	.84	.52	7.29	.06	52	0	.08
0	41	4.66	166	486	6	3.52	0	.54	.26	7.64	.41	53	0	1.48
98	116	2.17	43	517	102	.94	40	.1	.1	1.72	.16	19	2	1.13
86	10	.7	48	539	87	1.19	155	.08	.11	8.22	.53	2	0	1.13
68	9	.6	42	468	76	1.02	136	.07	.09	6.24	.41	2	<1	2.6
92	40	1.44	34	576	597	1.03	32	.4	.22	3.2	.22	19	<1	2.48
38	52	15.9	10	355	63	1.54	102	.09	.24	2	.07	18	15	1.13
76	104	31.6	20	707	127	3.1	194	.17	.48	3.81	.12	33	25	1.13
60	83	25.2	16	565	101	2.46	154	.13	.38	3.02	.1	26	20	1.8
68	23	.56	48	278	254	.66	34	.1	.09	2.85	.32	11	<1	.41
64	43	.9	36	443	124	.61	17	.12	.12	2.54	.23	10	1	.92
61	23	.54	41	496	69	.64	14	.09	.08	2.48	.28	8	1	.32
113	118	1.03	37	367	316	4.79	2	.11	.06	3.74	.2	57	4	1.13
86	67	.49	66	461	427	6.21	35	.06	.23	4.11	.2	48	4	.79
100	114	.95	44	423	378	4.56	2	.09	.09	1.55	.17	48	3	1.13
23	15	.44	49	102	951	.37	23	.04	.03	.2	.03	2	0	.11
64	11	.42	14	148	331	.38	18	.07	.1	1.21	.03	10	0	.78
91	21	.37	67	363	193	.71	72	.09	.13	2.47	.27	13	1	2.51
73	21	.37	67	364	201	.71	92	.09	.13	2.47	.27	13	1	3.14

(For purposes of calculations, use "0" for t, <1, <.1, <.01, etc.)

Table A–1
Food Composition

Computer Code Number	Food Description	Measure	Wt (g)	H₂O (%)	Ener (cal)	Prot (g)	Carb (g)	Dietary Fiber (g)	Fat (g)	Fat Breakdown (g)		
										Sat	Mono	Poly
MEATS: FISH and SHELLFISH—Cont.												
572	Without added fat	4 oz	113	73	133	27	0	0	2	.4	.3	.5
1599	Grouper, baked or broiled	4 oz	113	73	133	28	0	0	1	.3	.3	.5
573	Haddock, breaded, fried[1]	4 oz	113	55	264	22	14	1	13	3.2	5.4	3.3
1050	Haddock, smoked	4 oz	113	72	131	29	0	0	1	.2	.2	.4
	Halibut:											
1600	Baked or broiled	4 oz	113	72	158	30	0	0	3	.5	1.1	1.1
574	Baked with butter & lemon juice	4 oz	113	69	186	29	0	0	7	2.7	2.1	1.1
1051	Smoked	1 oz	28	49	63	6	0	0	4	.7	1.3	1.9
1054	Raw	4 oz	113	78	124	24	0	0	3	.4	.7	.9
575	Herring, pickled	3 oz	85	55	223	12	8	0	15	2	10.1	1.4
1052	Lobster meat, cooked w/moist heat	1 c	145	76	142	30	2	0	1	.2	.2	.1
1687	Ocean perch, baked/broiled	4 oz	113	73	137	27	0	0	2	.4	.9	.6
576	Ocean perch, breaded/fried	4 oz	113	59	249	22	9	1	13	3.2	5.7	3.4
1056	Octopus, raw	4 oz	113	80	93	17	3	0	1	.3	.2	.3
	Oysters:											
577	Raw, Eastern	1 c	248	85	169	18	10	0	6	1.9	.8	2.4
578	Raw, Pacific	1 c	248	82	201	23	12	0	6	1.3	.9	2.2
	Cooked:											
579	Eastern, breaded, fried, medium	6 ea	88	65	173	8	10	<1	11	2.8	4.1	2.9
580	Western, simmered	4 oz	113	64	184	21	11	0	5	1.2	.8	2
581	Pollock, baked or broiled	4 oz	113	74	128	27	0	0	1	.3	.2	.6
1055	Pollock, moist heat, poached	4 oz	113	74	128	27	0	0	1	.3	.2	.6
	Salmon:											
582	Canned pink, solids and liquid	4 oz	113	69	157	22	0	0	7	1.7	2.1	2.3
583	Broiled or baked	4 oz	113	62	244	31	0	0	13	2.2	6	2.7
584	Smoked	4 oz	113	72	132	21	0	0	5	1	2.3	1.1
585	Atlantic sardines, canned, drained, 2 = 24 g	4 oz	113	60	235	28	0	0	13	1.7	4.4	5.8
586	Scallops, breaded, cooked from frozen	6 ea	93	58	199	17	9	<1	10	2.5	4.2	2.7
1588	Scallops, imitation, from surimi	4 oz	113	74	112	14	12	0	<1	.1	.1	.2
1688	Scallops, steamed/boiled	½ c	60	81	64	10	1	0	2	.3	.7	.6
	Shrimp:											
587	Cooked, boiled, 2 large = 11 g	16 ea	86	77	85	18	0	0	1	.2	.2	.4
588	Canned, drained	½ c	64	73	77	15	1	0	1	.2	.2	.5
589	Fried, 2 large = 15 g[1]	12 ea	90	53	218	19	10	<1	11	1.9	3.6	4.6
1057	Raw, large, about 7 g each	14 ea	100	76	106	20	1	0	2	.3	.3	.7
1589	Shrimp, imitation, from surimi	4 oz	113	75	114	14	10	0	2	.3	.2	.9
1053	Snapper, baked or broiled	4 oz	113	70	145	30	0	0	2	.4	.4	.7
1060	Squid, fried in flour[2]	4 oz	113	65	198	20	9	<1	8	2.1	3.1	2.4
1590	Surimi[3]	4 oz	113	76	112	17	8	0	1	.2	.2	.5
1058	Swordfish, raw	4 oz	113	76	137	22	0	0	5	1.2	1.8	1
1059	Swordfish, baked or broiled	4 oz	113	69	176	29	0	0	6	1.6	2.2	1.3
590	Trout, baked or broiled	4 oz	113	71	170	26	0	0	7	1.8	2	2.1
	Tuna, light, canned, drained solids:											
591	Oil pack	3 oz	85	60	168	25	0	0	7	1.3	2.5	2.4
592	Water pack	3 oz	85	74	98	22	0	0	1	.2	.1	.3
1061	Bluefin tuna, fresh	4 oz	113	68	163	26	0	0	6	1.4	1.8	1.9

[1]Dipped in egg, bread crumbs, and flour; fried in vegetable shortening.

[2]Recipe is 94.6% squid, 4.9% flour, and 0.6% salt.

[3]Surimi is processed from Walleye (Alaska) pollock. Also see Imitation crab, shrimp, scallops.

(Computer code number is for West Diet Analysis program)

Chol (mg)	Calc (mg)	Iron (mg)	Magn (mg)	Pota (mg)	Sodi (mg)	Zinc (mg)	VT-A (RE)	Thia (mg)	Ribo (mg)	Niac (mg)	V-B6 (mg)	Fola (μg)	VT-C (mg)	VT-E α-TE (mg)
77	20	.39	66	390	119	.72	13	.09	.13	2.47	.27	10	2	2.14
53	24	1.29	42	537	60	.58	57	.09	.01	.43	.4	12	0	2.26
96	63	1.93	46	346	524	.59	33	.08	.14	4.51	.28	19	<1	1.56
87	56	1.59	61	469	862	.57	25	.05	.06	5.75	.45	17	0	.45
47	68	1.21	121	652	78	.6	61	.08	.1	8.07	.45	16	0	1.23
54	66	1.17	116	636	112	.57	93	.08	.1	7.69	.43	16	5	1.27
28	14	.24	23	128	136	.12	13	.01	.02	1.64	.09	1	<1	.27
36	53	.95	94	510	61	.48	53	.07	.08	6.62	.39	14	0	.96
11	65	1.04	7	59	740	.45	219	.03	.12	2.81	.14	2	0	.85
104	88	.57	51	510	551	4.23	38	.01	.1	1.55	.11	16	0	1.45
61	155	1	44	395	109	.7	16	.15	.15	2.77	.31	12	1	.23
71	136	1.58	38	324	432	.67	23	.14	.18	2.69	.24	15	1	2.41
54	60	6.01	34	395	261	1.91	51	.03	.04	2.38	.41	18	6	1.36
131	112	16.5	117	387	523	225	74	.25	.24	3.42	.15	25	9	2.11
124	20	12.6	55	417	263	41.2	201	.17	.58	4.98	.12	25	20	2.11
71	55	6.12	51	214	366	76.7	79	.13	.18	1.45	.06	12	3	2.01
113	18	10.4	50	342	240	37.6	169	.14	.5	4.11	.1	17	15	1.81
108	7	.32	83	437	132	.68	26	.08	.09	1.87	.08	4	0	.23
108	7	.32	83	437	132	.68	26	.08	.09	1.87	.08	4	0	.23
62	242[4]	.95	38	368	626	1.04	19	.03	.21	7.42	.34	17	0	1.53
99	8	.62	35	425	75	.58	71	.24	.19	7.56	.25	6	0	2.83
26	12	.96	20	197	885	.35	29	.03	.11	5.35	.31	2	0	1.53
160	433[4]	3.31	44	450	572	1.5	76	.09	.26	5.95	.19	13	0	.34
57	39	.76	55	309	431	.99	20	.04	.1	1.4	.13	17	2	2.23
25	9	.35	49	117	899	.37	23	.01	.02	.35	.03	2	0	.11
19	15	.15	33	168	246	.55	31	.01	.04	.6	.08	7	1	.81
167	33	2.65	29	156	192	1.34	57	.03	.03	2.22	.11	3	2	.44
110	38	1.75	26	135	108	.8	11	.02	.02	1.76	.07	1	1	.6
159	60	1.13	36	202	309	1.24	50	.12	.12	2.76	.09	7	1	3.58
152	52	2.41	37	185	148	1.11	54	.03	.03	2.55	.1	3	2	.82
41	21	.68	49	101	797	.37	23	.03	.04	.19	.03	2	0	.11
53	45	.27	42	590	65	.5	40	.06	<.01	.39	.52	7	2	.45
295	44	1.15	43	316	347	1.97	12	.06	.52	2.95	.07	6	5	2.2
34	10	.29	49	127	162	.37	22	.02	.02	.25	.03	2	0	2.14
44	5	.92	31	326	102	1.3	41	.04	.11	11	.37	2	1	.57
57	7	1.18	38	417	130	1.67	46	.05	.13	13.3	.43	3	1	.81
78	97	.43	35	507	63	.58	17	.17	.11	6.54	.39	22	2	.57
15	11	1.18	26	175	301	.77	20	.03	.1	10.5	.09	5	0	1.02
25	9	1.3	23	201	287	.65	14	.03	.06	11.3	.3	3	0	.45
43	9	1.16	57	286	44	.68	740	.27	.28	9.81	.52	2	0	1.13

[4]If bones are discarded, calcium value is greatly reduced.

(For purposes of calculations, use "0" for t, <1, <.1, <.01, etc.)

Table A–1
Food Composition

Computer Code Number	Food Description	Measure	Wt (g)	H$_2$O (%)	Ener (cal)	Prot (g)	Carb (g)	Dietary Fiber (g)	Fat (g)	Fat Breakdown (g) Sat	Mono	Poly
	MEATS: BEEF, LAMB, PORK, and others											
	BEEF, cooked:[1]											
	Braised, simmered, pot roasted:											
	Relatively fat, choice chuck blade:											
593	Lean and fat, piece 2½ x 2½ x ¾"	4 oz	113	47	393	30	0	0	29	11.6	12.6	1.1
594	Lean only	4 oz	113	55	297	35	0	0	16	6.3	7	.5
	Relatively lean, like choice round:											
595	Lean and fat, pce 4⅛ x 2½ x ¾"	4 oz	113	52	311	32	0	0	19	7.2	8.3	.7
596	Lean only	4 oz	113	57	249	36	0	0	11	3.6	4.7	.4
	Ground beef, broiled, patty 3 x ⅝":											
597	Extra lean, about 16% fat	4 oz	113	54	299	32	0	0	18	7	7.8	.7
598	Lean, 21% fat	4 oz	113	53	316	32	0	0	20	7.9	8.7	.7
	Roasts, oven cooked, no added liquid:											
	Relatively fat, prime rib:											
601	Lean and fat, pce 4⅛ x 2¼ x ½"	4 oz	113	46	425	25	0	0	35	14.3	15.2	1.3
602	Lean only	4 oz	113	58	274	31	0	0	16	6.6	6.8	.5
	Relatively lean, choice round:											
603	Lean and fat, pce 2½ x 2½ x ¾"	4 oz	113	59	273	30	0	0	16	6.2	6.9	.6
604	Lean only	4 oz	113	65	198	33	0	0	6	2.3	2.7	.2
1701	Steak, rib, broiled, lean	4 oz	113	58	250	32	0	0	13	5	5	.4
	Steak, broiled, relatively lean, choice sirloin:											
605	Lean and fat, pce 2½ x 2½ x ¾"	4 oz	113	52	320	31	0	0	21	8.7	9.3	.8
606	Lean only	4 oz	113	62	228	34	0	0	9	3.5	3.9	.4
	Steak, broiled, relatively fat, choice T-bone:											
1063	Lean and fat	4 oz	113	53	337	28	0	0	24	9.7	10.1	.9
1064	Lean only	4 oz	113	60	242	32	0	0	12	4.7	4.7	.4
	Variety meats:											
1086	Brains, panfried	4 oz	113	71	221	15	0	0	18	4.2	4.5	2.6
599	Heart, simmered	4 oz	113	64	197	33	<1	0	6	1.9	1.4	1.5
600	Liver, fried	4 oz	113	56	245	30	9	0	9	3	1.8	1.9
1062	Tongue, cooked	4 oz	113	56	320	25	<1	0	23	10.3	11	.9
607	Beef, canned, corned	4 oz	113	58	282	31	0	0	17	7	6.8	.7
608	Beef, dried, cured	1 oz	28	57	46	8	<1	0	1	.5	.5	.1
	LAMB, domestic, cooked:											
	Chop, arm, braised (5.6 oz raw w/bone):											
609	Lean and fat	1 ea	70	44	242	21	0	0	17	6.9	7.1	1.2
610	Lean only	1 ea	55	49	153	20	0	0	8	2.8	3.4	.5
	Chop, loin, broiled (4.2 oz. raw w/bone):											
611	Lean and fat	1 ea	64	52	202	16	0	0	15	6.3	6.2	1.1
612	Lean only	1 ea	46	61	99	14	0	0	4	1.6	2	.3
1067	Cutlet, avg of lean cuts, cooked	4 oz	113	54	330	28	0	0	23	9.9	9.9	1.7
	Leg, roasted, 3 oz = 4⅛ x 2¼ x ½":											
613	Lean and fat	4 oz	113	57	292	29	0	0	19	7.8	7.9	1.3
614	Lean only	4 oz	113	64	216	32	0	0	9	3.1	3.8	.6
615	Rib, roasted, lean and fat	4 oz	113	48	406	24	0	0	34	14.5	14.2	2.5
616	Rib, roasted, lean only	4 oz	113	60	262	30	0	0	15	5.4	6.6	1
1065	Shoulder, roasted, lean and fat	4 oz	113	56	312	25	0	0	23	9.6	9.2	1.8

[1]Outer layer of fat removed to about ½" of the lean. Deposits of fat within the cut remain.

(Computer code number is for West Diet Analysis program)

PAGE KEY: A–4 = BEV   A–6 = DAIRY   A–12 = EGGS   A–14 = FAT/OIL   A–18 = FRUIT   A–26 = BAKERY   A–36 = GRAIN   A–44 = FISH   A–48 = MEATS   A–50 = POULTRY   A–54 = SAUSAGE   A–56 = MIXED/FAST   A–64 = NUTS/SEEDS   A–68 = SWEETS   A–70 = VEG/LEG   A–84 = MISC   A–88 = SOUPS/SAUCES   A–90 = FAST   A–106 = FRZN ENTREE   A–112 = BABY FOODS

Chol (mg)	Calc (mg)	Iron (mg)	Magn (mg)	Pota (mg)	Sodi (mg)	Zinc (mg)	VT-A (RE)	Thia (mg)	Ribo (mg)	Niac (mg)	V-B6 (mg)	Fola (µg)	VT-C (mg)	VT-E α-TE (mg)
112	11	3.46	22	274	67	7.61	0	.08	.27	3.55	.32	10	0	.26
120	15	4.17	26	297	81	11.7	0	.09	.32	3.03	.33	7	0	.16
109	7	3.54	25	319	57	5.57	0	.08	.27	4.23	.37	11	0	.22
109	6	3.92	28	348	58	6.21	0	.08	.29	4.63	.41	12	0	.2
112	10	3.14	28	418	93	7.29	0	.08	.36	6.63	.36	12	0	.2
114	14	2.78	27	396	101	7.03	0	.07	.27	6.77	.34	12	0	.23
96	12	2.62	22	334	71	5.94	0	.08	.19	3.81	.26	8	0	.27
90	11	2.96	28	422	81	7.87	0	.09	.24	4.67	.34	9	0	.14
81	7	2.09	27	405	67	4.89	0	.09	.18	3.93	.4	7	0	.23
78	6	2.21	31	447	70	5.38	0	.1	.19	4.25	.43	8	0	.12
90	15	3	31	445	78	8	0	.11	.25	5.92	.45	9	0	.16
102	12	3.4	32	407	70	6.5	0	.13	.3	4.38	.45	10	0	.28
101	12	3.81	36	456	75	7.39	0	.15	.33	4.85	.51	11	0	.16
94	9	3.01	28	401	69	5.31	0	.11	.25	4.63	.39	8	0	.24
91	8	3.4	33	460	74	6.12	0	.13	.28	5.26	.44	9	0	.16
2253	10	2.52	17	400	178	1.53	0	.15	.29	4.29	.44	7	4	2.37
219	7	8.52	28	264	71	3.55	0	.16	1.75	4.62	.24	2	2	.81
545	12	7.12	26	411	120	6.18	12123[2]	.24	4.69	16.4	1.63	249	26	.72
121	8	3.84	19	204	68	5.44	0	.03	.4	2.44	.18	6	1	.4
97	14	2.36	16	153	1136	4.04	0	.02	.17	2.77	.15	10	2	.17
12	2	1.28	9	126	972	1.49	0	.02	.06	1.55	.1	3	4	.04
84	18	1.68	18	214	50	4.26	0	.05	.18	4.67	.08	13	0	.11
67	14	1.49	16	186	42	4.01	0	.04	.15	3.48	.07	12	0	.1
64	13	1.16	15	209	49	2.23	0	.06	.16	4.54	.08	12	0	.08
44	9	.92	13	173	39	1.9	0	.05	.13	3.15	.07	11	0	.07
110	12	2.27	25	340	77	4.68	0	.13	.32	7.51	.16	19	0	.15
105	12	2.25	27	355	75	4.99	0	.11	.31	7.47	.17	23	0	.17
101	9	2.4	29	383	77	5.6	0	.13	.33	7.19	.19	26	0	.2
110	25	1.81	23	307	83	3.96	0	.1	.24	7.65	.13	17	0	.11
100	24	2.01	26	356	92	5.07	0	.1	.26	6.99	.17	25	0	.17
104	23	2.22	26	285	75	5.94	0	.1	.27	6.97	.15	24	0	.16

[2] Value varies widely.

(For purposes of calculations, use "0" for t, <1, <.1, <.01, etc.)

Table A–1
Food Composition

Computer Code Number	Food Description	Measure	Wt (g)	H$_2$O (%)	Ener (cal)	Prot (g)	Carb (g)	Dietary Fiber (g)	Fat (g)	Fat Breakdown (g) Sat	Mono	Poly
	MEATS: BEEF, LAMB, PORK, and others—Cont.											
1066	Shoulder, roasted, lean only	4 oz	113	63	231	28	0	0	12	4.6	4.9	1.1
	Variety meats:											
1069	Brains, panfried	4 oz	113	76	164	14	0	0	12	2.9	2.1	1.2
1068	Heart, braised	4 oz	113	64	209	28	2	0	9	3.6	2.5	.9
1070	Sweetbreads, cooked	4 oz	113	60	264	26	0	0	17	7.8	6.2	.8
1071	Tongue, cooked	4 oz	113	58	311	24	0	0	23	8.9	11.3	1.4
	PORK, cured, cooked (see also #669–672):											
617	Bacon, medium slices	3 pce	19	13	109	6	<1	0	9	3.3	4.5	1.1
1087	Breakfast strips, cooked	2 pce	23	27	106	7	<1	0	8	2.9	3.7	1.3
618	Canadian-style bacon	2 pce	47	62	87	11	1	0	4	1.3	1.9	.4
	Ham, roasted:											
619	Lean and fat, 2 pces 4⅛ x 2¼ x ¼"	4 oz	113	65	275	24	0	0	19	6.8	8.9	2.1
620	Lean only	4 oz	113	68	177	24	0	0	6	2	3	.7
621	Ham, canned, roasted, 8% fat	4 oz	113	69	189	24	1	0	10	3.2	4.6	1
	PORK, fresh, cooked:											
	Chops, loin (cut 3 per lb with bone):											
1291	Braised, lean and fat	1 ea	71	44	170	19	0	0	10	3.6	4.3	1
1292	Braised, lean only	1 ea	55	51	112	16	0	0	5	1.9	2.3	1
622	Broiled, lean and fat	1 ea	87	50	211	24	0	0	12	4.6	5.4	1
623	Broiled, lean only	1 ea	72	57	151	21	0	0	7	2.6	3.4	1
624	Panfried, lean and fat	1 ea	89	45	247	27	0	0	15	5.4	6.3	1.7
625	Panfried, lean only	1 ea	67	53	161	17	0	0	10	3.5	4	1.7
626	Leg, roasted, lean and fat	4 oz	113	53	308	30	0	0	20	7	9	2
627	Leg, roasted, lean only	4 oz	113	59	233	35	0	0	9	3	4	1
628	Rib, roasted, lean and fat	4 oz	113	51	288	31	0	0	17	6.7	7.9	1
629	Rib, roasted, lean only	4 oz	113	57	252	32	0	0	13	4.9	5.9	1
630	Shoulder, braised, lean and fat	4 oz	113	47	391	32	0	0	26	9.6	11.8	2.6
631	Shoulder, braised, lean only	4 oz	113	54	281	37	0	0	14	4.8	6.5	1.3
1088	Spareribs, cooked, yield from 1 lb raw with bone	4 oz	113	40	450	33	0	0	34	12.5	15	3
1095	Rabbit, roasted (1 cup meat = 140 g)	4 oz	113	61	223	33	0	0	9	2.7	2.5	1.8
	VEAL, cooked:											
632	Cutlet, braised or broiled, 4⅛ x 2¼ x ½"	4 oz	113	52	322	34	0	0	19	7.6	7.6	1.3
633	Rib roasted, lean, 2 pieces 4⅛ x 2¼ x ¼"	4 oz	113	60	257	27	0	0	16	6.1	6.2	1.1
634	Liver, panfried	4 oz	113	67	187	24	3	0	8	2.9	1.7	1.2
1096	Venison (deer meat), roasted	4 oz	113	65	179	34	0	0	4	1.4	1	.7
	MEATS: POULTRY and POULTRY PRODUCTS											
	CHICKEN, cooked:											
	Fried, batter dipped:[1]											
635	Breast (5.6 oz with bones)	1 ea	140	52	364	35	13	<1	18	4.9	7.6	4.3
636	Drumstick (3.4 oz with bones)	1 ea	72	53	192	16	6	<1	11	3	4.6	2.7
637	Thigh	1 ea	86	51	238	19	8	<1	14	3.8	5.8	3.3
638	Wing	1 ea	49	46	158	10	5	<1	11	2.9	4.4	2.5
	Fried, flour coated:[1]											
639	Breast (4.2 oz with bones)	1 ea	98	57	217	31	2	<1	9	2.4	3.4	1.9

[1]Fried in vegetable shortening.

(Computer code number is for West Diet Analysis program)

PAGE KEY: A–4 = BEV   A–6 = DAIRY   A–12 = EGGS   A–14 = FAT/OIL   A–18 = FRUIT   A–26 = BAKERY   A–36 = GRAIN   A–44 = FISH
A–48 = MEATS   A–50 = POULTRY   A–54 = SAUSAGE   A–56 = MIXED/FAST   A–64 = NUTS/SEEDS   A–68 = SWEETS   A–70 = VEG/LEG
A–84 = MISC   A–88 = SOUPS/SAUCES   A–90 = FAST   A–106 = FRZN ENTREE   A–112 = BABY FOODS

Chol (mg)	Calc (mg)	Iron (mg)	Magn (mg)	Pota (mg)	Sodi (mg)	Zinc (mg)	VT-A (RE)	Thia (mg)	Ribo (mg)	Niac (mg)	V-B6 (mg)	Fola (μg)	VT-C (mg)	VT-E α-TE (mg)
99	21	2.42	28	301	77	6.48	0	.1	.29	6.53	.17	28	0	.2
2309	14	1.91	16	232	152	1.54	0	.12	.27	2.8	.12	6	14	1.73
281	16	6.26	27	213	71	4.17	0	.19	1.35	4.94	.34	2	8	.79
452	14	2.4	21	328	59	3.04	0	.02	.24	2.9	.06	15	23	.77
213	11	2.99	18	179	76	3.39	0	.09	.48	4.18	.19	3	8	.36
16	2	.31	5	92	303	.62	0	.13	.05	1.39	.05	1	6²	.1
24	3	.45	6	107	483	.83	0	.17	.08	1.72	.08	1	10	.07
27	5	.38	10	183	726	.8	0	.39	.09	3.25	.21	2	10²	.12
70	8	1	21	323	1341	2.6	0	.68	.25	5.04	.43	3	0	.29
62	8	1	25	357	1500	2.9	0	.77	.29	5.67	.53	5	0	.29
46	8	1	23	397	1207	2.6	0	1.09	.28	5.68	.45	6	26²	.29
57	15	.77	13	266	34	1.7	2	.43	.18	3	.26	2	<1	.19
43	15	.77	13	266	34	1.7	1	.38	.2	3	.25	2	<1	.14
70	17	.76	24	368	54	2	3	.76	.28	4.37	.35	4	<1	.18
57	12	.66	21	315	46	1.8	1	.66	.22	3.99	.34	4	<1	.14
82	24	.81	26	378	71	2	3	.91	.27	5	.35	5	<1	.23
55	15	.7	17	245	52	2.6	1	.49	.25	3.03	.27	3	<1	.17
106	16	1.15	25	398	68	3.36	3	.72	.35	5.16	.45	11	<1	.29
108	8	1.29	33	442	73	3.41	3	.91	.4	5.56	.38	3	<1	.24
82	32	1.01	24	476	52	2.34	2	.82	.34	7	.34	3	<1	.23
80	29	1.13	25	494	53	2.4	2	.86	.35	7	.39	3	<1	.23
123	20	1.83	21	417	99	4.7	3	.61	.35	6	.4	5	<1	.29
129	9	2.22	25	458	115	5.64	2	.68	.41	6.74	.46	6	<1	.29
137	53	2.1	27	362	105	5.22	3	.46	.43	6.2	.4	5	0	.29
93	21	2.57	24	433	53	2.59	0	.1	.24	9.56	.53	12	0	.68
134	32	1.24	27	316	91	4.13	0	.04	.34	10.3	.29	16	0	.45
125	12	1.1	25	333	104	4.64	0	.06	.31	7.92	.28	15	0	.4
635	8	2.97	22	232	60	10.8	9095³	.15	2.2	9.62	.56	858	35	.38
127	8	5.07	27	379	61	3.12	0	.2	.68	7.61	.43⁴	5⁴	0	.02
119	28	1.75	34	281	385	1.33	28	.16	.2	14.7	.6	8	0	1.48
62	12	.97	14	133	193	1.68	19	.08	.15	3.67	.19	6	0	.59
80	15	1.25	18	165	247	1.75	25	.1	.19	4.91	.22	8	0	.74
39	10	.63	8	68	156	.68	17	.05	.07	2.58	.15	3	0	.54
87	16	1.17	29	253	74	1.08	15	.08	.13	13.5	.57	4	0	.45

(2)Values based on products containing added ascorbic acid or sodium ascorbate. If none added, ascorbic acid content would be negligible.

(3)Value varies widely.

(4)Values estimated from other game meat.

(For purposes of calculations, use "0" for t, <1, <.1, <.01, etc.)

Table A–1
Food Composition

Computer Code Number	Food Description	Measure	Wt (g)	H₂O (%)	Ener (cal)	Prot (g)	Carb (g)	Dietary Fiber (g)	Fat (g)	Fat Breakdown (g)		
										Sat	Mono	Poly
	MEATS: POULTRY and POULTRY PRODUCTS—Cont.											
	CHICKEN—Cont.											
1212	Breast, without skin	1 ea	86	60	160	29	<1	<1	4	1.1	1.5	.9
640	Drumstick (2.6 oz with bones)	1 ea	49	57	120	13	1	<1	7	1.8	2.7	1.6
641	Thigh	1 ea	62	54	162	17	2	<1	9	2.5	3.6	2.1
1099	Thigh, without skin	1 ea	52	59	113	15	1	<1	5	1.4	2	1.3
642	Wing	1 ea	32	49	102	8	1	<1	7	1.9	2.8	1.6
	Roasted:											
643	All types of meat	1 c	140	64	266	40	0	0	10	2.9	3.7	2.4
644	Dark meat	1 c	140	63	287	38	0	0	14	3.7	5	3.2
645	Light meat	1 c	140	65	242	43	0	0	6	1.8	2.2	1.4
646	Breast, without skin	1 ea	86	65	141	27	0	0	3	.9	1.1	.7
647	Drumstick	1 ea	44	67	95	12	0	0	5	1.4	2	1
1703	Leg, without skin	1 ea	95	65	163	26	0	0	5	1.4	2	1
648	Thigh	1 ea	62	59	153	15	0	0	10	2.7	3.8	2.1
1100	Thigh, without skin	1 ea	52	63	108	13	0	0	6	1.6	2.2	1.3
649	Stewed, all types:	1 c	140	67	248	38	0	0	9	2.6	3.3	2.2
656	Canned, boneless chicken	4 oz	113	69	187	25	0	0	9	2.5	3.6	2
1102	Gizzards, simmered	3 ea	66	67	101	18	1	0	2	.7	.6	.7
1101	Hearts, simmered	8 ea	25	65	45	6	<1	0	2	.6	.5	.6
2300	Liver, simmered: Ounce	3 oz	85	68	133	21	1	0	5	1.6	1.1	.8
1098	Liver, simmered: Piece = 20 g	6 ea	120	68	187	29	1	0	7	2.2	1.6	1.1
	DUCK, roasted:											
1293	Meat with skin, about 2.7 cups	½ ea	382	52	1287	73	0	0	108	36.9	49.3	13.9
651	Meat only, about 1.5 cups	½ ea	221	64	444	52	0	0	25	9.2	8.2	3.2
	GOOSE, domesticated, roasted:											
1294	Meat only, 4.2 cups	½ ea	591	57	1406	171	0	0	75	26.9	25.6	9.1
1295	Meat with skin, about 5.5 cups	½ ea	774	52	2360	194	0	0	169	53.2	78.9	19.5
	TURKEY:											
	Roasted, meat only:											
652	Dark meat	4 oz	113	63	250	31	0	0	13	4	4	3.5
653	Light meat	4 oz	113	66	223	32	0	0	9	2.7	3.8	2.3
654	All types, chopped or diced	1 c	140	65	238	41	0	0	7	2.3	1.5	2
655	All types, sliced	4 oz	113	65	193	33	0	0	6	1.9	1.2	1.6
1103	Ground, cooked	4 oz	113	59	266	31	0	0	15	3.8	5.5	3.7
1106	Gizzard, cooked	2 ea	134	65	218	39	1	0	5	1.5	1	1.5
1107	Heart, cooked	4 ea	64	64	113	17	1	0	4	1.1	.8	1.1
1108	Liver, cooked	1 ea	75	66	126	18	3	0	4	1.4	1.1	.8
	POULTRY FOOD PRODUCTS (see also items in Sausages and Lunchmeats section):											
658	Chicken roll, light meat	2 pce	57	69	91	11	1	0	4	1.1	1.7	.9
1567	Chicken patty, breaded, cooked	1 ea	75	49	213	12	11	<1	13	4	6	1.7
659	Turkey and gravy, frozen package	3 oz	85	85	57	5	4	<1	2	.7	.8	.4
	Turkey breast, Louis Rich:											
1104	Barbecued	2 oz	57	69	72	11	2	0	2	.6	.6	.4
1943	Hickory smoked	1 pce	80	–	80	16	2	0	1	0	–	–

(Computer code number is for West Diet Analysis program)

PAGE KEY: A–4 = BEV   A–6 = DAIRY   A–12 = EGGS   A–14 = FAT/OIL   A–18 = FRUIT   A–26 = BAKERY   A–36 = GRAIN   A–44 = FISH   A–48 = MEATS   A–50 = POULTRY   A–54 = SAUSAGE   A–56 = MIXED/FAST   A–64 = NUTS/SEEDS   A–68 = SWEETS   A–70 = VEG/LEG   A–84 = MISC   A–88 = SOUPS/SAUCES   A–90 = FAST   A–106 = FRZN ENTREE   A–112 = BABY FOODS

Chol (mg)	Calc (mg)	Iron (mg)	Magn (mg)	Pota (mg)	Sodi (mg)	Zinc (mg)	VT-A (RE)	Thia (mg)	Ribo (mg)	Niac (mg)	V-B6 (mg)	Fola (μg)	VT-C (mg)	VT-E α-TE (mg)
78	14	.98	27	237	68	.93	6	.07	.11	12.7	.55	3	0	.36
44	6	.66	11	112	44	1.42	12	.04	.11	2.96	.17	4	0	.35
60	9	.92	16	146	55	1.56	18	.06	.15	4.31	.2	5	0	.48
53	7	.76	14	134	49	1.45	11	.05	.13	3.7	.2	5	0	.24
26	5	.4	6	57	25	.56	12	.02	.04	2.14	.13	1	0	.38
124	21	1.69	35	340	120	2.94	22	.1	.25	12.8	.66	8	0	.37
130	21	1.86	32	336	130	3.92	31	.1	.32	9.17	.5	11	0	.37
119	21	1.48	38	346	107	1.72	13	.09	.16	17.4	.84	6	0	.37
73	13	.89	25	220	64	.86	5	.06	.1	11.8	.52	3	0	.23
41	5	.57	10	101	40	1.4	8	.03	.1	2.67	.15	4	0	.12
88	11	1.26	23	234	90	3.03	18	.07	.22	5.8	.35	9	0	.25
58	7	.83	14	137	52	1.46	30	.04	.13	3.95	.19	4	0	.16
49	6	.68	12	123	46	1.34	10	.04	.12	3.39	.18	4	0	.14
116	20	1.64	29	252	98	2.79	21	.07	.23	8.55	.36	8	0	.37
70	16	1.79	14	155	570	1.6	39	.02	.15	7.18	.4	5	2	.24
128	7	2.74	13	118	44	2.89	37	.02	.16	2.63	.08	35	1	.79
61	5	2.22	5	33	12	1.8	2	.01	.18	.69	.08	20	<1	.4
536	12	7.23	18	119	42	3.68	4177	.13	1.49	3.78	.5	655	13	1.22
757	17	10.2	25	168	61	5.21	5894	.18	2.1	5.34	.7	924	19	1.73
320	42	10.3	61	779	225	7.11	241	.66	1.03	18.4	.69	23	0	2.67
196	26	5.97	44	557	143	5.75	51	.57	1.04	11.3	.55	22	0	1.55
567	83	17	147	2293	449	18.7	71	.54	2.3	24.1	2.78	71	0	5.91
704	100	21.9	170	2546	541	20.3	163	.6	2.5	32.3	2.86	15	0	13.5
101	37	2.64	27	310	86	4.7	0	.07	.28	3.99	.36	10	0	.72
86	24	1.53	29	322	71	2.31	0	.07	.15	7.11	.53	7	0	.1
106	35	2.49	36	417	98	4.34	0	.09	.25	7.62	.64	10	0	.46
86	28	2.02	29	338	79	3.52	0	.07	.21	6.17	.52	8	0	.37
116	28	2.2	27	306	121	3.25	0	.06	.19	5.47	.44	8	0	.38
310	20	7.28	25	281	72	5.57	75	.04	.44	4.11	.16	69	2	.21
145	8	4.4	14	117	35	3.37	5	.04	.56	2.08	.2	50	1	.1
469	8	5.85	11	145	48	2.32	2805	.04	1.07	4.46	.39	500	1	2.18
28	24	.55	11	129	332	.41	14	.04	.07	3.02	.12	1	0	.11
45	7	.86	18	208	352	.61	21	.11	.1	5.18	.26	8	<1	1.46
15	12	.79	7	52	471	.59	11	.02	.11	1.53	.08	3	0	.3
22	10	.4	12	166	609	.5	0	.02	.06	5.45	.22	2	<1	–
35	0	.72	–	–	1060	–	0	–	–	–	–	–	0	–

(For purposes of calculations, use "0" for t, <1, <.1, <.01, etc.)

Table A–1
Food Composition

Computer Code Number	Food Description	Measure	Wt (g)	H₂O (%)	Ener (cal)	Prot (g)	Carb (g)	Dietary Fiber (g)	Fat (g)	Fat Breakdown (g)		
										Sat	Mono	Poly
MEATS: POULTRY and POULTRY PRODUCTS TURKEY—Cont.												
1947	Honey roasted	1 pce	80	–	80	16	3	0	1	.5	–	–
1945	Oven roasted	1 pce	80	–	70	16	–	0	1	0	–	–
660	Turkey loaf, breast meat	4 oz	113	72	125	25	0	0	2	.5	.5	.3
661	Turkey patty, breaded, fried	2 oz	57	50	160	8	9	<1	10	2.7	4.2	2.7
662	Turkey, frozen, roasted, seasoned	4 oz	113	68	175	24	3	0	7	2.2	1.4	1.9
1704	Turkey roll, light meat	1 pce	28	72	42	5	<1	0	2	.6	.7	.5
MEATS: SAUSAGES and LUNCHMEATS (see also Poultry Food Products)												
1072	Beerwurst/beer salami, beef	1 oz	28	53	93	4	<1	0	8	3.7	4	.3
1074	Beerwurst/beer salami, pork	1 oz	28	61	67	4	1	0	5	1.8	2.5	.7
1075	Berliner sausage	1 oz	28	61	65	4	1	0	5	1.7	2.3	.4
	Bologna:											
1297	Beef	1 pce	23	55	72	3	<1	0	7	2.8	3.2	.3
2115	Beef, light, Oscar Mayer	1 pce	28	–	60	3	2	0	4	1.5	–	–
663	Beef & pork	1 pce	28	54	88	3	1	0	8	3	3.8	.7
2155	Healthy Favorites	2 ea	46	–	45	7	2	0	1	0	–	–
1298	Pork	1 pce	23	61	57	4	<1	0	5	1.6	2.2	.5
2114	Regular, light, Oscar Mayer	1 pce	28	–	60	3	2	0	4	1.5	–	–
664	Turkey	1 pce	28	65	56	4	<1	0	4	1.4	1.4	1.2
1970	Turkey, Louis Rich	1 pce	28	–	50	3	1	0	4	1	–	–
665	Braunschweiger sausage	2 pce	57	48	205	8	2	0	18	6.2	8.5	2.1
1073	Bratwurst, link	1 ea	70	51	226	10	2	0	19	6.9	9.3	2
666	Brown & serve sausage links, cooked	2 ea	26	45	102	4	1	0	10	3.4	4.4	1
1089	Cheesefurter/cheese smokie	2 ea	86	52	280	12	1	0	25	9	11.8	2.6
2157	Chicken breast, Healthy Favorites	4 pce	52	–	40	9	1	0	0	0	0	0
1556	Chorizo, pork & beef	3 oz	85	32	387	20	2	0	33	12.2	15.6	2.9
1950	Coldcuts, fat free, deli thin	1 pce	13	–	10	2	1	0	0	0	0	0
1090	Corned beef loaf, jellied	1 pce	28	69	43	6	0	0	2	.7	.8	.1
	Frankfurters:											
1077	Beef, large link, 8/package	1 ea	57	55	180	7	1	0	16	6.9	7.7	.8
1078	Beef and pork, large link, 8/package	1 ea	57	54	182	6	1	0	17	6.2	7.8	1.6
667	Beef and pork, small link, 10/pkg	1 ea	45	54	144	5	1	0	13	4.9	6.2	1.2
657	Chicken frankfurter, 10/package	1 ea	45	57	115	6	3	0	9	2.5	3.8	1.8
668	Turkey frankfurter, 10/package	1 ea	45	63	101	6	1	0	8	2.7	2.5	2.2
1968	Turkey/chicken frank 8/pkg	1 ea	43	–	80	6	1	0	6	2	–	–
	Ham:											
669	Ham lunchmeat, canned, 3 x 2 x ½"	1 pce	21	52	70	3	<1	0	6	2.3	3	.7
670	Chopped ham, packaged	2 pce	42	64	76	7	1	0	5	1.4	2.1	.5
671	Ham lunchmeat, regular	2 pce	57	65	103	10	2	0	6	1.9	2.8	.7
672	Ham lunchmeat, extra lean	2 pce	57	71	74	11	1	0	3	.9	1.3	.3
2156	Honey ham, Healthy Favorites	4 pce	52	–	50	9	2	0	2	.5	–	–
2113	Oscar Mayer lower sodium ham	1 pce	21	–	23	3	1	0	1	.3	–	–
673	Turkey ham lunchmeat	2 pce	57	71	73	11	<1	0	3	1	.7	.9
1091	Kielbasa sausage	1 pce	26	54	81	3	1	0	7	2.6	3.4	.8
1092	Knockwurst sausage, link	1 ea	68	55	209	8	1	0	19	6.9	8.7	2
1093	Mortadella lunchmeat	2 pce	30	52	93	5	1	0	8	2.9	3.4	.9
1097	Olive loaf lunchmeat	2 pce	57	58	134	7	5	<1	9	3.3	4.5	1.1

(Computer code number is for West Diet Analysis program)

PAGE KEY: A–4 = BEV   A–6 = DAIRY   A–12 = EGGS   A–14 = FAT/OIL   A–18 = FRUIT   A–26 = BAKERY   A–36 = GRAIN   A–44 = FISH
A–48 = MEATS   A–50 = POULTRY   A–54 = SAUSAGE   A–56 = MIXED/FAST   A–64 = NUTS/SEEDS   A–68 = SWEETS   A–70 = VEG/LEG
A–84 = MISC   A–88 = SOUPS/SAUCES   A–90 = FAST   A–106 = FRZN ENTREE   A–112 = BABY FOODS

Chol (mg)	Calc (mg)	Iron (mg)	Magn (mg)	Pota (mg)	Sodi (mg)	Zinc (mg)	VT-A (RE)	Thia (mg)	Ribo (mg)	Niac (mg)	V-B6 (mg)	Fola (μg)	VT-C (mg)	VT-E α-TE (mg)
35	0	.72	–	–	940	–	0	–	–	–	–	–	0	–
35	0	–	–	–	910	–	0	–	–	–	–	–	0	–
46	8	.45	23	315	1617	1.28	0	.04	.12	9.45	.41	5	0[1]	.43
35	8	1.25	9	156	456	.82	6	.06	.11	1.3	.11	5	0	1.36
60	6	1.86	25	338	768	2.88	0	.05	.19	7.11	.31	6	0	.43
12	11	.37	4	71	137	.45	0	.03	.06	1.98	.09	1	0	.04
17	3	.43	3	49	288	.69	0	.02	.03	.96	.05	1	4	.05
17	2	.22	4	72	347	.49	0	.16	.05	.92	.1	1	8	.06
13	3	.33	4	80	363	.7	0	.11	.06	.88	.06	1	2	.06
13	3	.38	3	36	226	.5	0	.01	.02	.55	.03	1	5	.06
10	–	–	–	–	310	–	–	–	–	–	–	–	–	–
15	3	.43	3	51	288	.55	0	.05	.04	.73	.05	1	6[1]	.06
15	–	.36	–	–	510	–	–	–	–	–	–	–	–	–
14	3	.18	3	65	272	.47	0	.12	.04	.9	.06	1	8	.06
15	–	–	–	–	310	–	–	–	–	–	–	–	–	–
28	24	.43	4	56	246	.49	0	.02	.05	1	.06	2	0	.15
20	20	.36	–	–	250	–	0	–	–	–	–	–	0	–
89	5	5.34	6	113	652	1.6	2405	.14	.87	4.77	.19	25	6[1]	.2
44	34	.72	11	196	778	1.47	0	.17	.16	2.31	.09	4	20	.19
16	2	.62	4	70	248	.3	0	.21	.09	.96	.06	1	0	.06
58	50	.93	11	177	930	1.94	33	.21	.14	2.5	.11	3	17	.27
25	–	.72	–	–	620	–	–	–	–	–	–	–	–	–
75	7	1.35	15	338	1049	2.9	0	.54	.25	4.36	.45	2	0	.19
4	0	.18	–	–	153	–	0	–	–	–	–	–	0	–
13	3	.58	3	29	267	1.16	0	0	.03	.5	.03	2	2	.05
35	11	.81	2	95	585	1.24	0	.03	.06	1.38	.07	2	14	.11
28	6	.66	6	95	638	1.05	0	.11	.07	1.5	.07	2	15	.14
22	5	.52	4	75	504	.83	0	.09	.05	1.18	.06	2	12[1]	.11
45	43	.9	6	38	616	.47	17	.03	.05	1.39	.14	2	0	.09
39	48	.83	6	81	641	1.4	0	.02	.08	1.86	.1	4	0	.28
40	60	1.08	–	–	480	–	0	–	–	–	–	–	0	–
13	1	.15	2	45	270	.31	0	.08	.04	.65	.04	1	<1	.06
21	3	.35	7	134	576	.9	0	.36	.09	2.2	.15	1	12[1]	.11
32	4	.56	11	188	746	1.21	0	.49	.14	2.98	.19	2	16[1]	.17
27	4	.43	10	198	810	1.09	0	.53	.13	2.74	.26	2	15[1]	.09
25	–	.72	–	–	630	–	–	–	–	–	–	–	–	–
10	–	.24	–	–	173	–	–	–	–	–	–	–	–	–
32	6	1.57	9	185	567	1.68	0	.03	.14	2.01	.14	3	0	.37
17	11	.38	4	70	279	.52	0	.06	.06	.75	.05	1	5	.06
39	7	.62	7	135	687	1.13	0	.23	.09	1.86	.12	1	18	.39
17	5	.42	3	49	374	.63	0	.04	.05	.8	.04	1	8	.07
22	62	.31	11	169	846	.79	11	.17	.15	1.05	.13	1	5	.14

[1]Values based on products containing added ascorbic acid or sodium ascorbate. If none added, ascorbic acid content would be negligible.

(For purposes of calculations, use "0" for t, <1, <.1, <.01, etc.)

Table A–1
Food Composition

Computer Code Number	Food Description	Measure	Wt (g)	H₂O (%)	Ener (cal)	Prot (g)	Carb (g)	Dietary Fiber (g)	Fat (g)	Fat Breakdown (g)		
										Sat	Mono	Poly
	MEATS: SAUSAGES and LUNCHMEATS (see also Poultry Food Products)—Cont.											
1952	Turkey breast, fat free	1 pce	28	–	25	4	1	0	0	0	0	0
1080	Turkey pastrami	2 pce	57	71	80	10	1	0	4	1	1.2	.9
1969	Turkey salami	1 pce	28	–	45	5	0	0	3	1	–	–
1081	Pepperoni sausage	2 pce	11	27	54	2	<1	0	5	1.8	2.3	.5
1094	Pickle & pimento loaf	2 pce	57	57	149	7	3	<1	12	4.5	5.5	1.5
1082	Polish sausage	1 oz	28	53	92	4	<1	0	8	2.9	3.9	.9
674	Pork sausage, cooked,[1] link, small	2 ea	26	45	96	5	<1	0	8	2.8	3.6	1
1079	Pork sausage, cooked, patty	4 oz	113	45	418	22	1	0	35	12.2	15.8	4.3
675	Salami, pork and beef	2 pce	57	60	143	8	1	0	11	4.6	5.2	1.1
676	Salami, turkey	2 pce	57	66	111	9	<1	0	8	2.3	2.6	2
677	Beef & pork, dry	3 pce	30	35	125	7	1	0	10	3.7	5.1	1
	Sandwich spreads:											
1300	Ham salad spread	1 c	240	63	518	21	26	0	37	12.2	17.3	6.5
678	Pork and beef	2 tbs	30	60	70	2	4	<1	5	1.8	2.3	.8
1296	Chicken/turkey	2 tbs	26	66	52	3	2	0	4	.9	.8	1.6
1084	Smoked link sausage, beef and pork	1 ea	68	52	228	9	1	0	21	7.2	9.7	2.2
1083	Smoked link sausage, pork	1 ea	68	39	265	15	1	0	22	7.7	9.9	2.6
1085	Summer sausage	2 pce	46	51	154	7	<1	0	14	5.5	6	.6
1076	Turkey breakfast sausage	1 pce	28	60	65	6	0	0	5	1.6	1.8	1.2
679	Vienna sausage, canned	2 ea	32	60	89	3	1	0	8	3	4	.5
	MIXED DISHES and FAST FOODS											
	MIXED DISHES:											
1445	Almond chicken	1 c	242	77	275	20	18	4	14	2	5.3	5.8
1981	Baked beans, fat free, honey	½ oz	120	74	110	7	24	7	0	0	0	0
1454	Bean cake	1 ea	32	23	130	2	16	1	7	1	2.9	2.6
680	Beef stew w/ vegetables, homemade	1 c	245	82	218	16	15	2	10	4.9	4.5	.5
1109	Beef stew w/ vegetables, canned	1 c	245	82	194	14	17	2	8	2.4	3.1	.3
1116	Beef, macaroni, tomato sauce casserole	1 c	226	73	284	21	25	3	11	4.2	4.7	.6
2295	Beef fajita	1 ea	189	63	347	15	39	3	15	4.3	6.4	1
1265	Beef flauta	1 ea	113	49	360	17	13	2	27	4.9	11.6	9.1
681	Beef pot pie, homemade[2]	1 pce	210	55	517	21	39	3	31	8.4	14.9	7.4
1898	Broccoli, batter fried	1 c	85	74	123	3	9	2	9	1.3	2.2	4.9
1462	Buffalo wings/spicy chicken wings	2 ea	32	53	98	8	<1	<1	7	1.8	2.8	1.6
1675	Carrot raisin salad	½ c	88	58	202	1	21	3	14	2.1	3.9	7.1
2248	Cheeseburger deluxe	1 ea	219	53	563	28	38	–	33	15	12.6	2
682	Chicken à la king, homemade	1 c	245	68	468	27	12	1	34	12.7	14.3	6.2
683	Chicken & noodles, homemade	1 c	240	71	367	22	26	2	18	5.9	7.1	3.5
684	Chicken chow mein, canned	1 c	250	89	95	6	18	2	1	0	.1	.8
685	Chicken chow mein, homemade	1 c	250	78	255	31	10	1	10	2.4	4.3	3.1
1266	Chicken fajitas	1 ea	223	61	405	22	50	4	13	2.5	6	3.5
1264	Chicken flauta	1 ea	113	53	343	14	13	2	27	4.3	11.1	9.6
686	Chicken pot pie, homemade (⅓)	1 pce	232	57	545	23	42	3	33	10.9	15.5	6.6
1672	Chili con carne	½ c	127	77	128	12	11	2	4	1.7	1.7	.3
1112	Chicken salad with celery	2 c	78	53	268	11	1	<1	25	4	7.2	12.1
1382	Chicken teriyaki, breast	1 pce	128	67	176	26	7	<1	4	.9	1	.9
687	Chili with beans, canned	1 c	255	76	286	15	30	11	14	6	5.9	.9
1479	Chinese pastry	1 oz	28	46	67	1	13	<1	1	.2	.4	.8
688	Chop suey with beef & pork	1 c	250	63	483	26	35	4	25	5.7	9.8	3.9

[1] Cooked weight is half the weight of raw sausage.

[2] Crust made with vegetable shortening and enriched flour.

(Computer code number is for West Diet Analysis program)

PAGE KEY: A–4 = BEV   A–6 = DAIRY   A–12 = EGGS   A–14 = FAT/OIL   A–18 = FRUIT   A–26 = BAKERY   A–36 = GRAIN   A–44 = FISH
A–48 = MEATS   A–50 = POULTRY   A–54 = SAUSAGE   A–56 = MIXED/FAST   A–64 = NUTS/SEEDS   A–68 = SWEETS   A–70 = VEG/LEG
A–84 = MISC   A–88 = SOUPS/SAUCES   A–90 = FAST   A–106 = FRZN ENTREE   A–112 = BABY FOODS

Chol (mg)	Calc (mg)	Iron (mg)	Magn (mg)	Pota (mg)	Sodi (mg)	Zinc (mg)	VT-A (RE)	Thia (mg)	Ribo (mg)	Niac (mg)	V-B6 (mg)	Fola (µg)	VT-C (mg)	VT-E α-TE (mg)
10	0	0	–	–	310	–	0	–	–	–	–	–	0	–
31	5	.95	8	148	595	1.23	0	.03	.14	2.01	.15	3	0	.12
20	0	0	–	–	290	–	0	–	–	–	–	–	0	–
9	1	.15	2	38	224	.27	0	.03	.03	.54	.03	<1	0	.02
21	54	.58	10	194	792	.8	4	.17	.14	1.17	.11	3	8	.14
20	3	.41	4	67	245	.55	0	.14	.04	.97	.05	1	<1	.06
22	8	.32	4	94	336	.65	0	.19	.07	1.18	.09	1	<1	.07
94	36	1.42	19	409	1462	2.84	0	.84	.29	5.13	.37	2	2	.29
37	7	1.51	9	112	607	1.21	0	.14	.21	2.01	.12	1	7³	.13
47	11	.92	9	139	572	1.03	0	.04	.1	2.01	.14	2	0	.33
24	2	.45	5	113	558	.97	0	.18	.09	1.46	.15	1	8³	.08
89	19	1.42	24	360	2188	2.64	0	1.04	.29	5.04	.36	2	14	4.18
11	4	.24	2	33	304	.31	3	.05	.04	.52	.04	1	0	.52
8	3	.16	3	48	98	.27	11	.01	.02	.43	.03	1	<1	.57
48	7	.99	8	128	642	1.43	0	.18	.12	2.19	.12	1	13	.15
46	20	.79	13	228	1020	1.92	0	.48	.17	3.08	.24	3	1	.17
33	6	1.17	6	125	571	1.18	0	.07	.15	1.98	.12	1	9	.1
23	5	.52	6	76	188	.97	0	.03	.08	1.42	.08	1	0	.14
17	3	.28	2	32	304	.51	0	.03	.03	.51	.04	1	0	.07
35	81	2.12	59	550	615	1.56	75	.08	.19	8.59	.4	31	10	2.64
0	40	2.7	–	–	135	–	–	–	–	–	–	–	12	–
0	3	.65	6	56	55	.15	0	.06	.04	.49	.02	9	0	1.14
64	29	2.94	40	613	292	5.29	568	.15	.17	4.66	.28	37	17	.49
34	29	2.21	39	426	1006	4.24	262	.07	.12	2.45	.2	31	7	.34
57	28	3.11	42	559	841	4.3	93	.23	.25	5.22	.33	22	13	.51
22	64	3	32	362	721	2	44	.3	.26	4	.27	21	24	1.77
45	50	2.15	29	292	187	4.18	15	.07	.15	2.13	.25	10	14	4.01
44	29	3.78	6	334	596	3.17	519	.29	.29	4.83	.24	29	6	3.78
16	67	.94	20	242	62	.38	102	.08	.13	.75	.11	43	53	2.1
26	5	.4	6	59	61	.56	17	.01	.04	2.06	.13	1	<1	.24
10	26	.74	14	317	117	.18	1462	.08	.05	.63	.22	9	5	4.94
88	206	4.69	44	445	1108	5	129	.39	.46	7.4	.29	29	8	1.18
186	127	2.45	20	404	760	1.8	272	.1	.42	5.39	.23	11	12	.98
96	26	2.16	26	149	600	1.53	10	.05	.17	4.32	.19	10	0	–
8	45	1.25	14	418	725	1.3	28	.05	.1	1	.09	12	12	.05
78	57	2.5	28	473	718	2.12	50	.07	.22	4.25	.41	19	10	.75
41	83	3.7	51	532	439	1.77	56	.48	.37	6.6	.35	41	22	2.05
37	52	.97	28	243	189	1.18	21	.05	.1	3.21	.22	8	14	4.05
72	70	3.02	25	343	594	2	735	.32	.32	4.87	.46	29	5	3.25
67	34	2.62	23	347	506	1.8	84	.06	.57	1.25	.17	15	<1	.81
47	16	.62	11	138	201	.8	31	.03	.07	3.27	.34	8	1	7.52
80	27	1.75	36	309	1866	1.94	16	.08	.2	8.69	.46	13	3	.35
43	120	8.75	115	931	1331	5.1	87	.12	.27	.91	.34	58	4	1.87
0	7	.55	6	28	3	.2	<1	.04	<.01	.35	.02	1	0	.254
52	44	4.45	61	586	930	3.9	152	.42	.42	6.4	.47	50	23	2.07

(3)Values based on products containing added ascorbic acid or sodium ascorbate. If none added, ascorbic acid content would be negligible.

(For purposes of calculations, use "0" for t, <1, <.1, <.01, etc.)

Table A–1
Food Composition

Computer Code Number	Food Description	Measure	Wt (g)	H$_2$O (%)	Ener (cal)	Prot (g)	Carb (g)	Dietary Fiber (g)	Fat (g)	Fat Breakdown (g)		
										Sat	Mono	Poly
	MIXED DISHES and FAST FOOD—Cont.											
	MIXED DISHES—Cont.											
690	Coleslaw[1]	1 c	120	74	178	2	15	2	13	2	2.9	7.7
689	Corn pudding[2]	1 c	250	76	273	11	32	4	13	6.3	4.3	1.7
1110	Corned beef hash, canned	1 c	220	67	398	19	24	1	25	11.9	10.9	.9
1255	Deviled egg (½ egg + filling)	1 ea	31	69	63	4	<1	0	5	1.24	1.7	1.5
	Egg foo yung patty:											
1467	Meatless	1 ea	86	94	26	3	<1	0	1	.4	.5	.2
1458	With beef	1 ea	86	74	129	9	3	<1	9	2.2	3.2	2.4
1465	With chicken	1 ea	86	74	130	9	4	<1	9	2.1	3.1	2.5
1602	Egg roll, meatless	1 ea	64	70	101	3	10	1	6	1.2	2.5	1.6
1550	Egg roll, with meat	1 ea	64	66	114	5	9	1	6	1.6	2.9	1.6
1113	Egg salad	1 c	183	57	586	17	3	0	56	10.6	17.5	24.2
691	French toast w/wheat bread, homemade[3]	1 pce	65	54	151	5	16	<1	7	2	3	1.7
1355	Green pepper, stuffed	1 ea	172	74	236	11	20	2	12	5.3	5.3	.6
1487	Hot & sour soup (Chinese)	1 c	244	88	133	12	5	<1	6	2	2.9	1.2
2242	Hamburger deluxe	1 ea	110	49	279	13	27	–	14	4.1	5.3	2.6
1997	Hummous/hummus	¼ c	62	64	105	3	12	2	5	.8	2.2	2
	Lasagna:											
1346	With meat, homemade	1 pce	245	66	382	22	39	3	15	7.7	5	.8
1111	Without meat, homemade	1 pce	218	68	298	15	39	3	9	5.4	2.4	.6
1117	Frozen entree	1 pce	205	74	235	15	25	3	9	4	3.3	.5
1606	Lo mein, meatless	1 c	200	83	123	6	23	3	1	.3	.3	.4
1607	Lo mein, with meat	1 c	200	71	284	16	27	3	13	2.9	4.2	4.7
692	Macaroni & cheese, canned[4]	1 c	240	80	228	9	26	1	10	4.2	3.1	1.4
693	Macaroni & cheese, homemade[5]	1 c	200	58	430	17	40	1	22	8.9	8.8	3.6
1115	Macaroni salad, no cheese	1 c	141	60	363	3	21	3	30	4.4	8.5	15.5
1120	Meat loaf, beef	1 pce	87	62	185	14	5	<1	11	4	4.8	.6
1119	Meat loaf, beef and pork (⅓)	1 pce	87	57	221	17	4	<1	15	5.4	6.4	1.2
1303	Moussaka (lamb & eggplant)	1 c	250	83	209	18	14	3	9	2.7	3.7	1.5
1899	Mushrooms, batter fried	5 ea	70	66	148	2	8	1	12	2.1	3	6.4
715	Potato salad with mayonnaise and eggs[6]	½ c	125	76	179	3	14	2	10	1.8	3.1	4.7
1674	Pizza, combination, ½ of 12" round	1 pce	53	48	123	9	14	–	4	1	1.7	.6
1673	Pizza, pepperoni, ½ of 12" round	1 pce	47	46	121	7	13	–	5	1.5	2.1	.8
694	Quiche Lorraine, ⅛ of 8" quiche[7]	1 pce	176	54	508	20	20	1	39	18	13.8	4.9
1449	Ramen noodles, cooked	1 c	227	83	156	5	29	3	2	.4	.4	.4
1671	Ravioli, meat	½ c	125	68	194	11	18	1	9	3	3.6	1
1597	Fried rice (meatless)	1 c	166	68	264	5	34	1	11	1.7	2.9	6.2
2142	Roast beef hash	½ c	95	68	158	11	10	1	8	2.5	2.9	1.7
	Spaghetti (enriched) in tomato sauce:											
	With cheese:											
695	Canned	1 c	250	80	190	5	38	2	1	0	.4	.5
696	Homemade	1 c	250	77	260	9	37	2	9	2	5.4	1.2

[1]Recipe: 41% cabbage; 12% celery; 12% table cream; 12% sugar; 7% green pepper; 6% lemon juice; 4% onion; 3% pimento; 3% vinegar; 2% each for salt, dry mustard, and white pepper.
[2]Recipe: 55% yellow corn, 23% whole milk, 14% egg, 4% sugar, 3% salt, and 1% pepper.
[3]Recipe: 35% whole milk, 32% white bread, 29% egg, and cooked in 4% margarine.
[4]Made with corn oil.
[5]Made with margarine.
[6]Recipe: 62% potatoes; 12% egg; 8% mayonnaise; 7% celery; 6% sweet pickle relish; 2% onion; 1% each for green pepper, pimento, salt, and dry mustard.
[7]Crust made with vegetable shortening and enriched flour.

(Computer code number is for West Diet Analysis program)

PAGE KEY: A–4 = BEV   A–6 = DAIRY   A–12 = EGGS   A–14 = FAT/OIL   A–18 = FRUIT   A–26 = BAKERY   A–36 = GRAIN   A–44 = FISH
A–48 = MEATS   A–50 = POULTRY   A–54 = SAUSAGE   A–56 = MIXED/FAST   A–64 = NUTS/SEEDS   A–68 = SWEETS   A–70 = VEG/LEG
A–84 = MISC   A–88 = SOUPS/SAUCES   A–90 = FAST   A–106 = FRZN ENTREE   A–112 = BABY FOODS

Chol (mg)	Calc (mg)	Iron (mg)	Magn (mg)	Pota (mg)	Sodi (mg)	Zinc (mg)	VT-A (RE)	Thia (mg)	Ribo (mg)	Niac (mg)	V-B6 (mg)	Fola (μg)	VT-C (mg)	VT-E α-TE (mg)
6[8]	41	.88	11	215	324	.24	60	.05	.04	.1	.13	47	10	4.8
250	100	1.4	37	403	138	1.25	90	1.03	.32	2.47	.29	63	7	.53
73	29	4.4	36	440	1188	3.3	0	.02	.2	4.62	.43	20	0	.48
121	15	.35	3	37	94	.3	49	.02	.14	.02	.05	13	0	.86
37	7	.26	2	77	257	.17	14	.01	.07	1.07	.02	5	0	1.57
180	26	1.1	11	143	185	1.16	92	.05	.24	.73	.16	22	3	1.79
182	28	.85	12	143	188	.81	95	.05	.24	.95	.13	22	3	1.87
30	12	.74	9	97	307	.25	15	.07	.1	.75	.05	13	3	.81
38	12	.77	10	124	305	.5	14	.13	.12	1.31	.09	8	2	.79
574	74	1.8	13	180	666	1.44	262	.08	.66	.08	.47	61	0	8.87
76	64	1.09	11	86	311	.44	81	.13	.21	1.06	.05	15	<1	.31
38	17	1.88	20	230	203	2.2	44	.14	.09	2.91	.31	17	55	.77
22	29	1.87	27	351	1562	1.15	2	.19	.22	4.56	.15	12	1	.12
26	63	2.64	22	227	504	2	9	.23	.2	3.7	.12	18.7	2	.83
0	31	.97	18	107	150	.68	2	.06	.03	.25	.24	37	5	.62
56	258	3.43	50	461	745	3.19	158	.21	.33	4	.21	19	16	1.15
31	252	2.5	44	375	714	1.7	156	.2	.28	2.49	.17	17	15	1.07
33	158	2.17	39	453	496	2.19	149	.16	.24	3.06	.19	17	25	2.08
22	48	2.18	30	396	624	.91	163	.18	.23	2.48	.18	41	13	.35
61	25	2.2	34	260	276	1.85	38	.42	.27	3.4	.26	39	9	1.51
24	199	.96	31	139	730	1.2	73	.12	.24	.96	.02	8	<1	.15
42	362	1.8	37	240	1086	1.2	234	.2	.4	1.8	.05	10	1	.13
22	27	.67	16	137	289	.38	39	.08	.05	.75	.26	16	3	10.1
72	35	1.61	18	236	329	2.92	14	.07	.22	3.36	.11	10	1	.32
91	35	1.55	16	236	389	3.12	23	.2	.22	3.18	.19	11	1	.33
101	104	2.2	38	578	400	2.84	105	.21	.31	4.01	.26	45	6	.88
14	54	.77	8	180	121	.423	10	.07	.22	1.65	.05	8	1	.92
85	24	.81	19	318	661	.39	41	.1	.07	1.11	.18	8	13	.233
14	68	1.03	12	119	255	.75	68	.14	.12	1.31	.06	18	1	–
10	43	.63	6	102	178	.35	36	.09	.16	2.04	.04	35	1	–
205	201	1.9	27	271	549	1.48	243	.22	.45	4.71	.1	17	3	1.91
38	20	1.78	24	51	1349	.61	204	.22	.09	1.42	.07	8	<1	.09
84	33	1.99	20	259	619	1.67	94	.13	.20	2.85	.15	13	11	–
42	30	1.84	24	134	286	.84	62	.21	.11	2.25	.1	22	4	2.46
29	10	1.24	18	294	427	2.43	<1	.08	.1	1.89	.25	10	4	–
8	40	2.75	21	303	955	1.12	120	.35	.27	4.5	.13	6	10	2.12
8	80	2.25	26	408	955	1.3	140	.25	.17	2.25	.2	8	12	2.75

[8]From dairy cream in recipe.

(For purposes of calculations, use "0" for t, <1, <.1, <.01, etc.)

Table A–1
Food Composition

Computer Code Number	Food Description	Measure	Wt (g)	H$_2$O (%)	Ener (cal)	Prot (g)	Carb (g)	Dietary Fiber (g)	Fat (g)	Fat Breakdown (g) Sat	Mono	Poly
	MIXED DISHES and FAST FOODS—Cont.											
	MIXED DISHES—Cont.											
	With meatballs:											
697	Canned	1 c	250	78	258	12	28	6	10	2.1	3.9	3.9
698	Homemade	1 c	248	70	332	19	39	8	12	3.3	6.3	2.2
716	Spinach soufflé[1]	1 c	136	74	219	11	3	4	18	7.1	6.8	3.1
1553	Sweet & sour pork	1 c	226	76	231	14	25	1	8	2.8	3.8	2.9
1263	Sweet & sour chicken breast	1 ea	131	79	117	8	15	1	3	.6	.8	1.5
1515	Three bean salad	1 ea	340	82	316	9	30	7	19	2.8	4.3	11.1
717	Tuna salad[2]	1 c	205	63	383	33	19	1	19	3.2	5.9	8.4
1121	Tuna noodle casserole, homemade	1 c	202	75	238	17	25	2	7	1.9	1.5	3.2
1270	Waldorf salad	1 c	142	59	411	3	13	2	41	5.4	10.9	22.2
	FAST FOODS and SANDWICHES (see end of this appendix for additional Fast Foods):											
699	Burrito,[3] beef & bean	1 ea	175	52	385	17	50	4	14	6.3	5.3	.9
700	Burrito, bean	1 ea	174	53	358	11	57	7	11	5.5	3.8	1
2106	Burrito, chicken con queso	1 ea	306	77	280	12	53	5	6	1.5	–	–
701	Cheeseburger with bun, regular	1 ea	112	55	261	13	20	–	14	6.7	5.2	1.1
702	Cheeseburger with bun, 4-oz patty	1 ea	194	51	487	25	41	–	25	10.2	9.1	3.1
703	Chicken patty sandwich	1 ea	157	47	444	21	33	1	25	7.4	9	7.2
704	Corndog	1 ea	111	47	292	11	35	–	12	3.3	5.8	2.2
1922	Corndog, chicken	1 ea	113	59	272	13	26	–	13	–	–	–
705	Enchilada	1 ea	230	63	451	14	40	–	27	15	8.9	1.1
706	English muffin with egg, cheese, bacon	1 ea	138	49	362	19	30	1	19	8.6	6.4	1.9
	Fish sandwich:											
707	Regular, with cheese	1 ea	140	45	400	16	36	<1	22	6.2	6.8	7.2
708	Large, no cheese	1 ea	170	47	464	18	44	<1	24	5.6	8.3	8.9
709	Hamburger with bun, regular	1 ea	98	45	252	12	30	1	9	3.2	3.4	1.6
710	Hamburger with bun, 4-oz patty	1 ea	174	51	466	26	31	–	26	9.7	11.4	2.2
711	Hot dog/frankfurter with bun	1 ea	85	54	210	9	16	–	13	4.4	5.9	1.5
	Lunchables:											
2129	Bologna & American cheese	1 ea	128	–	450	18	19	0	34	15	–	–
2130	Ham & cheese	1 ea	128	–	320	22	19	0	17	8	–	–
2117	Honey ham & Amer. w/choc pudding	1 ea	176	–	390	18	34	1	20	9	–	–
2118	Honey turkey & cheddar w/Jello	1 ea	163	–	320	17	27	1	16	9	–	–
2131	Pepperoni & American cheese	1 ea	128	–	480	20	19	0	36	17	–	–
2125	Salami & American cheese	1 ea	128	–	430	18	18	0	32	15	–	–
2127	Turkey & cheddar cheese	1 ea	128	–	360	20	20	1	22	11	–	–
712	Pizza, cheese, ⅛ of 15" round[4]	1 pce	120	49	268	15	39	2	6	2.9	1.9	.9
	SANDWICHES:											
	Avocado, cheese, tomato, & lettuce:											
1276	On white bread, firm	1 ea	205	57	489	15	40	4	32	9	12.7	8
1278	On part whole wheat	1 ea	195	58	454	14	33	5	31	9	12.6	8
1277	On whole wheat	1 ea	209	57	481	16	39	7	32	9	12.9	8

[1] Recipe: 29% whole milk, 26% spinach, 13% egg white, 13% cheddar cheese, 7% egg yolk, 7% butter, 4% flour, 1% salt and pepper.

[2] Made with drained chunk light tuna, celery, onion, pickle relish, and mayonnaise-type salad dressing.

[3] Made with a 10½"-diameter flour tortilla.

[4] Crust made with vegetable shortening and enriched flour.

(Computer code number is for West Diet Analysis program)

PAGE KEY: A–4 = BEV   A–6 = DAIRY   A–12 = EGGS   A–14 = FAT/OIL   A–18 = FRUIT   A–26 = BAKERY   A–36 = GRAIN   A–44 = FISH
A–48 = MEATS   A–50 = POULTRY   A–54 = SAUSAGE   A–56 = MIXED/FAST   A–64 = NUTS/SEEDS   A–68 = SWEETS   A–70 = VEG/LEG
A–84 = MISC   A–88 = SOUPS/SAUCES   A–90 = FAST   A–106 = FRZN ENTREE   A–112 = BABY FOODS

Chol (mg)	Calc (mg)	Iron (mg)	Magn (mg)	Pota (mg)	Sodi (mg)	Zinc (mg)	VT-A (RE)	Thia (mg)	Ribo (mg)	Niac (mg)	V-B6 (mg)	Fola (μg)	VT-C (mg)	VT-E α-TE (mg)
22	52	3.25	20	245	1220	2.39	100	.15	.17	2.25	.12	5	5	1.5
74	124	3.72	40	665	1009	2.45	159	.25	.3	3.97	.2	10	22	1.64
184	230	1.35	38	201	763	1.29	676	.09	.3	.48	.12	62	3	1.22
38	28	1.49	34	390	1220	1.7	27	.55	.22	3.62	.35	11	23	.62
23	16	.8	21	187	732	.66	20	.06	.08	3.06	.18	6	12	.4
0	80	3.21	57	508	1164	1.22	52	.16	.21	.91	.1	120	10	4.43
27	35	2.05	39	365	824	1.15	55	.06	.14	13.7	.17	15	5	1.95
41	34	2.3	31	182	775	1.21	13	.18	.15	7.81	.2	10	1	1.19
22	42	.85	36	268	250	.59	41	.09	.05	.35	.37	27	6	10.8
37	80	3.71	63	497	1011	2.91	49	.4	.63	4.1	.28	56	1	1.05
3	90	3.62	70	524	790	1.22	26	.5	.49	3.25	.24	94	2	1.39
10	40	.72	–	–	600	–	40	–	–	–	–	–	15	–
38	132	1.93	19	167	710	1.9	51	.23	.17	4.64	.11	16	2	.97
70	200	4	35	392	1228	4.07	76	.41	.33	9.41	.21	27	2	–
52	52	4.03	30	305	826	1.62	27	.28	.2	5.87	.17	25	8	.47
50	64	3.92	11	167	617	.83	23	.18	.44	2.64	.06	38	0	.44
65	–	–	–	–	670	–	–	–	–	–	–	–	–	–
62	458	1.86	71	338	1106	3.54	262	.11	.6	2.69	.55	48	1	2.07
221	196	3.11	32	201	741	1.71	149	.45	.5	3.71	.15	41	1	.57
52	141	2.67	28	270	718	.9	74	.35	.32	3.23	.08	24	2	1.4
60	90	2.81	36	366	661	1.07	32	.36	.24	3.66	.12	48	3	.94
39	47	2.25	21	197	516	1.88	12	.23	.29	4.3	.12	16	2	.39
84	75	4.49	37	426	600	4.7	3	.28	.33	5.45	.3	37	1	1.31
38	20	2.01	11	124	581	1.72	0	.2	.24	3.16	.04	26	<1	.24
85	300	2.7	–	–	1620	–	60	–	–	–	–	–	0	–
60	300	1.8	–	–	1770	–	80	–	–	–	–	–	–	–
55	250	2.7	–	–	1540	–	–	–	–	–	–	–	–	–
50	20	6	–	–	1360	–	–	–	–	–	–	–	–	–
95	250	2.7	–	–	1840	–	–	–	–	–	–	–	–	–
80	250	2.7	–	–	1740	–	60	–	–	–	–	–	–	–
70	300	1.8	–	–	1650	–	60	–	–	–	–	–	–	–
18	222	1.1	30	209	640	1.56	140	.35	.31	4.73	.08	112	2	.55
35	282	2.98	52	554	552	1.67	146	.36	.38	3.59	.3	77	11	5.26
32	277	3.01	64	584	525	1.85	136	.33	.37	3.73	.36	76	11	5.22
33	269	3.45	97	648	594	2.63	137	.34	.36	4.18	.41	88	11	4.89

(For purposes of calculations, use "0" for t, <1, <.1, <.01, etc.)

Table A–1
Food Composition

Computer Code Number	Food Description	Measure	Wt (g)	H$_2$O (%)	Ener (cal)	Prot (g)	Carb (g)	Dietary Fiber (g)	Fat (g)	Fat Breakdown (g)		
										Sat	Mono	Poly
	FAST FOODS and SANDWICHES (see end of this appendix for additional Fast Foods)—Cont.											
	SANDWICHES—Cont.											
	Bacon, lettuce & tomato:											
1137	On white bread, soft	1 ea	135	46	401	12	34	2	24	6	9	8
1139	On part whole wheat	1 ea	136	47	398	13	32	3	25	6	9.5	8
1138	On whole wheat	1 ea	149	47	421	14	37	6	26	6	9.6	8
	Cheese, grilled:											
1140	On white bread, soft	1 ea	117	37	393	17	29	1	23	12.2	7.6	2.1
1142	On part whole wheat	1 ea	117	37	389	18	27	2	24	12.3	7.7	2.2
1141	On whole wheat	1 ea	131	38	416	19	33	5	24	12.5	8	2.4
1596	Chicken fillet	1 ea	182	47	515	24	39	1	29	8.5	10.4	8.4
	Chicken salad:											
1143	On white bread, soft	1 ea	105	39	371	10	28	1	24	4	7.3	12
1145	On part whole wheat	1 ea	105	40	366	10	27	2	25	4	7	12
1144	On whole wheat	1 ea	118	40	389	12	32	5	25	4	7.6	12
1146	Corned beef & swiss on rye	1 ea	147	45	457	28	25	3	28	9.8	9	6.4
	Egg salad:											
1147	On white bread, soft	1 ea	111	42	380	9	29	1	26	4.5	8	11.8
1149	On part whole wheat	1 ea	111	42	375	9	27	2	26	4.5	8	11.8
1148	On whole wheat	1 ea	125	42	403	11	33	5	27	4.7	8	12
	Ham:											
1279	On rye bread	1 ea	116	56	241	16	20	3	10	2.2	3.8	3.6
1151	On white bread, soft	1 ea	122	55	260	17	23	1	11	2.3	4.1	3.6
1153	On part whole wheat	1 ea	122	55	257	17	22	2	11	2.3	4.1	3.7
1152	On whole wheat	1 ea	136	54	284	19	27	4	12	2.5	4.4	3.9
	Ham & cheese:											
1280	On white bread, soft	1 ea	151	49	388	21	29	1	20	7.8	6.8	4.6
1282	On part whole wheat	1 ea	151	50	384	22	27	3	21	7.8	6.9	4.7
1281	On whole wheat	1 ea	165	49	411	24	33	5	22	8	7.1	4.9
1150	Ham & swiss on rye	1 ea	145	50	368	23	25	3	19	7.2	6.2	4.6
	Ham salad:											
1154	On white bread, soft	1 ea	125	46	365	10	34	1	21	5	8	7.5
1156	On part whole wheat	1 ea	125	46	360	10	33	2	22	5	8	7.5
1155	On whole wheat	1 ea	139	46	387	12	38	5	22	5	8	7.8
1157	Patty melt: Ground beef & cheese on rye	1 ea	177	42	600	36	24	3	40	13.8	14.5	7.9
	Peanut butter & jelly:											
1158	On white bread, soft	1 ea	100	27	345	10	47	3	14	2.7	6.6	3.9
1160	On part whole wheat	1 ea	100	27	341	11	46	4	14	2.8	6.6	4
1159	On whole wheat	1 ea	114	28	368	13	51	7	15	2.9	6.9	4.2
1161	Reuben, grilled: Corned beef, swiss cheese, sauerkraut on rye	1 ea	233	51	639	29	40	5	40	13.7	12.8	9.7
	Roast beef:											
713	On a bun	1 ea	150	49	374	23	36	–	15	3.9	7.3	1.8
1162	On white bread, soft	1 ea	122	46	315	23	27	1	13	2.7	4.3	4.9
1164	On part whole wheat	1 ea	122	47	311	23	25	2	13	2.8	4.3	5
1163	On whole wheat	1 ea	136	46	339	25	30	4	14	3	4.6	5.3
	Tuna salad:											
1165	On white bread, soft	1 ea	116	45	331	13	32	2	17	3	5	8
1167	On part whole wheat	1 ea	116	46	326	13	30	3	17	3	5	8

(Computer code number is for West Diet Analysis program)

PAGE KEY: A–4 = BEV   A–6 = DAIRY   A–12 = EGGS   A–14 = FAT/OIL   A–18 = FRUIT   A–26 = BAKERY   A–36 = GRAIN   A–44 = FISH
A–48 = MEATS   A–50 = POULTRY   A–54 = SAUSAGE   A–56 = MIXED/FAST   A–64 = NUTS/SEEDS   A–68 = SWEETS   A–70 = VEG/LEG
A–84 = MISC   A–88 = SOUPS/SAUCES   A–90 = FAST   A–106 = FRZN ENTREE   A–112 = BABY FOODS

Chol (mg)	Calc (mg)	Iron (mg)	Magn (mg)	Pota (mg)	Sodi (mg)	Zinc (mg)	VT-A (RE)	Thia (mg)	Ribo (mg)	Niac (mg)	V-B6 (mg)	Fola (μg)	VT-C (mg)	VT-E α-TE (mg)
28	60	2.33	22	252	731	1.16	35	.4	.23	3.8	.19	31	13	4.37
27	73	2.6	38	313	753	1.43	35	.4	.25	4.3	.23	35	14	4.84
26	62	3.18	75	378	818	2.29	35	.4	.23	4.6	.29	47	13	4.38
55	393	1.79	26	152	1129	2.03	209	.28	.39	2.27	.08	24	<1	1.17
53	405	2.08	38	206	1143	2.27	209	.25	.36	2.35	.09	27	<1	1.56
53	398	2.53	73	269	1219	3.05	211	.26	.34	2.72	.16	39	<1	1.2
60	60	4.68	35	353	957	1.87	31	.33	.24	6.81	.2	29	9	–
32	56	1.98	17	129	447	.73	26	.23	.17	3.36	.25	24	<1	7.21
31	67	2.13	30	181	461	.98	26	.24	.18	3.78	.29	27	<1	7.59
31	58	2.58	63	240	526	1.72	26	.25	.17	4.17	.34	39	<1	7.26
79	307	2.75	39	193	1064	3.69	80	.23	.35	3.26	.19	32	1	3.93
147	65	2.21	15	106	507	.69	73	.24	.29	1.82	.2	34	0	7.31
146	77	2.36	29	161	521	.93	73	.26	.32	2.25	.24	38	0	7.68
147	69	2.81	61	217	592	1.68	74	.27	.31	2.61	.3	49	0	7.41
35	38	1.72	29	303	1289	1.76	6	.78	.28	4.66	.38	23	17	2.21
36	47	1.86	24	287	1263	1.59	6	.8	.25	4.67	.36	19	17	2.25
35	56	2.09	34	329	1274	1.79	6	.8	.27	5.03	.39	21	17	2.56
36	50	2.5	62	389	1364	2.45	6	.83	.27	5.45	.46	31	18	2.33
59	224	2.2	29	304	1564	2.26	87	.78	.35	4.47	.34	24	14	2.94
57	236	2.49	43	356	1578	2.5	87	.75	.37	4.92	.38	27	14	3.32
57	228	2.93	77	419	1655	3.27	88	.76	.36	5.29	.45	39	14	2.98
56	309	1.99	41	313	1289	2.74	77	.73	.38	4.52	.37	29	14	2.89
31	53	1.93	17	148	872	.98	11	.47	.26	3	.18	20	3	4.61
29	64	2.2	31	200	886	1.22	11	.48	.23	3.45	.2	24	3	4.98
28	57	2.65	64	262	961	1.98	11	.49	.21	3.82	.29	36	3	4.67
116	219	3.76	43	369	895	6.79	137	.28	.47	6.39	.35	39	<1	4.62
2	61	2.23	51	256	290	1.02	<1	.3	.17	5.17	.13	43	<1	2.06
0	73	2.52	65	309	305	1.26	<1	.27	.19	5.63	.17	47	<1	2.45
0	64	2.97	99	374	375	2.04	<1	.28	.18	6.03	.24	59	<1	2.09
114	411	3.68	47	318	1685	5.44	130	.25	.41	4	.3	39	15	5.32
55	58	4.56	33	341	855	3.66	22	.4	.33	6.33	.28	43	2	.21
34	47	3.21	23	335	1243	2.95	9	.26	.28	5	.32	23	10	3.08
34	56	3.33	33	377	1254	3.14	9	.24	.25	5.36	.33	26	10	3.39
34	50	3.77	61	438	1343	3.85	9	.25	.25	5.78	.4	36	10	3.18
16	56	2	21	149	543	.62	24	.23	.17	5	.13	23	1	4.06
14	67	2.35	34	200	557	.86	24	.25	.19	5	.17	27	1	4.43

(For purposes of calculations, use "0" for t, <1, <.1, <.01, etc.)

Table A–1
Food Composition

Computer Code Number	Food Description	Measure	Wt (g)	H$_2$O (%)	Ener (cal)	Prot (g)	Carb (g)	Dietary Fiber (g)	Fat (g)	Fat Breakdown (g) Sat	Mono	Poly
	FAST FOODS and SANDWICHES (see end of this appendix for additional Fast Foods)—Cont.											
1166	On whole wheat	1 ea	130	45	353	15	36	5	18	3	5	8
	Turkey:											
1168	On white bread, soft	1 ea	122	54	270	19	22	1	11	2	3.5	5
1170	On part whole wheat	1 ea	122	54	267	19	21	2	11	2	3.5	5
1169	On whole wheat	1 ea	136	53	294	21	26	4	12	2.2	3.8	5.3
	Turkey ham:											
1272	On rye bread	1 ea	116	57	239	16	19	3	10	2.2	3.1	4.3
1273	On white bread, soft	1 ea	122	55	259	17	23	1	11	2.3	3.3	4.4
1275	On part whole wheat	1 ea	122	56	255	17	22	2	11	2.4	3.3	4.4
1274	On whole wheat	1 ea	136	55	282	19	27	4	12	2.6	3.6	4.7
714	Taco	1 ea	78	58	168	9	12	–	9	5.2	3	.4
	Tostada:											
1114	With refried beans	1 ea	157	66	243	10	29	8	11	5.9	3.3	.8
1118	With beans & beef	1 ea	192	70	284	14	25	3	14	9.8	3	.5
1354	With beans & chicken	1 ea	157	67	253	19	19	3	11	4.5	4.4	1.6
	Vegetarian foods:											
1511	Baked beans, canned	½ c	127	73	118	6	26	6	1	.1	t	.2
1175	Breakfast links	1 ea	34	50	87	6	3	1	6	1	2	3.2
1171	Nuteena	1 pce	67	58	160	8	5	2	12	1.7	4.6	3.7
1173	Redi-burger	1 pce	68	57	130	14	5	1	6	.7	1.3	3.3
1174	Vege-burger	½ c	108	73	110	22	4	1	1	.1	.1	.4
	Vegetarian foods, Worthington											
1854	Burger, no salt added	½ c	113	–	150	22	7	–	4	–	–	–
1846	Chik slices, canned	2 pce	60	–	90	4	2	–	8	–	–	–
1833	Chili, canned	½ c	106	–	144	8	11	–	8	–	–	–
1835	Choplets, canned slices	2 pce	92	–	100	18	4	–	2	–	–	–
1831	Country stew, canned	1 ea	269	–	219	1	23	–	10	–	–	–
1836	Non-meat balls, canned	3 ea	54	–	100	6	5	–	6	–	–	–
1838	Numete, canned slices	1 pce	68	–	150	7	7	–	11	–	–	–
1839	Prime stakes, canned	1 pce	92	–	160	10	7	–	10	–	–	–
1840	Protose, canned slices	1 pce	76	–	180	17	9	–	8	–	–	–
1842	Saucettes, canned links	2 pce	67	–	150	10	3	–	11	–	–	–
1844	Savory slices, canned	2 pce	56	–	100	8	4	–	6	–	–	–
1849	Skallops, no salt added, canned	½ c	85	–	80	13	4	–	1	–	–	–
1847	Turkee slices, canned	2 pce	63	–	130	9	3	–	9	–	–	–
	NUTS, SEEDS, and PRODUCTS											
	Almonds:											
1365	Dry roasted, salted	1 c	138	3	810	22	33	14	71	6.7	46.2	14.9
718	Slivered, packed, unsalted	1 c	135	4	795	27	27	13[1]	70	6.7	45.8	14.9
719	Whole, dried, unsalted:	1 c	142	4	836	28	29	13[1]	74	7	48.1	15.6
720	Ounce	1 oz	28	4	165	6	6	3[1]	15	1.4	9.6	3.1
721	Almond butter	1 tbs	16	1	101	2	3	1	9	.9	6.1	2
722	Brazil nuts, dry (about 7)	1 oz	28	3	184	4	4	2	19	4.6	6.5	6.8
	Cashew nuts, salted:											
723	Dry roasted:	1 c	137	2	786	21	45	4	64	12.5	37.4	10.7
724	Ounce	1 oz	28	2	161	4	9	1	13	2.6	7.7	2.2

[1]Values reported for dietary fiber in almonds vary from 7.0 to 14.3 g/100 g.

(Computer code number is for West Diet Analysis program)

PAGE KEY: A–4 = BEV   A–6 = DAIRY   A–12 = EGGS   A–14 = FAT/OIL   A–18 = FRUIT   A–26 = BAKERY   A–36 = GRAIN   A–44 = FISH
A–48 = MEATS   A–50 = POULTRY   A–54 = SAUSAGE   A–56 = MIXED/FAST   A–64 = NUTS/SEEDS   A–68 = SWEETS   A–70 = VEG/LEG
A–84 = MISC   A–88 = SOUPS/SAUCES   A–90 = FAST   A–106 = FRZN ENTREE   A–112 = BABY FOODS

Chol (mg)	Calc (mg)	Iron (mg)	Magn (mg)	Pota (mg)	Sodi (mg)	Zinc (mg)	VT-A (RE)	Thia (mg)	Ribo (mg)	Niac (mg)	V-B6 (mg)	Fola (µg)	VT-C (mg)	VT-E α-TE (mg)
14	59	2.79	67	262	629	1.66	24	.26	.18	6	.22	39	1	4.12
34	44	1.57	24	236	1238	1.05	9	.2	.18	7	.33	19	0	3.21
34	53	1.8	34	279	1249	1.24	9	.21	.19	7.39	.35	22	0	3.52
35	47	2.19	62	336	1339	1.89	9	.22	.19	7.88	.41	32	0	3.31
41	40	3.03	28	287	1004	2.43	6	.2	.29	3.81	.23	24	0	2.45
43	49	3.29	23	271	976	2.27	6	.21	.27	3.81	.23	20	0	2.49
41	58	3.42	33	313	987	2.46	6	.22	.29	4.17	.25	23	0	2.79
43	52	3.86	61	371	1069	3.15	6	.23	.28	4.57	.31	33	0	2.57
26	101	1.1	32	216	366	1.79	67	.07	.2	1.47	.11	11	1	.86
33	229	2.06	64	440	592	2.07	93	.11	.36	1.44	.17	82	1	1.26
63	161	2.09	58	419	743	2.71	148	.08	.42	2.44	.21	83	3	1.54
53	171	1.81	49	367	435	2.29	87	.11	.2	4.49	.32	54	3	1.89
0	63	.37	41	376	504	1.78	22	.19	.08	.54	.17	30	4	.673
0	21	1.27	12	79	302	.5	22	.8	.14	3.8	.2	9	0	–
0	21	1.2	40	200	120	.87	10	.47	.58	.14	.45	60	<1	–
0	19	1.4	13	120	370	1.2	10	.6	.4	6.7	.8	17	<1	–
0	32	2.7	24	110	190	1.1	10	.53	.68	5	.56	27	<1	–
–	–	1.8	–	40	170	–	–	.3	.1	8	.5	–	–	–
–	–	.72	–	20	330	–	–	.03	.34	.8	.12	–	–	–
–	–	.82	–	136	417	–	–	.11	.05	3.79	.15	–	–	–
–	–	.36	–	10	440	–	–	–	–	–	–	–	–	–
–	40	2.69	–	299	758	–	–	.38	.03	7.98	.3	–	–	–
–	20	.72	–	30	210	–	–	.9	.03	.2	–	–	–	–
–	20	–	–	150	410	–	–	.09	–	6	.04	–	–	–
–	–	1.08	–	35	410	–	–	.15	.17	3	.12	–	–	–
–	20	1.8	–	120	470	–	–	.23	.17	8	.3	–	–	–
–	–	–	–	15	430	–	–	.03	.03	.14	.12	–	–	–
–	–	.36	–	35	340	–	–	.03	.07	.2	.08	–	–	–
–	–	.72	–	5	80	–	–	–	–	–	–	–	–	–
–	–	.72	–	25	430	–	–	.9	.07	3	.16	–	–	–
0	389	5.24	420	1062	1076	6.76	0	.18	.83	3.89	.1	88	1	7.66
0	359	4.94	400	988	15	3.94	0	.28	1.05	4.54	.15	79	1	32.4
0	378	5.2	420	1039	16[2]	4.15	0	.3	1.11	4.77	.16	83	1	34.1
0	75	1.04	84	205	3[2]	.83	0	.06	.22	.95	.03	17	<1	6.72
0	43	.59	48	121	2[3]	.49	0	.02	.1	.46	.01	10	<1	3.25
0	50	.96	64	170	1	1.3	0	.28	.03	.46	.07	1	<1	2.13
0	62	8.22	356	774	877[4]	7.67	0	.27	.27	1.92	.35	95	0	.78
0	13	1.7	74	158	179[4]	1.59	0	.06	.06	.4	.07	19	0	.16

[2]Salted almonds contain 1108 mg sodium per cup, 221 mg per ounce.

[3]Salted almond butter contains 72 mg sodium per tablespoon.

[4]Dry-roasted cashews without salt contain 21 mg sodium per cup, or 4 mg per ounce.

(For purposes of calculations, use "0" for t, <1, <.1, <.01, etc.)

Table A–1
Food Composition

Computer Code Number	Food Description	Measure	Wt (g)	H$_2$O (%)	Ener (cal)	Prot (g)	Carb (g)	Dietary Fiber (g)	Fat (g)	Fat Breakdown (g) Sat	Mono	Poly
	NUTS, SEEDS, and PRODUCTS—Cont.											
725	Oil roasted:	1 c	130	4	748	21	37	4	63	12.4	36.9	10.6
726	Ounce	1 oz	28	4	161	5	8	1	14	2.7	8	2.3
1366	Cashew nuts, unsalted, dry roasted	1 c	137	2	786	21	45	4	64	12.5	37.4	10.7
1367	Cashew nuts, unsalted, oil roasted	1 c	130	4	748	21	37	4	63	12.4	36.9	10.6
727	Cashew butter, unsalted	1 tbs	16	3	94	3	4	1	8	1.6	4.7	1.3
728	Chestnuts, European, roasted (1 cup = approx 17 kernels)	1 c	143	40	350	5	76	9	3	.6	1.1	1.2
	Coconut, raw:											
729	Piece 2 x 2 x ½"	1 pce	45	47	159	2	7	4	15	13.4	.6	.2
730	Shredded/grated, unpacked[1]	½ c	40	47	142	1	6	4	13	11.9	.6	.2
	Coconut, dried, shredded/grated:											
731	Unsweetened	1 c	78	3	514	5	19	13	50	44.6	2.1	.6
732	Sweetened	1 c	93	13	465	3	44	4	33	29.3	1.4	.4
733	Filberts/hazelnuts, chopped:	1 c	115	5	726	15	18	9	72	5.3	56.4	6.9
734	Ounce	1 oz	28	5	177	4	4	2	18	1.3	13.9	1.7
735	Macadamias, oil roasted, salted:	1 c	134	2	962	10	17	12	102	15.3	80.9	1.8
736	Ounce	1 oz	28	2	201	2	4	3	21	3.2	16.9	.4
1368	Macadamias, oil roasted, unsalted	1 c	134	2	962	10	17	12	102	15.3	80.9	1.8
	Mixed nuts:											
737	Dry roasted, salted	1 c	137	2	814	24	35	12	71	9.4	43	14.7
738	Oil roasted, salted	1 c	142	2	876	24	30	13	80	12.4	45	18.9
1369	Oil roasted, unsalted	1 c	142	2	876	24	30	13	80	12.4	45	18.9
	Peanuts:											
739	Oil roasted, salted:	1 c	144	2	837	38	27	10	71	9.8	35.3	22.5
740	Ounce	1 oz	28	2	163	7	5	2	14	1.9	6.9	4.4
1370	Oil roasted, unsalted	1 c	144	2	837	38	27	9	71	9.8	35.3	22.5
741	Dried, unsalted:	1 c	146	2	854	35	31	10	73	10.1	36.1	22.9
742	Ounce	1 oz	28	2	166	7	6	2	14	2	7	4.4
743	Peanut butter:	½ c	129	1	759	32	27	8	64	12.3	30.4	18.6
1371	Tablespoon	2 tbs	32	1	188	8	7	2	16	3.1	7.6	4.6
744	Pecan halves, dried, unsalted:	1 c	108	5	720	8	20	5[2]	73	5.8	45.5	18.1
745	Ounce	1 oz	28	5	187	2	5	1[2]	19	1.5	11.9	4.8
1372	Pecan halves, dry roasted, salted	¼ c	28	1	185	2	6	1	18	1.5	11.4	4.5
746	Pine nuts/piñons, dried	1 oz	28	6	159	3	5	3	17	2.7	6.5	7.3
747	Pistachios, dried, shelled	1 oz	28	4	162	6	7	3	14	1.7	9.3	2.1
1373	Pistachios, dry roasted, salted, shelled	1 c	128	2	776	19	35	14	68	8.6	45.6	10.2
748	Pumpkin kernels, dried, unsalted	1 oz	28	7	151	7	5	4	13	2.5	4	5.9
1374	Pumpkin kernels, roasted, salted	1 c	227	7	1184	75	30	15	96	18.1	29.7	43.6
749	Sesame seeds, hulled, dried	¼ c	38	5	223	10	4	.3	21	2.9	7.9	9.1
	Sunflower seed kernels:											
750	Dry	¼ c	36	5	205	8	7	2	18	1.9	3.4	11.8
751	Oil roasted	¼ c	34	3	209	7	5	2	19	2	3.7	12.9
752	Tahini (sesame butter)	1 tbs	15	3	91	3	3	1	8	1.2	3.2	3.7
1334	Trail Mix w/chocolate chips	1 c	146	7	707	21	66	–	47	8.9	19.8	16.5
753	Black walnuts, chopped:	1 c	125	4	758	30	15	6	71	4.5	15.9	46.9

[1]½ cup packed = 65 g.

[2]Dietary fiber data calculated/derived from data on other nuts.

PAGE KEY: A–4 = BEV   A–6 = DAIRY   A–12 = EGGS   A–14 = FAT/OIL   A–18 = FRUIT   A–26 = BAKERY   A–36 = GRAIN   A–44 = FISH
A–48 = MEATS   A–50 = POULTRY   A–54 = SAUSAGE   A–56 = MIXED/FAST   A–64 = NUTS/SEEDS   A–68 = SWEETS   A–70 = VEG/LEG
A–84 = MISC   A–88 = SOUPS/SAUCES   A–90 = FAST   A–106 = FRZN ENTREE   A–112 = BABY FOODS

Chol (mg)	Calc (mg)	Iron (mg)	Magn (mg)	Pota (mg)	Sodi (mg)	Zinc (mg)	VT-A (RE)	Thia (mg)	Ribo (mg)	Niac (mg)	V-B6 (mg)	Fola (µg)	VT-C (mg)	VT-E α-TE (mg)
0	53	5.33	332	689	813[3]	6.18	0	.55	.23	2.34	.32	88	0	2.03
0	11	1.16	72	148	175[3]	1.35	0	.12	.05	.51	.07	19	0	.437
0	62	8.22	356	774	22	7.67	0	.27	.27	1.92	.35	95	0	.78
0	53	5.33	332	689	22	6.18	0	.55	.23	2.34	.32	88	0	2.03
0	7	.8	41	87	2[4]	.83	0	.05	.03	.26	.04	11	0	.25
0	41	1.3	47	847	3	.81	3	.35	.25	1.92	.71	100	37	1.72
0	6	1.09	14	160	9	.49	0	.03	.01	.24	.02	12	1	.33
0	6	.97	13	142	8	.44	0	.03	.01	.22	.02	11	1	.29
0	20	2.59	70	423	29	1.57	0	.05	.08	.47	.23	7	1	1.05
0	14	1.79	46	313	243	1.69	0	.03	.02	.44	.25	8	1	1.26
0	216	3.76	327	511	3	2.76	8	.57	.13	1.31	.7	83	1	27.5
0	53	.93	80	126	1	.68	2	.14	.03	.32	.17	20	<1	6.7
0	60	2.41	157	440	348[5]	1.47	1	.28	.15	2.71	.26	21	0	.55
0	13	.5	32	92	73[5]	.31	<1	.06	.03	.57	.05	4	0	.12
0	60	2.41	155	440	9	1.47	1	.28	.15	2.71	.26	21	0	.55
0	96	5.07	308	817	917[6]	5.21	1	.27	.27	6.44	.41	69	1	8.22
0	153	4.56	334	825	926[6]	7.21	3	.71	.31	7.19	.34	118	1	8.5
0	153	4.56	334	825	16	7.21	3	.71	.31	7.19	.34	118	1	8.5
0	126	2.64	266	982	624[7]	9.55	0	.36	.16	20.4	.37	181	0	10.7
0	25	.52	52	193	123[7]	1.88	0	.07	.03	4.03	.07	36	0	2.07
0	126	2.64	266	982	9	9.55	0	.36	.16	20.4	.37	181	0	10.7
0	79	3.3	256	961	9	4.83	0	.64	.14	19.7	.37	212	0	10.8
0	15	.64	49	187	2	.94	0	.12	.03	3.83	.07	41	0	2.07
0	44	2.15	203	930	617[8]	3.24	0	.18	.13	16.9	.48	101	0	10.4
0	11	.54	50	232	153[8]	.81	0	.04	.03	4.22	.12	25	0	3.2
0	39	2.3	138	423	1[9]	5.91	14	.92	.14	.96	.2	42	2	3.35
0	10	.6	36	111	<1[9]	1.55	4	.24	.04	.25	.05	11	1	.87
0	10	.62	38	105	218	1.61	4	.09	.03	.26	.05	11	1	.84
0	2	.87	66	176	20	1.22	1	.35	.06	1.24	.03	16	1	.98
0	38	1.92	45	306	2[10]	.38	7	.23	.05	.31	.07	16	2	1.46
0	90	4.06	166	1241	998	1.74	31	.54	.31	1.8	.33	76	9	8.26
0	12	4.24	152	226	5[11]	2.12	11	.06	.09	.49	.06	16	1	.28
0	98	33.8	1212	1829	1305	16.9	86	.48	.72	3.95	.2	130	4	2.27
0	50	2.96	132	155	15	3.91	3	.27	.03	1.78	.05	36	0	.86
0	42	2.44	127	248	1[12]	1.82	2	.82	.09	1.62	.28	82	1	18.1
0	19	2.28	43	164	1[12]	1.77	2	.11	.09	1.4	.27	80	<1	17.1
0	21	.95	53	69	<1	1.58	1	.24	.02	.85	.02	15	0	.341
5.84	159	4.96	253	946	177	4.28	6	.6	.33	6.44	.38	95	2	–
0	73	3.85	253	655	1	4.58	37	.27	.14	.26	.69	82	4	3.28

[3] Oil-roasted cashews without salt contain 22 mg sodium per cup, or 5 mg per ounce.
[4] Salted cashew butter contains 98 mg sodium per tablespoon.
[5] Macadamia nuts without salt contain 9 mg sodium per cup, or 2 mg per ounce.
[6] Mixed nuts without salt contain about 15 mg sodium per cup.
[7] Peanuts without salt contain 22 mg sodium per cup, or 4 mg per ounce.

[8] Peanut butter without added salt contains 3 mg sodium per tablespoon.
[9] Salted pecans contain 816 mg sodium per cup, or 214 mg per ounce.
[10] Salted pistachios contain approx 221 mg sodium per ounce.
[11] Salted pumpkin/squash kernels contain approximately 163 mg sodium per ounce.
[12] Unsalted sunflower seeds contain 1 mg sodium per ¼ cup.

(For purposes of calculations, use "0" for t, <1, <.1, <.01, etc.)

Table A–1
Food Composition

Computer Code Number	Food Description	Measure	Wt (g)	H₂O (%)	Ener (cal)	Prot (g)	Carb (g)	Dietary Fiber (g)	Fat (g)	Fat Breakdown (g)		
										Sat	Mono	Poly
	NUTS, SEEDS, and PRODUCTS—Cont.											
754	Ounce	1 oz	28	4	170	7	3	1	16	1	3.6	10.6
755	English walnuts, chopped:	1 c	120	4	770	17	22	5	74	6.7	17	47
756	Ounce	1 oz	28	4	180	4	5	1	17	1.6	4	11.1
	SWEETENERS and SWEETS (see also Dairy [milk desserts] and Baked Goods)											
757	Apple butter	2 tbs	35	52	64	<1	17	<1	<1	t	t	.1
1124	Butterscotch topping	2 tbs	41	32	103	1	27	<1	<1	t	t	0
1125	Caramel topping	2 tbs	41	32	103	1	27	<1	<1	t	t	0
	Cake frosting, creamy vanilla:											
1127	Canned	2 tbs	31	13	131	<1	22	0	5	1.5	2.7	.7
1123	From mix	2 tbs	31	12	132	<1	22	0	5	1	2.1	1.8
	Cake frosting, lite:											
2061	Milk chocolate	1 tbs	29	18	105	0	21	1	2	.7	–	–
2062	Vanilla	1 tbs	29	15	110	0	22	<1	2	.6	–	–
	Candy:											
1128	Almond Joy candy bar	1 oz	28	8	130	1	16	2	8	4.7	1.5	.7
2069	Butterscotch morsels	¼ c	43	1	243	0	29	0	12	12	–	–
758	Caramel, plain or chocolate	1 oz	28	8	107	1	22	<1	2	1.9	.2	.1
1961	Chewing gum, sugarless	1 pce	3	–	5	0	2	–	0	–	0	0
	Chocolate (see also #784, 785, 971):											
	Milk chocolate:											
759	Plain	1 oz	28	1	143	2	17	1	9	5.2	2.8	.3
760	With almonds	1 oz	28	2	147	3	15	2	10	4.8	3.8	.6
761	With peanuts	1 oz	28	5	155	5	11	2	12	3.4	5.1	2.6
762	With rice cereal	1 oz	28	2	139	2	18	1	7	4.5	2.4	.2
763	Semisweet chocolate chips	1 c	170	1	811	7	108	10	50	29.8	16.9	1.6
764	Sweet dark chocolate (candy bar)	1 oz	28	1	133	1	17	2	8	5.9	3.3	.3
1133	SKOR English toffee candy bar	1 ea	32	4	169	1	18	<1	11	7	2.5	2
765	Fondant candy, uncoated (mints, candy corn, other)	1 oz	28	7	100	0	26	0	<1	.1	0	–
1697	Fruit Roll-up (small)	1 ea	14	21	41	<1	11	<1	<1	t	t	.1
766	Fudge, chocolate	1 oz	28	10	107	<1	22	<1	2	1.5	.7	.1
767	Gumdrops	1 oz	28	1	108	0	28	0	<1	0	t	.1
768	Hard candy, all flavors	1 oz	28	1	104	0	28	0	0	0	0	0
769	Jellybeans	1 oz	28	6	104	0	26	0	<1	0	t	.1
1134	M&M's plain chocolate candy	1 pkg	48	1	228	3	33	1	11	5	3	.3
1135	M&M's peanut chocolate candy	1 pkg	47	2	234	5	28	2	13	5	5.1	2
1130	Mars almond bar	1 ea	50	5	234	4	31	1	11	4.8	4.4	.8
1129	Milky Way candy bar	1 ea	60	2	251	3	43	1	9	4.7	3.3	.3
1708	Milk chocolate-coated peanuts	½ c	85	2	441	11	42	4	29	12.4	11	3.7
1709	Peanut brittle, recipe	½ c	74	2	335	6	51	1	14	3.7	6.2	3.5
1132	Reese's peanut butter cup	2 ea	45	8	218	5	21	2	14	10.4	.9	.9
1131	Snickers candy bar (2.2oz)	1 ea	61	6	278	6	37	2	14	7.3	4.1	.5
1482	Fruit juice bar (2.5 fl oz)	1 ea	77	78	63	1	16	–	<1	–	–	–
771	Gelatin dessert/Jello, prepared	½ c	120	85	71	1	17	0	0	0	0	0
1702	SugarFree	½ c	113	98	8	1	1	0	0	0	0	0
772	Honey:	1 c	339	17	1030	1	279	0	0	0	0	0
773	Tablespoon	1 tbs	21	17	64	<1	17	<1	0	0	0	0

(Computer code number is for West Diet Analysis program)

PAGE KEY: A–4 = BEV   A–6 = DAIRY   A–12 = EGGS   A–14 = FAT/OIL   A–18 = FRUIT   A–26 = BAKERY   A–36 = GRAIN   A–44 = FISH
A–48 = MEATS   A–50 = POULTRY   A–54 = SAUSAGE   A–56 = MIXED/FAST   A–64 = NUTS/SEEDS   A–68 = SWEETS   A–70 = VEG/LEG
A–84 = MISC   A–88 = SOUPS/SAUCES   A–90 = FAST   A–106 = FRZN ENTREE   A–112 = BABY FOODS

Chol (mg)	Calc (mg)	Iron (mg)	Magn (mg)	Pota (mg)	Sodi (mg)	Zinc (mg)	VT-A (RE)	Thia (mg)	Ribo (mg)	Niac (mg)	V-B6 (mg)	Fola (µg)	VT-C (mg)	VT-E α-TE (mg)
0	16	.87	57	149	<1	.97	9	.06	.03	.2	.16	18	1	.73
0	113	2.93	203	602	12	3.28	15	.46	.18	1.25	.67	79	4	3.14
0	27	.69	48	142	3	.77	4	.11	.04	.29	.16	18	1	.73
0	2	.05	1	32	0	.02	0	0	<.01	.03	.01	0	1	.01
<1	22	.07	3	34	143	.08	11	0	.04	.02	.01	1	<1	–
<1	22	.07	3	34	143	.08	11	0	.04	.02	.01	1	<1	–
0	1	.03	<1	11	28	0	70	0	<.01	<.01	0	0	0	.63
0	3	.07	1	7	69	.03	33	.01	.01	.11	<.01	0	0	–
0	3	.43	–	–	72	–	0	–	–	–	–	–	0	–
0	1	.03	–	–	53	–	0	–	–	–	–	–	0	–
1	22	.34	19	105	38	.23	3	.01	.04	.13	.02	2	<1	–
0	0	0	–	79	45	–	0	.03	.04	.03	–	–	0	–
2	39	.04	5	61	69	.12	2	<.01	.05	.07	.01	1	<1	.13
–	–	–	–	0	0	–	–	–	–	–	–	–	–	–
6	54	.39	17	109	23	.39	14	.02	.08	.09	.01	2	<1	.35
5	63	.46	25	124	21	.38	4	.02	.12	.21	.01	3	<1	.53
3	33	.53	35	150	11	.69	6	.08	.05	2.14	.04	23	0	1.3
5	48	.21	14	97	41	.32	3	.02	.08	.13	.02	3	<1	.35
0	54	5.32	196	621	19	2.75	3	.09	.15	.73	.08	5	0	2.02
0	5	.59	33	96	3	.42	1	.01	.07	.19	.01	1	0	.28
19	36	.13	11	76	74	.24	22	.01	.11	.03	.01	2	<1	.438
0	1	.02	<1	4	11	.01	0	<.01	<.01	<.01	<.01	0	0	0
0	6	.55	13	12	2	.01	<1	<.01	.01	.2	.03	0	<1	.01
4	12	.14	7	29	18	.11	13	<.01	.02	.03	<.01	1	<1	.03
0	1	.11	<1	1	12	0	0	0	<.01	<.01	0	0	0	0
0	1	.08	1	1	11	<.01	0	<.01	<.01	<.01	<.01	0	0	0
0	1	.31	1	10	7	.01	0	0	0	0	0	0	0	0
0	81	.73	32	188	49	.61	12	.03	.12	.26	.03	4	0	.41
0	63	.7	39	184	44	.72	5	.03	.1	1.51	.08	26	0	1.01
4	84	.55	36	163	85	.55	22	.02	.16	.47	.03	7	1	.3
12	78	.46	20	145	144	.43	28	.02	.13	.21	.03	5	1	.39
8	88	1.12	77	427	35	1.61	0	.1	.15	3.61	.18	7	0	2.17
10	22	1.02	37	153	334	.71	35	.14	.04	2.57	.08	52	0	1.21
7	35	.49	38	180	131	.63	9	.02	.09	1.79	.04	13	0	.6
7	70	.48	37	200	164	.7	19	.03	.11	1.83	.11	24	<1	.93
0	4	.15	3	41	3	.04	2	.01	.01	.12	.02	5	7	0
0	2	.04	1	1	50	.04	0	0	<.01	<.01	<.01	0	0	0
0	2	.01	1	0	54	.03	0	0	<.01	<.01	<.01	0	0	0
0	20	1.42	7	176	14	.75	0	0	.13	.41	.08	7	8	0
0	1	.09	<1	11	1	.05	0	0	.01	.03	.01	<1	<1	0

(For purposes of calculations, use "0" for t, <1, <.1, <.01, etc.)

Table A–1
Food Composition

Computer Code Number	Food Description	Measure	Wt (g)	H$_2$O (%)	Ener (cal)	Prot (g)	Carb (g)	Dietary Fiber (g)	Fat (g)	Fat Breakdown (g) Sat	Mono	Poly
	SWEETENERS and SWEETS (see also Dairy [milk desserts] and Baked Goods)—Cont.											
774	Jams or preserves:	1 tbs	20	35	48	<1	13	<1	<1	0	t	0
775	Packet	1 ea	14	34	34	<1	9	<1	<1	t	t	0
776	Jellies:	1 tbs	18	28	49	<1	13	<1	<1	t	t	t
777	Packet	1 ea	14	28	38	<1	10	<1	<1	t	t	t
1136	Marmalade	2 tbs	40	33	98	<1	26	<1	0	0	0	0
770	Marshmallows	4 ea	28	16	90	1	23	<1	<1	0	0	0
1126	Marshmallow creme topping	3 tbs	50	18	155	1	40	0	<1	0	0	0
778	Popsicle/ice pops	1 ea	95	80	68	0	18	0	0	0	0	0
	Sugars:											
779	Brown sugar	1 c	220	2	827	0	214	0	0	0	0	0
780	White sugar, granulated:	1 c	200	<1	774	0	200	0	0	0	0	0
781	Tablespoon	1 tbs	12	<1	46	0	12	0	0	0	0	0
782	Packet	1 ea	6	<1	23	0	6	0	0	0	0	0
783	White sugar, powdered, sifted	1 c	100	<1	389	0	100	0	<1	0	0	0
	Sweeteners:											
1711	Equal, packet	1 ea	1	5	4	1	0	0	0	0	0	0
1712	Sweet 'N Low, packet	1 ea	1	<1	4	0	1	0	0	0	0	0
	Syrups:											
	Chocolate:											
785	Hot fudge type	2 tbs	38	22	131	2	22	<1	5	2.2	1.4	1.2
784	Thin type	2 tbs	38	37	83	1	22	1	<1	.2	.1	<.1
786	Molasses, blackstrap[1]	2 tbs	40	29	94	0	24	0	0	0	0	0
1710	Light cane	1 tbs	21	26	56	0	14	0	<1	0	0	0
787	Pancake table syrup (corn and maple)	¼ c	79	24	227	0	60	0	0	0	0	0
	VEGETABLES and LEGUMES											
788	Alfalfa sprouts	1 c	33	91	10	1	1	1	<1	t	t	.1
1815	Amaranth leaves, raw, chopped	1 c	28	93	7	1	1	<1	<1	<.1	<.1	<.1
1816	Amaranth leaves, raw, each	1 ea	14	93	4	0	1	<1	<1	<.1	<.1	<.1
1817	Amaranth leaves, cooked	1 c	132	92	29	3	5	2	<.1	.1	.1	.1
1987	Arugula, raw, chopped	5 ea	10	92	3	0	0	–	0	–	–	–
789	Artichokes, cooked globe (300 g w/refuse)	1 ea	120	84	60	4	13	6	<1	t	t	.1
1177	Artichoke hearts, cooked from frozen	9 oz	240	86	108	7	22	13	1	.3	t	.5
1176	Artichoke hearts, marinated	6 oz	170	59	168	4	13	8	14	2	3	7.7
2021	Artichoke hearts, in water	⅔ c	101	86	44	2	10	6	0	<.1	<.1	.1
	Asparagus, green, cooked:											
	From fresh:											
790	Cuts and tips	½ c	90	92	22	2	4	2	<1	.1	t	.1
791	Spears, ½" diam at base	6 ea	90	92	22	2	4	2	<1	.1	t	.1
	From frozen:											
792	Cuts and tips	½ c	90	91	25	3	4	2	<1	.1	t	.2
793	Spears, ½" diam at base	6 ea	90	91	25	3	4	2	<1	.1	t	.2
794	Canned, spears, ½" diam at base	6 ea	120	94	23	3	3	2	1	.2	t	.3
795	Bamboo shoots, canned, drained slices	1 c	131	94	25	2	4	3	1	.1	t	.2
1795	Bamboo shoots, raw slices	1 c	151	91	41	4	8	3	<1	.1	0	.2
1798	Bamboo shoots, cooked slices	1 c	120	96	14	2	2	1	0	.1	<.1	.1

[1]Light molasses would contain about 66 mg calcium, 2.1 mg iron, 18 mg magnesium, and 366 mg potassium for 2 tbsp.

(Computer code number is for West Diet Analysis program)

Chol (mg)	Calc (mg)	Iron (mg)	Magn (mg)	Pota (mg)	Sodi (mg)	Zinc (mg)	VT-A (RE)	Thia (mg)	Ribo (mg)	Niac (mg)	V-B6 (mg)	Fola (μg)	VT-C (mg)	VT-E α-TE (mg)
0	4	.2	1	15	8	.01	<1	0	<.01	.01	<.01	7	2	.02
0	3	.07	1	11	6	.01	<1	0	<.01	.01	<.01	5	1	0
0	1	.04	1	12	6	.01	<1	<.01	<.01	.01	<.01	<1	<1	0
0	1	.03	1	9	5	.01	<1	<.01	<.01	.01	<.01	<1	<1	0
0	15	.06	1	15	22	.02	2	<.01	<.01	.02	.01	14	2	0
0	1	.06	1	1	13	.01	<1	<.01	<.01	.02	<.01	<1	0	0
0	2	.11	1	3	23	.02	<1	<.01	<.01	.04	<.01	1	0	0
0	0	0	1	4	11	.02	0	0	0	0	0	0	0	0
0	187	4.2	64	761	86	.4	0	.02	.01	.18	.06	2	0	0
0	2	.13	0	4	2	.07	0	0	.04	0	0	0	0	0
0	<1	.01	0	<1	<1	<.01	0	0	<.01	0	0	0	0	0
0	<1	<.01	0	<1	<1	<.01	0	0	<.01	0	0	0	0	0
0	1	.06	1	2	1	.03	0	0	0	0	0	0	0	0
0	<1	.02	–	<1	<1	–	0	0	0	0	–	–	0	–
0	<1	–	<1	1	1	–	–	–	–	–	–	–	–	–
5	38	.46	18	82	49	.3	8	.01	.08	.08	.01	2	<1	0
0	5	.81	25	85	36	.28	1	<.01	.02	.12	<.01	2	<1	–
0	344[2]	7[1]	86[1]	997[1]	22	.4	0	.01	.02	.43	.28	<1	0	0
0	43	.99	51	307	8	.06	0	.01	<.01	.2	.14	0	0	0
0	1	.07	2	2	66	.03	0	.01	.01	.02	0	0	0	0
0	11	.32	9	26	2	.3	5	.03	.04	.16	.01	12	3	.01
0	61	.66	16	174	6	.26	83	.01	.04	.19	.05	24	12	.22
0	30	.32	8	86	3	.13	41	0	.02	.09	.03	12	6	.11
0	276	2.98	73	846	28	1.16	366	.03	.18	.74	.23	75	54	.66
0	16	.15	5	37	3	.05	24	0	.01	.03	.01	10	2	.43
0	54	1.55	72	425	114	.59	21	.08	.08	1.2	.13	61	12	.23
0	50	1.34	74	634	127	.86	39	.15	.38	2.2	.21	286	12	.46
0	39	1.62	48	439	899	.54	28	.06	.17	1.38	.15	149	52	1.87
0	40	1.36	40	265	66	.3	15	.06	.05	.59	.09	45	7	.2
0	18	.66	9	144	10	.38	49	.11	.11	.97	.11	131	10	.34
0	18	.66	9	144	10	.38	49	.11	.11	.97	.11	131	10	.34
0	21	.58	12	196	4	.5	74	.06	.09	.94	.02	122	22	1.13
0	21	.58	12	196	4	.5	74	.06	.09	.94	.02	122	22	1.13
0	19	2.2	12	206	468[2]	.48	64	.07	.12	1.14	.13	115	22	.52
0	10	.42	5	105	9	.85	1	.03	.03	.18	.18	4	1	.5
0	20	.76	5	805	6	1.68	3	.23	.11	.91	.36	11	6	1.51
0	14	.29	4	640	5	.56	0	.02	.06	.36	.12	3	0	.84

[2]Low sodium pack contains 3 mg sodium.

(For purposes of calculations, use "0" for t, <1, <.1, <.01, etc.)

Table A–1
Food Composition

Computer Code Number	Food Description	Measure	Wt (g)	H_2O (%)	Ener (cal)	Prot (g)	Carb (g)	Dietary Fiber (g)	Fat (g)	Sat	Mono	Poly
	VEGETABLES AND LEGUMES—Cont.											
	Beans (see also alphabetical listing in this section):											
1990	Adzuki beans, cooked	½ c	115	66	147	9	29	1	.12	.04	.01	.02
796	Black beans, cooked	½ c	86	66	114	8	20	7	<1	.1	t	.2
	Canned beans (white/navy):											
803	With pork and tomato sauce	½ c	126	73	123	7	24	6	1	.5	.6	.2
804	With sweet sauce	1 c	253	71	281	13	53	11	4	1.4	1.6	.5
805	With frankfurters	1 c	257	69	365	17	40	18	17	6	7.3	2.2
	Lima beans:											
797	Thick seeded (Fordhooks), cooked from frozen	½ c	85	74	85	5	16	6	<1	.1	t	.1
798	Thin seeded (Baby), cooked from frozen	½ c	90	72	95	6	18	6	<1	.1	t	.1
799	Cooked from dry, drained	½ c	94	70	108	7	20	7	<1	.1	t	.2
1998	Red Mexican, cooked f/dry	1 c	224	70	252	15	47	18	1	.2	.2	.3
	Snap bean/green string beans cuts and french style:											
800	Cooked from fresh	½ c	62	89	22	1	5	2	<1	t	t	.1
801	Cooked from frozen	½ c	67	92	17	1	4	2	<1	t	t	.1
802	Canned, drained	½ c	67	93	13	1	3	1	<1	t	t	t
1713	Snap bean, yellow, cooked f/fresh	½ c	63	89	22	1	5	1	<1	t	t	.1
	Bean sprouts (mung):											
806	Raw	1 c	104	90	31	3	6	2	<1	.1	t	.1
807	Cooked, stir-fried	1 c	124	84	62	5	13	4	<1	.1	.1	.1
808	Cooked, boiled, drained	1 c	124	93	26	3	5	1	<1	t	t	t
1788	Canned, drained	1 c	125	96	15	2	3	1	0	<.1	<.1	<.1
	Beets, cooked from fresh:											
809	Sliced or diced	½ c	85	87	37	1	8	1	<1	t	t	.1
810	Whole beets, 2" diam	2 ea	100	87	44	2	10	2	<1	t	t	.1
	Beets, canned:											
811	Sliced or diced	½ c	85	91	26	1	6	2	<1	t	t	t
812	Pickled slices	½ c	114	82	74	1	19	2	<1	t	t	t
813	Beet greens, cooked, drained	½ c	72	89	19	2	4	2	<1	t	t	.1
	Broccoli, raw:											
817	Chopped	1 c	88	91	25	3	5	3	<1	.1	t	.2
818	Spears	1 ea	151	91	42	4	8	5	1	.1	t	.3
	Broccoli, cooked from fresh:											
819	Spears	1 ea	180	91	50	5	9	5	1	.1	t	.3
820	Chopped	1 c	156	91	44	5	8	5	1	.1	t	.3
	Broccoli, cooked from frozen:											
821	Spear, small piece	3 ea	90	91	25	3	5	2	<1	t	t	.1
822	Chopped	1 c	184	91	51	6	10	5	<1	t	t	.1
1603	Broccoflower, steamed	3½ oz	100	90	32	3	6	3	<1	t	t	.1
823	Brussels sprouts, cooked from fresh	½ c	78	87	30	2	7	4	<1	.1	t	.2
824	Brussels sprouts, cooked from frozen	½ c	77	87	33	3	6	3	<1	.1	t	.2
	Cabbage, common varieties:											
825	Raw, shredded or chopped	1 c	70	92	17	1	4	1	<1	t	t	.1

(Computer code number is for West Diet Analysis program)

Chol (mg)	Calc (mg)	Iron (mg)	Magn (mg)	Pota (mg)	Sodi (mg)	Zinc (mg)	VT-A (RE)	Thia (mg)	Ribo (mg)	Niac (mg)	V-B6 (mg)	Fola (µg)	VT-C (mg)	VT-E α-TE (mg)
0	32	2.3	60	612	9	2	.69	.13	.07	.82	.11	139	0	–
0	23	1.81	60	305	1	.97	1	.21	.05	.43	.06	128	0	.07
9	71	4.15	44	378	554	7.4	16	.07	.06	.63	.09	28	4	.7
18	154	4.23	86	673	850	3.82	29	.12	.15	.89	.22	95	8	1.37
15	123	4.47	72	604	1105	4.83	40	.15	.14	2.32	.12	77	6	1.21
0	19	1.16	29	347	45	.37	16	.06	.05	.91	.1	18	11	.25
0	25	1.76	50	370	26	.5	15	.06	.05	.69	.1	14	5	.58
0	16	2.26	40	478	2	.89	0	.15	.05	.4	.15	78	0	.17
0	84	3.72	96	738	481	1.74	1	.27	.13	.75	.23	188	4	.15
0	29	.79	16	185	2	.22	41[1]	.05	.06	.38	.03	21	6	.09
0	30	.55	14	75	9	.42	35[2]	.03	.05	.28	.04	5	5	.09
0	17	.6	9	73	168[3]	.19	23[4]	.01	.04	.13	.02	21	3	.09
0	29	.8	16	188	2	.23	5	.05	.06	.39	.04	21	6	.18
0	14	.95	22	154	6	.43	2	.09	.13	.78	.09	63	14	.01
0	16	2.36	41	272	11	1.12	4	.17	.22	1.49	.16	86	20	.01
0	15	.81	17	125	12	.58	2	.06	.13	1.01	.07	36	14	.01
0	18	.54	11	34	175	.35	3	.04	.09	.28	.04	12	<1	.01
0	14	.67	20	259	65	.3	3	.02	.03	.28	.06	68	3	.26
0	16	.79	23	305	77	.35	4	.03	.04	.33	.07	80	4	.3
0	13	1.55	14	125	232[5]	.18	1	.01	.03	.13	.05	26	3	.23
0	13	.47	17	168	301	.3	1	.01	.05	.29	.06	30	3	.342
0	82	1.37	49	654	174	.36	367	.08	.21	.36	.09	10	18	.22
0	42	.77	22	286	24	.35	136[6]	.06	.1	.56	.14	62	82	1.46
0	72	1.33	38	491	41	.6	233[6]	.1	.18	.96	.24	107	141	2.51
0	83	1.51	43	526	47	.68	250[6]	.1	.2	1.03	.26	90	134	3.04
0	72	1.31	37	456	41	.59	217[6]	.09	.18	.89	.22	78	116	2.64
0	46	.55	18	162	22	.27	170[6]	.05	.07	.41	.12	27	36	.93
0	94	1.12	37	331	44	.55	348[6]	.1	.15	.84	.24	103	74	3.04
0	32	.7	20	322	23	.5	67	.07	.09	.76	.18	48	63	.3
0	28	.94	16	247	16	.26	56	.08	.06	.47	.14	47	48	.66
0	19	.57	19	252	18	.28	46	.08	.09	.42	.22	78	35	.45
0	33	.41	10	172	13	.13	9	.03	.03	.21	.07	30	22	.07

[1]Data is for green varieties; yellow beans contain 10 RE per cup.

[2]Data is for green varieties; yellow beans contain 15 RE per cup.

[3]Low sodium pack contains 3 mg sodium per cup.

[4]For green varieties; yellow beans contain 14 RE per cup.

[5]Low sodium pack contains 39 mg sodium.

[6]Vitamin A for whole plant: leaves are 1600 RE/100 g raw; flower clusters are 300/100 g raw;

(For purposes of calculations, use "0" for t, <1, <.1, <.01, etc.)

Table A–1
Food Composition

Computer Code Number	Food Description	Measure	Wt (g)	H₂O (%)	Ener (cal)	Prot (g)	Carb (g)	Dietary Fiber (g)	Fat (g)	Fat Breakdown (g)		
										Sat	Mono	Poly
	VEGETABLES AND LEGUMES—Cont.											
826	Cooked, drained	1 c	150	94	33	2	7	4	1	.1	t	.3
	Cabbage, Chinese:											
1178	Bok choy, raw, shredded	1 c	70	95	9	1	2	1	<1	t	t	.1
827	Bok choy, cooked, drained	1 c	170	96	20	3	3	3	<1	t	t	.1
1937	Kim chee style	1 c	150	92	31	2	6	2	0	<.1	<.1	.2
828	Pe tsai, raw, chopped	1 c	76	94	12	1	2	1	<1	t	t	.1
1796	Pe tsai, cooked	1 c	119	95	17	2	3	2	0	<.1	<.1	.1
	Cabbage, red, coarsely chopped:											
829	Raw	1 c	70	92	19	1	4	2	<1	t	t	.1
830	Cooked, drained	½ c	75	94	16	1	3	2	<1	t	t	.1
831	Cabbage, savoy, coarsely chopped, raw	1 c	70	91	19	1	4	2	<1	t	t	t
1785	Cabbage, savoy, cooked	1 c	145	92	35	3	8	4	0	<.1	<.1	.1
1896	Capers	1 tsp	5	86	0	0	0	0	0	–	–	–
	Carrots, raw:											
832	Whole, 7 ½ x 1 ⅛"	1 ea	72	88	31	1	7	2	<1	t	t	.1
833	Grated	½ c	55	88	24	1	6	2	<1	t	t	t
	Carrots, cooked, sliced, drained:											
834	From fresh	½ c	78	87	35	1	8	2	<1	t	t	.1
835	From frozen	½ c	73	90	26	1	6	3	<1	t	t	t
836	Carrots, canned, sliced, drained	½ c	73	93	17	<1	4	2	<1	t	t	.1
837	Carrot juice, canned	½ c	123	89	49	1	11	2	<1	t	t	.1
	Cauliflower, flowerets:											
838	Raw	½ c	50	92	12	1	3	1	<1	t	t	.1
839	Cooked from fresh, drained	½ c	62	93	14	1	3	1	<1	.1	t	.1
840	Cooked, from frozen, drained	½ c	90	94	17	1	3	2	<1	t	t	.1
	Celery, pascal type, raw:											
841	Large outer stalk, 8 x 1½" (root end)	1 ea	40	95	6	<1	1	1	<1	t	t	t
842	Diced	1 c	120	95	19	1	4	2	<1	t	t	.1
1789	Celeriac/celery root, cooked	3½ oz	99	93	25	1	6	4	<1	<.1	<.1	.1
1179	Chard, swiss, raw, chopped	1 c	36	93	7	1	1	1	<1	t	t	t
1180	Chard, swiss, cooked	1 c	175	93	35	3	7	4	<1	t	t	.1
1855	Chayote fruit, raw	1 ea	203	93	49	2	11	6	1	–	–	–
1856	Chayote fruit, cooked	1 c	160	93	38	1	8	1	1	–	–	–
	Chickpeas (see Garbanzo Beans #854)											
	Collards, cooked, drained:											
843	From fresh	½ c	64	95	17	1	4	2	<1	t	t	.1
844	From frozen	½ c	85	88	31	3	6	3	<1	.1	t	.1
	Corn, cooked, drained:											
845	From fresh, on cob, 5" long	1 ea	77	70	83	3	19	2	1	.2	.3	.5
846	From frozen, on cob, 3½" long	1 ea	63	73	59	2	14	2	<1	.1	.1	.2
847	Kernels, cooked from frozen	½ c	82	76	66	2	17	2	<1	t	t	t
	Corn, canned:											
848	Cream style	½ c	128	79	92	2	23	2	1	.1	.2	.3
849	Whole kernel, vacuum pack	½ c	105	77	83	3	20	6	1	.1	.2	.3
	Cowpeas (see Black-eyed peas #814–816)											
850	Cucumber slices with peel	7 pce	28	96	4	<1	1	<1	<1	t	t	t
1948	Cucumber, kim chee style	1 c	150	91	32	2	7	2	<1	.1	0	.1

(Computer code number is for West Diet Analysis program)

Chol (mg)	Calc (mg)	Iron (mg)	Magn (mg)	Pota (mg)	Sodi (mg)	Zinc (mg)	VT-A (RE)	Thia (mg)	Ribo (mg)	Niac (mg)	V-B6 (mg)	Fola (µg)	VT-C (mg)	VT-E α-TE (mg)
0	46	.25	12	146	12	.13	19	.09	.08	.42	.17	30	30	.16
0	73	.56	13	176	45	.13	210	.03	.05	.35	.14	46	31	.08
0	158	1.77	19	631	58	.29	437	.05	.11	.73	.28	69	44	.2
0	145	1.28	28	375	995	.35	426	.07	.1	.75	.34	88	80	.24
0	58	.24	10	180	7	.17	91	.03	.04	.3	.18	60	20	.09
0	38	.36	12	268	11	.21	115	.05	.05	.6	.21	64	19	.12
0	36	.34	11	144	8	.15	3	.03	.02	.21	.15	14	40	.07
0	28	.26	8	105	6	.11	2	.03	.01	.15	.1	9	26	.09
0	24	.28	20	161	20	.19	70	.05	.02	.21	.13	56	22	.07
0	44	.55	35	267	35	.33	129	.07	.03	.03	.22	67	25	.24
0	2	.05	–	–	105	–	1	–	–	–	–	–	0	–
0	19	.36	11	232	25	.14	2024	.07	.04	.67	.11	10	7	.33
0	15	.27	8	177	19	.11	1546	.05	.03	.51	.08	8	5	.25
0	24	.48	10	177	51	.23	1913	.03	.04	.39	.19	11	2	.33
0	20	.34	7	115	43	.17	1291	.02	.03	.32	.09	8	2	.31
0	18	.47	6	130	175[1]	.19	1004	.01	.02	.4	.08	7	2	.31
0	29	.57	17	359	36	.22	3166	.11	.07	.47	.27	5	10	.01
0	11	.22	7	152	15	.14	1	.03	.03	.26	.11	28	23	.02
0	10	.2	6	88	9	.11	1	.03	.03	.25	.11	27	27	.03
0	15	.37	8	125	16	.12	2	.03	.05	.28	.08	37	28	.04
0	16	.16	4	115	35	.05	5	.02	.02	.13	.03	11	3	.14
0	48	.48	13	344	104	.16	16	.06	.05	.39	.1	34	8	.43
0	26	.43	12	172	61	.2	0	.03	.04	.42	.1	3	4	.2
0	18	.65	29	136	77	.13	119	.01	.03	.14	.04	5	11	.68
0	101	3.96	150	961	313	.58	550	.06	.15	.63	.15	15	31	3.31
0	39	.81	28	305	8	.71	11	.06	.08	1.02	.27	56	22	.24
0	21	.35	19	277	2	.5	8	.04	.06	.67	.19	29	13	.144
0	15	.1	4	83	10	.07	175	.01	.03	.19	.03	4	8	.56
0	179	.95	25	213	42	.23	508	.04	.1	.54	.1	64	22	.43
0	2	.47	25	193	13	.37	17[2]	.17	.06	1.24	.05	36	5	.07
0	2	.38	18	158	3	.4	13[2]	.11	.04	.96	.14	19	3	.06
0	2	.25	15	113	4	.29	20[2]	.06	.06	1.05	.08	19	2	.07
0	4	.49	22	172	364[3]	.68	12[2]	.03	.07	1.23	.08	57	6	.12
0	5	.44	24	195	286[4]	.48	25[2]	.04	.08	1.23	.06	51	9	.1
0	4	.07	3	41	1	.06	6	.01	.01	.06	.01	4	2	.02
0	14	7.23	12	176	1532	.77	50	.05	.05	.69	.17	35	5	.24

[1]Low sodium pack contains 31 mg sodium.

[2]For yellow varieties; white varieties contain only a trace of vitamin A.

[3]Low sodium pack contains 4 mg sodium per ½ cup.

[4]Low sodium pack contains 6 mg sodium per cup.

(For purposes of calculations, use "0" for t, <1, <.1, <.01, etc.)

Table A–1
Food Composition

Computer Code Number	Food Description	Measure	Wt (g)	H$_2$O (%)	Ener (cal)	Prot (g)	Carb (g)	Dietary Fiber (g)	Fat (g)	Fat Breakdown (g) Sat	Mono	Poly
	VEGETABLES AND LEGUMES—Cont.											
	Dandelion greens:											
851	Raw	1 c	55	86	25	1	5	2	<1	.1	t	.2
852	Chopped, cooked, drained	1 c	105	90	35	2	7	3	1	.1	.1	.4
853	Eggplant, cooked	1 c	160	92	45	1	11	4	<1	.1	t	.2
1714	Endive, fresh, chopped	¼ c	13	94	2	<1	<1	<1	<1	t	t	t
856	Escarole/curly endive, chopped	1 c	50	94	8	1	2	1	<1	t	t	t
854	Garbanzo beans (chickpeas), cooked	1 c	164	60	269	15	45	8	4	.4	1	1.9
1939	Grape leaves, raw	10 g	10	79	7	0	1	–	0	–	–	–
855	Great northern beans, cooked	1 c	177	69	209	15	37	10	1	.3	t	.3
857	Jerusalem artichoke, raw slices	1 c	150	78	114	3	26	2	<1	0	t	t
1794	Jicama	1 c	120	90	46	1	11	6	0	<.1	0	.1
	Kale, cooked, drained:											
858	From fresh	½ c	65	91	21	1	4	1	<1	t	t	.1
859	From frozen	½ c	65	90	19	2	3	1	<1	t	t	.2
860	Kidney beans, canned	1 c	256	77	217	13	40	16	1	.1	.1	.5
1181	Kohlrabi, raw slices	1 c	140	91	38	2	9	5	<1	t	t	.1
861	Kohlrabi, cooked	1 c	165	90	48	3	11	3	<1	t	t	.1
1183	Leeks, raw, chopped	1 c	104	83	63	2	15	3	<1	t	t	.2
1182	Leeks, cooked, chopped	½ c	52	91	16	<1	4	2	<1	t	t	.1
862	Lentils, cooked from dry	½ c	99	70	115	9	20	5	<1	.1	.1	.2
1288	Lentils, sprouted, stir-fried	4 oz	113	69	115	10	24	4	1	.1	.1	.2
1289	Lentils, sprouted, raw	1 c	77	67	82	7	17	3	<1	t	.1	.2
	Lettuce:											
	Butterhead/Boston types:											
863	Head, 5" diameter	¼ ea	41	96	5	1	1	1	<1	t	t	.1
864	Leaves, inner or outer	4 ea	30	96	4	<1	1	<1	<1	t	t	t
	Iceberg/crisphead:											
865	Head, 6" diameter	¼ ea	135	96	17	1	3	1	<1	t	t	.1
866	Wedge, ¼ head	1 ea	135	96	18	1	3	1	<1	t	t	.1
867	Chopped or shredded	1 c	56	96	7	1	1	1	<1	t	t	.1
868	Looseleaf, chopped	½ c	28	94	5	<1	1	<1	<1	t	t	t
869	Romaine, chopped	½ c	28	95	4	<1	1	<1	<1	t	t	t
870	Romaine, inner leaf	3 ea	30	95	5	<1	1	<1	<1	t	t	t
1930	Luffa, cooked (Chinese okra)	1 c	178	89	57	3	13	6	0	.1	<.1	.1
	Mushrooms:											
871	Raw, sliced	½ c	35	92	9	1	2	<1	<1	t	t	.1
872	Cooked from fresh, pieces	½ c	78	91	21	2	4	2	<1	t	t	.1
1962	Stir fried, shitake slices	1 c	145	83	80	2	21	3	<1	.1	.1	<.1
873	Canned, drained	½ c	78	91	19	1	4	2	<1	t	t	.1
1951	Mushroom caps, pickled	8 ea	47	92	11	1	2	1	<1	<.1	0	.1
	Mustard greens:											
874	Cooked from fresh	½ c	70	95	11	2	1	1	<1	t	.1	t
875	Cooked from frozen	½ c	75	94	14	2	2	2	<1	t	.1	t
876	Navy beans, cooked from dry	1 c	182	63	258	16	48	16	1	.3	.1	.4
	Okra, cooked:											
877	From fresh pods	8 ea	85	90	27	2	6	2	<1	t	t	t
878	From frozen slices	½ c	92	91	34	2	8	3	<1	.1	t	.1
1236	Batter fried from fresh	1 c	92	69	175	3	12	2	13	2.1	3.4	7.1
1930	Chinese, (Luffa), cooked	1 c	178	89	57	3	13	6	0	.1	<.1	.1

(Computer code number is for West Diet Analysis program)

PAGE KEY: A–4 = BEV   A–6 = DAIRY   A–12 = EGGS   A–14 = FAT/OIL   A–18 = FRUIT   A–26 = BAKERY   A–36 = GRAIN   A–44 = FISH
A–48 = MEATS   A–50 = POULTRY   A–54 = SAUSAGE   A–56 = MIXED/FAST   A–64 = NUTS/SEEDS   A–68 = SWEETS   A–70 = VEG/LEG
A–84 = MISC   A–88 = SOUPS/SAUCES   A–90 = FAST   A–106 = FRZN ENTREE   A–112 = BABY FOODS

Chol (mg)	Calc (mg)	Iron (mg)	Magn (mg)	Pota (mg)	Sodi (mg)	Zinc (mg)	VT-A (RE)	Thia (mg)	Ribo (mg)	Niac (mg)	V-B6 (mg)	Fola (µg)	VT-C (mg)	VT-E α-TE (mg)
0	102	1.71	20	218	42	.23	770	.1	.14	.44	.14	15	19	1.38
0	147	1.89	25	243	46	.29	1229	.14	.18	.54	.17	13	19	2.63
0	10	.56	21	397	5	.24	10	.12	.03	.96	.14	23	2	.05
0	7	.10	2	41	3	.1	27	.01	.01	.05	<.01	18	1	.06
0	26	.41	8	157	11	.39	103	.04	.04	.2	.01	71	3	.22
0	80	4.74	79	477	11	2.51	4	.19	.1	.86	.23	282	2	.57
0	72	.69	–	26	2	–	86	.02	.01	.12	–	–	3	–
0	120	3.77	88	692	4	1.56	<1	.28	.1	1.21	.21	181	2	.53
0	21	5.1	25	644	6	.18	3	.3	.09	1.95	.12	20	6	.29
0	14	.72	14	180	5	.19	2	.02	.03	.24	.05	14	24	5.48
0	47	.58	12	148	15	.16	481	.03	.05	.32	.09	9	27	.55
0	90	.61	12	209	10	.12	413	.03	.07	.44	.06	9	16	.12
0	61	3.23	72	658	873	1.41	<1	.27	.22	1.17	.06	129	3	.13
0	34	.56	27	490	28	.04	5	.07	.03	.56	.21	22	87	.67
0	41	.66	31	561	35	.51	6	.07	.03	.64	.25	20	89	2.76
0	61	2.18	29	187	21	.12	10	.06	.03	.42	.24	67	12	.96
0	16	.57	7	45	5	.03	2	.01	.01	.1	.06	13	2	.36
0	19	3.3	36	365	2	1.26	1	.17	.07	1.05	.18	178	1	.11
0	16	3.52	40	322	11	1.81	5	.25	.1	1.36	.19	76	14	.27
0	19	2.47	28	247	8	1.16	3	.18	.1	.87	.15	77	13	.22
0	13	.12	5	104	2	.07	40	.02	.02	.12	.02	30	3	.18
0	10	.09	4	76	2	.05	29	.02	.02	.09	.01	22	2	.13
0	25	.67	12	213	12	.3	45	.06	.04	.25	.05	76	5	.38
0	25	.67	12	213	12	.3	45	.06	.04	.25	.05	76	5	.38
0	11	.28	5	88	5	.12	18	.03	.02	.1	.02	31	2	.16
0	19	.39	3	74	3	.08	53	.01	.02	.11	.01	14	5	.12
0	10	.31	2	81	2	.07	73	.03	.03	.14	.01	38	7	.12
0	11	.33	2	87	2	.07	78	.03	.03	.15	.01	41	7	.13
0	112	.8	101	570	420	.97	103	.23	.1	1.54	.33	81	29	1.22
0	2	.43	3	129	1	.26	0	.04	.16	1.44	.03	7	1	.04
0	5	1.36	9	277	2	.68	0	.06	.23	3.48	.07	14	3	.09
0	4	.64	20	170	6	1.94	0	.05	.25	2.18	.23	30	.44	.17
0	9	.62	12	101	331	.56	0	.07	.02	1.24	.05	10	0	.09
0	2	.5	5	139	95	.28	0	.03	.16	1.42	.03	6	1	.05
0	51	.49	11	141	11	.08	212	.03	.04	.3	.07	51	18	1.41
0	76	.84	10	104	19	.15	335	.03	.04	.19	.08	52	10	1.31
0	127	4.51	107	670	2	1.93	<1	.37	.11	.97	.3	255	2	.55
0	54	.38	48	273	4	.47	49	.11	.05	.74	.16	39	14	.59
0	88	.62	47	215	3	.57	47	.09	.11	.72	.04	133	11	.64
15	104	.77	37	214	137	.5	43	.13	.1	.75	.13	37	10	3.08
0	112	.8	101	570	420	.97	103	.23	.1	1.54	.33	81	29	1.22

(For purposes of calculations, use "0" for t, <1, <.1, <.01, etc.)

Table A–1
Food Composition

Computer Code Number	Food Description	Measure	Wt (g)	H₂O (%)	Ener (cal)	Prot (g)	Carb (g)	Dietary Fiber (g)	Fat (g)	Fat Breakdown (g)		
										Sat	Mono	Poly
	VEGETABLES AND LEGUMES—Cont.											
	Onions:											
879	Raw, chopped	1 c	160	90	61	2	14	3	<1	t	t	.1
880	Raw, sliced	1 c	115	90	44	1	10	2	<1	t	t	.1
881	Cooked, drained, chopped	½ c	105	88	46	1	11	1	<1	t	t	.1
882	Dehydrated flakes	¼ c	14	4	45	1	12	1	<1	t	t	t
1934	Onions, pearl, cooked	1 c	185	87	81	3	19	3	<1	.1	.1	.1
	Spring/green onions, chopped:											
883	Bulb and top	½ c	50	90	16	1	4	1	<1	t	t	t
1185	Green tops only	1 c	100	92	34	2	6	3	<1	.1	.1	.2
1184	White part only	½ c	50	92	25	1	5	1	<1	t	t	t
884	Onion rings, breaded, heated f/frozen	2 ea	20	28	81	1	8	<1	5	1.7	2.2	1
1917	Palm hearts, cooked slices	1 c	146	70	150	4	39	2	<1	.1	.1	<.1
	Parsley:											
885	Raw, chopped	½ c	30	88	11	1	2	1	<1	t	.1	t
886	Raw, sprigs	5 ea	5	88	2	<1	<1	<1	<1	t	t	t
888	Parsnips, sliced, cooked	½ c	78	78	63	1	15	3	<1	t	.1	t
	Peas:											
	Black-eyed, cooked:											
814	From dry, drained	½ c	85	70	99	7	18	6	<1	.1	t	.2
815	From fresh, drained	½ c	82	76	80	3	17	4	<1	.1	t	.1
816	From frozen, drained	½ c	85	66	112	7	20	7	1	.2	.1	.2
889	Edible pod peas, cooked	1 c	160	89	67	5	11	4	<1	.1	t	.2
890	Green, canned, drained	½ c	85	82	59	4	11	3	<1	.1	t	.1
891	Green, cooked from frozen	½ c	80	80	62	4	11	4	<1	t	t	.1
1786	Snow peas, raw	1 c	145	89	61	4	11	4	0	.1	<.1	.1
1787	Snow peas, raw	10 ea	29	89	12	1	2	1	0	<.1	<.1	<.1
892	Split, green, cooked from dry	½ c	98	70	116	8	21	3	<1	.1	.1	.2
1187	Peas & carrots, cooked from frozen	½ c	80	86	38	2	8	3	<1	.1	t	.2
1186	Peas & carrots, canned w/liquid	½ c	128	88	49	3	11	4	<1	.1	t	.2
	Peppers, hot:											
893	Hot green chili, canned	½ c	68	93	17	1	4	1	<1	t	t	t
894	Hot green chili, raw	1 ea	45	88	18	1	4	1	<1	t	t	.1
1715	Hot red chili, raw, diced	1 tbs	9	88	4	<1	1	<1	<1	t	t	t
1988	Jalapeno, raw	2 oz	57	90	25	–	–	–	–	–	–	–
895	Jalapeno, chopped, canned	½ c	68	89	16	1	3	2	<1	t	t	.2
1918	Jalapeno wheels, in brine (Ortega)	2 tbs	29	–	10	0	2	–	0	0	0	0
	Peppers, sweet, green:											
896	Whole pod (90 g with refuse), raw	1 ea	74	92	20	1	5	1	<1	t	t	.1
897	Cooked, chopped (1 pod cooked = 73 g)	½ c	68	92	19	1	5	1	<1	t	t	.1
	Peppers, sweet, red:											
1286	Raw, chopped	1 c	100	92	27	1	6	2	<1	t	t	.1
1807	Raw, each	1 ea	74	92	20	1	5	1	<1	<.1	<.1	.1
1287	Cooked, chopped	½ c	68	92	19	1	5	1	<1	t	t	.1
	Peppers, sweet, yellow:											
1872	Raw, large	1 ea	186	92	50	2	12	4	<1	<.1	<.1	.2
1873	Strips	10 pce	52	92	14	1	3	1	<1	0	<.1	.6
898	Pinto beans, cooked from dry	½ c	85	64	116	7	22	7	<1	t	.1	.2

(Computer code number is for West Diet Analysis program)

PAGE KEY: A–4 = BEV   A–6 = DAIRY   A–12 = EGGS   A–14 = FAT/OIL   A–18 = FRUIT   A–26 = BAKERY   A–36 = GRAIN   A–44 = FISH
A–48 = MEATS   A–50 = POULTRY   A–54 = SAUSAGE   A–56 = MIXED/FAST   A–64 = NUTS/SEEDS   A–68 = SWEETS   A–70 = VEG/LEG
A–84 = MISC   A–88 = SOUPS/SAUCES   A–90 = FAST   A–106 = FRZN ENTREE   A–112 = BABY FOODS

Chol (mg)	Calc (mg)	Iron (mg)	Magn (mg)	Pota (mg)	Sodi (mg)	Zinc (mg)	VT-A (RE)	Thia (mg)	Ribo (mg)	Niac (mg)	V-B6 (mg)	Fola (μg)	VT-C (mg)	VT-E α-TE (mg)
0	32	.35	16	251	5	.3	0	.07	.03	.24	.19	30	10	.21
0	23	.25	12	181	3	.22	0	.05	.02	.17	.13	22	7	.15
0	23	.25	12	174	3	.22	0	.04	.02	.17	.13	16	5	.14
0	36	.22	13	227	3	.26	0	.07	.01	.14	.22	23	10	.19
0	41	.44	20	305	433	.39	0	.08	.04	.30	.24	28	10	.24
0	36	.74	10	138	8	.19	19	.03	.04	.26	.03	32	9	.07
0	56	2.2	21	260	7	.22	40	.07	.1	.6	0	80	51	.3
0	20	.44	8	115	3	.12	<1	.03	.02	.17	.05	18	13	.06
0	6	.34	4	26	75	.08	5	.06	.03	.72	.01	3	<1	.14
0	26	2.47	15	2637	20	5.45	10	.07	.25	1.25	1.06	30	10	.73
0	41	1.86	15	166	17	.32	156	.03	.03	.39	.03	46	40	.54
0	6	.31	3	27	3	.04	26	<.01	<.01	.02	<.01	8	7	.09
0	29	.45	23	286	8	.2	0	.06	.04	.56	.07	45	10[1]	.78
0	20	2.15	45	238	3	1.1	1	.17	.05	.42	.09	177	<1	.24
0	106	.92	43	343	3	.85	65	.08	.12	1.16	.05	104	2	.18
0	20	1.8	43	319	4	1.21	6	.22	.05	.62	.08	120	2	.33
0	67	3.15	42	384	6	.59	21	.2	.12	.86	.23	47	77	.62
0	17	.81	14	147	186[2]	.6	65	.1	.07	.62	.05	38	8	.32
0	19	1.26	23	134	70	.75	54	.23	.08	1.18	.09	47	8	.14
0	62	3.02	35	290	6	.39	21	.22	.12	.87	.23	60	87	.57
0	12	.6	7	58	1	.08	4	.04	.02	.17	.05	12	17	.11
0	14	1.26	35	355	2	.98	1	.19	.05	.87	.05	64	<1	.38
0	18	.75	13	126	54	.36	621	.18	.05	.92	.07	21	6	.26
0	29	.96	18	128	332	.74	739	.09	.07	.74	.11	23	8	.54
0	5	.34	10	127	797	.12	41[3]	.01	.03	.54	.1	7	46	.47
0	8	.54	11	153	3	.13	35[3]	.04	.04	.43	.13	11	109	.31
0	2	.11	2	32	1	.03	101	.01	.01	.09	.03	2	22	.06
–	–	–	–	3	3	–	38	–	–	–	–	–	66	.47
0	18	1.9	8	92	995	.13	116	.02	.03	.34	.14	9	9	.47
0	–	–	–	55	390	–	–	–	–	–	–	–	21	.2
0	7	.34	7	131	1	.09	47	.05	.02	.38	.18	16	66	.51
0	6	.31	7	113	1	.08	40	.04	.02	.32	.16	11	51	.47
0	9	.46	10	177	2	.12	570	.07	.03	.51	.25	22	190	.69
0	7	.34	7	131	1	.09	422	.05	.02	.38	.18	16	141	.51
0	6	.31	7	112	1	.08	256	.04	.02	.32	.16	11	116	.47
0	20	.86	22	394	4	.32	44	.05	.05	1.66	.31	48	342	.56
0	6	.24	6	110	1	.09	12	.01	.01	.46	.09	14	96	.16
0	41	2.23	47	398	2	.92	<1	.16	.08	.34	.13	147	2	.8

[1] Value for Vitamin C is highest right after harvest and drops after that.

[2] Low sodium pack contains 1.7 mg sodium.

[3] Data is for green chili peppers; red varieties contain 809 RE vitamin A per ½ cup; 484 RE per whole pepper.

(For purposes of calculations, use "0" for t, <1, <.1, <.01, etc.)

Table A–1
Food Composition

Computer Code Number	Food Description	Measure	Wt (g)	H$_2$O (%)	Ener (cal)	Prot (g)	Carb (g)	Dietary Fiber (g)	Fat (g)	Fat Breakdown (g)		
										Sat	Mono	Poly
	VEGETABLES AND LEGUMES—Cont.											
1191	Poi, two finger	¼ c	60	72	67	<1	16	<1	<1	t	t	t
	Potatoes:[1]											
	Baked in oven, 4¾" x 2⅓" diam:											
899	With skin	1 ea	202	71	220	5	51	5	<1	.1	1	.1
900	Flesh only	1 ea	156	75	145	3	34	2	<1	t	t	.1
901	Skin only	1 ea	58	47	115	2	27	2	<1	t	t	t
	Baked in microwave, 4¾" x 2⅓" diam:											
902	With skin	1 ea	202	72	212	5	49	5	<1	.1	t	.1
903	Flesh only	1 ea	156	74	156	3	36	2	<1	t	t	.1
904	Skin only	1 ea	58	64	77	3	17	2	<1	t	t	t
	Boiled, about 2½" diam:											
905	Peeled after boiling	1 ea	136	77	118	3	27	2	<1	t	t	.1
906	Peeled before boiling	1 ea	135	78	116	2	27	2	<1	t	t	.1
	French fried, strips 2–3½" long:											
907	Oven heated	10 pce	50	35	163	2	19	1	9	3.8	4.2	.9
908	Fried in vegetable oil	10 ea	50	40	155	2	19	2	8	2.5	4	1.2
1188	Fried in veg and animal oil	10 ea	50	38	158	2	20	2	8	3.4	4	.5
909	Hashed browns from frozen	1 c	156	56	340	5	44	3	18	7	8	2.1
	Mashed:											
910	Home recipe with whole milk[2]	½ c	105	79	81	2	18	2	1	.3	.2	.1
911	Home recipe with milk and marg	½ c	105	76	111	2	18	2	4	1.1	1.9	1.3
912	Prepared from flakes; water, milk, margarine, salt added	½ c	110	76	124	2	17	1	6	1.6	2.5	1.7
	Potato products, prepared:											
	Au gratin:											
913	From dry mix	½ c	122	79	114	3	16	2	5	3.2	1.4	.2
914	From home recipe[3]	½ c	122	74	162	6	14	2	9	4.3	3.2	1.3
	Scalloped:											
915	From dry mix	½ c	122	79	114	3	16	1	5	3.2	1.5	.2
916	From home recipe[4]	½ c	122	81	105	4	13	1	5	1.7	1.6	.9
	Potato salad (see Mixed Dishes #715)											
1192	Potato puffs, cooked from frozen	½ c	62	61	107	1	16	1	6	1.1	1.9	0
918	Pumpkin, cooked from fresh, mashed	1 c	245	94	49	2	12	2	<1	.1	t	t
919	Pumpkin, canned	½ c	123	90	42	1	10	3	<1	.2	.1	t
1891	Radicchio, raw, shredded	½ c	20	93	5	0	1	–	<1	–	–	–
1894	Radicchio, raw, leaf	10 ea	80	93	18	1	4	–	<1	–	–	–
920	Red radishes	10 ea	45	95	8	<1	2	<1	<1	t	t	t
1793	Daikon radishes (Chinese) raw	½ c	44	95	8	<1	2	1	<.1	<.1	<.1	<.1
921	Refried beans, canned	½ c	126	72	135	8	23	7	1	.5	.6	.2
1375	Rutabaga, cooked cubes	½ c	85	89	33	1	7	2	<1	t	t	.1
922	Sauerkraut, canned with liquid	½ c	118	93	22	1	5	3	<1	t	t	.1
923	Seaweed, kelp, raw	1 oz	28	82	12	<1	3	<1	<1	.1	t	t
924	Seaweed, spirulina, dried	1 oz	28	5	81	16	7	1	2	.8	.2	.6
1866	Shallots, raw, chopped	1 tbs	10	80	7	0	2	0	<1	0	0	0

[1]Vitamin C varies with length of storage. After 3 months of storage approximately two-thirds of the ascorbic acid remains; after 6 to 7 months, about one-third remains.

[2]Recipe: 84% potatoes, 15% whole milk, 1% salt.

[3]Recipe: 55% potatoes, 30% whole milk, 9% cheddar cheese, 3% butter, 2% flour, 1% salt.

[4]Recipe: 59% potatoes, 36% whole milk, 2% butter, 2% flour, 1% salt.

(Computer code number is for West Diet Analysis program)

Chol (mg)	Calc (mg)	Iron (mg)	Magn (mg)	Pota (mg)	Sodi (mg)	Zinc (mg)	VT-A (RE)	Thia (mg)	Ribo (mg)	Niac (mg)	V-B6 (mg)	Fola (µg)	VT-C (mg)	VT-E α-TE (mg)
0	10	.53	14	110	7	.13	1	.08	.02	.66	.16	13	2	.11
0	20	2.75	55	844	16	.65	0	.22	.07	3.31	.7	22	26[1]	.1
0	8	.55	39	610	8	.45	0	.16	.03	2.18	.47	14	20[1]	.06
0	20	4.08	25	332	12	.28	0	.07	.06	1.78	.36	13	8[1]	.02
0	22	2.5	55	903	16	.73	0	.24	.06	3.45	.69	24	30[1]	.1
0	8	.64	39	641	11	.51	0	.2	.04	2.54	.5	19	24[1]	.06
0	27	3.45	21	377	9	.3	0	.04	.04	1.29	.28	10	9[1]	.02
0	7	.42	30	515	5	.41	0	.14	.03	1.96	.41	14	18[1]	.07
0	11	.42	27	443	7	.36	0	.13	.03	1.77	.36	12	10[1]	.07
0	6	.83	11	270	306	.2	0	.04	.02	1.33	.11	11	3	.25
0	8	.68	17	356	82	.26	1	.07	.02	1.14	.12	17	3	.25
6	10	.38	17	366	108	.19	0	.09	.01	1.63	.12	15	5	.25
0	23	2.36	26	680	53	.5	0	.17	.03	3.78	.2	10	10	.3
2	27	.28	19	314	318	.3	6	.09	.04	1.18	.24	9	7[1]	.5
2[5]	27	.27	19	303	310	.28	57	.09	.04	1.13	.23	8	6[1]	.32
4[5]	54	.24	20	256	365	.2	59	.12	.05	.73	.01	8	11	3.08
6	102	.39	18	268	536	.29	38	.02	.1	1.15	.05	8	4	.12
18[6]	146	.78	24	483	528	.84	47	.08	.14	1.22	.21	10	12	.64
13	44	.47	17	249	416	.31	54	.02	.07	1.26	.05	12	4	.18
7[7]	70	.7	23	463	410	.49	38	.08	.11	1.29	.22	11	13	.4
0	19	0	12	162	251	.19	1	.12	.01	1.05	.14	10	1	.03
0	37	1.4	22	564	2	.56	2651	.08	.19	1.01	.11	21	12	2.6
0	32	1.71	28	253	6	.21	2712	.03	.07	.45	.07	15	5	1.3
0	4	.11	3	60	4	.12	1	0	.01	.05	.01	12	2	.45
0	15	.45	10	242	18	.5	2	.01	.02	.2	.05	48	6	1.81
0	9	.13	4	104	11	.13	<1	<.01	.02	.13	.03	12	10	0
0	12	.18	7	100	9	.07	0	.01	.01	.09	.02	12	10	<.01
0	58	2.24	49	495	534	1.73	<1	.06	.07	.61	.13	105	8	0
0	41	.45	20	277	17	.3	48	.07	.03	.61	.09	13	16	.13
0	35	1.73	15	201	780	.22	2	.02	.03	.17	.15	28	17	.12
0	48	.81	34	25	66	.35	3	.01	.04	.13	<.01	50	<1	.24
0	34	8.08	55	382	293	.57	16	.67	1.04	3.63	.1	26	3	1.4
0	4	.12	2	33	1	.04	0	.01	0	.02	.03	3	1	.01

[5] Data is for margarine; if butter is used, cholesterol = 25 mg for 29 total mg.

[6] Data is for butter; if margarine is used, cholesterol = 37 mg.

[7] Data is for butter; if margarine is used cholesterol = 15 mg.

(For purposes of calculations, use "0" for t, <1, <.1, <.01, etc.)

Table A–1
Food Composition

Computer Code Number	Food Description	Measure	Wt (g)	H$_2$O (%)	Ener (cal)	Prot (g)	Carb (g)	Dietary Fiber (g)	Fat (g)	Fat Breakdown (g) Sat	Mono	Poly
	VEGETABLES AND LEGUMES—Cont.											
1557	Snow peas, stir-fried	1 c	165	89	69	5	12	4	<1	.1	t	.1
925	Soybeans, cooked from dry	½ c	86	63	149	14	9	5	8	1.1	1.7	4.4
1996	Soybeans, dry roasted	½ c	86	0	387	34	28	7	19	2.7	4.1	10.5
	Soybean products:											
926	Miso	½ c	138	42	284	16	39	7	8	1.2	1.8	4.7
927	Tofu (soybean curd, regular)	½ c	124	85	94	10	2	1	6	.9	1.3	3.3
	Spinach:											
928	Raw, chopped	1 c	56	92	12	2	2	2	<1	t	t	.1
929	Cooked, from fresh, drained	½ c	90	91	21	3	3	2	<1	t	t	.1
930	Cooked from frozen (leaf)	½ c	95	90	27	3	5	2	<1	t	t	.1
931	Canned, drained solids	½ c	107	92	25	3	4	3	1	.1	t	.2
	Spinach soufflé (see Mixed Dishes)											
	Squash, summer varieties, cooked:											
932	Varieties averaged	½ c	90	94	18	1	4	1	<1	.1	t	.1
933	Crookneck	½ c	90	94	18	1	4	1	<1	.1	t	.1
934	Zucchini	½ c	90	95	14	1	4	1	<1	t	t	t
	Squash, winter varieties, cooked:											
	Average of all varieties, baked:											
935	Mashed	1 c	245	89	96	2	21	7	2	.3	.1	.7
936	Cubes	1 c	205	89	80	2	18	6	1	.3	.1	.5
937	Acorn, baked, mashed	½ c	122	83	68	1	18	5	<1	t	t	.1
1218	Acorn, boiled, mashed	½ c	122	90	41	1	11	3	<1	t	t	t
	Butternut:											
938	Baked cubes	1 c	205	88	82	2	22	6	<1	t	t	.1
1219	Baked, mashed	½ c	122	88	49	1	13	3	<1	t	t	t
1193	Cooked from frozen	½ c	120	88	47	1	12	3	<1	t	t	t
1194	Hubbard, baked, mashed	½ c	120	85	60	3	13	3	1	.2	.1	.3
1195	Hubbard, boiled, mashed	½ c	118	91	35	2	8	3	<1	.1	t	.2
1196	Spaghetti, baked or boiled	½ c	77	92	22	1	5	1	<1	t	t	.1
1189	Succotash, cooked from frozen	½ c	85	74	79	4	17	5	1	.1	.1	.4
	Sweet potatoes:											
939	Baked in skin, peeled, 5 x 2" diam	1 ea	114	67	140	3	28	4	<1	t	t	.1
940	Boiled without skin, 5 x 2" diam	1 ea	151	73	159	3	37	3	<1	.1	t	.2
941	Candied, 2½ x 2"	1 pce	105	67	143	1	29	2	3	1.4	.7	.2
	Canned:											
942	Solid pack	½ c	128	74	129	3	30	2	<1	.1	t	.1
943	Vacuum pack, mashed	½ c	127	76	116	2	27	4	<1	.1	t	.1
944	Vacuum pack, 3¾ x 1"	2 pce	80	76	73	1	17	2	<1	t	t	.1
1940	Taro shoots, cooked slices	1 c	140	95	20	1	4	–	0	<.1	<.1	<.1
1941	Taro, tahitian, cooked slices	1 c	137	86.5	60	6	9	–	.93	.19	.08	.39
	Tomatillos:											
1877	Raw, each	1 ea	34	92	11	0	2	1	<1	–	–	–
1875	Raw, chopped	½ c	66	92	21	1	4	1	1	–	–	–
	Tomatoes:											
945	Raw, whole, 2⅗" diam	1 ea	123	94	26	1	6	1	<1	.1	.1	.2
946	Raw, chopped	1 c	180	94	38	2	8	2	1	.1	.1	.2

(Computer code number is for West Diet Analysis program)

PAGE KEY: A–4 = BEV   A–6 = DAIRY   A–12 = EGGS   A–14 = FAT/OIL   A–18 = FRUIT   A–26 = BAKERY   A–36 = GRAIN   A–44 = FISH
A–48 = MEATS   A–50 = POULTRY   A–54 = SAUSAGE   A–56 = MIXED/FAST   A–64 = NUTS/SEEDS   A–68 = SWEETS   A–70 = VEG/LEG
A–84 = MISC   A–88 = SOUPS/SAUCES   A–90 = FAST   A–106 = FRZN ENTREE   A–112 = BABY FOODS

Chol (mg)	Calc (mg)	Iron (mg)	Magn (mg)	Pota (mg)	Sodi (mg)	Zinc (mg)	VT-A (RE)	Thia (mg)	Ribo (mg)	Niac (mg)	V-B6 (mg)	Fola (μg)	VT-C (mg)	VT-E α-TE (mg)
0	71	3.43	40	330	7	.45	21	.22	.12	.94	.25	55	84	.64
0	88	4.42	74	443	1	.99	1	.13	.24	.34	.2	46	1	1.68
0	232	3.41	196	1173	2	4.11	2	.37	.65	.91	.19	176	4	3.96
0	92	3.76	58	226	5033	4.57	12	.13	.34	1.19	.3	46	0	.01
0	130	6.65	126	150	9	.99	11	.1	.06	.24	.06	19	<1	.01
0	55	1.52	44	312	44	.3	376	.04	.11	.4	.11	109	16	1.06
0	122	3.21	78	419	63	.68	737	.09	.21	.44	.22	131	9	.86
0	139	1.44	65	283	82	.66	739	.06	.16	.4	.14	103	12	.91
0	136	2.46	81	370	29[1]	.49	939	.02	.15	.41	.11	105	15	1.39
0	24	.32	22	173	1	.35	26[2]	.04	.04	.46	.06	18	5	.11
0	24	.32	22	173	1	.35	26[2]	.04	.04	.46	.08	18	5	.11
0	12	.31	20	228	3	.16	22[2]	.04	.04	.38	.07	15	4	.11
0	34	.81	20	1070	2	.64	871	.21	.06	1.72	.18	69	24	.29
0	29	.68	16	896	2	.53	729	.17	.05	1.44	.15	57	20	.25
0	54	1.14	52	535	5	.21	52	.2	.02	1.08	.24	23	13	.04
0	32	.68	32	322	4	.13	31	.12	.01	.65	.14	14	8	.02
0	84	1.23	59	582	8	.27	1435	.15	.03	1.99	.25	39	31	.04
0	50	.73	35	348	5	.16	854	.09	.02	1.19	.15	23	18	.02
0	23	.69	11	160	2	.14	401	.06	.05	.56	.08	20	4	.01
0	20	.56	26	430	10	.18	725	.09	.06	.67	.21	19	11	.14
0	12	.33	15	253	6	.12	473	.05	.03	.39	.12	11	8	.14
0	16	.26	8	91	14	.15	8	.03	.02	.63	.08	6	3	.09
0	13	.75	20	225	38	.38	20	.06	.06	1.11	.08	28	5	.31
0	32	2	28	396	11	.33	1928	.08	.14	.69	.27	26	25	.32
0	32	.85	15	276	20	.41	2575	.08	.21	.97	.37	17	26	.42
8[3]	27	1.19	12	198	73	.16	440	.02	.04	.41	.04	12	7	3.99
0	38	1.7	31	268	96	.27	1937	.03	.11	1.22	.3	14	7	.35
0	28	1.13	28	398	67	.23	1013	.05	.07	.94	.24	21	34	.32
0	18	.71	18	250	42	.14	638	.03	.05	.59	.15	13	21	.2
0	20	.57	11	482	3	.76	7	.05	.07	1.13	.16	4	26	1.4
0	204	214	70	854	74	.14	241.7	.06	.27	.66	.16	9.9	52	4.11
0	2	.21	7	91	<1	.07	4	.01	.01	.63	.02	2	4	.13
0	5	.41	13	177	1	.15	8	.03	.02	1.22	.04	5	8	.25
0	6	.55	13	273	11	.11	76	.07	.06	.77	.1	18	23[4]	.47
0	9	.81	20	400	16	.16	112	.11	.09	1.13	.14	27	34[4]	.68

[1]Dietary pack contains 58 mg sodium.

[2]Applies to squash including skin; flesh has no appreciable vitamin A value.

[3]For recipe using butter.

[4]Year-round average. From June through October, ascorbic acid is approximately 32 mg and 47 mg, respectively, for one tomato and 1 c chopped tomato. From November through May, market samples average around 12 and 18 mg, respectively.

(For purposes of calculations, use "0" for t, <1, <.1, <.01, etc.)

Table A–1
Food Composition

Computer Code Number	Food Description	Measure	Wt (g)	H₂O (%)	Ener (cal)	Prot (g)	Carb (g)	Dietary Fiber (g)	Fat (g)	Fat Breakdown (g)		
										Sat	Mono	Poly
	VEGETABLES AND LEGUMES—Cont.											
	Tomatoes—Cont.:											
947	Cooked from raw	1 c	240	92	65	3	14	2	1	.1	.2	.4
948	Canned, solids and liquid	1 c	240	94	48	2	10	2	1	.1	.1	.2
1879	Tomatoes, sundried:	1 c	54	15	139	8	30	7	2	.2	.3	.6
1881	Pieces	10 pce	20	15	52	3	11	2	1	.1	.1	.2
1885	Oil pack, drained	33 ea	100	54	213	5	23	7	14	1.9	8.7	2.1
2020	Tomato, raw	1 ea	123	94	26	1	6	1	<1	.1	.1	.2
949	Tomato juice, canned	1 c	244	94	41	2	10	1	<1	t	t	.1
	Tomato products, canned:											
950	Paste	1 c	262	80	220	10	49	11	2	.3	.4	.9
951	Puree	1 c	250	87	102	4	25	6	<1	t	t	.1
952	Sauce	1 c	245	89	73	3	18	3	<1	.1	.1	.2
953	Turnips, cubes, cooked from fresh	½ c	78	94	14	1	4	2	<1	t	t	t
	Turnip greens, cooked:											
954	From fresh, leaves and stems	1 c	144	93	29	2	6	4	<1	.1	t	.1
955	From frozen, chopped	1 c	164	90	49	6	8	7	1	.2	.1	.3
956	Vegetable juice cocktail, canned	½ c	121	93	23	1	6	1	<1	t	t	t
	Vegetables, mixed:											
957	Canned, drained	½ c	81	87	38	2	8	3	<1	t	t	.1
958	Frozen, cooked, drained	½ c	91	83	53	3	12	5	<1	t	t	.1
1818	Water chestnuts, Chinese, raw	½ c	62	74	66	1	15	2	0	<.1	<.1	<.1
959	Water chestnuts, canned, slices	½ c	70	86	35	1	9	2	<1	t	t	t
960	Water chestnuts, canned, whole	4 ea	28	86	14	<1	3	1	<1	t	t	t
1190	Watercress, fresh, chopped	½ c	17	95	2	<1	<1	<1	<1	t	t	t
	MISCELLANEOUS											
	Baking powders for home use:											
	Sodium aluminum sulfate:											
962	With monocalcium phosphate monohydrate	1 tsp	3	2	4	<1	1	0	0	0	0	0
963	With monocalcium phosphate monohydrate, calcium sulfate	1 tsp	3	5	2	0	1	0	0	0	0	0
964	Straight phosphate	1 tsp	4	4	2	<1	1	0	0	0	0	0
965	Low sodium	1 tsp	4	6	4	<1	2	0	<1	0	0	0
1204	Baking soda	1 tsp	3	<1	0	0	0	0	0	0	0	0
966	Basil, dried	1 tbs	4	6	10	1	2	1	<1	–	–	–
2068	Cajun seasoning	1 tsp	3	5	6	<1	1	<1	<1	–	–	–
961	Carob flour	1 c	103	4	394	5	92	41	1	.1	.2	.2
967	Catsup:	¼ c	61	67	64	1	17	1	<1	t	t	.1
968	Tablespoon	1 tbs	15	67	16	<1	4	<1	<1	t	t	t
1200	Cayenne/red pepper	1 tbs	5	8	16	1	3	1	1	.2	.1	.4
969	Celery seed	1 tsp	2	6	8	<1	1	<1	1	t	.3	.1
1203	Chili powder:	1 tbs	8	8	25	1	4	3	1	.3	.3	.6
970	Teaspoon	1 tsp	3	8	8	<1	2	1	<1	.1	.1	.2
	Chocolate:											
971	Baking, unsweetened, square	1 oz	28	1	146	3	8	4	15	9.2	5.2	.5

(Computer code number is for West Diet Analysis program)

PAGE KEY: A–4 = BEV   A–6 = DAIRY   A–12 = EGGS   A–14 = FAT/OIL   A–18 = FRUIT   A–26 = BAKERY   A–36 = GRAIN   A–44 = FISH
A–48 = MEATS   A–50 = POULTRY   A–54 = SAUSAGE   A–56 = MIXED/FAST   A–64 = NUTS/SEEDS   A–68 = SWEETS   A–70 = VEG/LEG
A–84 = MISC   A–88 = SOUPS/SAUCES   A–90 = FAST   A–106 = FRZN ENTREE   A–112 = BABY FOODS

Chol (mg)	Calc (mg)	Iron (mg)	Magn (mg)	Pota (mg)	Sodi (mg)	Zinc (mg)	VT-A (RE)	Thia (mg)	Ribo (mg)	Niac (mg)	V-B6 (mg)	Fola (μg)	VT-C (mg)	VT-E α-TE (mg)
0	14	1.34	34	670	26	.26	178	.17	.14	1.8	.23	31	55	.91
0	62[1]	1.46	29	530	391[2]	.38	144	.11	.07	1.76	.22	19	36	.77
0	59	4.91	105	1851	1131	1.08	47	.29	.26	4.89	.18	37	21	<.01
0	22	1.82	39	685	419	.4	17	.11	.1	1.81	.07	14	8	<.01
0	47	2.68	81	1565	266	.78	129	.19	.38	3.63	.32	23	102	–
0	6	.55	14	273	11	.11	77	.07	.06	.77	.1	18	23	.47
0	22	1.42	27	537	881[3]	.34	137	.11	.08	1.64	.27	49	45	2.22
0	92	7.83	133	2441	2070[4]	2.1	647	.41	.5	8.44	1	59	110	11.3
0	37	2.33	60	1050	998[5]	.55	340	.18	.13	4.3	.38	27	88	6.3
0	34	1.89	47	909	1482[6]	.61	240	.16	.14	2.82	.38	23	32	3.43
0	17	.17	6	105	39	.16	0	.02	.02	.23	.05	7	9	.02
0	197	1.15	32	292	42	.2	792	.06	.1	.59	.26	170	39	2.48
0	248	3.18	43	366	25	.67	1308	.09	.12	.77	.11	65	36	4.79
0	13	.51	13	234	442	.24	142	.05	.03	.88	.17	25	33	.39
0	22	.86	13	237	121	.33	944	.04	.04	.47	.06	19	4	.49
0	23	.74	20	154	32	.45	389	.06	.11	.77	.07	17	3	.33
0	7	.04	14	362	9	.31	0	.09	.12	.62	.20	10	2	.74
0	3	.61	3	83	6	.27	<1	.01	.02	.25	.11	4	1	.35
0	1	.25	1	33	2	.11	<1	<.01	.01	.1	.04	2	<1	.14
0	20	.03	4	56	7	.02	80	.01	.02	.03	.02	2	7	.17
0	58	0	<1	4	328	0	0	0	0	0	0	0	0	–
0	176	.32	1	1	318	<.01	0	0	0	0	0	0	0	0
0	295	.43	1	<1	316	<.01	0	0	0	0	0	0	0	0
0	173	.35	1	434	4	.03	0	0	0	0	0	0	0	<.01
0	0	0	0	0	821	0	0	0	0	0	0	0	0	0
0	85	1.68	19	154	2	.26	38	.01	.01	.31	–	–	2	.07
–	–	–	–	30	474	–	–	–	–	–	–	–	–	–
0	358	3.04	56	852	36	.95	1	.05	.47	1.96	.38	30	<1	.65
0	12	.43	13	295	723	.14	62	.05	.04	.84	.11	9	9	.9
0	3	.1	3	72	178	.03	15	.01	.01	.21	.03	2	2	.22
0	8	.41	8	106	2	.13	209	.02	.05	.44	–	–	4	.24
0	35	.9	9	28	3	.14	<1	.01	.01	.1	–	–	<1	.02
0	22	1.12	14	149	81	.21	279	.03	.06	.61	–	4	5	.08
0	7	.43	5	50	30	.07	105	.01	.02	.2	–	2	2	.03
0	21	1.79	88	233	4	1.14	3	.02	.05	.31	.03	2	0	.34

(1) Calcium is added as a firming agent.

(2) Dietary pack contains 31 mg sodium.

(3) If no salt is added, sodium content is 24 mg.

(4) If salt is added, sodium content is 2070 mg.

(5) If salt is added, sodium content is 998 mg.

(6) With salt added.

(For purposes of calculations, use "0" for t, <1, <.1, <.01, etc.)

Table A–1
Food Composition

Computer Code Number	Food Description	Measure	Wt (g)	H$_2$O (%)	Ener (cal)	Prot (g)	Carb (g)	Dietary Fiber (g)	Fat (g)	Fat Breakdown (g) Sat	Mono	Poly
	MISCELLANEOUS—Cont.											
	For other chocolate items, see Sweeteners & Sweets											
972	Cilantro/coriander, fresh	1 tbs	1	93	<1	<1	<1	<1	<1	t	t	t
1197	Cornstarch	1 tbs	8	8	30	<1	7	<1	<1	t	t	t
2287	Cinnamon	1 tsp	2	10	5	<1	2	1	<1	t	t	t
2239	Curry powder	1 tsp	2	10	7	<1	1	1	<1	t	.2	t
1202	Dill weed, dried	1 tbs	3	7	8	1	2	1	<1	–	–	–
1705	Dip, french onion	1 tbs	14	70	31	<1	<1	<1	3	1.9	.9	.1
975	Garlic cloves	1 ea	3	59	4	<1	1	<1	<1	t	0	t
2238	Garlic powder	1 tsp	3	6	9	<1	2	<1	<1	t	t	t
977	Gelatin, dry, unsweetened: Envelope	1 ea	7	13	23	6	0	0	<1	t	t	t
978	Ginger root, slices, raw	2 pce	4	81	3	<1	1	<1	<1	t	t	t
1198	Horseradish, prepared	1 tbs	15	87	6	<1	1	<1	<1	t	t	t
1997	Hummous/hummus	1 c	246	65	421	12	50	10	21	3	9	8
1909	Mustard, country dijon	1 tsp	5	–	5	0	0	0	0	0	0	0
2019	Mustard, gai choy chinese	1 tbs	15.6	94	33	2	6	–	.27	–	–	–
979	Mustard, prepared (1 packet = 1 tsp)	1 tsp	5	80	4	<1	<1	<1	<1	t	.2	t
	Miso (see #926 under Vegetables and Legumes, Soybean products)											
2067	No MSG seasoned salt	1 tsp	5	<1	3	<1	1	<1	<1	–	–	–
980	Olives, green	5 ea	19	78	22	<1	<1	<1	2	.3	1.9	.2
981	Olives, ripe, pitted	5 ea	22	80	25	<1	1	1	2	.3	1.8	.2
2288	Onion powder	1 tsp	2	5	7	<1	2	<1	<1	t	t	t
2237	Oregano, ground	1 tsp	1	7	5	<1	1	<1	<1	t	t	.1
2066	Oriental seasoning blend	1 tsp	3	<1	10	<1	2	<1	<1	–	–	–
2236	Paprika	1 tsp	2	10	6	<1	1	<1	<1	t	t	.2
887	Parsley, freeze dried	¼ c	1	2	3	<1	<1	<1	<1	t	t	t
	Parsley, fresh (see #885 and #886)											
985	Pepper, black	1 tsp	2	11	5	<1	1	1	<1	t	t	t
	Pickles:											
986	Dill, medium, 3¾ x 1¼" diam	1 ea	65	92	12	<1	3	1	<1	t	t	.1
987	Fresh pack, slices, 1½" diam x ¼"	2 pce	15	92	3	<1	3	<1	<1	t	t	t
988	Sweet, medium	1 ea	35	65	41	<1	11	<1	<1	t	t	t
989	Pickle relish, sweet	2 tbs	30	63	41	<1	10	1	<1	.1	t	.1
	Popcorn (see Grain Products #539–541)											
917	Potato chips	14 ea	28	2	150	2	15	1	10	3.1	2.8	3.5
1201	Sage, ground	1 tsp	1	8	3	<1	1	<1	<1	.1	t	t
1347	Salsa, from recipe	1 tbs	14	93	3	<1	1	<1	<1	t	t	t
2218	Salsa, pico de gallo, medium	2 tbs	30	92	5	0	2	<1	0	0	0	0
990	Salt	1 tsp	5	<1	0	0	0	0	0	0	0	0
	Salt substitutes:											
1205	Morton, salt substitute	1 tsp	2	2	<1	0	<1	0	0	0	0	0
1207	Morton, light salt	1 tsp	6	0	0	0	0	0	0	0	0	0
2289	Norcliff Thayer, no salt, packet	1 ea	1	0	0	0	0	0	0	0	0	0
991	Vinegar, cider	½ c	120	94	17	0	7	0	0	0	0	0
2172	Balsamic	1 tbs	15	64	21	0	5	0	0	0	0	0
2176	Malt	1 tbs	15	90	5	0	<1	0	0	0	0	0
2182	Tarragon	1 tbs	15	95	3	0	<1	0	0	0	0	0
2181	White wine	1 tbs	15	89	5	0	<1	0	0	0	0	0

(Computer code number is for West Diet Analysis program)

PAGE KEY: A–4 = BEV   A–6 = DAIRY   A–12 = EGGS   A–14 = FAT/OIL   A–18 = FRUIT   A–26 = BAKERY   A–36 = GRAIN   A–44 = FISH   A–48 = MEATS   A–50 = POULTRY   A–54 = SAUSAGE   A–56 = MIXED/FAST   A–64 = NUTS/SEEDS   A–68 = SWEETS   A–70 = VEG/LEG   A–84 = MISC   A–88 = SOUPS/SAUCES   A–90 = FAST   A–106 = FRZN ENTREE   A–112 = BABY FOODS

Chol (mg)	Calc (mg)	Iron (mg)	Magn (mg)	Pota (mg)	Sodi (mg)	Zinc (mg)	VT-A (RE)	Thia (mg)	Ribo (mg)	Niac (mg)	V-B6 (mg)	Fola (µg)	VT-C (mg)	VT-E α-TE (mg)
0	1	.02	<1	5	<1	<.01	3	<.01	<.01	.01	<.01	<1	<1	.25
0	<1	.04	<1	<1	1	<.01	0	0	0	0	0	0	0	0
0	25	.76	1	10	1	.04	1	<.01	<.01	.03	.02	–	1	–
0	10	.59	5	31	1	.08	2	<.01	.01	.07	–	–	<1	<.01
0	54	1.46	14	99	6	.1	0	.01	.01	.09	.04	–	–	–
6	17	.01	2	22	27	.04	28	.01	.02	.02	<.01	2	<1	.08
0	5	.05	1	12	1	.03	0	.01	<.01	.02	.04	<1	1	0
0	2	.08	2	33	1	.07	0	.01	<.01	.02	.61	2	<1	<.01
0	4	.08	2	1	14	.01	0	<.01	.02	.01	<.01	2	0	0
0	1	.02	2	17	1	.01	0	<.01	<.01	.03	.01	<1	<1	.01
0	9	.13	4	44	14	.18	0	0	0	0	.01	2	0	<.01
0	123	4	71	428	600	2.7	6	.23	.13	1	.98	146	19	2.46
0	–	–	–	10	120	–	–	–	–	–	–	–	–	–
–	–	–	–	–	–	–	–	–	–	–	–	–	–	–
0	4	.1	2	6	63	.03	0	0	0	0	<.01	0	0	.09
–	–	–	–	13	1390	–	–	–	–	–	–	–	–	–
0	12	.31	4	10	456	.01	6	0	0	0	<.01	<1	0	.57
0	19	.74	1	2	192	.05	9	<.01	0	.01	<.01	0	<1	.66
0	8	.06	2	19	1	.05	0	.01	<.01	.01	.03	3	<1	–
0	16	.44	3	17	<1	.04	7	<.01	<.01	.06	–	–	1	.02
–	–	–	–	12	107	–	–	–	–	–	–	–	–	–
0	4	.5	4	47	1	.08	121	.01	.04	.32	–	–	1	.01
0	2	.54	4	63	4	.06	63	.01	.03	.15	.02	21	1	–
0	9	.58	4	25	1	.03	<1	<.01	<.01	.02	0	–	0	.02
0	6	.34	7	75	833	.09	21	.01	.02	.04	.01	1	1	.1
0	5	.08	2	17	192	.02	5	<.01	<.01	.01	<.01	<1	<1	.02
0	1	.21	1	11	328	.03	4	<.01	.01	.06	.01	<1	<1	.06
0	6	.24	1	60	214	.02	3	0	.01	0	<.01	0	2	.05
0	7	.46	19	357	166[1]	.31	0	.05	.06	1.07	.19	13	9	1.37
0	17	.28	4	11	<1	.05	6	.01	<.01	.06	–	–	<1	.02
0	1	.06	1	23	55	.02	21	.01	<.01	.06	.01	2	5	.04
0	–	–	–	–	260	–	–	–	–	–	–	–	–	–
0	1	.01	<1	<1	1938	0	0	0	0	0	0	0	0	0
0	11	–	<1	1006	<1	–	0	–	–	–	–	–	–	–
0	3	0	4	1500	1099	0	0	0	0	0	0	0	0	0
0	–	–	–	385	0	–	0	0	0	0	0	0	0	–
0	7	.7	26	120	1	0	0	0	0	0	0	0		0
–	2	.07	–	11	3	–	–	.07	.07	.07	–	–	<1	–
–	2	.07	–	14	5	–	–	.07	.07	.07	–	–	2	–
–	<1	.07	–	2	1	–	–	.07	.07	.07	–	–	<1	–
–	1	.07	–	12	1	–	–	.07	.07	.07	–	–	<1	–

(1)If no salt added, sodium = 2 mg.

(For purposes of calculations, use "0" for t, <1, <.1, <.01, etc.)

A

Table A–1
Food Composition

Computer Code Number	Food Description	Measure	Wt (g)	H$_2$O (%)	Ener (cal)	Prot (g)	Carb (g)	Dietary Fiber (g)	Fat (g)	Fat Breakdown (g)		
										Sat	Mono	Poly
MISCELLANEOUS—Cont.												
	Yeast:											
992	Baker's, dry, active, package	1 ea	7	8	21	3	3	2	<1	t	.2	t
993	Brewer's, dry	1 tbs	8	5	23	3	3	3	<1	t	t	0
SOUPS, SAUCES, AND GRAVIES												
	SOUPS, canned, condensed:											
	Unprepared, condensed:											
1210	Cream of celery	1 c	251	85	181	3	18	2	11	2.8	2.6	5
1215	Cream of chicken	1 c	251	82	233	7	19	1	15	4.2	6.5	3
1216	Cream of mushroom	1 c	251	81	259	4	19	1	19	5.1	3.6	8.9
1220	Onion	1 c	246	86	113	8	16	2	4	.5	1.5	1.3
	Prepared w/equal volume whole milk:											
994	Clam chowder, New England	1 c	248	85	164	9	17	1	7	2.9	2.3	1.1
1209	Cream of celery	1 c	248	87	164	6	15	1	10	3.9	2.5	2.6
995	Cream of chicken	1 c	248	85	191	7	15	<1	11	4.6	4.5	1.6
996	Cream of mushroom	1 c	248	85	203	6	15	1	14	5.1	3	4.6
1214	Cream of potato	1 c	248	87	149	6	17	1	6	3.8	1.7	.6
1213	Oyster stew	1 c	245	89	135	6	10	0	8	5	2.1	.3
997	Tomato	1 c	248	85	161	6	22	1	6	2.9	1.6	1.1
	Prepared with equal volume of water:											
998	Bean with bacon	1 c	253	84	172	8	23	9	6	1.5	2.2	1.8
999	Beef broth/bouillon/consommé	1 c	240	98	17	3	<1	0	1	.3	.2	t
1000	Beef noodle	1 c	244	92	83	5	9	1	3	1.1	1.2	.5
1001	Chicken noodle	1 c	241	92	75	4	9	1	2	.7	1.1	.6
1002	Chicken rice	1 c	241	94	60	4	7	1	2	.5	.9	.4
1208	Chili beef	1 c	250	85	170	7	21	9	7	3.3	2.8	.3
1003	Clam chowder, Manhatten	1 c	244	92	78	2	12	1	2	.4	.4	1.3
1004	Cream of chicken	1 c	244	91	117	3	9	<1	7	2.1	3.3	1.5
1005	Cream of mushroom	1 c	244	90	129	2	9	<1	9	2.4	1.7	4.2
1006	Minestrone	1 c	241	91	82	4	11	1	3	.6	.7	1.1
1211	Onion	1 c	241	93	58	4	8	1	2	.3	.8	.7
1007	Split pea & ham	1 c	253	82	190	10	28	5	4	1.8	1.8	.6
1008	Tomato	1 c	244	90	85	2	17	<1	2	.4	.4	1
1009	Vegetable beef	1 c	244	92	78	6	10	<1	2	.9	.8	.1
1010	Vegetarian vegetable	1 c	241	92	72	2	12	<1	2	.3	.8	.7
1707	Ready to serve											
	Chunky chicken soup	½ c	126	84	89	6	9	<1	3	1	1.5	.7
	SOUPS, dehydrated:											
	Unprepared, dry products:											
1011	Beef bouillon, packet	1 ea	6	3	14	1	1	<1	1	.3	.2	t
1012	Onion soup, packet	1 ea	34	4	100	4	18	4	2	.5	1.2	.2
	Prepared with water:											
1299	Beef broth/bouillon	1 c	244	97	20	1	2	0	1	.3	.3	t
1376	Chicken broth	1 c	244	97	22	1	1	0	1	.3	.4	.4
1013	Chicken noodle	1 c	251	94	53	3	8	<1	1	.3	.5	.4
1122	Cream of chicken	1 c	261	91	107	2	13	1	5	3.4	1.2	.4
1014	Onion	1 c	246	96	27	1	5	<1	1	.1	.3	.1
1217	Split pea	1 c	255	87	125	7	21	3	1	.4	.7	.3
1015	Tomato vegetable	1 c	252	93	55	2	10	1	1	.4	.3	.1

(Computer code number is for West Diet Analysis program)

PAGE KEY: A–4 = BEV   A–6 = DAIRY   A–12 = EGGS   A–14 = FAT/OIL   A–18 = FRUIT   A–26 = BAKERY   A–36 = GRAIN   A–44 = FISH
A–48 = MEATS   A–50 = POULTRY   A–54 = SAUSAGE   A–56 = MIXED/FAST   A–64 = NUTS/SEEDS   A–68 = SWEETS   A–70 = VEG/LEG
A–84 = MISC   A–88 = SOUPS/SAUCES   A–90 = FAST   A–106 = FRZN ENTREE   A–112 = BABY FOODS

Chol (mg)	Calc (mg)	Iron (mg)	Magn (mg)	Pota (mg)	Sodi (mg)	Zinc (mg)	VT-A (RE)	Thia (mg)	Ribo (mg)	Niac (mg)	V-B6 (mg)	Fola (µg)	VT-C (mg)	VT-E α-TE (mg)
0	4	1.16	7	140	4	.45	<1	.16	.38	2.79	.11	164	<1	.01
0	17[1]	1.38	18	151	10	.63	0	1.25	.34	3.03	.4	313	0	–
28	80	1.26	13	245	1900	.3	60	.06	.1	.66	.02	5	1	.38
20	68	1.2	5	175	1972	1.26	113	.06	.12	1.64	.03	3	<1	.33
3	65	1.05	10	168	2033	1.19	0	.06	.17	1.62	.02	8	2	2.6
0	54	1.35	5	137	2115	1.23	0	.07	.05	1.21	.1	30	2	.57
22	186	1.49	22	300	992	.8	40	.07	.24	1.03	.13	10	3	.15
32	186	.69	22	310	1009	.2	67	.07	.25	.44	.06	8	1	.97
27	181	.67	17	273	1047	.67	94	.07	.26	.92	.07	8	1	.24
20	179	.59	20	270	1076	.64	37	.08	.28	.91	.06	10	2	1.34
22	166	.55	17	322	1061	.67	67	.08	.24	.64	.09	9	1	.1
32	166	1.05	20	235	1041	10.3	44	.07	.23	.34	.06	10	4	.49
17	159	1.81	22	449	932	.29	109	.13	.25	1.52	.16	21	68	2.6
3	81	2.05	46	402	951	1.03	89	.09	.03	.57	.04	32	2	.08
0	14	.41	5	130	782	0	0	<.01	.05	1.87	.02	5	0	0
5	15	1.1	5	100	952	1.54	63	.07	.06	1.07	.04	4	<1	.02
7	17	.77	5	55	1106	.39	71	.05	.06	1.39	.03	2	<1	.07
7	17	.75	0	101	815	.26	66	.02	.02	1.13	.02	1	<1	.05
13	43	2.13	30	525	1035	1.4	151	.06	.07	1.07	.16	18	4	.18
2	27	1.63	12	187	578	.98	96	.03	.04	.82	.1	10	4	.73
10	34	.61	2	88	986	.63	56	.03	.06	.82	.02	2	<1	.2
2	46	.51	5	100	1032	.59	0	.05	.09	.72	.01	5	1	1.24
2	34	.92	7	313	911	.73	234	.05	.04	.94	.1	16	1	.07
0	27	.67	2	67	1053	.61	0	.03	.02	.6	.05	15	1	.29
8	23	2.28	48	400	1006	1.32	45	.15	.08	1.47	.07	3	2	.15
0	12	1.76	7	264	871	.24	69	.09	.05	1.42	.11	15	66	2.49
5	17	1.12	5	173	956	1.54	189	.04	.05	1.03	.08	10	2	.32
0	22	1.08	7	210	822	.46	301	.05	.05	.92	.05	11	1	.8
15	13	.87	4	88	446	.5	65	.04	.09	2.21	.03	2	1	.09
1	4	.06	3	27	1019	0	<1	<.01	.01	.27	.01	2	0	.01
2	48	.51	22	226	3044	.2	1	.1	.21	1.73	.03	6	1	.37
0	10	.02	7	37	1362	.07	1	<.01	.02	.36	0	0	0	.02
0	15	.07	5	24	1484	.01	12	.01	.03	.19	0	2	0	.02
3	32	.5	7	31	1278	.2	6	.07	.06	.88	.01	2	<1	.03
3	76	.26	5	214	1185	1.57	123	.1	.2	2.61	.05	5	1	.15
0	12	.15	5	64	849	.06	<1	.03	.06	.48	0	1	<1	.103
3	20	.94	43	224	1148	.56	5	.21	.14	1.26	.05	40	0	.13
0	8	.63	20	104	1142	.17	19	.06	.04	.79	.05	10	7	.81

(For purposes of calculations, use "0" for t, <1, <.1, <.01, etc.)

Table A–1
Food Composition

Computer Code Number	Food Description	Measure	Wt (g)	H₂O (%)	Ener (cal)	Prot (g)	Carb (g)	Dietary Fiber (g)	Fat (g)	Fat Breakdown (g)		
										Sat	Mono	Poly
	SAUCES											
	From dry mixes, prepared with milk:											
1016	Cheese sauce	1 c	279	77	307	16	23	1	17	9.3	5.3	1.6
1017	Hollandaise	1 c	259	84	240	5	14	<1	20	11.6	5.9	.9
1018	White sauce	1 c	264	82	240	10	21	<1	13	6.4	4.7	1.7
	From home recipe:											
1019	White sauce, medium¹	1 c	250	77	355	9	20	<1	27	7.8	9.1	8.8
1206	Lowfat cheese sauce	¼ c	61	73	85	6	4	0	5	2.1	1.9	.9
	Ready to serve:											
2202	Alfredo sauce, reduced fat	¼ c	69	–	170	5	16	0	10	6	–	–
1020	Barbeque sauce	1 tbs	16	81	10	<1	1	<1	<1	t	.1	.1
1706	Chili sauce, tomato base	1 tbs	17	68	18	<1	4	<1	<1	t	t	t
2126	Creole sauce	¼ c	62	–	25	1	4	1	1	0	–	–
2124	Hoisin sauce	2 tbs	34	47	70	1	14	0	2	0	–	–
2199	Pesto sauce	2 tbs	29	21	155	5	2	<1	14	3.6	9.1	1.1
1021	Soy sauce	1 tbs	18	71	10	<1	2	0	<1	t	t	t
2123	Szechuan sauce	2 tbs	31	82	23	1	4	<1	1	.1	.2	.2
1380	Teriyaki sauce	1 tbs	18	68	15	<1	3	0	0	0	0	0
	Spaghetti sauce, canned:											
1377	Plain	1 c	249	75	271	5	40	8	12	1.7	6.1	3.3
1378	With meat	1 c	257	74	309	9	39	8	15	2.8	7.2	3.3
1379	With mushrooms	½ c	123	75	108	2	13	1	3	.4	1.5	.8
	GRAVIES											
	Canned:											
1022	Beef	1 c	233	88	123	9	11	1	6	2.7	2	.2
1023	Chicken	1 c	238	85	188	5	13	<1	14	3.4	6.1	3.5
1024	Mushroom	1 c	238	89	119	3	13	<1	6	1	2.8	2.4
1025	From dry mix, brown	1 c	258	92	75	2	13	<1	2	.8	.7	.1
1026	From dry mix, chicken	1 c	260	91	83	3	14	<1	2	.5	.9	.4
	FAST FOOD RESTAURANTS											
	ARBY'S											
1402	Bac'n cheddar deluxe	1 ea	226	59	501	21	38	<1	31	8.5	12.4	11.2
	Roast beef sandwiches:											
1403	Regular	1 ea	147	47	363	21	34	1	17	6.6	7.6	2.4
1404	Junior	1 ea	86	48	275	11	22	<1	10	3.9	5	1.7
1405	Super	1 ea	234	58	509	22	50	1	26	7	11	5.4
1407	Beef 'n cheddar	1 ea	197	34	516	25	44	1	27	7.6	12.1	7.1
1408	Chicken breast sandwich	1 ea	184	52	401	20	47	1	20	3	8.8	10.3
1412	Ham'n cheese sandwich	1 ea	156	54	328	23	32	<1	13	4.7	5.4	2.7
1726	Italian sub sandwich	1 ea	297	–	671	34	47	–	39	12.8	15.7	8.5
1413	Turkey sandwich, deluxe	1 ea	197	61	263	20	33	<1	6	1.6	2.3	7.8
1680	Turkey sub sandwich	1 ea	277	62	486	33	47	–	19	5.3	6	7
	Milk shakes:											
1419	Chocolate	1 ea	340	74	451	10	77	<1	12	2.8	7	1.7
1420	Jamocha	1 ea	326	75	368	9	59	0	11	2.5	6.4	1.6
1421	Vanilla	1 ea	312	75	330	11	46	0	12	3.9	5.3	2.3
1728	Salad, roast chicken	1 ea	400	89	204	24	12	–	7	3.3	.9	.9
1729	Sports drink, Upper Ten	1 ea	358	88	169	0	42	–	0	0	0	0

Source: Arby's Inc. for the basic nutrients. Values for some nutrients from known values of major ingredients.

⁽¹⁾Made with enriched flour, margarine, and whole milk.

(Computer code number is for West Diet Analysis program)

Chol (mg)	Calc (mg)	Iron (mg)	Magn (mg)	Pota (mg)	Sodi (mg)	Zinc (mg)	VT-A (RE)	Thia (mg)	Ribo (mg)	Niac (mg)	V-B6 (mg)	Fola (µg)	VT-C (mg)	VT-E α-TE (mg)
53	569	.28	47	552	1565	.97	117	.15	.56	.32	.14	13	2	.34
52	124	.9	8	124	1564	.7	220	.04	.18	.06	.5	22	<1	.26
34	425	.26	264	444	797	.55	92	.08	.45	.53	.07	16	3	1.58
29	261	.73	32	344	369	.94	310	.19	.42	.98	.1	14	2	3.4
11	165	.25	10	99	387	.73	58	.03	.14	.16	.03	4	0	.55
30	150	0	–	80	600	–	80	0	.1	0	–	–	0	–
0	3	.12	1	27	128	.03	14	<.01	<.01	.06	.01	1	1	.18
0	3	.14	2	63	227	.05	24	.02	.01	.27	.02	1	3	.05
0	20	0	–	–	340	–	40	–	–	–	–	–	0	–
0	0	0	–	–	500	–	0	–	–	–	–	–	0	–
9	209	1.22	17	103	211	.52	43	.01	.05	.22	.04	8	3	–
0	3	.36	6	32	1029	.07	0	.01	.02	.6	.03	3	3	0
0	6	.28	6	54	255	.06	27	.01	.01	.28	.02	1	2	–
0	4	.31	11	41	690	.02	0	.01	.01	.23	.02	4	0	0
0	70	1.62	60	956	1235	.52	306	.14	.15	3.76	.88	54	28	4.98
16	69	2	61	978	1213	1.41	299	.14	.17	4.64	.9	54	27	6.08
0	15	1	15	333	494	.34	242	.08	.08	.93	.16	13	9	1.35
7	14	1.63	5	188	1304	2.33	0	.07	.08	1.54	.02	5	0	.15
5	48	1.12	5	259	1373	1.9	264	.04	.1	1.05	.02	5	0	.37
0	17	1.57	5	252	1356	1.67	0	.08	.15	1.6	.05	29	0	.19
3	67	.23	10	57	1075	.31	0	.04	.08	.81	0	0	0	.05
3	39	.26	10	62	1133	.32	0	.05	.15	.78	.03	3	3	.05
37	108	4.5	–	422	1672	3	39	.34	.45	9.4	–	–	11	–
41	57	4.6	15	400	888	3.56	1	.28	.46	10.4	.2	13	1	–
21	39	2.6	8	194	502	1.5	–	.17	.25	6.4	.1	7	–	–
40	83	6	23	491	1082	3.45	28	.36	.5	11.4	.3	19	8	–
53	152	6.2	24	326	1184	3.05	–	.43	.64	10	–	19	1	–
41	54	2.6	27	298	919	.14	–	.2	.51	8	.34	16	5	–
51	157	2.7	29	353	1292	.83	37	.77	.34	7	.31	24	22	–
69	410	4.32	–	565	2062	–	100	.92	.49	8.2	–	–	11	–
33	131	2.7	30	357	1275	1.5	40	.08	.43	15.6	.52	20	12	–
51	400	4.68	–	500	2033	–	–	13.2	.54	18.8	–	–	–	–
36	250	2.7	48	410	341	1.5	40	.06	.85	.8	.14	14	5	–
35	250	2.7	36	525	262	1.5	60	.06	.77	5	.14	14	2	–
32	300	2.7	36	686	281	1.5	100	.23	.85	4	.14	37	2	–
43	170	1.98	–	877	508	–	485	.33	.54	5.6	–	–	51	–
0	–	–	–	0	40	–	–	–	–	–	–	–	–	–

(For purposes of calculations, use "0" for t, <1, <.1, <.01, etc.)

Table A–1
Food Composition

Computer Code Number	Food Description	Measure	Wt (g)	H₂O (%)	Ener (cal)	Prot (g)	Carb (g)	Dietary Fiber (g)	Fat (g)	Fat Breakdown (g)		
										Sat	Mono	Poly
	BURGER KING											
	Croissant sandwiches:											
1422	Egg, bacon, & cheese	1 ea	119	50	353	15	18	<1	24	8.1	12.1	3
1423	Egg, sausage, & cheese	1 ea	163	47	543	21	22	1	42	14	20.5	5.1
1424	Egg, ham, & cheese	1 ea	145	57	352	18	19	<1	22	7	11.1	2
	Whopper sandwiches:											
1425	Whopper	1 ea	265	58	618	27	44	3	38	10.8	10.8	12.8
1426	Whopper with cheese	1 ea	289	57	708	32	44	3	45	15.7	12.8	12.8
1427	Double beef	1 ea	351	57	860	46	45	3	56	19	19	13
1428	Double beef & cheese	1 ea	374	57	947	52	45	3	63	23.9	21.9	14
1431	Hamburger	1 ea	109	47	275	15	30	1	11	4	5	1
1432	Cheeseburger	1 ea	120	49	313	18	29	1	15	6.3	6.3	1
1433	Double cheeseburger with bacon	1 ea	159	49	460	32	20	1	28	13	12.9	2
1434	Chicken sandwich	1 ea	230	45	703	26	54	2	43	8	11	20.1
1629	BK broiler chicken sandwich	1 ea	248	59	540	30	41	2	29	6	–	–
1435	Chicken tenders	1 ea	95	50	270	17	15	2	13	3.2	5.3	3.2
1436	Ham & cheese sandwich	1 ea	230	59	471	24	44	<1	23	10	8	4
1437	Ocean catch fish fillet	1 ea	189	47	534	19	44	1	36	6	5.8	12.7
1439	French fries (salted)	1 svg	74	38	255	3	27	2	13	3	6	1
1630	French toast sticks	1 svg	141	33	500	4	60	1	27	–	–	–
1440	Onion rings	1 svg	79	51	198	3	26	3	9	1.3	5.1	2.6
1441	Milk shakes, chocolate	1 ea	273	75	298	9	52	3	7	3.9	3.9	0
1442	Milk shakes, vanilla	1 ea	273	75	298	9	51	1	7	3.9	2.9	0
1443	Fried apple pie	1 ea	125	47	343	3	43	2	17	3.3	8.9	1

Source: Burger King Corporation.

	DAIRY QUEEN											
	Ice cream cones:											
1446	Small vanilla	1 ea	85	64	140	4	22	0	4	3	1	–
1447	Regular vanilla	1 ea	142	65	230	6	36	0	7	5	1	1
1448	Large vanilla	1 ea	213	66	340	9	53	0	10	7	1	1
1450	Chocolate dipped	1 ea	156	60	330	6	40	<1	16	8	4	3
1453	Chocolate sundae	1 ea	177	62	300	6	54	<1	7	5	1	1
1455	Banana split	1 ea	383	68	529	9	97	2	11	8.3	3.1	.4
1456	Peanut Buster Parfait	1 ea	305	53	710	16	94	1	32	10	10	9
1457	Hot Fudge Brownie Delight	1 ea	266	53	619	10	89	1	25	12.2	10.5	1.7
1459	Buster bar	1 ea	149	45	450	11	40	<1	29	9	10	8
1645	Breeze, strawberry, regular	1 ea	354	70	420	12	90	–	1	–	–	–
1460	Dilly bar	1 ea	85	55	210	3	21	<1	13	6	3	3
1461	DQ ice cream sandwich	1 ea	60	48	138	3	24	<1	4	2	1	1
2265	Float	1 ea	397	76	410	5	82	0	7	5	1	1
2266	Freeze	1 ea	397	72	500	9	89	0	12	7.5	3.4	.4
1463	Milk shakes, regular	1 ea	418	71	548	13	93	<1	15	8.4	2.1	2.1
1464	Milk shakes, large	1 ea	489	72	636	14	107	<1	17	10.6	2.1	2.1
1466	Milk shakes, malted	1 ea	418	68	610	13	106	<1	14	8	2	2
1470	Misty slush, small	1 ea	454	88	220	0	56	0	0	0	0	0
2250	Starkiss	1 ea	85	75	80	0	21	0	0	0	0	0
2267	Sundae, waffle cone, strawberry	1 ea	173	–	173	8	56	–	12	5	3	3

(Computer code number is for West Diet Analysis program)

Chol (mg)	Calc (mg)	Iron (mg)	Magn (mg)	Pota (mg)	Sodi (mg)	Zinc (mg)	VT-A (RE)	Thia (mg)	Ribo (mg)	Niac (mg)	V-B6 (mg)	Fola (μg)	VT-C (mg)	VT-E α-TE (mg)
227	151	1.8	–	–	797	–	81	.32	.3	2.02	.11	–	2	–
261	154	2.97	–	–	1025	–	82	.37	.33	4.1	.12	–	<1	–
232	151	1.8	–	–	1400	–	81	.49	.32	3.02	.22	–	10	–
88	59	4.4	–	–	834	–	98	.32	.4	6.87	.34	–	9	–
113	246	4.4	–	–	1248	–	147	.33	.47	6.88	.32	–	9	–
169	80	7.3	–	–	920	–	100	.34	.56	10	–	–	9	–
193	249	7.28	–	–	1336	–	150	.35	.63	9.97	–	–	9	–
32	42	1.9	–	–	529	–	21	.23	.25	4.23	–	–	3	–
47	104	1.88	–	–	741	–	63	.23	.29	4.17	–	–	3	–
104	144	3.24	–	–	863	–	58	.22	.3	4.32	–	–	1	–
60	100	3.62	–	–	1406	–	13	.45	.31	10	–	–	1	–
80	40	5.4	–	–	480	–	40	–	–	–	–	–	6	–
38	19	.78	–	–	571	–	5	.08	.08	7.56	–	–	<1	–
70	195	3.2	–	–	1534	–	85	.87	.42	6	–	–	7	–
45	44	2.67	–	–	808	–	15	.21	.2	2.96	–	–	1	–
0	6	.69	–	–	153	–	0	.06	.2	5	–	–	2	–
0	60	2.7	–	–	490	–	–	–	–	–	–	–	–	–
0	79	.51	–	–	516	–	0	.04	.03	.46	–	–	<1	–
19	192	1.73	–	–	221	–	58	.12	.53	.12	–	–	0	–
19	288	–	–	–	221	–	58	.11	.55	.12	–	–	3	–
0	17	1.6	–	–	254	–	4	.27	.18	.6	–	–	7	–
15	100	.4	–	150	60	–	20	.03	.17	.06	–	–	<1	–
20	150	.7	–	260	95	–	40	.06	.26	.11	.09	–	0	–
30	200	1.4	–	380	140	–	60	.12	.34	.17	–	–	0	–
20	300	.7	–	290	100	–	40	.06	.26	.11	.09	–	0	–
20	150	1.1	–	290	140	–	40	.06	.26	.3	.14	–	0	–
31	311	3.74	–	893	259	–	156	.16	.27	.41	.21	–	16	–
30	350	3.6	–	660	410	–	60	.15	.51	3	.22	–	2	–
30	262	4.71	–	445	297	–	70	.1	.6	.26	.16	–	1	–
15	300	1.1	–	400	220	–	20	.12	.17	3	.08	–	1	–
–	500	1.8	–	490	170	–	–	.12	.68	–	–	–	24	–
10	250	.72	–	170	50	–	20	.03	.14	–	.06	–	1	–
5	59	.71	–	103	133	–	15	.03	.26	.39	.05	–	<1	–
20	200	1.1	–	–	85	–	40	.06	.26	.05	.09	–	<1	–
30	300	1.8	–	–	180	–	98	.15	.51	–	.15	–	2	–
47	421	1.52	–	600	242	–	84	.24	.63	.84	.2	–	0	–
53	477	1.53	–	700	276	–	212	.16	.72	.85	–	–	0	–
45	400	1.44	–	570	230	–	80	.12	.66	.8	.19	–	0	–
0	0	0	–	–	20	–	–	–	–	–	–	–	0	–
0	0	0	–	–	10	–	0	–	–	–	–	–	0	–
20	150	1.44	–	330	220	–	40	.09	.26	–	–	–	6	–

(For purposes of calculations, use "0" for t, <1, <.1, <.01, etc.)

Table A–1
Food Composition

Computer Code Number	Food Description	Measure	Wt (g)	H₂O (%)	Ener (cal)	Prot (g)	Carb (g)	Dietary Fiber (g)	Fat (g)	Fat Breakdown (g) Sat	Mono	Poly
	DAIRY QUEEN—Cont.											
	Yogurt:											
1641	Yogurt cone, regular	1 ea	142	67	180	6	38	–	1	–	–	–
1643	Yogurt sundae, strawberry	1 ea	170	70	200	6	43	–	1	–	–	–
	Sandwiches:											
1474	Chicken	1 ea	202	56	455	25	39	<1	21	4.2	7.4	8.5
1647	Chicken fillet, grilled	1 ea	184	63	300	25	33	–	8	2	2	3
1475	Fish fillet	1 ea	177	58	385	17	41	<1	17	3.1	5.2	8.3
1476	Fish fillet with cheese	1 ea	191	56	436	20	42	<1	22	6.2	7.3	8.3
1477	Hamburger, single	1 ea	148	55	323	18	30	<1	17	6.2	6.2	1
1478	Hamburger, double	1 ea	210	57	488	33	31	<1	26	12.7	11.7	2.1
1480	Cheeseburger, single	1 ea	162	55	379	21	31	<1	19	9.3	7.3	1
1481	Cheeseburger, double	1 ea	239	54	603	39	33	<1	36	19	13.7	2.1
	Hot dog:											
1483	Regular	1 ea	100	51	283	9	23	<1	16	6.1	7.1	2
1484	With cheese	1 ea	114	49	333	12	24	<1	21	9.1	8.1	2
1485	With chili	1 ea	128	53	323	11	26	2	19	7.1	8.1	2
1489	French fries, small	1 ea	71	38	210	3	29	1	10	2	5	3
1490	French fries, large	1 ea	113	50	344	4	46	2	16	3.5	7.1	5.3
1491	Onion rings	1 ea	85	46	240	4	29	<1	12	3	5	4
	Source: International Dairy Queen.											
	HARDEE'S											
1734	Frisco burger hamburger	1 ea	242	–	760	36	43	–	50	18	–	–
1735	Frisco grilled chicken sandwich	1 ea	244	–	620	35	44	–	34	10	–	–
1736	Frisco grilled chicken salad	1 ea	278	–	120	18	2	–	4	1	–	–
1737	Peach shake	1 ea	345	–	390	10	77	–	4	3	–	–
	JACK IN THE BOX											
	Breakfast items:											
1492	Breakfast Jack sandwich	1 ea	126	50	312	19	31	–	13	5.2	5	2.5
1494	Sausage crescent	1 ea	156	39	580	22	28	–	43	15.5	21.5	5.7
1495	Supreme crescent	1 ea	146	39	506	22	32	–	31	13.2	18.9	7.8
1496	Pancake platter	1 ea	231	45	610	15	87	–	22	8.6	7.6	3.5
1497	Scrambled egg platter	1 ea	249	52	655	21	58	–	37	10.2	19.4	5.1
	Sandwiches:											
1654	Bacon cheeseburger	1 ea	242	49	710	35	41	0	45	15	15.7	8.7
1498	Hamburger	1 ea	98	39	283	13	31	0	11	4.1	4.9	2
1499	Cheeseburger	1 ea	113	39	339	16	33	0	14	6	6	2.3
1739	Chicken caesar pita sandwich	1 ea	237	59	520	27	44	4	26	6	–	–
1500	Jumbo Jack burger	1 ea	205	55	501	23	37	0	31	9	11.6	7.4
1501	Jumbo Jack burger with cheese	1 ea	246	55	620	29	42	0	37	12	15.2	9.1
1655	Chicken sandwich	1 ea	160	52	400	20	38	0	18	4	–	–
1505	Chicken supreme	1 ea	228	55	577	23	45	0	34	10	13.8	10.6

(Computer code number is for West Diet Analysis program)

PAGE KEY: A–4 = BEV   A–6 = DAIRY   A–12 = EGGS   A–14 = FAT/OIL   A–18 = FRUIT   A–26 = BAKERY   A–36 = GRAIN   A–44 = FISH
A–48 = MEATS   A–50 = POULTRY   A–54 = SAUSAGE   A–56 = MIXED/FAST   A–64 = NUTS/SEEDS   A–68 = SWEETS   A–70 = VEG/LEG
A–84 = MISC   A–88 = SOUPS/SAUCES   A–90 = FAST   A–106 = FRZN ENTREE   A–112 = BABY FOODS

Chol (mg)	Calc (mg)	Iron (mg)	Magn (mg)	Pota (mg)	Sodi (mg)	Zinc (mg)	VT-A (RE)	Thia (mg)	Ribo (mg)	Niac (mg)	V-B6 (mg)	Fola (μg)	VT-C (mg)	VT-E α-TE (mg)
–	200	.72	–	190	80	–	–	.06	.26	–	–	–	–	–
–	250	.72	–	240	80	–	–	.06	.34	–	–	–	12	–
58	42	1.9	–	370	804	–	21	.4	.36	12	–	–	3	–
50	60	3.6	–	330	800	–	20	.3	1.02	12	–	–	2	–
47	42	1.9	–	292	656	–	16	.3	.24	3	–	–	–	–
62	104	1.9	–	301	882	–	83	.3	.27	5	–	–	–	–
47	104	3.75	–	271	605	–	21	.31	.27	4	–	–	1	–
101	42	5.7	–	440	668	–	21	.3	.46	7	–	–	1	–
62	156	3.74	–	280	831	–	83	.31	.35	4	–	–	1	–
127	212	5.7	–	465	1132	–	159	.3	.54	7.4	–	–	1	–
25	40	1.41	–	172	707	–	0	.23	.14	2	–	–	<1	–
35	101	1.41	–	182	928	–	89	.23	.17	2	–	–	<1	–
30	40	1.45	–	262	726	–	60	.23	.14	3	–	–	<1	–
0	10	.72	–	430	115	–	0	.09	.02	2	–	–	5	–
0	13	1.27	–	689	177	–	0	.13	.03	2.65	–	–	8	–
0	20	.72	–	90	135	–	15	.09	.05	.4	–	–	2	–
70	–	–	–	–	1280	–	–	–	–	–	–	–	–	–
95	–	–	–	–	1730	–	–	–	–	–	–	–	–	–
60	–	–	–	–	520	–	–	–	–	–	–	–	–	–
25	–	–	–	–	290	–	–	–	–	–	–	–	–	–
193	208	2.8	–	229	927	–	83	.47	.41	3	–	–	9	–
185	150	2.7	–	260	1010	–	100	.6	.51	4.6	–	–	0	–
200	143	3.4	–	258	887	–	143	.65	.54	4.2	–	–	11	–
100	100	1.8	–	310	890	–	80	.03	.85	7	–	–	6	–
444	175	5.73	–	526	1239	–	175	–	.77	5.85	–	–	11	–
110	250	5.4	–	540	1240	–	80	.24	.48	8.8	.39	–	9	–
26	101	1.8	–	–	556	–	–	.15	.26	2	–	–	–	–
41	205	2.72	–	–	753	–	40	.23	.23	3.03	–	–	–	–
55	250	2.7	–	490	1050	–	80	–	–	–	–	–	2	–
67	80	2.86	–	–	677	–	–	.33	.27	1.66	–	–	–	–
104	203	3.86	–	–	1108	–	–	.37	.45	1.63	–	–	–	–
45	150	1.8	–	180	1290	–	40	–	–	–	–	–	0	–
79	186	2.7	–	–	1368	–	74	.36	.3	10.2	–	–	6	–

(For purposes of calculations, use "0" for t, <1, <.1, <.01, etc.)

Table A–1
Food Composition

Computer Code Number	Food Description	Measure	Wt (g)	H₂O (%)	Ener (cal)	Prot (g)	Carb (g)	Dietary Fiber (g)	Fat (g)	Fat Breakdown (g)		
										Sat	Mono	Poly
	JACK IN THE BOX—Cont.											
1656	Chicken sandwich, sourdough ranch	1 ea	225	73	205	14	41	7	0	0	0	0
1583	Double cheeseburger	1 ea	149	41	441	24	34	0	27	11.8	11.6	3.1
1651	Grilled sourdough burger	1 ea	223	48	670	32	39	0	43	16	17.8	7.9
1740	Monterey roast beef sandwich	1 ea	238	57	540	30	40	3	30	9	–	–
1508	Tacos, regular	1 ea	81	58	191	7	16	2	11	4.2	–	–
1509	Tacos, super	1 ea	135	59	300	13	24	3	17	6.4	–	–
2268	Taco salad	1 ea	402	76	503	34	28	–	31	13.4	11.9	1.6
	Teriyaki bowl:											
1668	Chicken	1 ea	440	62	580	28	115	6	2	–	–	–
1679	Beef	1 ea	440	62	640	28	124	7	3	1	–	–
1516	French fries	1 ea	109	37	351	5	45	5	17	4	11	.6
1517	Hash browns	1 ea	62	51	174	1	15	1	12	2.8	7.4	.3
1518	Onion rings	1 ea	108	34	398	5	40	0	24	6.3	15.9	.9
	Milk shakes:											
1519	Chocolate	1 ea	322	72	390	9	74	0	6	3.5	2.1	–
1520	Strawberry	1 ea	328	67	363	10	66	0	8	4.3	2	–
1521	Vanilla	1 ea	317	73	365	9	65	0	7	4.2	1.8	–
1522	Apple turnover	1 ea	119	34	379	3	52	0	21	4.3	11.5	1.8
	Source: Jack in the Box Restaurant, Inc.											
	KENTUCKY FRIED CHICKEN											
	Rotisserie Gold:											
1472	Dark qtr, no skin	1 ea	117	60	217	27	0	–	12	3.5	–	–
1473	Dark qtr, w/skin	1 ea	146	54	333	30	1	–	24	6.6	–	–
1513	White qtr with wing, w/skin	1 ea	176	59	335	40	1	–	19	5.4	–	–
1525	White qtr with wing, no skin	1 ea	117	20	199	37	0	–	6	1.7	–	–
	Original recipe:											
1253	Center breast	1 ea	95	52	240	23	8	<1	13	3.5	7.2	1.8
1251	Side breast	1 ea	69	47	204	14	7	<1	12	3.5	7.3	1.7
1250	Drumstick	1 ea	47	51	125	11	2	<1	7	1.8	3.4	1.1
1252	Thigh	1 ea	88	49	266	17	7	<1	19	4.9	8.7	2.6
1249	Wing	1 ea	42	41	136	9	4	<1	9	2.3	4.6	1.4
	Dinners:											
2269	2-pce dinner, white	1 ea	322	59	702	32	56	2	39	9.5	18.4	7.9
2270	2-pce dinner, dark	1 ea	346	71	721	33	57	1	40	10.1	17.9	8.5
2271	2-pce dinner, combo	1 ea	341	47	741	32	58	1	42	10.7	19.3	8.8
	Hot & spicy:											
1451	Center breast	1 ea	125	48	360	28	13	–	22	5	–	–
1452	Side breast	1 ea	120	43	400	22	16	–	28	6	–	–
1430	Thigh	1 ea	119	47	370	24	10	–	27	6	–	–
1471	Wing	1 ea	61	38	220	14	5	–	16	4	–	–
	Extra crispy recipe:											
1261	Center breast	1 ea	104	48	291	25	9	<1	17	4	9.5	1.9
1259	Side breast	1 ea	84	40	290	17	11	<1	20	4.2	9.3	1.7
1258	Drumstick	1 ea	58	48	170	11	5	<1	11	3	6.8	1.5
1260	Thigh	1 ea	107	43	373	18	13	<1	29	7.6	15.7	4
1257	Wing	1 ea	53	32	216	10	8	<1	15	4	9.6	2
	Dinners:											
2272	2-pce dinner, white	1 ea	348	57	829	34	62	1	49	11.8	25.6	8.6
2273	2-pce dinner, dark	1 ea	375	59	878	36	62	1	54	13.3	26.9	9.9

(Computer code number is for West Diet Analysis program)

Chol (mg)	Calc (mg)	Iron (mg)	Magn (mg)	Pota (mg)	Sodi (mg)	Zinc (mg)	VT-A (RE)	Thia (mg)	Ribo (mg)	Niac (mg)	V-B6 (mg)	Fola (µg)	VT-C (mg)	VT-E α-TE (mg)
0	0	4.91	–	–	136	–	341	–	–	–	–	–	82	–
72	245	2.7	–	–	842	–	98	.15	.34	6	–	–	–	–
110	200	4.5	–	510	1140	–	150	.65	.48	8	.33	–	6	–
75	300	3.6	–	500	1270	–	80	–	–	–	–	–	5	–
21	104	1.1	35	249	426	1.2	0	.07	.17	1	.13	–	0	–
37	161	1.6	45	316	771	1.8	0	.12	.08	1.4	.18	–	3	–
92	410	3.8	–	–	1600	–	270	.29	.53	5.8	–	–	9	–
30	100	1.8	–	380	1220	–	1100	–	–	–	–	–	9	–
25	150	4.5	–	430	930	–	1000	–	–	–	–	–	6	–
0	0	1.3	–	–	194	–	–	.18	.03	3.8	–	–	29	–
0	0	.39	–	–	339	–	0	.05	–	1.09	–	–	7	–
0	31	2.31	–	–	473	–	–	.3	.18	2.73	–	–	3	–
25	300	.72	–	680	210	–	–	.15	.6	.4	–	–	0	–
33	330	.36	–	605	198	–	–	.15	.43	.4	–	–	0	–
31	313	–	–	594	188	–	–	.15	.34	.4	–	–	0	–
0	0	2.12	–	87	498	–	–	.24	.14	2.12	–	–	10	–
128	10	.18	–	–	772	–	15	–	–	–	–	–	1	–
163	10	.18	–	–	980	–	15	–	–	–	–	–	1	–
157	10	.18	–	–	1104	–	15	–	–	–	–	–	1	–
97	10	.18	–	–	667	–	15	–	–	–	–	–	1	–
85	28	.83	–	–	562	–	14	.07	.14	9.5	–	–	–	–
65	57	.92	–	–	502	–	12	.05	.1	5.29	–	–	–	–
62	17	.91	–	–	222	–	12	.04	.1	2.64	–	–	–	–
104	37	1.1	–	–	547	–	29	.07	.25	4.65	–	–	–	–
47	24	.92	–	–	304	–	12	.02	.06	2.83	–	–	–	–
119	215	3.71	–	–	1854	–	76	.22	.38	11.8	.5	–	36	–
164	197	3.84	–	–	1738	–	76	.25	.57	10.6	.46	–	37	–
160	217	3.88	–	–	1801	–	57	.24	.53	10.9	.47	–	38	–
80	20	.72	–	–	750	–	15	–	–	–	–	–	6	–
80	40	1.08	–	–	850	–	15	–	–	–	–	–	6	–
100	20	1.08	–	–	670	–	15	–	–	–	–	–	6	–
65	20	.72	–	–	440	–	30	–	–	–	–	–	–	–
66	29	.62	–	–	652	–	13	.08	.1	11.5	–	–	–	–
54	14	.61	–	–	514	–	11	.07	.08	6.49	–	–	–	–
58	12	.59	–	–	277	–	27	.05	.1	3.11	–	–	–	–
88	48	1.08	–	–	510	–	29	.09	.19	6.38	–	–	–	–
58	18	.05	–	–	287	–	27	–	.03	.05	2.69	–	–	–
125	161	2.51	–	–	1915	–	76	.31	.34	12.8	.56	–	36	–
176	180	3.48	–	–	1869	–	77	.32	.5	12	.53	–	36	–

(For purposes of calculations, use "0" for t, <1, <.1, <.01, etc.)

Table A–1
Food Composition

Computer Code Number	Food Description	Measure	Wt (g)	H₂O (%)	Ener (cal)	Prot (g)	Carb (g)	Dietary Fiber (g)	Fat (g)	Fat Breakdown (g)		
										Sat	Mono	Poly
	KENTUCKY FRIED CHICKEN—Cont.											
2274	2-pce dinner, combo	1 ea	371	57	919	35	65	1	58	14.1	29.4	10.6
2275	Mashed potatoes	⅓ c	80	81	60	2	12	1	1	.2	.4	t
1526	Breadstick	1 ea	33	10	110	3	17	0	3	0	–	–
1268	Corn-on-the-cob	1 ea	143	70	210	5	32	8	11	.5	1	1.5
1527	Cornbread	1 pce	56	26	228	3	25	1	13	2	–	–
1269	Coleslaw	⅓ c	79	75	100	1	12	<1	5	.9	1.5	3
1429	Chicken, hot wings	1 svg	119	38	415	24	16	–	29	–	–	–
1381	Kentucky nuggets	6 ea	96	41	287	16	15	<1	18	4	8.7	2.2
	Kentucky nugget sauce:											
2276	Barbeque	2 tsp	30	68	37	<1	8	–	1	.1	–	.3
2277	Sweet & sour	2 tbs	30	48	61	<1	14	–	1	.1	–	.3
2278	Honey	2 tbs	30	8	104	0	26	–	–	–	–	–
2279	Mustard	2 tbs	30	69	38	1	6	–	1	.1	–	1.2
1386	Kentucky fries	1 svg	119	42	352	5	40	5	18	5	12.5	1.1
1534	Macaroni & cheese	1 svg	114	71	162	7	15	0	8	3	–	–
1387	Mashed potatoes & gravy	⅓ c	86	80	74	1	11	<1	4	.4	.4	.2
1388	Buttermilk biscuit	1 ea	75	28	270	6	32	<1	15	3.7	6.7	2.5
1530	Pasta salad	1 svg	108	78	135	2	14	1	8	1	–	–
1389	Potato salad	⅓ c	90	74	130	2	13	1	8	1.4	2.8	3.5
1383	Potato wedges	1 svg	92	55	192	3	25	3	9	3	–	–
1390	Baked beans	⅓ c	89	70	107	4	19	3	2	.4	.5	.2
1391	Chicken Little sandwich	1 ea	57	32	205	7	17	1	12	2.4	–	4.1
1535	Red beans & rice	1 svg	111	76	113	4	18	3	3	1	–	–
1529	Vegetable medley salad	1 ea	114	77	126	1	21	3	4	1	–	–

Source: Kentucky Fried Chicken Corporation.

	LONG JOHN SILVER'S											
	Fish, batter fried:											
1523	Fish & Fryes (fries), 3 piece	1 ea	350	54	893	28	84	–	46	10	26	9
1524	Fish & Fryes, 2 piece	1 ea	260	54	608	27	52	–	37	8	23	5
2280	Fish dinner, 3 piece	1 ea	540	60	1180	47	93	–	70	–	–	–
2240	Fish and lemon crumb dinner, 3 piece	1 ea	493	71.3	610	39	86	–	13	2.2	3.9	5.3
2241	Fish and lemon crumb dinner, 2 piece	1 ea	334	76.8	330	24	46	–	5	.9	1.6	1.2
	Chicken:											
1528	Chicken Plank dinner, 3 piece	1 ea	370	56	825	30	94	–	41	9	23	9
2281	Chicken Plank dinner, 4 piece	1 ea	440	60	1037	41	82	–	59	–	–	–
2282	Chicken Nugget dinner, 6 piece	1 ea	300	60	699	23	54	–	45	–	–	–
1531	Clam chowder	1 ea	185	86	131	10	9	1	6	2	2	2
1532	Clam dinner	1 ea	460	47	1262	31	145	–	66	14	40	13
1533	Fish & chicken dinner	1 ea	460	52	1014	38	109	–	52	11	31	10
2243	Oysters, breaded and fried	1 svg	139	67	368	19	40	<1	18	4.5	6.9	4.6
2283	Scallop dinner	1 ea	320	60	747	17	66	–	45	–	–	–
2284	Seafood platter	1 ea	410	60	976	29	85	–	58	–	–	–
1537	Shrimp dinner, batter fried	1 ea	300	54	761	16	80	–	43	9	25	8
2285	Fish sandwich platter	1 ea	400	59	835	30	84	–	42	–	–	–
	Salads:											
1539	Ocean chef salad	1 ea	320	89	150	16	18	3	1	.6	.6	.3
1540	Seafood salad	1 ea	480	89	656	26	21	3	54	9	14	30

(Computer code number is for West Diet Analysis program)

PAGE KEY: A–4 = BEV   A–6 = DAIRY   A–12 = EGGS   A–14 = FAT/OIL   A–18 = FRUIT   A–26 = BAKERY   A–36 = GRAIN   A–44 = FISH   A–48 = MEATS   A–50 = POULTRY   A–54 = SAUSAGE   A–56 = MIXED/FAST   A–64 = NUTS/SEEDS   A–68 = SWEETS   A–70 = VEG/LEG   A–84 = MISC   A–88 = SOUPS/SAUCES   A–90 = FAST   A–106 = FRZN ENTREE   A–112 = BABY FOODS

Chol (mg)	Calc (mg)	Iron (mg)	Magn (mg)	Pota (mg)	Sodi (mg)	Zinc (mg)	VT-A (RE)	Thia (mg)	Ribo (mg)	Niac (mg)	V-B6 (mg)	Fola (μg)	VT-C (mg)	VT-E α-TE (mg)
172	183	2.96	–	–	1949	–	76	.31	.45	11.7	.49	–	36	–
<1	21	.28	14	218	228	.16	5	.01	.04	.96	.11	7	4	–
0	30	.18	–	–	15	–	0	–	–	–	–	–	0	–
688	0	.34	–	72	–	–	19	.14	.11	1.8	–	–	2	–
42	60	.72	–	–	194	–	10	–	–	–	–	–	–	–
4	26	.32	–	–	155	–	28	.03	.03	.17	–	–	24	–
132	35	2.86	–	–	1084	–	13	–	–	–	–	–	5	–
67	2	.1	–		874	–	15	.02	.02	1	.05	–	<1	–
–	6	.21	–	–	477	–	39	–	.01	.2	–	–	–	–
–	5	.21	–	–	157	–	60	–	.02	.04	–	–	–	–
–	1	.21	–	–	–	–	0	–	.01	.08	–	–	–	–
–	11	.32	–	–	367	–	1	–	.01	.17	–	–	–	–
7	17	1.5	–	–	826	–	0	.23	.08	3.09	–	–	0	–
16	120	.72	–	–	531	–	–	–	–	–	–	–	0	–
<1	14	.3	–	–	278	–	11	–	.03	.86	–	–	–	–
3	49	2.2	–	–	652	–	32	.28	.22	3	–	–	–	–
1	20	1.08	–	–	663	–	110	–	–	–	–	–	7	–
8	7	1.6	11	184	305	.29	58	.05	.02	.4	.14	5	–	–
3	–	–	–	–	428	–	–	–	–	–	–	–	–	–
2	32	1.2	23	185	433	1.29	40	.05	.04	.4	.07	26	2	–
21	27	2.05	–	–	401	–	6	.19	.14	2.65	–	–	–	–
4	10	.71	–	–	312	–	–	–	–	–	–	–	–	–
0	20	.36	–	–	240	–	375	–	–	–	–	–	5	–
64	182	4	–	1021	1395	2.7	36	.41	.39	7.3	–	–	14	–
60	40	2	–	897	1474	1.2	–	.38	.34	8	–	–	9	–
119	–	–	–	–	2797	–	–	–	–	–	–	–	–	–
125	200	5.4	–	990	1420	2.25	700	.75	.6	24	–	–	6	–
75	80	1.8	–	440	640	.9	1000	.3	.26	14	–	–	18	–
51	185	4	–	1085	1855	2.78	37	.49	.47	14.8	–	–	8	–
25	–	–	–	–	2433	–	–	–	–	–	–	–	–	–
25	–	–	–	–	853	–	–	–	–	–	–	–	–	–
19	187	1.68	–	355	551	.56	140	.1	.24	1.87	–	–	–	–
96	255	5.73	–	1160	2332	3.8	51	.96	.55	15	–	–	15	–
80	213	4.8	–	1366	2231	3	43	.64	.64	15	–	–	10	–
108	28	4.48	24	182	677	15.7	108	.3	.34	4.4	–	13	4	–
37	–	–	–	–	1579	–	–	–	–	–	–	–	–	–
95	–	–	–	–	2161	–	–	–	–	–	–	–	–	–
91	181	3.26	–	761	1477	2.7	36	.41	.4	8	–	–	8	–
75	–	–	–	–	1402	–	–	–	–	–	–	–	–	–
55	137	5	–	130	998	.4	684	.16	.2	4	–	–	29	–
95	259	8	–	224	1692	1.5	345	.26	.45	5	–	–	36	–

(For purposes of calculations, use "0" for t, <1, <.1, <.01, etc.)

Table A–1
Food Composition

Computer Code Number	Food Description	Measure	Wt (g)	H₂O (%)	Ener (cal)	Prot (g)	Carb (g)	Dietary Fiber (g)	Fat (g)	Fat Breakdown (g)		
										Sat	Mono	Poly
	LONG JOHN SILVER'S—Cont.											
1541	Coleslaw	1 ea	98	70	140	1	20	1	6	1	1.5	3.5
1542	Fryes (fries) serving	1 ea	85	43	250	3	28	1	15	2.5	7.4	5
1543	Hush puppies	1 ea	47	38	137	4	20	<1	4	.8	2.6	1.4

Source: Long John Silver's, Lexington, KY.

Computer Code Number	Food Description	Measure	Wt (g)	H₂O (%)	Ener (cal)	Prot (g)	Carb (g)	Dietary Fiber (g)	Fat (g)	Sat	Mono	Poly
	McDONALD'S											
	Sandwiches:											
1221	Big Mac	1 ea	215	53	508	25	46	3	26	9	7.4	4.1
1444	McChicken	1 ea	187	52	486	17	41	2	28	5	8.4	10
1591	McLean deluxe	1 ea	206	64	332	23	36	2	11	4	3.5	1
1438	McLean deluxe with cheese	1 ea	219	63	382	25	37	2	15	7	4	1.3
1222	Quarter-pounder	1 ea	166	52	403	22	34	2	20	8	7	1
1223	Quarter-pounder with cheese	1 ea	194	50	507	27	34	2	28	12	1	2
1224	Filet-O-Fish	1 ea	142	49	357	13	40	2	16	3.6	4	5
1225	Hamburger	1 ea	102	49	251	12	33	2	8	3	2.7	.9
1226	Cheeseburger	1 ea	116	55	302	14	34	2	12	5	3.6	1
1227	French fries, small serving	1 ea	68	40	207	3	26	2	10	1.7	3.1	2.5
1228	Chicken McNuggets	6 ea	112	51	303	19	16	0	18	3.8	5.7	3.7
	Sauces (packet):											
1229	Hot mustard	1 ea	30	60	63	5	8	<1	4	.47	1.1	2
1230	Barbecue	1 ea	32	58	53	<1	12	<1	<1	.1	.1	.2
1231	Sweet & sour	1 ea	32	57	55	<1	14	<1	<1	.1	.1	.3
	Low-fat (frozen yogurt) milk shakes:											
1232	Chocolate	1 ea	293	71	346	13	62	<1	5	3.5	.1	.7
1233	Strawberry	1 ea	293	72	342	12	63	<1	5	3.4	.1	.6
1234	Vanilla	1 ea	293	75	308	12	54	<1	5	3.3	.1	.6
	Low-fat (frozen yogurt) sundaes:											
1237	Hot caramel	1 ea	168	56	283	6	58	<1	3	2	.5	1.5
1235	Hot fudge	1 ea	168	60	275	8	50	2	5	4.5	.5	2
1267	Strawberry	1 ea	168	65	226	6	49	1	1	.7	.2	.5
1238	Vanilla	1 ea	80	65	100	4	21	<1	1	.3	.2	.5
1239	Pie, apple	1 ea	83	35	286	3	34	1	14	3.7	4.5	2.8
	Muffins (fat-free)											
2290	Blueberry	1 ea	75	41	170	3	40	–	0	0	0	0
1240	Apple bran	1 ea	85	39	206	4	46	2	<1	.2	.1	.4
1241	Cookies, McDonaldland	1 ea	56	3	258	<1	41	<1	9	4.5	.9	.9
1242	Cookies, Chocolaty chip	1 ea	56	3	282	3	36	1	14	.7	.9	3.6
	Breakfast items:											
1243	English muffin with spread	1 ea	59	41	146	5	27	2	2	2.3	.6	.6
1244	Egg McMuffin	1 ea	138	57	292	18	29	1	13	6.1	1	4.1
1245	Hotcakes with marg & syrup	1 ea	176	44	442	8	80	2	11	1.9	4	4.6
1246	Scrambled eggs	1 ea	100	73	166	12	1	0	12	2	5	2
1247	Pork sausage	1 ea	48	45	193	8	<1	0	18	6	7	2
1248	Hashbrown potatoes	1 ea	53	55	130	1	15	1	8	1.4	7.3	2
1392	Sausage McMuffin	1 ea	117	42	377	13	28	2	24	8.6	8.5	3
1393	Sausage McMuffin with egg	1 ea	167	53	452	22	28	2	29	10	13.9	4
1394	Biscuit with biscuit spread	1 ea	75	32	257	5	32	1	13	9	1	3

(Computer code number is for West Diet Analysis program)

Chol (mg)	Calc (mg)	Iron (mg)	Magn (mg)	Pota (mg)	Sodi (mg)	Zinc (mg)	VT-A (RE)	Thia (mg)	Ribo (mg)	Niac (mg)	V-B6 (mg)	Fola (μg)	VT-C (mg)	VT-E α-TE (mg)
15	60	.72	–	190	260	.6	40	.06	.07	2	–	–	–	–
0	200	.72	–	370	500	.4	–	.09	–	1.6	–	–	6	–
–	78	1.4	–	127	49	.6	–	.12	.06	1.6	–	–	–	–
76	201	4.3	45	454	928	4.8	–	.49	.43	6	.25	49	3	1.01
52	127	2.5	32	316	789	1	–	.9	.24	7.6	.39	36	1	6.09
57	126	4	38	517	780	4.7	–	.38	.34	7	.28	42	8	.6
70	134	4	42	537	1005	–	150	.38	.34	7	–	–	6	.82
68	123	4	33	394	672	–	40	.38	.26	7	.32	–	4	.35
94	139	4	–	–	1132	–	150	.38	.34	7	.32	–	4	.79
36	121	1.81	31	260	735	–	20	.3	.14	9.06	.1	–	<1	1.49
27	119	2.7	23	245	490	–	40	.3	.17	4	–	–	2	.22
40	127	2.7	26	267	725	–	80	.3	.26	4	–	–	2	.44
0	9	.53	26	469	110	–	0	.15	0	2	.18	–	9	.83
65	15	1.08	26	323	580	–	0	.12	.14	8	.36	–	0	1.48
3	7	.8	–	29	85	–	2	.01	.01	.15	–	–	<1	–
0	4	0	–	51	277	–	40	.01	.01	.17	–	–	2	–
0	2	.17	–	8	158	–	60	0	.01	.08	–	–	1	–
24	369	.84	–	539	240	–	60	.12	.51	.4	.1	–	0	–
24	365	.29	–	540	169	–	60	.12	.51	.4	.11	–	0	–
24	360	.1	–	533	171	–	60	.12	.51	.31	–	–	0	–
7	227	.14	–	318	180	–	60	.09	.34	.27	–	–	0	–
5	242	.55	–	414	170	–	40	.09	.34	.29	–	–	0	–
5	209	.16	–	307	109	–	40	.06	.34	.25	–	–	1	–
3	95	.23	–	–	76	–	19	.03	.16	.38	–	–	0	–
0	17	1.2	7	68	175	.16	10	.12	.09	1.02	.03	3	1	1.58
0	80	.72	–	–	220	.37	–	.12	.14	.8	–	–	1	–
0	39	1.22	15	–	227	–	1	.17	.19	2.27	–	–	1	0
0	10	1.63	11	–	271	–	0	.13	.15	1.81	.03	–	0	.99
3	28	1.6	4	–	249	–	0	.13	.15	1.78	–	–	0	.92
6	126	2	13	65	362	.39	31	.24	.29	2.45	.03	16	1	.12
235	152	2.76	4	–	726	–	102	.48	.34	3.79	.08	–	0	.86
9	86	1.57	22	–	693	–	40	.3	.34	3.03	.11	–	0	.95
416	49	1.8	10	–	290	–	100	.07	.26	.05	–	–	0	.9
36	8	.6	7	–	346	–	0	.26	.11	2.23	–	–	0	.29
0	7	.27	11	–	330	–	0	.06	.02	.8	–	–	1	.58
49	138	2.34	23	–	667	–	35	.46	.22	4.33	.13	–	0	.69
264	160	3.78	27	–	966	–	105	.56	.45	5.25	.21	–	0	1.14
0	67	1.44	9	–	730	–	0	.23	.1	1.65	.03	–	0	.8

(For purposes of calculations, use "0" for t, <1, <.1, <.01, etc.)

Table A–1
Food Composition

Computer Code Number	Food Description	Measure	Wt (g)	H₂O (%)	Ener (cal)	Prot (g)	Carb (g)	Dietary Fiber (g)	Fat (g)	Fat Breakdown (g)		
										Sat	Mono	Poly
	McDONALD'S—Cont.											
	Breakfast items—Cont.:											
1395	Biscuit with sausage	1 ea	123	37	448	12	33	1	30	9	10	3
1396	Biscuit with sausage & egg	1 ea	180	48	548	19	34	1	37	11	14	4
1397	Biscuit with bacon, egg, cheese	1 ea	156	46	462	15	34	1	28	9	9	3
	Salads:											
1398	Chef salad	1 ea	283	86	186	18	8	3	10	4	3	1
1400	Garden salad	1 ea	213	92	77	5	6	2	4	1	1	1
1401	Chunky chicken salad	1 ea	250	86	138	24	7	3	4	1	1	1
	Source: McDonald's Corporation.											
	PIZZA HUT											
	Pan pizza:											
1657	Cheese	2 pce	205	48	492	30	57	5	18	8.6	5.5	2.7
1658	Pepperoni	2 pce	211	45	540	29	62	5	22	9.2	9.3	3.4
1659	Supreme	2 pce	255	54	589	32	53	7	30	13.8	11.9	4.3
1660	Super supreme	2 pce	257	55	563	33	53	6	26	12	–	–
	Thin 'n crispy:											
1649	Cheese pizza	2 pce	148	43	398	28	37	4	17	10	4.6	2.3
1623	Pepperoni pizza	2 pce	146	42	413	26	36	4	20	11	–	–
1622	Supreme pizza	2 pce	200	53	459	28	41	5	22	11	–	–
1620	Super supreme pizza	2 pce	203	52	463	29	44	5	21	10	–	–
	Hand tossed:											
1619	Cheese pizza	2 pce	220	50	518	34	55	7	20	13.6	–	–
1618	Pepperoni pizza	2 pce	197	47	500	28	50	6	23	12.9	–	–
1648	Supreme pizza	2 pce	239	54	540	32	50	7	26	13.8	–	–
1617	Super supreme pizza	2 pce	243	53	556	33	54	7	25	13	–	–
	Personal pan pizza:											
1610	Pepperoni	1 ea	256	43	675	37	76	8	29	12.5	12.1	4.5
1609	Supreme	1 ea	264	47	647	33	76	9	28	11.2	12.4	4.4
	Source: Pizza Hut.											
	TACO BELL											
	Breakfast burrito:											
1601	Bacon breakfast burrito	1 ea	99	48	291	11	23	–	17	4	–	–
1627	Country breakfast burrito	1 ea	113	53	281	10	26	–	16	5	–	–
1626	Fiesta breakfast burrito	1 ea	92	47	275	9	23	–	16	6	–	–
1625	Grande breakfast burrito	1 ea	177	52	457	14	46	–	24	8	–	–
1604	Sausage breakfast burrito	1 ea	106	49	303	11	23	–	19	6	–	–
	Burritos:											
1544	Bean with red sauce	1 ea	191	54	414	14	58	11	13	6.4	4.4	1.1
1545	Beef with red sauce	1 ea	191	53	457	23	44	4	19	9.7	6.9	.8
1546	Beef & bean with red sauce	1 ea	191	59	393	17	44	5	15	4.8	5.8	1.9
1569	Big beef supreme	1 ea	298	64	525	25	51	–	25	11	–	–
1552	Chicken burrito	1 ea	171	58	345	17	41	–	13	5	–	–
1547	Supreme with red sauce	1 ea	241	61	475	19	52	5	21	7.3	7.5	1.9
1571	7 layer burrito	1 ea	234	60	458	14	55	8	20	5.9	–	–
1538	Chilito	1 ea	156	49	391	17	41	–	18	9	–	–
1549	Chilito, steak	1 ea	257	62	496	26	47	–	23	10	–	–

(Computer code number is for West Diet Analysis program)

PAGE KEY: A–4 = BEV   A–6 = DAIRY   A–12 = EGGS   A–14 = FAT/OIL   A–18 = FRUIT   A–26 = BAKERY   A–36 = GRAIN   A–44 = FISH   A–48 = MEATS   A–50 = POULTRY   A–54 = SAUSAGE   A–56 = MIXED/FAST   A–64 = NUTS/SEEDS   A–68 = SWEETS   A–70 = VEG/LEG   A–84 = MISC   A–88 = SOUPS/SAUCES   A–90 = FAST   A–106 = FRZN ENTREE   A–112 = BABY FOODS

Chol (mg)	Calc (mg)	Iron (mg)	Magn (mg)	Pota (mg)	Sodi (mg)	Zinc (mg)	VT-A (RE)	Thia (mg)	Ribo (mg)	Niac (mg)	V-B6 (mg)	Fola (µg)	VT-C (mg)	VT-E α-TE (mg)
34	78	1.88	16	–	1084	–	0	.47	.18	4.17	.21	–	0	1.11
259	106	3	22	–	1244	–	62	.46	.36	4.1	.21	–	0	1.62
244	105	2.75	21	–	1238	–	102	.39	.35	2.04	.13	–	0	1.53
161	142	1.54	36	–	427	–	1067	.32	.28	4.27	–	–	22	1.31
27	48	1.62	22	–	79	–	1014	.1	.11	.45	–	–	24	.87
64	45	1.06	37	–	225	–	1666	.22	.17	8.82	–	–	26	1.08
34	630	5.4	60	320	940	4.1	90	.56	.6	5.2	.17	–	7	–
42	520	6.3	56	405	1127	4.2	100	.63	.49	5.4	.17	0	8	–
48	500	5	76	580	1363	5.6	120	.81	.8	6	.31	–	10	–
55	540	6.7	72	532	1447	5.4	120	.75	.66	6.4	–	–	11	–
33	660	3.2	48	261	867	3.6	70	.39	.39	4.8	.16	–	5	–
46	450	3.2	44	287	986	3.5	70	.42	.43	5.2	–	–	6	–
42	430	5.9	68	544	1328	4.7	100	.6	.49	5.4	–	–	10	–
56	460	4.9	60	463	1336	4.5	100	.59	.44	5.4	–	–	8	–
55	750	5.4	72	396	1276	4.7	100	.48	.49	5.4	–	–	10	–
50	440	5	60	415	1267	3.8	100	.54	.53	5.6	–	–	7	–
55	480	8.1	80	578	1470	5.7	110	.69	.53	7.2	–	–	12	–
54	440	6.8	76	516	1648	4.8	110	.71	.58	7.4	–	–	12	–
53	730	5.8	60	408	1335	3.8	120	.56	.66	8.2	.2	–	10	–
49	520	6.7	60	487	1313	3.8	120	.59	.66	8	.32	–	11	–
181	80	1.8	–	–	652	–	310	–	–	–	–	–	–	–
173	80	3.42	–	–	627	–	310	–	–	–	–	–	–	–
27	60	1.44	–	–	680	–	260	–	–	–	–	–	–	–
183	200	3.6	–	–	1053	–	630	–	–	–	–	–	1	–
183	80	1.8	–	–	661	–	320	–	–	–	–	–	–	–
9	136	3.22	–	459	1064	–	46	.03	1.87	1.84	.29	–	49	–
53	106	3.46	–	352	1215	–	67	.37	1.98	3.19	.3	–	2	–
32	107	2.07	48	426	1095	2.58	77	.47	.4	2.98	.57	37	2	–
72	200	4.5	–	–	1418	–	840	–	–	–	–	–	8	–
57	140	2.52	–	–	854	–	440	–	–	–	–	–	1	–
31	145	3.4	47	473	1116	–	118	.39	2	2.73	.33	–	24	–
17	85	2.29	–	–	983	–	297	–	–	–	–	–	5	–
47	300	3.06	–	–	980	–	950	–	–	–	–	–	–	–
78	200	2.70	–	–	1313	–	970	–	–	–	–	–	2	–

(For purposes of calculations, use "0" for t, <1, <.1, <.01, etc.)

A

Table A–1
Food Composition

Computer Code Number	Food Description	Measure	Wt (g)	H₂O (%)	Ener (cal)	Prot (g)	Carb (g)	Dietary Fiber (g)	Fat (g)	Fat Breakdown (g)		
										Sat	Mono	Poly
	TACO BELL—Cont											
2286	Enchirito with red sauce	1 ea	213	62	382	20	31	5	20	9.3	4.9	1.5
	Tacos:											
1551	Taco	1 ea	78	59	183	10	11	1	11	4.6	4.5	.8
2252	Taco Bellgrande	1 ea	163	63	355	18	18	1	23	10.9	9	1.3
1554	Soft taco	1 ea	92	54	225	12	18	1	12	5.4	4.3	1.2
1536	Soft taco supreme	1 ea	124	60	262	13	20	2	15	7.3	–	–
1568	Soft taco, chicken	1 ea	128	65	223	14	20	–	10	4	–	–
1572	Soft taco, steak	1 ea	100	56	217	12	21	–	9	4	–	–
1555	Tostada with red sauce	1 ea	156	69	243	9	27	5	11	4.1	5.5	.8
1558	Mexican pizza	1 ea	223	55	575	21	40	2	37	11.4	14	9.7
1559	Taco salad with salsa	1 ea	595	73	939	36	60	8	62	19	26.6	12.3
1560	Nachos, regular	1 ea	107	39	349	8	38	3	19	6.1	7.6	2.1
1561	Nachos, Bellgrande	1 ea	287	58	649	22	61	–	35	12.3	–	2.6
1562	Pintos & cheese with red sauce	1 ea	128	69	190	9	19	7	9	3.6	4	.8
1563	Taco sauce, packet	1 ea	4	96	1	<1	<1	<1	<1	0	0	0
1564	Salsa	1 ea	10	42	18	1	4	–	<1	0	0	0
1565	Cinnamon twists	1 ea	47	3	231	3	32	1	11	5.4	3.5	1.2
1628	Caramel roll	1 ea	85	19	353	6	46	–	16	4	–	–
	Border Light menu:											
1749	Bean burrito	1 ea	198	–	330	14	55	8	6	2	–	–
1750	Burrito supreme	1 ea	248	–	350	20	50	4	8	3	–	–
1744	7 layer burrito	1 ea	276	–	440	19	67	10	9	3.5	–	–
1745	Taco	1 ea	78	–	140	11	11	2	5	1.5	–	–
1746	Taco supreme	1 ea	106	–	160	13	14	2	5	1.5	–	–
1747	Soft taco	1 ea	99	–	180	13	19	2	5	2.5	–	–
1748	Soft taco supreme	1 ea	128	–	200	14	23	2	5	2.5	–	–
1742	Taco salad without chips	1 ea	464	–	330	30	35	10	9	4.5	–	–
1743	Taco salad with chips	1 ea	535	–	680	35	81	10	25	8	–	–
	Source: Taco Bell Corporation.											
	WENDY'S											
	Hamburgers:											
1566	Single on white bun, no toppings	1 ea	119	44	350	21	29	<1	16	–	–	–
2253	Double on white bun, no toppings	1 ea	197	44	560	41	32	<1	34	7.4	12.5	8
2296	Big Classic	1 ea	241	63	470	26	36	–	25	–	–	–
	Cheeseburgers:											
1570	Bacon cheeseburger	1 ea	147	46	460	29	23	<1	28	13	13	2
2297	Double with lettuce & tomato	1 ea	215	50	548	30	32	2	33	12.9	11.8	5.4
2254	Double with all toppings	1 ea	291	50	735	48	27	2	47	18.4	18	5.9
1730	Chicken sandwich, grilled	1 ea	177	62	290	24	35	2	7	1.5	–	–
	Baked potatoes:											
1573	Plain	1 ea	250	75	250	6	52	4	<1	t	t	.1
1574	With bacon & cheese	1 ea	350	71	570	19	57	4	30	11.8	11.4	5.6
1575	With broccoli & cheese	1 ea	365	74	500	13	54	5	25	9.2	8.3	4.5
1576	With cheese	1 ea	350	71	590	16	55	4	34	12.5	12.7	7.1
1577	With chili & cheese	1 ea	400	72	510	22	63	8	20	13	6.8	.9
1578	With sour cream & chives	1 ea	310	71	460	6	53	4	24	10	7.9	3.3
1579	Chili	1ea	256	81	230	21	16	–	9	–	–	–

(Computer code number is for West Diet Analysis program)

PAGE KEY: A–4 = BEV   A–6 = DAIRY   A–12 = EGGS   A–14 = FAT/OIL   A–18 = FRUIT   A–26 = BAKERY   A–36 = GRAIN   A–44 = FISH
A–48 = MEATS   A–50 = POULTRY   A–54 = SAUSAGE   A–56 = MIXED/FAST   A–64 = NUTS/SEEDS   A–68 = SWEETS   A–70 = VEG/LEG
A–84 = MISC   A–88 = SOUPS/SAUCES   A–90 = FAST   A–106 = FRZN ENTREE   A–112 = BABY FOODS

A

Chol (mg)	Calc (mg)	Iron (mg)	Magn (mg)	Pota (mg)	Sodi (mg)	Zinc (mg)	VT-A (RE)	Thia (mg)	Ribo (mg)	Niac (mg)	V-B6 (mg)	Fola (µg)	VT-C (mg)	VT-E α-TE (mg)
54	269	2.84	–	423	1243	–	100	.26	.42	2.3	1	–	28	–
32	84	1.07	–	159	276	–	24	.05	.14	1.2	.12	–	1	–
56	182	1.9	–	334	472	–	40	.11	.29	2.02	.21	–	5	–
32	116	2.27	–	196	554	–	30	.39	.22	2.74	.1	–	1	–
44	78	1.74	–	–	533	–	291	–	–	–	–	–	2	–
58	60	1.44	–	–	553	–	540	–	–	–	–	–	2	–
31	50	1.08	–	–	569	–	130	–	–	–	–	–	–	–
16	179	1.53	–	401	596	–	95	.06	.17	.63	.26	–	45	–
52	257	3.74	80	408	1031	5.4	215	.32	.33	2.96	1.11	60	31	–
82	405	7.22	–	1066	1307	–	407	.52	.77	4.88	.57	–	78	–
9	193	.91	52	161	403	1.7	88	.17	.16	.69	.19	10	2	–
36	297	3.48	–	674	997	–	40	.1	.34	2.17	–	–	58	–
16	156	1.42	110	384	642	2.17	87	.05	.15	.4	.21	68	52	–
0	1	.02	–	4	42	–	6	0	<.01	.02	<.01	–	<1	–
0	36	.6	–	376	376	–	7	.02	.14	0	–	–	2	–
1	37	.49	–	36	316	–	0	.14	.05	.96	.05	–	1	–
15	60	1.44	–	–	312	–	330	–	–	–	–	–	4	–
5	100	3.6	–	–	1340	–	400	–	–	–	–	–	2	–
25	80	2.7	–	–	1300	–	600	–	–	–	–	–	9	–
5	250	4.5	–	–	1430	–	350	–	–	–	–	–	5	–
20	0	0	–	–	280	–	40	–	–	–	–	–	0	–
20	0	0	–	–	340	–	100	–	–	–	–	–	2	–
25	40	1.08	–	–	550	–	40	–	–	–	–	–	0	–
25	40	1.08	–	–	610	–	100	–	–	–	–	–	2	–
50	100	2.7	–	–	1610	–	1200	–	–	–	–	–	27	–
50	250	3.6	–	–	1620	–	1800	–	–	–	–	–	27	–
65	100	4.5	–	265	420	–	0	.38	.34	6	–	–	–	–
125	48	6.3	42	431	575	8.35	0	.22	.43	9	.47	29	<1	–
80	40	4.5	–	470	900	–	60	.3	.25	5	–	–	12	–
65	136	3.6	33	332	860	5.14	82	.26	.28	5.7	.23	25	1	–
84	177	4	33	430	864	4.41	111	.34	.35	5.29	.25	28	5	–
165	180	5.4	50	620	883	8.8	112	.36	.53	10	.46	31	5	–
55	100	2.8	–	–	720	–	20	–	–	–	–	–	6	–
0	40	2.7	66	1360	60	.65	0	.27	.1	3.82	.7	67	36	–
22	200	3.7	80	1380	180	2.53	150	.22	.17	4.64	.87	33	36	–
22	250	3.6	83	1550	430	.86	350	.3	.25	4	.86	66	90	–
22	350	3.6	78	1380	450	.61	200	.22	.25	3.3	.8	33	36	–
22	250	6.13	111	1590	810	3.78	172	.3	.26	4.1	.9	50	36	–
15	40	2.7	70	1420	230	.9	100	.22	.14	3	.79	32	36	–
–	60	4.5	–	565	960	–	200	.12	.17	3	–	–	9	–

(For purposes of calculations, use "0" for t, <1, <.1, <.01, etc.)

Table A–1
Food Composition

Computer Code Number	Food Description	Measure	Wt (g)	H₂O (%)	Ener (cal)	Prot (g)	Carb (g)	Dietary Fiber (g)	Fat (g)	Fat Breakdown (g)		
										Sat	Mono	Poly
	WENDY'S—Cont.											
1580	French fries	1 ea	106	43	306	4	38	1	15	7	5	2
1581	Frosty dairy dessert	1 c	216	35	354	7	53	0	13	5	3	2
1582	Chocolate chip cookies	1 ea	64	4	320	3	40	1	17	5.5	5.8	4.9
	Source: Wendy's International.											
	CONVENIENCE FOODS & MEALS											
	ALPINE LACE											
	Cheese spread, free'n lean:											
1926	Cheddar	1 oz	28	–	30	5	1	–	0	0	0	0
1928	Cream cheese	1 oz	28	–	30	5	1	–	0	0	0	0
1929	Garden vegetable	1 oz	28	–	30	5	1	–	0	0	0	0
1932	Garlic herb	1 oz	28	–	30	5	1	–	0	0	0	0
1933	Horseradish	1 oz	28	–	30	5	1	–	0	0	0	0
	BUDGET GOURMET											
1695	Chicken cacciatore	1 ea	312	80	300	20	27	–	13	–	–	–
1694	Sweet & sour chicken with rice	1 ea	284	72	350	18	53	–	7	–	–	–
1689	Teriyaki chicken	1 ea	340	77	360	20	44	–	12	–	–	–
1692	Linguini & shrimp	1 ea	284	77	330	15	33	–	15	–	–	–
1691	Scallops & shrimp	1 ea	326	79	320	16	43	–	9	–	–	–
2245	Seafood Newburg	1 ea	284	74	350	17	43	–	12	–	–	–
1693	Sirloin tips with country gravy	1 ea	284	80	310	16	21	–	18	–	–	–
1690	Veal parmigiana	1 ea	340	75	440	26	39	–	20	–	–	–
1696	Yankee pot roast	1 ea	312	77	380	27	22	–	21	–	–	–
	Source: The All American Gourmet Company.											
	HAAGEN DAZS											
1755	Ice cream bar, vanilla almond	1 ea	107	–	370	6	26	–	27	14	10	3
	Sorbet:											
1758	Lemon	½ c	113	–	140	0	35	–	0	0	0	0
1760	Orange	½ c	113	–	140	0	36	–	0	0	0	0
1759	Raspberry	½ c	113	–	110	0	27	–	0	0	0	0
	Yogurt, frozen:											
1753	Chocolate	½ c	98	–	170	8	26	–	4	2	2	0
1754	Strawberry	½ c	98	–	170	6	27	–	4	2	2	0
	Yogurt extra, frozen:											
1752	Brownie nut	½ c	101	–	220	8	29	–	9	4	4	1
1751	Raspberry rendezvous	½ c	101	–	132	4	26	–	2	1	1	0
	HEALTHY CHOICE											
	Entrees:											
2255	Chicken Chow Mein	1 ea	241	78	220	18	31	–	3	.8	–	.8
2112	Fish, lemon pepper	1 ea	303	78	290	14	47	7	5	1	–	–
1624	Lasagna	1 ea	284	78	260	18	37	–	5	–	–	–
2111	Meatloaf, traditional, entree	1 ea	340	79	320	16	46	7	8	4	–	–
2293	Spaghetti	1 ea	284	77	280	14	42	–	6	–	–	–
2104	Zucchini lasagna	1 ea	397	80	330	20	58	11	2	1	–	–

(Computer code number is for West Diet Analysis program)

PAGE KEY: A–4 = BEV   A–6 = DAIRY   A–12 = EGGS   A–14 = FAT/OIL   A–18 = FRUIT   A–26 = BAKERY   A–36 = GRAIN   A–44 = FISH   A–48 = MEATS   A–50 = POULTRY   A–54 = SAUSAGE   A–56 = MIXED/FAST   A–64 = NUTS/SEEDS   A–68 = SWEETS   A–70 = VEG/LEG   A–84 = MISC   A–88 = SOUPS/SAUCES   A–90 = FAST   A–106 = FRZN ENTREE   A–112 = BABY FOODS

Chol (mg)	Calc (mg)	Iron (mg)	Magn (mg)	Pota (mg)	Sodi (mg)	Zinc (mg)	VT-A (RE)	Thia (mg)	Ribo (mg)	Niac (mg)	V-B6 (mg)	Fola (µg)	VT-C (mg)	VT-E α-TE (mg)
15	13	1.02	45	689	105	.51	0	.15	.04	2.96	.26	33	12	–
44	257	.86	43	518	194	.92	143	.11	.45	.31	.12	17	<1	–
5	10	1.09	15	100	235	.46	0	.06	.07	.4	.03	6	0	–
5	100	–	–	30	165	–	–	–	–	–	–	–	–	–
5	100	–	–	30	165	–	–	–	–	–	–	–	–	–
5	100	–	–	30	165	–	–	–	–	–	–	–	–	–
5	100	–	–	30	165	–	–	–	–	–	–	–	–	–
5	100	–	–	30	165	–	–	–	–	–	–	–	–	–
60	150	1.8	–	–	810	–	40	.23	.51	5	–	–	21	–
40	60	.72	–	–	640	–	80	.12	.34	3	–	–	2	–
55	80	1.4	–	–	610	–	300	.15	.34	6	–	–	12	–
75	10	3.6	–	–	1250	–	1000	.3	.17	3	–	–	2	–
70	150	.72	–	–	690	–	150	–	.26	3	–	–	12	–
70	100	.72	–	–	660	–	40	.23	.26	2	–	–	–	–
40	60	.36	–	–	570	–	150	.15	.17	4	–	–	2	–
165	30	4.5	–	–	1160	–	1000	.45	.6	6	–	–	6	–
70	150	1.8	–	–	690	–	600	.15	.43	7	–	–	6	–
90	160	.38	–	220	85	–	160	–	.18	–	–	–	–	–
0	–	–	–	30	20	–	–	–	–	–	–	–	7	–
0	–	–	–	80	20	–	–	–	––	–	–	–	20	–
0	–	–	–	60	15	–	–	–	–	–	–	–	7	–
40	146	.7	–	240	45	–	20	–	.17	–	–	–	5	–
50	146	–	–	140	45	–	20	.03	.17	–	–	–	–	–
55	152	.73	–	250	60	–	20	–	.14	–	–	–	–	–
20	81	–	–	97	25	–	0	–	.1	–	–	–	5	–
45	20	1.4	–	290	440	–	81	.15	.14	4	–	–	4	–
25	20	1.08	–	–	360	–	100	–	–	–	–	–	30	–
20	100	2.7	–	500	420	–	150	.3	.26	2	–	–	2	–
35	40	1.8	–	–	460	–	150	–	–	–	–	–	54	–
20	6	3.6	–	540	480	–	250	.38	.26	2	–	–	5	–
10	200	2.7	–	–	310	–	250	–	–	–	–	–	0	–

(For purposes of calculations, use "0" for t, <1, <.1, <.01, etc.)

Table A–1
Food Composition

Computer Code Number	Food Description	Measure	Wt (g)	H₂O (%)	Ener (cal)	Prot (g)	Carb (g)	Dietary Fiber (g)	Fat (g)	Fat Breakdown (g)		
										Sat	Mono	Poly
	HEALTHY CHOICE—Cont.											
	Dinners:											
2110	Pasta shells marinara	1 ea	340	74	360	25	59	5	3	1.5	–	–
2292	Sirloin tips	1 ea	334	81	280	23	30	–	8	–	–	–
2291	Sole au gratin	1 ea	312	80	270	16	40	–	5	–	–	–
	Low-fat ice milk:											
2257	Berry	½ c	113	–	120	3	23	–	2	1	–	0
2258	Chocolate	½ c	113	–	130	3	24	–	2	1	–	0
1608	Cookie & cream	½ c	113	–	130	4	24	–	2	–	–	0
1621	Vanilla	½ c	113	–	120	4	21	–	2	1	–	0
	Low-fat ice cream:											
973	Brownie	½ c	71	61	120	3	22	2	2	1	–	.7
650	Chocolate chip	½ c	71	62	120	3	21	1	2	1	–	0
259	Butter pecan	½ c	71	61	120	3	22	1	2	1	–	.7
45	Rocky road	½ c	71	53	140	3	28	2	2	1	–	0
391	Vanilla fudge	½ c	71	62	120	3	21	1	2	1.5	–	.7
	Source: ConAgra Frozen Foods, Omaha, NE.											
	HEALTH VALLEY											
	Soups, fat-free:											
2001	Beef broth, no salt added	6.9 oz	196	98	15	4	0	0	0	0	0	0
2073	Beef broth, w/salt	6.9 oz	196	98	15	4	0	0	0	0	0	0
2016	Black bean & vegetable	7.5 oz	213	85	70	7	12	11	0	0	0	0
2017	Chicken broth	7.5 oz	213	97	22	4	1	0	0	0	0	0
2018	14 garden vegetable	7.5 oz	213	92	50	5	6	5	0	0	0	0
2015	Lentil & carrot	7.5 oz	213	86	90	8	14	7	0	0	0	0
2014	Split pea & carrot	7.5 oz	213	86	90	8	14	7	0	0	0	0
2013	Tomato vegetable	7.5 oz	213	90	50	5	8	6	0	0	0	0
	LA CHOY											
2100	Egg rolls, mini, chicken	1 svg	106	53	220	8	35	3	6	1.5	–	–
2099	Egg rolls, mini, shrimp	1 svg	106	56	210	7	35	3	4	1	–	–
	LEAN CUISINE											
	Dinners:											
1639	Baked cheese ravioli	1 ea	241	77	240	13	30	3	8	3	3	.5
1640	Chicken cacciatore	1 ea	308	80	280	22	31	4	7	2	–	1
1632	Chicken chow mein	1 ea	255	78	240	14	34	–	5	1	–	1
1633	Lasagna	1 ea	291	79	260	19	34	2	5	2	2	.5
1634	Macaroni & cheese	1 ea	255	74	290	15	37	–	9	4	–	.5
1631	Spaghetti w/meatballs	1 ea	269	75	280	19	35	11	7	2	2.6	1
2256	Fillet of fish florentine, entree	1 ea	273	80	220	26	13	–	7	3	–	2
	Pizza:											
1635	French bread cheese pizza	1 ea	145	52	300	17	38	<1	9	3	5	.5
1638	French bread deluxe pizza	1 ea	174	56	320	22	39	2	8	3	3	.5
1637	French bread pepperoni pizza	1 ea	149	51	330	19	38	2	11	3	5.4	1
1636	French bread sausage pizza	1 ea	170	55	330	22	40	2	9	3	4.3	.5
	Source: Stouffer's Foods Corp, Solon, OH.											
	TASTE ADVENTURE SOUPS											
1905	Black bean	1 c	227	–	130	6	26	6	1	–	–	–
1904	Curry lentil	1 c	227	–	130	6	28	5	1	–	–	–
1906	Lentil chili	1 c	227	–	170	10	31	6	1	–	–	–
1903	Split pea	1 c	227	–	130	5	25	5	1	–	–	–

(Computer code number is for West Diet Analysis program)

PAGE KEY: A–4 = BEV   A–6 = DAIRY   A–12 = EGGS   A–14 = FAT/OIL   A–18 = FRUIT   A–26 = BAKERY   A–36 = GRAIN   A–44 = FISH
A–48 = MEATS   A–50 = POULTRY   A–54 = SAUSAGE   A–56 = MIXED/FAST   A–64 = NUTS/SEEDS   A–68 = SWEETS   A–70 = VEG/LEG
A–84 = MISC   A–88 = SOUPS/SAUCES   A–90 = FAST   A–106 = FRZN ENTREE   A–112 = BABY FOODS

Chol (mg)	Calc (mg)	Iron (mg)	Magn (mg)	Pota (mg)	Sodi (mg)	Zinc (mg)	VT-A (RE)	Thia (mg)	Ribo (mg)	Niac (mg)	V-B6 (mg)	Fola (µg)	VT-C (mg)	VT-E α-TE (mg)
25	400	1.8	–	–	390	–	100	–	–	–	–	–	4	–
65	20	2.7	–	540	370	–	700	.15	.17	5	.35	–	42	–
55	80	1.1	–	430	470	–	–	.23	.17	1.6	–	–	6	–
5	100	–	–	160	60	–	–	.03	.17	–	–	–	–	–
5	100	–	–	191	70	–	–	.03	.17	–	–	–	–	–
5	150	–	–	180	80	–	–	.03	.17	–	–	–	–	–
5	150	–	–	180	60	–	–	.06	.25	–	–	–	–	–
3	80	0	–	268	55	–	40	–	–	–	–	–	0	–
3	100	0	–	240	50	–	40	–	–	–	–	–	0	–
3	100	0	–	212	60	–	40	–	–	–	–	–	0	–
3	100	0	–	168	60	–	40	.03	.15	–	–	–	0	–
3	100	0	–	296	50	–	40	–	–	–	–	–	0	–
0	–	–	–	160	60	–	–	–	–	.8	–	–	–	–
0	–	–	–	160	290	–	–	–	–	.8	–	–	–	–
0	60	4.5	–	600	290	–	1000	.3	.1	1.2	.2	120	0	–
0	–	.39	–	130	315	–	–	–	.03	2.17	–	–	–	–
0	40	1.08	–	360	250	–	1000	.23	.07	2	.16	24	6	–
0	60	4.5	–	390	270	–	1000	.09	.14	5	.4	24	0	–
0	60	4.5	–	390	270	–	1000	.09	.14	5	.4	–	0	–
0	40	.72	–	540	230	–	1000	.09	.07	2	.12	32	9	–
5	20	1.44	–	–	460	–	20	–	–	–	–	–	0	–
5	20	1.44	–	–	510	–	20	–	–	–	–	–	0	–
55	200	1.44	42	380	590	1.5	60	.06	.25	1.2	.2	48	36	–
45	40	1.44	47	560	570	.97	100	.22	.17	6	–	–	9	–
30	40	1.08	30	350	530	1.1	60	.15	.17	5	–	–	6	–
25	150	1.8	44	700	590	2.9	100	.15	.25	3	.32	–	6	–
30	250	.72	–	160	550	–	20	.12	.25	1.2	–	–	0	–
35	100	1.8	47	500	490	2.5	60	.15	.25	3	.2	–	4	–
65	150	.72	58	780	590	1.2	500	.15	.34	2	.14	<1	1	–
15	250	2.7	34	320	590	1.6	60	.37	.34	4	.1	–	6	–
40	200	1.44	38	440	860	2.08	150	.45	.51	5	.16	–	6	–
25	200	3.6	34	390	790	1.8	100	.45	.42	5	.07	–	6	–
40	250	2.7	39	440	860	2.2	80	.45	.51	5	.07	–	6	–
–	–	–	–	609	530	–	–	–	–	–	–	–	–	–
–	–	–	–	440	550	–	–	–	–	–	–	–	–	–
–	–	–	–	609	420	–	–	–	–	–	–	–	–	–
–	–	–	–	450	550	–	–	–	–	–	–	–	–	–

(For purposes of calculations, use "0" for t, <1, <.1, <.01, etc.)

Table A–1
Food Composition

Computer Code Number	Food Description	Measure	Wt (g)	H₂O (%)	Ener (cal)	Prot (g)	Carb (g)	Dietary Fiber (g)	Fat (g)	Fat Breakdown (g)		
										Sat	Mono	Poly
	WEIGHT WATCHERS											
	Cheese, fat-free slices:											
1978	Cheddar, sharp	2 pce	21	60	30	5	2	0	0	0	0	0
1980	Swiss	2 pce	21	59	30	5	2	0	0	0	0	0
1977	White	2 pce	21	59	30	5	2	0	0	0	0	0
1979	Yellow	2 pce	21	59	30	5	2	0	0	0	0	0
	Dinners:											
2259	Beef stroganoff	1 ea	238	73	290	22	26	3	9	4	3	2
1646	Oven fried fish	1 ea	198	79	240	20	23	–	7	–	5	2
2260	Fried chicken patty	1 pce	184	73	270	16	14	–	16	8	6	2
2261	Chicken burrito w/vegetable	1 ea	216	68	330	15	36	–	14	4	6	3
2029	Chicken chow mein	1 ea	255	81	200	12	34	3	2	.5	–	–
2262	Pasta primavera	1 ea	238	75	260	15	22	2	11	.8	8	3
1972	Margarine, reduced fat	1 tbs	14	50	60	0	0	0	7	1.5	–	–
	Pizza:											
1653	Cheese pizza	1 ea	164	56	300	22	37	2	7	3	3	1
1650	Deluxe combination pizza	1 ea	200	64	330	26	35	3	10	3	5	2
2294	Sausage pizza	1 ea	175	60	320	24	35	2	10	2	6	2
1652	Pepperoni pizza	1 ea	171	56	320	26	31	–	10	3	5	2
	Desserts:											
2263	Apple pie	1 ea	98	49	200	2	39	–	5	1	2	2
2264	Boston cream pie	1 ea	85	48	170	4	35	1	4	1	1	2
1644	Chocolate brownie	1 ea	35	29	100	3	17	<1	4	1	2	1
2024	Chocolate eclair	1 ea	60	45	150	3	24	2	5	1.5	–	–
1642	Strawberry cheesecake	1 ea	109	62	180	7	28	–	5	1	1	2
2027	Triple chocolate cheesecake	1 ea	89	52	200	7	32	1	5	2.5	–	–
2247	Chocolate mousse	1 ea	78	44	190	6	33	3	4	1.5	–	–
	SWEET SUCCESS:											
	Drinks, prepared:											
1776	Chocolate chip	1 c	265	81	180	15	30	6	3	1.6	–	–
1777	Chocolate fudge	1 c	265	81	180	15	30	6	2	–	–	–
1774	Chocolate mocha	1 c	265	81	180	15	30	6	1	1	–	–
1778	Milk chocolate	1 c	265	81	180	15	30	6	2	1	–	–
1775	Vanilla	1 c	265	81	180	15	33	6	1	.6	–	–
	Drinks, ready to drink:											
2147	Chocolate mint	1¼ c	284	82	179	11	34	5	3	0	–	–
2148	Strawberry	1¼ c	284	82	179	11	34	5	3	0	–	–
	Shakes:											
1771	Chocolate almond	1¼ c	313	82	200	12	38	6	3	1.1	1.6	.3
1773	Chocolate fudge	1¼ c	313	82	200	12	38	6	5	1.1	1.6	.3
1768	Chocolate mocha	1¼ c	313	82	200	12	38	6	3	.8	.8	1.3
1769	Chocolate raspberry truffle	1¼ c	313	82	200	12	38	6	3	1.1	1.6	.3
1770	Vanilla creme	1¼ c	313	82	200	12	38	6	3	.8	1.8	.4
	Snack bars:											
1767	Chocolate brownie	1 ea	33	8	120	2	23	3	4	2	.5	.6
1766	Chocolate chip	1 ea	33	8	120	2	23	3	4	2	.4	.5
1765	Peanut butter	1 ea	33	8	120	2	23	3	4	2	.6	.6
1921	Oatmeal raisin	1 ea	33	7	120	2	23	3	4	2	–	–

Source: Foodway National Inc., Boise, ID.

(Computer code number is for West Diet Analysis program)

PAGE KEY: A–4 = BEV   A–6 = DAIRY   A–12 = EGGS   A–14 = FAT/OIL   A–18 = FRUIT   A–26 = BAKERY   A–36 = GRAIN   A–44 = FISH
A–48 = MEATS   A–50 = POULTRY   A–54 = SAUSAGE   A–56 = MIXED/FAST   A–64 = NUTS/SEEDS   A–68 = SWEETS   A–70 = VEG/LEG
A–84 = MISC   A–88 = SOUPS/SAUCES   A–90 = FAST   A–106 = FRZN ENTREE   A–112 = BABY FOODS

Chol (mg)	Calc (mg)	Iron (mg)	Magn (mg)	Pota (mg)	Sodi (mg)	Zinc (mg)	VT-A (RE)	Thia (mg)	Ribo (mg)	Niac (mg)	V-B6 (mg)	Fola (µg)	VT-C (mg)	VT-E α-TE (mg)
0	100	0	–	65	310	–	57	–	–	–	–	–	0	–
0	100	0	–	75	280	–	57	–	–	–	–	–	0	–
0	100	0	–	65	310	–	57	–	–	–	–	–	0	–
0	100	0	–	65	310	–	57	–	–	–	–	–	0	–
25	80	2.7	–	350	600	–	60	.23	.26	4	.32	–	4	–
15	20	.72	–	340	380	–	100	.09	.14	1.6	–	–	5	–
70	39	1.7	–	350	610	–	75	.19	.18	4	–	–	6	–
65	56	2.3	–	390	800	–	38	.52	.39	5.9	–	–	3	–
25	40	.72	–	360	430	–	300	–	–	–	–	–	36	–
5	300	1.8	–	260	800	–	350	.23	.26	3	.18	–	18	–
0	0	0	–	5	130	–	50	–	–	–	–	–	0	–
35	450	1.4	–	420	630	–	200	.3	.51	3	.06	–	12	–
25	350	1.8	–	490	650	–	350	.3	.51	3	.2	–	21	–
35	300	1.8	–	470	630	–	250	.3	.51	3	.06	–	18	–
35	400	1.8	–	420	710	–	200	.23	.51	3	–	–	15	–
5	20	1.1	–	80	280	–	–	.06	.07	.4	–	–	1	–
5	65	.6	–	120	290	–	14	.03	.02	.3	.08	–	1	–
10	19	.9	–	120	150	–	14	.06	.03	.2	.03	–	1	–
0	40	0	–	65	150	–	0	–	–	–	–	–	0	–
20	80	.36	–	140	210	–	40	.06	.07	1.6	–	–	2	–
10	80	1.08	–	170	200	–	0	–	–	–	–	–	0	–
5	60	1.8	–	320	150	–	0	–	–	–	–	–	0	–
6	500	6.3	140	600	288	5.25	–	.53	.6	7	.7	140	21	7.05
6	500	6.3	140	750	336	5.25	–	.53	.6	7	.7	140	21	7.05
6	500	6.3	140	800	336	5.25	–	.53	.6	7	.7	140	21	7.05
6	500	6.3	140	750	336	5.25	–	.53	.6	7	.7	140	21	7.05
6	500	6.3	140	830	312	5.25	–	.53	.6	7	.7	140	21	7.05
6	449	5.67	125	502	215	4.82	314	.48	.54	6.24	.62	125	19	6.28
6	449	5.67	125	502	188	4.82	314	.48	.54	6.24	.62	125	19	6.28
5	500	6.3	140	540	240	5.25	–	.53	.6	7	.7	140	21	6.92
4	500	6.3	140	520	220	5.25	–	.53	.6	7	.7	140	21	6.92
5	500	6.3	140	1490	220	5.25	–	.53	.6	7	.7	140	21	6.92
5	500	6.3	140	520	220	5.25	–	.53	.6	7	.7	140	21	6.92
5	500	6.3	140	350	220	5.25	–	.53	.6	7	.7	140	21	6.92
5	150	2.71	8	140	35	.01	–	.22	.25	3	.3	60	9	3.01
5	150	2.71	8	110	40	.01	–	.22	.25	3	.3	60	9	3.01
5	150	2.71	8	125	35	.01	–	.22	.25	3	.3	60	9	3.01
5	2	2.71	–	–	30	–	–	–	–	–	–	–	9	3.01

(For purposes of calculations, use "0" for t, <1, <.1, <.01, etc.)

Table A–1
Food Composition

Computer Code Number	Food Description	Measure	Wt (g)	H$_2$O (%)	Ener (cal)	Prot (g)	Carb (g)	Dietary Fiber (g)	Fat (g)	Fat Breakdown (g)		
										Sat	Mono	Poly
BABY FOODS												
1720	Apple juice	4 fl oz	125	88	59	0	15	–	<1	–	–	–
1721	Applesauce, strained	1 tbs	14	89	6	<1	2	–	<1	–	–	–
1716	Carrots, strained	1 tbs	14	92	4	<1	1	–	<1	–	–	–
1718	Cereal, mixed, millk added	1 tbs	14	75	16	1	2	–	<1	–	–	–
1719	Cereal, rice, milk added	1 tbs	14	75	16	1	2	–	<1	–	–	–
1723	Chicken and noodles, strained	1 tbs	14	88	7	<1	1	–	<1	–	–	–
1722	Peas, strained	1 tbs	14	88	6	1	1	–	<1	–	–	–
1717	Teething biscuits	1 ea	11	6	43	1	8	–	<1	–	–	–

(Computer code number is for West Diet Analysis program)

PAGE KEY: A–4 = BEV   A–6 = DAIRY   A–12 = EGGS   A–14 = FAT/OIL   A–18 = FRUIT   A–26 = BAKERY   A–36 = GRAIN   A–44 = FISH
A–48 = MEATS   A–50 = POULTRY   A–54 = SAUSAGE   A–56 = MIXED/FAST   A–64 = NUTS/SEEDS   A–68 = SWEETS   A–70 = VEG/LEG
A–84 = MISC   A–88 = SOUPS/SAUCES   A–90 = FAST   A–106 = FRZN ENTREE   A–112 = BABY FOODS

Chol (mg)	Calc (mg)	Iron (mg)	Magn (mg)	Pota (mg)	Sodi (mg)	Zinc (mg)	VT-A (RE)	Thia (mg)	Ribo (mg)	Niac (mg)	V-B6 (mg)	Fola (μg)	VT-C (mg)	VT-E α-TE (mg)
–	5	.71	4	114	4	.04	3	.01	.02	.1	.04	<1	72	.75
–	1	.03	<1	10	<1	<.01	<1	<.01	<.01	.01	<.01	<1	6	.08
–	3	.05	1	28	5	.02	164	<.01	.01	.07	.01	2	1	.07
–	31	1.49	4	28	7	.1	3	.06	.08	.82	.01	2	–	–
–	34	1.73	6	27	7	.09	4	.07	.07	.74	.02	1	–	–
–	3	.06	1	6	2	.04	16	<.01	.01	.07	.01	1	<1	.03
–	3	.14	2	16	<1	.05	8	.01	.01	.14	.01	4	1	.07
–	29	.39	4	36	40	.1	1	.03	.06	.48	.01	2	1	.05

(For purposes of calculations, use "0" for t, <1, <.1, <.01, etc.)

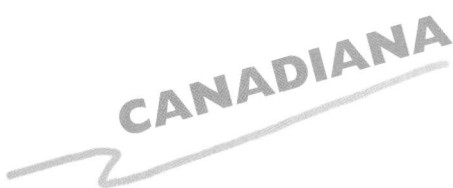

CONTENTS

RECOMMENDED NUTRIENT INTAKES (RNI) FOR CANADIANS

Like the RDA on the inside front cover pages, the Recommended Nutrient Intakes (RNI) for Canadians make recommendations for intakes of vitamins, minerals, protein, and energy. The RNI are presented in Tables B-1 and B-2.

CANADA'S GUIDELINES FOR HEALTHY EATING

Canada's Guidelines for Healthy Eating provide general recommendations about diet for consumers. They state that people should:

- Enjoy a variety of foods.
- Emphasize cereals, breads, other grain products, vegetables, and fruits.
- Choose lower-fat dairy products, leaner meats, and foods prepared with little or no fat.
- Achieve and maintain a healthy body weight by enjoying regular physical activity and healthy eating.
- Limit salt, alcohol, and caffeine.

In addition, Table 2-2 in Chapter 2 presents the *Nutrition Recommendations for Canadians*, developed as key nutrition messages for scientists and professionals to support the health of Canadians over two years of age.

CANADA'S FOOD GUIDE TO HEALTHY EATING

The 1992 *Canada's Food Guide to Healthy Eating* gives consumers detailed information for selecting foods to meet the *Nutrition Recommendations* and the *Guidelines for Healthy Eating* (1990). The *Food Guide* was designed to meet the nutritional needs of all Canadians four years of age and older and takes a total diet approach, covering all foods and beverages rather than a foundation diet which gives minimum servings of food groups.

The rainbow side of the Food Guide (Figure B-1) shows the four food groups with their names and pictorial examples of foods in each group. Key statements direct consumers about selecting foods generally from all the groups, and more specifically within each group. The bar side shows the number of servings recommended for each group, using a range of servings instead of a single minimum number. Also on the bar side, sample serving sizes are provided for some foods.

FOOD LABELS IN CANADA

By law, labels must conform to standards with regard to nutrition information. Table B-3 offers some definitions of terms seen on food labels, and Figure B-2 illustrates where label information is located.

TABLE B-1

Recommended Nutrient Intakes for Canadians, 1990

AGE	SEX	WEIGHT (kg)	PROTEIN (g/day)[a]	FAT-SOLUBLE VITAMINS		
				Vitamin A (RE/day)[b]	Vitamin D (µg/day)[c]	Vitamin E (mg/day)[d]
Infants (months)						
0–4	Both	6	12[f]	400	10	3
5–12	Both	9	12	400	10	3
Children and Adults (years)						
1	Both	11	13	400	10	3
2–3	Both	14	16	400	5	4
4–6	Both	18	19	500	5	5
7–9	M	25	26	700	2.5	7
	F	25	26	700	2.5	6
10–12	M	34	34	800	2.5	8
	F	36	36	800	5	7
13–15	M	50	49	900	5	9
	F	48	46	800	5	7
16–18	M	62	58	1,000	5	10
	F	53	47	800	2.5	7
19–24	M	71	61	1,000	2.5	10
	F	58	50	800	2.5	7
25–49	M	74	64	1,000	2.5	9
	F	59	51	800	2.5	6
50–74	M	73	63	1,000	5	7
	F	63	54	800	5	6
75+	M	69	59	1,000	5	6
	F	64	55	800	5	5
Pregnancy (additional amount needed)						
1st trimester			5	0	2.5	2
2nd trimester			20	0	2.5	2
3rd trimester			24	0	2.5	2
Lactation (additional amount needed)			20	400	2.5	3

NOTE: Recommended intakes of energy and of certain nutrients are not listed in this table because of the nature of the variables upon which they are based. The figures for energy are estimates of average requirements for expected patterns of activity. For nutrients not shown, the following amounts are recommended based on at least 2,000 kcalories per day and body weights as given: thiamin, 0.4 milligrams per 1,000 kcalories (0.48 milligrams/5,000 kilojoules); riboflavin, 0.5 milligrams per 1,000 kcalories (0.6 milligrams/5,000 kilojoules); niacin, 7.2 niacin equivalents per 1,000 kcalories (8.6 niacin equivalents/5,000 kilojoules); vitamin B_6, 15 micrograms, as pyridoxine, per gram of protein. Recommended intakes during periods of growth are taken as appropriate for individuals representative of the midpoint in each age group. All recommended intakes are designed to cover individual variations in essentially all of a healthy population subsisting upon a variety of common foods available in Canada.

SOURCE: Health and Welfare Canada, *Nutrition Recommendations: The Report of the Scientific Review Committee* (Ottawa: Canadian Government Publishing Centre, 1990), Table 20, p. 204.

TABLE B-1

Recommended Nutrient Intakes for Canadians, 1990 continued

WATER-SOLUBLE VITAMINS			MINERALS					
Vitamin C (mg/day)e	Folate (µg/day)	Vitamin B$_{12}$ (µg/day)	Calcium (mg/day)	Phosphorus (mg/day)	Magnesium (mg/day)	Iron (mg/day)	Iodine (µg/day)	Zinc (mg/day)
20	25	0.3	250	150	20	0.3[g]	30	2[h]
20	40	0.4	400	200	32	7	40	3
20	40	0.5	500	300	40	6	55	4
20	50	0.6	550	350	50	6	65	4
25	70	0.8	600	400	65	8	85	5
25	90	1.0	700	500	100	8	110	7
25	90	1.0	700	500	100	8	95	7
25	120	1.0	900	700	130	8	125	9
25	130	1.0	1,100	800	135	8	110	9
30	175	1.0	1,100	900	185	10	160	12
30	170	1.0	1,000	850	180	13	160	9
40	220	1.0	900	1,000	230	10	160	12
30	190	1.0	700	850	200	12	160	9
40	220	1.0	800	1,000	240	9	160	12
30	180	1.0	700	850	200	13	160	9
40	230	1.0	800	1,000	250	9	160	12
30	185	1.0	700	850	200	13[i]	160	9
40	230	1.0	800	1,000	250	9	160	12
30	195	1.0	800	850	210	8	160	9
40	215	1.0	800	1,000	230	9	160	12
30	200	1.0	800	850	210	8	160	9
0	200	0.2	500	200	15	0	25	6
10	200	0.2	500	200	45	5	25	6
10	200	0.2	500	200	45	10	25	6
25	100	0.2	500	200	65	0	50	6

[a]The primary units are expressed per kilogram of body weight. The figures shown here are examples.

[b]One retinol equivalent (RE) corresponds to the biological activity of 1 microgram of retinol, 6 micrograms of beta-carotene, or 12 micrograms of other carotenes.

[c]Expressed as cholecalciferol or ergocalciferol.

[d]Expressed as δ-α-tocopherol equivalents, relative to which β- and γ-tocopherol and α-tocotrienol have activities of 0.5, 0.1, and 0.3, respectively.

[e]Cigarette smokers should increase intake by 50 percent.

[f]The assumption is made that the protein is from breast milk or is of the same biological value as that of breast milk, and that between 3 and 9 months, adjustment for the quality of the protein is made.

[g]Based on the assumption that breast milk is the source of iron.

[h]Based on the assumption that breast milk is the source of zinc.

[i]After menopause, the recommended intake is 8 milligrams per day.

B

TABLE B-2

Average Energy Requirements for Canadians

AGE	SEX	AVERAGE HEIGHT (cm)	AVERAGE WEIGHT (kg)	AVERAGE REQUIREMENTS[a]					
				(kcal/kg)[b]	(MJ/kg)[b]	(kcal/day)	(MJ/day)	(kcal/cm)	(MJ/cm)
Infants (months)									
0–2	Both	55	4.5	120–100	0.50–0.42	500	2.0	9	0.04
3–5	Both	63	7.0	100–95	0.42–0.40	700	2.8	11	0.05
6–8	Both	69	8.5	95–97	0.40–0.41	800	3.4	11.5	0.05
9–11	Both	73	9.5	97–99	0.41	950	3.8	12.5	0.05
Children and Adults (years)									
1	Both	82	11	101	0.42	1,100	4.8	13.5	0.06
2–3	Both	95	14	94	0.39	1,300	5.6	13.5	0.06
4–6	Both	107	18	100	0.42	1,800	7.6	17	0.07
7–9	M	126	25	88	0.37	2,200	9.2	17.5	0.07
	F	125	25	76	0.32	1,900	8.0	15	0.06
10–12	M	141	34	73	0.30	2,500	10.4	17.5	0.07
	F	143	36	61	0.25	2,200	9.2	15.5	0.06
13–15	M	159	50	57	0.24	2,800	12.0	17.5	0.07
	F	157	48	46	0.19	2,200	9.2	14	0.06
16–18	M	172	62	51	0.21	3,200	13.2	18.5	0.08
	F	160	53	40	0.17	2,100	8.8	13	0.05
19–24	M	175	71	42	0.18	3,000	12.6		
	F	160	58	36	0.15	2,100	8.8		
25–49	M	172	74	36	0.15	2,700	11.3		
	F	160	59	32	0.13	1,900	8.0		
50–74	M	170	73	31	0.13	2,300	9.7		
	F	158	63	29	0.12	1,800	7.6		
75+	M	168	69	29	0.12	2,000	8.4		
	F	155	64	23	0.10	1,500	6.3		

[a]Requirements can be expected to vary within a range of ±30 percent.
[b]First and last figures are averages at the beginning and end of the three-month period.

SOURCE: Health and Welfare Canada, *Nutrition Recommendations: The Report of the Scientific Review Committee* (Ottawa: Canadian Government Publishing Centre, 1990), Tables 5 and 6, pp. 25, 27.

THE CANADIAN EXCHANGE SYSTEM

The *Good Health Eating Guide* is the Canadian exchange system of meal planning.[a] It contains several features similar to those of the U.S. exchange system including the following:

- Foods are divided into lists according to carbohydrate, protein, and fat content.
- Foods are interchangeable within a group.
- Most foods are eaten in measured amounts.
- An energy value is given for each food group.

Tables B-4 through B-11 present the Canadian exchange system.

TABLE B-3

Terms on Food Labels

Energy

- **kcalorie reduced** 50% or fewer kcalories than the regular version.
- **light** term may be used to describe anything (for example, light in colour, texture, flavour, taste, or kcalories); read the label to find out what is "light" about the product.
- **low kcalorie** kcalorie-reduced and no more than 15 kcalories per serving.

Fat and Cholesterol

- **low cholesterol** no more than 3 mg of cholesterol per 100 g of the food and low in saturated fat; *does not* always mean low in total fat.
- **low fat** no more than 3 g of fat per serving; *does not* always mean low in kcalories.
- **lower fat** at least 25% less fat than the comparison food; be aware that 80% fat-free still means the food is 20% fat.

Carbohydrates: Fibre and Sugar

- **carbohydrate reduced** not more than 50% of the carbohydrate found in the regular version; *does not* always mean the product is lower in kcalories because other ingredients such as fat may have increased.
- **source of dietary fibre** a product that provides 2–4 g of fibre.
- **high source of dietary fibre** a product that provides 4–6 g of fibre.
- **very high source of fibre** a product that provides 6 g (or more) of fibre.
- **sugar free** low in carbohydrates and kcalories; can be used as an extra food in the exchange system.
- **unsweetened or no sugar added** no sugar was added to the product; sugar may be found naturally in the food (for example, fruit canned in its own juice).

---

[a]The tables for the Canadian exchange system are adapted from the *Good Health Eating Guide Resource,* copyright 1994, with permission of the Canadian Diabetes Association.

B

FIGURE B-1

CANADA'S FOOD GUIDE TO HEALTHY EATING

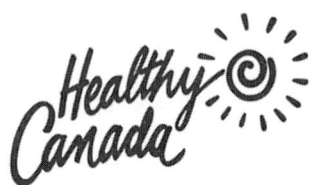

Healthy Canada
Health and Welfare Canada
Santé et Bien-être social Canada
CANADA'S
Food Guide
TO HEALTHY EATING
Enjoy a variety of foods from each group every day.
Choose lower-fat foods more often.
YOGOURT 2.2%
0.1%
SKIM MILK CHEESE
EVAP MILK
POWDER
2%
SKIM
TOFU
Grain Products
Choose whole grain and enriched products more often.
Vegetables & Fruit
Choose dark green and orange vegetables and orange fruit more often.
Milk Products
Choose lower-fat milk products more often.
Meat & Alternatives
Choose leaner meats, poultry and fish, as well as dried peas, beans and lentils more often.

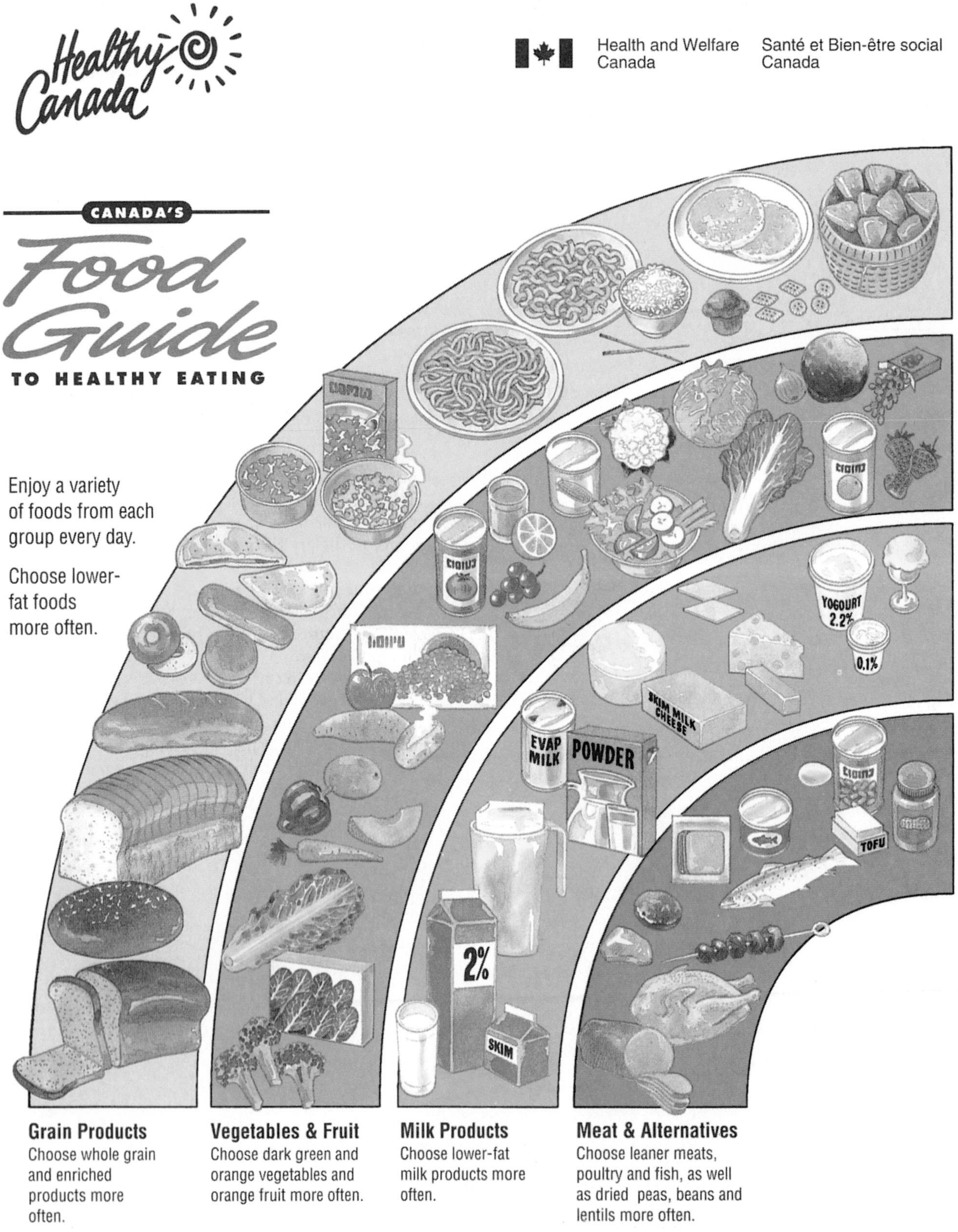

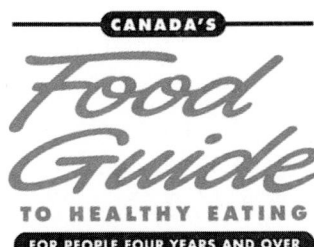

Different People Need Different Amounts of Food

The amount of food you need every day from the 4 food groups and other foods depends on your age, body size, activity level, whether you are male or female and if you are pregnant or breast-feeding. That's why the Food Guide gives a lower and higher number of servings for each food group. For example, young children can choose the lower number of servings, while male teenagers can go to the higher number. Most other people can choose servings somewhere in between.

B

Grain Products
5-12
SERVINGS PER DAY

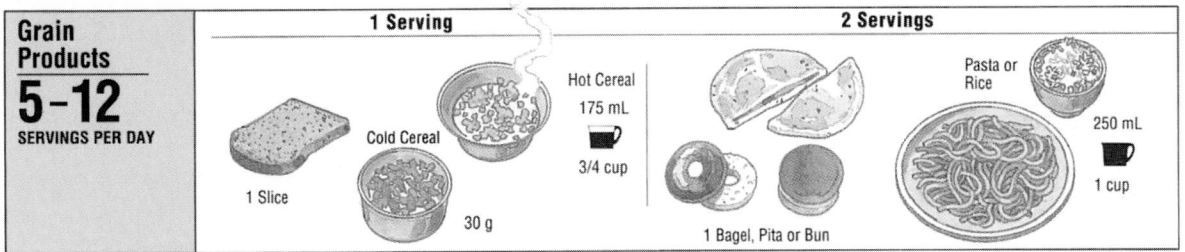

1 Serving
1 Slice
Cold Cereal
30 g
Hot Cereal
175 mL
3/4 cup

2 Servings
1 Bagel, Pita or Bun
Pasta or Rice
250 mL
1 cup

Vegetables & Fruit
5-10
SERVINGS PER DAY

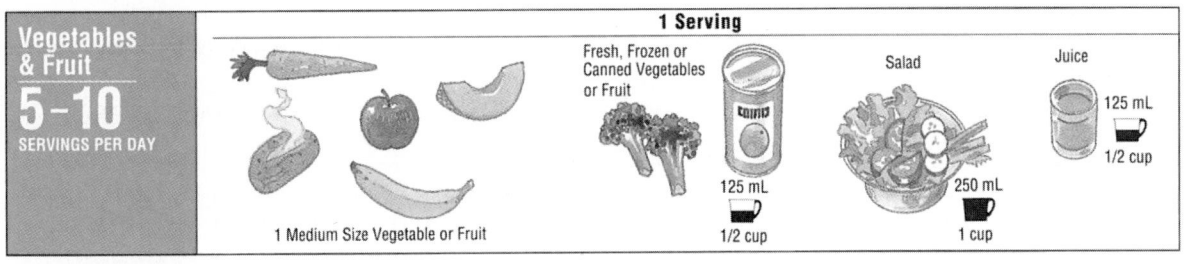

1 Serving
1 Medium Size Vegetable or Fruit
Fresh, Frozen or Canned Vegetables or Fruit
125 mL
1/2 cup
Salad
250 mL
1 cup
Juice
125 mL
1/2 cup

Milk Products
SERVINGS PER DAY
Children 4–9 years: 2–3
Youth 10–16 years: 3–4
Adults: 2–4
Pregnant & Breast-feeding Women: 3–4

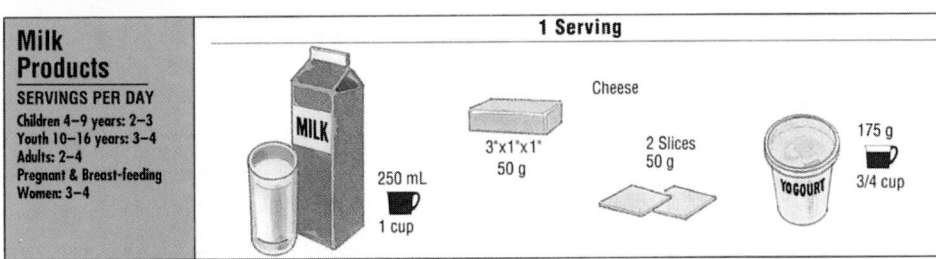

1 Serving
MILK
250 mL
1 cup
Cheese
3"x1"x1"
50 g
2 Slices
50 g
175 g
3/4 cup
YOGOURT

Other Foods

Taste and enjoyment can also come from other foods and beverages that are not part of the 4 food groups. Some of these foods are higher in fat or Calories, so use these foods in moderation.

Meat & Alternatives
2-3
SERVINGS PER DAY

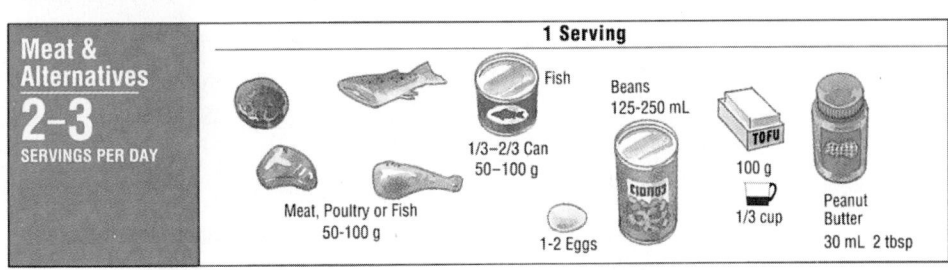

1 Serving
Meat, Poultry or Fish
50-100 g
Fish
1/3–2/3 Can
50–100 g
1-2 Eggs
Beans
125-250 mL
TOFU
100 g
1/3 cup
Peanut Butter
30 mL 2 tbsp

Enjoy eating well, being active and feeling good about yourself. That's VITALITĒ

FIGURE B-2

READING CANADIAN FOOD LABELS

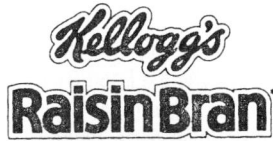

OUR COMMITMENT TO QUALITY

Kellogg's is committed to providing foods of outstanding quality and freshness. If this product in any way falls below the high standards you've come to expect from Kellogg's, please send your comments and both top flaps to:

Consumer Affairs
KELLOGG CANADA INC.
Etobicoke, Ontario M9W 5P2

IF IT DOESN'T SAY *Kellogg's* ON THE BOX,
IT'S NOT *Kellogg's* IN THE BOX.
SI LE NOM *Kellogg's* N'EST PAS SUR LA BOÎTE,
CE N'EST PAS *Kellogg's* DANS LA BOÎTE.

- HIGH IN FIBRE
- LOW IN FAT
- PRESERVATIVE FREE

- SOURCE ÉLEVÉE DE FIBRES
- FAIBLE EN MATIÈRES GRASSES
- SANS AGENT DE CONSERVATION

NUTRITION INFORMATION
APPORT NUTRITIONNEL

	Per 40 g serving cereal (175 mL, ¾ cup) Par ration de 40 g de céréale (175 mL, ¾ tasse)	Per 40 g serving cereal with 125 mL Partly Skimmed Milk (2%) Par ration de 40 g de céréale avec 125 mL de lait partiellement écrémé (2.0 %)	
ENERGY	130Cal 540kJ	195Cal 810kJ	ÉNERGIE
PROTEIN	3.0g	7.3g	PROTÉINES
FAT	0.4g	2.9g	MATIÈRES GRASSES
CARBOHYDRATE	32g	38g	GLUCIDES
SUGARS*	11g	18g	*SUCRES
STARCH	16g	16g	AMIDON
DIETARY FIBRE	4.6g	4.6g	FIBRES ALIMENTAIRES
SODIUM	235mg	300mg	SODIUM
POTASSIUM	240mg	440mg	POTASSIUM

% of Recommended Daily Intake
% de l'apport quotidien conseillé

VITAMIN A	0%	7%	VITAMINE A
VITAMIN D	0%	23%	VITAMINE D
VITAMIN B1	62%	66%	VITAMINE B1
VITAMIN B2	3%	16%	VITAMINE B2
NIACIN	13%	18%	NIACINE
VITAMIN B6	13%	16%	VITAMINE B6
FOLACIN	11%	14%	FOLACINE
VITAMIN B12	0%	25%	VITAMINE B12
PANTOTHENATE	9%	15%	PANTOTHENATE
CALCIUM	1%	15%	CALCIUM
PHOSPHORUS	12%	23%	PHOSPHORE
MAGNESIUM	20%	27%	MAGNÉSIUM
IRON	38%	39%	FER
ZINC	16%	22%	ZINC

*Approximately half of the sugars occur naturally in the raisins.
Environ la moitié des sucres se retrouvent à l'état naturel dans les fruits.

Canadian Diabetes Association Food Choice Values
40 g (175 mL, ¾ cup) cereal Système des choix d'aliments de l'Association canadienne du diabète 40 g (175 mL, ¾ tasse)
cereale = 1 ■ + ¼ ▲ + ½ ✹ choices/choix

INGREDIENTS / INGRÉDIENTS

WHOLE WHEAT, RAISINS (COATED WITH SUGAR, HYDROGENATED VEGETABLE OIL), WHEAT BRAN, SUGAR, GLUCOSE-FRUCTOSE, SALT, MALT (CORN FLOUR, MALTED BARLEY), VITAMINS (THIAMIN HYDROCHLORIDE, PYRIDOXINE HYDROCHLORIDE, FOLIC ACID, d-CALCIUM PANTOTHENATE), MINERALS (IRON, ZINC OXIDE).

BLÉ ENTIER, RAISINS SECS (ENROBÉS DE SUCRE, D'HUILE VÉGÉTALE HYDROGÉNÉE), SON DE BLÉ, SUCRE, GLUCOSE-FRUCTOSE, SEL, MALT (FARINE DE MAÏS, ORGE MALTÉ), VITAMINES (CHLORHYDRATE DE THIAMINE, CHLORHYDRATE DE PYRIDOXINE, ACIDE FOLIQUE, PANTOTHÉNATE DE d-CALCIUM), MINÉRAUX (FER, OXYDE DE ZINC).

Made by / Produit par
KELLOGG CANADA INC.
ETOBICOKE, ONTARIO
CANADA M9W 5P2
*Registered trademark of /
*Marque déposée de
KELLOGG CANADA INC. © 1994

00094

WHAT YOU WILL FIND ON A LABEL:

Nutrition Claims

- in Canada, it is optional for a company to decide to use claims,
- when claims appear on a label, they must follow government laws

Nutrition Information

- gives detailed nutrition facts about the product, including serving size and core list
- does not have to appear by law on food products in Canada
- refers to the food as packaged, so if you add milk, eggs or other food, the nutritional content of the food you eat can be very different

Serving Size

- the amount of food for which the information is given
- check the serving size: the serving size on the label may not be the same as the serving size you would actually eat (for example, the serving size of cereal may be ¾ cup, much smaller than your regular serving

Core List

- the energy (in Calories and kilojoules), grams of protein, fat and carbohydrate for each serving
- some products break down fat into monounsaturates, polyunsaturates, saturates, and cholesterol (to find out what these mean, look at the Fats & Oils section)
- carbohydrates may include the amount of sugars, starch and fibre, or may list these items separately

Sodium and Potassium (in milligrams)

Vitamins and Minerals (as percent of your recommended daily intake)

Canadian Diabetes Association Food Choice Values and Symbols

- the Values and Symbols are tools to help you fit the food into your meal plan, they are not an endorsement by CDA
- it is up to the food company to decide if they want their foods analyzed and assigned symbols
- when they are on a label, they have been assigned by a dietitian working for CDA, so you can be sure the information is correct

Ingredients

- must be found on all food labels by law
- ingredients are listed in decreasing order by weight, so what you see first is what you get the most of

TABLE B-4

Canadian Exchange System: Starch Foods

1 starch choice = 15 g carbohydrate (starch), 2 g protein, 290 kJ (68 kcal)

Food	Measure	Mass (Weight)
Breads		
Bagels	½	30 g
Bread crumbs	50 mL (¼ c)	30 g
Bread cubes	250 mL (1 c)	30 g
Bread sticks	2	20 g
Brewis, cooked	50 mL (¼ c)	45 g
Chapati	1	20 g
Cookies, plain	2	20 g
English muffins, crumpets	½	30 g
Flour	40 mL (2½ tbs)	20 g
Hamburger buns	½	30 g
Hot dog buns	½	30 g
Kaiser rolls	½	30 g
Matzo, 15 cm	1	20 g
Melba toast, rectangular	4	15 g
Melba toast, rounds	7	15 g
Pita, 20 cm (8") diameter	¼	30 g
Pita, 15 cm (6") diameter	½	30 g
Plain rolls	1 small	30 g
Pretzels	7	20 g
Raisin bread	1 slice	30 g
Rice cakes	2	30 g
Roti	1	20 g
Rusks	2	20 g
Rye, coarse or pumpernickel	½ slice	30 g
Soda crackers	6	20 g
Tortillas, corn (taco shell)	1	30 g
Tortilla, flour	1	30 g
White (French and Italian)	1 slice	25 g
Whole-wheat, cracked-wheat, rye, white enriched	1 slice	30 g
Cereals		
Bran flakes, 100% bran	125 mL (½ c)	30 g
Cooked cereals, cooked	125 mL (½ c)	125 g
Dry	30 mL (2 tbs)	20 g
Cornmeal, cooked	125 mL (½ c)	125 g
Dry	30 mL (2 tbs)	20 g
Ready-to-eat unsweetened cereals	125 mL (½ c)	20 g
Shredded wheat biscuits, rectangular or round	1	20 g
Shredded wheat, bite size	125 mL (½ c)	20 g
Wheat germ	75 mL (⅓ c)	30 g
Cornflakes	175 mL (⅔ c)	20 g
Rice Krispies	175 mL (⅔ c)	20 g
Cheerios	200 mL (¾ c)	20 g
Muffets	1	20 g
Puffed rice	300 mL (1¼ c)	15 g
Puffed wheat	425 mL (1⅔ c)	20 g

(continued on next page)

TABLE B-4

Canadian Exchange System: Starch Foods continued

1 starch choice = 15 g carbohydrate (starch), 2 g protein, 290 kJ (68 kcal)

Food	Measure	Mass (Weight)
Grains		
Barley, cooked	125 mL (½ c)	120 g
Dry	30 mL (2 tbs)	20 g
Bulgur, kasha, cooked, moist	125 mL (½ c)	70 g
Cooked, crumbly	75 mL (1/3 c)	40 g
Dry	30 mL (2 tbs)	20 g
Couscous, cooked moist	125 mL (½ c)	70 g
Dry	30 mL (tbs)	20 g
Quinoa, cooked moist	125 mL (½ c)	70 g
Dry	30 mL (2 tbs)	20 g
Rice, cooked, brown & white (short & long grain)	125 mL (½ c)	70 g
Rice, cooked, wild	75 mL (⅓ c)	70 g
Tapioca, pearl and granulated, quick cooking, dry	30 mL (2 tbs)	15 g
Pastas		
Macaroni, cooked	125 mL (½ c)	70 g
Noodles, cooked	125 mL (½ c)	80 g
Spaghetti, cooked	125 mL (½ c)	70 g
Starchy Vegetables		
Beans and peas, dried, cooked	125 mL (½ c)	80 g
Breadfruit	1 slice	75 g
Corn, canned, whole kernel	125 mL (½ c)	85 g
Corn on the cob	½ medium cob	140 g
Cornstarch	30 mL (2 tbs)	15 g
Plantains	⅓ small	50 g
Popcorn, air-popped, unbuttered	750 mL (3 c)	20 g
Potatoes, whole (with or without skin)	½ medium	95 g
Yams, sweet potatoes, (with or without skin)	½	75 g

Food	Exchanges per serving	Measure	Mass (Weight)
Note: Food items found in this category provide more than 1 starch exchange:			
Bran flakes	1 starch + ½ sugar	150 mL (⅔ c)	24 g
Cheese puffs	1 starch + 2 fats	27 chips	30 g
Cheese twists	1 starch + 1½ fats	30 chips	30 g
Corn, canned creamed	1 starch + 1½ fruits and vegetables	12 mL (½ c)	113 g
Corn chips	1 starch + 2 fats	30 chips	30 g
Croissant, small	1 starch + 1½ fats	1 small	35 g
Large	1 starch + 1½ fats	½ large	30 g
Pancakes, homemade using 50 mL (¼ c) batter (6" diameter)	1½ starches + fat	1 medium	50 g
Potatoes, french fried (homemade or frozen)	1 starch + 1 fat	10 regular size	35 g
Potato chips	1 starch + 2 fats	15 chips	30 g
Soup, canned,* (prepared with equal volume of water)	1 starch	250 mL (1 c)	260 g
Tea biscuit	1 starch + 2 fats	1	30 g
Tortilla chips (nachos)	1 starch + 1½ fats	13 chips	20 g
Waffles, packaged	1 starch + 1 fat	1	35 g

*Soup can vary according to brand and type. Check the label for Food Choice Values and Symbols or the core nutrient listing.

TABLE B-5

Canadian Exchange System: Fruits and Vegetables

1 fruits and vegetables choice = 10 g carbohydrate, 1 g protein, 190 kJ (44 kcal)

Food	Measure	Mass (Weight)
Fruits (fresh, frozen, without sugar, canned in water)		
Apples, raw (with or without skin)	½ medium	75 g
Sauce unsweetened	125 mL (½ c)	120 g
Sweetened	see *Combined Food Choices*, Table B-12	
Apple butter	20 mL (4 tsp)	20 g
Apricots, raw	2 medium	115 g
Canned, in water	4 halves, plus 30 mL (2 tbs) liquid	110 g
Bake-apples (cloudberries), raw	125 mL (½ c)	120 g
Bananas, with peel	½ small	75 g
Peeled	½ small	50 g
Berries (blackberries, blueberries, boysenberries, huckleberries, loganberries, raspberries)		
Raw	125 mL (½ c)	70 g
Canned, in water	125 mL (½ c), plus 30 mL (2 tbs) liquid	100 g
Cantaloupe, wedge with rind	¼	240 g
Cubed or diced	250 mL (1 c)	160 g
Cherries, raw, with pits	10	75 g
Raw, without pits	10	70 g
Canned, in water, with pits	75 mL (⅓ c), plus 30 mL (2 tbs) liquid	90 g
Canned, in water, without pits	75 mL (⅓ c), plus 30 mL (2 tbs) liquid	85 g
Crabapples, raw	1 small	55 g
Cranberries, raw	250 mL (1 c)	100 g
Figs, raw	1 medium	50 g
Canned, in water	3 medium, plus 30 mL (2 tbs) liquid	100 g
Foxberries, raw	250 mL (1 c)	100 g
Fruit cocktail, canned, in water	125 mL (½ c), plus 30 mL (2 tbs) liquid	120 g
Fruit, mixed, cut-up	125 mL (½ c)	120 g
Gooseberries, raw	250 mL (1 c)	150 g
Canned, in water	250 mL (1 c), plus 30 mL (2 tbs) liquid	230 g
Grapefruit, raw, with rind	½ small	185 g
Raw, sectioned	125 mL (½ c)	100 g
Canned, in water	125 mL (½ c), plus 30 mL (2 tbs) liquid	120 g
Grapes, raw, slip skin	125 mL (½ c)	75 g
Raw, seedless	125 mL (½ c)	75 g
Canned, in water	75 mL (⅓ c), plus 30 mL (2 tbs) liquid	115 g
Guavas, raw	½	50 g
Honeydew melon, raw, with rind	½	225 g
Cubed or diced	250 mL (1 c)	170 g
Kiwis, raw, with skin	2	155 g
Kumquats, raw	3	60 g
Loquats, raw	8	130 g
Lychee fruit, raw	8	120 g
Mandarin oranges, raw, with rind	1	135 g
Raw, sectioned	125 mL (½ c)	100 g
Canned, in water	125 mL (½ c), plus 30 mL (2 tbs) liquid	100 g
Mangoes, raw, without skin and seed	⅓	65 g

(continued on next page)

Food	Measure	Mass (Weight)
Diced	75 mL (⅓ c)	65 g
Nectarines	½ medium	75 g
Oranges, raw, with rind	1 small	130 g
Raw, sectioned	125 mL (½ c)	95 g
Papayas, raw, with skin and seeds	¼ medium	150 g
Raw, without skin and seeds	¼ medium	100 g
Cubed or diced	125 mL (½ c)	100 g
Peaches, raw, with seed and skin	1 large	100 g
Raw, sliced or diced	125 mL (½ c)	100 g
Canned in water, halves or slices	125 mL (½ c), plus 30 mL (2 tbs) liquid	120 g
Pears, raw, with skin and core	½	90 g
Raw, without skin and core	½	85 g
Canned, in water, halves	1 half plus 30 mL (2 tbs) liquid	90 g
Persimmons, raw, native	1	30 g
Raw, Japanese	¼	50 g
Pineapple, raw	1 slice	75 g
Raw, diced	125 mL (½ c)	75 g
Canned, in juice, diced	75 mL (⅓ c), plus 15 mL (1 tbs) liquid	55 g
Canned, in juice, sliced	1 slice, plus 15 mL (1 tbs) liquid	55 g
Canned, in water, diced	125 mL (½ c), plus 30 mL (2 tbs) liquid	100 g
Canned, in water, sliced	2 slices, plus 15 mL (1 tbs) liquid	100 g
Plums, raw	2 small	60 g
Damson	6	65 g
Japanese	1	70 g
Canned, in apple juice	2, plus 30 mL (2 tbs) liquid	70 g
Canned, in water	3, plus 30 mL (2 tbs) liquid	100 g
Pomegranates, raw	½	140 g
Strawberries, raw	250 mL (1 c)	150 g
Frozen/canned, in water	250 mL (1 c), plus 30 mL (2 tbs) liquid	240 g
Rhubarb	250 mL (1 c)	150 g
Tangelos, raw	1	205 g
Tangerines, raw	1 medium	115 g
Raw, sectioned	125 mL (½ c)	100 g
Watermelon, raw, with rind	1 wedge	310 g
Cubed or diced	250 mL (1 c)	160 g
Dried Fruit		
Apples	5 pieces	15 g
Apricots	4 halves	15 g
Banana flakes	30 mL (2 tbs)	15 g
Currants	30 mL (2 tbs)	15 g
Dates, without pits	2	15 g
Peaches	½	15 g
Pears	½	15 g
Prunes, raw, with pits	2	15 g
Raw, without pits	2	10 g
Stewed, no liquid	2	20 g
Stewed, with liquid	2, plus 15 mL (1 tbs) liquid	35 g
Raisins	30 mL (2 tbs)	15 g
Juices (no sugar added or unsweetened)		
Apricot, grape, guava, mango, prune	50 mL (¼ c)	55 g
Apple, carrot, papaya, pear, pineapple, pomegranate	75 mL (⅓ c)	80 g
Cranberry (see *Sugars*, Table B-8)		
Clamato (see *Sugars*, Table B-8)		

(continued on next page)

TABLE B-5

Canadian Exchange System: Fruits and Vegetables continued

Food	Measure	Mass (Weight)
Grapefruit, loganberry, orange, raspberry, tangelo, tangerine	125 mL (½ c)	130 g
Tomato, tomato-based mixed vegetables	250 mL (1 c)	255 g
Vegetables (fresh, frozen, or canned)		
Artichokes, French, globe	2 small	50 g
Beets, diced or sliced	125 mL (½ c)	85 g
Carrots, diced, cooked or uncooked	125 mL (½ c)	75 g
Chestnuts, fresh	5	20 g
Parsnips, mashed	125 mL (½ c)	80 g
Peas, fresh or frozen	125 mL (½ c)	80 g
Canned	75 mL (⅓ c)	55 g
Pumpkin, mashed	125 mL (½ c)	45 g
Rutabagas, mashed	125 mL (½ c)	85 g
Sauerkraut	250 mL (1 c)	235 g
Snow peas	250 mL (1 c)	135 g
Squash, yellow or winter, mashed	125 mL (½ c)	115 g
Succotash	75 mL (⅓ c)	55 g
Tomatoes, canned	250 mL (1 c)	240 g
Tomato paste	50 mL (¼ c)	55 g
Tomato sauce*	75 mL (⅓ c)	100 g
Turnips, mashed	125 mL (½ c)	115 g
Vegetables, mixed	125 mL (½ c)	90 g
Water chestnuts	8 medium	50 g

*Tomato sauce varies according to brand name. Check the label or discuss with your dietitian.

TABLE B-6

Canadian Exchange System: Milk

Type of Milk	Carbohydrate (g)	Protein (g)	Fat (g)	Energy
Nonfat (0%)	6	4	0	170 kJ (40 kcal)
1%	6	4	1	206 kJ (49 kcal)
2%	6	4	2	244 kJ (58 kcal)
Whole (4%)	6	4	4	319 kJ (76 kcal)

Food	Measure	Mass (Weight)
Buttermilk (higher in salt)	125 mL (½ c)	125 g
Evaporated milk	50 mL (¼ c)	50 g
Milk	125 mL (½ c)	125 g
Powdered milk, regular	30 mL (2 tbs)	15 g
Instant	50 mL (¼ c)	15 g
Yogurt, plain	125 mL (½ c)	125 g

Food	Exchanges per Serving	Measure	Mass (Weight)
Note: Food items found in this category provide more than 1 milk exchange:			
Chocolate milk, 2%	2 milks 2% + 1 sugar	250 mL (1 c)	300 g
Frozen yogurt	1 milk + 1 sugar	125 mL (½ c)	125 g
Milkshake	1 milk + 3 sugars + ½ protein	250 mL (1 c)	300 g

TABLE B-7

Canadian Exchange System: Sugars

1 sugar choice = 10 g carbohydrate (sugar), 167 kJ (40 kcal)

Food	Measure	Mass (Weight)
Beverages		
Condensed milk	15 mL (1 tbs)	
Flavoured fruit crystals*	75 mL (⅓ c)	
Iced tea mixes*	75 mL (⅓ c)	
Regular soft drinks	125 mL (½ c)	
Sweet drink mixes*	75 mL (⅓ c)	
Tonic water	125 mL (½ c)	

*These beverages have been made with water.

Food	Measure	Mass (Weight)
Miscellaneous		
Bubble gum (large square)	1 piece	5 g
Cranberry cocktail	75 mL (⅓ c)	80 g
Cranberry cocktail, light	350 mL (1⅓ c)	260 g
Cranberry sauce	30 mL (2 tbs)	
Hard candy mints	2	5 g
Honey, molasses, corn & cane syrup	10 mL (2 tsp)	15 g
Jelly bean	4	10 g
Licorice	1 short stick	10 g
Marshmallows	2 large	15 g
Popsicle	1 stick (½ popsicle)	
Powdered gelatin mix (Jello®) (reconstituted)	50 mL (¼ c)	
Regular jam, jelly, marmalade	15 mL (1 tbs)	
Sugar, white, brown, icing, maple	10 mL (2 tsp)	10 g
Sweet pickles	2 small	100 g
Sweet relish	30 mL (2 tbs)	

Food	Exchanges per Serving	Measures	Mass (Weight)
The following food items provide more than 1 sugar exchange:			
Aero® bar	2½ sugars + 2½ fats	1 bar	43 g
Brownie	1 sugar + 1 fat	1	20 g
Clamato juice	1½ sugars	175 mL (⅔ c)	
Fruit salad, light syrup	1 sugar + 1 fruits & vegetables	125 mL (½ c)	130 g
Sherbet	3 sugars + ½ fat	125 mL (½ c)	95 g
Smarties®	4½ sugars + 2 fats	1 box	60 g

TABLE B-8

Canadian Exchange System: Protein Foods

1 protein choice = 7 g protein, 3 g fat, 230 kJ (55 kcal)

Food	Measure	Mass (Weight)
Cheese		
Low-fat cheese, about 7% milk fat	1 slice	30 g
Cottage cheese, 2% milkfat or less	50 mL (¼ c)	55 g
Ricotta, about 7% milkfat	50 mL (¼ c)	60 g
Fish		
Anchovies (see *Extras*, Table B-11)		
Canned, drained (e.g., mackerel, salmon, tuna packed in water)	(⅓ of 6.5 oz can)	30 g
Cod tongues, cheeks	75 mL (⅓ c)	50 g
Fillet or steak (e.g., Boston blue, cod, flounder, haddock, halibut, mackerel, orange roughy, perch, pickerel, pike, salmon, shad, snapper, sole, swordfish, trout, tuna, whitefish)	1 piece	30 g
Herring	⅓ fish	30 g
Sardines, smelts	2 medium or 3 small	30 g
Squid, octopus	50 mL (¼ c)	40 g
Shellfish		
Clams, mussels, oysters, scallops, snails	3 medium	30 g
Crab, lobster, flaked	50 mL (¼ c)	30 g
Shrimp, fresh	5 large	30 g
Frozen	10 medium	30 g
Canned	18 small	30 g
Dry pack	50 mL (¼ c)	30 g
Meat and Poultry (e.g., beef, chicken, goat, ham, lamb, pork, turkey, veal, wild game)		
Back, peameal bacon	3 slices, thin	30 g
Chop	½ chop, with bone	40 g
Minced or ground, lean or extra-lean	30 mL (2 tbs)	30 g
Sliced, lean	1 slice	30 g
Steak, lean	1 piece	30 g
Organ Meats		
Hearts, liver	1 slice	30 g
Kidneys, sweetbreads, chopped	50 mL (¼ c)	30 g
Tongue	1 slice	30 g
Tripe	5 pieces	60 g
Soyabean		
Bean curd or tofu	½ block	70 g
Eggs		
In shell, raw or cooked	1 medium	50 g
Without shell, cooked or poached in water	1 medium	45 g
Scrambled	50 mL (¼ c)	55 g

(continued on next page)

TABLE B-8

Canadian Exchange System: Protein Foods continued

1 protein choice = 7 g protein, 3 g fat, 230 kJ (55 kcal)

Food	Exchanges per Serving	Measures	Mass (Weight)
Note: The following choices provide more than 1 protein exchange:			
Cheese			
Cheeses	1 protein + 1 fat	1 piece	25 g
Cheese, coarsely grated (e.g., cheddar)	1 protein + 1 fat	50 mL (¼ c)	25 g
Cheese, dry, finely grated (e.g., parmesan)	1 protein + 1 fat	45 mL	15 g
Cheese, ricotta, high fat	1 protein + 1 fat	50 mL (¼ c)	55 g
Fish			
Eel	1 protein + 1 fat	1 slice	50 g
Meat			
Bologna	1 protein + 1 fat	1 slice	20 g
Canned lunch meats	1 protein + 1 fat	1 slice	20 g
Corned beef, canned	1 protein + 1 fat	1 slice	25 g
Corned beef, fresh	1 protein + 1 fat	1 slice	25 g
Ground beef, medium-fat	1 protein + 1 fat	30 mL (2 tbs)	25 g
Meat spreads, canned	1 protein + 1 fat	45 mL	35 g
Mutton chop	1 protein + 1 fat	½ chop, with bone	35 g
Paté (see *Fats and Oils,* Table B-10)			
Sausages, garlic, Polish or knockwurst	1 protein + 1 fat	1 slice	50 g
Sausages, pork, links	1 protein + 1 fat	1 link	25 g
Spareribs or shortribs, with bone	1 protein + 1 fat	1 large	65 g
Stewing beef	1 protein + 1 fat	1 cube	25 g
Summer sausage or salami	1 protein + 1 fat	1 slice	40 g
Weiners, hot dogs	1 protein + 1 fat	½ medium	25 g
Miscellaneous			
Blood pudding	1 protein + 1 fat	1 slice	25 g
Peanut butter	1 protein + 1 fat	15 mL (1 tbs)	15 g

TABLE B-9

Canadian Exchange System: Fats and Oils

1 fat choice = 5 g fat, 190 kJ (45 kcal)

Food	Measure	Mass (Weight)	Food	Measure	Mass (Weight)
Avocado*	⅛	30 g	Nuts (continued):		
Bacon, side, crisp*	1 slice	5 g	Sesame seeds	15 mL (1 tbs)	10 g
Butter*	5 mL (1 tsp)	5 g	Sunflower seeds		
Cheese spread	15 mL (1 tbs)	15 g	Shelled	15 mL (1 tbs)	10 g
Coconut, fresh*	45 mL (3 tbs)	15 g	In shell	45 mL (3 tbs)	15 g
Coconut, dried*	15 mL (1 tbs)	10 g	Walnuts	4 halves	10 g
Cream, Half and half			Oil, cooking and salad	5 mL (1 tsp)	5 g
(cereal), 10%*	30 mL (2 tbs)	30 g	Olives, green	10	45 g
Light (coffee), 20%*	15 mL (1 tbs)	15 g	Ripe black	7	57 g
Whipping, 32 to 37%*	15 mL (1 tbs)	15 g	Pâté, liverwurst,	15 mL (1 tbs)	15 g
Cream cheese*	15 mL (1 tbs)	15 g	meat spreads		
Gravy*	30 mL (2 tbs)	30 g	Salad dressing: blue,	10 mL (2 tsp)	10 g
Lard*	5 mL (1 tsp)	5 g	French, Italian,		
Margarine	5 mL (1 tsp)	5 g	mayonnaise,		
Nuts, shelled:			Thousand Island	5 mL (1 tsp)	5 g
Almonds	8	5 g	Salad dressing,	30 mL (2 tbs)	30 g
Brazil nuts	2	10 g	low-calorie		
Cashews	5	10 g	Salt pork, raw	5 mL (1 tsp)	5 g
Filberts, hazelnuts	5	10 g	or cooked*		
Macadamia	3	5 g	Sesame oil	5 mL (1 tsp)	5 g
Peanuts	10	10g	Sour cream		
Pecans	5 halves	5 g	12% milkfat	30 mL (2 tbs)	30 g
Pignolias, pine nuts	25 mL (5 tsp)	10 g	7% milkfat	60 mL (4 tbs)	60 g
Pistachios, shelled	20	10 g	Shortening*	5 mL (1 tsp)	5 g
Pistachios, in shell	20	20 g			
Pumpkin and squash seeds	20 mL (4 tsp)	10 g			

*These items contain higher amounts of saturated fat.

B

TABLE B-10

Canadian Exchange System: Extras

Extras have no more than 2.5 g carbohydrate, 60 kJ (14 kcal)

Vegetables 125 mL (½ c)
Artichokes
Asparagus
Bamboo shoots
Bean sprouts, mung or soya
Beans, string, green, or yellow
Bitter melon (balsam pear)
Bok choy
Broccoli
Brussels sprouts
Cabbage
Cauliflower
Celery
Chard
Cucumbers
Eggplant
Endive
Fiddleheads
Greens: beet, collard, dandelion, mustard, turnip, etc.
Kale
Kohlrabi
Leeks
Lettuce
Mushrooms
Okra
Onions, green or mature
Parsley
Peppers, green, yellow or red
Radishes
Rapini
Rhubarb
Sauerkraut
Shallots
Spinach
Sprouts: alfalfa, radish, etc.
Tomato wedges
Watercress
Zucchini

Free Foods (may be used without measuring)

Artificial sweetener, such as cyclamate or aspartame	Lime juice or lime wedges
	Marjoram, cinnamon, etc.
Baking powder, baking soda	Mineral water
Bouillon from cube, powder, or liquid	Mustard
	Parsley
Bouillon or clear broth	Pimentos
Chowchow, unsweetened	Salt, pepper, thyme
Coffee, clear	Soda water, club soda
Consommé	Soya sauce
Dulse	Sugar-free Crystal Drink
Flavorings and extracts	Sugar-free Jelly Powder
Garlic	Sugar-free soft drinks
Gelatin, unsweetened	Tea, clear
Ginger root	Vinegar
Herbal teas, unsweetened	Water
Horseradish, uncreamed	Worcestershire sauce
Lemon juice or lemon wedges	

Condiments

Food	Measure
Anchovies	2 fillets
Barbecue sauce	15 mL (1 tbs)
Bran, natural	30 mL (2 tbs)
Brewer's yeast	5 mL (1 tsp)
Carob powder	5 mL (1 tsp)
Catsup	5 mL (1 tsp)
Chili sauce	5 mL (1 tsp)
Cocoa powder	5 mL (1 tsp)
Cranberry sauce, unsweetened	15 mL (1 tbs)
Dietetic fruit spreads	5 mL (1 tsp)
Maraschino cherries	1
Nondairy coffee whitener	5 mL (1 tsp)
Nuts, chopped pieces	5 mL (1 tsp)
Pickles	
Unsweetened dill	2
Sour mixed	11
Sugar substitutes, granular	5 mL (1 tsp)
Whipped toppings	15 mL (1 tbs)

TABLE B-11

Canadian Exchange System: Combined Food Choices

Food	Exchanges per Serving	Measure	Mass (Weight)
Angel food cake	½ starch + 2½ sugars	¹⁄₁₂ cake	50 g
Apple crisp	½ starch + 1½ fruits & vegetables		
	1 + sugar + 1–2 fats	125 mL (½ c)	
Applesauce, sweetened	1 fruits & vegetables + 1 sugar	125 mL (½ c)	
Beans and pork in	1 starch + ½ fruits & vegetables		
tomato sauce	+ ½ sugar + 1 protein	125 mL (½ c)	135 g
Beef burrito	2 starches + 3 proteins + 3 fats		110 g
Brownie	1 sugar + 1 fat	1	20 g
Cabbage rolls*	1 starch + 2 proteins	3	310 g
Caesar salad	2–4 fats	20 mL dressing (4 tsp)	
Cheesecake	½ starch + 2 sugars + ½ protein + 5 fats	1 piece	80 g
Chicken fingers	1 starch + 2 proteins + 2 fats	6 small	100 g
Chicken and snow pea	2 starches + ½ fruits & vegetables		
Oriental	+ 3 proteins + 1 fat	500 mL (2 c)	
Chili	1½ starches + ½ fruits & vegetables		
	+ 3½ protein	300 mL (1¼ c)	325 g
Chips			
Potato chips	1 starch + 2 fats	15 chips	30 g
Corn chips	1 starch + 2 fats	30 chips	30 g
Tortilla chips	1 starch + 1½ fats	13 chips	
Cheese twist	1 starch + 1½ fats	30 chips	30 g
Chocolate bar			
Aero®	2½ sugars + 2½ fats	bar	43 g
Smarties®	4½ sugars + 2 fats	package	60 g
Chocolate cake (without icing)	1 starch + 2 sugars + 3 fats	¹⁄₁₀ of a 8" pan	
Chocolate devil's food cake	2 starches + 2 sugars	¹⁄₁₂ of a	
(without icing)	+ 3 fats	9" pan	
Chocolate milk	2 milks 2% + 1 sugar	250 mL (1 c)	300 g
Clubhouse (triple-decker)	3 starches + 3 proteins		
sandwich	+ 4 fats		
Cookies			
Chocolate chip	½ starch + ½ sugar + 1½ fats	2	22 g
Oatmeal	1 starch + 1 sugar + 1 fat	2	40 g
Donut (chocolate glazed)	1 starch + 1½ sugars + 2 fats	1	65 g
Egg roll	1 starch + ½ protein + 1 fat		75 g
Four bean salad	1 starch + ½ protein + 1 fat	125 mL (½ c)	
French toast	1 starch + ½ protein + 2 fats	1 slice	65 g
Fruit in heavy syrup	1 fruits & vegetables + 1½ sugars	125 mL (½ c)	
Granola bar	½ starch + 1 sugar + 1–2 fats		30 g
Granola cereal	1 starch + 1 sugar + 2 fats	125 mL (½ c)	45 g
Hamburger	2 starches + 3 proteins + 2 fats	junior size	
Ice cream and cone, plain flavour			
Ice cream	½ milk + 2–3 sugars + 1–2 fats		100 g
Cone	½ sugar		4 g
Lasagna			
Regular cheese	1 starch + 1 fruits & vegetables + 3 proteins + 2 fats	3" × 4" piece	
Low-fat cheese	1 starch + 1 fruits & vegetables + 3 proteins	3" × 4" piece	

* If eaten with sauce, add ½ fruits & vegetables exchange.

(continued on next page)

TABLE B-11

Canadian Exchange System: Combined Food Choices continued

Food	Exchanges per Serving	Measure	Mass (Weight)
Legumes			
Dried beans (kidney, navy, pinto, fava, chick peas)	2 starches + 1 protein	250 mL (1 c)	180 g
Dried peas	2 starches + 1 protein	250 mL (1 c)	210 g
Lentils	2 starches + 1 protein	250 mL (1 c)	210 g
Macaroni and cheese	2 starches + 2 proteins + 2 fats	250 mL (1 c)	210 g
Minestrone soup	1½ starches + ½ fruits & vegetables + ½ fat	250 mL (1 c)	
Muffin	1 starch + ½ sugar + 1 fat	1 small	45 g
Nuts (dry or roasted without any oil added)			
Almonds, dried sliced	½ protein + 2 fats	50 mL (¼ c)	22 g
Brazil nuts, dried unblanched	½ protein + 2½ fats	5 large	23 g
Cashew nuts, dry roasted	½ starch + ½ protein + 2 fats	50 mL (¼ c)	28 g
Filbert hazelnut, dry	½ protein + 3½ fats	50 mL (¼ c)	30 g
Macadamia nuts, dried	½ protein + 4 fats	50 mL (¼ c)	28 g
Peanuts, raw	1 protein + 2 fats	50 mL (¼ c)	30 g
Pecans, dry roasted	½ fruits & vegetables + 3 fats	50 mL (¼ c)	22 g
Pine nuts, pignolia dried	1 protein + 3 fats	50 mL (¼ c)	34 g
Pistachio nuts, dried	½ fruits & vegetables + ½ protein + 2 ½ fats	50 mL (¼ c)	27 g
Pumpkin seeds, roasted	2 proteins + 2½ fats	50 mL (¼ c)	47 g
Sesame seeds, whole dried	½ fruits & vegetables + ½ protein + 2½ fats	50 mL (¼ c)	30 g
Sunflower kernel, dried	½ protein + 1½ fats	50 mL (¼ c)	17 g
Walnuts, dried chopped	½ protein + 3 fats	50 mL (¼ c)	26 g
Perogies	2 starches + 1 protein + 1 fat	3	
Pie, fruit	1 starch + 1 fruits & vegetables + 2 sugars + 3 fats	1 piece	120 g
Pizza, cheese	1 starch + 1 protein + 1 fat	1 slice (⅛ of a 12")	50 g
Pork stir-fry	½ to 1 fruits & vegetables + 3 proteins	200 mL (¾ c)	
Potato salad	1 starch + 1 fat	125 mL (½ c)	130 g
Potatoes, scalloped	2 starches + 1 milk + 1–2 fats	200 mL (¾ c)	210 g
Pudding, bread or rice	1 starch + 1 sugar + 1 fat	125 mL (½ c)	
Pudding, vanilla	1 milk + 2 sugars	125 mL (½ c)	
Raisin bran cereal	1 starch + ½ fruits & vegetables + ½ sugar	175 mL (⅔ c)	40 g
Rice krispie squares	½ starch + 1½ sugars + ½ fat	1 square	30 g
Shepherd's pie	2 starches + 1 fruits & vegetables + 3 proteins	325 mL (1⅓ c)	
Sherbet, orange	3 sugars + ½ fat	125 mL (½ c)	
Spaghetti and meat sauce	2 starches + 1 fruits & vegetables + 2 proteins + 3 fats	250 mL (1 c)	
Stew	2 starches + 2 fruits & vegetables + 3 proteins + ½ fat	200 mL (¾ c)	
Sundae	4 sugars + 3 fats	125 mL (½ c)	
Tuna casserole	1 starch + 2 proteins + ½ fat	125 mL (½ c)	
Yogurt, fruit bottom	1 fruits & vegetables + 1 milk + 1 sugar	125 mL (½ c)	125 g
Yogurt, frozen	1 milk + 1 sugar	125 mL (½ c)	125 g

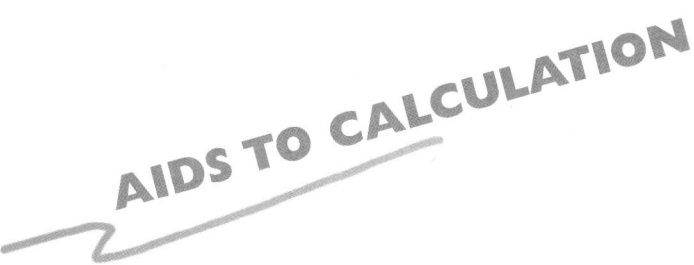

AIDS TO CALCULATION

C

CONTENTS

Mathematical problems have been worked out for you as examples at appropriate places in the text. This appendix aims to help with the use of the metric system and with those problems not fully explained elsewhere.

CONVERSION FACTORS

Conversion factors are useful mathematical tools in everyday calculations, like the ones encountered in the study of nutrition. A conversion factor is a fraction in which the numerator (top) and the denominator (bottom) express the same quantity in different units. For example, 2.2 pounds (lb) and 1 kilogram (kg) are equivalent; they express the same weight. The conversion factor used to change pounds to kilograms or vice versa is:

$$\frac{2.2 \text{ lb}}{1 \text{ kg}} \quad \text{or} \quad \frac{1 \text{ kg}}{2.2 \text{ lb}}$$

Because both factors equal 1, measurements can be multiplied by the factor without changing the value of the measurement. Thus the units can be changed.

The correct factor to use in a problem is the one with the unit you are seeking in the numerator (top) of the fraction. Following are two examples of problems commonly encountered in nutrition study; they illustrate the usefulness of conversion factors.

EXAMPLE 1

Convert the weight of 130 pounds to kilograms.

1. Choose the conversion factor in which the unit you are seeking is on top:

$$\frac{1 \text{ kg}}{2.2 \text{ lb}}$$

2. Multiply 130 pounds by the factor:

$$130 \text{ lb} \times \frac{1 \text{ kg}}{2.2 \text{ lb}} = \frac{130 \text{ kg}}{2.2}$$

= 59 kg (rounded off to the nearest whole number).

EXAMPLE 2

How many grams (g) of saturated fat are contained in a 3-ounce (oz) hamburger?

1. Appendix A shows that a 4-ounce hamburger contains 7 grams of saturated fat. You are seeking grams of saturated fat; therefore, the conversion factor is:

$$\frac{7 \text{ g saturated fat}}{4 \text{ oz hamburger}}$$

2. Multiply 3 ounces of hamburger by the conversion factor:

$$3 \text{ oz hamburger} \times \frac{7 \text{ g saturated fat}}{4 \text{ oz hamburger}} = \frac{3 \times 7}{4} = \frac{21}{4}$$

= 5 g saturated fat (rounded off to the nearest whole number)

C-1

Energy Units

1 cal[a] = 4.2 kJ

1 MJ = 240 cal

1 kJ = 0.24 cal

1 g carbohydrate = 4 cal = 17 kJ

1 g fat = 9 cal = 37 kJ

1 g protein = 4 cal = 17 kJ

1 g alcohol = 7 cal = 29 kJ

PERCENTAGES

A percentage is a comparison between a number of items (perhaps your intake of energy) and a standard number (perhaps the number of calories recommended for your age and sex—your energy RDA). The standard number is the number you divide by. The answer you get after the division must be multiplied by 100 to be stated as a percentage (*percent* means "per 100").

EXAMPLE 3

What percentage of the RDA for energy is your energy intake?

1. Find your energy RDA (inside front cover). We'll use 2,100 calories to demonstrate.

2. Total your energy intake for a day—for example, 1,200 calories.

3. Divide your calorie intake by the RDA calories:

1,200 cal (your intake) ÷ 2,100 cal (RDA) = 0.571

4. Multiply your answer by 100 to state it as a percentage:

0.571 × 100 = 57.1 = 57% (rounded off to the nearest whole number)

In some problems in nutrition, the percentage may be more than 100. For example, suppose your daily intake of vitamin A is 3,200 RE and your RDA (male) is 1,000 RE. Your intake as a percentage of the RDA is more than 100 percent (that is, you consume more than 100 percent of your vitamin A RDA). The following calculations show your vitamin A intake as a percentage of the RDA:

3,200 ÷ 1,000 = 3.2

3.2 × 100 = 320% of RDA

EXAMPLE 4

Food labels express nutrients and energy contents of foods as percentages of the Daily Values. If a serving of a food contains 200 mg of calcium, for example, what percentage of the calcium Daily Value does the food provide?

---

[a]Note: Throughout this book and in the Appendixes, the term *calorie* is used to mean kilocalorie. Thus, when converting the calories of foods listed in Appendixes A or D to kilojoules, do not enlarge the calorie values—they are kilocalorie values.

1. Find the calcium Daily Value on the inside front cover, page c.

2. Divide the milligrams of calcium in the food by the Daily Value, standard.

$$\frac{200}{1,000} = 0.2$$

3. Multiply by 100.

0.2 × 100 = 20% of the Daily Value.

EXAMPLE 5

This example demonstrates how to calculate the percentage of fat in a day's meals.

1. Recall the general formula for finding percentages of calories from a nutrient

(one nutrient's calories ÷ total calories) × 100 = the percentage of calories from that nutrient

Say a day's meals provides 1,754 calories and 54 grams of fat. First, convert fat grams to fat calories:

54g × 9 cal per g = 486 cal from fat

Then apply the general formula for finding percentages of calories from fat:

(fat calories ÷ total calories) × 100 = percentage of calories from fat

(486 ÷ 1,754) × 100 = 27. 7 (28 percent, rounded)

RATIOS

A ratio is a comparison of two or three values in which one of the values is reduced to 1. A ratio compares identical units and so is expressed without units. For example, Table 8-7 in Chapter 8 compares the milligrams of potassium to the milligrams of sodium in selected foods.

EXAMPLE 6

Find the potassium-to-sodium ratio of your diet.

1. Using Appendix A and your diet record from the Do It section of Chapter 2, find how many milligrams of potassium and sodium you consumed. For this exercise, we assume 3,000 milligrams potassium and 2,500 milligrams sodium.

2. Divide the potassium milligrams by the sodium milligrams:

3,000 mg potassium ÷ 2,500 mg sodium = 1.2

3. The potassium-to-sodium ratio is usually expressed as correct to one decimal point: 1.2.

The potassium-to-sodium ratio of this diet is 1.2:1 (read as "one point two to one" or simply "one point two"). A ratio greater than 1 means that the first value (in this case, milligrams of potassium) is greater than the second (sodium). When the second value is larger, the ratio is less than 1.

WEIGHTS AND MEASURES

Length
1 inch (in) = 2.54 centimeters (cm)
1 foot (ft) = 30.48 centimeters
1 meter (m) = 39.37 inches

Temperature

Steam___	100° C	212° F___	Steam
Body temperature___	37° C	98.6° F___	Body temperature
Ice___	0° C	32° F___	Ice
Celsius[b]		Fahrenheit	

To convert Fahrenheit temperature (t_F) to Celsius:

$$t_C = \frac{5}{9}\ (t_F - 32)$$

To convert Celsius temperature (t_C) to Fahrenheit:

$$t_F = \frac{9}{5}\ t_C + 32$$

Volume
1 liter (l) = 1.06 quarts (qt) or 0.85 imperial quart
1 liter = 1,000 milliliters (ml)
1 milliliter = 0.034 fluid ounces
1 gallon = 3.79 liters
1 quart = 0.95 liter or 32 fluid ounces
1 cup (c) = 8 fluid ounces, or about 250 milliliters
1 tablespoon (tbs) = 15 milliliters
3 teaspoons (tsp) = 1 tablespoon
1 teaspoon (tsp) = about 5 g or 5 ml
16 tablespoons = 1 cup
4 cups = 1 quart

Weight
1 ounce (oz) = approximately 28 grams (g)
16 ounces = 1 pound (lb)
1 pound = 454 grams
1 kilogram (kg) = 1,000 grams or 2.2 pounds
1 gram = 1,000 milligrams (mg)
1 milligram = 1,000 micrograms (μg)

International Units (IU)
To convert IU to:

■ RE:[c] from animal sources, divide by 3.33; and from vegetables and fruits, divide by 10
■ μg vitamin D: divide by 40 or multiply by 0.025
■ mg α-TE:[d] divide by 1.5

Sodium
To convert milligrams of sodium to grams of salt:

$$mg\ sodium \div 400 = g\ of\ salt$$

The reverse is also true:

$$g\ salt \times 400 = mg\ sodium$$

C

---

[b]Also known as centigrade.

[c]Retinol equivalents (vitamin A).
[d]Alpha-tocopherol equivalents (vitamin E).

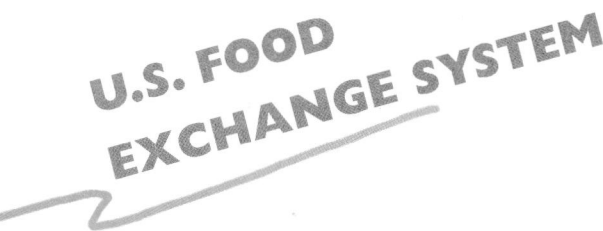

U.S. FOOD
EXCHANGE SYSTEM

D

CONTENTS

The U.S. food exchange system is intended to help people with diabetes control the levels of glucose and lipids in the blood by controlling the grams of carbohydrate and fat they consume. Other diet planners have found the system invaluable for achieving calorie control and moderation.

PLANNING A DIET

Unlike the Daily Food Guide of Chapter 2, which sorts foods primarily by their protein, vitamin, and mineral contents, the exchange system sorts foods into three main groups by their proportions of carbohydrate, fat, and protein. These three groups—the carbohydrate group, the fat group, and the meat and meat substitute group (protein)—are each subdivided into several exchange lists of foods (Table D-1, see page D-2).

PORTION SIZES All of the food portions in a given list provide approximately the same amounts of energy nutrients (carbohydrate, fat, and protein) and the same number of calories. Portion sizes are strictly defined so that every item on a given list provides roughly the same amount of energy. Any food on a list can then be exchanged, or traded, for any other food on that same list without affecting a plan's balance or total calories.

To apply the system successfully, users must become familiar with portion sizes. A convenient way to remember the portion sizes and energy values is to keep in mind a typical item from each list. Table D-1 includes some representa-

tive portion sizes; Figure D-1 shows the foods on each of the exchange lists and their accurate portion sizes.

THE FOODS ON THE LISTS Foods are not always on the exchange list where you might first expect them to be because they are grouped according to their energy-nutrient contents rather than by their source (such as milks), their outward appearance, or their vitamin and mineral contents. For example, cheeses are grouped with meats in the exchange system because, like meats, cheeses contribute energy from protein and fat but provide negligible carbohydrate. (In the food group plans presented earlier, cheeses are classed with milk because they are milk products with a similar calcium content.)

For similar reasons, starchy vegetables such as corn, green peas, and potatoes are listed on the starch list in the exchange system, rather than with the vegetables. Likewise, olives are not classed as a "fruit" as a botanist would claim; they are classified as a "fat" because their fat content makes them more similar to butter than to berries. Bacon is also on the fat list to remind users of its high fat content. These groupings permit you to see the characteristics of foods that are significant to energy intake.

Users of the exchange lists learn to view mixtures of foods, such as casseroles and soups, as combinations of foods from different exchange lists. They also learn to interpret food labels with the exchange system in mind. Knowing that foods on the starch list provide 15 grams of carbohydrate and those on the vegetable list provide 5, you can interpret the label of a

TABLE D-1

Exchange Groups and Lists

List	Portion Size	Carbohydrate (g)	Protein (g)	Fat (g)	Energy (cal)
Carbohydrate Group					
Starch	1 slice; ½ c	15	3	1 or less	80
Fruit	varies	15	—	—	60
Milk	1 c				
Skim		12	8	0–3	90
Low-fat		12	8	5	120
Whole		12	8	8	150
Other carbohydrates	varies	15	varies	varies	varies
Vegetable	½ c	5	2	—	25
Meat and Meat Substitute Group 1 oz					
Very Lean		—	7	0–1	35
Lean		—	7	3	55
Medium-fat		—	7	5	75
High-fat		—	7	8	100
Fat Group	1 tsp pure fat	—	—	5	45

lasagna dinner that lists 37 grams of carbohydrate as "2 starches" (mostly noodles) and "1 vegetable" (the sauce).

CONTROLLING ENERGY, FAT, AND SODIUM The exchange system helps people control their energy intakes by paying close attention to portion sizes. A portion of any food on a given list provides roughly the same amount of energy nutrients and total calories. The portion sizes have been adjusted so that all portions have the same energy value. For example, 17 grapes count as one fruit portion, as does ½ grapefruit. A whole grapefruit counts as two portions.

A *portion* in the exchange system is not the same as a *serving* in the Daily Food Guide, especially when it comes to meats. The exchange system lists meats and most cheeses in single ounces; that is , 1 *portion* (or *exchange*) of meat is 1 ounce, whereas one *serving* is 2 to 3 ounces. Calculating meat by the ounce encourages the planner to keep close track of the exact amounts eaten. This in turn helps control energy and fat intakes.

By allocating items like bacon and avocados to the fat list, the exchange system alerts consumers to foods that are unexpectedly high in fat. Even the starch list specifies which grain products contain added fat (such as biscuits, muffins, and waffles). In addition, the exchange system encourages users to think of nonfat milk as milk and of whole milk as milk with added fat, and to think of very lean meats as meats and of lean, medium-fat, and high-fat meats as meats

with added fat. To that end, foods on the milk and meat lists are separated into categories based on their fat contents.

Control of food energy and fat intake can be highly successful with the exchange system. Exchange plans do not, however, guarantee adequate intakes of vitamins and minerals. Food group plans work better from that standpoint because the food groupings are based on similarities in vitamin-mineral content. In the exchange system, for example, meats are grouped with cheeses, yet the meats are iron-rich and calcium-poor, whereas the cheeses are iron-poor and calcium-rich. To take advantage of the strengths of both food group plans and exchange patterns, and to compensate for their weaknesses, diet planners often combine these two diet-planning tools, as the following section shows.

People wishing to control the sodium in their diets can begin by eliminating any foods bearing this symbol [🖊] found on any exchange list. The symbol identifies each food that, in one exchange, provides 400 mg or more of sodium. Other foods may also contribute substantially to sodium, however (consult Chapter 8 for details).

COMBINING FOOD GROUP PLANS AND EXCHANGE LISTS

A diet planner may find that using a food group plan together with the exchange lists eases the task of choosing foods that will provide all the nutrients. The food group plan ensures that all classes of nutritious foods are included, thus

TABLE D-2

Diet Planning with the Exchange System Using the Daily Food Guide Pattern

Pattern from Daily Food Guide Plan	Selections Made Using the Exchange System	Energy Cost (cal)
Grains (breads and cereals)—6 to 11 servings	Starch list—select 9 exchanges	720
Vegetables—3 to 5 servings	Vegetable list—select 4 exchanges	100
Fruits—2 to 4 servings	Fruit list—select 3 exchanges	180
Meat—2 to 3 servings[a]	Meat list—select 6 lean exchanges	330
Milk—2 servings	Milk list—select 2 nonfat exchanges	180
	Fat list—select 5 exchanges	225
Total		1,735

[a]In the food group plan, 1 serving is 2 to 3 ounces; in the exchange system, 1 exchange is 1 ounce. The Daily Food Guide suggests that amounts should total 5 to 7 ounces of meat daily.

promoting adequacy, balance, and variety. The exchange system classifies the food selections by their energy-yielding nutrients, thus controlling energy and fat intakes.

Table D-2 shows how to use the Daily Food Guide plan together with the exchange lists to plan a diet. The Daily Food Guide ensures that a certain number of servings is chosen from each of the five food groups (see the first column of the table). The second column translates the number of servings (using the midpoint) into exchanges. With the addition of a small amount of fat, this sample diet plan provides about 1,750 calories. Most people can meet their needs for all the nutrients within this reasonable energy allowance. (Table D-3 shows patterns for other energy intakes.) The next step in diet planning is to assign the exchanges to meals and snacks. The final plan might look like the one in Table D-4. To aid you in the development of your own diet plan, Tables D-5 through D-13 pre-sent the U.S. exchange system in detail.

Next, a person could begin to fill in the plan with real foods to create a menu. For example, the breakfast plan calls for 2 starches, 1 fruit, and 1 nonfat milk. A person might select a bowl of shredded wheat with banana slices and milk (1 cup shredded wheat = 2 starches, 1 small banana = 1 fruit, and 1 cup nonfat milk = 1 milk); or a bagel and a bowl of cantaloupe pieces topped with yogurt (1 bagel = 2 starches, ⅓ cantaloupe melon = 1 fruit, and ¾ cup nonfat plain yogurt = 1 milk). A person who wanted butter on the bagel could move a fat exchange or two from dinner to breakfast. If willing to use two fat exchanges at breakfast, the person could have pancakes with strawberries and milk (4 small pancakes = 2 starches plus 2 fats, 1¼ cup strawberries = 1 fruit, and a cup of nonfat milk = 1 milk). Then the person could move on to complete the menu for lunch, dinner and snacks.

U.S. EXCHANGE LISTS FOR MEAL PLANNING[a]

SOURCE: *Exchange Lists for Meal Planning* (Alexandria, Va.: American Diabetes Association and American Dietetic Association). For a copy of the 33-page booklet, call (800) 232-3472 or (800) 366-1655.

TABLE D-3

Diet Patterns for Different Energy Intakes

EXCHANGE	ENERGY LEVEL (cal)						
	1,200	1,500	1,800	2,000	2,200	2,600	3,000
Starch	6	7	8	9	11	13	15
Meat (lean)	4	5	6	6	6	7	8
Vegetable	3	4	5	5	5	6	6
Fruit	2	3	4	4	4	5	6
Milk (nonfat)	2	2	2	3	3	3	3
Fat	3	5	6	7	8	10	12

NOTE: These patterns follow the Daily Food Guide plan and supply less than 30 percent of calories as fat.

FIGURE D-1

THE EXCHANGE SYSTEM: EXAMPLE FOODS, PORTION SIZES, AND ENERGY-NUTRIENT CONTRIBUTIONS

THE CARBOHYDRATE GROUP

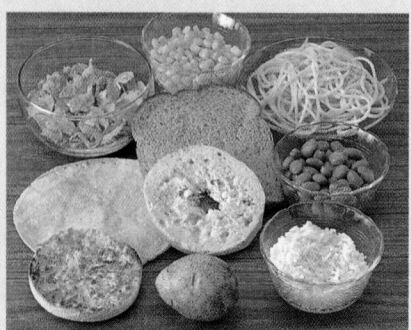

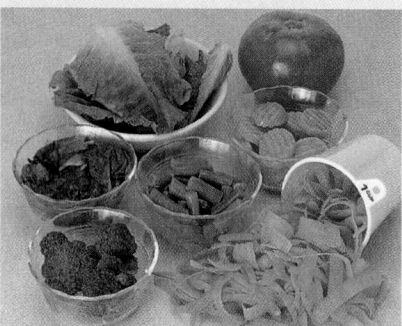

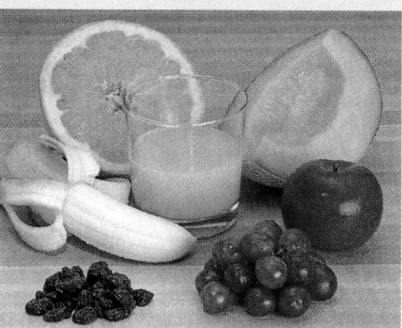

Starch
1 starch exchange is like:
1 slice bread
¾ c ready-to-eat cereal
½ c cooked pasta
⅓ c cooked rice
½ c cooked beansᵃ
½ c corn, peas, or yams
1 small (3 oz) potato
½ bagel, English muffin, or bun
1 tortilla, waffle, or roll
(1 starch = 15 g carbohydrate, 3 g
protein, 0–1 g fat, and 80 cal)

   ᵃ ½ c cooked beans = 1 very lean meat exchange *plus* 1 starch exchange.

Vegetables
1 vegetable exchange is like:
½ c cooked carrots, greens, green
beans, brussels sprouts, beets, broccoli,
cauliflower, or spinach
1 c raw carrots, radishes, or salad
greens
1 lg tomato
(1 vegetable = 5 g carbohydrate, 2 g
protein, and 25 cal)

Fruits
1 fruit exchange is like:
1 small banana, nectarine, apple, or
orange
½ large grapefruit or pear
½ c orange, apple, or grapefruit juice
17 small grapes
⅓ cantaloupe (or 1 c cubes)
2 tbs raisins
(1 fruit = 15 g carbohydrate and 60
cal)

THE MEAT AND MEAT SUBSTITUTES GROUP (PROTEIN)

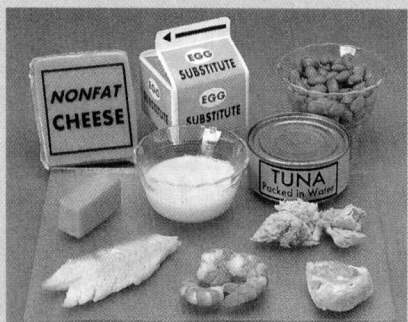

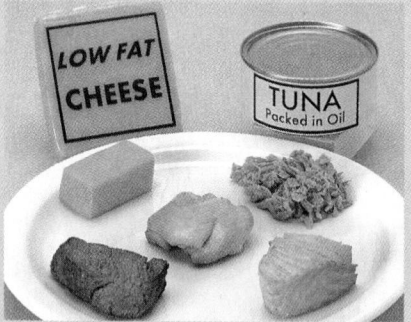

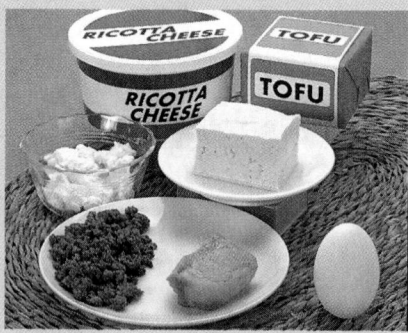

Meat and substitutes (very lean)
1 very lean meat exchange is like:
1 oz chicken (white meat, no skin)
1 oz cod, flounder, or trout
1 oz tuna (canned in water)
1 oz clams, crab, lobster, scallops,
shrimp, or imitation seafood
1 oz fat-free cheese
½ c cooked beans, peas, or lentils
¼ c nonfat or low-fat cream cheese
2 egg whites (or ¼ c egg substitute)
(1 very lean meat = 7 g protein, 0–1 g
fat, and 35 cal)

Meats and substitutes (lean)
1 lean meat exchange is like:
1 oz beef or pork tenderloin
1 oz chicken (dark meat, no skin)
1 oz herring or salmon
1 oz tuna (canned in oil, drained)
1 oz low-fat cheese or luncheon meats
(1 lean meat = 7 g protein, 3 g fat, and
55 cal)

Meats and substitutes (medium-fat)
1 medium-fat meat exchange is like:
1 oz ground beef
1 oz pork chop
1 egg
¼ c ricotta
4 oz tofu
(1 medium-fat meat = 7 g protein, 5 g
fat, and 75 cal)

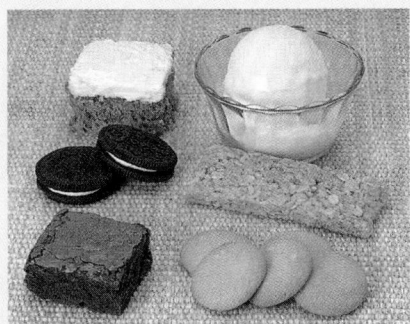

Other carbohydrates
1 other carbohydrates exchange is like:
2 small cookies
1 small brownie or cake
5 vanilla wafers
1 granola bar
½ c ice cream
(1 other carbohydrate = 15 g
carbohydrate and may be exchanged
for 1 starch, 1 fruit, or 1 milk. Because
many items on this list contain added
sugar and fat, their fat and calorie
values vary and their portion sizes are
small.)

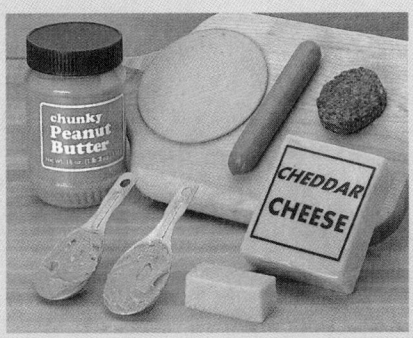

Meats and substitutes (high-fat)
1 high-fat meat exchange is like:
1 oz pork sausage
1 oz luncheon meat (such as bologna)
1 oz regular cheese (such as cheddar
or Swiss)
1 small hot dog (turkey or chicken)[b]
2 tbs peanut butter[c]
(1 high-fat meat = 7 g protein, 8 g fat,
and 100 cal)

[b]A beef or pork hot dog counts as 1 high-fat meat
exchange *plus* 1 fat exchange.
[c]Peanut butter counts as 1 high-fat meat exchange
plus 1 fat exchange.

Milks (nonfat and very-low fat)
1 nonfat milk exchange is like:
1 c nonfat milk
¾ c nonfat yogurt, plain
1 c nonfat or lowfat buttermilk
½ c evaporated nonfat milk
⅓ c dry nonfat milk
(1 nonfat milk = 12 g carbohydrate,
8 g protein, 0–3 g fat, and 90 cal)

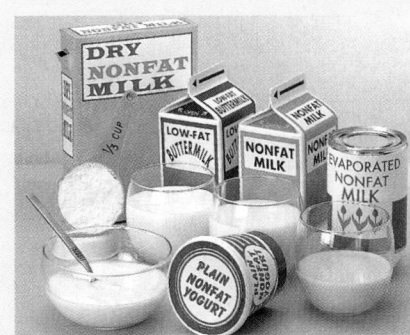

Milks (low-fat)
1 low-fat milk exchange is like:
1 c 2% milk
¾ c low-fat yogurt, plain
(1 low-fat milk = 12 g carbohydrate,
8 g protein, 5 g fat, and 120 cal)

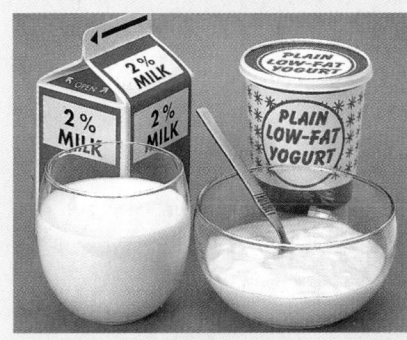

Milks (whole)
1 whole milk exchange is like:
1 c whole milk
½ c evaporated whole milk
(1 whole milk = 12 g carbohydrate,
8 g protein, 8 g fat, and 150 cal)

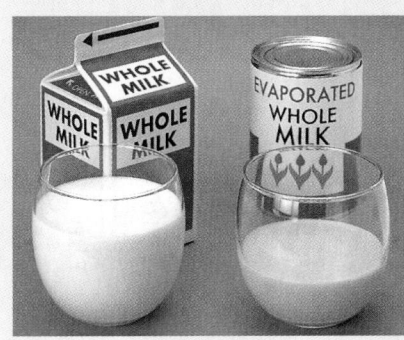

THE FAT GROUP

Fats
1 fat exchange is like:
1 tsp butter
1 tsp margarine or mayonnaise
(1 tbs reduced fat)
1 tsp any oil
1 tbs salad dressing (2 tbs reduced
fat)
8 large black olives
10 large peanuts
⅛ medium avocado
1 slice bacon
2 tbs shredded coconut
1 tbs cream cheese (2 tbs reduced fat)
(1 fat = 5 g fat and 45 cal)

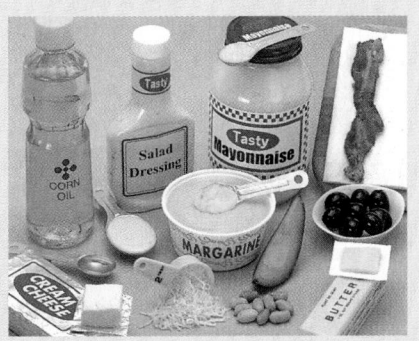

TABLE D-4

A Sample Diet Plan

Exchange	Breakfast	Lunch	Snack	Dinner	Evening Snack
9 starch	2	2	1	3	1
4 vegetable				4	
3 fruit	1	1	1		
6 lean meat		2		4	
2 nonfat milk	1	1			1
5 fat		1		4	

NOTE: This diet plan is one of many possibilities. It follows the number of servings suggested by the Daily Food Guide and meets dietary recommendations to provide 55 to 60 percent of its kcalories from carbohydrate, 15 to 20 percent from protein, and less than 30 percent from fat.

TABLE D-5

U.S. Exchange System: Starch List

1 starch exchange = 15 g carbohydrate, 3 g protein, 0–1 g fat, and 80 cal
Note: In general, a starch serving is ½ c cereal, grain, pasta, or starchy vegetable; 1 oz of bread; ¾ to 1 oz snack food.

Serving Size	Food	Serving Size	Food
Bread		½ c	Plantains
½ (1 oz)	Bagels	1 small (3 oz)	Potatoes, baked or boiled
2 slices (1½ oz)	Bread, reduced-calorie	½ c	Potatoes, mashed
1 slice (1 oz)	Bread, white (including French and Italian), whole-wheat, pumpernickel, rye	1 c	Squash, winter (acorn, butternut)
		½ c	Yams, sweet potatoes, plain
2 (⅔ oz)	Bread sticks, crisp, 4" × ½"	**Crackers and Snacks**	
½	English muffins	8	Animal crackers
½ (1 oz)	Hot dog or hamburger buns	3	Graham crackers, 2½" square
½	Pita, 6" across	¾ oz	Matzoh
1 (1 oz)	Plain rolls, small	4 slices	Melba toast
1 slice (1 oz)	Raisin bread, unfrosted	24	Oyster crackers
1	Tortillas, corn, 6" across	3 c	Popcorn (popped, no fat added or low-fat microwave)
1	Tortillas, flour, 7–8" across		
1	Waffles, 4½" square, reduced-fat	¾ oz	Pretzels
Cereals and Grains		2	Rice cakes, 4" across
½ c	Bran cereals	6	Saltine-type crackers
½ c	Bulgur, cooked	15–20 (¾ oz)	Snack chips, fat-free (tortilla, potato)
½ c	Cereals, cooked		
¾ c	Cereals, unsweetened, ready-to-eat	2–5 (¾ oz)	Whole-wheat crackers, no fat added
3 tbs	Cornmeal (dry)	**Dried Beans, Peas, and Lentils**	
⅓ c	Couscous	½ c	Beans and peas, cooked (garbanzo, lentils, pinto, kidney, white, split, black-eyed)
3 tbs	Flour (dry)		
¼ c	Granola, low-fat		
¼ c	Grape nuts	⅔ c	Lima beans
½ c	Grits, cooked	3 tbs	Miso 🖊
½ c	Kasha	**Starchy Foods Prepared with Fat**	
¼ c	Millet	**Count as 1 starch + 1 fat exchange.**	
¼ c	Muesli	1	Biscuit, 2½" across
½ c	Oats	½ c	Chow mein noodles
½ c	Pasta, cooked	1 (2 oz)	Corn bread, 2" cube
1½ c	Puffed cereals	6	Crackers, round butter type
½ c	Rice milk	1 c	Croutons
⅓ c	Rice, white or brown, cooked	16–25 (3 oz)	French-fried potatoes
½ c	Shredded wheat	¼ c	Granola
½ c	Sugar-frosted cereal	1 (1½ oz)	Muffin, small
3 tbs	Wheat germ	2	Pancake, 4" across
Starchy Vegetables		3 c	Popcorn, microwave
⅓ c	Baked beans	3	Sandwich crackers, cheese or peanut butter filling
½ c	Corn		
1 (5 oz)	Corn on cob, medium	⅓ c	Stuffing, bread (prepared)
1 c	Mixed vegetables with corn, peas, or pasta	2	Taco shell, 6" across
		1	Waffle, 4½" square
½ c	Peas, green	4–6 (1 oz)	Whole-wheat crackers, fat added

🖊 = 400 mg or more of sodium per serving.

TABLE D-6

U.S. Exchange System: Fruit List

1 fruit exchange = 15 g carbohydrate and 60 cal

Note: In general, a fruit serving is 1 small to medium fresh fruit; ½ c canned or fresh fruit or fruit juice; ¼ c dried fruit. The weights given include skin, core, seeds, and rind.

Serving Size	Food
1 (4 oz)	Apples, unpeeled, small
½ c	Applesauce, unsweetened
4 rings	Apples, dried
4 whole (5½ oz)	Apricots, fresh
8 halves	Apricots, dried
½ c	Apricots, canned
1 (4 oz)	Bananas, small
¾ c	Blackberries
¾ c	Blueberries
⅓ melon (11 oz) or 1 c cubes	Cantaloupe, small
12 (3 oz)	Cherries, sweet, fresh
½ c	Cherries, sweet, canned
3	Dates
1½ large or 2 medium (3½ oz)	Figs, fresh
1½	Figs, dried
½ c	Fruit cocktail
½ (11 oz)	Grapefruit, large
¾ c	Grapefruit sections, canned
17 (3 oz)	Grapes, small
1 slice (10 oz) or 1 c cubes	Honeydew melon
1 (3½ oz)	Kiwi
¾ c	Mandarin oranges, canned
½ (5½ oz) or ½ c	Mangoes, small
1 (5 oz)	Nectarines, small
1 (6½ oz)	Oranges, small

Serving Size	Food
½ (8 oz) or 1 c cubes	Papayas
1 (6 oz)	Peaches, medium, fresh
½ c	Peaches, canned
½ (4 oz)	Pears, large, fresh
½ c	Pears, canned
¾ c	Pineapple, fresh
½ c	Pineapple, canned
2 (5 oz)	Plums, small
½ c	Plums, canned
3	Prunes, dried
2 tbs	Raisins
1 c	Raspberries
1¼ c whole berries	Strawberries
2 (8 oz)	Tangerines, small
1 slice (13½ oz) or 1¼ c cubes	Watermelon
Fruit Juice	
½ c	Apple juice/cider
⅓ c	Cranberry juice cocktail
1 c	Cranberry juice cocktail, reduced-calorie
⅓ c	Fruit juice blends, 100% juice
⅓ c	Grape juice
½ c	Grapefruit juice
½ c	Orange juice
½ c	Pineapple juice
⅓ c	Prune juice

TABLE D-7

U.S. Exchange System: Milk List

Serving Size	Food
Nonfat and Very Low-Fat Milk	
1 nonfat/low-fat milk exchange = 12 g carbohydrate, 8 g protein, 0–3 g fat, 90 cal	
1 c	Nonfat milk
1 c	½% milk
1 c	1% milk
1 c	Nonfat or low-fat buttermilk
½ c	Evaporated nonfat milk
⅓ c dry	Dry nonfat milk
¾ c	Plain nonfat yogurt
1 c	Nonfat or low-fat fruit-flavored yogurt sweetened with aspartame or with a nonnutritive sweetener

Serving Size	Food
Low-Fat Milk	
1 low-fat milk exchange = 12 g carbohydrate, 8 g protein, 5 g fat, 120 cal	
1 c	2% milk
¾ c	Plain low-fat yogurt
1 c	Sweet acidophilus milk
Whole Milk	
1 whole milk exchange = 12 g carbohydrate, 8 g protein, 8 g fat, 150 cal	
1 c	Whole milk
½ c	Evaporated whole milk
1 c	Goat's milk
1 c	Kefir

TABLE D-8

U.S. Exchange System: Other Carbohydrates List

1 other carbohydrate exchange = 15 g carbohydrate, or 1 starch, or 1 fruit, or 1 milk exchange

Food	Serving Size	Exchanges per Serving
Angel food cake, unfrosted	¹⁄₁₂ cake	2 carbohydrates
Brownies, small, unfrosted	2″ square	1 carbohydrate, 1 fat
Cake, unfrosted	2″ square	1 carbohydrate, 1 fat
Cake, frosted	2″ square	2 carbohydrates, 1 fat
Cookie, fat-free	2 small	1 carbohydrate
Cookies or sandwich cookies	2 small	1 carbohydrate, 1 fat
Cupcakes, frosted	1 small	2 carbohydrates, 1 fat
Cranberry sauce, jellied	¼ c	2 carbohydrates
Doughnuts, plain cake	1 medium, (1½ oz)	1½ carbohydrates, 2 fats
Doughnuts, glazed	3¾″ across (2 oz)	2 carbohydrates, 2 fats
Fruit juice bars, frozen, 100% juice	1 bar (3 oz)	1 carbohydrate
Fruit snacks, chewy (pureed fruit concentrate)	1 roll (¾ oz)	1 carbohydrate
Fruit spreads, 100% fruit	1 tbs	1 carbohydrate
Gelatin, regular	½ c	1 carbohydrate
Gingersnaps	3	1 carbohydrate
Granola bars	1 bar	1 carbohydrate, 1 fat
Granola bars, fat-free	1 bar	2 carbohydrates
Hummus	⅓ c	1 carbohydrate, 1 fat
Ice cream	½ c	1 carbohydrate, 2 fats
Ice cream, light	½ c	1 carbohydrate, 1 fat
Ice cream, fat-free, no sugar added	½ c	1 carbohydrate
Jam or jelly, regular	1 tbs	1 carbohydrate
Milk, chocolate, whole	1 c	2 carbohydrates, 1 fat
Pie, fruit, 2 crusts	⅙ pie	3 carbohydrates, 2 fats
Pie, pumpkin or custard	⅛ pie	1 carbohydrate, 2 fats
Potato chips	12–18 (1 oz)	1 carbohydrate, 2 fats
Pudding, regular (made with low-fat milk)	½ c	2 carbohydrates
Pudding, sugar-free (made with low-fat milk)	½ c	1 carbohydrate
Salad dressing, fat-free 🖉	¼ c	1 carbohydrate
Sherbet, sorbet	½ c	2 carbohydrates
Spaghetti or pasta sauce, canned 🖉	½ c	1 carbohydrate, 1 fat
Sweet roll or danish	1 (2½ oz)	2½ carbohydrates, 2 fats
Syrup, light	2 tbs	1 carbohydrate
Syrup, regular	1 tbs	1 carbohydrate
Syrup, regular	¼ c	4 carbohydrates
Tortilla chips	6–12 (1 oz)	1 carbohydrate, 2 fats
Vanilla wafers	5	1 carbohydrate, 1 fat
Yogurt, frozen, low-fat, fat-free	⅓ c	1 carbohydrate, 0–1 fat
Yogurt, frozen, fat-free, no sugar added	½ c	1 carbohydrate
Yogurt, low-fat with fruit	1 c	3 carbohydrates, 0–1 fat

🖉 = 400 mg or more sodium per exchange.

TABLE D-9

U.S. Exchange System: Vegetable List

1 vegetable exchange = 5 g carbohydrate, 2 g protein, 25 cal
Note: In general, a vegetable serving is ½ c cooked vegetables or vegetable juice; 1 c raw vegetables. Starchy vegetables such as corn, peas, and potatoes are on the starch list.

Artichokes
Artichoke hearts
Asparagus
Beans (green, wax, Italian)
Bean sprouts
Beets
Broccoli
Brussels sprouts
Cabbage
Carrots
Cauliflower
Celery
Cucumbers
Eggplant
Green onions or scallions
Greens (collard, kale, mustard, turnip)
Kohlrabi
Leeks
Mixed vegetables (without corn, peas, or pasta)

Mushrooms
Okra
Onions
Pea pods
Peppers (all varieties)
Radishes
Salad greens (endive, escarole, lettuce, romaine, spinach)
Sauerkraut ✎
Spinach
Summer squash (crookneck)
Tomatoes
Tomaties, canned
Tomato sauce ✎
Tomato/vegetable juice ✎
Trunips
Water chestnuts
Watercress
Zucchini

✎ = 400 mg or more sodium per exchange.

TABLE D-10

U.S. Exchange System: Meat and Meat Substitutes List

Note: In general, a meat serving is 1 oz meat, poultry, or cheese; ½ c dried beans (weigh meat and poultry and measure beans after cooking).

Serving Size	Food	Serving Size	Food
Very Lean Meat and Substitutes		2 tbs	Grated Parmesan
1 very lean meat exchange = 7 g protein, 0–1 g fat, 35 cal		1 oz	Cheeses with ≤ 3 g fat/oz
1 oz	Poultry: Chicken or turkey (white meat, no skin), Cornish hen (no skin)		Other:
		1½ oz	Hot dogs with ≤ 3 g fat/oz 🖊
1 oz	Fish: Fresh or frozen cod, flounder, haddock, halibut, trout; tuna, fresh or canned in water	1 oz	Processed sandwich meat with ≤ 3 g fat/oz (turkey pastrami or kielbasa)
1 oz	Shellfish: Clams, crab, lobster, scallops, shrimp, imitation shellfish	1 oz	Liver, heart (high in cholesterol)
1 oz	Game: Duck or pheasant (no skin), venison, buffalo, ostrich	**Medium-Fat Meat and Substitutes**	
	Cheese with ≤ 1 g fat/oz:	1 medium-fat meat exchange = 7 g protein, 5 g fat, and 75 cal	
¼ c	Nonfat or low-fat cottage cheese	1 oz	Beef: Most beef products (ground beef, meat loaf, corned beef, short ribs, Prime grades of meat trimmed of fat, such as prime rib)
1 oz	Fat-free cheese		
	Other:	1 oz	Pork: Top loin, chop, Boston butt, cutlet
1 oz	Processed sandwich meats with ≤ 1 g fat/oz (such as deli thin, shaved meats, chipped beef 🖊 , turkey ham)	1 oz	Lamb: Rib roast, ground
		1 oz	Veal: Cutlet (ground or cubed, unbreaded)
2	Egg whites	1 oz	Poultry: Chicken dark meat (with skin), ground turkey or ground chicken, fried chicken (with skin)
¼ c	Egg substitutes, plain		
1 oz	Hot dogs with ≤ 1 g fat/oz	1 oz	Fish: Any fried fish product
1 oz	Kidney (high in cholesterol)		Cheese with ≤ 5 g fat/oz:
1 oz	Sausage with ≤ 1 g fat/oz 🖊	1 oz	Feta
Count as one very lean meat and one starch exchange:		1 oz	Mozzarella
½ c	Dried beans, peas, lentils (cooked)	¼ c (2 oz)	Ricotta
Lean Meat and Substitutes			Other:
1 lean meat exchange = 7 g protein, 3 g fat, 55 cal		1	Egg (high in cholesterol, limit to 3/week)
1 oz	Beef: USDA Select or Choice grades of lean beef trimmed of fat (round, sirloin, and flank steak); tenderloin; roast (rib, chuck, rump); steak (T-bone, porterhouse, cubed), ground round	1 oz	Sausage with ≤ 5 g fat/oz
		1 c	Soy milk
		¼ c	Tempeh
		4 oz or ½ c	Tofu
1 oz	Pork: Lean pork (fresh ham); canned, cured, or boiled ham; Canadian bacon 🖊 ; tenderloin, center loin chop	**High-Fat Meat and Substitutes**	
		1 high-fat meat exchange = 7 g protein, 8 g fat, 100 cal	
		1 oz	Pork: Spareribs, ground pork, pork sausage
1 oz	Lamb: Roast, chop, leg		
1 oz	Veal: Lean chop, roast	1 oz	Cheese: All regular cheeses (American 🖊 , cheddar, Monterey Jack, swiss)
1 oz	Poultry: Chicken, turkey (dark meat, no skin), chicken white meat (with skin), domestic duck or goose (well-drained of fat, no skin)		Other:
		1 oz	Processed sandwich meats with ≤ 8 g fat/oz (bologna, pimento loaf, salami)
	Fish:	1 oz	Sausage (bratwurst, Italian, knockwurst, Polish, smoked)
1 oz	Herring (uncreamed or smoked)	1 (10/lb)	Hot dog (turkey or chicken) 🖊
6 medium	Oysters	3 slices (20 slices/lb)	Bacon
1 oz	Salmon (fresh or canned), catfish	Count as one high-fat meat plus one fat exchange:	
2 medium	Sardines (canned)	1 (10/lb)	Hot dog (beef, pork, or combination) 🖊
1 oz	Tuna (canned in oil, drained)	2 tbs	Peanut butter (contains unsaturated fat)
1 oz	Game: Goose (no skin), rabbit		
	Cheese:		
¼ c	4.5%-fat cottage cheese		

🖊 = 400 mg or more sodium per exchange.

TABLE D-11

U.S. Exchange System: Fat List

1 fat exchange = 5 g fat, 45 cal

Note: In general, a fat serving is 1 tsp regular butter, margarine, or vegetable oil; 1 tbs regular salad dressing. Many fat-free and reduced fat foods are on the Free Foods List.

Serving Size	Food
Monounsaturated Fats	
⅛ medium (1 oz)	Avocadoes
1 tsp	Oil (canola, olive, peanut)
8 large	Olives, ripe (black)
10 large	Olives, green, stuffed 🖊
6 nuts	Almonds, cashews
6 nuts	Mixed nuts (50% peanuts)
10 nuts	Peanuts
4 halves	Pecans
2 tsp	Peanut butter, smooth or crunchy
1 tbs	Sesame seeds
2 tsp	Tahini paste
Polyunsaturated Fats	
1 tsp	Margarine, stick, tub, or squeeze
1 tbs	Margarine, lower-fat (30% to 50% vegetable oil)
1 tsp	Mayonnaise, regular
1 tbs	Mayonnaise, reduced-fat
4 halves	Nuts, walnuts, English
1 tsp	Oil (corn, safflower, soybean)
1 tbs	Salad dressing, regular
2 tbs	Salad dressing, reduced-fat
2 tsp	Mayonnaise-type salad dressing, regular 🖊
1 tbs	Mayonnaise-type salad dressing, reduced-fat
1 tbs	Seeds: pumpkin, sunflower
Saturated Fats[a]	
1 slice (20 slices/lb)	Bacon, cooked
1 tsp	Bacon, grease
1 tsp	Butter, stick
2 tsp	Butter, whipped
1 tbs	Butter, reduced-fat
2 tbs (½ oz)	Chitterlings, boiled
2 tbs	Coconut, sweetened, shredded
2 tbs	Cream, half and half
1 tbs (½ oz)	Cream cheese, regular
2 tbs (1 oz)	Cream cheese, reduced-fat
	Fatback or salt pork[b]
1 tsp	Shortening or lard
2 tbs	Sour cream, regular
3 tbs	Sour cream, reduced-fat

🖊 = 400 mg or more sodium per exchange

[a]Saturated fats can raise blood cholesterol levels.

[b]Use a piece 1" × 1" × ¼" if you plan to eat the fatback cooked with vegetables. Use a piece 2" × 1" × ½" when eating only the vegetables with the fatback removed.

TABLE D-12

U.S. Exchange System: Free Foods List

Note: A serving of free food contains fewer than 20 calories; those with serving sizes should be limited to three servings a day whereas those without serving sizes can be eaten freely.

Serving Size	Food	Serving Size	Food
Fat-Free or Reduced-Fat Foods			Bouillon or broth, low-sodium
1 tbs	Cream cheese, fat-free		Carbonated or mineral water
1 tbs	Creamers, nondairy, liquid	1 tbs	Cocoa powder, unsweetened
2 tsp	Creamers, nondairy, powdered		Coffee
1 tbs	Mayonnaise, fat-free		Club soda
1 tsp	Mayonnaise, reduced-fat		Diet soft drinks, sugar-free
4 tbs	Margarine, fat-free		Drink mixes, sugar-free
1 tsp	Margarine, reduced-fat		Tea
1 tbs	Mayonnaise type salad dressing, nonfat		Tonic water, sugar-free
1 tsp	Mayonnaise type salad dressing, reduced-fat	**Condiments**	
	Nonstick cooking spray	1 tbs	Catsup
1 tbs	Salad dressing, fat-free		Horseradish
2 tbs	Salad dressing, fat-free, Italian		Lemon juice
¼ c	Salsa		Lime juice
1 tbs	Sour cream, fat-free, reduced-fat		Mustard
2 tbs	Whipped topping, regular or light	1½ large	Pickles, dill 🖊
			Soy sauce, regular or light 🖊
Sugar-Free or Low-Sugar Foods		1 tbs	Taco sauce
1 piece	Candy, hard, sugar-free		Vinegar
	Gelatin dessert, sugar-free	**Seasonings**	
	Gelatin, unflavored		Flavoring extracts
	Gum, sugar-free		Garlic
2 tsp	Jam or jelly, low-sugar or light		Herbs, fresh or dried
	Sugar substitutes		Pimento
2 tbs	Syrup, sugar-free		Spices
Drinks			Hot pepper sauces
	Bouillon, broth, consommé 🖊		Wine, used in cooking
			Worcestershire sauce

🖊 = 400 mg or more sodium per exchange.

D

TABLE D-13

U.S. Exchange System: Combination Foods List

Food	Serving Size	Exchanges per Serving
Entrées		
Tuna noodle casserole, lasagna, spaghetti with meatballs, chili with beans, macaroni and cheese ✐	1 c (8 oz)	2 carbohydrates, 2 medium-fat meats
Chow mein (without noodles or rice)	2 c (16 oz)	1 carbohydrate, 2 lean meats
Pizza, cheese, thin crust ✐ (5 oz)	¼ of 10"	2 carbohydrates, 2 medium-fat meats, 1 fat
Pizza, meat topping, thin crust ✐ (5 oz)	¼ of 10"	2 carbohydrates, 2 medium-fat meats, 2 fats
Pot pie ✐	1 (7 oz)	2 carbohydrates, 1 medium-fat meat, 4 fats
Frozen Entrées		
Salisbury steak with gravy, mashed potato	1 (11 oz)	2 carbohydrates, 3 medium-fat meats, 3–4 fats
Turkey with gravy, mashed potato, dressing ✐	1 (11 oz)	2 carbohydrates, 2 medium-fat meats, 2 fats
Entree with less than 300 kcalories ✐	1 (8 oz)	2 carbohydrates, 3 lean meats
Soups		
Bean ✐	1 c	1 carbohydrate, 1 very lean meat
Cream (made with water) ✐	1 c (8 oz)	1 carbohydrate, 1 fat
Split pea (made with water) ✐	½ c (4 oz)	1 carbohydrate
Tomato (made with water) ✐	1 c (8 oz)	1 carbohydrate
Vegetable beef, chicken noodle, or other broth-type ✐	1 c (8 oz)	1 carbohydrate
Fast Foods		
Burritos with beef ✐	2	4 carbohydrates, 2 medium-fat meats, 2 fats
Chicken nuggets ✐	6	1 carbohydrate, 2 medium-fat meats, 1 fat
Chicken breast and wing, breaded and fried ✐	1	1 carbohydrate, 4 medium-fat meats, 2 fats
Fish sandwich/tartar sauce ✐	1	3 carbohydrates, 1 medium-fat meat, 3 fats
French fries, thin	20–25	2 carbohydrates, 2 fats
Hamburger, regular	1	2 carbohydrates, 2 medium-fat meats
Hamburger, large ✐	1	2 carbohydrates, 3 medium-fat meats, 1 fat
Hot dog with bun ✐	1	1 carbohydrate, 1 high-fat meat, 1 fat
Individual pan pizza ✐	1	5 carbohydrates, 3 medium-fat meats, 3 fats
Soft serve cone	1 medium	2 carbohydrates, 1 fat
Submarine sandwich ✐	1 (6")	3 carbohydrates, 1 vegetable, 2 medium-fat meats, 1 fat
Taco, hard shell ✐	1 (6 oz)	2 carbohydrates, 2 medium-fat meats, 2 fats
Taco, soft shell ✐	1 (3 oz)	1 carbohydrate, 1 medium-fat meat, 1 fat

✐ = 400 mg or more sodium per exchange.

NUTRITION RESOURCES

E

CONTENTS

Books

Journals

Addresses and Internet Addresses

People interested in nutrition often want to know where they can find reliable nutrition information. Wherever you live, there are several sources you can turn to:

■ The Department of Health may have a nutrition expert.
■ The local extension agent is often an expert.
■ The food editor of your local paper may be well informed.
■ The dietitian at the local hospital had to fulfill a set of qualifications before he or she became an RD (see Controversy 1).
■ There may be knowledgeable professors of nutrition or biochemistry at a nearby college or university.
■ The Internet may lead you to the information you seek.

Should you wish to search the Internet for topics in nutrition and health, try these search engines: Webcrawler (http://webcrawler.com) or Yahoo (http://yahoo.com/Health/Medicine)
You may also be interested in building a nutrition library of your own. Books you can buy, journals you can subscribe to, and mailing and Internet addresses (when available) you can use to obtain general information are given below.

BOOKS

For students seeking to establish a personal library of nutrition references, the authors of this text recommend the following books:

■ *Present Knowledge in Nutrition* (Washington, D.C.: International Life Sciences Institute—Nutrition Foundation).

This large paperback has chapters on more than 50 topics, including energy, obesity, each of the nutrients, several diseases, malnutrition, growth and its assessment, immunity, alcohol, fiber, exercise, drugs, and toxins. Watch for an update; new editions come out every few years.

■ M. E. Shils, J. A. Olson, and M. Shike, eds., *Modern Nutrition in Health and Disease,* 8th ed. (Philadelphia: Lea & Febiger, 1994).

This two-volume set is a major technical reference on nutrition topics. It contains encyclopedic articles on the nutrients, foods, the diet, metabolism, malnutrition, age-related needs, and nutrition in disease.

■ Food and Nutrition Board, *Recommended Dietary Allowances,* 10th ed. (Washington, D.C.: National Academy Press, 1989).

This book reviews the functions of each nutrient, dietary sources, and deficiency and toxicity symptoms as well as recommendations for intakes. The Canadian equivalent is *Nutrition Recommendations,* available by mail from the Canadian Government Publishing Centre, Supply and Services Canada, Ottawa, Ontario K1A OS9, Canada.

■ Food and Nutrition Board, *Diet and Health: Implications for Reducing Chronic Disease Risk* (Washington, D.C.: National Academy Press, 1989).

This 749-page book presents the integral relationship between diet and chronic disease prevention. Its nutrient chapters provide evidence on how diet influences disease development, and its disease chapters review the dietary patterns implicated in each chronic disease.

■ E. M. N. Hamilton and S. A. S. Gropper, *The Biochemistry of Human Nutrition: A Desk Reference* (St. Paul, Minn.: West, 1987).

This 324-page paperback presents the biochemical concepts necessary for an understanding of nutrition. It is a handy reference book for those who have forgotten the basics of biochemistry or for those who are learning biochemistry for the first time.

We also recommend three of our own books that explore topics in nutrition, fitness, and the life span:

■ E. N. Whitney and S. R. Rolfes, *Understanding Nutrition,* 7th ed. (St. Paul, Minn.: West, 1996).

■ L. K. DeBruyne, F. S. Sizer, and E. N. Whitney, *The Fitness Triad: Motivation, Nutrition, and Training* (St. Paul, Minn.: West, 1991).

■ S. R. Rolfes, L. K. DeBruyne, and E. N. Whitney, *Life Span Nutrition: Conception through Life* (St. Paul, Minn.: West, 1990).

JOURNALS

Nutrition Today is an enjoyable magazine for the interested layperson. It makes a point of raising controversial issues and providing a forum for conflicting opinions. Six issues per year are published. Order from Williams and Wilkins, 428 East Preston Street, Baltimore, MD 21202.

The *Journal of the American Dietetic Association,* the official publication of the ADA, contains articles of interest to dietitians and nutritionists, news of legislative action on food and nutrition, and a very useful section of abstracts of articles from many other journals of nutrition and related areas. There are 12 issues per year, available from the American Dietetic Association (see "Addresses," below).

Nutrition Reviews, a publication of the International Life Sciences Institute, does much of the work for the library researcher, compiling recent evidence on current topics and presenting extensive bibliographies. Twelve issues per year are available from Springer-Verlag New York, 175 Fifth Avenue, New York, NY 10010.

Nutrition and the M.D. is a monthly newsletter that provides up-to-date, easy-to-read, practical information on nutrition for health-care providers. It is available from PM, Inc., 7100 Hayven Hurst Avenue, Suite 107, Van Nuys, CA 91406.

Other journals that deserve mention here are *Food Technology, Journal of Nutrition, American Journal of Clinical Nutrition,* and *Journal of Nutrition Education. FDA Consumer,* a government publication with many articles of interest to the consumer, is available from the Food and Drug Administration (see "Addresses," below).

ADDRESSES AND INTERNET ADDRESSES

U.S. GOVERNMENT

■ Federal Trade Commission (FTC)
Public Reference Branch
(202) 326-2222

■ Food and Drug Administration (FDA)
Office of Consumer Affairs
HFE 881 Room 16–63
5600 Fishers Lane
Rockville, MD 20857
Internet address: http://www.fda.gov/

■ FDA Consumer Information Line
(301) 443-3170

■ FDA Office of Food Labeling (HFS-150)
200 C Street SW
Washington, DC 20204
(202) 205-4561; fax: (202) 205-4564

■ FDA Office of Nutrition and Food Sciences
200 C Street SW
Washington, DC 20204
(202) 205-4561

■ FDA Office of Plant and Dairy Foods
and Beverages (HFS-300)
200 C Street SW
Washington, DC 20204
(202) 205-4064; fax: (202) 205-4422

■ FDA Office of Special Nutritionals (HFS-450)
200 C Street SW
Washington, DC 20204
(202) 205-4168; fax: (202) 205-5295

■ Food and Nutrition Information Center
National Agricultural Library, Room 304
10301 Baltimore Blvd.
Beltsville, MD 20705-2351
(301) 504-5719; fax: (301) 504-6409
Internet address: fnic@nalusda.gov

■ Food Research and Action Center
1875 Connecticut Avenue, NW, Suite 540
Washington, DC 20009
(202) 986-2200

■ Superintendent of Documents
U.S. Government Printing Office
Washington, DC 20402

- U.S. Department of Agriculture (USDA)
  14th Street SW and Independence Avenue
  Washington, DC 20250
  Internet address: http://www.usda.gov/fcs/cnpp
  (202) 720-2791
- USDA Center for Nutrition Policy and Promotion
  1120 20th Street, NW, Suite 200, North Lobby
  Washington, DC 20036
  (202) 418-2321
- USDA Food Safety and Inspection Service
  Food Safety Education office
  Room 1180–S
  Washington, DC 20250
  (202) 690-0351
- USDA Health Inspection Service
  4700 River Road
  Riverdale, MD 20737-1228
- USDA Meat and Poultry Hotline
  (800) 535-4555
- U.S. Department of Education (DOE)
  Accreditation Agency Evaluation Branch
  7th and D Street SW
  Building 3, Room 336
  Washington, DC 20202
  (202) 708-7417
- U.S. Environmental Protection Agency (EPA)
  401 M Street NW
  Washington, DC 20460
  (202) 382-3535
- U.S. EPA Safe Drinking Water Hotline
  (800) 426-4791
- U.S. Public Health Service Public Affairs Office
  Hubert H. Humphrey Building
  Room 725–H
  200 Independence Avenue SW
  Washington, DC 20201
  (202) 245-6867

CANADIAN GOVERNMENT
Federal

- Bureau of Nutritional Sciences, Food Directorate
  Health Protection Branch
  Department Health Canada
  Banting Building
  Tunney's Pasture, Ottawa, Ontario K1A 0L2
- Nutrition Programs Unit
  Health Promotion Directorate
  Health Canada
  4th Floor, Jeanne Mance Building
  Tunney's Pasture, Ottawa, Ontario K1A 1B4
- Food Production and Inspection Branch
  Agriculture and Agri-Food Canada
  59 Camelot Drive
  Nepean, Ontario KIA OY9
- Nutrition Specialist, Health Support Services
  Indian and Northern Health Services Directorate
  Health Canada
  11th Floor, Jeanne Mance Building
  Tunney's Pasture, Ottawa, Ontario K1A 0L3

Provincial & Territorial

- Special Services Coordinator
  Health & Community Services Agency
  P.O. Box 2000, 4 Sydney Street
  Charlottetown, Prince Edward Island, Canada C1A 7N8
- Director
  Health Promotion Division
  Department of Health
  P.O. Box 8700
  Confederation Bldg, West Block
  St. John's, Newfoundland, AIB 4J6
- Senior Nutrition Consultant
  Public Health Services
  Department of Health and Community Services
  P.O. Box 5100
  Fredericton, New Brunswick E3B 5G8
- Nutrition Coordinator, Nutrition Program Planning,
  Public Health and Health Promotion
  Department of Health
  P.O. Box 488
  Halifax, Nova Scotia B3J 2R8
- Responsable des programmes de nutrition
  Direction de la Santé
  Ministère de la Santé et des Services sociaux
  3e étage, 1075 chemin Saint-Foy
  Québec, Québec G1S 2M1
- Senior Nutrition Consultant
  Public Health Branch
  Ministry of Health, 8th Floor
  5700 Yonge Street
  New York, Ontario M2M4K2
- Program Specialist Nutrition
  Program Development Branch
  Healthy Public Policy Program Division
  Manitoba Health
  599 Empress Street
  Box 925
  Winnipeg, Manitoba R3C2T6
- Provincial Nutritionist, Health Promotion Unit
  Population Health
  Saskatchewan Health Branch
  3475 Albert Street
  Regina, Saskatchewan S4S 6X6
- Population Health and Program Development,
  Prevention and Promotion Branch, Alberta Heath
  Jasper Avenue Building, 24th Floor
  10025 Jasper Avenue
  Edmonton, Alberta TSJ2P4
- Ministry of Health
  Nutrition Section
  1520 Blanshard Street, 1st Floor
  Victoria, British Columbia V8W 3C8
- Director Nutrition Services, Yukon Hospital Corporation
  Department of Health and Social Services
  5 Hospital Road
  Whitehorse, Yukon Y1A 2C6

■ Consultant, Infant/Child Nutrition, Community Health
Program
Department of Health and Social Services
6th Floor, P.O. Box 1320
Yellowknife, Northwest Territories X1A 2L9

INTERNATIONAL AGENCIES

■ Food and Agriculture Organization of the United Nations
(FAO)
Liaison Office for North America
1001 22nd Street NW
Washington, DC 20437
(202) 653-2400
■ World Health Organization (WHO)
Regional Office
525 23rd Street NW
Washington, DC 20037
(202) 861-3200
■ Internet Health Resources
Internet address: http://www.ihr.com/

CONSUMER ORGANIZATIONS

■ Center for Science in the Public Interest (CSPI)
1875 Connecticut Avenue NW, Suite 300
Washington, DC 20009
■ Choice in Dying, Inc.
200 Varick Street, Suite 1001
New York, NY 10014
(212) 366-5540; fax: (212) 366-5337
■ Consumer' Association of Canada
P.O. Box 9300
Ottawa, Ontario K1G 3T9
■ Consumer Information Catalog
Pueblo, CO 81009
■ Consumer's Union
101 Truman Avenue
Yonkers, NY 10703-1057
(914) 378-2000
■ National Council Against Health Fraud, Inc.
P.O. Box 1276
Loma Linda, CA 92354
Internet address: http://www.primenet.com/~ncahf/

FOOD SAFETY

■ Alliance for Food & Fiber
Food Safety Hotline
(800) 266-0200
■ FDA Seafood Hotline
(800) FDA-4010
■ National Lead Information Center
(800) LEAD-FYI (532-3394)
(800) 424-LEAD (424-5323)
■ National Pesticide Telecommunications Network
Texas Tech University
Thompson Hall, Room S129
Lubbock, TX 79430
NPTN Hotline (800) 858-PEST

■ USDA/FDA Foodborne Illness Education
Information Center
c/o Food and Nutrition Information Center
National Agricultural Library/USDA
Beltsville, MD 20705-2351
(301) 504-5719

INFANCY AND CHILDHOOD

■ American Academy of Pediatrics
P.O. Box 927
141 Northwest Point Boulevard
Elk Grove Village, IL 60009-0927
■ Association of Birth Defect Children, Inc.
827 Irma Street
Orlando, FL 32803
(407) 245-7035
■ Canadian Paediatric Society
410 Smyth Rd.
Ottawa, Ontario K1H 8L1
■ National Center for Education in Maternal & Child
Health
2000 15th Street North, Suite 701
Arlington, VA 22201-2617
(703) 524-7802
■ National Maternal and Child Health Clearinghouse
8201 Greensboro Drive
Suite 600
McLean, VA 22102
(703) 821-8955, Ext. 254 or 255
■ Nurture/Center to Prevent Childhood Malnutrition
1840 18th Street, NW
Washington, DC 20009
(202) 797-9244; fax: (202) 797-9257

PROFESSIONAL NUTRITION ORGANIZATIONS

■ American Dietetic Association (ADA)
216 West Jackson Boulevard, Suite 800
Chicago, IL 60606–6995
(312) 899-0040
■ ADA, The National Center for Nutrition and Dietetics'
Food and Nutrition Information Hotline
(800) 366–1655
■ American Institute of Nutrition
American Society for Clinical Nutrition
9650 Rockville Pike
Bethesda, MD 20814-3998
■ Dietitians of Canada
480 University Avenue, Suite 604
Toronto, Ontario M5G 1V2, Canada
(416) 596-0857

- National Academy of Sciences/National Research Council (NAS/NRC)
  2101 Constitution Avenue NW
  Washington, DC 20418
- National Institute of Nutrition
  302–265 Carling Avenue
  Ottawa, Ontario K1S 2E1
- Nutrition Foundation, Inc. (INACG)
  1126 Sixteenth Street NW, Suite 111
  Washington, DC 20036
- Nutrition Information Service
  University of Alabama at Birmingham
  Room 447 Webb Building
  UAB Station
  Birmingham, AL 35294-3360

ALCOHOL AND DRUG ABUSE

- Al-Anon Family Group Headquarters
  P.O. Box 862
  Midtown Station
  New York, NY 10018–0862
  (800) 356-9996
- Alateen
  1372 Broadway
  New York, NY 10018
  (800) 356-9996
- Alcohol & Drug Abuse Information Line
  (800) 252-6465
- Alcoholics Anonymous (AA)
  General Service Office
  475 Riverside Drive
  New York, NY 10115
  (212) 870-3400
- Narcotics Anonymous (NA)
  P.O. Box 9999
  Van Nuys, CA 91409
  (818) 780-3951
- National Clearinghouse for Alcohol and Drug Information (NCADI)
  P.O. Box 2345
  Rockville, MD 20847-2345
  (800) 729-6686
- National Council on Alcoholism and Drug Dependence
  12 West 21st Street
  New York, NY 10010
  (800) NCA-CALL
- OSAP's National Clearinghouse for Alcohol and Drug Information (ONCADI)
  P.O. Box 2345
  Rockville, MD 20847-2345
  (800) 729-6686

BODY SIZE ACCEPTANCE

- Grace-Full Eating (Newsletter)
  Terry Garrison
  Annabel Taylor Hall
  Cornell University
  Ithaca, NY 14853
- National Association to Advance Fat Acceptance (NAAFA)
  P.O. Box 188620
  Sacramento, CA 95818
  (916) 558-6880
- Radiance Magazine
  P.O. Box 30246
  Oakland, CA 94604
  (510) 482-0680

WEIGHT CONTROL AND EATING DISORDERS

- American Anorexia & Bulimia Association, Inc.
  418 East 76th Street
  New York, NY 10021
  (212) 734-1114
- Anorexia Nervosa and Related Eating Disorders (ANRED)
  P.O. Box 5102
  Eugene, OR 97405
  (503) 344-1144
- National Association of Anorexia Nervosa and Associated Disorders, Inc. (ANAD)
  P.O. Box 7
  Highland Park, IL 60035
  (708) 831-3438
- National Eating Disorder Information Centre
  200 Elizabeth St., College Wing 1-328
  Toronto, Ontario M5G 2C4
- Overeaters Anonymous (OA)
  383 Van Ness Avenue, Suite 1601
  Torrace, CA 90501
- T.O.P.S. (Take Off Pounds Sensibly)
  P.O. Box 07360
  Milwaukee, WI 53207

FITNESS

- American College of Sports Medicine
  P.O. Box 1440
  Indianapolis, IN 46204
  (317) 637-9200
- President's Council on Physical Fitness and Sports
  701 Pennsylvania Avenue NW
  Suite 250
  Washington, DC 20004
  (202) 272-3421
- Sport Medicine and Science Council of Canada
  1600 James Naismith Drive
  Gloucester, Ontario K1B 5N4

E

PREGNANCY

- American College of Obstetricians and Gynecologists
  Resource Center
  409 12th Street SW
  Washington, DC 20024-2188
- La Leche League International, Inc.
  1400 N. Meacham Rd.
  P.O. Box 4079
  Schaumburg, IL 60168-4079
  (847) 519-7730
- March of Dimes Birth Defects Foundation
  (National Headquarters)
  1275 Mamaroneck Avenue
  White Plains, NY 10605

TRADE ORGANIZATIONS

- Beech-Nut
  Checkerboard Square, 1B
  St. Louis, MO 63164
  (800) 523-6633
- Borden Farm Products
  Product Publicity
  180 East Broad Street
  Columbus, OH 43215
- Campbell Soup Company
  Food Service Division
  Campbell Place
  Camden, NJ 08103-1799
- Elan Pharma, Nutrition Division
  2 Thurber Blvd.
  Smithfield, RI 02917
- General Mills, Inc.
  Nutrition Department
  Number One General Mills Boulevard
  Minneapolis, MN 55426
- Kraft Foods
  Consumer Response and Information Center
  One Kraft Court
  Glenview, Illinois 60025
- Kellogg Company
  P.O. Box CAMB
  Battle Creek, MI 49016-1986
- Mead Johnson Nutritionals
  2400 West Lloyd Expressway
  Evansville, IN 47721
- Nabisco Consumer Affairs
  100 DeForest Avenue
  East Hanover, NJ 07936
  (800) 932-7800
  (800) NABISCO
- National Dairy Council
  O'Hare International Center
  10255 West Higgins Road, Suite 900
  Rosemond, IL 60018

- NutraSweet Simplesse Company
  P.O. Box 830
  Deerfield, IL 60015
  (800) 321-7254
- Pillsbury Company
  Consumer Relations
  P.O. Box 550
  Minneapolis, MN 55440-9843
- Procter and Gamble Company
  One Procter and Gamble Plaza
  Cincinnati, OH 45202
- Ross Laboratories
  Abbot Laboratory
  625 Cleveland Avenue
  Columbus, OH 43216
- Sherwood Medical
  1915 Olive Street
  St. Louis, MO 63103
- Sunkist Growers, Inc.
  Consumer Affairs Department
  P.O. Box 7888
  Van Nuys, CA 91409-7888
- United Fresh Fruit and Vegetable Association
  727 North Washington Street
  Alexandria, VA 22314
  (800) 336-3065
- USA Rice Council
  P.O. Box 740123
  Houston, TX 77274
- Vitamin Nutrition Information Service (VNIS)
  Hoffmann-LaRoche, Inc.
  340 Kingsland Street
  Nutley, NJ 07110
- Weight Watchers Food Company
  Consumer Affairs Department
  P.O. Box 10
  Boise, ID 83707-0010

WORLD HUNGER

- Bread for the World
  802 Rhode Island Avenue NE
  Washington, DC 20018
- Center on Hunger, Poverty and Nutrition Policy
  Tufts University School of Nutrition
  11 Curtis Avenue
  Medford, MA 02155
  (617) 627-3956
- Freedom from Hunger
  P.O. Box 2000
  1644 DaVinci Court
  Davis, CA 95617
  (916) 758-6200
- Oxfam America
  115 Broadway
  Boston, MA 02116

◼ SEEDS Magazine
P.O. Box 6170
Waco, TX 76706
◼ Worldwatch Institute
1776 Massachusetts Avenue NW
Washington, DC 20036

HEALTH AND DISEASE

◼ Alzheimer's Disease Education and Referral Center
P.O. Box 8250
Silver Spring, Maryland 20907-8250
(800) 438-4380
◼ National Institutes of Health (NIH)
9000 Rockville Pike
Bethesda, MD 20892
(301) 496-2433
Internet address: http://www.nih.gov
◼ Alzheimer's Disease Information and Referral Service
919 North Michigan Avenue
Chicago, IL 60611
(800) 272-3900
◼ American Academy of Allergy, Asthma, and Immunology
611 East Wells Street
Milwaukee, WI 53202
(414) 272-6071; fax: (414) 276-3349
◼ American Cancer Society
Cancer Information Center
1701 Rickenbacker Drive, Suite 5B
Sun City Center, FL 33573-5361
(800) ACS-2345
Internet address: http://www.cancer.org
◼ American Council on Science and Health
1995 Broadway, 16th Floor
New York, NY 10023-5860
◼ American Dental Association
Division of Communications
211 East Chicago Avenue
Chicago, IL 60611-2678
◼ American Diabetes Association
1660 Duke Street
Alexandria, VA 22314
(703) 549-1500
(800) 232-3472
◼ American Heart Association
Box BHG, National Center
7320 Greenville Avenue
Dallas, TX 75231
(800) 242-8721
Internet address: http://www.amhrt.org
◼ American Institute for Cancer Research
1759 R Street NW
Washington, DC 20009

◼ American Medical Association
515 North State Street
Chicago, IL 60610
(312) 464-5000
Internet address: http://www.ama-assn.org
◼ American Public Health Association
1015 Fifteenth Street NW
Washington, DC 20005
◼ American Red Cross AIDS Education Office
1730 D Street NW
Washington, DC 20006
(202) 737-8300
◼ Canadian Diabetes Association
15 Toronto St., Suite 1001
Toronto, Ontario M5C 2E3
(416) 362-4440
◼ Canadian Public Health Association
Publications, Suite 400
1565 Carling Ave.
Ottawa, Ontario K1Z 8R1
◼ Centers for Disease Control and Prevention (CDC)
Information Hotline
(404) 332-4555
Internet address: http://www.cdc.gov
◼ Disease Prevention and Health Promotion's National Health Information Center, Office of
(800) 336-4797
◼ The Food Allergy Network
4744 Holly Avenue
Fairfax, VA 22030-5647
(703) 691-3179
◼ National AIDS Hotline (CDC)
(800) 342-AIDS (English)
(800) 344-SIDA (Spanish)
(800) 2437-TTY (Deaf)
(900) 820-2437
◼ National Cancer Institute
Office of Cancer Communications
Building 31, Room 10824
Bethesda, MD 20892
(800) 4-CANCER
Internet address: http://www.nci.nih.gov
◼ National Digestive Disease Information Clearinghouse (NDOIC)
2 Information Way
Bethesda, MD 20892-3570
(301) 654-3810
◼ National Heart, Lung, and Blood Institute
National High Blood Pressure Education Program
Information Center
P.O. Box 30105
Bethesda, MD 20824-0105
(301) 951-3260

- National Institute of Allergy and Infectious Diseases
  Office of Communications, Building 31, Room 7A50
  31 Center Drive, MSC 2520
  Bethesda, MD 20892-2520
  (301) 496-5717
- National Institute of Dental Research (NIDR)
  Building 31, Room 2C35
  31 Center Drive, MSC 2290
  Bethesda, MD 20892
  (301) 496-4261
- National Osteoporosis Foundation
  2100 M Street NW, Suite 602
  Washington, DC 20037
  (202) 223-2226

- New England Journal of Medicine
  Internet address: http://www.nejm.org
- ODPHP National Health Information Center (ONHIC)
  (800) 336-4797
  Internet address: http://NHIC-NT.Health.org
- Smoking and Health Office (CDC)
  Technical Information Center
  Mail Stop K-12
  1600 Clifton Road NE
  Atlanta, GA 30333

E

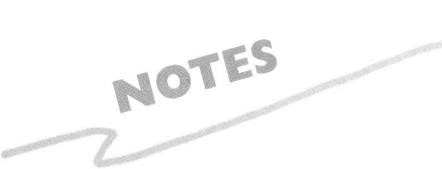

NOTES

CHAPTER I

1. J. Anderson, Making nutrition sense from nutrition headlines, *Food Insight Reports from the International Food Information Council Foundation,* 1100 Connecticut Avenue NW, Suite 430, Washington, D.C. 20036, 1992.

2. D. Woznicki and H. Nguyen, We are what we read: Shaping the nation's nutrition IQ through the media, *Priorities* 7 (1995): 20–23.

3. J. P. Goldberg, Nutrition and health communication: The message and the media over half a century, *Nutrition Reviews* 50 (1992): 71–77.

4. C. M. Ripsin and coauthors, Oat products and lipid lowering: A meta-analysis, *Journal of the American Medical Association* 267 (1992): 3317–3325.

5. G. B. Abernathy and coauthors, Efficacy of tube feedings in supplying estimated energy requirements of hospitalized patients, *Journal of Parenteral and Enteral Nutrition* 13 (1989): 387–391.

6. E. N. Whitney, C. B. Cataldo, L. K. DeBruyne, and S. R. Rolfes, *Nutrition for Health and Health Care* (St. Paul: West, 1995), p. 555.

7. V. Woolf, *A Room of One's Own* (New York: Harcourt Brace, 1929), p. 30.

8. J. Avorn and coauthors, Reduction of bacteriuria and pyuria after ingestion of cranberry juice, *Journal of the American Medical Association* 271 (1994): 751–754.

9. *Teaching Tolerance,* Southern Poverty Law Center, 400 Washington Avenue, Montgomery, AL 36104.

10. U.S. Department of Agriculture, *Dietary Guidelines for Americans,* Garden Bulletin No. 232 (Washington, D.C.: Government Printing Office, 1995), p. 8.

11. A. A. Hertzler and R. Frary, Dietary status and eating out practices of college students, *Journal of the American Dietetic Association* 92 (1992): 867–869.

12. National Center for Health Statistics, *Healthy People 2000 Review: Health United States 1992* (Hyattsville, Md.: Public Health Service, 1993), p. 252.

13. N. S. Scrimshaw, Nutrition and health from womb to tomb, *Nutrition Today,* March/April 1996, pp. 55–67.

14. *Healthy People 2000: National Health Promotion and Disease Prevention Objectives* (Washington, D.C.: U.S. Department of Health and Human Services, 1990).

15. J. M. McGinnis and P. R. Lee, Healthy People 2000 at mid decade, *Journal of the American Medical Association* 273 (1995): 1123–1129.

16. B. Ervin and D. Reed, eds., Fruit and vegetable consumption, *Nutrition Monitoring in the United States: Chartbook I* (Hyattsville, Md.: Public Health Service, 1993), p. 30.

17. Fast food and the American diet, Chapter 7 in *Issues in Nutrition* (New York: American Council on Science and Health, 1991): 26-29.

18. The single food fallacy, Chapter 2 in *Issues in Nutrition* (New York: American Council on Science and Health, 1991), pp. 46–47.

19. S. P. Murphy, D. Rose, M. Hudes, and F. E. Viteri, Demographic and economic factors associated with dietary quality for adults in the 1987–88 Nationwide Food Consumption Survey, *Journal of the American Dietetic Association* 92 (1992): 1352–1357.

20. Convenient food and the new household economics, *Journal of the American Dietetic Association* 92 (1992): 981.

21. R. G. Hansen, Why calories count: Communicating moderation and a balanced diet, *Food Technology,* October 1991, pp. 86–93.

CONTROVERSY I

1. D. M. Eisenberg and coauthors, Unconventional medicine in the United States: Prevalence, costs, and patterns of use, *New England Journal of Medicine* 328 (1993): 246–252.

2. P. Kurtzweil, Phony doctor sentenced, *FDA Consumer,* March 1995, p. 32.

3. J. M. Ashley and W. T. Jarvis, Position of the American Dietetic Association: Food and nutrition misinformation, *Journal of the American Dietetic Association* 95 (1995): 705–707.

4. R. Wyden, *Deception and Fraud in the Diet Industry,* part I, serial no. 101-50 (Washington, D.C.: Government Printing Office, 1990), p. 1.

5. E. A. Young, National Dairy Council award for excellence in medical/dental nutrition education lecture, 1992: Perspective on nutrition in medical education, *American Journal of Clinical Nutrition* 56 (1992): 745–751.

6. A. G. Swanson, 1990 ASCN Nutrition educators' symposium and information exchange: Nutrition sciences in medical-student education, *American Journal of Clinical Nutrition* 53 (1991): 587–588.

7. National Nutrition Monitoring and Related Research Act of 1990, Public Law 101-445, as quoted in C. H. Halstead, Toward standardized training of physicians in clinical nutrition, *American Journal of Clinical Nutrition* 56 (1992): 1–3.

8. Position of the American Dietetic Association: Nutrition education of health professionals, *Journal of the American Dietetic Association* 91 (1991): 611–613.

9. M. T. Kane and coauthors, Role delineation for dietetic practitioners: Empirical results, *Journal of the American Dietetic Association* 90 (1990): 1124–1133.

10. B. Haughton and J. Shaw, Functional roles of today's public health nutritionist, *Journal of the American Dietetic Association* 92 (1992): 1218–1222.

11. D. A. Dougherty and J. Garey, President's page: ADA support for licensing, *Journal of the American Dietetic Association* 89 (1989): 1508–1510.

CHAPTER 2

1. USDA Center for Nutrition Policy and Promotion, *The Healthy Eating Index* (Washington, D.C.: Government Printing Office, 1995).

2. Food and Nutrition Board, *Recommended Dietary Allowances*, 10th ed. (Washington, D.C.: National Academy of Sciences, 1989).

3. Food and Nutrition Board, How Should the Recommended Dietary Allowances Be Revised? (booklet) (Washington, D.C.: National Academy Press, 1994).

4. L. J. Machlin and H. E. Sauberlich, New views on the function and health effects of vitamins, *Nutrition Today*, January/February 1994, pp. 25–29; Food and Nutrition Board, 1994.

5. J. Hallfrisch and coauthors, Acceptability of a 7-day higher-carbohydrate, lower-fat menu: The Beltsville Diet Study, *Journal of the American Dietetic Association* 88 (1988): 163–168.

6. J. Dollahite, D. Franklin, and R. McNew, Problems encountered in meeting the Recommended Dietary Allowances for menus designed according to the Dietary Guidelines for Americans, *Journal of the American Dietetic Association* 95 (1995): 341–345.

7. E. N. Siguel, Role of essential fatty acids: Dangers in the U.S. Department of Agriculture dietary recommendations and in low-fat diets, *American Journal of Clinical Nutrition* (1994): 973–974.

8. L. R. Young and M. Nestle, Portion sizes in dietary assessment: Issues and policy implications, *Nutrition Reviews* 53 (1995): 149–158.

9. J. E. Foulke, Cooking up the new food label, *FDA Consumer*, May 1993, pp. 33–38.

10. P. Kurtzweil, Food label makes good eating easier, *FDA Consumer*, September 1995, pp. 16–19.

CONTROVERSY 2

1. F. Berrino and P. Muti, Mediterranean diet and cancer, *European Journal of Clinical Nutrition* 43 (1989): 49–55.

2. A. Trichopoulou, Correspondence, *New England Journal of Medicine* 327 (1992): 53.

3. World Health Organization, Life expectancy, number of survivors, and chances in 1000 of eventually dying from specified causes, at selected ages, by sex, latest available year, in *World Health Statistics Annual* (Geneva: World Health Organization, 1989), pp. 158–163.

4. World Health Organization, 1989.

5. F. M. Sacks and W. W. Willet, More on chewing the fat: The good fat and the good cholesterol (editorial), *New England Journal of Medicine* 325 (1991): 1740–1742.

6. M. Nestle, Mediterranean diets: Historical and research overview, *American Journal of Clinical Nutrition* 61 (1995): 1313S–1320S.

7. A. P. Simopoulos, The Mediterranean Food Guide, *Nutrition Today*, March/April 1995, pp. 54–61.

8. The Mediterranean diet and food culture—a symposium, *European Journal of Clinical Nutrition* (Supplement) 43 (1989).

9. L. Masana and coauthors, The Mediterranean-type diet: Is there a need for further modification? *American Journal of Clinical Nutrition* 53 (1991): 886–889.

10. J. C. Waterlow, Diet of the classical period of Greece and Rome, *European Journal of Clinical Nutrition* 43 (1989): 3–12.

11. D. Kromhout and coauthors, Food consumption patterns in the 1960s in seven countries, *American Journal of Clinical Nutrition* 49 (1989): 889–894.

12. J. W. Anderson, B. M. Smith, and N. J. Gustafson, Health benefits and practical aspects of high-fiber diets, *American Journal of Clinical Nutrition* 59 (1994): 1242S–1247S.

13. D. E. Thomas, J. R. Brotherhood, and J. C. Brand, Carbohydrate feeding before exercise: Effect of glycemic index, *International Journal of Sports Medicine* 12 (1991): 180–186.

14. P. B. Geil and J. W. Anderson, Nutrition and health implications of dry beans: A review, *Journal of the American College of Nutrition* 13 (1994): 549–558; American Dietetic Association, Nutrition recommendations and principles for people with diabetes mellitus, *Diabetes Care* 17 (1994): 519.

15. S. Mackay and J. J. Ball, Do beans and oat bran add to the effectiveness of a low-fat diet? *European Journal of Clinical Nutrition* 46 (1992): 641–648.

16. J. W. Anderson and coauthors, Meta-analysis of the effects of soy protein intake on serum lipids, *New England Journal of Medicine* 333 (1995); 276–282.

17. L. Schweigerer and J. Fotis, Genistein, a dietary-derived inhibitor of in vitro angiogenesis, *Proceedings of the National Academy of Sciences*, 90 (1993): 2690–2694.

18. P. Leatherwood and P. Pollet, as cited by Geil and Anderson, 1994.

19. Sacks and Willett, 1991.

20. T. W. A. de Bruin and coauthors, Different postprandial metabolism of olive oil and soybean oil: A possible mechanism of the high-density lipoprotein conserving effect of olive oil, *American Journal of Clinical Nutrition* 58 (1993): 477–483.

21. S. M. Grundy and M. A. Denke, Dietary influences on serum lipids and lipoproteins, *Journal of Lipid Research* 31 (1990): 1149–1172; P. Mata and coauthors, Effects of long-term monounsaturated- vs polyunsaturated-enriched diets on lipoproteins in healthy men and women, *American Journal of Clinical Nutrition* 55 (1992): 846–850; M. B. Katan, P. L. Zock, and R. P. Mensink, Effects of fats and fatty acids on blood lipids in humans: An overview, *American Journal of Clinical Nutrition* 60 (1994): 1017S–1022S.

22. B. Halliwell and S. Chirico, Lipid peroxidation: Its mechanism, measurement, and significance, *American Journal of Clinical Nutrition* 57 (1993): 715S–725S; P. Reaven and coauthors, Feasibility of using an oleate-rich diet to reduce the susceptibility of low-density lipoprotein to oxidative modification in humans, *American Journal of Clinical Nutrition* 54 (1991): 701–706.

23. D. M. Hegsted, Dietary fat and serum lipids: An evaluation of the experimental data, *American Journal of Clinical Nutrition* 57 (1993): 875–883.

24. B. R. Goldin, Anticarcinogenic properties of cultured dairy products (abstract), *Supplement to the Journal of the American Dietetic Association* (1989): A157.

25. E. Hilton and coauthors, Ingestion of yogurt containing *Lactobacillus acidophilus* as prophylaxis for candidal vaginitis, *Annals of Internal Medicine* 116 (1992): 353–357.

26. Yogurt and the immune system, *Tallahassee Democrat*, December 12, 1992.

27. J. M. Gaziano and coauthors, Moderate alcohol intake, increased levels of high-density lipoprotein and its subfractions, and decreased risk of myocardial infarction, *New England Journal of Medicine* 329 (1993): 1829–1834; P. R. Ridker and coauthors, Association of moderate alcohol consumption and plasma concentration of endogenous tissue-type plasminogen activator, *Journal of the American Medical Association* 272 (1994): 929–933.

28. C. S. Fuchs and coauthors, Alcohol consumption and mortality among women, *New England Journal of Medicine* 332 (1995): 1245–1250.

29. T. A. Pearson and P. Terry, What to advise patients about drinking alcohol—The clinician's conundrum, *Journal of the American Medical Association* 272 (1994): 967–968.

30. W. P. T. James, G. G. Duthie, and K. W. J. Wahle, The Mediterranean diet: Protective or simply nontoxic? *European Journal of Clinical Nutrition* 43 (1989): 31–41.

31. K. Meister, The not-so-great Mediterranean diet pyramid, *Priorities* 7 (1995): 14–18.

CHAPTER 3

1. J. E. Benson and coauthors, Relationship between nutrient intake, body mass index, menstrual function, and ballet injury, *Journal of the American Dietetic Association* 89 (1989): 58–63.

2. G. A. Falciglia and P. A. Norton, Evidence for a genetic influence on preference for some foods, *Journal of the American Dietetic Association* 94 (1994): 154–158.

3. D. R. Morse and coauthors, Oral digestion of a complex-carbohydrate cereal: Effects of stress and relaxation of physiological and salivary measures, *American Journal of Clinical Nutrition* 49 (1989): 97–105.

4. P. M. Brannon, Adaptation of the exocrine pancreas to diet, *Annual Review of Nutrition* 10 (1990): 85–105.

5. Brannon, 1990.

6. J. L. Jeraci, B. A. Lewis, and P. J. Van Soest, Interaction between human gut bacteria and fiberous structures, in G. A. Spiller, ed., *Dietary Fiber in Human Nutrition* (Boca Raton: CRC Press, 1993), pp. 371–376.

7. J. H. Meyer, The stomach and nutrition, in M. E. Shils, J. A. Olson, and M. Shike, eds., *Modern Nutrition in Health and Diseases* (Philadelphia: Lea & Febiger, 1994), pp. 1029–1035.

CONTROVERSY 3

1. A. E. Harper, 1990 Atwater Lecture: The science and the practice of nutrition: Reflections and directions, *American Journal of Clinical Nutrition* 53 (1991): 413–420.

2. S. M. Garn and W. R. Leonard, What did our ancestors eat? *Nutrition Reviews* 47 (1989): 337–345.

3. Garn and Leonard, 1989.

4. J. C. Brand and coauthors, Plasma glucose and insulin responses to traditional Pima Indian meals, *American Journal of Clinical Nutrition* 51 (1990): 416–420.

5. B. A. Swinburn, Deterioration in carbohydrate metabolism and lipoprotein changes induced by modern, high-fat diet in Pima Indians and Caucasians, *Journal of Clinical Endocrinology and Metabolism* 73 (1991): 156–165.

6. L. Seachrist, Gene ups obesity, accelerates diabetes, *Science News* 148 (1995): 103.

7. W. Hoy, A. Light, and D. Megill, Cardiovascular disease in Navajo Indians with type 2 diabetes, *Public Health Reports* 100 (1995): 87–94.

8. N. J. Murphy and coauthors, Dietary change and obesity associated with glucose intolerance in Alaskan natives, *Journal of the American Dietetic Association* 95 (1995): 676–682.

9. R. Fabsitz, Administrator of the Strong Heart Study, as quoted by K. A. Fackelmann, *Science News* 142 (1992): 168–170.

10. M. Segal, Native food preparation fosters botulism, *FDA Consumer*, January/February 1992, pp. 23–26.

CHAPTER 4

1. G. Annison and D. L. Topping, Nutritional role of resistant starch: Chemical structures vs physiological function, *Annual Review of Nutrition* 14 (1994): 297–320.

2. J. L. Jeraci, B. A. Lewis, and P. J. Van Soest, Interaction between human gut bacteria and fibrous substrates, in G. A. Spiller, ed., *Dietary Fiber in Human Nutrition* (Boca Raton: CRC Press, 1993), pp. 371–376.

3. C. M. Ripsin and coauthors, Oat products and lipid lowering: A meta-analysis, *Journal of the American Medical Association* 267 (1992): 3317–3325; S. R. Glore and coauthors, Soluble fiber and serum lipids: A literature review, *Journal of the American Dietetic Association* 94 (1994): 425–436; E. B. Rinim and coauthors, Vegetable, fruit, and cereal fiber intake and risk of coronary heart disease among men, *Journal of the American Medical Association* 275 (1996): 447–451.

4. M. A. Eastwood, The physiological effects of dietary fiber: An update, *Annual Review of Nutrition* 12 (1992): 19–35.

5. J. F. Swain and coauthors, Comparison of the effects of oat bran and low-fiber wheat on serum lipoprotein levels and blood pressure, *New England Journal of Medicine* 322 (1990): 147–152.

6. Dietary fibre: Importance of function as well as amount, *Lancet* 340 (1992): 1133–1134.

7. L. Cara and coauthors, Effects of oat bran, rice bran, wheat fiber, and wheat germ on postprandial lipemia in healthy adults, *American Journal of Clinical Nutrition* 55 (1992): 81–88.

8. L. U. Thompson, Antioxidants and hormone-mediated health benefits of whole grains, *Food Science and Nutrition* 34 (1994): 473–497.

9. S. Welsh and J. F. Guthrie, Changing American diets, in A. Bendich and C. E. Butterworth, Jr., eds., *Micronutrients in Health and in Disease Prevention* (New York: Marcel Dekker, 1991), pp. 381–408.

10. Food and Nutrition Board, *Recommended Dietary Allowances,* 10th ed. (Washington, D.C.: National Academy of Sciences, 1989), p. 42.

11. WHO Study Group on Diet, Nutrition, and Prevention of Noncommunicable Diseases, Diet, nutrition, and the prevention of chronic diseases, *Nutrition Reviews* 49 (1991): 291–301.

12. S. G. Cooper and E. J. Tracey, Small-bowel obstruction caused by oat-bran bezoar, *New England Journal of Medicine* 320 (1989): 1148–1149.

13. R. J. Hine, What practitioners need to know about folic acid, *Journal of the American Dietetic Association* 96 (1996): 451–452.

14. K. R. Silvester, H. N. Englyst, and J. H. Cummings, Ileal recovery of starch from whole diets containing resistant starch measured in vitro and fermentation of ileal efferent, *American Journal of Clinical Nutrition* 62 (1995): 403–411.

15. D. A. T. Southgate, Digestion and metabolism of sugars, *American Journal of Clinical Nutrition* 62 (1995): 203S–211S.

F

16. Eastwood, 1992.

17. Annison and Topping, 1994.

18. J. M. Saavedra and J. A. Perman, Current concepts in lactose malabsorption and intolerance, *Annual Review of Nutrition* 9 (1989): 475–502.

19. F. L. Suarez, D. A. Savaiano, and M. D. Levitt, A comparison of symptoms after the consumption of milk or lactose-hydrolyzed milk by people with self-reported severe lactose intolerance, *New England Journal of Clinical Nutrition* 333 (1995): 1–4; A. O. Johnson and coauthors, Adaptation of lactose maldigesters to continued milk intakes, *American Journal of Clinical Nutrition* 58 (1993); 879–881.

20. Food and Nutrition Board, 1989, p. 41.

21. J. C. B. Miller, Importance of glycemic index in diabetes, *American Journal of Clinical Nutrition* (supplement) 59 (1994): 747S–752S.

22. K. Indar-Brown, C. Noreberg, and Z. Madar, Glycemic and insulinemic responses after ingestion of ethnic foods by NIDDM and healthy subjects, *American Journal of Clinical Nutrition* 55 (1992): 89–95: T. M. Wolever and coauthors, The glycemic index: Methodology and clinical implications, *American Journal of Clinical Nutrition* 54 (1991): 846–854.

23. E. Jequier, Carbohydrates as a source of energy, *American Journal of Clinical Nutrition* (supplement) 59 (1994): 682S–685S.

24. M. F. Saad and coauthors, A two-step model for development of non-insulin-dependent diabetes, *American Journal of Medicine* 90 (1991): 229–235.

25. L. Ressetti, A. Giaccari, and R. A. DeFronzo, Glucose toxicity, *Diabetes Care* 13 (1990): 610–630.

26. G. A. Colditz and coauthors, Weight gain as a risk factor for clinical diabetes mellitus in women, *Annals of Internal Medicine* 122 (1995): 481–486.

27. H. Shimokata and coauthors, Age as independent determinant of glucose tolerance, *Diabetes* 40 (1991): 44–51; M. J. Busby, Glucose tolerance in women: The effects of age, body composition, and sex hormones, *Journal of the American Geriatric Society* 40 (1992): 497–502.

28. T. L. Holbrook, E. Barrett-Connor, and D. L. Wingard, A prospective population-based study of alcohol use and non-insulin-dependent diabetes mellitus, *American Journal of Epidemiology* 132 (1990): 902–909.

29. E. T. Skarfos, K. I. Selinus, and H. O. Lithell, Risk factors for developing non-insulin dependent diabetes: A 10 year follow-up of men in Uppsala, *British Medical Journal* 303 (21 September 1991): 755–760.

30. J. Randal, Insulin key to diabetes but not a full cure, *FDA Consumer*, May 1992, pp. 15–19.

31. D. M. Nathan, Long-term complications of diabetes mellitus, *New England Journal of Medicine* 328 (1993): 1676–1685.

32. M. W. Steffes and S. M. Mauer, Toward a basic understanding of diabetic complications, *New England Journal of Medicine* 325 (1991): 883–884.

33. Position statement: Nutrition recommendations and principles for people with diabetes mellitus, *Diabetes Care* 17 (1994): 519–522; A. Monk and coauthors, Practice guidelines for medical nutrition therapy provided by dietitians for persons with non-insulin-dependent diabetes mellitus, *Journal of the American Dietetic Association* 95 (1995): 999–1006.

34. B. Vessby, Dietary carbohydrates in diabetes, *American Journal of Clinical Nutrition* (supplement) 59 (1994): 742S–746S.

35. Position statement: Nutrition recommendations and principles for people with diabetes mellitus, 1994.

36. S. P. Helmrich and coauthors, Physical activity and reduced occurrence of non-insulin-dependent diabetes mellitus, *New England Journal of Medicine* 325 (1991): 147–152; A dissenting view appears in a letter by R. S. Surwitt and J. D. Lane, Physical activity and non-insulin-dependent diabetes mellitus, *New England Journal of Medicine* 325 (1991): 1887.

37. F. J. Service, Hypoglycemia and the postprandial syndrome, *New England Journal of Medicine* 321 (1989): 1472–1474.

38. K. S. Polonsky, A practical approach to fasting hypoglycemia, *New England Journal of Medicine* 326 (1992): 1020–1021.

39. J. Palardy and coauthors, Blood glucose measurements during symptomatic episodes in patients with suspected postprandial hypoglycemia, *New England Journal of Medicine* 3211 (1989): 1421–1425.

40. R. Lozano, S. A. Chalew, and A. A. Kowarski, Cornstarch ingestion after oral glucose loading: Effect on glucose concentrations, hormone response, and symptoms in patients with postprandial hypoglycemic syndrome, *American Journal of Clinical Nutrition* 52 (1990): 667–670.

41. Palardy and coauthors, 1989.

42. D. J. A. Jenkins and coauthors, Low glycemic index: Lente carbohydrates and physiological effects of altered food frequency, *American Journal of Clinical Nutrition* (supplement) 59 (1994): 706S–709S.

43. W. H. Glinsmann and Y. K. Park, Perspective on the 1986 Food and Drug Administration assessment of the safety of carbohydrate sweeteners: Uniform definitions and recommendations for future assessments, *American Journal of Clinical Nutrition* 62 (1995): 161S–169S.

44. Position of the American Dietetic Association: Health implications of dietary fiber, *Journal of the American Dietetic Association* 93 (1993): 1446–1447.

CONTROVERSY 4

1. U.S. Department of Agriculture, Sugar and sweetener situation and outlook report, March 1996, p. 3–4.

2. W. H. Glinsmann and Y. K. Park, Perspective on the 1986 Food and Drug Administration assessment of the safety of carbohydrate sweeteners: Uniform definitions and recommendations for future assessments, *American Journal of Clinical Nutrition* 62 (1995): 1615–1695.

3. U.S. Department of Agriculture, 1996, p. 6.

4. C. J. Lewis and coauthors, Nutrient intakes and body weights of persons consuming high and moderate levels of added sugars, *Journal of the American Dietetic Association* 92 (1992): 708–713.

5. A. L. Peters, M. B. Davidson, and K. Eisenberg, Effect of isocaloric substitution of chocolate cake for potato in type 1 diabetic patients, *Diabetes Care* 13 (1990): 888–892.

6. C. A. Beebe and coauthors, Nutrition management for individuals with noninsulin-dependent diabetes mellitus in the 1990s: A review by the Diabetes Care and Education Dietetic Practice Group, *Journal of the American Dietetic Association* 91 (1991): 196–202, 205–207; Nutrition Subcommittee of the British Diabetic Association's Professional Advisory Committee, Dietary recommendations for people with diabetes: An update for the 1990s, *Diabetes Medicine* 9 (1992): 189–202.

7. M. K. Lockwood and C. D. Eckhert, Sucrose-induced lipid, glucose, and insulin elevations, microvascular injury, and selenium, *American Journal of Physiology* 262 (1992): R144–R149.

8. K. N. Frayn and S. M. Kingman, Dietary sugars and lipid metabolism in humans, *American Journal of Clinical Nutrition* 62 (1995): 250S–263S.

9. Frayn and Kingman, 1995.

10. American Heart Association Nutrition Committee, Dietary guidelines for healthy American adults, *Circulation* 94 (1996): 1795–1800.

11. T. W. Jones and coauthors, Oral glucose provokes excessive adrenomedullary and symptomatic responses in normal children, *Pediatric Notes* 14 (1990): 86.

12. E. H. Wender and M. V. Solunto, Effects of sugar on aggressive and inattentive behavior in children with attention deficit disorder with hyperactivity and normal children, *Pediatrics* 88 (1991): 960–966.

13. S. Saravis, Aspartame: Effects on learning, behavior, and mood, *Pediatrics* 86 (1990): 75–83.

14. J. Bachorowski and coauthors, Sucrose and delinquency behavioral assessment, *Pediatrics* 86 (1990): 244–253.

15. J. W. White and M. Wolraich, Effect of sugar on behavior and mental performance, *American Journal of Clinical Nutrition* 62 (1995): 242S–249S.

16. A. Sheiham, Why free sugar consumption should be below 15 kg per person per year in industrial countries: The dental evidence, *British Dental Journal* 171 (1991): 63–65.

17. K. G. König and J. M. Navia, Nutritional role of sugars in oral health, *American Journal of Clinical Nutrition* 62 (1995): 275S–283S.

18. Dr. Thomas Truhe as quoted in E. Whitford, Dentists target starch as real cavity friend, *Atlanta Constitution*, 26 March 1991, pp. D1, D10.

19. Sheiham, 1991.

20. National Research Council Committee on Diet and Health, *Diet and Health: Implications for Reducing Chronic Disease Risk* (Washington, D.C., National Academy Press, 1989), p. 279.

21. B. Szepesi, Carbohydrates, *Present Knowledge in Nutrition*, 6th ed. (Washington, D.C.: ILSI Press, 1996), pp. 33–43.

22. WHO study group on Diet, Nutrition and Preventing Noncommunicable Diseases, Diet, nutrition and the prevention of chronic diseases, *Nutrition Reviews* 49 (1991): 291.

23. F. R. J. Bonet, Undigestible sugars in food products, *American Journal of Clinical Nutrition* 59 (1994): 763S–769S.

24. W. L. Dills, Sugar alcohols as bulk sweeteners, *Annual Review of Nutrition* (1989): 161–186.

25. E. K. Salminen and coauthors, Xylitol vs glucose: Effect on the rate of gastric emptying and motilin, insulin, and gastric inhibitory polypeptide release, *American Journal of Clinical Nutrition* 49 (1989): 1228–1232.

26. Position of the American Dietetic Association: Use of nutritive and nonnutritive sweeteners, *Journal of the American Dietetic Association* 93 (1993): 816–821.

27. S. Cohen and coauthors, Saccharin and urothelial proliferation: A threshold phenomenon, *FASEB Journal* 6 (1992): A1594.

28. Quantitative Regulation (180.37), D. Plumb, FDA Center for Food and Nutrition Safety, *Personal Communication*, 6 July 1992.

29. A bibliography of 167 research articles on aspartame can be found in J. Van de Kamp, Adverse effects of aspartame, *Current Bibliographies in Medicine* (Washington, D.C.: Government Printing Office, 1991).

30. Aspartame, *FDA Consumer,* October 1991, p. 35.

31. L. Tollefson and R. J. Barnard, An analysis of FDA passive surveillance reports of seizures associated with consumption of aspartame, *Journal of the American Dietetic Association* 92 (1992): 598–601.

32. Health and Welfare Canada, *Nutrition Recommendations* (Ottawa: Canadian Government Printing Centre, 1990), p. 190.

33. M. G. Tordoff and M. I. Friedman, Drinking saccharin increases food intake and preference—I. Comparison with other drinks, *Appetite* 12 (1989): 1–10; M. G. Tordoff and M. I. Friedman, Drinking saccharin increases food intake and preference—II. Hydrational factors, *Appetite* 12 (1989): 11–21; M. G. Tordoff and M. I. Friedman, Drinking saccharin increases food intake and preference—III. Sensory and associative factors, *Appetite* 12 (1989): 23–36; M. G. Tordoff and M. I. Friedman, Drinking saccharin increases food intake and preference—IV. Cephalic phase and metabolic factors, Appetite 12 (1989): 37–56.

34. D. J. Canty and M. M. Chan, Effects of consumption of caloric vs noncaloric sweet drinks on indices of hunger and food consumption in normal adults, *American Journal of Clinical Nutrition* 53 (1991): 1159–1164; B. J. Rolls, Effects of intense sweeteners on hunger, food intake, and body weight: A review, *American Journal of Clinical Nutrition* 53 (1991): 872–878; L. A. Chen and E. S. Parham, College students' use of high-intensity sweeteners is not consistently associated with sugar consumption, *Journal of the American Dietetic Association* 91 (1991): 686–690.

35. A. Drewnowski and coauthors, Comparing the effects of aspartame and sucrose on motivational ratings, taste preferences, and energy intake in humans, *American Journal of Clinical Nutrition* 59 (1994): 338–345.

36. A. Drewnowski, Intense sweeteners and control of appetite, *Nutrition Reviews* 53 (1995): 1–7.

37. Cantry and Chan, 1991; G. H. Anderson, Sugars, sweetness, and food intake, *American Journal of Clinical Nutrition* 62 (1995): 195S–202S.

38. Position of the American Dietetic Association, 1993.

39. Position of the American Dietetic Association, 1993.

CHAPTER 5

1. R. L. Leibel, Fat as fuel and metabolic signal, *Nutrition Reviews* 50 (1992): II12–II16.

2. J. E. Blundell and coauthors, Control of human appetite: Implications for the intake of dietary fat, *Annual Review of Nutrition* 16 (1996): 285–319.

3. D. Kritchevsky, Preface to the PORIM International Palm Oil Development Conference, *American Journal of Clinical Nutrition* 53 (1991): v.

4. M. B. Katan, P. L. Zock, and R. P. Mensink, Effects of fats and fatty acids on blood lipids in humans: An overview, *American Journal of Clinical Nutrition* 60 (1994): 1017S–1022S.

5. M. Hamosh, *Lingual and Gastric Lipases: Their Role in Fat Digestion* (Boston: CRC Press, 1990).

6. A. B. R. Thompson, Intestinal aspects of lipid absorption, *Nutrition Today*, July/August 1989, pp. 16–20.

7. D. R. Saunders and J. K. Sillery, Absorption of triglyceride by human small intestine: Dose-response relationship, *American Journal of Clinical Nutrition* 48 (1988): 988–991.

F

8. NIH Consensus Conference, Triglyceride, high-density lipoprotein, and coronary heart disease, *Journal of the American Medical Association* 269 (1993): 505–510.

9. All major nutrition, health, and governmental agencies concur on this point. For a dissenting view, see T. L. V. Ulbright and D. A. T. Southgate, Coronary heart disease: Seven dietary factors, *Lancet* 338 (1991): 985–992.

10. K. K. Carroll, Dietary fats and cancer, *American Journal of Clinical Nutrition* 53 (1991): 1064S–1067S; D. F. Birt, The influence of dietary fat on carcinogenesis: Lessons from experimental models, *Nutrition Reviews* 48 (1990): 1–5; K. L. Erickson and N. E. Hubbard, Dietary fat and tumor metastasis, *Nutrition Reviews* 48 (1990): 6–14.

11. D. M. Hegsted, Dietary fatty acids, serum cholesterol and coronary heart disease, in G. J. Nelson, ed., *Health Effects of Dietary Fatty Acids* (Champaign, Ill.: American Oil Chemists Society, 1991), pp. 50–68.

12. NIH Consensus Development Panel, Triglyceride, high-density lipoprotein, and coronary heart disease, *Journal of the American Medical Society* 269 (1993): 505–510.

13. Hegsted, 1991; Ulbright and Southgate, 1991.

14. D. J. McNamara, Cardiovascular disease, in M. E. Shils, J. A. Olson, and M. Shike, eds., *Modern Nutrition in Health and Disease* (Philadelphia: Lea & Febiger, 1994), pp. 1533–1544.

15. B. Halliwell, Oxidation of low-density lipoproteins: Questions of initiation, propagation, and the effect of antioxidants, *American Journal of Clinical Nutrition* 61 (1995): 670S–677S.

16. C. A. Drevon, Marine oils and their effects, *Nutrition Reviews* 50 (1992): 38–45; A. P. Simopoulos, Omega-3 fatty acids in health and disease and in growth and development, *American Journal of Clinical Nutrition* 54 (1991): 438–463.

17. J. Dyerberg, Linolenate-derived polyunsaturated fatty acids and prevention of atherosclerosis, *Nutrition Reviews* 44 (1986): 125–134; J. P. Middaugh, Cardiovascular deaths among Alaskan Natives, 1980–1986, *American Journal of Public Health* 80 (1990): 282–285.

18. M. D. Boudreau and coauthors, Lack of dose response by dietary ω-3 fatty acids at a constant ratio of ω-3 to ω-6 fatty acids in suppressing eicosanoid biosynthesis from arachidonic acid, *American Journal of Clinical Nutrition* 54 (1991): 111–117.

19. M. B. Katan, Fish and heart disease: What is the real story? *Nutrition Reviews* 53 (1995): 228–230.

20. D. S. Siscovick and coauthors, Dietary intake and cell membrane levels of long-chain ω-3 polyunsaturated fatty acids and the risk of primary cardiac arrest, *Journal of the American Medical Association* 274 (1995): 1363–1367; R. F. Gillum, M. E. Mussolino, and J. H. Madans, The relationship between fish consumption and stroke incidence: The NHANES I Epidemiologic Follow-up Study, *Archives of Internal Medicine* 156 (1996): 537–542.

21. Fish oil supplements, *FDA Consumer*, October 1990, p. 32.

22. K. N. Seidelin, B. Myrup, and B. Fischer-Hanson, ω-3 fatty acids in adipose tissue and coronary artery disease are inversely related, *American Journal of Clinical Nutrition* 55 (1992): 1117–1119; K. H. Bønaa, K. S. Bjerve, and A. Nordøy, Habitual fish consumption, plasma phospholipid fatty acids, and serum lipids: The Tromsø, Study, *American Journal of Clinical Nutrition* 55 (1992): 1126–1134.

23. Katan, 1995.

24. S. J. Bhathena and coauthors, Effects of ω-3 fatty acids and vitamin E on hormones involved in carbohydrate and lipid metabolism in men, *American Journal of Clinical Nutrition* 54 (1991): 684–688.

25. C. D. Berdanier, ω-3 Fatty acids: A panacea?, *Nutrition Today,* July/August 1994, pp. 28–32.

26. O. Haglund and coauthors, The effects of fish oil on triglycerides, cholesterol, fibrinogen, and malondialdehyde in humans supplemented with vitamin E, *Journal of Nutrition* 121 (1991): 165–169.

27. A. P. Simopoulos and coauthors, Conferences, Symposia, and Reports, *Nutrition Today*, July/August 1994, pp. 24–27.

28. D. A. Hughes and coauthors, Fish oil supplementation inhibits the expression of major histocompatibility complex class II molecules and adhesion molecules on human monocytes, *American Journal of Clinical Nutrition* 63 (1996): 267–272.

29. G. T. Gerhard and coauthors, Comparison of three species of dietary fish: Effects on serum concentrations of low-density-lipoprotein cholesterol and apolipoprotein in normotriglyceridemic subjects, *American Journal of Clinical Nutrition* 54 (1991): 334–339; K. L. Radack, C. C. Deck, and G. A. Huster, ω-3 fatty acid effects on lipids, lipoproteins, and apolipoproteins at very low doses: Results of a randomized controlled trial in hypertriglyceridemic subjects, *American Journal of Clinical Nutrition* 51 (1990): 599–605.

30. E. A. Emken, *Trans*-fatty acids and coronary heart disease: Physiochemical properties, intake, and metabolism, *American Journal of Clinical Nutrition* 62 (1995): 655S–708S.

31. ASCN/AIN Task Force on *Trans*-fatty acids, Position paper on *trans*-fatty acids, *American Journal of Clinical Nutrition* 63 (1996): 663–670.

32. J. T. Judd and coauthors, Dietary *trans* fatty acids: Effects on plasma lipids and lipoproteins of healthy men and women, *American Journal of Clinical Nutrition* 59 (1994): 861–868; A. Ascherio and coauthors, *Trans*-fatty acid intake and risk of myocardial infarction, *Circulation* 89 (1994): 94–101; M. B. Katan, P. L. Zock, and R. P. Mensink, *Trans*-fatty acid and their effects on lipoproteins in humans, *Annual Review of Nutrition* 15 (1995): 473–493; M. B. Katan, Commentary on the supplement *trans*-fatty acids and coronary heart disease risk, *American Journal of Clinical Nutrition* 62 (1995): 518–519.

33. M. B. Katan and R. P. Mensink, Isomeric fatty acids and serum lipoproteins, *Nutrition Reviews* 50 (1992): 46–48; S. S. Jonnalagadda and coauthors, Effects of individual fatty acids on chronic diseases, *Nutrition Today*, May/June 1996, pp. 90–106.

34. M. G. Enig and coauthors, Isomeric *trans*-fatty acids in the U.S. diet, *Journal of the American College of Nutrition* 9 (1990): 471–486.

35. J. E. Hunter and T. H. Applewhite, Reassessment of *trans*-fatty acid availability in the U.S. diet, *American Journal of Clinical Nutrition* 54 (1991): 363–369.

36. W. C. Willett and A. Ascherio, *Trans*-fatty acids: Are the effects only marginal? *American Journal of Public Health* 84 (1994): 722–724. M. B. Katan, European researcher calls for reconsideration of *trans*-fatty acid, *Journal of the American Dietetic Association* 94 (1994): 1097–1098; W. C. Willett and A. Ascherio, Response to the International Life Sciences Institute report on *trans*-fatty acids, *American Journal of Clinical Nutrition* 62 (1995): 524–526.

37. S. N. Gersholt, Nutrition evaluation of dietary fat substitutes, *Nutrition Reviews* 53 (1995): 305–313.

38. J. A. Westrate and K. H. van het Hof, Sucrose polyester and plasma carotenoid concentrations in healthy subjects, *American Journal of Clinical Nutrition* 62 (1995): 591–597.

39. Position of the American Dietetic Association: Fat replacements, *Journal of the American Dietetic Association* 91 (1991): 1285–1288.

40. A. R. Kristal, A. L. Shattuck, and H. J. Henry, Patterns of dietary behavior associated with selecting diets low in fat: Reliability and validity of a behavioral approach to dietary assessment, *Journal of the American Dietetic Association* 90 (1990): 214–220 present a validated food questionnaire that correlates well with fat intake. Similar principles for reduction of fat by way of meat and milk intakes are found in L. M. Smith-Schneider, M. J. Sigman-Grant, and P. M. Kris-Etherton, Dietary fat reduction strategies, *Journal of the American Dietetic Association* 92 (1992): 34–38.

41. A. R. Kristal and coauthors, Long-term maintenance of a low-fat diet: Durability of fat-related dietary habits in the Women's Health Trial, *Journal of the American Dietetic Association* 92 (1992): 553–559.

CONTROVERSY 5

1. K. R. Westerterp, Food quotient, respiratory quotient, and energy balance, *American Journal of Clinical Nutrition* 57 (1993): 759S–765S.

2. Some of the earliest reports of this effect were from E. B. Forbes and coauthors (1946); the study described here is L. B. Oscai, M. M. Brown, and W. C. Miller, Effect of dietary fat on food intake, growth and body composition in rats, *Growth* 48 (1984): 415–424.

3. G. A. Bray, The nutrient balance approach to obesity, *Nutrition Today* 28 (1993): 13–18.

4. Food and Nutrition Board, *Recommended Dietary Allowances,* 10th ed. (Washington, D.C.: National Academy of Sciences, 1989), p. 33.

5. T. E. Prewitt and coauthors, Changes in body weight, body composition, and energy intakes in women fed high- and low-fat diets, *American Journal of Clinical Nutrition* 54 (1991): 304–310.

6. B. Heitmann, Dietary fat intake and weight gain in women genetically predisposed for obesity, *American Journal of Clinical Nutrition* 61 (1995): 1213–1217.

7. C. Bennet and coauthors, Short-term effects of dietary-fat ingestion on energy expenditure and nutrient balance, *American Journal of Clinical Nutrition* 55 (1992): 1071–1077.

8. W. C. Miller and coauthors, Diet composition, energy intake, and exercise in relation to body fat in men and women, *American Journal of Clinical Nutrition* 52 (1990): 426–430.

9. J. Gregory and coauthors, *The Dietary and Nutritional Survey of British Adults* (London: Office of Population Censuses Survey, HMSO, 1990) as cited in J. E. Blundell and coauthors, Control of human appetite: Implications for the intake of dietary fat, *Annual Review of Nutrition* 16 (1996): 285–319.

10. R. L. Atkinson, Role of diet in obesity treatment, an address presented at the North American Association for the Study of Obesity and Emory University School of Medicine conference Obesity Update: Pathophysiology, Clinical Consequences, and Therapeutic Options, Atlanta, Georgia, August 31–September 2, 1992.

11. R. J. Stubbs and coauthors, Covert manipulation of dietary fat and energy density effect on substrate flux and food intake in men eating ad libitum, *American Journal of Clinical Nutrition* 62 (1995): 316–329.

12. R. J. Stubbs and coauthors, Covert manipulation of the ratio of dietary fat to carbohydrate and energy density: Effect on food intakes and energy balance in free-living men eating ad libitum, *American Journal of Clinical Nutrition* 62 (1995): 330–337.

13. A. Tremblay and coauthors, Impact of dietary fat content and fat oxidation on energy intake in humans, *American Journal of Clinical Nutrition* 49 (1989): 799–805.

14. B. J. Rolls and coauthors, Satiety after preloads with different amounts of fat and carbohydrate: Implications for obesity, *American Journal of Clinical Nutrition* 60 (1994): 476–487.

15. B. J. Rolls and V. A. Hammer, Fat, carbohydrate, and the regulation of energy intake, *American Journal of Clinical Nutrition* 62 (1995): 1086S–1095S.

16. J. P. Flatt, Use and storage of carbohydrate and fat, *American Journal of Clinical Nutrition* 61 (1995): 952S–959S; J. P. Flatt, Carbohydrate balance and food intake regulation (letter), *American Journal of Clinical Nutrition* 62 (1995): 155–156; A. M. Prentice and coauthors, Reply to JP Flatt (letter), *American Journal of Clinical Nutrition* 62 (1995): 156–157.

17. T. J. Horton and coauthors, Fat and carbohydrate overfeeding in humans: Different effects on energy storage, *American Journal of Clinical Nutrition* 62 (1995): 19–29.

18. Flatt, Use and storage of carbohydrate and fat, 1995.

19. Horton and coauthors, 1995.

20. D. E. Larson and coauthors, Ad libitum food intake on a "cafeteria diet" in Native American women: Relations with body composition and 24-h energy expenditure, *American Journal of Clinical Nutrition* 62 (1995): 911–917.

21. G. W. Reed and J. O. Hill, Measuring the thermic effect of food, *American Journal of Clinical Nutrition* 63 (1996): 164–169.

22. M. K. Hellerstein and coauthors, Measurement of de novo hepatic lipogenesis in humans using stable isotopes, *Journal of Clinical Investigation* 87 (1991): 1841–1852; B. Swinburn and E. Ravussin, Energy balance or fat balance? *American Journal of Clinical Nutrition* 57 (1993): 766S–771S.

23. M. K. Hellerstein, J. M. Schwarz, and R. A. Neese, Regulation of hepatic de novo lipogenesis in humans, *Annual Review of Nutrition* 16 (1996): 523–557.

24. J. B. Allred, personal communication, 1996; J. B. Allred and D. F. Bowers, Regulation of acetyl CoA carboxylase and gene expression, in C. D. Berdanier and J. L. Hargrove, eds., *Nutrition and Gene Expression* (Boca Raton: CRC Press, 1992), pp. 269–295.

25. Interagency Board for Nutrition Monitoring and Related Research, *Third Report on Nutrition Monitoring in the United States* (Washington, D.C.: Government Printing Office, 1995), p. 149.

26. Interagency Board for Nutrition Monitoring and Related Research, 1995, pp. 194–195.

CHAPTER 6

1. V. R. Young and J. S. Marchini, Mechanisms and nutritional significance of metabolic responses to altered intakes of protein and amino acids with reference to nutritional adaptation in humans, *American Journal of Clinical Nutrition* 51 (1990): 270–289.

2. Young and Marchini, 1990.

3. D. J. Clauw and P. Katz, Treatment of the eosinophilia-myalgia syndrome, *New England Journal of Medicine* 323 (1990): 417–418; E. A. Belongia, A. N. Mayeno, and M. T. Osterholm, The eosinophilia-myalgia syndrome and tryptophan, *Annual Review of Nutrition* 12 (1992): 235–256; Dietary supplements: Recent chronology and legislation, *Nutrition Reviews* 53 (1995): 31–36.

4. L-Tryptophan recall expanded, *FDA Consumer,* June 1991, pp. 38–39.

5. H. N. Christensen, Amino acid nutrition: A two-step absorptive process, *Nutrition Reviews* 51 (1993): 95–100.

F

6. S. A. Anderson and D. J. Raiten, eds., *Safety of Amino Acids Used as Supplements* (Bethesda, Md.: Federation of American Societies for Experimental Biology, 1992).

7. M. C. Crim and H. N. Munro, Proteins and amino acids, in M. E. Shils, J. A. Olson, and M. Shike, eds., *Modern Nutrition in Health and Disease* (Philadelphia: Lea & Febiger, 1994), p. 31.

8. Young and Marchini, 1990.

9. V. R. Young, Soy protein in relation to human protein and amino acid nutrition, *Journal of the American Dietetic Association* 91 (1991): 828–835.

10. V. R. Young and P. L. Pellett, Plant proteins in relation to human protein and amino acid nutrition, *American Journal of Clinical Nutrition* 59 (1994): 1203S–1212S; Position of the American Dietetic Association: Vegetarian diets, *Journal of the American Dietetic Association* 93 (1993): 1317–1319.

11. Protein Quality Evaluation: Report of a Joint FAO/WHO Expert Consultation, Food and Nutrition paper no. 51 (Rome, Italy: FAO and WHO, 1990).

12. A thorough review of methodology in whole-body protein turnover is provided by J. C. Waterlow, Whole-body protein turnover in humans—past, present, and future, *Annual Review of Nutrition* 15 (1995): 57–92.

13. H. W. Lane and coauthors, Nutrition and human physiological adaptations to space flight, *American Journal of Clinical Nutrition* 58 (1993): 583–588.

14. A full discussion of PEM appears in B. Torun and F. Chew, Protein-energy malnutrition, in M. E. Shils, J. A. Olson, and M. Shike, eds., *Modern Nutrition in Health and Disease* (Philadelphia: Lea & Febiger, 1994), pp. 950–976.

15. C. Gopalan, The contribution of nutrition research to the control of undernutrition: The Indian experience, *Annual Review of Nutrition* 12 (1992): 1–17; D. B. Jelliffe and E. F. P. Jelliffe, Causations of kwashiorkor: Toward a multifactorial consensus, *Pediatrics* 90 (1992): 376–379.

16. J. C. Waterlow, Childhood malnutrition in developing nations: Looking back and forward, *Annual Review of Nutrition* 14 (1994): 1–19.

17. A. P. Delahoussaye and J. L. Jorizzo, Cutaneous manifestations of nutritional disorders, *Dermatologic Clinics* 7 (1989): 559–570.

18. B. D. Woodward and R. G. Miller, Depression of thymus-dependent immunity in wasting protein-energy malnutrition does not depend on an altered ratio of helper (CD4+) to suppressor (CD8+) cells or on a disproportionately large atrophy of the T-cell relative to the B-cell pool, *American Journal of Clinical Nutrition* 53 (1991): 1329–1335; H. P. Redmond and coauthors, Impaired macrophage function in severe protein-energy malnutrition, *Journal of the American Dietetic Association* 91 (1991): 192–195.

19. R. K. Chandra, 1990 McCollum Award Lecture: Nutrition and immunity: Lessons from the past and new insights into the future, *American Journal of Clinical Nutrition* 53 (1991): 1087–1101.

20. M. A. Dhansay, A. J. Benade, and P. R. Donald, Plasma lecithin-cholesterol acyltransferase activity and plasma lipoprotein composition and concentrations in kwashiorkor, *American Journal of Clinical Nutrition* 53 (1991): 512–519.

21. J. C. Wolgemuth and coauthors, Wasting malnutrition and inadequate nutrient intakes identified in a multiethnic homeless population, *Journal of the American Dietetic Association* 92 (1992): 834–839; M. Nestle and S. Guttmacher, Hunger in the United States: Rationale, methods, and policy implications of state hunger surveys, *Journal of Nutrition Education* 24 (1992): 18S–22S; M. Mowe,

T. Bohmer, and E. Kindt, Reduced nutritional status in an elderly population (>70 yrs) is probable before disease and possibly contributes to the development of disease, *American Journal of Clinical Nutrition* 59 (1994): 317–324; J. Dye, Malnourished children in the United States: Caught in the cycle of poverty, *Journal of the American Dietetic Association* 94 (1994): 218; M. L. Taylor, and S. A. Koblinsky, Dietary intake and growth status of young homeless children, *Journal of the American Dietetic Association* 93 (1993): 464–466; Nutritional status of poor children in the United States, *Journal of the American Dietetic Association* 95 (1995): 248–250.

22. J. M. Dodds, S. L. Parker, and P. S. Haines, Hunger in the 80's and 90's: A challenge for nutrition educators, *Journal of Nutrition Education* 24 (1992): 2S.

23. J. W. Anderson and coauthors, Meta-analysis of the effects of soy protein intake on serum lipids, *New England Journal of Medicine* 333 (1995): 276–282.

24. F. E. Ahmed, Effect of diet on progression of chronic renal disease, *Journal of the American Dietetic Association* 91 (1991): 1266–1270.

25. W. H. Chow and coauthors, Protein intake and renal cell cancer, *Journal of the National Cancer Institute* 86 (1994): 1131–1139.

26. J. Hu and coauthors, Dietary intakes and urinary excretion of calcium and acids: A cross-sectional study of women in China, *American Journal of Clinical Nutrition* 58 (1993): 398–406.

27. Food and Nutrition Board, *Recommended Dietary Allowances*, 10th ed. (Washington, D.C.: National Academy of Sciences, 1989), pp. 72–73; C. D. Arnaud and S. D. Danchez, The role of calcium in osteoporosis, *Annual Review of Nutrition* 10 (1990): 397–414; R. P. Heaney, Protein intake and the calcium economy, *Journal of the American Dietetic Association* 93 (1993): 1259–1260.

28. J. A. Metz, J. J. B. Anderson, and P. N. Gallagher, Intakes of calcium, phosphorus, and protein, and physical activity levels are related to radial bone mass in young adult women, *American Journal of Clinical Nutrition* 58 (1993): 537–542; Heaney, 1993.

29. R. R. Recker and coauthors, Bone gain in young adult women, *Journal of the American Medical Association* 268 (1992): 2403–2408.

CONTROVERSY 6

1. U.S. Department of Agriculture, *Dietary Guidelines for Americans*, Home and Garden Bulletin No. 232 (Washington, D.C.: Government Printing Office, 1995), p. 8.

2. M. Thorogood, The epidemiology of vegetarianism and health, *Nutrition Research Reviews* 8 (1995): 179–192.

3. Position of the American Dietetic Association, Vegetarian diets, *Journal of the American Dietetic Association* 93 (1993): 1317–1319.

4. M. J. Toth and E. F. Poehlman, Sympathetic nervous system activity and resting metabolic rate in vegetarians, *Metabolism: Clinical and Experimental* 43 (1994): 621–625.

5. Thorogood, 1995.

6. L. J. Beilin, Vegetarian and other complex diets, fats, fiber, and hypertension, *American Journal of Clinical Nutrition* 59 (1994): 1130S–1135S.

7. G. E. Fraser, Diet and coronary heart disease: Beyond dietary fats and low-density lipoprotein cholesterol, *Journal of the American Dietetic Association* 59 (1994): 1117S–1123S.

8. M. Kestin and coauthors, Cardiovascular disease risk factors in free-living men: Comparison of two prudent diets, one based on lacto-ovo vegetarianism and the other allowing meat, *American Journal of Clinical Nutrition* 50 (1989): 280–287.

9. S. A. Morgan, A. J. Sinclair, and K. O'Dea, Effect on serum lipids of addition of safflower oil or olive oil to very-low-fat diets rich in lean beef, *Journal of the American Dietetic Association* 93 (1993): 644–648.

10. C. L. Melby, M. L. Toohey, and J. Cebrick, Blood pressure and blood lipids among vegetarian, semivegetarian, and nonvegetarian African Americans, *American Journal of Clinical Nutrition* 59 (1994): 103–109.

11. K. K. Carroll, Review of clinical studies on cholesterol-lowering response to soy protein, *Journal of the American Dietetic Association* 91 (1991): 820–827.

12. J. W. Anderson, B. M. Johnstone, and M. E. Cook-Newell, Meta-analysis of the effects of soy protein intake on serum lipids, *New England Journal of Medicine* 333 (1995): 276–282.

13. P. K. Mills and coauthors, Cancer incidence among California Seventh-Day Adventists, 1976–1982, *American Journal of Clinical Nutrition* 59 (1994): 1136S–1142S.

14. U. G. Allinger and coauthors, Shift from a mixed to a lactovegetarian diet: Influence on acidic lipids in fecal water—A potential risk factor for colon cancer, *American Journal of Clinical Nutrition* 50 (1989): 992–996; R. Frentzel-Beyme and J. Chang-Claude, Vegetarian diets and colon cancer: The German experience, *American Journal of Clinical Nutrition* 59 (1994): 1143S–1152S.

15. B.C.-H. Chiu and coauthors, Diet and risk of non-Hodgkins lymphoma in older women, *Journal of the American Medical Association* 275 (1996): 1315–1321.

16. L. H. Allen and coauthors, Interactive effects of dietary quality on the growth and attained size of young Mexican children, *American Journal of Clinical Nutrition* 56 (1992): 329–333.

17. T. A. B. Sanders and S. Reddy, Vegetarian diets and children, *American Journal of Clinical Nutrition* 59 (1994): 1176S–1181S.

18. L. H. Allen, The nutrition CRSP: What is marginal malnutrition, and does it affect human function?, *Nutrition Reviews* 51 (1993): 255–267.

19. P. C. Dagneles, High prevalence of rickets in infants on macrobiotic diets, *American Journal of Clinical Nutrition* 51 (1990): 202–208.

20. J. Sabate and coauthors, Attained height of lacto-ovo vegetarian children and adolescents, *European Journal of Clinical Nutrition* 45 (1991): 51–58; M. S. Tayter and K. C. Stanek, Anthropometric and dietary assessment of omnivore and lacto-ovo-vegetarian children, *Journal of the American Dietetic Association* 89 (1989): 1661–1663.

21. V. R. Young and P. L. Pellett, Plant proteins in relation to human protein and amino acid nutrition, *American Journal of Clinical Nutrition* 59 (1994): 1203S–1212S; Position of the American Dietetic Association, 1993.

22. C. Lamgerg-Allardt and coauthors, Low serum 25-hydroxyvitamin D concentrations and secondary hyperparathyroidism in middle-aged white strict vegetarians, *American Journal of Clinical Nutrition* 58 (1993): 684–689.

23. D. R. Miller and coauthors, Vitamin B-12 status in a macrobiotic community, *American Journal of Clinical Nutrition* 53 (1991): 524–529.

CHAPTER 7

1. W. Mertz, A balanced approach to nutrition for health: The need for biologically essential minerals and vitamins, *Journal of the American Dietetic Association* 94 (1994): 1259–1262.

2. Food and Nutrition Board, *Recommended Dietary Allowances,* 10th ed. (Washington, D.C.: National Academy of Sciences, 1989), p. 20.

3. K. Fackelmann, Olestra: Too good to be true? *Science News,* 27 January 1996, p. 61.

4. A. C. Ross and M. E. Ternus, Vitamin A as a hormone: Recent advances in understanding the actions of retinol, retinoic acid, and beta carotene, *Journal of the American Dietetic Association* 93 (1993): 1285–1290; J. A. Olson, Vitamin A, in E. E. Ziegler and L. J. Filer, eds., *Present Knowledge in Nutrition,* 7th ed. (Washington, D.C.: ILSI Press, 1996), pp. 109–119.

5. K. P. West, G. R. Howard, and A. Sommer, Vitamin A and infection: Public health implications, *Annual Review of Nutrition* 9 (1989): 63–86.

6. W. W. Fawzi and coauthors, Vitamin A supplementation and dietary vitamin A in relation to the risk of xerophthalmia, *American Journal of Clinical Nutrition* 58 (1993): 385–391.

7. L. M. DeLuca, Vitamin A in epithelial differentiation and skin carcinogenesis, *Nutrition Reviews* (supplement) 52 (1994): S45–S52.

8. West, Howard, and Sommer, 1989.

9. J. C. Butler and coauthors, Measles severity and serum retinol (vitamin A) concentration among children in the United States, *Pediatrics* 91 (1993): 1176–1181.

10. C. B. Stephensen and coauthors, Vitamin A is excreted in the urine during acute infection, *American Journal of Clinical Nutrition* 60 (1994): 388–392.

11. West, Howard, and Sommer, 1989.

12. C. Carlier and coauthors, Prevalence of malnutrition and vitamin A deficiency in the Diourbel, Fatik, and Kolack regions of Senegal: Epidemiological study, *American Journal of Clinical Nutrition* 53 (1991): 70–73; J. A. Olson, 1992 Atwater Lecture: The irresistible fascination of carotenoids and vitamin A, *American Journal of Clinical Nutrition* 57 (1993): 833–839.

13. World-wide vitamin A deficiency targeted as a public health problem, *Nutrition Today* 30 (1995): 53.

14. N. M. P. Daulaire and coauthors, Childhood mortality after a high dose of vitamin A in high risk populations, *British Medical Journal* 304 (1992): 207–210; W. W. Fawzi and coauthors, Dietary vitamin A intake and risk of mortality among children, *American Journal of Clinical Nutrition* 59 (1994): 401–408.

15. J. N. Hathcock and coauthors, Evaluation of vitamin A toxicity, *American Journal of Clinical Nutrition* 52 (1990): 183–202.

16. K. J. Rothman and coauthors, Teratogenicity of high vitamin intake, *New England Journal of Medicine* 333 (1995): 1369–1373.

17. Hathcock and coauthors, 1990.

18. A. T. Diplock, Antioxidant nutrients and disease prevention: An overview, *American Journal of Clinical Nutrition* 53 (1991): 189S–193S.

19. E. R. Greenberg and coauthors, Mortality associated with low plasma concentration of beta carotene and effect of oral supplementation, *Journal of the American Medical Association* 275 (1996): 699–703.

20. S. S. Hannah and A. W. Norman, 1α, 25 (OH)$_2$ vitamin D$_3$-regulated expression of the eukaryotic genome, *Nutrition Reviews* 52 (1994): 376–382; H. F. DeLuca, Vitamin D: 1993, *Nutrition Today,* November/December 1993, pp. 6–11.

21. H. Reichel, H. P. Koeffler, and A. W. Norman, The role of the vitamin D endocrine system in health and disease, *New England Journal of Medicine* 320 (1989): 980–991; J. W. Pike, Vitamin D$_3$ receptors: Structure and function in transcription, *Annual Review of Nutrition* 11 (1991): 189–216.

22. Single day therapy for nutritional rickets, *Pediatric Notes* 16 (1992): 66.

23. Food and Nutrition Board, 1989, pp. 94–95.

24. S. Blank and coauthors, An outbreak of hypervitaminosis D associated with the overfortification of milk from a home-delivery dairy, *American Journal of Public Health* 85 (1995): 656–659.

25. M. F. Holick, Vitamin D, in M. E. Shils, J. A. Olson, and M. Shike, eds., *Modern Nutrition in Health and Disease* (Philadelphia: Lea & Febiger, 1994) p. 313.

26. L. Packer, Protective role of vitamin E in biological systems, *American Journal of Clinical Nutrition* 53 (1991): 1050S–1055S.

27. S. N. Meydani, M. Hayek, and L. Coleman, Influence of vitamin E and B_6 on immune response, *Annals of the New York Academy of Science* 669 (1992): 125–139; S. N. Meydani and coauthors, Vitamin E supplementation enhances cell-mediated immunity in healthy elderly subjects, *American Journal of Clinical Nutrition* 52 (1990): 557–563.

28. J. Raloff, Vitamin E fights radicals—again and again, *Science News* 27 (1989): 327.

29. S. N. Meydani and coauthors, Assessment of the safety of high-dose, short-term supplementation with vitamin E in healthy older adults, *American Journal of Clinical Nutrition* 60 (1994): 704–709.

30. S. P. Murphy, A. F. Subar, and G. Block, Vitamin E intakes and sources in the United States, *American Journal of Clinical Nutrition* 52 (1990): 361–367.

31. D. A. Bender, *Nutritional Biochemistry of the Vitamins* (Cambridge: Cambridge University Press, 1992), pp. 106–127.

32. J. W. Suttie, Vitamin K and human nutrition, *Journal of the American Dietetic Association* 92 (1992): 590.

33. Food and Nutrition Board, 1989, pp. 107–114.

34. Food and Nutrition Board, 1989, p. 20.

35. R. S. Rivlin and P. Dutta, Vitamin B_2 (riboflavin), *Nutrition Today* 30 (1995): 62–67.

36. R. B. Colletti and coauthors, Niacin treatment of hypercholesterolemia in children, *Pediatrics* 92 (1993): 78–82; D. R. Illingworth and coauthors, Comparative effects of lovastatin and niacin in primary hypercholesterolemia, *Archives of Internal Medicine* 154 (1994): 1557–1559.

37. M. T. Behme, Nicotinamide and diabetes prevention, *Nutrition Reviews* 53 (1995): 137–139.

38. Y. Henkin, K. C. Johnson, and J. P. Segrest, Rechallenge with crystalline niacin after drug-induced hepatitis from sustained-release niacin, *Journal of the American Medical Association* 264 (1990): 241–243.

39. L. B. Bailey, The role of folate in human nutrition, *Nutrition Today,* September/October 1990, pp. 12–19.

40. Folic acid fights heart risk factor, *Science News* 148 (1995): 264.

41. N. Pancharuniti and coauthors, Plasma homocyst(e)ine, folate, and vitamin B_{12} concentrations and risk for early-onset coronary artery disease, *American Journal of Clinical Nutrition* 59 (1994): 940–948; J. Selhub and coauthors, Vitamin status and intake as primary determinants of homocysteinemia in an elderly population, *Journal of the American Medical Association* 270 (1993): 2693–2698.

42. Centers for Disease Control and Prevention, Recommendations for use of folic acid to reduce number of spina bifida cases and other neural tube defects, *Journal of the American Medical Association* 269 (1993): 1233, 1236, 1238.

43. J. M. Scott, P. N. Kirke, and D. G. Weir, The role of nutrition in neural tube defects, *Annual Review of Nutrition* 10 (1990): 277–295.

44. J. L. Mills and coauthors, Maternal vitamin levels during pregnancies producing infants with neural tube defects, *Journal of Pediatrics* 120 (1992): 863–871; A. E. Czeil and I. Dudaas, Prevention of the first occurrence of neural-tube defects by periconceptional vitamin supplementation, *New England Journal of Medicine* 327 (1992): 1832–1835; Scott, Kirke, and Weir, 1990.

45. R. J. Hine, What practitioners need to know about folic acid, *Journal of the American Dietetic Association* 96 (1996): 451–452; a full discussion of folate and neural tube defects is found in C. E. Butterworth and A. Bendich, Folic acid and the prevention of birth defects, *Annual Review of Nutrition* 16 (1996): 73–97.

46. M. Nestle, Folate fortification and neural tube defects: Policy implications, *Journal of Nutrition Education* 26 (1994): 287–293; A. Bendich, Folic acid and prevention of neural tube birth defects: Critical assessment of FDA proposals to increase folic acid intakes, *Journal of Nutrition Education* 26 (1994): 294–299.

47. J. F. Gregory, Chemical and nutritional aspects of folate research: Analytical procedures, methods of folate synthesis, stability, and bioavailability of dietary folates, *Advances in Food and Nutrition Research* 33 (1989): 1–101 as cited in L. B. Bailey, Evaluation of a new Recommended Dietary Allowance for folate, *Journal of the American Dietetic Association* 92 (1992): 463–468, 471; How do foods affect folate bioavailability? *Nutrition Reviews* 48 (1990): 326–328.

48. N. Swiatlo and coauthors, Relative folate bioavailability from diets containing human, bovine, and goat milk, *Journal of Nutrition* 120 (1990): 172–177.

49. L. C. Rall and S. N. Meydani, Vitamin B_6 and immune competence, *Nutrition Reviews* 51 (1993): 217–225; S. N. Meydani and coauthors, Vitamin B_6 deficiency impairs interleukin 2 production and lymphocyte proliferation in elderly adults, *American Journal of Clinical Nutrition* 53 (1991): 1275–1280.

50. T. R. Guilarte, Vitamin B_6 and cognitive development: Recent research findings from human and animal studies, *Nutrition Reviews* 51 (1993): 193–198.

51. J. E. Leklem, Vitamin B-6, in E. E. Ziegler and L. J. Filer, eds., *Present Knowledge in Nutrition,* 7th ed. (Washington, D.C.: ILSI Press, 1996), pp. 174–183.

52. W. O. Song, Pantothenic acid: How much do we know about this B-complex vitamin? *Nutrition Today,* March/April 1990, pp. 19–25.

53. D. A. Bender, Ascorbic acid, in *Nutritional Biochemistry of the Vitamins* (New York: Cambridge University Press, 1992), pp. 360–389; Food and Nutrition Board, 1989, p. 117.

54. Food and Nutrition Board, 1989, p. 119.

55. M. Levine and coauthors, Vitamin C pharmacokinetics in healthy volunteers: Evidence for a Recommended Dietary Allowance, *Proceedings of the National Academy of Sciences* 93 (1996): 3704–3709.

56. D. L. Tibble, L. J. Giuliano, and S. P. Fortmann, Reduced plasma ascorbic acid concentrations in nonsmokers regularly exposed to environmental tobacco smoke, *American Journal of Clinical Nutrition* 58 (1993): 886–890.

57. Food and Nutrition Board, 1989, pp. 115-124.

58. C. S. Johnston, L. J. Martin, and X. Cai, Antihistamine effect of supplemental ascorbic acid and neutrophil chemotaxis, *Journal of the American College of Nutrition* 11 (1992): 172–176.

59. A. R. Sherman and N. A. Hallquist, Immunity, in M. L. Brown, ed., *Present Knowledge in Nutrition,* 6th ed. (Washington, D.C.: Nutrition Foundation, 1990), pp. 463–476.

F

60. C. Bucca, G. Rolla, and J. C. Farina, Effect of vitamin C on transient increase of bronchial responsiveness in conditions affecting the airways, *Annals of the New York Academy of Sciences* 669 (1992): 175–186; E. M. Peters and coauthors, Vitamin C supplementation reduces the incidence of postrace symptoms of upper-respiratory-tract infection in ultramarathon runners, *American Journal of Clinical Nutrition* 57 (1993): 170–174.

61. B. J. Rolls, Aging and appetite, *Nutrition Reviews* 50 (1992): 422–426; Are older Americans making better food choices to meet diet and health recommendations? *Nutrition Reviews* 51 (1993): 20–22.

62. C. S. Johnson and M. F. Yen, Megadose of vitamin C delays insulin response to a glucose challenge in normoglycemic adults, *American Journal of Clinical Nutrition* 60 (1994): 735–738.

63. R. A. Jacob, Vitamin C, in M. E. Shils, J. A. Olson, and M. Shike, eds., *Modern Nutrition in Health and Disease* (Philadelphia: Lea & Febiger, 1994), pp. 432–448.

64. V. Herbert, Vitamin C supplements are dangerous for iron-overloaded persons, *Journal of the American Dietetic Association* 93 (1993): 526–527.

65. M. M. Bender and coauthors, Trends in prevalence and magnitude of vitamin and mineral supplement usage and correlation with health status, *Journal of the American Dietetic Association* 92 (1992): 1096–1101.

66. L. H. Allen, The Nutrition CRSP: What is marginal malnutrition, and does it affect human function? *Nutrition Reviews* 51 (1993): 255–267.

67. R. Oren and Y. Ilan, Reversible hepatic injury induced by long-term vitamin A ingestion, *American Journal of Medicine* 93 (1992): 703–704.

68. T. E. Kowalski and coauthors, Vitamin A hepatotoxicity: A cautionary note regarding 25,000 IU supplements, *American Journal of Medicine* 97 (1994): 523–528.

69. J. N. Hathcock, Safety limits for nutrient intakes: Concepts and data requirements, *Nutrition Reviews* 51 (1993): 278–285.

70. I. H. Rosenburg and coauthors, Dietary supplements: Recent chronology and legislation, *Nutrition Reviews* 53 (1995): 31–36.

71. C. Hasler, Nutritional implications of dietary phytochemicals, 1995 ADA annual meeting, Chicago.

72. Adverse events associated with ephedrine-containing products—Texas, December 1993–September 1995, *Morbidity and Mortality Weekly Report* 45 (1996): 689–693.

73. For details about legalities in supplement marketing, see Dietary supplements: Recent chronology and legislation, *Nutrition Reviews* 53 (1995): 31–36.

74. C. S. Johnston and B. Luo, Comparison of the absorption and excretion of three commercially available sources of vitamin C, *Journal of the American Dietetic Association* 94 (1994): 779–781.

CONTROVERSY 7

1. B. Halliwell, Antioxidants in human health and disease, *Annual Review of Nutrition* 16 (1996): 33–50; J. D. Morrow and coauthors, increase in circulating products of lipid peroxidation (F_2-isoprostanes) in smokers—Smoking as a cause of oxidative damage, *New England Journal of Medicine* 332 (1995): 1198–1203.

2. G. W. Burton and M. G. Traber, Vitamin E: Antioxidant activity, biokinetics, and bioavailability, *Annual Review of Nutrition* 10 (1990): 357–382.

3. C. L. Rock, R. A. Jacob, and P. E. Bowen, Update on the biological characteristics of the antioxidant micronutrient: Vitamin C, vitamin E, and the carotenoids, *Journal of the American Dietetic Association* 96 (1996): 693–702.

4. B. Caballero, Vitamin E improves the action of insulin, *Nutrition Reviews* 51 (1993): 339–340; G. Paolisso and coauthors, Pharmacologic doses of vitamin E improve insulin action in healthy subjects and non-insulin-dependent diabetic subjects, *American Journal of Clinical Nutrition* 57 (1993): 650–656;

5. B. Halliwell, Free radicals and antioxidants: A personal view, *Nutrition Reviews* 52 (1994): 253–265.

6. D. Zava, Nutritional implications of dietary phytochemicals, a lecture given at the American Dietetic Association annual meeting, Chicago, 1995.

7. I. T. Johnson, G. Williamson, and S. R. R. Musk, Anticarcinogenic factors in plant foods: A new class of nutrients? *Nutrition Research Reviews* 7 (1994): 175–204; B. N. Ames, M. K. Shigenaga, and T. M. Hagen, Oxidants, antioxidants, and the degenerative diseases of aging, *Proceedings of the National Academy of Sciences* 90 (1993): 7915–7922.

8. N. I. Krinsky, Effects of carotenoids in cellular and animal systems, *American Journal of Clinical Nutrition* 52 (1991): 238S–246S; T. Byers and G. Perry, Dietary carotenes, vitamin C, and vitamin E as protective antioxidants in human cancers, *Annual Review of Nutrition* 12 (1992): 139–159.

9. R. G. Ziegler, Vegetables, fruits, and carotenoids and the risk of cancer, *American Journal of Clinical Nutrition* 53 (1991): 251S–259S.

10. H. B. Stahalein and coauthors, Beta-carotene and cancer prevention: The Basel Study, *American Journal of Clinical Nutrition* 53 (1991): 265S–269S; N. Potischman and coauthors, Breast cancer and dietary and plasma concentrations of carotenoids and vitamin A, *American Journal of Clinical Nutrition* 52 (1990): 909–915.

11. E. R. Greenberg and coauthors, A clinical trial of antioxidant vitamins to prevent colorectal adenoma, *New England Journal of Medicine* 33 (1994): 141–147.

12. O. P. Heinonen, J. K. Huttunen, and D. Albanes (and other participants in the alpha-tocopherol, beta carotene cancer prevention study group), The effect of vitamin E and beta carotene on the incidence of lung cancer and other cancers in male smokers, *New England Journal of Medicine* 330 (1994): 1029–1035.

13. K. Smigel, Beta-carotene fails to prevent cancer in two major studies; CARET intervention stopped, *Journal of the National Cancer Institute* 88 (1996): 145; G. S. Omenn and coauthors, Effects of a combination of beta-carotene and vitamin A on lung cancer and cardiovascular disease, *New England Journal of Medicine* 334 (1996): 1150–1155.

14. C. H. Hennekens and coauthors, Lack of effect of long-term supplementation with beta-carotene on the incidence of malignant neoplasms and cardiovascular disease, *New England Journal of Medicine* 334 (1996): 1145–1149.

15. P. James, K. Norum, and I. Rosenberg, Meeting summary, *Nutrition Reviews* (supplement) 52 (1994): S87–S90.

16. G. Block, Vitamin C and cancer prevention: The epidemiologic evidence, *American Journal of Clinical Nutrition* 53 (1991): 270S–282S.

17. M. A. Wagstaff and coauthors, Malignant melanoma: Diet, alcohol, and obesity, *Journal of the American Dietetic Association* 94 (1994): 1210.

18. E. R. Greenberg and coauthors, 1994; Heinonen, Huttunen, and Albanes, 1994.

F

19. L. A. Levin, Opthalmology, *Journal of the American Medical Association* 273 (1995): 1703–1705.

20. T. Byers, Vitamin E supplements and coronary heart disease, *Nutrition Reviews* 51 (1993): 333–336; K. F. Gey and coauthors, Increased risk of cardiovascular disease at suboptimal plasma concentrations of essential antioxidants: An epidemiological update with special attention to carotene and vitamin C, *American Journal of Clinical Nutrition* 57 (1993): 787S–797S.

21. B. Halliwell, Oxidation of low-density lipoproteins: Questions of initiation, propagation, and the effect of antioxidants, *American Journal of Clinical Nutrition* 61 (1995): 670S–677S.

22. K. F. Gey and coauthors, Inverse correlation between plasma vitamin E and mortality from ischemic heart disease in cross-cultural epidemiology, *American Journal of Clinical Nutrition* 53 (1991): 326S–334S; Gey and coauthors, 1993.

23. M. J. Stampfer and coauthors, Vitamin E consumption and the risk of coronary disease in women, *New England Journal of Medicine* 328 (1993): 1444–1449; E. B. Rimm and coauthors, Vitamin E consumption and the risk of coronary disease in men, *New England Journal of Medicine* 328 (1993): 1450–1456.

24. H. N. Hodis and coauthors, Serial coronary angiographic evidence that antioxidant vitamin intake reduces progression of coronary artery atherosclerosis, *Journal of the American Medical Association* 273 (1995): 1849–1854.

25. L. H. Kushi and coauthors, Dietary antioxidant vitamins and death from coronary heart disease in postmenopausal women, *New England Journal of Medicine* 334 (1996): 1156–1162.

26. N. G. Stephens and coauthors, Randomised controlled trial of vitamin E in patients with coronary disease: Cambridge Heart Antioxidant Study (CHAOS), *Lancet* 347 (1996): 781–786.

27. P. Dowd and Z. B. Zheng, On the mechanism of the anticlotting action of vitamin E quinone, *Proceedings of the National Academy of Sciences* 92 (1995): 8171–8175.

28. Gey and coauthors, 1993; D. L. Trout, Vitamin C and cardiovascular risk factors, *American Journal of Clinical Nutrition* 53 (1991): 322S–325S; Stampfer and coauthors, 1993; Rimm and coauthors, 1993.

29. D. Kritchevsky, Antioxidant vitamins in the prevention of cardiovascular disease, *Nutrition Today*, January/February 1992, pp. 30–33.

30. Trout, 1991; J. P. Moran and coauthors, Plasma ascorbic acid concentrations relate inversely to blood pressure in human subjects, *American Journal of Clinical Nutrition* 57 (1993): 213–217.

31. M. Abbey, M. Noakes, and P. J. Nestel, Dietary supplementation with orange and carrot juice in cigarette smokers lowers oxidation products in copper-oxidized low-density lipoproteins, *Journal of the American Dietetic Association* 95 (1995): 671–675.

32. T. Repka and R. P. Hebbel, Hydroxyl radical formation by sickle erythrocyte membranes: Role of pathological iron deposits and cytoplasmic reducing agents, *Blood* 78 (1991): 2753–2758; V. Herbert, The antioxidant supplement myth, *American Journal of Clinical Nutrition* 60 (1994): 157–158; B. Halliwell, Antioxidants: Sense or speculation? *Nutrition Today*, November/December 1994, pp. 15–19.

33. Heinonen, Huttunen, and Albanes, 1994.

34. H. C. W. De Vet and coauthors, The role of beta-carotene and other dietary factors in the etiology of cervical dysplasia, *International Journal of Epidemiology* 20 (1991): 603–610.

35. Herbert, 1994.

36. Greenberg and coauthors, 1994.

37. W. A. Pryor, The antioxidant nutrients and disease prevention—What do we know and what do we need to find out? *American Journal of Clinical Nutrition* 53 (1991): 391S–393S.

CHAPTER 8

1. Food and Nutrition Board, *Recommended Dietary Allowances*, 10th ed. (Washington, D.C.: National Academy of Sciences, 1989), pp. 247–261.

2. S. H. Swan and coauthors, Is drinking water related to spontaneous abortion? Reviewing the evidence from the California Department of Health Services Studies, *Epidemiology* 3 (1992): 83–93; M. A. McGeehin and coauthors, Case-control studies of bladder cancer and water disinfection methods in Colorado, *American Journal of Epidemiology* 138 (1993): 492–501.

3. R. Lipin, Electron beam cleans dirty water, *Science News* 148 (1995): 171.

4. V. Lambert, Bottled water: New trends, new rules, *FDA Consumer*, June 1993, pp. 9–11.

5. Food and Drug Administration, Quality standards for foods with no identity standards: Bottled waters, *Federal Register* 59 (1994): 61529–61538.

6. V. Matkovic, Calcium metabolism and calcium requirements during skeletal modeling and consolidation of bone mass, *American Journal of Clinical Nutrition* 54 (1991): 245S–260S.

7. C. C. Arnaud and S. D. Sanchez, The role of calcium in osteoporosis, *Annual Review of Nutrition* 10 (1990): 397–414.

8. C. M. Weaver and coauthors, Differences in calcium metabolism between adolescent and adult females, *American Journal of Clinical Nutrition* 61 (1995): 577–581.

9. Food and Nutrition Board, 1989, pp. 174–184.

10. Food and Nutrition Board, 1989, p. 176.

11. J. L. Groff, S. S. Gropper, and S. M. Hunt, Macrominerals, in *Advanced Nutrition and Human Metabolism*, 2nd ed. (St. Paul, MN: West Publishing Company, 1995), pp. 325–351.

12. Food and Nutrition Board, 1989, pp. 190–191.

13. B. C. Coleman, Too many Maalox moments can kill, *Tallahassee Democrat*, 30 August 1995.

14. Diet, nutrition and the prevention of chronic diseases: A report of the WHO study group on diet, nutrition, and prevention of noncommunicable diseases, *Nutrition Reviews* 49 (1991): 291–301.

15. Food and Nutrition Board, 1989, p. 253.

16. H. S. Wright and coauthors, The 1987–88 Nationwide Food Consumption Survey: An update on the nutrient intake of respondents, *Nutrition Today*, May/June 1991, pp. 21–27.

17. Committee on Diet and Health, Food and Nutrition Board, *Diet and Health: Implications for Reducing Chronic Disease Risk* (Washington, D.C.: National Academy Press, 1989), pp. 99–135.

18. M. E. Reusser and D. A. McCarron, Micronutrient effects on blood pressure regulation, *Nutrition Reviews* (1994): 367–375.

19. V. C. Tritto and coauthors, Abnormalities of sodium handling and of cardiovascular adaptations during high salt diet in patients with mild heart failure, *Circulation* 88 (1993): 1620–1627.

20. H. Hwang, J. Dwyer, and R. M. Russell, Diet, *Heliobacter pylori* infection, food preservation and gastric cancer risk: Are there new roles for preventative factors? *Nutrition Reviews* 52 (1994): 75–83.

21. A. J. Knox, Salt and asthma, *British Medical Journal* 307 (1993): 1159–1160.

22. Food and Nutrition Board, 1989, p. 251.

23. C. Xue-Yi and coauthors, Timing of vulnerability of the brain to iodine deficiency in endemic cretinism, *New England Journal of Medicine* 331 (1994): 1739–1744; N. Bleichrodt and coauthors, The benefits of adequate iodine intake, *Nutrition Reviews* 5 (1996): S72–S78.

24. G. R. DeLong, Effects of nutrition on brain development in humans, *American Journal of Clinical Nutrition* 57 (1993): 286S–290S.

25. B. S. Hetzel, Iodine deficiency and fetal brain damage, *New England Journal of Medicine* 331 (1994): 1770–1771.

26. J. A. Pennington, A review of iodine toxicity reports, *Journal of the American Dietetic Association* 90 (1990): 1571–1581.

27. H. C. Holt, B. J. Demott, and J. A. Bacon, The iodine concentration of market milk in Tennessee, 1981–1986, *Journal of Food Protection* 52 (1989): 115–118.

28. D. C. Rocky and J. P. Cello, Evaluation of the gastrointestinal tract in patients with iron-deficiency anemia, *New England Journal of Medicine* 329 (1993): 1691–1695.

29. R. Yip and P. R. Dallman, Iron, in E. E. Ziegler and L. J. Filer, eds., *Present Knowledge in Nutrition,* 7th ed. (Washington, D.C.: ILSI Press, 1996), pp. 277–292.

30. Iron deficiency, *Nutrition and the M.D.,* August 1994, p. 3.

31. R. Yip, The changing characteristics of childhood iron nutritional status in the United States, in L. J. Filer, ed., *Dietary Iron: Birth to Two Years* (New York: Raven Press, 1989), pp. 37–56.

32. Yip, 1989.

33. V. Herbert, Everyone should be tested for iron disorders (abstract), *Journal of the American Dietetic Association* 92 (1992): 1502.

34. J. M. McCord, Effects of positive iron status at a cellular level, *Nutrition Reviews* 54 (1996): 85–88.

35. D. P. Mascotti, D. Rup, and R. E. Thach, Regulation of iron metabolism, *Annual Review of Nutrition* 15 (1995): 239–261.

36. J. T. Salonen and coauthors, High stored iron levels are associated with excess risk of myocardial infarction in Eastern Finnish men, *Circulation* 86 (1992): 803–811.

37. C. T. Sempos, A. C. Looker, and R. F. Gillum, Iron and heart disease: The epidemiological data, *Nutrition Reviews* 54 (1996): 73–84.

38. R. L. Nelson and coauthors, Body iron stores and risk of colonic neoplasia, *Journal of the National Cancer Institute* 86 (1994): 455–460.

39. P. Idjradinata, W. E. Watkins, and E. Pollit, Adverse effect of iron supplementation on weight gain of iron-replete young children, *Lancet* 343 (1994): 1252–1254.

40. V. Herbert, S. Shaw, and E. Jayatilleke, Vitamin C supplements are harmful to lethal for the over 10% of Americans with high iron stores, *FASEB Journal* 8 (1994): A678.

41. T. Yancy, quoting the American Association of Poison Control Centers, in Parents are urged to watch for iron poisoning in children as deaths rise, *Tallahassee Democrat,* 29 September 1993.

42. FDA wants warnings on labels for iron supplements, *Journal of the American Dietetic Association* 95 (1995): 7.

43. R. D. Baynes and T. H. Bothwell, Iron deficiency, *Annual Review of Nutrition* 10 (1990): 133–148.

44. A. S. Prasad, Discovery of human zinc deficiency and studies in an experimental human model, *American Journal of Clinical Nutrition* 53 (1991): 403–412.

45. H. H. Sandstead, Requirements and toxicity of essential trace elements, illustrated by zinc and copper, *American Journal of Clinical Nutrition* 61 (1995): 621S–624S.

46. R. W. Crofton and coauthors, Inorganic zinc and the intestinal absorption of ferrous iron, *American Journal of Clinical Nutrition* 50 (1989): 141–144.

47. J. Zheng and coauthors, Measurement of zinc bioavailability from beef and a ready-to-eat high-fiber breakfast cereal in humans: Application of a whole-gut lavage technique, *American Journal of Clinical Nutrition* 58 (1993): 902–907.

48. O. A. Levander and R. F. Burk, Selenium, in E. E. Ziegler and L. J. Filer, *Present Knowledge in Nutrition,* 7th ed. (Washington, D.C.: ILSI Press, 1996), pp. 320–328.

49. P. R. Larsen and M. J. Berry, Nutritional and hormonal regulation of thyroid hormone deiodases, *Annual Review of Nutrition* 15 (1995): 323–352.

50. Food and Nutrition Board, 1989, p. 219.

51. Acute and chronic selenium toxicity (Diet Therapy/Obesity Update), *Nutrition and the M.D.,* January 1991, p. 7.

52. Food and Nutrition Board, 1989, p. 219.

53. D. Schultz, Fluoride: Cavity-fighter on tap, *FDA Consumer,* January/February 1992, pp. 34–38.

54. Position of the American Dietetic Association: The impact of fluoride on dental health, *Journal of the American Dietetic Association* 94 (1994): 1428–1431.

55. B. D. Gessner and coauthors, Acute fluoride poisoning from a public water system, *New England Journal of Medicine* 330 (1994): 95–99.

56. American Academy of Pediatrics, Fluoride supplementation for children: Interim policy recommendations, *Pediatrics* 95 (1995): 777.

57. R. A. Anderson and coauthors, Supplemental-chromium effects on glucose, insulin, glucagon, and urinary chromium losses in subjects consuming controlled low-chromium diets, *American Journal of Clinical Nutrition* 54 (1991): 909–916.

58. D. Littlefield, Chromium decreases blood glucose in a patient with diabetes (letter), *Journal of the American Dietetic Association* 94 (1994): 1368.

59. Anderson and coauthors, 1991.

60. H. C. Lukaski and coauthors, Chromium supplementation and resistance training: Effects on body composition, strength, and trace element status of men, *American Journal of Clinical Nutrition* 63 (1996): 954–965.

61. J. McBride, Chromium supplementation helps keep blood glucose levels in check, *Journal of the American Dietetic Association* 91 (1991): 178.

62. D. S. Kelly and coauthors, Effects of low-copper diets on human immune response, *American Journal of Clinical Nutrition* 62 (1995): 412–416; Decreased dietary copper impairs vascular function, *Nutrition Reviews* 51 (1993): 188–189.

63. Sandstead, 1995.

64. F. H. Nielsen, Facts and fallacies about boron, *Nutrition Today,* May/June 1992, pp. 6–12.

65. R. A. Goyer, Nutrition and metal toxicity, *American Journal of Clinical Nutrition* 61 (1995): 646S–650S.

CONTROVERSY 8

1. J. D. Zuckerman, Hip fracture, *New England Journal of Medicine* 334 (1996): 1519–1525.

2. National Research Council, *Diet and Health: Implications for Reducing Chronic Risk* (Washington, D.C.: National Academy Press, 1991), p. 121.

3. C. C. Johnson and coauthors, Calcium supplementation and increases in bone mineral density in children, *New England Journal*

F

of Medicine 327 (1992): 82–87; Maximizing peak bone mass: Calcium supplementation increases bone mineral density in children, *Nutrition Reviews* 50 (1992): 335–337.

4. A. Devine and coauthors, A longitudinal study of the effect of sodium and calcium intakes on regional bone density in post-menopausal women, *American Journal of Clinical Nutrition* 62 (1995): 740–745.

5. B. L. Riggs and L. J. Melton, The prevention and treatment of osteoporosis, *New England Journal of Medicine* 327 (1992): 620–627.

6. S. R. Cummings and coauthors, Risk factors for hip fractures in white women, *New England Journal of Medicine* 332 (1995): 767–773; J. Lutz and R. Tesar, Mother-daughter pairs: Spinal and femoral bone densities and dietary intakes, *American Journal of Clinical Nutrition* 52 (1990): 878–888.

7. A history of racial and ethnic differences in regard to bone health appears in W. S. Pollitzer and J. J. B. Anderson, Ethnic and genetic differences in bone mass: A review with a hereditary vs environmental perspective, *American Journal of Clinical Nutrition* 50 (1989): 1244–1259.

8. C. N. Meridith, Exercise in the prevention of osteoporosis, in H. Munro and G. Schlierf, eds., *Nutrition of the Elderly* (New York: Raven Press, 1992), pp. 169–175.

9. E. S. Orwoll and coauthors, The relationship of swimming exercise to bone mass in men and women, *Archives of Internal Medicine* 149 (1989): 2197–2200.

10. J. E. Benson and coauthors, Relationship between nutrient intake, body mass index, menstrual function, and ballet injury, *Journal of the American Dietetic Association* 89 (1989): 58–63.

11. J. F. Aloia and coauthors, To what extent is bone mass determined by fat-free or fat mass? *American Journal of Clinical Nutrition* 61 (1995): 1110–1114; Cummings and coauthors, 1995; S. L. Edelstein and E. Barrett-Connor, Relation between body size and bone mineral density in elderly men and women, *American Journal of Epidemiology* 138 (1993): 160–169; I. R. Reid and coauthors, Determinants of total body and regional bone mineral density in normal post-menopausal women—A key role for fat mass, *Journal of Clinical Endocrinology and Metabolism* 75 (1992): 45–51.

12. R 271. J. A. Langlow and coauthors, *Archives of Internal Medicine* 156 (1996): 989–994.

13. G. Saggese and coauthors, Hypomagnesemia and the parathyroid hormone–vitamin D endocrine system in children with insulin– dependent diabetes mellitus, *Journal of Pediatrics* 118 (1991): 220–225.

14. J. L. Hopper and E. Seeman, The bone density of female twins discordant for tobacco use, *New England Journal of Medicine* 330 (1994): 387–392.

15. C. W. Slemenda, Cigarettes and the skeleton, *New England Journal of Medicine* 330 (1994): 430–431.

16. S. S. Harris and B. Dawson-Hughes, Caffeine and bone loss in healthy postmenopausal women, *American Journal of Clinical Nutrition* 60 (1994): 573–578.

17. E. Fernandez-Repollet, P. Van Loon, and M. Martinez-Maldonado, Renal and systemic effects of short-term high protein feeding in normal rats, *American Journal of the Medical Sciences* 297 (1989): 348–354; J. C. Howe, Postprandial response of calcium metabolism in post menopausal women to meals varying in protein level/source, *Metabolism: Clinical and Experimental* 39 (1990): 1246–1252; R. P. Heaney, Protein intake and the calcium economy, *Journal of the American Dietetic Association* 93 (1993): 1259–1260.

18. R. Tesar and coauthors, Axial peripheral bone density and nutrient intakes of post menopausal vegetarian and omnivorous women, *American Journal of Clinical Nutrition* 56 (1992): 699–704.

19. Howe, 1990.

20. J. Bonjour and coauthors, Hip fracture, femoral bone mineral density, and protein supply in elderly patients, in H. Munro and G. Schlierf, eds., *Nutrition of the Elderly* (New York: Raven Press 1992), pp. 151–159.

21. V. Matkovic and J. Z. Ilich, Calcium requirements for growth: Are current recommendations adequate? *Nutrition Reviews* 51 (1993): 171–180.

22. D. V. Porter, Washington update: NIH Consensus Development Conference Statement Optimal Calcium Intake, *Nutrition Today*, September/October 1994, pp. 37–40; R. P. Heaney, Thinking straight about calcium, *New England Journal of Medicine* 328 (1993): 503–505.

23. B. Dawson-Hughes, Calcium supplementation and bone loss: A review of controlled clinical trials, *American Journal of Clinical Nutrition* 54 (1991): 2745–2805; I. R. Reid and coauthors, Effect of calcium supplementation on bone loss in postmenopausal women, *New England Journal of Medicine* 328 (1993): 460–464.

24. D. I. Levenson and R. S. Bockman, A review of calcium preparations, *Nutrition Reviews*, 52 (1994): 221–232.

25. Committee on Diet and Health, *Diet and Health: Implications for Reducing Chronic Disease Risk* (Washington, D.C.: National Academy Press, 1989), p. 17.

CHAPTER 9

1. Y. Schutz and E. Jéquier, Energy needs: Assessment and requirements, in M. E. Shils, J. A. Olson, and M. Shike, eds., *Modern Nutrition in Health and Disease* (Philadelphia: Lea & Febiger, 1994), pp. 101–111.

2. L. O. Schulz and D. A. Schoeller, A compilation of total daily energy expenditures and body weights in healthy adults, *American Journal of Clinical Nutrition* 60 (1994): 676–681.

3. T. J. Horton and C. A. Geissler, Effect of habitual exercise on daily energy expenditure and metabolic rate during standardized activity, *American Journal of Clinical Nutrition* 59 (1994): 13–19.

4. C. G. Solomon, W. C. Willett, and J. E. Manson, Body weight and mortality, in T. B. Van Itallie and A. P. Simopoulos, eds., *Obesity: New Directions in Assessment and Management* (Philadelphia: Charles Press, 1995), pp. 1–11.

5. G. A. Colditz and coauthors, Weight gain as a risk factor for clinical diabetes mellitus in women, *Annals of Internal Medicine* 122 (1995): 481–486.

6. D. A. McCarron and M. E. Reusser, Body weight and blood pressure regulation, *American Journal of Clinical Nutrition* 63 (1996): 423S–425S.

7. J. E. Manson and coauthors, Body weight and mortality among women, *New England Journal of Medicine* 333 (1995): 677–685.

8. R. J. Kuczmarski and coauthors, Increasing prevalence of overweight among US adults: The National Health and Nutrition Examination Surveys, 1960 to 1991, *Journal of the American Medical Association* 272 (1994): 205–211; Data from the 1988–1991 National Health and Nutrition Examination Survey (NHANES III), as reported in National Heart, Lung, and Blood Institute Obesity Education Summary Report, September 1994; Prevalence of overweight among adolescents—United States, 1988–1991, *Morbidity and Mortality Weekly Report* 43 (1994): 818–821.

9. A. Must and coauthors, Long-term morbidity and mortality of overweight adolescents, *New England Journal of Medicine* 327 (1992): 1350–1355; G. A. Bray, Adolescent overweight may be tempting fate, *New England Journal of Medicine* 327 (1992): 1378–1380.

10. T. K. Young and D. E. Gelskey, Is noncentral obesity metabolically benign? Implications for prevention from a population survey, *Journal of the American Medical Association* 274 (1995): 1939–1941.

11. C. Ley, B. Lees, and J. C. Stevenson, Sex- and menopause-associated changes in body fat distribution, *American Journal of Clinical Nutrition* 55 (1992): 950–954.

12. R. J. Troisi, Cigarette smoking, dietary intake, and physical activity: Effects on body fat distribution—The Normative Aging Study, *American Journal of Clinical Nutrition* 53 (1991): 1104–1111.

13. M. E. Mohs, R. R. Watson, and T. Leonard-Green, Nutritional effects of marijuana, heroin, cocaine, and nicotine, *Journal of the American Dietetic Association* 90 (1990): 1261–1267; D. F. Williamson and coauthors, Smoking cessation and severity of weight gain in a national cohort, *New England Journal of Medicine* 324 (1991): 739–745; K. M. Flegal and coauthors, The influence of smoking cessation on the prevalence of overweight in the United States, *New England Journal of Medicine* 333 (1995): 1165–1170.

14. G. E. Swan and D. Carmelli, Characteristics associated with excessive weight gain after smoking cessation in men, *American Journal of Public Health* 85 (1995): 73–77.

15. S. L. Gortmaker and coauthors, Social and economic consequences of overweight in adolescence and young adulthood, *New England Journal of Medicine* 329 (1993): 1008–1012.

16. W. C. Willett and coauthors, Weight, weight change, and coronary heart disease in women, *Journal of the American Medical Association* 273 (1995): 461–465.

17. R. Roubenolt, G. E. Dallal, and P. W. F. Wilson, Predicting body fatness: The body mass index vs estimation by bioelectrical impedance, *American Journal of Public Health* 85 (1995): 726–728.

18. M. E. J. Lean, H. S. Han, and C. E. Morrison, Waist circumference as a measure for indicating need for weight management, *British Medical Journal* 311 (1995): 158–161.

19. O. Ortiz and coauthors, Differences in skeletal muscle and bone mineral mass between black and white females and their relevance to estimates of body composition, *American Journal of Clinical Nutrition* 55 (1992): 8–13.

20. C. Orphanidou and coauthors, Accuracy of subcutaneous fat measurement: Comparison of skinfold calipers, ultrasound, and computed tomography, *Journal of the American Dietetic Association* 94 (1994): 855–858.

21. G. A. Bray, An approach to the classification and evaluation of obesity, in P. Björntorp and B. N. Brodoff, eds., *Obesity* (Philadelphia: J. B. Lippincott, 1992), pp. 294–308.

22. N. Read, S. French, and K. Cunningham, The role of the gut in regulating food intake in man, *Nutrition Reviews* 52 (1994): 1–10; P. Norton, G. Falciglia, and D. Gist, Physiologic control of food intake by neural and chemical mechanisms, *Journal of the American Dietetic Association* 93 (1993): 450–454; D. J. Shide and coauthors, Accurate energy compensation for intragastric and oral nutrients in lean males, *American Journal of Clinical Nutrition* 61 (1995): 754–764; J. E. Blundell and coauthors, Control of human appetite: Implications for the intake of dietary fat, *Annual Review of Nutrition* 16 (1996): 285–319.

23. C. Bouchard and L. Pérusse, Genetics of obesity, *Annual Review of Nutrition* 13 (1993): 337–354 is an in-depth review of the topic.

24. Y. Zhang and coauthors, Positional cloning of the mouse obese gene and its human homologue, *Nature* 372 (1994): 425–431.

25. Fifth obesity gene found in mice, *Science News* 149 (1996): 257–272.

26. F. Rohner-Jeanrenaud and B. Jeanrenaud, Obesity, leptin and the brain, *New England Journal of Medicine* 334 (1996): 324–325.

27. R. V. Considine and coauthors, Serum immunoreactive–leptin concentrations in normal-weight and obese humans, *New England Journal of Medicine* 334 (1996): 292–295.

28. A. J. Stunkard, Body weight regulation, an address presented at the conference, *Obesity Update: Pathophysiology, Clinical Consequences and Therapeutic Options*, in Atlanta, Georgia, August 31–September 2, 1992.

29. R. L. Leibel, M. Rosenbaum, and J. Hirsch, Changes in energy expenditure resulting from altered body weight, *New England Journal of Medicine* 332 (1995): 621–628; E. Saltzman and S. B. Roberts, The role of energy expenditure in energy regulation: Findings from a decade of research, *Nutrition Reviews* 53 (1995): 209–220.

30. P. Lönnroth and U. Smith, Intermediary metabolism with an emphasis on lipid metabolism, adipose tissue, and fat cell metabolism, in P. Björntorp and B. N. Brodoff, eds., *Obesity* (Philadelphia: J. B. Lippincott, 1992), pp. 3-14.

31. R. H. Eckel, Lipoprotein lipase regulation in obesity and after weight loss, an address given at the conference, *Obesity Update*, 1992.

32. Lönnroth and Smith, 1992.

33. K. Clément and coauthors. Genetic variation in the ß$_3$-adrenergic receptor and an increased capacity to gain weight in patients with morbid obesity, *New England Journal of Medicine* 333 (1995): 352–354.

34. S. Welle and coauthors, Energy expenditure under free-living conditions in normal-weight and overweight women, *American Journal of Clinical Nutrition* 55 (1992): 14–21.

35. A. J. Hill, C. F. Weaver, and J. E. Blundell, Food craving, dietary restraint and mood, *Appetite* 17 (1991): 187–197.

36. P. J. Rogers, Why a palatability construct is needed, *Appetite* 14 (1990): 159–161.

37. T. A. Spiegel, E. E. Shrager, and E. Stellar, Responses of lean and obese subjects to preloads, deprivation, and palatability, *Appetite* 13 (1989): 45–69.

38. D. J. Mela and D. A. Sacchetti, Sensory preferences for fats: Relationships with diet and body composition, *American Journal of Clinical Nutrition* 53 (1991): 908–915.

39. Blundell, 1996.

40. R. Rising and coauthors, Determinants of total daily energy expenditure: Variability in physical activity, *American Journal of Clinical Nutrition* 59 (1994): 800–804.

41. R. C. Klesges, M. L. Shelton, and L. M. Klesges, Effects of television on metabolic rate: Potential implications for childhood obesity, *Pediatrics* 91 (1993): 281–286.

42. L. R. Young and M. Nestle, Portion sizes in dietary assessment: Issues and implications, *Nutrition Reviews* 53 (1995): 149–158.

43. P. M. Suter, Y. Schutz, and E. Jéquier, The effect of ethanol on fat storage in healthy subjects, *New England Journal of Medicine* 326 (1992): 983–985.

44. J. Polivy, Psychological consequences of food restriction, *Journal of the American Dietetic Association* 96 (1996): 589–592.

45. M. E. Sweeny and coauthors, Severe vs moderate energy restriction with and without exercise in the treatment of obesity: Efficiency of weight loss, *American Journal of Clinical Nutrition* 57 (1993): 127–134.

46. J. J. Gleysteen, J. J. Barboriak, and E. A. Sasse, Sustained coronary-risk-factor reduction after bypass for morbid obesity, *American Journal of Clinical Nutrition* 51 (1990): 774–778.

47. F. Pollner, Obesity surgery regaining favor, *Medical World News*, May 1991, p. 37, a report of the NIH Symposium Gastrointestinal Surgery for Severe Obesity, March 1991.

48. J. D. Halverson, Metabolic risk of obesity surgery and long-term follow-up, *American Journal of Clinical Nutrition* 55 (1992): 602S–605S.

49. R. L. Atkinson, Treatment of obesity (editorial), *Nutrition Reviews* (1992): 338–345.

50. T. Cramer, Cal-Ban banned, *FDA Consumer*, June 1992, pp. 39–40.

51. S. Alger and coauthors, Effect of phenylpropalamine on energy expenditure and weight loss in overweight women, *American Journal of Clinical Nutrition* 57 (1993): 120–126.

52. G. Haus and coauthors, Key modifiable factors in weight maintenance: Fat intake, exercise, and weight cycling, *Journal of the American Dietetic Association* 94 (1994): 409–413.

53. D. G. Schlundt and coauthors, The role of breakfast in the treatment of obesity: A randomized clinical trial, *American Journal of Clinical Nutrition* 55 (1992): 645–651.

54. W. D. McArdle, F. I. Katch, and V. L. Katch, *Exercise Physiology: Energy, Nutrition, and Human Performance*, 3rd ed. (Philadelphia: Lea & Febiger, 1991), pp. 651–652.

CONTROVERSY 9

1. F. X. Pi-Sunyer, Health implications of obesity, *American Journal of Clinical Nutrition* 53 (1991): 1595S–1603S; L. I. Katzel and coauthors, Effects of weight loss vs aerobic exercise training on risk factors for coronary disease in healthy, obese, middle aged, and older men, *Journal of the American Medical Association* 274 (1995): 1915–1921.

2. A. M. Wolf and G. A. Colditz, Social and economic effects of body weight in the United States, *American Journal of Clinical Nutrition* 63 (1996): 466S–469S.

3. J. E. Manson and coauthors, Body weight and mortality among women, *New England Journal of Medicine* 333 (1995): 677–685.

4. R. P. Troiano, The relationship between body weight and mortality: A quantitative analysis of combined information from existing studies, *International Journal of Obesity* 20 (1996): 63–75.

5. M. Stern, Epidemiology of obesity and its link to heart disease, *Metabolism: Clinical and Experimental* 44 (1995): 1–3.

6. J. G. Meisler and S. St. Jeor, Summary and recommendations from the American Health Foundation's Expert Panel on Healthy Weight, *American Journal of Clinical Nutrition* 63 (1996): 474S–477S.

7. A. Gott, relating 1989 findings of the Michigan Health Council, in Deception and Fraud in the Diet Industry, Part I, serial no. 101–50 (Washington, D.C.: Government Printing Office, 1990), p. 2.

8. L. Lissner and coauthors, Variability of body weight and health outcomes in the Framingham population, *New England Journal of Medicine* 324 (1991): 1839–1844.

9. A. Frank, Accreditation and certification: The rationalization of obesity-management services, *American Journal of Clinical Nutrition*, 62 (1995): 439–440.

10. G. L. Blackburn, Treatment of obesity is imperative: Physicians can make a difference, an address presented at the conference, *Obesity Update*, 1992.

11. T. A. Wadden and coauthors, Treatment of obesity by very low calorie diet, behavior therapy, and their combination: A five year perspective, *International Journal of Obesity* 13 (1989): 39–46.

12. F. X. Pi-Sunyer, The role of very-low-calorie diets in obesity, *American Journal of Clinical Nutrition* 56 (1992): 240S–245S.

13. D. M. Garner, Positive alternatives to weight loss in selected patients, an address presented at the conference, *Obesity Update*, 1992.

14. S. C. Wooley and D. M. Garner, Obesity treatment: The high cost of false hope, *Journal of the American Dietetic Association* 91 (1991): 1248–1251.

15. E. S. Parham, Applying a philosophy of nutrition education to weight control, *Journal of Nutrition Education* 22 (1990): 194–197.

16. Parham, 1990.

CHAPTER 10

1. S. N. Blair and coauthors, Changes in physical fitness and all-cause mortality, *Journal of the American Medical Association* 263 (1995): 1093–1098; R. S. Paffenbarger and coauthors, The association of changes in physical-activity level and other lifestyle characteristics with mortality among men, *New England Journal of Medicine* 328 (1993): 538–545.

2. American Heart Association Position Statement on Exercise Benefits and recommendations for physical activity programs for all Americans, *Circulation* 86 (1992): 340–344; A. M. Bovens and coauthors, Physical activity, fitness, and selected risk factors for CHD in active men and women, *Medicine and Science in Sports and Exercise* 25 (1993): 572–576; R. R. Pate and coauthors, Physical activity and public health: A recommendation from the Centers for Disease Control and Prevention and the American College of Sports Medicine, *Journal of the American Medical Association* 273 (1995): 402–407.

3. American College of Sports Medicine, The recommended quality and quantity of exercise for developing and maintaining fitness in healthy adults, *Medicine and Science in Sports and Exercise* 22 (1990): 265–274.

4. Physical activity and cardiovascular health: NIH Consensus Development Panel on Physical Activity and Cardiovascular Health, *Journal of the American Medical Association* 276 (1996): 241–246.

5. P. T. Williams, High-density lipoprotein cholesterol and other risk factors for coronary heart disease in female runners, *New England Journal of Medicine* 334 (1996): 1298–1303.

6. I. M. Lee, C. C. Hsieh, and R. S. Paffenbarger, Exercise intensity and longevity in men: The Harvard alumni study, *Journal of the American Medical Association* 272 (1995): 1179–1184; Paffenbarger and coauthors, 1993.

7. R. R. Recker and coauthors, Bone gain in young adult women, *Journal of the American Medical Association* 268 (1992): 2403–2408; A. M. Fehily and coauthors, Factors affecting bone density in young adults, *American Journal of Clinical Nutrition* 56 (1992): 579–586; B. P. Conroy and coauthors, Bone mineral density in elite junior Olympic weightlifters, *Medicine and Science in Sports and Exercise* 25 (1993): 1103–1109.

8. J. A. Woods and J. M. Davis, Exercise, monocyte/macrophage function, and cancer, *Medicine and Science in Sports and Exercise* 26 (1994): 147–157.

9. D. C. Nieman, Exercise, upper respiratory tract infection, and the immune system, *Medicine and Science in Sports and Exercise* 26 (1994): 128–139.

10. J. A. Smith, Guidelines, standards, and perspectives in exercise immunology, *Medicine and Science in Sports and Exercise* 27 (1995): 497–506.

11. W. D. McArdle, F. I. Katch, and V. L. Katch, *Exercise Physiology: Energy, Nutrition, and Human Performance*, 3rd ed. (Philadelphia: Lea & Febiger, 1991), pp. 199–232.

12. K. B. Schechtman and coauthors, Measuring physical activity with a single question, *American Journal of Public Health* 81 (1991): 771–773.

13. P. Astrand, Something old and something new . . . very new, *Nutrition Today*, June 1968, pp. 9–11.

14. E. F. Coyle, Substrate utilization during exercise in active people, *American Journal of Clinical Nutrition* (supplement) 61 (1995): 968–974.

15. E. F. Coyle, Timing and method of increased carbohydrate intake to cope with heavy training, competition, and recovery, in C. Williams and J. T. Devlin, eds., *Foods, Nutrition and Sports Performance: An International Scientific Consensus* (London: E & FN Spon, 1992), pp. 35–63.

16. M. Hargreaves, Carbohydrate and exercise, in Williams and Devlin, 1992, pp. 19–33.

17. L. J. Hoffer, Cori cycle contribution to plasma glucose appearance in man, *Journal of Parenteral and Enteral Nutrition* 14 (1990): 646–648.

18. D. C. Nieman, *Fitness and Sports Medicine* (Palo Alto, Calif.: Bull, 1990), p. 231.

19. E. F. Coyle, Substrate utilization during exercise in active people, *American Journal of Clinical Nutrition* (supplement) 61 (1995): 968–979.

20. Coyle, 1995.

21. Coyle, 1995.

22. P. W. R. Lemon, Effect of exercise on protein requirements, in Williams and Devlin, 1992, pp. 65–86.

23. Lemon, 1992.

24. Position of the American Dietetic Association and the Canadian Dietetic Association: Nutrition for physical fitness and athletic performance for adults, *Journal of the American Dietetic Association* 93 (1993): 691–695.

25. Lemon, 1992.

26. J. R. Berring and S. N. Steen, *Sports Nutrition for the 90s: The Health Professional's Handbook* (Gaithersburg, Md.: Aspen, 1991), pp. 8–9.

27. K. P. G. Kempen, W. H. M. Saris, and K. R. Westerterp, Energy balance during an 8-wk energy-restricted diet with and without exercise in obese women, *American Journal of Clinical Nutrition* 62 (1995): 722–729.

28. C. J. Zelasko, Exercise for weight loss: What are the facts? *Journal of the American Dietetic Association* 95 (1995): 1414–1417.

29. A. Singh, F. M. Moses, and P. A. Deuster, Chronic multivitamin-mineral supplementation does not enhance physical performance, *Medicine and Science in Sports and Exercise* 24 (1992): 726–732.

30. G. M. Fogelholm, Dietary and biochemical indices of nutritional status in male athletes, *Journal of the American College of Nutrition* 11 (1992): 181–191.

31. E. J. van der Beek, Vitamin supplementation and physical exercise performance, in Williams and Devlin, 1992, pp. 95–112.

32. E. J. van der Beek and coauthors, Controlled vitamin C restriction and physical performance in volunteers, *Journal of the American College of Nutrition* 9 (1990): 332–339.

33. I. Gillam, S. Skinner, and R. Telford, Effect of antioxidant supplements on indices of muscle damage and regeneration (abstract), *Medicine and Science in Sports and Exercise* 24 (1992): S17; A. H. Goldfarb, Antioxidants: Role of supplementation to prevent exercise-induced oxidative stress, *Medicine and Science in Sports and Exercise* 25 (1993): 232–236.

34. S. K. Sumida and coauthors, Exercise-induced lipid peroxidation and leakage of enzymes before and after vitamin E supplementation, *International Journal of Biochemistry* 21 (1989): 835–838, as cited in Goldfarb, 1993.

35. J. D. Robertson and coauthors, Influence of vitamin E supplementation on muscle damage following endurance exercise, *International Journal for Vitamin and Nutrition Research* 60 (1990): 171–172.

36. ACSM position stand on osteoporosis and exercise, *Medicine and Science in Sports and Exercise* 27 (1995): i–vii.

37. P. M. Clarkson and E. M. Haymes, Exercise and mineral status of athletes: Calcium, magnesium, phosphorus, and iron, *Medicine and Science in Sports and Exercise* 27 (1995): 831–843.

38. A. A. Skolnick, "Female athlete triad": Risk for women, *Journal of the American Medical Association* 270 (1993): 775–777.

39. D. Benardot, M. Schwartz, and D. Heller, Nutrient intake in young, highly competitive gymnasts, *Journal of the American Dietetic Association* 89 (1989): 401–403.

40. P. M. Clarkson, Minerals: Exercise performance and supplementation in athletes, in Williams and Devlin, 1992, pp. 113–146.

41. A. C. Snyder, L. L. Dvorak, and J. B. Roepke, Influence of dietary iron source on measures of iron status among female runners, *Medicine and Science in Sports and Exercise* 21 (1989): 7–10; E. Coleman, Nutritional concerns of vegetarian athletes, *Sports Medicine Digest*, February 1995, pp. 1–3.

42. Clarkson and Haymes, 1995.

43. Food and Nutrition Board, *Recommended Dietary Allowances*, 10th ed. (Washington, D.C.: National Academy of Sciences, 1989), p. 200.

44. Clarkson, 1992.

45. Clarkson and Haymes, 1995.

46. L. R. Brilla and T. F. Haley, Effect of magnesium supplementation on strength training in humans, *Journal of the American College of Nutrition* 11 (1992): 326–329.

47. R. M. Philen and coauthors, Survey of advertising for nutritional supplements in health and bodybuilding magazines, *Journal of the American Medical Association* 268 (1992): 1008–1011.

48. K. L. Ropp, No-win situation for athletes, *FDA Consumer*, December 1992, pp. 8–12.

49. A. J. M. Wagenmakers, J. H. Coakley, and R. H. T. Edwards, Metabolism of branched-chain amino acids and ammonia during exercise: Clues from McArdle's disease, *International Journal of Sports Medicine* 11 (1990): S101–S113.

50. J. E. Greenleaf, Problems: Thirst, drinking behavior, and involuntary dehydration, *Medicine and Science in Sports and Exercise* 24 (1992): 645–656.

51. E. F. Coyle and S. J. Montain, Carbohydrate and fluid ingestion during exercise: Are there trade-offs? *Medicine and Science in Sports and Exercise* 24 (1992): 671–678.

52. R. J. Maughan, Fluid and electrolyte loss and replacement in exercise, in Williams and Devlin, 1992, pp. 147–178.

53. N. Clark, J. Tobin, and C. Ellis, Feeding the ultraendurance athlete: Practical tips and a case study, *Journal of the American Dietetic Association* 92 (1992): 1258–1262.

54. N. Clark, Revving up with sugar and caffeine, *Physician and Sports Medicine,* November 1991, pp. 15–16.

55. B. H. Sung and coauthors, Effects of caffeine on blood pressure response during exercise in normotensive healthy young men, *American Journal of Cardiology* 65 (1990): 909–913.

56. J. M. Duthel and coauthors, Caffeine and sport: Role of physical exercise upon elimination, *Medicine and Science in Sports and Exercise* 23 (1991): 980–985.

57. S. A. Tilgner and M. R. Schiller, Dietary intakes of female college athletes: The need for nutrition education, *Journal of the American Dietetic Association* 89 (1989): 967–969; D. R. Green and coauthors, An evaluation of dietary intakes of triathletes: Are RDA's being met? *Journal of the American Dietetic Association* 89 (1989): 1653–1654.

58. L. Houtkooper, as quoted in Sports nutrition expert shares secrets of success, *Journal of the American Dietetic Association* 92 (1992): 420.

59. N. Clark, Breakfast is for champions, *Physician and Sports Medicine,* July 1992, pp. 29–30.

60. M. St. Louis and coauthors, The emergence of grade A eggs as a major source of Salmonella enteritidis infections, *Journal of the American Medical Association* 259 (1988): 2103–2107.

CONTROVERSY 10

1. Task force on DSM-IV, 307.50 Eating Disorders Not Otherwise Specified, *DSM-IV Draft Criteria* (Washington, D.C.: American Psychiatric Association, 1993), p. P:2.

2. L. M. Mellin, C. E. Irwin, and S. Scully, Prevalence of disordered eating in girls: A survey of middle-class children, *Journal of the American Dietetic Association* 92 (1992): 851–853.

3. D. C. Moore, Body image and eating behavior in adolescents, *Journal of the American College of Nutrition* 12 (1993): 975–980.

4. D. Neumark-Sztainer, R. Butler, and H. Palti, Dieting and binge eating: Which dieters are at risk? *Journal of the American Dietetic Association* 95 (1995): 586–588.

5. D. Neumark-Sztainer, Excessive weight preoccupation, *Nutrition Today,* March/April 1995, pp. 68–74.

6. A. A. Skolnick, "Female athlete triad" risk for women, *Journal of the American Medical Association* 270 (1993): 921–923.

7. J. H. Wilson, Nutrition, physical activity and bone health in women, *Nutrition Research Reviews* 7 (1994): 67–91.

8. K. K. Yeager and coauthors, The female athlete triad: Disordered eating, amenorrhea, osteoporosis, *Medicine and Science in Sports and Exercise* 25 (1993): 775–777.

9. Yeager and coauthors, 1993.

10. C. L. Otis, American College of Sports Medicine's Ad Hoc Task Force on Women's Issues in Sports Medicine, as quoted in Skolnick, 1993.

11. J. E. Benson and coauthors, Relationship between nutrient intake, body mass index, menstrual function, and ballet injury, *Journal of the American Dietetic Association* 89 (1989): 58–63.

12. J. T. Baer and L. J. Taper, Amenorrheic and eumenorrheic adolescent runners: Dietary intake and exercise training status, *Journal of the American Dietetic Association* 92 (1992): 89–91; P. M. Howat and coauthors, The influence of diet, body fat, menstrual cycling, and activity upon the bone density of females, *Journal of the American Dietetic Association* 89 (1989): 1305–1307.

13. N. T. Frusztajer and coauthors, Nutrition and the incidence of stress fractures in ballet dancers, *American Journal of Clinical Nutrition* 51 (1990): 779–783.

14. "Anorexia athletica," Special report on nutrition and the athlete, *Sports Medicine Digest,* 1989, p. 10; S. N. Steen and K. D. Brownell, Patterns of weight loss and regain in wrestlers: Has the tradition changed? *Medicine and Science in Sports and Exercise* 22 (1990): 762–768.

15. B. J. Larson, Relationship of family communication patterns to Eating Disorder Inventory scores in adolescent girls, *Journal of the American Dietetic Association* 91 (1991): 1065–1067.

16. G. Szmukler and C. Dare, Family therapy of early-onset, short-history anorexia nervosa, in D. B. Woodside and L. Shekter-Wolfson, eds., *Family Approaches in Treatment of Eating Disorders* (Washington, D.C.: American Psychiatric Press, 1991), pp. 25–47.

17. R. C. Casper and coauthors, Total daily energy expenditure and activity level in anorexia nervosa, *American Journal of Clinical Nutrition* 53 (1991): 1143–1150; L. Scalfi and coauthors, Bioimpedance analysis and resting energy expenditure in undernourished and refed anorectic patients, *European Journal of Clinical Nutrition* 47 (1993): 61–67.

18. Position of the American Dietetic Association: Nutrition intervention in the treatment of anorexia nervosa, bulimia nervosa, and binge eating, *Journal of the American Dietetic Association* 94 (1994): 902–907.

19. J. T. Dwyer, Adolescence, in E. E. Ziegler and L. J. Filer, eds., *Present Knowledge in Nutrition* (Washington, D.C.: ILSI Press, 1996), pp. 404–413.

20. L. G. Tolstoi, The role of pharmacotherapy in anorexia nervosa and bulimia, *Journal of the American Dietetic Association* 89 (1989): 1640–1646.

21. American Psychiatric Association Workgroup on Eating Disorders, Practice guidelines for eating disorders, I. Disease definition, epidemiology, and natural history, *American Journal of Psychiatry* 150 (1993): 212–228.

22. D. M. Stein, The prevalence of bulimia: A review of empirical research, *Journal of Nutrition Education* 23 (1991): 205–213.

23. L. G. Roberto, Impasses in the family treatment of bulimia, in D. B. Woodside and L. Shekter-Wolfson, eds., *Family Approaches in Treatment of Eating Disorders* (Washington, D.C.: American Psychiatric Press, 1991), pp. 69–85.

24. P. W. Meilman, F. A. von Hippel, and M. S. Gaylor, Self-induced vomiting in college women: Its relation to eating, alcohol use, and Greek life, *College Health* 40 (1991): 39–41.

25. C. M. Bulik and coauthors, Drug use in women with anorexia and bulimia nervosa, *International Journal of Eating Disorders* 11 (1992): 213–225.

26. G. T. Wilson, Do obese patients have eating disorders? An address presented at the North American Association for the Study of Obesity and Emory University School of Medicine conference on Obesity Update: Pathophysiology, Clinical Consequences, and Therapeutic Options, Atlanta, Georgia, August 31–September 2, 1992.

27. R. L. Spitzer and coauthors, Binge eating disorder: A multisite field trial of the diagnostic criteria, *International Journal of Eating Disorders* 11 (1992): 191–203.

28. E. LeShan, *Winning the Losing Game: Why I Will Never Be Fat Again* (New York: Crowell, 1979).

CHAPTER 11

1. A Platt, The resurgence of infectious diseases, *World Watch,* July/August 1995, pp. 26–32; R. Lewis, The rise of antibiotic-resistant infections, *FDA Consumer,* September 1995, pp. 11–15.

2. WHO Study Group, Diet, nutrition, and the prevention of chronic diseases, *World Health Organization Technical Report Series 797* (Geneva: WHO Office of Publications, 1990), p. 55.

3. P. M. Newberne and M. Lockniskar, Nutrition and immune status, in I. R. Rowland, ed., *Nutrition, Toxicity, and Cancer* (Boca Raton, Fla.: CRC Press, 1991), pp. 301–378.

4. R. K. Chandra, Effect of vitamin and trace-element supplementation on immune response and infection in elderly subjects, *Lancet* 340 (1992): 1124–1127.

5. P. M. Newberne and M. Lockniskar, Nutrition and immune status, in I. R. Rowland, ed., *Nutrition, Toxicity, and Cancer* (Boca Raton, Fla.: CRC Press, 1991), pp. 301–378; S. S. Hannah and A. W. Norman, $1\alpha25(OH)_2$ vitamin D_3-regulated expression of the eukaryotic genome, *Nutrition Reviews* 52 (1994): 376–382; M. C. Goldschmidt, Reduced bactericidal activity in neutrophils from scorbutic animals and the effect of ascorbic acid on these target bacteria in vivo and in vitro, *American Journal of Clinical Nutrition* 54 (1991): 1214S–1220S; S. N. Gershoff, Vitamin C (ascorbic acid): New roles, new requirements? *Nutrition Reviews* 51 (1993): 313–326; L. C. Rall and S. N. Meydani, Vitamin B_6 and immune competence, *Nutrition Reviews* 51 (1993): 217–225; R. K. Chandra and coauthors, Nutrition and immunity in the elderly: Clinical significance, *Nutrition Reviews* 53 (1995): S80–S85; B. L. O'Dell, Interleukin-2 production is altered by copper deficiency, *Nutrition Reviews* 51 (1993): 307–309; H. McCoy and M. A. Kenny, Magnesium and immune function: Recent findings, *Magnesium Research* 5 (1992): 281–293.

6. A. E. Platt, Confronting infectious diseases, in L. R. Brown, ed., *State of the World 1996: A Worldwatch Institute Report on Progress toward a Sustainable Society* (New York: Norton, 1996), pp. 114–132.

7. Position of the American Dietetic Association and the Canadian Dietetic Association: Nutrition intervention in the care of persons with human immunodeficiency virus infection, *Journal of the American Dietetic Association* 94 (1994): 1042–1045.

8. D. C. Macallan and coauthors, Energy expenditure and wasting in human immunodeficiency virus infection, *New England Journal of Medicine* 333 (1995): 83–88.

9. U. Süttmann and coauthors, Weight gain and increased concentrations of receptor proteins for tumor necrosis factor after patients with symptomatic HIV injection received fortified nutrition support, *Journal of the American Dietetic Association* 96 (1996): 565–569.

10. D. Farley, Food safety crucial for people with lowered immunity, *FDA Consumer,* July/August 1990, pp. 7–9.

11. J. Henkel, Battling AIDS fraud, *FDA Consumer,* March 1996, p. 30.

12. National Research Council, *Diet and Health: Implications for Reducing Chronic Disease Risk* (Washington, D.C.: National Academy Press, 1989), pp. 665–710.

13. An excellent review of atherogenesis appears in P. D. Reaven and J. L. Witztum, Oxidized low density lipoproteins in atherogenesis: Role of dietary modification, *Annual Review of Nutrition* 16 (1996): 51–71.

14. D. S. Siscovick and coauthors, Dietary intake and cell membrane levels of long-chain n-3 polyunsaturated fatty acids and the risk of primary cardiac arrest, *Journal of the American Medical Association* 274 (1995): 1363–1367.

15. L. Kuller and coauthors, Prevalence of subclinical atherosclerosis and cardiovascular disease and association with risk factors in the Cardiovascular Health Study, *American Journal of Epidemiology* 139 (1994): 1164–1179.

16. C. L. Johnson and coauthors, Declining serum total cholesterol levels among US adults—The National Health and Nutrition Examination Surveys, *Journal of the American Medical Association* 269 (1993): 3002–3008.

17. Johnson and coauthors, 1993.

18. J. P. Despres and coauthors, Hyperinsulinemia as an independent risk factor for ischemic heart disease, *New England Journal of Medicine* 334 (1996): 952–957.

19. B. A. Griffin and A. Zampelas, Influence of dietary fatty acids on the atherogenic lipoprotein phenotype, *Nutrition Research Reviews* 8 (1995): 1–26.

20. NIH Consensus Conference, Triglyceride, high-density lipoprotein, and coronary heart disease, *Journal of the American Medical Association* 269 (1993): 505–510.

21. M. J. Stampfer and coauthors, A prospective study of cholesterol, apolipoproteins, and the risk of myocardial infarction, *New England Journal of Medicine* 325 (1991): 373–381; NIH Consensus Conference, 1993.

22. M. J. Klag and coauthors, Serum cholesterol in young men and subsequent cardiovascular disease, *New England Journal of Medicine* 328 (1993): 313–318.

23. WHO Study Group, 1990, p. 55.

24. W. M. M. Verschuren, Serum total cholesterol and long-term coronary heart disease mortality in different cultures, *Journal of the American Medical Association* 274 (1995): 131–136.

25. D. M. Hegsted, Dietary fatty acids, serum cholesterol, and coronary heart disease, in G. J. Nelson, ed., *Health Effects of Dietary Fatty Acids* (Champaign, Ill: American Oil Chemists' Society, 1991), pp. 50–68; D. J. McNamara, Cardiovascular disease, in M. E. Shils, J. A. Olson, and M. Shike, eds., *Modern Nutrition in Health and Disease* (Philadelphia: Lea & Febiger, 1994), pp. 1533–1544.

26. Report of the Expert Panel on Population Strategies for Blood Cholesterol Reduction, *Circulation* 83 (1991): 2156–2161.

27. Verschuren, 1995.

28. E. B. Rimm and coauthors, Vegetable, fruit, and cereal fiber intake and risk of coronary heart disease among men, *Journal of the American Medical Association* 275 (1996): 447–451.

29. R. E. Andersen and coauthors, Relation of weight loss to changes in serum lipids and lipoproteins in obese women, *American Journal of Clinical Nutrition* 62 (1995): 350–357.

30. J. S. Stamler and A. Slivka, Biological chemistry of thiols in vascular-related disease, *Nutrition Reviews* 54 (1996): 1–30; J. B. Ubbink, Homocysteine—an atherogenic and thrombogenic factor? *Nutrition Reviews* 53 (1995): 323–332.

31. A. L. Macnair, Physical activity, not diet, should be the focus of measures for the primary prevention of cardiovascular disease, *Nutrition Research Reviews* 7 (1994): 43–65; S. N. Blair and coauthors, Influences of cardiorespiratory fitness and other precursors on cardiovascular disease and all-cause mortality in men and women, *Journal of the American Medical Association* 276 (1996): 205–210.

32. R. R. Wind and coauthors, Change in waist-hip ratio with weight loss and its association with change in cardiovascular risk factors, *American Journal of Clinical Nutrition* 55 (1992): 1086–1092.

33. C. Bouchard, G. A. Bray, and V. S. Hubbard, Basic and clinical aspects of regional fat distribution, *American Journal of Clinical Nutrition* 52 (1990): 946–950; G. A. Bray, Obesity, in E. E. Ziegler and L. J. Filer, ed., *Present Knowledge in Nutrition,* 7th ed. (Washington, D.C.: ILSI Press, 1996), pp. 19–32.

34. D. Ornish and coauthors Can lifestyle changes reverse coronary heart disease? The Lifestyle Heart Trial, *Lancet* 336 (1990):

129–133; K. K. Gould and coauthors, Changes in myocardial perfusion abnormalities by positron emission tomography after long-term, intense risk factor modification, *Journal of the American Medical Association* 274 (1995): 894–901.

35. J. M. Gaziano and coauthors, Moderate alcohol intake, increased levels of high-density lipoprotein and its subfractions, and decreased risk of myocardial infarction, *New England Journal of Medicine* 329 (1993): 1829–1834; P. R. Ridker and coauthors, Association of moderate alcohol consumption and plasma concentration of endogenous tissue–type plasminogen activator, *Journal of the American Medical Association* 272 (1994): 929–933.

36. C. S. Fuchs and coauthors, Alcohol consumption and mortality among women, *New England Journal of Medicine* 332 (1995): 1245–1250; H. O. Hein, P. Suadicani, and F. Gyntelberg, Alcohol consumption, serum low density lipoprotein cholesterol concentrations, and risk of ischemic heart disease: Six year followup to the Copenhagen male study, *British Medical Journal* 312 (1996): 736–741.

37. T. A. Pearson and P. Terry, What to advise patients about drinking alcohol—the clinician's conundrum, *Journal of the American Medical Association* 272 (1994): 967–968.

38. The Expert Panel, Summary of the second report of the National Cholesterol Education Program (NCEP) Expert Panel on Detection, Evaluation, and Treatment of High Blood Cholesterol in Adults (Adult Treatment Panel II), *Journal of the American Medical Association* 269 (1993): 3015–3023.

39. J. R. DiPalma and W. S. Thayer, Use of niacin as a drug, *Annual Review of Nutrition* 11 (1991): 169–187.

40. National Center for Health Statistics Data Line, *Public Health Reports* 109 (1994): 713.

41. From presentations at the American Heart Association's Scientific Sessions, 1992, as reported in Syndrome X: Insulin resistance, hypertension, dyslipidemia, obesity, and CAD, *Nutrition Close-Up* 9 (1992).

42. R. F. Murray, Skin color and blood pressure: Genetics or environment, *Journal of the American Medical Association* 266 (1991): 2049.

43. W. B. Kannel, Blood pressure as a cardiovascular risk factor, *Journal of the American Medical Association* 275 (1996): 1571–1575.

44. S. A. Corrigan and coauthors, Weight reduction in the prevention and treatment of hypertension: A review of representative clinical trials, *American Journal of Health Promotion* 5 (1991): 208–214.

45. D. A. McCarron and M. E. Reusser, Body weight and blood pressure regulation, *American Journal of Clinical Nutrition* 63 (1996): 423S–425S.

46. P. F. Kokkinos and coauthors, Effects of regular exercise on blood pressure and left ventricular hypertrophy in African-American men with severe hypertension, *New England Journal of Medicine* 333 (1995): 1462–1467.

47. G. Kelly and Z. V. Tran, Aerobic exercise and normotensive adults: A meta-analysis, *Medicine and Science in Sports and Exercise* 27 (1995): 1371–1377.

48. U.S. Department of Agriculture, *Nutrition and Your Health: Dietary Guidelines for Americans*, Home and Garden Bulletin no. 232 (Washington, D.C.: Government Printing Office, 1995); R. G. Victor and J. Hansen, Alcohol and blood pressure—a drink a day . . . , *New England Journal of Medicine* 332 (1995): 1782–1783.

49. M. E. Reusser and D. A. McCauon, Micronutrient effects on blood pressure regulation, *Nutrition Reviews* 52 (1994): 367–375.

50. D. A. McCarron, Dietary calcium and lower blood pressure: We can all benefit, *Journal of the American Medical Association* 275 (1996): 1128–1129.

51. P. T. Strickland and J. D. Groopman, Biomarkers for assessing environmental exposure to carcinogens in the diet, *American Journal of Clinical Nutrition* 61 (1995): 710S–720S.

52. K. E. Anderson and A. Kappas, Dietary regulation of cytochrome P450, *Annual Review of Nutrition* 11 (1991): 141–167.

53. Committee on Comparative Toxicity of Naturally Occurring Carcinogens, *Carcinogens and Anticarcinogens in the Human Diet* (Washington, D.C.: National Academy Press, 1996), pp. 1–18.

54. American Medical Association's Council on Scientific Affairs, Diet and cancer: Where do matters stand? *Archives of Internal Medicine* 153 (1993): 50–56.

55. WHO Study Group, 1990, p. 65; H. S. Black, Effect of a low-fat diet on the incidence of actinic keratosis, *New England Journal of Medicine* 330 (1994): 1272–1275.

56. B. C.-H. Chiu and coauthors, Diet and risk of non-Hodgkin lymphoma in older women, *Journal of the American Medical Association* 275 (1996): 1315–1321.

57. D. J. Hunter and coauthors, Cohort studies of fat intake and the risk of breast cancer—a pooled analysis, *New England Journal of Medicine* 334 (1996): 356–361.

58. J. Raloff, Eco cancers: Do environmental factors underlie a breast cancer epidemic? *Science News* 144 (1993): 10–13.

59. R. A. Karmall, Fatty acid metabolism and biochemical mechanisms in cancer, in G. J. Nelson, ed., *Health Effects of Dietary Fatty Acids* (Champaign, Ill.: American Oil Chemists' Society, 1991), pp. 150–156.

60. M. A. Belury, Conjugated dienoic linoleate: A polyunsaturated fatty acid with unique chemoprotective properties, *Nutrition Reviews* 53 (1995): 83–89.

61. L. A. Sauer, R. T. Cauchy, and A. S. Hurtubise, Effects of omega-6 and omega-3 fatty acids on the rate of 3H-thymidine incorporation (3H-TI) in hepatoma 7288CTC performed in situ, *FASEB Journal* 43 (1990): A508; K. K. Carroll, Nutrition and cancer: Fat, in I. R. Rowland, ed., *Nutrition, Toxicity, and Cancer* (Boca Raton, Fla.: CRC Press, 1991), pp. 439–453.

62. Anderson and Kappas, 1991.

63. Committee on Comparative Toxicity of Nationally Occurring Carcinogens, 1996, pp. 35–126.

64. J. Dwyer, Dietary fiber and colorectal cancer risk, *Nutrition Reviews* 51 (1993): 147–148.

65. D. Kritchevsky, Dietary fiber and colon cancer, in I. R. Rowland, ed., *Nutrition, Toxicity, and Cancer* (Boca Raton, Fla.: CRC Press, 1991), pp. 481–489.

66. B. J. Trock, E. Lanza, and P. Greenwald, High-fiber diet and colon cancer: A critical review, in *Recent Progress in Research on Nutrition and Cancer* (New York: Wiley-Liss, 1990), pp. 145–157.

67. R. R. Watson and coauthors, Effect of beta carotene on lymphocyte subpopulations in elderly humans: Evidence for a dose-response relationship, *American Journal of Clinical Nutrition* 53 (1990): 90–94.

68. C. S. Muir as cited in C. E. Butterworth and coauthors, Folate deficiency and cervical dysplasia, *Journal of the American Medical Association* 267 (1992): 528–533.

69. National Research Council, 1991, pp. 356–357.

70. L. W. Wattenberg, Inhibition of carcinogenesis by minor dietary constituents, *Cancer Research* 52 (1992): 2085S–2091S.

71. E. Giovannucci and coauthors, Intake of carotinoids and retinol in relation to risk of prostate cancer, *Journal of the National Cancer Institute* 87 (1995): 1767–1776.

72. M. A. Wagstaff and coauthors, Oregano flavonoids as lipid antioxidants, Journal of the American Dietetic Association 93 (1993): 1217.

73. M. Messina and S. Barnes, The role of soy products in reducing risk of cancer, *Journal of the National Cancer Institute* 83 (1991): 541–546.

74. A. Cassidy, S. Bingham, and K. D. R. Setchell, Biological effects of a diet of soy protein rich in isoflavones on the menstrual cycle of premenopausal women, *American Journal of Clinical Nutrition* 60 (1994): 333–340.

75. D. Kostie, W. S. White, and J. A. Olson, Intestinal absorption, serum clearance, and interactions between lutein and β-carotene when administered to human adults in separate or combined oral doses, *American Journal of Clinical Nutrition* 62 (1995): 604–610.

76. J. N. Hathcock, Safety and regulatory issues for photochemical sources: "Designer foods," *Nutrition Today*, November/December 1993, pp. 23–25; L. U. Thompson, Antioxidants and hormone-mediated health benefits of whole grains, *Critical Reviews in Food Science and Nutrition* 34 (1994): 473–497.

77. K. Smigel, Beta-carotene fails to prevent cancer in two major studies, CARET intervention stopped, *Journal of the National Cancer Institute* 88 (1996): 145.

78. Dietary flavonoids and risk of coronary heart disease, *Nutrition Reviews* 52 (1994): 59–61.

79. J. H. Weisburger, Nutritional approach to cancer prevention with emphasis on vitamins, antioxidants, and carotenoids, *American Journal of Clinical Nutrition* (supplement) 53 (1991): 226–237; R. G. Ziegler, Vegetables fruits, and carotenoids and the risk of cancer, *American Journal of Clinical Nutrition* (supplement) 53 (1991): 251–259.

80. G. Block, The data support a role for antioxidants in reducing cancer risk, *Nutrition Reviews* 50 (1992) 207–213.

81. K. McNutt, Medicinals in food, Part I: Is Science coming full circle? *Nutrition Today*, September/October 1995, pp. 218–222.

82. National Academy of Sciences, quoted in First International Conference on East-West Perspectives on Functional Foods, Nutrition Today, March/April 1996, pp. 70–73.

83. Position of the American Dietetic Association: Phytochemicals and functional foods, Journal of the American Dietetic Association 95 (1995): 493–496; E. A. Decker, The role of phenolics, conjugated linoleic acid, carnosine, and pyrroloquinoline quinone as nonessential dietary antioxidants, *Nutrition Reviews* 53 (1995): 49–58.

84. W. Mertz, A balanced approach to nutrition for health, *Journal of the American Dietetic Association* 94 (1994): 1259–1262.

85. *The Surgeon General's Report on Nutrition and Health, Summary and Recommendations* (Washington, D.C.: Department of Health and Human Services—Public Health Service publication no. 88-50211, 1988).

86. A. K. Kant, A. Shatzkin, and R. G. Ziegler, Dietary diversity and subsequent cause-specific mortality in the NHANES I Epidemiologic Follow-up Study, *Journal of the American College of Nutrition* 14 (1995): 233–238.

CONTROVERSY 11

1. Inhibition of LDL oxidation by phenolic substances in red wine: A clue to the French paradox? *Nutrition Reviews* 51 (1993): 185–187.

2. E. B. Rimm and coauthors, Review of moderate alcohol consumption and reduced risk of coronary heart disease: The effect due to beer, wine, or spirits? *British Medical Journal* 321 (1996): 731–736.

3. R. N. Amarasuriya and coauthors, Ethanol stimulates apolipoprotein A-1 secretion by human hepatocytes: Implications for a mechanism for atherosclerosis prevention, *Metabolism* 41 (1992): 827–832; NIH Consensus Development Panel on Triglyceride, High-Density Lipoprotein, and Coronary Heart Disease, Triglyceride, high-density lipoprotein, and coronary heart disease, *Journal of the American Medical Association* 269 (1993): 505–510; Ethanol stimulates apo A-1 secretion in human hepatocytes: A possible mechanism underlying the cardioprotective effect of ethanol, *Nutrition Reviews* 51 (1993): 151–152.

4. H. Wechsler and coauthors, Health and behavioral consequences of binge drinking in college: A national survey of students at 140 campuses, *Journal of the American Medical Association* 272 (1994): 1672–1677.

5. M. Frezza and coauthors, High blood alcohol levels in women: The role of decreased gastric alcohol dehydrogenase activity and first-pass metabolism, *New England Journal of Medicine* 322 (1990): 95–99.

6. J. P. Flatt, Body weight, fat storage, and alcohol metabolism, *Nutrition Reviews* 50 (1992): 267–270.

7. B. B. Duncan and coauthors, Association of the waist-to-hip ratio is different with wine than with beer or hard liquor consumption, *American Journal of Epidemiology* 142 (1995): 1034–1038.

8. A. Urbano-Marquez and coauthors, The effects of alcoholism on skeletal and cardiac muscle, *New England Journal of Medicine* 320 (1989): 409–415.

9. M. Russell and coauthors, Alcohol drinking patterns and blood pressure, *American Journal of Public Health* 81 (1991): 452–457.

10. R. J. Rubin and coauthors, *The Cost of Disorders of the Brain* (Washington, D.C.: National Foundation for Brain Research, 1992), pp. 45–49.

11. B. N. Ames, R. Magaw, and L. S. Gold, Ranking possible carcinogenic hazards, *Science* 236 (1987): 271–280.

12. J. E. Foulke, Urethane in alcoholic beverages under investigation, *FDA Consumer,* January/February 1993, pp. 19–23.

13. T. L. Holbrook, E. Barrett-Connor, and D. L. Wingard, A prospective population-based study of alcohol use and non-insulin-dependent diabetes mellitus, *American Journal of Epidemiology* 132 (1990): 902–909.

14. A. L. Klatsky, M. A. Armstrong, and G. D. Friedman, Alcohol and mortality, *Annals of Internal Medicine* 117 (1992): 646–654.

15. M. V. Singer, S. Teyssen, and V. E. Eysselein, Action of beer and its ingredients on gastric acid secretion and release of gastrin in humans, *Gastroenterology* 10 (1991): 935–942.

16. Committee on Substance Abuse, Alcohol use and abuse: A pediatric concern, *Pediatrics* 95 (1995): 439–442.

CHAPTER 12

1. D. J. P. Barker, Growth in utero and coronary heart disease, *Nutrition Reviews* 54 (1996): S1–S7; L. A. Hanson and coauthors, Early dietary influence on later immunocompetence, *Nutrition Reviews* 54 (1996): S23–S30.

2. National Academy of Sciences, Food and Nutrition Board, *Nutrition during Pregnancy* (Washington, D.C.: National Academy Press, 1990), pp. 176–211.

3. S. J. Ventura and coauthors, Advance report of final natality statistics, 1994, *Monthly Vital Statistics Report,* June 1996, p. 1.

4. Transplacental nutrient transfer and intrauterine growth retardation, *Nutrition Reviews* 50 (1992): 56–57.

5. B. Torun and F. Chew, Protein-energy malnutrition, in M. E. Shils, J. A. Olson, and M. Shike, eds., *Modern Nutrition in Health and Disease* (Philadelphia: Lea & Febiger, 1994), pp. 950–976 presents a full discussion of PEM.

6. D. J. P. Barker and coauthors, Relation of fetal and infant growth to plasma fibrinogen and factor VII concentrations in adult life, *British Medical Journal* 304 (1992): 148–152.

7. National Academy of Sciences, 1990, p. 137.

8. J. A. Nettleton, Are N-3 fatty acids essential nutrients for fetal development? *Journal of the American Dietetic Association* 93 (1993): 58–64.

9. S. F. Olsen and coauthors, Randomised controlled trial of effect of fish-oil supplementation on pregnancy duration, *Lancet* 339 (1992): 1003–1006.

10. G. J. Cuskelly, H. McNulty, and J. M. Scott, Effect of increasing dietary folate on red-cell folate: Implications for prevention of neural tube defects, *Lancet* 347 (1996): 657–659.

11. National Academy of Sciences, 1990, pp. 96–120.

12. K. G. Dewey and M. A. McCrory, Effects of dieting and physical activity on pregnancy and lactation, *American Journal of Clinical Nutrition* (supplement) 59 (1994): 446S–453S.

13. B. Luke and coauthors, The association between occupational factors and preterm birth: A United States nurses' study, *American Journal of Obstetrics and Gynecology* 173 (1995): 849–862.

14. A. M. Fraser, J. E. Brockert, and R. H. Ward, Association of young maternal age with adverse reproductive outcomes, *New England Journal of Medicine* 332 (1995): 1113–1117.

15. J. D. Skinner and B. R. Carruth, Dietary quality of pregnant and nonpregnant adolescents, *Journal of the American Dietetic Association* 91 (1991): 718–720.

16. Position of the American Dietetic Association: Nutrition care for pregnant adolescents, *Journal of the American Dietetic Association* 94 (1994): 449–450; P. A. Flanagan and coauthors, Adolescent development and transitions to motherhood, *Pediatrics* 96 (1995): 273–277.

17. E. Erikson, *Childhood and Society* (New York: Norton, 1963).

18. M. Erick, Battling morning (noon and night) sickness: New approaches for treating an age-old problem, *Journal of the American Dietetic Association* 94 (1994): 147–148.

19. D. L. Olds, C. R. Henderson, Jr., and R. Tatelbaum, Intellectual impairment in children of women who smoke cigarettes during pregnancy, *Pediatrics* 93 (1994): 221–227; M. Weitzman, S. Gortmaker, and A. Sobol, Maternal smoking and behavior problems of children, *Pediatrics* 90 (1992): 342–349.

20. H. S. Klonoff-Cohen and coauthors, The effect of passive smoking and tobacco exposure through breast milk on sudden infant death syndrome, *Journal of the American Medical Association* 273 (1995): 795–798.

21. T. A. King and coauthors, Neurologic manifestations of in utero cocaine exposure in near-term infants, *Pediatrics* 96 (1995): 259–264; J. J. Volpe, Effect of cocaine use on the fetus, *New England Journal of Medicine* 327 (1992): 399–407.

22. D. B. Petitti and C. Coleman, Cocaine and the risk of low birth weight, *American Journal of Public Health* 80 (1990): 25–28; S. Parker and coauthors, Jitteriness in full-term neonates: Prevalence and correlates, *Pediatrics* 85 (1990): 17–23; M. van de Bor, F. J. Walther,

and M. Ebrahimi, Decreased cardiac output in infants of mothers who abused cocaine, *Pediatrics* 85 (1990): 30–32; L. N. Eisen and coauthors, Perinatal cocaine effects on neonatal stress behavior and performance on the Brazelton Scale, *Pediatrics* 88 (1991): 477–480; M. Mirochnick and coauthors, Circulating catecholamine concentrations in cocaine-exposed neonates: A pilot study, *Pediatrics* 88 (1991): 481–485.

23. K. J. Rothman and coauthors, Teratogenicity of high vitamin intake, *New England Journal of Medicine* 333 (1995): 1369–1373.

24. National Academy of Sciences, 1990; J. L. Mills and coauthors, Moderate caffeine use and the risk of spontaneous abortion and intrauterine growth retardation, *Journal of the American Medical Association* 269 (1993): 593–597.

25. J. O. Beattie, Alcohol exposure and the fetus, *European Journal of Clinical Nutrition* 46 (1992): S7–S17.

26. Committee on Substance Abuse and Committee on Children with Disabilities, American Academy of Pediatrics, Fetal alcohol syndrome and fetal alcohol effects, *Pediatrics* 91 (1993): 1004–1006; K. Strömand and A. Hellström, Fetal alcohol syndrome: An opthalmological and socioeducational prospective study, *Pediatrics* 97 (1996): 845–850.

27. Update: Trends in fetal alcohol syndrome—United States, 1979–1993, *Morbidity and Mortality Weekly Reports* 44 (1995): 249–251.

28. Committee on Substance Abuse and Committee on Children with Disabilities, 1993.

29. C. D. Naylor and coauthors, Cesarean delivery in relation to birth weight and gestational glucose tolerance: Pathophysiology or practice style? *Journal of the American Medical Association* 17 (1996): 1165–1170.

30. F. G. Cummingham and M. D. Lindheimer, Hypertension in pregnancy, *New England Journal of Medicine* 326 (1992): 927–932.

31. Position of the American Dietetic Association: Promotion and support of breast feeding, *Journal of the American Dietetic Association* 93 (1993): 467–469.

32. A. C. Goedhart and J. G. Bindels, The composition of human milk as a model for the design of infant formulas: Recent findings and possible applications, *Nutrition Research Reviews* 7 (1994): 1–23.

33. J. S. Forsyth, Is breastfeeding worthwhile? *European Journal of Clinical Nutrition* 46 (1992): S19–S25.

34. National Academy of Sciences, 1990, pp. 151–152.

35. S-J. Chang, Antimicrobial proteins of maternal and cord sera and human milk in relation to maternal nutrition status, *American Journal of Clinical Nutrition* 51 (1990): 183–187.

36. Breast milk and subsequent intelligence quotient in children born preterm, *Nutrition Reviews* 50 (1992): 334–335.

37. National Academy of Sciences, Food and Nutrition Board, *Nutrition during Lactation* (Washington, D.C.: National Academy Press, 1991), pp. 28–49.

38. C. R. Howard and coauthors, Antenatal formula advertising: Another potential threat to breast-feeding, *Pediatrics* 94 (1994): 102–104.

39. C. I. Dungy and coauthors, Effect of discharge samples on duration of breast-feeding, *Pediatrics* 90 (1992): 233–237.

40. S. Charles and B. Prystowsky, Early discharge, in the end: Maternal abuse, child neglect, and physician harassment, *Pediatrics* 96 (1995): 746–747.

41. J. B. Schwartz and coauthors, Does WIC participation improve breastfeeding practices? *American Journal of Public Health* 85 (1995): 729–731.

F

42. WIC Program, *ADA Legislative Newsletter*, January/February 1993, p. 2.

43. I. B. Stehlin, Infant formula: Second best but good enough, *FDA Consumer*, June 1996, p. 17–20.

44. L. B. Dusdieker and coauthors, Prolonged maternal fluid supplementation in breast-feeding, *Pediatrics* 86 (1990): 737–740.

45. J. A. Mennella and G. K. Beauchamp, The transfer of alcohol to human milk: Effects on flavor and the infant's behavior, *New England Journal of Medicine* 325 (1991): 981–985.

46. Postprandial thermogenesis in lactating women, *Nutrition Reviews* 49 (1991): 209–210; National Academy of Sciences, 1991, pp. 14–15; F. M. Kramer and coauthors, Breast feeding reduces maternal lower-body fat, *Journal of the American Dietetic Association* 93 (1993): 429–433.

47. K. G. Dewey and coauthors, A randomized study of the effects of aerobic exercise by lactating women on breast-milk volume and composition, *New England Journal of Medicine* 330 (1994): 449–453; A. Prentice, Should lactating women exercise? *Nutrition Reviews* 52 (1994): 358–360.

48. R. F. Black, Transmission of HIV-1 in the breast-feeding process, *Journal of the American Dietetic Association* 96 (1996): 267–274.

49. American Academy of Pediatrics, Committee on Drugs, The transfer of drugs and other chemicals into human milk, *Pediatrics* 93 (1994): 137–150.

50. L. A. Barness, ed., Committee on Nutrition, *Pediatric Nutrition Handbook* (Elk Grove, Ill.: American Academy of Pediatrics, 1993), pp. 11–22.

51. American Academy of Pediatrics Work Group on Cow's Milk Protein and Diabetes Mellitus, Infant feeding practices and their possible relationship to the etiology of diabetes mellitus, *Pediatrics* 94 (1994): 752–754; C. Lévy-Marchal and coauthors, Antibodies against bovine albumin and other diabetes markers in French children, *Diabetes Care* 18 (1995): 1089–1094.

52. G. J. Fuchs and coauthors, Iron status and intake of older infants fed formula vs cow milk with cereal, *American Journal of Clinical Nutrition* 58 (1993): 343–348.

53. S. M. Garn and M. La Velle, as quoted by A. P. Simopoulos, Characteristics of obesity, in P. Björntorp and B. N. Brodoff, eds., *Obesity* (Philadelphia: Lippincott, 1992), pp. 309–319.

54. E. M. Widdowson, Mental contentment and physical growth, *Lancet* 1 (1951): 1316–1318.

CONTROVERSY 12

1. J. E. Henningfield and coauthors, Drinking coffee and carbonated beverages blocks absorption of nicotine from nicotine polacrilex gum, *Journal of the American Medical Association* 264 (1990): 1560–1564.

2. J. J. Murray and M. D. Healy, Drug-mineral interactions: A new responsibility for the hospital dietitian, *Journal of the American Dietetic Association* 91 (1991): 66–70, 73.

3. Why food and medicine don't always make a good mix, *Tufts University Diet and Nutrition Letter*, July 1989, pp. 3–6.

4. S. M. Vaziri and coauthors, The impact of female hormone usage on the lipid profile: The Framingham Offspring Study, *Archives of Internal Medicine* 153 (1993): 2200–2206.

5. R. A. Hatcher and coauthors, *Contraceptive Technology* (New York: Irvington, 1992), pp. 240–241.

6. Hatcher, and coauthors, 1992, p. 146.

7. K. Amatayakul and coauthors, Oral contraceptives: Effect of long-term use on liver vitamin A storage assessed by the relative dose response test, *American Journal of Clinical Nutrition* 49 (1989): 845–848.

8. Hatcher, and coauthors, 1992, pp. 284–285.

9. Murray and Healy, 1991.

10. K. Silverman and coauthors, Withdrawal syndrome after the double-blind cessation of caffeine consumption, *New England Journal of Medicine* 327 (1992): 1109–1114.

11. E. C. Strain and coauthors, Caffeine dependence syndrome: Evidence from case histories and experimental evaluations, *Journal of the American Medical Association* 272 (1994): 1043–1048.

12. M. R. Joesoef and coauthors, Are caffeinated beverages risk factors for delayed conception? *Lancet* 335 (1990): 136–137.

13. Grounds for breaking the coffee habit? *Tufts University Diet and Nutrition Letter*, February 1990, pp. 3–6; C. E. Lewis and coauthors, Inconsistent associations of caffeine-containing beverages with blood pressure and with lipoproteins, *American Journal of Epidemiology* 138 (1993): 502–507; W. C. Willett and coauthors, Coffee consumption and coronary heart disease in women: A ten-year follow up, *Journal of the American Medical Association* 275 (1996): 458–462.

14. A. G. Dulloo and coauthors, Normal caffeine consumption: Influence on thermogenesis and daily energy expenditure in lean and postobese human volunteers, *American Journal of Clinical Nutrition* 49 (1989): 44–50.

15. S. S. Harris and B. Dawson-Hughes, Caffeine and bone loss in healthy postmenopausal women, *American Journal of Clinical Nutrition* 60 (1994): 573–578.

16. A. F. Subar, L. C. Harlan, and M. E. Mattson, Food and nutrient intake differences between smokers and nonsmokers in the U.S., *American Journal of Public Health* 80 (1990): 1323–1329.

17. G. van Poppel, S. Spanhaak, and T. Ockhuizen, Effects of beta carotene on immunological indexes in healthy male smokers, *American Journal of Clinical Nutrition* 57 (1993): 402–407.

18. G. Schectman, J. C. Byrd, and H. W. Gruchow, The influence of smoking on vitamin C status in adults, *American Journal of Public Health* 79 (1989): 158–162.

19. Food and Nutrition Board, *Recommended Dietary Allowances*, 10th ed. (Washington, D.C.: National Academy of Sciences, 1989), pp. 115–124.

CHAPTER 13

1. S. Shea and coauthors, Variability and self regulation of energy intake in young children in their everyday environment, *Pediatrics* 90 (1992): 542–546.

2. R. C. Klesges and coauthors, Parental influence on food selection in young children and its relationships to childhood obesity, *American Journal of Clinical Nutrition* 53 (1991): 859–864.

3. F. Lifshitz and N. Moss, Nutritional dwarfing: Growth, dieting, and fear of obesity, *Journal of the American College of Nutrition* 7 (1988): 367–376.

4. M. L. Burroughs and R. D. Terry, Parents' perspectives toward their children's eating behavior, *Topics in Clinical Nutrition* 8 (1992): 45–52.

5. American Red Cross Standard First Aid Workbook (American National Red Cross, 1991), p. 28.

F

6. D. Benton and G. Roberts, Effects of Vitamin and mineral supplementation on intelligence of a sample of schoolchildren, *Lancet,* 23 January 1988, pp. 140–143. U.S. data from E. Kennedy and J. Goldberg, What are American children eating & implications for public policy, *Nutrition Reviews* 53 (1995): 111–126.

7. P. L. Splett and M. Story, Child nutrition: Objectives for the decade, *Journal of the American Dietetic Association* 91 (1991): 665–668; N. S. Scrimshaw, Iron deficiency, *Scientific American,* October 1991, pp. 46–52.

8. J. D. Haas and M. W. Fairchild, Summary and conclusions of the International Conference on Iron Deficiency and Behavioral Development, October 10–12, 1988, *American Journal of Clinical Nutrition* 50 (1989): 703–705.

9. P. Mushak and A. F. Crocetti, Lead and nutrition, *Nutrition Today,* February 1996, pp. 12–17.

10. D. E. Glotzer and H. Bauchner, Management of childhood lead poisoning: A survey, *Pediatrics* 89 (1992): 614–618.

11. H. L. Needleman and coauthors, The long-term effects of exposure to low doses of lead in childhood: An 11-year follow-up report, *New England Journal of Medicine* 322 (1990): 83–88.

12. H. L. Needleman and coauthors, Bone lead levels and delinquent behavior, *Journal of the American Medical Association* 275 (1996): 363–369.

13. Centers for Disease Control, as cited by H. Pearson, Stepped-up lead screenings urged, *AAP News,* April 1993, pp. 1, 8.

14. R. W. Miller, The metal in our mettle, *FDA Consumer,* December 1988/January 1989, pp. 24–27.

15. J. Raloff, Lead effects show in child's balance, *Science News* 135 (1989): 54.

16. K. N. Dietrich, O. G. Berger, and P. A Succop, Lead exposure and the motor development status of urban six-year-old children in Cincinnati: Prospective study, *Pediatrics* 91 (1993): 301–307.

17. Environmental exposure to lead and cognitive deficits in children, *New England Journal of Medicine* 320 (1989): 595–596.

18. R. A. Goyer, Nutrition and metal toxicity, *American Journal of Clinical Nutrition* 61 (1995): 646S–650S.

19. H. A. Sampson and A. W. Burks, Mechanisms of food allergy, *Annual Review of Nutrition* 16 (1996): 161–177.

20. S. A. Bock and F. M. Atkins, Patterns of food hypersensitivity during sixteen years of double-blind, placebo-controlled food challenges, *Journal of Pediatrics* 117 (1990): 561–567.

21. H. A. Sampson and D. D. Metcalfe, Food allergies, *Journal of the American Medical Association* 268 (1992): 2840–2844.

22. K. S. Rowe and K. J. Rowe, Synthetic food coloring and behavior: A dose response effect in a double-blind, placebo-controlled, repeated-measures study, *Journal of Pediatrics* 124 (1994): 691–698.

23. Kids get up and go—not! International Food Information Council, *Press Release,* 11 August 1992.

24. R. C. Klesges, M. L. Shelton, and L. M. Klesges, Effects of television on metabolic rate: Potential implications for childhood obesity, *Pediatrics* 91 (1993): 281–286.

25. W. H. Dietz and S. L. Gortmaker, TV or not TV: Fat is the question, *Pediatrics* 91 (1993): 499–501.

26. N. D. Wong and coauthors, Television viewing and pediatric hypercholesterolemia, *Pediatrics* 90 (1992): 75–79.

27. Timely statement on NCEP report on children and adolescents, *Journal of the American Dietetic Association* 91 (1991): 983; N. A. Holtzman, The great god cholesterol, *Pediatrics* 87 (1991): 943–945.

28. C. L. Williams, Importance of dietary fiber in childhood, *Journal of the American Dietetic Association* 95 (1991): 1140–1146, 1149; Report of the Expert Panel on Blood Cholesterol Levels in Children and Adolescents, *Pediatrics* 89 (1992): entire supplement.

29. Position of the American Dietetic Association: Nutrition standards for child care programs, *Journal of the American Dietetic Association* 94 (1994): 323.

30. A. F. Meyers and coauthors, School breakfast program and school performance, *American Journal of Diseases of Children* 143 (1989): 1234–1239.

31. T. A. Nicklas and coauthors, Breakfast consumption affects adequacy of total daily intakes in children, *Journal of the American Dietetic Association* 93 (1993): 886–891.

32. B. A. Bidgood and C. Gameron, Meal/snack missing and dietary adequacy of primary school children, *Journal of the Canadian Dietetic Association* 53 (1992): 164–168.

33. J. Anding and coauthors, Blood lipids, cardiovascular fitness, obesity, and blood pressure: The presence of potential coronary heart disease risk factors in adolescents, *Journal of the American Dietetic Association* 96 (1996): 238–242.

34. K. Schuster, Feds put schools on a lowfat diet, *Food Management,* August 1994, pp. 78–84. Evidence that children grow well on a low-fat diet was provided by L. Van Horn, the principal investigator of the Dietary Intervention Study in Children (DISC), which follows children up to age 18, as cited in Kids grow well on low-fat diet, *Nutrition and the M.D.,* January 1996, pp. 6–7.

35. L. L. Birch, Children's preferences for high-fat foods, *Nutrition Reviews* 50 (1992): 249–255.

36. The Writing Group for the DISC Collaborative Research Group, Efficacy and safety of lowering dietary intake of fat and cholesterol in children with elevated low-density lipoprotein cholesterol: The Dietary Intervention Study in Children (DISC), *Journal of the American Medical Association* 273 (1995): 1429–1435.

37. Timely statement of the American Dietetic Association: Dietary guidance for healthy children, *Journal of the American Dietetic Association* 95 (1995): 370.

38. M. Story, M. Hayes, and B. Kalina, Availability of foods in high schools: Is there cause for concern? *Journal of the American Dietetic Association* 96 (1996): 123–126.

39. Kids make the nutritional grade, *IFIC Review,* October 1992.

40. S. M. Ott, Bone density in adolescents, *New England Journal of Medicine* 325 (1991): 1646–1647.

41. S. L. Barr, Associations of social and demographic variables with calcium intakes of high school students, *Journal of the American Dietetic Association* 94 (1994): 260–266, 269.

42. V. Matkovic, Diet, genetics, and peak bone mass of adolescent girls, *Nutrition Today,* March/April 1991, pp. 21–24.

43. L. E. Underwood, Normal adolescent growth and development, *Nutrition Today,* March/April, 1991, pp. 11–16.

44. G. A. L. Meijer and coauthors, Sleeping metabolic rate in relation to body composition and the menstrual cycle, *American Journal of Clinical Nutrition* 55 (1992): 637–640; M. Tai and coauthors, Resting metabolic rate during four phases of the menstrual cycle (abstract), *American Journal of Clinical Nutrition* 56 (1992): 101.

45. V. Tarasuk and G. H. Beaton, Menstrual-cycle patterns in energy and macronutrient intake, *American Journal of Clinical Nutrition* 53 (1991): 442–447.

46. R. S. London, L. Bradley, and N. Y. Chiamori, Effect of a nutritional supplement on premenstrual syndrome: A double-blind longitudinal study, *Journal of the American College of Nutrition* 10 (1991): 494–499.

47. A. M. Rossignol and H. Bonnlander, Caffeine-containing beverages, total fluid consumption, and premenstrual syndrome, *American Journal of Public Health* 80 (1990): 1106–1110.

48. S. Snider, Acne: Taming that age-old adolescent affliction, *FDA Consumer*, October 1990, pp. 16–19.

49. A reference providing in-depth coverage of these and other topics in women's nutrition is D. A. Krummel and P. M. Kris-Etherton, *Nutrition in Women's Health* (Gaitherburg, M.D.: Aspen, 1996).

50. Position of the American Dietetic Association and the Canadian Dietetic Association: Women's health and nutrition, *Journal of the American Dietetic Association* 95 (1995): 362–366.

51. R. Chernoff, Demographics of aging, in R. Chernoff, ed., *Geriatric Nutrition: The Health Professional's Handbook* (Gaithersburg, Md.: Aspen Publishers, 1991), pp. 1–9.

52. K. G. Kinsella, Changes in life expectancy 1900–1990, *American Journal of Clinical Nutrition* 55 (1992): 1196S–1202S.

53. N. B. Belloc and L. Breslow, Relationship of physical health status and health practices, *Preventive Medicine* 1 (1972): 409–421.

54. R. Weindruch, Caloric restriction and aging, *Scientific American*, January 1996, pp. 46–52.

55. E. J. Masoro, Assessment of nutritional component in prolongation of life and health by diet, *Proceedings of the Society for Experimental Biology and Medicine* 193 (1990): 31–34; Energy intake restriction and oxidant defense, *Nutrition Reviews* 49 (1991): 278–280.

56. N. S. Scrimshaw, Nutrition and health from womb to tomb, *Nutrition Today*, March/April 1996, pp. 55–67.

57. E. T. Poehlman and E. S. Horton, Regulation of energy expenditure in aging humans, *Annual Review of Nutrition* 10 (1990): 255–275.

58. L. Di Pietro, The epidemiology of physical activity and physical function in older people, *Medicine & Science in Sports & Exercise* 28 (1996): 596–660.

59. A. M. Egbert, The dwindles: Failure to thrive in older patients, *Nutrition Reviews* 54 (1996): S25–S30.

60. I. H. Rosenberg, Nutrition in the elderly, *Nutrition Reviews* 50 (1992): 349–350.

61. M. A. Fiatrone and coauthors, High-intensity strength training in nonagenarians, *Journal of the American Medical Association* 263 (1990): 3029–3034.

62. J. V. G. A. Durnin, Energy metabolism in the elderly, in H. Munro and G. Schlierf, eds., *Nutrition of the Elderly* (New York: Raven Press, 1992), pp. 51–63.

63. WHO Study Group on Diet, Nutrition, and Prevention of Noncommunicable Diseases, Diet, nutrition, and the prevention of chronic diseases, *Nutrition Reviews* 49 (1991): 291–301.

64. P. Merry and coauthors, Oxidative damage to lipids within the inflamed human joint provides evidence of radical-mediated hypoxic-reperfusion injury, *American Journal of Clinical Nutrition* 53 (1991): 362S–369S.

65. R. Roubenoff and L. C. Rall, Humoral mediation of changing body composition during aging and chronic inflammation, *Nutrition Reviews* 51 (1993): 1–11.

66. Merry and coauthors, 1991.

67. Processing of dietary retinoids is slowed in the elderly, *Nutrition Reviews* 49 (1991): 116–118.

68. K. Tucker, Micronutrient status and aging, *Nutrition Reviews* 53 (1995): (II) S9–S15.

69. H. J. Naurath and coauthors, Effects of vitamin B_{12}, folate and vitamin B_6 supplements in elderly people with normal serum vitamin concentrations, *Lancet* 346 (1995): 85–89.

70. G. E. Bunce, J. Kinoshita, and J. Horwitz, Nutritional factors in cataract, *Annual Review of Nutrition* 10 (1990): 233–254.

71. B. J. Rolls and P. A. Phillips, Aging and disturbances of thirst and fluid balance, *Nutrition Reviews* 48 (1990): 137–144.

72. H. Sato, T. Saito, and K. Yoshinaga, Renal function and histopathology in the elderly, in H. Munro and G. Schlierf, eds., *Nutrition of the Elderly* (New York: Raven Press, 1992), pp. 29–36.

73. H. Mertz, Trace elements in aging, in H. Munro and G. Schlierf, eds., *Nutrition of the Elderly* (New York: Raven Press, 1992), pp. 145–149.

74. R. J. Cousins and J. M. Hempe, Zinc, in M. L. Brown, ed., *Present Knowledge in Nutrition*, 6th ed. (Washington, D.C.: International Life Sciences Institute—Nutrition Foundation, 1990), pp. 251–260.

75. G. J. Fosmire, Trace mineral requirements, in R. Chernoff, ed., *Geriatric Nutrition: The Health Professional's Handbook* (Gaithersburg, Md.: Aspen Publishers, 1991), pp. 77–105.

76. Health report, *Time*, 29 August 1994, p. 21.

77. M. S. Claggett, Nutritional factors relevant to Alzheimer's disease, *Journal of the American Dietetic Association* 89 (1989): 392–396.

78. National Institute of Aging, *Progress Report on Alzheimer's Disease*, NIH publication no. 94–3885 (Washington, D.C.: Government Printing Office, 1994); E. M. Reiman and coauthors, Preclinical evidence of Alzheimer's disease in persons homozygous for the ϵ4 allele for apolipoprotein E, *New England Journal of Medicine* 334 (1996): 752–758.

79. D. Drachman of the University of Massachusetts, as reported by R. Wurtman in Food and mood, an interview, *Nutrition Action Healthletter*, September 1992, pp. 1, 5–7.

80. Wurtman, 1992.

81. S. Gauthier and coauthors, Progress report on the Canadian multicentre trial of tetrahydroaminoacridine with lecithin in Alzheimer's disease, *Canadian Journal of Neurological Sciences* 16 (1989): S543–S546.

82. First Alzheimer's drug approved, *FDA Consumer*, November 1993, p. 2.

83. K. M. Riggs and coauthors, Relations of vitamin B_{12}, vitamin B_6, folate, and homocysteine to cognitive performance in the Normative Aging Study, *American Journal of Clinical Nutrition* 63 (1996): 306–314.

84. A. Sorenson, N. Chapman, and D. N. Sundwall, Health promotion and disease prevention in the elderly, in R. Chernoff, ed., *Geriatric Nutrition: The Health Professional's Handbook* (Gaithersburg, Md.: Aspen Publishers, 1991), pp. 449–483; Are older Americans making better food choices to meet diet and health recommendations? *Nutrition Reviews* 51 (1993): 20–23.

85. R. K. Chandra, Effect of vitamin and trace-element supplementation on immune responses and infection in elderly subjects, *Lancet* 340 (1992): 1124–1127.

86. J. V. White and coauthors, Consensus of the Nutrition Screening Initiative: Risk factors and indicators of poor nutritional status in older Americans, *Journal of the American Dietetic Association* 91 (1991): 783–787.

87. An excellent review of the many problems associated with alcoholism in the elderly is found in AMA Council on Scientific Affairs, Alcoholism in the elderly, *Journal of the American Medical Association* 275 (1996): 797–801.

F

88. M. A. Davis and coauthors, Living arrangements and dietary quality of older U.S. adults, *Journal of the American Dietetic Association* 90 (1990): 1667–1672.

89. B. J. Rolls and T. M. McDermott, Effects of age on sensory-specific satiety, *American Journal of Clinical Nutrition* 54 (1991): 988–996.

90. F. Torres-Gil, Malnutrition and hunger in the elderly, *Nutrition Reviews* 54 (1996): (II) S7–S8.

91. J. Weinberg, Psychologic implications of the nutritional needs of the elderly, *Journal of the American Dietetic Association* 60 (1972): 293–296.

92. P. Kurtzweil, Growing older, eating better, *FDA Consumer,* March 1996, pp. 12–16.

CONTROVERSY 13

1. T. W. Castonguay and J. S. Stern, Hunger and appetite, in M. L. Brown, ed., *Present Knowledge in Nutrition,* 6th ed. (Washington, D.C.: International Life Sciences Institute—Nutrition Foundation, 1990), pp. 13–22.

2. C. Erlanson-Albertsson, Enterostatin: The pancreatic procolipase activation peptide—a signal for regulation of fat intake, *Nutrition Reviews* 50 (1992): 307–310.

3. P. Norton, G. Falciglia, and D. Gist, Physiologic control of food intake by neural and chemical mechanisms, *Journal of the American Dietetic Association* 93 (1993): 450–454.

4. J. D. Fernstrom, Dietary amino acids and brain function, *Journal of the American Dietetic Association* 94 (1994): 71–77.

5. P. J. Rogers, Food, mood, and appetite, *Nutrition Research Reviews* 8 (1995): 243–269.

6. P. J. Rogers and H. M. Lloyd, Nutrition and mental performance, *Proceedings of the Nutrition Society* 53 (1994): 443–456.

7. Rogers and Lloyd, 1994.

8. I. Blum and coauthors, Food preferences, body weight, and platelet-poor plasma serotonin and catecholamines, *American Journal of Clinical Nutrition* 57 (1993): 486–489.

9. M. W. Green and P. J. Rogers, Impaired cognitive functioning during spontaneous dieting, *Psychological Medicine* 25 (1995): 1003–1010.

10. Brain neurochemistry and macronutrient selection: A role for serotonin feedback? *Nutrition Reviews* 50 (1992): 21–22.

11. C. Benkelfat and coauthors, Mood-lowering effect of tryptophan depletion, *Archives of General Psychiatry* 51 (1994): 687–697.

12. Blum and coauthors, 1993.

13. Benkelfat and coauthors, 1994.

14. C. Greenwood, The role of diet in modulating brain metabolism and behavior, *Contemporary Nutrition* 14 (1989): whole issue.

15. M. L. Brown, ed., *Present Knowledge in Nutrition* (Washington, D.C.: International Life Sciences Institute—Nutrition Foundation, 1990).

16. G. Weidner and coauthors, Improvements in hostility and depression in relation to dietary change and cholesterol lowering, *Annals of Internal Medicine* 117 (1992): 820–823.

17. M. F. Muldoon, S. B. Manuck, and K. A. Matthews, Lowering cholesterol concentrations and mortality: A quantitative review of primary prevention trials, *British Medical Journal* 301 (1990): 309–314.

18. J. R. Kaplan and coauthors, Demonstration of an association among dietary cholesterol, central serotonergic activity, and social behavior in monkeys, *Psychosomatic Medicine* 56 (1994): 479–484.

19. Kaplan, 1994.

20. T. Hamazaki and coauthors, The effect of docosa hexaenoic acid on aggression in young adults: A placebo-controlled double-blind study, *Journal of Clinical Investigation* 97 (1996): 1129–1133.

21. Dr. James McGaugh, director of the center for neurobiology and memory at the University of California at Irvine, as quoted in A. Purvis, Ultra think fast, *Time,* 8 June 1992, p. 80.

22. V. Lambert, Using "smart" drugs and drinks may not be smart, *FDA Consumer,* April 1993, pp. 24–26.

23. P. F. Smith, C. L. Darlington, and K. Maclennan, Gingko biloba: An ancient Chinese tree with neuroprotective properties, *Asia Pacific Journal of Pharmacology* 10 (1995), and supplements 1, 3–4; S. Stoll and coauthors, Ginkgo biloba extract (EGB761) independently improves changes in passive-avoidance learning and brain membrane fluidity in the aging mouse, *Pharmacopsychiatry* 29 (1996): 144–149.

24. Sweet remembrances, *Science News,* 22 September 1990, p. 189; S. E. Gowans and H. P. Weingarten, Elevations of plasma glucose do not support taste-to-postingestive consequences of learning, *American Journal of Physiology* 261 (1991): 1407–1409.

25. Rogers, 1995.

26. E. diTomaso, M. Beltramo, and D. Piomelli, Brain cannabinoids in chocolate (scientific correspondence), *Nature* 382 (1996): 677–678.

27. Rogers, 1995.

28. Rogers and Lloyd, 1994, 447.

29. H. M. Lloyd and P. J. Rogers, Acute effects of breakfasts of differing fat and carbohydrate content on morning mood and cognitive performance, *Proceedings of the Nutrition Society* 53 (1994): 239A.

30. Rogers and Lloyd, 1994, 446.

CHAPTER 14

1. D. O. Cliver, *Eating Safely: Avoiding Foodborne Illnesses* (New York: American Council on Science and Health, 1993), p. 3.

2. R. L. Hall, Food safety and biotechnology, *Nutrition Today,* May/June 1991, pp. 15–20.

3. I. D. Wolf, Critical issues in food safety, 1991–2000, *Food Technology,* January 1992, pp. 64–70.

4. M. P. Doyle, Reducing foodborne diseases—What are the priorities? *Nutrition Reviews* 51 (1993): 346–347.

5. Other features of the botulinum toxin are in L. Vangelova, Botulinum toxin: A poison that can heal, *FDA Consumer,* December 1995, pp. 16–19.

6. B. P. Bell and coauthors, A multistate outbreak of *Escherichia coli* 0157:H7–associated bloody diarrhea and hemolytic uremic syndrome from hamburgers, *Journal of the American Medical Association* 272 (1994): 1349–1353.

7. M. Van Schothorst and N. Jardine, eds. *A Simple Guide to Understanding and Applying the Hazard Analysis Critical Control Point Concept* (Washington, D.C.: International Life Science Press, 1993).

8. New regulations for seafood, *FDA Consumer,* March 1996, pp. 2–3.

9. Outbreaks of *Salmonella* serotype Enteritidis infection associated with consumption of raw shell eggs—United States, 1994–1995, *Morbidity and Mortality Weekly Report* 45 (1996): 737–742.

10. V. Modeland, Fishing for facts on fish safety, *FDA Consumer,* February 1989, pp. 16–24.

11. Cliver, 1993.

12. J. A. Desenclos and coauthors, The protective effect of alcohol on the occurrence of epidemic oyster-borne hepatitis A, *Epidemiology* 3 (1992): 371–374.

13. Y. Sun and J. D. Oliver, Hot Sauce: No elimination of *Vibrio vulnificus, Journal of Food Protection* 58 (1995): 441–442.

14. Seafood safety: Highlights of the executive summary of the 1991 report by the Committee on Evaluation of the Safety of Fishery Products of the Food and Nutrition Board, Institute of Medicine, National Academy of Sciences, *Nutrition Reviews* 49 (1991): 357–363.

15. J. H. T. Luong, C. A. Groom, and K. B. Male, The potential role of biosensors in the food and drink industries, *Biosensors and Bioelectronics* 6 (1991): 547–554.

16. P. I. Peterkin, E. S. Idziak, and A. N. Sharpe, Detection of *Listeria monocytogenes* by direct colony hybridization on hydrophobic grid-membrane filters by using a chromogen-labeled DNA probe, *Applied and Environmental Microbiology* 57 (1991): 586–591; M. Hoshi, Y. Sasamoto, and M. Nonaka, Microbial sensor system for nondestructive evaluation of fish meat quality, *Biosensors and Bioelectronics* 6 (1991): 15–20.

17. R. D. Williams, Boil it, cook it, peel it or forget it, *FDA Consumer,* September 1991, p. 17.

18. K. E. Anderson and A. Kappas, Dietary regulation of cytochrome P450, *Annual Review of Nutrition* 11 (1991): 141–167.

19. A. Levin, Pesticides: How dangerous are they? *Building Economic Alternatives* (a quarterly publication of Co-op America, 2100 M Street, NW, Suite 310, Washington, DC 20063), Summer 1989, p. 16.

20. C. F. Chaisson, B. Petersen, and J. S. Douglass, *Pesticides in Foods: A Guide for Professionals* (Chicago: American Dietetic Association, 1991), pp. 2–3.

21. National Academy of Sciences Committee, as quoted by J. Raloff and D. Pendick, Pesticides in produce may threaten kids, *Science News,* 3 July 1993, pp. 4–5.

22. P. Weber, A place for pesticides? *World Watch,* May/June 1992, pp. 18–25.

23. Food and Drug Administration Pesticide Program, *Residues in Foods 1990* (Washington, D.C.: Food and Drug Administration, 1991).

24. Food and Drug Administration Pesticide Program, 1991.

25. M. V. Polo, M. J. Lagarda, and R. Farré, The effect of freezing on mineral element content of vegetables, *Journal of Food Composition and Analysis* 5 (1992): 77–78.

26. C. K. Winter, Pesticide residues and the Delaney Clause, *Food Technology* 47 (1993): 81–86; Government regulation of food safety: Interaction of scientific and societal forces, *Food Technology* 46 (1992): 73–80.

27. Federal update: Delaney Clause called "scientifically unmanageable," *Journal of the American Dietetic Association* 93 (1993): 268.

28. Wolf, 1992.

29. J. Hotchkiss and R. Cassens, Nitrate, nitrite, and nitroso compounds in foods (a scientific status summary by the Institute of Food Technologists' Expert Panel on Food Safety and Nutrition), April 1987, available from Institute of Food Science, Department of Food Science, Cornell University, Ithaca, NY 14853.

30. One honey of an alternative to sulfites, *Science News* 134 (1988): 218.

31. New "food freshener," *Nutrition Forum* 5 (1988): 49.

32. M. Naim and coauthors, Interaction of MSG taste with nutrition: Perspectives in consummatory behavior and digestion, *Physiology and Behavior* 49 (1991): 1019–1024.

33. D. J. Raiten, J. M. Talbot, and K. D. Fisher, eds., Executive summary from the report: Analysis of adverse reactions to monosodium glutamate (MSG), *Journal of Nutrition* (1995): 2892S–2906S.

34. D. Farley, Keeping up with the microwave revolution, *FDA Consumer,* March 1990, pp. 17–21.

35. D. Blumenthal, Deciding about dioxins, *FDA Consumer,* February 1990, pp. 11–13.

36. T. D. Etherton, P. M. Kris-Etherton, and E. W. Mills, Recombinant bovine and porcine somatotropin: Safety and benefits of these biotechnologies, *Journal of the American Dietetic Association* 93 (1993): 177–180.

37. Etherton, Kris-Etherton, and Mills, 1993.

38. Bovine somatotropin and the safety of cow's milk: National Institutes of Health Technology Assessment Conference Statement, *Nutrition Reviews* 49 (1991): 227–232.

39. Bovine somatotropin and the safety of cow's milk, 1991.

40. K. L. Ropp, New animal drug increases milk production, *FDA Consumer,* May 1994, pp. 24–27.

41. B. Corey, Bovine growth hormone harmless for humans, *FDA Consumer,* April 1990, pp. 17–18.

42. J. C. Juskevich and C. G. Guyer, Bovine growth hormone: Human food safety evaluation, *Science* 249 (1990): 875–884; R. W. Rhein, *BST = A Safe, More Plentiful Milk Supply* (booklet) (New York: American Council on Science and Health, 1990).

43. Bovine somatotropin and the safety of cow's milk, 1991.

CONTROVERSY 14

1. A. L. Owen, The impact of future foods on nutrition and health, *Journal of the American Dietetic Association* 90 (1990): 1217–1222.

2. H. L. Miller and S. J. Ackerman, Perspective on food biotechnology, *FDA Consumer,* March 1990, pp. 8–13.

3. J. Henkel, Genetic engineering: Fast forwarding to future foods, *FDA Consumer,* April 1995, pp. 6–11.

4. First biotech tomato marketed, *FDA Consumer,* September 1994, pp. 3–4.

5. Bioengineering regulations go public, *Science News,* 3 December 1994, p. 383; EPA proposes regulation of gene-altered pesticidal plants, *EDF Letter,* March 1995, p. 2.

6. American Medical Association Council on Scientific Affairs, Biotechnology and the American agricultural industry, *Journal of the American Medical Association* 265 (1991): 1429–1436.

7. J. A. Nordlee and coauthors, Identification of a brazil-nut allergen in transgenic soybeans, *New England Journal of Medicine* 334 (1996): 688–692.

8. D. D. Hopkins, R. J. Goldburg, and S. A. Hirsch, *A Mutable Feast: Assuring Food Safety in the Era of Genetic Engineering* (New York: Environmental Defense Fund, 1991).

9. Food and Drug Administration, Statement of policy: Foods derived from new plant varieties, *Federal Register,* 29 May 1992.

10. Biotechnology of food: Background information from the FDA, *Nutrition Today,* July/August 1994, pp. 19–20.

11. S. L. Huttner, Getting the products of biotechnology to market, *Priorities,* March 1995, pp. 11–14.

12. Position of the American Dietetic Association: Biotechnology and the future of food, *Journal of the American Dietetic Association* 95 (1995): 1429–1432.

13. Genetically engineered foods: Fears and facts, an interview with FDA's Jim Maryanski, *FDA Consumer,* January/February 1993, pp. 11–14.

14. WHO, *Safety and Nutritional Adequacy of Irradiated Foods* (Geneva, Switzerland: World Health Organization, 1994).

F

15. American Council on Science and Health, *Irradiated Foods* (booklet) (New York: American Council on Science and Health, 1988).

16. A. J. Swallow, Wholesomeness and safety of irradiated foods, in *Nutritional and Toxicological Consequences of Food Processing: Advances in Experimental Medicine and Biology* (New York: Plenum Press, 1991), pp. 11–31.

17. D. R. Murray, *Biology of Food Irradiation* (New York: John Wiley & Sons, 1990), pp. 105–106.

18. Food irradiation, Taped interview, National Public Radio broadcast, *Living on Earth*, 7 February 1992.

19. L. Heide and K. W. Bogl, Detection methods for irradiated foods—Luminescence and viscosity measures, *International Journal of Radiation Biology* 57 (1990): 201–219; T. Autio and S. Pinnioja, Identification of irradiated foods by the thermoluminescence of mineral contamination, *Zeitschrift für Lebensmittel-Untersuchung und -Forschung* 191 (1990): 177–180; A. M. Sjoberg and coauthors, Methods for detection of irradiation of spices, *Zeitschrift für Lebensmittel-Untersuchung und -Forschung* 190 (1990): 99–103.

20. Really rad radishes, *Earth Island Journal*, Summer 1991, p. 16.

21. Vijayalaxmi and S. G. Srikantia, A preview of the studies on the wholesomeness of irradiated wheat, conducted at the National Institute of Nutrition, India, *Radiation, Physics, and Chemistry* 34 (1989): 941–952.

22. Vijayalaxmi and Srikantia, 1989.

23. M. F. Jacobsen and S. Schmidt, Food irradiation: Zapping our troubles away? *Nutrition Action Health Letter*, April 1992, pp. 1, 5–7.

24. Anti-food irradiation (editorial), *Priorities*, Spring 1989, p. 41.

25. T. D. Etherton, The impact of biotechnology on animal agriculture and the consumer, *Nutrition Today*, July/August 1994, pp. 12–18.

26. Position of the American Dietetic Association: Food irradiation, *Journal of the American Dietetic Association* 96 (1996): 69–72.

CHAPTER 15

1. L. N. Burby, *World Hunger* (San Diego, Calif.: Lucent Books, 1995), pp. 13–16; P. L. Kutzner, *World Hunger: A Reference Handbook* (Santa Barbara, Calif.: ABC-CL10, 1991), pp. 158–159.

2. L. R. Brown, Facing food scarcity, *World Watch*, November/December 1995, pp. 10–20.

3. Position of the American Dietetic Association: World hunger, *Journal of the American Dietetic Association* 95 (1995): 1160–1162.

4. Examples: M. Countryman, Lessons of the divestment drive, *The Nation*, 26 March 1988, pp. 406–409; H. Orlans, The revolution at Gallaudet: Students provoke break with the past, *Change: The Magazine of Higher Learning*, January/February 1989, pp. 8–18; S. Conn, Thoughts on national service: An open letter to William F. Buckley, Jr., *Change: The Magazine of Higher Learning*, May/June 1991, pp. 6–7, 52; R. G. Braungart and M. M. Braungart, Youth movements in the 1980s: A global perspective, *International Sociology*, June 1990, pp. 157–181; E. Larsen, Youth environmental movement, *Utne Reader*, March/April 1991, pp. 30–31; J. Smith, The 1989 Chinese student movement: Lessons for nonviolent activists, *Peace and Change, A Journal of Peace Research*, January 1992, pp. 82–101; Windmill at Hamilton College generates heat, light, and a conservation campaign, *Chronicles of Higher Education*, 1 April 1992; A dollars-and-cents moral crusade in recycling, *Chronicles of Higher Education*, 15 April 1992, p. A5. Also, the Rainforest Action Network (450 San-some, Suite 700, San Francisco, CA 94111), which puts effective pressure on governments and corporations to stop destroying rainforests, originated and is maintained largely as a student effort.

5. L. R. Brown, Reexamining the world food prospect, in L. R. Brown, *State of the World 1989* (New York: W. W. Norton, 1989), pp. 41–58; L. R. Brown and J. E. Young, Feeding the world in the nineties, in L. R. Brown, *State of the World 1990* (New York: W. W. Norton, 1990), pp. 59–78.

6. C. Flavin and O. Tunali, Climate of hope: New strategies for stabilizing the world's atmosphere, *Worldwatch Paper* 130, June 1996, a 68-page monograph with several hundred references.

7. J. L. Jacobson, Abandoning homelands, in L. R. Brown and coauthors, *State of the World 1989* (New York: W. W. Norton, 1989), pp. 59–76.

8. S. Postel, Denial in the decisive decade, in L. R. Brown and coauthors, *State of the World 1992* (New York: W. W. Norton, 1992).

9. Postel, 1992.

10. United Nations Food and Agriculture Organization (FAO), *The State of Food and Agriculture, 1993* (Rome: 1993), as cited in L. R. Brown and H. Kane, *Full House* (New York: W. W. Norton, 1994), pp. 75–88.

11. Postel, 1992.

12. Position of the American Dietetic Association, 1995.

13. P. Uvin, The state of world hunger, *Nutrition Reviews* 52 (1994): 151–161.

14. Burby, 1995, p. 13.

15. Fact Sheet on Childhood Hunger and Poverty, (c. 1992), available from *Bread for the World*, 802 Rhode Island Avenue, NE, Washington, DC 20018.

16. S. Lewis, Food security, environment, poverty, and the world's children, *Journal of Nutrition Education* 24 (1 Supplement), January/February 1992, pp. 3S–5S.

17. M. Mudd, vice president, Kraft General Foods, quoted in *Journal of Nutrition Education* 24 (1 Supplement), January/February 1992, p. 1S.

18. L. D. McBean, ed., with D. Derelian, R. J. Fersh, and L. Parker, Hunger and undernutrition in America, *Dairy Council Digest*, March/April 1992.

19. L. V. E. Crawford, Rethinking domestic hunger policy: An interview with J. Larry Brown, *Seeds*, May/June 1990, pp. 6–9.

20. U.S. Department of Commerce, *Statistical Abstract of the United States, 1994* (Washington, D.C.: Bureau of the Census, 1994).

21. Fact Sheet on Childhood Hunger and Poverty, c. 1992.

22. M. Nestle and S. Guttmacher, Hunger in the United States: Rationale, methods, and policy implications of state hunger surveys, *Journal of Nutrition Education* 24 (1 Supplement), January/February 1992, pp. 18S–22S.

23. J. C. Wolgemuth and coauthors, Wasting malnutrition and inadequate nutrient intakes identified in a multiethnic homeless population, *Journal of the American Dietetic Association* 92 (1992): 834–839; M. A. Drake, The nutritional status and dietary adequacy of single homeless women and their children in shelters, *Public Health Reports* 107 (1992): 312–319; B. E. Cohen, N. Chapman, and M. R. Burt, Food sources and intake of homeless persons, *Journal of Nutrition Education* 24 (1 Supplement), January/February 1992, pp. 45S–51S.

24. World Bank, *World Development Report 1991* (New York: Oxford University Press, 1991); Postel, 1992, pp. 3–8.

25. L. Timberlake, *Only One Earth*, cited in Food for thought, *Seeds*, Sprouts edition, 1988.

26. R. W. Kates, Ending deaths from famine: The opportunity in Somalia, *New England Journal of Medicine* 328 (1993): 1055–1057.

27. *Tallahassee Democrat*, 14 October 1994; Burby, 1995.

28. Kates, 1993.

29. U.S. Department of Commerce, 1994, pp. 854–855.

30. L. R. Brown and coauthors, *State of the World 1995* (New York: W. W. Norton, 1995), p. 11; *Tallahassee Democrat*, 10 June 1995.

31. R. Green, Farm bill heavy on controversy, spending, *Tallahassee Democrat*, 25 February 1996, p. 3A.

32. B. Stutz, The landscape of hunger, *Audubon*, March/April 1993, pp. 54–57; Newsbreaks: Effects of environmental degradation on nutrition, *Nutrition Today*, March/April 1992, p. 4.

33. Brown and Young, 1990.

34. R. D. Kaplan, The coming anarchy, *Atlantic Monthly*, February 1994, pp. 44–76.

35. J. W. Clay and coauthors, *The Spoils of Famine: Ethiopian Famine Policy and Peasant Agriculture* (Cambridge, Mass.: Cultural Survival, 1988), as cited in Brown and Kane, 1994, pp. 146–157.

36. L. R. Brown, *Vital Signs 1993: The Trends That Are Shaping Our Future* (New York: W. W. Norton, 1993); L. R. Brown, A decade of discontinuity, *World Watch*, July/August 1993, pp. 19–26.

37. FAO, as cited in World Resources Institute (WRI), *World Resources 1992–93* (New York: Oxford University Press, 1992); bluefin tuna figure from D. Meadows and coauthors, *Beyond the Limits* (Post Mills, Vt.: Chelsea Green Publishing Company, 1992), as cited in Brown and Kane, 1994, pp. 75–88.

38. L. Brown, The Aral Sea: Going, going . . . , *World Watch*, January/February 1991.

39. Government of Canada, *The State of Canada's Environment* (Ottawa: 1991).

40. Brown and coauthors, 1995, p. 191.

41. J. W. M. la Riviere, Threats to the world's water, *Scientific American*, September 1989, pp. 80–94.

42. Brown and Young, 1990, pp. 64–65.

43. Population Reference Bureau (PRB), *1993 World Population Data Sheet* (Washington, D.C.: 1993), as cited in Brown and Kane, 1994, pp. 49–61.

44. Centers for Disease Control, Population based mortality assessment: Baidoa and Afgoi, Somalia, 1992, *Journal of the American Medical Association* (1993), as cited in L. R. Brown and H. Kane, *Full House* (New York: W. W. Norton, 1994), pp. 49–61.

45. P. S. Dasgupta, Population, poverty and the local environment, *Scientific American*, February 1995, pp. 40–45.

46. Postel, 1992.

47. L. R. Brown, *Who Will Feed China? Wake-up Call for a Small Planet* (New York: W. W. Norton, 1995).

48. Dasgupta, 1995.

49. Dasgupta, 1995.

50. Lewis, 1992.

51. Lewis, 1992.

52. Lewis, 1992.

53. J. Collins, The real roots of world hunger: Demand not supply, *Seeds*, March/April 1990, pp. 22–24.

54. Postel, 1992.

55. K. L. Clancy and J. Bowering, The need for emergency food: Poverty problems and policy responses, *Journal of Nutrition Education* 24 (1 Supplement), January/February 1992, pp. 12S–17S; J. M. Dodds, S. L. Parker, and P. S. Haines, Hunger in the 80s and 90s: A challenge for nutrition educators, *Journal of Nutrition Education* 24 (1 Supplement), January/February 1992, p. 2S.

56. C. Flavin and J. E. Young, Shaping the next industrial revolution, in L. R. Brown, *State of the World 1990* (New York: W. W. Norton, 1990), pp. 181–199.

57. Mudd, 1992.

58. J. Csete, Hunger and the Academy: Training nutritionists for the 1990s, *Journal of Nutrition Education* 24 (1 Supplement), January/February 1992, pp. 79S–83S.

59. W. L. Scheider, Fighting hunger and poverty: A strategy for nutrition educators, *Journal of Nutrition Education* 24 (1 Supplement), January/February 1992, pp. 84S–85S.

60. Position of the American Dietetic Association: Environmental issues, *Journal of the American Dietetic Association* 93 (1993): 589–591.

61. Position of the American Dietetic Association: Domestic hunger and inadequate access to food, *Journal of the American Dietetic Association* 90 (1990): 1427–1441.

62. P. Von Stackelberg, Whitewash: The dioxin coverup, *Greenpeace*, March/April 1989, pp. 7–11; National Wildlife Federation calls for ban on chlorine use, *International Wildlife*, January/February 1991, p. 26.

63. S. Smith, professor of nutrition, University of New Hampshire, Durham, N.H., personal communication, summer 1993.

CONTROVERSY 15

1. Committee on the Role of Alternative Farming Methods in Modern Production Agriculture, Board on Agriculture, National Research Council, *Alternative Agriculture* (Washington, D.C.: National Academy Press, 1989).

2. World Resources Institute, *The 1992 Information Please Environmental Almanac* (Boston: Houghton Mifflin, 1992), p. 13.

3. J. Dixon, Agency warns of threats posed by plant extinction, *Tallahassee Democrat*, 24 March 1992.

4. Dixon, 1992.

5. C. B. Heiser, Jr., *Seeds to Civilization: The Story of Food* (Cambridge, Mass.: Harvard University Press, 1990), p. 13.

6. P. Smith and J. Warrick, Boss hog: North Carolina's pork revolution, *Amicus Journal*, Spring 1996, pp. 36–42.

7. Committee on the Role of Alternative Farming Methods, 1989, p. 7.

8. U.S. Department of Commerce, *Statistical Abstract of the United States, 1994* (Washington, D.C.: Bureau of the Census, 1994), p. 668.

9. P. H. Raven, L. R. Berg, and G. B. Johnson, *Environment* (New York: Saunders, 1993), p. 407.

10. Committee on the Role of Alternative Farming Methods, 1989, p. 6.

11. A. B. Durning and H. B. Brough, Taking stock: Animal farming and the environment, *Worldwatch Paper 103*, July 1991, p. 35.

12. K. Mattes, Kicking the pesticide habit, *Amicus Journal*, Fall 1989, pp. 10–17.

13. Cheap food at any cost, *High Country News*, vol. 27, May 1, 1995.

14. C. Mitlo-Shartel and the Land Stewardship Project, Regenerating America's agriculture, *Building Economic Alternatives* (a quarterly publication of Co-op America, 2100 M. Street NW, Suite 310, Washington, D.C. 20063), Summer 1989, pp. 9–12.

15. Committee on the Role of Alternative Farming Methods, 1989.

16. Committee on the Role of Alternative Farming Methods, 1989, pp. 3–4.

17. Committee on the Role of Alternative Farming Methods, 1989, p. 5.

F

18. *Organic Agriculture: What the States Are Doing* (Washington, D.C.: Center for Science in the Public Interest, 1989), pp. 5, 14–15.

19. Florida voters will consider a penny-a-pound sugar tax on the 1996 ballot.

20. *Organic Agriculture: What the States Are Doing*, 1989, quoting from the assistant secretary of agriculture, Orville G. Bentley, in a USDA press release, February 1988.

21. Mitlo-Shartel and the Land Stewardship Project, 1989.

22. A. T. Durning and H. B. Brough, Reforming the livestock economy, in L. R. Brown and coauthors, *State of the World 1992* (New York: W. W. Norton, 1992), pp. 66–82.

23. S. Smith, professor of nutrition, University of New Hampshire, Durham, N.H., personal communication, August 1993.

24. A. Zorc, From family farm to agribusiness: The spoilage of America's meat industry, *Co-op America Quarterly*, Spring 1992, pp. 10–13, 19; Eating green, *Nutrition Action Health Letter*, January/February 1992, pp. 1, 5–7.

25. C. Flavin and J. E. Young, Shaping the next industrial revolution, in L. R. Brown, *State of the World 1993* (New York: W. W. Norton, 1993), pp. 180–199.

F

ANSWERS TO THE SELF-CHECK QUESTIONS

G

CHAPTER 1

1. d (p. 5)
2. a (p. 8)
3. a (p. 7)
4. c (p. 20)
5. b (p. 22)
6. False. At all meals, a vegan avoids eggs, bacon, and all other animal derived foods. (p. 13)
7. False. Heart disease and cancer are influenced by many factors with genetics and diet among them. (p. 14)
8. True (p. 8)
9. False. Only when a finding has been repeatedly confirmed by science is it wise to change your diet accordingly. (p. 3)
10. True (p. 30)

CHAPTER 2

1. d (p. 34)
2. d (p. 34)
3. b (p. 43)
4. d (p. 39)
5. d (p. 41)
6. True (p. 37)
7. False. The RDA are estimates of the needs of healthy persons only. Medical problems alter nutrient needs. (p. 35)
8. False. People who choose to eat no meats or products taken from animals can still use the Food Guide Pyramid to make their diets adequate. (p. 43)
9. False. By law, food labels must state as a percentage of the Daily Values the amounts of vitamins A and C present in a food. (p. 54)
10. True (p. 56)
11. False. The diets of the Mediterranean are generally low in animal protein and high in carbohydrates and fiber. (p. 67)

CHAPTER 3

1. c (p. 77)
2. d (p. 79)
3. a (p. 84)
4. c (p. 85)
5. d (p. 89)
6. True (p. 75)
7. False. The process of digestion occurs mainly in the small intestine. (p. 85)
8. False. The digestive tract works efficiently to digest all foods simultaneously, regardless of composition. (p. 86)
9. True (p. 85)
10. False. Absorption of the majority of nutrients takes place across the specialized cells of the small intestine. (p. 89)
11. False. Stone Age people achieved their abundant nutrient intakes using only the meats, fruits, and vegetables food groups. (p. 101)

CHAPTER 4

1. b (p. 105)
2. d (p. 106)
3. a (p. 107)
4. c (pp. 116, 117)
5. b (pp. 120, 121)
6. a (p. 120)
7. True (p. 106)
8. True (pp. 120, 122)
9. True (p. 124)
10. False. Type I diabetes is most often controlled with insulin injections. (p. 123)
11. True (p. 117)
12. False. Whole-grain bread remains more nutritious despite the enrichment of white flour. (p. 114)
13. True (p. 114)
14. False. The prevention of constipation and a lowered risk of colon cancer are achieved by eating a diet high in fiber. (p. 110)
15. False. Using artificial sweeteners has not been proven to help people lose weight. (p. 143)

CHAPTER 5

1. c (p. 146)
2. a (p. 151)

3. c (p. 151)
4. b (p. 154)
5. d (p. 173)
6. True (p. 155)
7. True (p. 157)
8. False. Consuming large amounts of *trans*-fatty acids elevates serum LDL cholesterol and thus raises the risk of heart disease and heart attack. (p. 165)
9. False. When olestra is present in the digestive tract, fat-soluble vitamins, including vitamin E, become unavailable for absorption. (p. 168)
10. True (p. 187)

CHAPTER 6

1. b (p. 190)
2. b (p. 194)
3. c (p. 198)
4. a (p. 210)
5. d (p. 220)
6. True (p. 202)
7. False. Excess protein in the diet may have adverse effects such as obesity, enlarged liver or kidneys, worsened kidney disease, and accelerated adult bone loss. (p. 214)
8. False. Impoverished people living on Indian reservations, in inner cities, and in rural areas of the United States, as well as some elderly, homeless, and ill people in hospitals, are often diagnosed with PEM. (p. 213)
9. True (p. 207)
10. True (p. 210)

CHAPTER 7

1. d (p. 227)
2. a (p. 234)
3. c (p. 229)
4. d (p. 233)
5. d (pp. 228, 247)
6. d (p. 227)
7. True (p. 256)
8. False. In general, nutrients are absorbed best from foods where they are dispersed among other ingredients that facilitate their absorption. (p. 255)
9. True (p. 259)
10. True (p. 258)
11. True (p. 275)

CHAPTER 8

1. d (p. 286)
2. c (p. 287)
3. b (p. 293)
4. d (p. 304)
5. a (p. 307)

6. False. The FDA requires that bottled water meets the same standards as those set for purity and sanitation of U.S. tap water. (p. 290)
7. False. You can survive being deprived of water for only a few days. (p. 285)
8. True (p. 300)
9. True (p. 290)
10. False. Butter, cream, and cream cheese are almost pure fat and poor sources of calcium, whereas vegetables such as broccoli, are good sources of available calcium. (p. 316)
11. False. Actions to prevent osteoporosis are best begun in childhood and adolescence, when the bones are growing most rapidly. (p. 328)

CHAPTER 9

1. b (p. 338)
2. d (p. 341)
3. c (p. 345)
4. a (p. 349)
5. d (p. 356)
6. d (p. 374)
7. False. The thermic effect of food is believed to have negligible effects on total energy expenditure. (p. 338)
8. True (p. 340)
9. True (p. 343)
10. False. There is no evidence that the body becomes internally "cleansed" during ketosis. Furthermore, the body slows its metabolism to conserve energy. (p. 354)

CHAPTER 10

1. c (p. 382)
2. b (p. 383)
3. d (p. 400)
4. d (p. 406)
5. a (p. 390)
6. False. The guidelines for developing physical fitness are more rigorous than those for obtaining health benefits. (p. 378)
7. False. The average resting pulse rate for adults is around 70 beats per minute, but the rate is lower for active people. (p. 382)
8. True (p. 404)
9. True (p. 397)
10. False. Anorexia nervosa occurs most often in women, but men account for about 1 in 20 eating disorder cases in the general population. (p. 416)

CHAPTER 11

1. b (p. 431)
2. d (p. 441)
3. c (p. 435)

4. d (p. 445)
5. d (p. 463)
6. False. The best way to plan a diet to support the immune system is to meet the RDA for each nutrient while not ingesting a dose from a supplement that would cause harm. (p. 426)
7. False. Vegetarians have lower mortality rates from cancer than the rest of the population, even when cancers linked to smoking and alcohol are taken out of the picture. (p. 444)
8. True (p. 438)
9. True (p. 433)
10. False. Hypertension is more severe and occurs earlier in life among African Americans than those of European or Asian descent. (p. 440)

CHAPTER 12

1. b (p. 477)
2. d (p. 483)
3. a (p. 489)
4. d (p. 493)
5. c (p. 475)
6. True (p. 473)
7. True (p. 486)
8. False. There is no proof for the theory that "stuffing the baby" at bedtime will promote sleeping through the night. (p. 499)
9. False. In general, the effect of nutritional deprivation of the mother is to reduce the quantity, not the quality, of her milk. (p. 492)
10. True (p. 509)

CHAPTER 13

1. d (p. 516)
2. c (p. 518)
3. c (p. 521)
4. d (pp. 530, 531)
5. b (p. 532)
6. False. Research to date does not support the idea that food allergies or intolerances cause hyperactivity in children, but studies continue. (p. 523)

7. True (p. 537)
8. False. Vitamin A absorption appears to increase with aging. (p. 538)
9. True (p. 524)
10. True (p. 550)

CHAPTER 14

1. b (p. 556)
2. c (p. 561)
3. d (p. 565)
4. a (p. 569)
5. d (p. 581)
6. False. Most hazardous contamination is not detectable by a food's odor, appearance, or taste. (p. 562)
7. False. Minerals are unaffected by heat processing because they cannot be destroyed, as vitamins can be. (p. 576)
8. True (p. 583)
9. False. The canning industry chooses treatments that employ the high-temperature–short-time [HTST] principle for canning. (p. 575)
10. True (p. 595)

CHAPTER 15

1. d (p. 608)
2. c (p. 615)
3. c (p. 606)
4. b (p. 604)
5. a (p. 623)
6. True (p. 601)
7. False. The number of people affected by famine is relatively small compared with the number suffering from less severe but chronic hunger. (p. 606)
8. False. The link between improved economic status and slowed population growth has been demonstrated in country after country. (p. 611)
9. False. Many more people need welfare and food assistance now than in the 1980s. (p. 604)
10. True. (p. 624)

GLOSSARY

A

absorb to take in, as nutrients are taken into the intestinal cells after digestion, the main function of the digestive tract with respect to nutrients.

acceptable daily intake (ADI) the estimated amount of sweetener that can be consumed daily over a person's lifetime without any adverse effects.

accredited approved; in the case of medical centers or universities, certified by an agency recognized by the U.S. Department of Education.

acesulfame (AY-sul-fame) **potassium**, also called **acesulfame-K** a zero-calorie sweetener approved by the FDA.

acetaldehyde (ass-et-AL-deh-hide) a substance to which ethanol is metabolized on its way to becoming harmless waste products that can be excreted.

acid reducers and **acid controllers** drugs that reduce the acid output of the stomach. They are most suitable for treating severe, persistent forms of heartburn, but are useless for neutralizing acid already present in the stomach. Previously sold as prescription ulcer medications, the drugs are now sold freely, but the packages bear warnings of side effects; some types interfere with the stomach's ability to destroy alcohol.

acidosis (acid-DOH-sis) blood acidity above normal, indicating excess acid (*osis* means "too much in the blood").

acids compounds that release hydrogens in a watery solution.

acid–base balance maintenance of the proper degree of acidity in each of the body's fluids.

acne chronic inflammation of the skin's follicles and oil-producing glands, which leads to an accumulation of oils inside the ducts that surround hairs; usually associated with the maturation of young adults.

added sugars sugars added to a food for any purpose, such as to add sweetness or bulk or to aid in browning (baked goods).

additives substances that are added to foods, but are not normally consumed by themselves as foods.

adequacy the dietary characteristic of providing all of the essential nutrients, fiber, and energy in amounts sufficient to maintain health and body weight.

aerobic (air-ROE-bic) requiring oxygen. Aerobic activity requires the heart and lungs to work harder than normal to deliver oxygen to the tissues, and therefore strengthens them.

agribusiness agriculture practiced on a massive scale by large corporations owning vast acreages and employing intensive technological, fuel, and chemical inputs.

AIDS acquired immune deficiency syndrome, caused by infection with HIV, a virus that is transmitted primarily by sexual contact, by contact with infected blood, by needles shared among drug users, or by materials transferred from an infected mother to her fetus or infant.

alcohol dehydrogenase (ADH) an enzyme system that breaks down alcohol. The antidiuretic hormone listed below is also abbreviated ADH.

alcoholism a dependency on alcohol marked by compulsive uncontrollable drinking with negative effects on physical health, family relationships, and social health.

alcohol-related birth defects see *fetal alcohol syndrome*.

alimentary canal see *digestive system*.

alitame a noncaloric sweetener formed from the amino acids L-aspartic acid and L-alanine. In the United States, the FDA is considering its approval.

alkalosis (al-kah-LOH-sis) blood alkalinity above normal (*alka* means "base"; *osis* means "too much in the blood").

allergy an immune reaction to a foreign substance, such as a component of food. Also called *hypersensitivity* by researchers.

aloe a tropical plant with widely claimed value as a topical treatment for minor skin injury. Some scientific evidence supports this claim; evidence against its use in severe wounds also exists.

alpha-lactalbumin (lact-AL-byoo-min) the chief protein in human breast milk. The chief protein in cow's milk is *casein* (CAY-seen).

alternative (low-input, or **sustainable) agriculture** agriculture practiced on a small scale using individualized approaches that vary with local conditions so as to minimize technological, fuel, and chemical inputs.

amenorrhea the absence or cessation of menstruation.

American Dietetic Association (ADA) the professional organization of dietitians in the United States. The Canadian equivalent is the Dietitians of Canada (DC), which operates similarly.

amine (a-MEEN) **group** the nitrogen-containing portion of an amino acid.

amino (a-MEEN-o) **acids** building blocks of protein. Each has an amine group at one end, an acid group at the other, and a distinctive side chain.

amino acid chelates compounds of minerals (such as calcium) combined with amino acids in a form that favors their absorption. Absorption approximates that of calcium from milk.

amino acid pools amino acids dissolved in cellular fluid that provide cells with ready raw materials from which to build new proteins or other molecules.

amniotic (am-nee-OTT-ic) **sac** the "bag of water" in the uterus in which the fetus floats.

anabolic steroid hormones chemical messengers related to the male sex hormone, testosterone, that stimulate building up of body tissues. *Anabolic* means *promoting growth; sterol* refers to compounds chemically related to cholesterol.

anaerobic (AN-air-ROE-bic) not requiring oxygen. Anaerobic activity may require strength but does not work the heart and lungs very hard for a sustained period.

anaphylactic (an-AFF-ill-LAC-tic) **shock** a life-threatening whole-body allergic reaction to an offending substance.

anecdotal evidence information based on interesting and entertaining, but not scientific, personal accounts of events.

anencephaly (an-en-SEFF-ah-lee) a severe neural tube defect that causes the brain not to form and leads to death soon after birth.

aneurysm (AN-you-rism) the ballooning out of an artery wall at a point that is weakened by deterioration.

anorexia nervosa an eating disorder characterized by a refusal to maintain a minimally normal body weight, self-starvation to the extreme, and a disturbed perception of body weight and shape; seen (usually) in teenage girls and young women (*anorexia* means "without appetite"; *nervos* means "of nervous origin").

antacids medications that react directly and immediately with the acid of the stomach, neutralizing it. Antacids are most suitable for treating occasional heartburn. Some preparations (such as Tums) contain the mineral calcium, but others do not.

antibodies (AN-tee-bod-ees) large proteins of the blood, produced by the immune system in response to invasion of the body by foreign substances (antigens). Antibodies combine with and inactivate the antigens.

antidiuretic hormone (ADH) a hormone produced by the pituitary gland in response to dehydration (or a high sodium concentration in the blood). It stimulates the kidneys to reabsorb more water and so to excrete less. (This hormone should not be confused with alcohol dehydrogenase, which is also abbreviated ADH.)

antigen a substance foreign to the body that elicits the formation of antibodies or an inflammation reaction from immune system cells. Food antigens are usually glycoproteins (large proteins with glucose molecules attached). Inflammation consists of local swelling and irritation and attracts white blood cells to the site.

antimicrobial agents preservatives that prevent spoilage by mold or bacterial growth. Familiar examples are acetic acid (vinegar) and sodium chloride (salt). Others are benzoic, propionic, and sorbic acids; nitrites and nitrates; and sulfur dioxide.

antioxidant (anti-OX-ih-dant) a compound that protects other compounds from oxygen by itself reacting with oxygen (*anti* means "against"; *oxy* means "oxygen").

antioxidants preservatives that prevent rancidity of fats in foods and other damage to food caused by oxygen. Examples are vitamins E and C, BHA, BHT, propyl gallate, and sulfites.

antipromoters compounds in foods that act in several ways to oppose the formation of cancer.

antisense gene the chemical opposite of a gene, which adheres to the native working gene and keeps it from producing proteins.

aorta (ay-OR-tuh) the large, primary artery that conducts blood from the heart to the body's smaller arteries.

Apgar score a system of scoring an infant's physical condition right after birth. Heart rate, respiration, muscle tone, response to stimuli, and color are ranked 0, 1, or 2. A low score indicates that medical attention is required to facilitate survival.

appendicitis inflammation and/or infection of the appendix, a sac protruding from the intestine.

appetite the psychological desire to eat; a learned motivation and a positive sensation that accompanies the sight, smell, or thought of appealing foods.

aquifers underground rock formations containing water that can be drawn to the surface for use.

arousal heightened activity of certain brain centers associated with attention, excitement, and anxiety.

arteries blood vessels that carry blood containing fresh oxygen supplies from the heart to the tissues.

artesian water water drawn from a well that taps a confined aquifer in which the water is under pressue.

arthritis a usually painful inflammation of joints caused by many conditions, including infections, metabolic disturbances, or injury; usually results in altered joint structure and loss of function.

artificial colors certified food colors, added to enhance appearance. (*Certified* means approved by the FDA). Vegetable dyes are extracted from vegetables such as beta-carotene from carrots. Food colors are a mix of vegetable dyes and synthetic dyes approved by the FDA for use in food.

artificial fats zero-energy fat replacers that are chemically synthesized to mimic the sensory and cooking qualities of naturally occurring fats, but are totally or partially resistant to digestion. Also called *fat analogues.*

artificial flavors, flavor enhancers chemicals that mimic natural flavors and those that enhance flavor.

ascorbic acid one of the active forms of vitamin C (the other is *dehydroascorbic acid*); an antioxidant nutrient.

aspartame a compound of phenylalanine and aspartic acid that tastes like the sugar sucrose but is much sweeter. It is used in both the United States and Canada.

atherosclerosis (ath-er-oh-scler-OH-sis) the most common form of cardiovascular disease, characterized by plaques along the inner walls of the arteries (*athero* means "porridge" or "soft"; *scleros* means "hard"; *osis* means "too much"). The related term *arteriosclerosis* refers to all forms of hardening of the arteries and includes some rare diseases.

atrophy (AT-tro-fee) a decrease in size of a muscle because of disuse.

attention deficit disorder see *hyperactivity*.

average a mathematical point foudn by adding a series of values and then dividing by the number of those values; also called the mean.

B

balance study a laboratory study in which a person is fed a controlled diet and the intake and excretion of a nutrient are measured. Balance studies are valid only for nutrients like calcium (chemical elements) that do not change while they are in the body.

balance the dietary characteristic of providing foods of a number of types in proportion to each other, such that foods rich in some nutrients do not crowd out of the diet foods that are rich in other nutrients. Also called *proportionality*.

basal metabolic rate (BMR) the rate at which the body uses energy to support its basal metabolism.

basal metabolism the sum total of all the involuntary activities that are necessary to sustain life, including circulation, respiration, temperature maintenance, hormone secretion, nerve activity, and new tissue synthesis, but excluding digestion and voluntary activities. Basal metabolism is the largest component of the average person's daily energy expenditure.

bases compounds that accept hydrogens from solutions.

basic foods milk and milk products; meats and similar foods such as fish and poultry; vegetables, including dried beans and peas; fruits; and grains. These foods are generally considered to form the basis of a nutritious diet. Also called *whole foods*.

bee pollen a product consisting of bee saliva, plant nectar, and pollen that confers no benefit on athletes and may cause an allergic reaction in individuals sensitive to it.

beer belly central body fatness associated with alcohol consumption.

behavior modification alteration of behavior using methods based on the theory that actions can be controlled by manipulating the environmental factors that cue, or trigger, the actions.

belladonna any part of the deadly nightshade plant; a fatal poison.

beriberi the thiamin-deficiency disease; characterized by loss of sensation in the hands and feet, muscular weakness, advancing paralysis, and abnormal heart action.

beta-carotene an orange pigment with antioxidant activity; a vitamin A precursor made by plants and stored in human fat tissue.

bicarbonate a common alkaline chemical; a secretion of the pancreas; also, the active ingredient of baking soda.

bile an emulsifier made by the liver from cholesterol and stored in the gallbladder. Bile does not digest fat as enzymes do but emulsifies it so that enzymes in the watery fluids may

contact it and split the fatty acids from their glycerol for absorption.

binge eating disorder a new eating disorder whose criteria are similar to those of bulimia nervosa, excluding purging or other compensatory behaviors.

bioaccumulation the accumulation of a contaminant in the tissues of living things at higher and higher concentrations along the food chain.

bioavailability absorbability; the individual differences in the proportion of a nutrient that is available for absorption from various sources.

bioelectrical impedance a technique to measure body fatness by measuring the body's electrical conductivity.

biosensor a genetically altered microbe that provides a rapid, low-cost, and accurate test for toxic products of microbial agents in foods.

biotechnology the science that manipulates biological systems or organisms to modify their products or components or create new products. See also *genetic engineering*.

biotin (BY-o-tin) a B vitamin; a coenzyme necessary for fat synthesis and other metabolic reactions.

bladder the sac that holds urine until time for elimination.

bleaching agents substances used to whiten foods such as flour and cheese. Peroxides are examples.

blood the fluid of the cardiovascular system, composed of water, red and white blood cells, other formed particles, nutrients, oxygen, and other constituents.

blood-brain barrier a barrier composed of the cells lining the blood vessels in the brain. These cells are so tightly glued to each other that blood-borne substances cannot get into the brain between the cells, but only by crossing the cell bodies themselves. Thus the cells, using all their sophisticated equipment, can screen substances for entry.

body composition the proportions of muscle, bone, fat, and other tissue that make up a person's total body weight.

body mass index (BMI) an indicator of obesity, calculated by dividing the weight of a person by the square of the person's height.

body system a group of related organs that work together to perform a function. Examples are the circulatory system, respiratory system, and nervous system.

bone density a measure of bone strength; the degree of mineralization of the bone matrix.

bone meal, powdered bone crushed or ground bone preparations intended to supply calcium to the diet, but not well absorbed and often contaminated with toxic materials.

boron a nonessential mineral that is promoted as a "natural" steroid replacement.

bottled water drinking water sold in bottles.

botulism an often-fatal food poisoning caused by botulinum toxin, a toxin produced by the *Clostridium botulinum* bacterium that grows without oxygen in nonacidic canned foods.

bovine somatotropin (BST) growth hormone of cattle, which can be produced for agricultural use by genetic engineering.

Also called *bovine growth hormone (BGH).*

bran the protective fibrous coating around a grain; the chief fiber donator of a grain.

branched-chain amino acids amino acids that, unlike the others, can provide energy directly to muscle tissue: leucine, isoleucine, and valine.

brewer's yeast see *nutritional* yeast.

brown fat adipose tissue abundant in hibernating animals and human infants. Brown fat cells are packed with pigmented, energy-burning enzymes that release heat rather than manufacturing fuels from fat. These enzymes give the cells a darkened appearance under a microscope.

brown sugar white sugar with molasses added, 95% pure sucrose.

buffers molecules that can help to keep the pH of a solution from changing by gathering or releasing H ions.

bulimia (byoo-LEEM-ee-uh) **nervosa** recurring episodes of binge eating combined with a morbid fear of becoming fat; usually followed by self-induced vomiting or purging.

C

caffeine a stimulant that in small amounts may produce alertness and reduced reaction time in some people, but that also creates fluid losses. Overdoses cause headaches, trembling, an abnormally fast heart rate, and other undesirable effects.

calcium citrate a calcium salt reported to have high absorbability. Other absorbable forms are calcium malate and calcium phosphate dibasic.

calcium pangamate a compound once thought to enhance aerobic metabolism, but now known to have no such effect.

calorie control control of energy intake, a feature of a sound diet plan.

calorie free as used on a food label, fewer than 5 calories per serving.

calories units of energy. Strictly speaking, the unit used to measure the energy in food is a kilocalorie (*kcalorie,* or *Calorie*): it is the amount of heat energy necessary to raise the temperature of a kilogram (a liter) of water 1 degree Celsius. This book follows the common practice of using the lowercase term *calorie* (abbreviated *cal*) to mean the same thing.

cancer a disease in which cells multiply out of control and disrupt normal functioning of one or more organs.

canning preservation by killing all microorganisms present in food and by then sealing out air. The food, container, and lid are heated until sterile; as the food cools, the lid makes an airtight seal, preventing contamination.

capillaries minute, weblike blood vessels that connect arteries to veins and permit transfer of materials between blood and tissues.

carbohydrate loading a regimen of performing exhausting exercise, followed by eating a high-carbohydrate diet, that enables muscles to store glycogen beyond their normal capacity; also called *glycogen loading* or *glycogen supercompensation.*

carbohydrate sweeteners ingredients composed of carbohydrates that contain sugars used for sweetening food products, including glucose, fructose, corn syrup, concentrated grape juice, and other sweet carbohydrates.

carbohydrates compounds composed of single or multiple sugars. The name means "carbon and water," and a chemical shorthand for carbohydrate is CHO, signifying carbon (C), hydrogen (H), and oxygen (O).

carbonated water water that contains carbon dioxide gas, either naturally occurring or added, that bubbles from it; also called *bubbling* or *sparkling* water. Seltzer, soda, or tonic waters are legally soft drinks and are not regulated as water.

carcinogen (car-SIN-oh-jen) a cancer-causing substance (*carcin* means "cancer"; *gen* means "gives rise to").

cardiac output the volume of blood discharged by the heart each minute.

cardiovascular disease (CVD) disease of the heart and blood vessels, also called *coronary heart disease.* The two most common forms of CVD are atherosclerosis and hypertension.

cardiovascular endurance the ability of the lungs and cardiovascular system to sustain effort over a period of time.

carnitine a nitrogen-containing compound formed in the body from glutamine and methionine that helps transport fatty acids across the mitochrondrial membrane. Carnitine supposedly "burns" fat and spares glycogen during endurance events, but it does neither.

carrying capacity the total number of living organisms that a given environment can support without deteriorating in quality.

case studies studies of individuals, usually in clinical settings where researchers can observe treatments and their apparent effects. To prove that a treatment has produced an effect requires simultaneous observation of an untreated similar subject (a *case control*).

casein or **sodium caseinate** the principal protein of cow's milk. Another milk protein, found in human milk's whey is **lactalbumin.**

cash crops crops grown for sale or export, as opposed to food crops grown for local consumption.

cat's claw an herb from the rain forests of Brazil and Peru, claimed, but not proved, to be an "all-purpose" remedy.

cataracts (CAT-uh-racts) thickening of the lens of the eye that can lead to blindness. Cataracts can be caused by injury, viral infection, toxic substances, genetic disorders, and possibly by some nutrient deficiencies or imbalances.

catecholamines neurotransmitters made from the amino acid tyrosine: dopamine, epinephrine, and norepinephrine.

cathartic a strong laxative.

CDC (Centers for Disease Control and Prevention) a branch of the Department of Health and Human Services that is responsible, among other things, for monitoring food-borne diseases.

cell salts a mineral preparation supposedly prepared from living cells.

cells the smallest units in which independent life can exist. All living things are single cells or organisms made of cells.

central obesity excess fat in the abdomen and around the trunk.

certified lactation consultant a health-care provider, often a registered nurse, with specialized training in breast and infant anatomy and physiology who teaches the mechanics of breast-feeding to new mothers. Certification is granted after passing a standardized post-training examination.

chamomile flowers that may provide some limited medical value in soothing menstrual, intestinal, and stomach discomforts.

chaparral an herbal product made from ground leaves of the creosote bush, and sold in tea or capsule form; supposedly, this herb has antioxidant effects, delays aging, "cleanses" the bloodstream, and treats certain skin conditions—all unproven claims. Chaparral has been found to cause acute toxic hepatitis, a severe liver illness.

chelating (KEE-late-ing) agents molecules that surround other molecules and are therefore useful in either preventing or promoting movement of substances from place to place. As food additives, they prevent discoloration, flavor changes, and rancidity that might occur because of processing. Examples are citric acid, malic acid, and tartaric acid (cream of tartar).

chlorophyll the green pigment of plants that captures energy from sunlight for use in photosynthesis.

Chinese restaurant syndrome see *MSG symptom complex.*

cholesterol (koh-LESS-ter-all) a member of the group of lipids known as sterols; a soft waxy substance manufactured in the body for a variety of purposes and also found in animal-derived foods.

cholesterol free on a food label, less than 2 mg cholesterol *and* 2 g or less saturated fat per serving.

choline (KOH-leen) a nonessential nutrient used to make the phospholipid lecithin and other molecules.

chromium picolinate a trace element supplement; falsely promoted to increase lean body mass, enhance energy, and burn fat.

chronic disease long-duration degenerative diseases characterized by deterioration of the body organs; examples include heart disease, cancer, and diabetes. Also called *degenerative disease* or *lifestyle disease.*

chylomicrons (KYE-low-MY-krons) clusters formed when lipids from a meal are combined with carrier proteins in the intestinal lining. Chylomicrons transport food fats through the watery body fluids to the liver and other tissues.

chyme (KIME) the fluid resulting from the actions of the stomach upon a meal.

cirrhosis (seer-OH-sis) advanced liver disease, often associated with alcoholism, in which liver cells have died, hardened, turned an orange color, and permanently lost their function.

coenzyme (co-EN-zime) a small molecule that works with an enzyme to promote the enzyme's activity. Many coenzymes have B vitamins as part of their structure (*co* means "with").

coenzyme Q10 a lipid found in cells (mitochondria) that has been shown to improve exercise performance in heart disease

patients, but is not effective in improving performance of healthy athletes.

collagen (COLL-a-jen) the chief protein of most connective tissues, including scars, ligaments, and tendons, and the underlying matrix on which bones and teeth are built.

colon the large intestine.

colostrum (co-LAHS-trum) a milklike secretion from the breast during the first day or so after delivery before milk appears; rich in protective factors.

comfrey leaves and roots of the comfrey plant; believed, but not proved, to have drug effects. Comfrey contains cancer-causing chemicals.

complementary proteins two or more proteins whose amino acid assortments complement each other in such a way that the essential amino acids missing from each are supplied by the other.

complete proteins proteins containing all the essential amino acids in the right balance to most human needs.

complex carbohydrates long chains of sugar units arranged to form starch or fiber; also called *polysaccharides.*

concentrated fruit juice sweetener a concentrated sugar syrup made from dehydrated, deflavored fruit juice, commonly grape juice; used to sweeten products that can then claim to be "all fruit."

condensed milk evaporated milk to which a large amount of sugar (sucrose) is added during processing; intended for making desserts, not for feeding babies. Accidental use of condensed milk in preparation of infant formula can cause dehydration.

confectioner's sugar finely powdered sucrose, 99.9% pure.

congeners (CON-jen-ers) chemical substances other than alcohol that account for some of the physiological effects of alcoholic beverages, such as taste and aftereffects.

constipation hardness and dryness of bowel movements, associated with discomfort in passing them from the body.

contaminant any substance occurring in food by accident; any food constituent that is not normally present.

control group a group of individuals who are similar in all possible respects to the group being treated in an experiment but who receive a sham treatment instead of the real one. Also called *control subjects.* See also *intervention studies.*

corn sweeteners corn syrup and sugar solutions derived from corn.

corn syrup a syrup, mostly glucose, partly maltose, produced by the action of enzymes on cornstarch. *High-fructose corn syrup (HFCS)* is mostly fructose; glucose (dextrose) and maltose make up the balance.

cornea (KOR-nee-uh) the hard, transparent membrane covering the outside of the eye.

correlation the simultaneous change of two factors, such as the increase of weight with increasing height (a *direct* or *positive* correlation) or the decrease of cancer incidence with increasing fiber intake (an *inverse* or *negative* correlation). A correlation between two factors suggests that one may cause the other, but does not rule out the possibility that both may be caused by a third factor. If the latter case turns out to be true, then the correlation is coincidental.

Correspondence school a school that offers courses and degrees by mail. Some correspondence schools are accredited; others are *diploma mills.*

cortex the outermost layer of something. The brain's cortex is the part of the brain where conscious thought takes place.

cortical bone the ivorylike outer bone layer that forms a shell surrounding trabecular bone and that comprises the shaft of a long bone.

creatine a nitrogen-containing compound that combines with phosphate to burn a high-energy compound stored in muscle. Claims that creatine enhances energy and stimulates muscle growth need further confirmation.

cretinism (CREE-tin-ism) severe mental and physical retardation of an infant caused by the mother's iodine deficiency during her pregnancy.

critical period a finite period during development in which certain events may occur that will have irreversible effects on later developmental stages. A critical period is usually a period of cell division in a body organ.

cruciferous vegetables vegetables with cross-shaped blossoms. Their intake is associated with low cancer rates in human populations. Examples are cauliflower, cabbage, brussels sprouts, broccoli, turnips, and rutabagas.

cuisine a style of cooking.

cyclamate a zero-calorie sweetener under consideration for use in the United States and used with restrictions in Canada.

D

Daily Values a set of nutrient intake standards designed for use on U.S. food labels.

degenerative disease chronic, irreversible disease characterized by degeneration of body organs due in part to such personal lifestyle elements as poor food choices, smoking, alcohol use, and lack of physical activity. Also called *lifestyle diseases, chronic diseases,* or the *disease of old age.*

dehydration loss of water. The symptoms progress rapidly, from thirst to weakness to exhaustion and delirium, and end in death.

denaturation the change in shape of a protein brought about by heat, acids, bases, alcohol, salts of heavy metals, or other agents.

dental caries decay of the teeth (*caries* means "rottenness").

desiccated liver a powder sold in health-food stores and supposed to contain in concentrated form all the nutrients found in liver. Possibly not dangerous, this supplement has no particular nutritional merit, and grocery store liver is considerably less expensive (*desiccated* means "totally dried").

dextrose an older name for glucose.

DHEA a hormone secretion of the adrenal gland whose level falls with advancing age. DHEA may protect antioxidant nutrients; low blood levels are associated with elevated risk of diseases. Theories that DHEA might stimulate hormone-responsive cancers such as breast or prostate are unproved.

diabetes (dye-uh-BEET-eez) a disease (technically termed *diabetes mellitus*) characterized by inadequate or ineffective insulin, which renders a person unable to regulate blood glucose normally. In Type I diabetes (also called *juvenile-onset*, or *insulin-dependent* diabetes) the pancreas produces no insulin; in Type II diabetes (also called *adult-onset* or *noninsulin-dependent* diabetes) the pancreas makes insulin, but the fat cells are resistant to its effects.

diarrhea frequent, watery bowel movements usually caused by diet, stress, or irritation of the colon. Severe, prolonged diarrhea robs the body of fluid and certain minerals, causing dehydration and imbalances that can be dangerous if left untreated.

diastolic (dye-as-TOL-ik) **pressure** the second figure in a blood pressure reading (the "lub" of the heartbeat), which reflects the arterial pressure when the heart is between beats.

diet the foods (including beverages) a person usually eats and drinks.

dietary supplement a product, other than tobacco, added to the diet that contains one of the following ingredients: a vitamin, mineral, herb, botanical (plant extract), amino acid, metabolite, constituent, extract, or combination of any of these ingredients.

diet-induced thermogenesis see *thermic effect of food.*

dietitian a person trained in nutrition, food science, and diet planning. See also *registered dietitian.*

digest to break molecules into smaller molecules, a main function of the digestive tract with respect to food.

digestive system the body system composed of organs that break down complex food particles into smaller, absorbable products. The *digestive tract* and *alimentary canal* are names for the tubular organs that extend from the mouth to the anus. The whole system, including the pancreas, liver, and gallbladder, is sometimes called the *gastrointestinal*, or *GI*, system.

dipeptides (dye-PEP-tides): protein fragments that are two amino acids long. A peptide is a strand of amino acids (*di* means "two").

diploma mill an organization that awards meaningless degrees without requiring its students to meet educational standards.

disaccharides pairs of single sugars linked together (*di* means "two").

distilled water water that has been vaporized and recondensed, leaving it free of dissolved minerals.

diuretics (dye-you-RET-ics) compounds, usually medications, causing increased urinary water excretion; "water pills".

diverticulosis (dye-ver-tic-you-LOH-sis) outpocketing or ballooning out of areas of the intestinal wall, caused by weakening of the muscle layers that encase the intestine.

DNA and RNA (deoxyribonucleic acid and **ribonucleic acid)** the genetic materials of cells necessary in protein synthesis; falsely promoted as ergogenic aids.

dolomite a compound of minerals (calcium magnesium carbonate) found in limestone and marble. Dolomite is powdered and is sold as a calcium-magnesium supplement, but may be contaminated with toxic minerals such as arsenic, cadmium, mercury, and lead and is not well absorbed.

drink a dose of any alcoholic beverage that delivers ½ ounce of pure ethanol.

drying preservation by removing sufficient water from food to inhibit microbial growth.

dysentery (DISS-en-terry) an infection of the digestive tract that causes diarrhea.

E

eating disorder a disturbance in eating behavior that jeopardizes a person's physical or psychological health.

echinacea an herb popular before the advent of antibiotics for its assumed "anti-infectious" properties and as an all-purpose remedy, especially for colds and allergy and for healing of wounds. A small body of research from the 1970s seems to lend preliminary support for some of the claims, but also pointed to an insecticidal property, leading to questions about its safety. Also called *cone-flower.*

edema (eh-DEEM-uh) swelling of body tissue caused by leakage of fluid from the blood vessels, seen in (among other conditions) protein deficiency.

electrolytes compounds that partly dissociate in water to form ions, such as the potassium ion (K$^+$) and the chloride ion (Cl$^-$).

electron part of an atom; a negatively charged particle. Stable atoms (and molecules, which are made of atoms) have even numbers of electrons in pairs. An atom or molecule with an unpaired electron is a *free radical.*

elemental calcium a term on supplement labels referring to the amount of calcium present among other constituents. For example, an antacid may contain 1,200 milligrams of calcium carbonate, but just 500 milligrams of calcium itself; the rest is made up of carbonate.

elemental diets diets composed of purified ingredients of known chemical composition; intended to supply all essential nutrients to people who cannot eat foods.

embolism an embolus that causes sudden closure of a blood vessel.

embolus (EM-boh-luss) a thrombus that breaks loose (*embol* means "to insert").

embryo (EM-bree-oh) the stage of human gestation from the third to eighth week after conception.

emetic (em-ETT-ic) an agent that causes vomiting.

emulsification the process of mixing lipid with water, by adding an emulsifier.

emulsifier a substance that mixes with both fat and water and permanently disperses fat in water, forming an emulsion.

endogenous opiates, endorphins compounds made in the brain whose actions mimic those of opiate drugs (morphine, heroin) in reducing pain and producing pleasure.

endosperm the bulk of the edible part of a grain, the starchy part.

energy the capacity to do work. The energy in food is chemical energy; it can be converted to mechanical, electrical, heat, or other forms of energy in the body. Food energy is measured in calories.

energy-yielding nutrients the nutrients the body can use for energy. They may also supply building blocks for body structures.

enriched foods and **fortified foods** foods to which nutrients have been added. If the starting material is a whole, basic food such as milk or whole grain, the result may be highly nutritious. If the starting material is a concentrated form of sugar or fat, the result may be less nutritious.

enriched, fortified refers to addition of nutrients to a refined food product. As defined by U.S. law, this term means that specified levels of thiamin, riboflavin, niacin, folate and iron have been added to refined grains and grain products. The terms *enriched* and *fortified* can refer to addition of more nutrients than just these five; read the label. Formerly, *enriched* and *fortified* carried distinct meanisngs with regard to the nutrient amounts added to foods. But a change in the law has made these terms virtually synonymous.

entertoxins poisons that act upon mucous membranes, such as those of the digestive tract.

enzymes (EN-zimes) protein catalysts. A catalyst is a compound that facilitates a chemical reaction without itself being altered in the process.

EPA (Environmental Protection Agency) a federal agency that is responsible, among other things, for regulating pesticides and establishing water quality standards.

EPA, DHA eicosapentaenoic acid, docosahexaenoic acid; omega-3 fatty acids made from linolenic acid in the tissues of fish.

ephedrine One of a chemically-related group of compounds with dangerous amphetamine-like stimulant effects; commonly added to herbal preparations such as Ma huang, to weight-loss products, and to products claimed to imitate the effects of illegal drugs of abuse. Dangerous side effects are likely, especially when ephedrine is combined with caffeine.

epidemiological studies studies of populations; often used in nutrition to search for correlations between dietary habits and disease incidence; a first step in seeking nutrition-related causes of diseases.

epinephrine the major hormone that elicits the stress response.

epithelial (ep-ih-THEE-lee-ull) **tissue** the layers of the body that serve as selective barriers to environmental factors. Examples are the cornea, the skin, the respiratory lining, and the lining of the digestive tract.

ergogenic the term implies "energy giving," but, in fact, no products impart such a quality (*ergo* means "work"; *genic* means "gives rise to").

erythrocyte (eh-REETH-ro-sight) **hemolysis** (he-MOLL-ih-sis) rupture of the red blood cells, caused by vitamin E deficiency (*erythro* means "red"; *cyte* means "cell"; *hemo* means "blood"; *lysis* means "breaking").

essential amino acids amino acids that either cannot be synthesized at all by the body or cannot be synthesized in amounts sufficient to meet physiological need. Also called *indispensable amino acids*.

essential fatty acids fatty acids that the body needs but cannot make in amounts sufficient to meet physiological needs.

essential nutrients the nutrients the body cannot make for itself (or cannot make fast enough) from other raw materials; nutrients that must be obtained from food to prevent deficiencies.

ethanol the alcohol of alcoholic beverages, produced by the action of microorganisms on the carbohydrates of grape juice or other carbohydrate-containing fluids.

ethnic foods foods associated with particular cultural subgroups within a population.

euphoria an inflated sense of well-being and pleasure brought on by a moderate dose of alcohol and some other drugs.

evaporated milk formula formula made at home from evaporated milk, sugar, and water, seldom used today and not recommended.

evaporated milk milk concentrated to half volume by evaporation. Adding water reconstitutes the milk; the taste is altered by the processing, however.

exchange system a diet planning tool that organizes foods with respect to their nutrient contents and calorie amounts. Foods on any single exchange list can be used interchangeably. See the Exchange System, Appendix D for details.

experimental group the people or animals participating in an experiment who receive the treatment under investigation. Also called *experimental subjects*. See also *intervention studies*.

externalities hidden costs that are not reflected in the prices of things, such as the costs of subsidies that permit agribusiness foods to be sold at artificially low prices.

extra lean on a food label, less than 5 g of fat, less than 2 g of saturated fat, *and* less than 95 mg of cholesterol per serving.

extracellular fluid fluid residing outside the cells.

extrusion a process by which the form of food is changed, such as changing corn to corn chips.

F

famine widespread scarcity of food in an area that causes starvation and death in a large portion of the population.

fast foods restaurant foods that are available within minutes after customers order them—traditionally, hamburgers, french fries, and milkshakes; more recently, salads and other vegetable dishes as well. These foods may or may not meet people's nutrient needs well, depending on the selections made and on the energy allowances and nutrient needs of the eaters.

fasting hypoglycemia hypoglycemia that occurs after 8 to 14 hours of fasting.

fat cells cells that specialize in the storage of fat and that form the fat tissue.

fat free less than 0.5 g of fat per serving.

fat replacer any substance added to a food that replaces some or all of the fat in the food.

fatfold test measurement of the thickness of a fold of skin on the back of the arm (over the triceps muscle), below the shoulder blade (subscapular), or in other places, using a caliper. Also called *skinfold test*.

fats lipids that are solid at room temperature (70°F or 25°C).

fatty acids organic acids composed of carbon chains of various lengths. Each fatty acid has an acid end and hydrogens attached to all of the carbon atoms of the chain.

fatty liver an early stage of liver deterioration seen in several diseases, including kwashiorkor and alcoholic liver disease in which fat accumulates in the liver cells.

FDA (Food and Drug Administration) a part of the Department of Health and Human Services' Public Health Service that is responsible for ensuring the safety and wholesomeness of all foods sold in interstate commerce except meat, poultry, and eggs (which are under the jurisdiction of the USDA); inspecting food plants and imported foods; and setting standards for food consumption.

feces waste material remaining after digestion and absorption are complete; eventually discharged from the body.

female athlete triad a potentially fatal triad of medical problems seen in women athlete: disordered eating, amenorrhea, and osteoporosis.

fetal alcohol effect (FAE) partial abnormalities from prenatal alcohol exposure, not sufficient for diagnosis with FAS, but impairing to the child. Also called *alcohol-related birth defects (ARBD)* or *subclinical FAS*.

fetal alcohol syndrome (FAS) the cluster of symptoms seen in an infant or child whose mother consumed excess alcohol during her pregnancy. FAS includes, but is not limited to, brain damage, growth retardation, mental retardation, and facial abnormalities.

fetus (FEET-us) the stage of human gestation from eight weeks after conception until birth of an infant.

feverfew an herb sold as a migraine headache preventive. Some evidence exists to support this claim.

fibers the indigestible polysaccharides in food, comprised mostly of cellulose, hemicellulose, and pectin. Also called *nonstarch polysaccharides*.

fibrosis (fye-BROH-sis) an intermediate stage of alcoholic liver deterioration in which liver cells lose their function and assume the characteristics of connective tissue cells (fibers).

fight-or-flight reaction the body's instinctive hormone- and nerve-mediated reaction to danger. Also known as the *stress response*.

filtered water water treated by filtration, usually through *activated carbon filters* that reduce the lead in tap water, or by *reverse osmosis* units that force pressurized water across a membrane removing lead, arsenic, and some microorganisms from tap water.

flexibility the capacity of the joints to move through a full range of motion; the ability to bend and recover without injury.

fluid and electrolyte balance maintenance of the proper amounts and kinds of fluids and minerals in each compartment of the body.

fluid and electrolyte imbalance failure to maintain the proper amount and kind of fluid in every body compartment; a medical emergency.

fluorapatite (floor-APP-uh-tight) a crystal of bones and teeth, formed when fluoride displaces the hydroxy portion of hydroxyapatite. Fluorapatite resists being dissolved back into body fluid.

fluorosis (floor-OH-sis) discoloration of the teeth due to ingestion of too much fluoride during tooth development.

folate (FOH-late) a B vitamin that acts as part of a coenzyme important in the manufacture of new cells. Other names for folate are *folacin* and *folic acid*.

food medically, any substance that the body can take in and assimilate that will enable it to stay alive and to grow; the carrier of nourishment; socially, a more limited number of such substances defined as acceptable by each culture.

food aversion an intense dislike of a food, possibly biological in nature, resulting from an illness or other negative experience associated with that food.

food group plans diet planning tools that sort foods into groups based on origin and nutrient content and then specify that people should eat certain minimum numbers of servings of foods from each group.

food insecurity the condition of uncertain access to food of sufficient quality or quantity.

food intolerance an adverse effect of a food or food additive not involving the immune response.

food poisoning illness transmitted to human beings through food; caused by a poisonous substance (*food intoxication*) or an infectious agent (*food-borne infection*). Also called *food-borne illness.*

food poverty hunger occurring when enough food exists in an area but some of the people cannot obtain it because they lack money, they are being deprived for political reasons, they live in a country at war, or because of other problems such as lack of transportation.[13]

food shortage hunger occurring when an area of the world lacks enough total food to feed its people.

foodways the sum of a culture's habits, customs, beliefs, and preferences concerning food.

formaldehyde a substance to which methanol is metabolized on the way to being converted to harmless waste products that can be excreted.

fortified (with respect to milk) milk to which vitamins A and D have been added.

fossil fuel coal, oil, and natural gas. These are nonrenewable fuels that pollute. Renewable or alternative fuels, such as solar and wind energy, pollute less or not at all.

foxglove a plant that contains a substance used in the heart medicine digoxin.

fraud or **quackery** the promotion, for financial gain, of devices, treatments, services, plans, or products (including diets and supplements) that alter or claim to alter a human condition without proof of safety or effectiveness. (The word *quackery* comes from the term *quacksalver,* meaning a person who quacks loudly about a miracle product—a lotion or a salve.)

free radical an atom or molecule with one or more unpaired electrons that make it unstable and highly reactive.

free, without, no, zero on a food label, none or a trivial amount. *Calorie free* means containing fewer than 5 calories per serving; *sugar free* or *fat free* means containing less than half a gram per serving.

freezing preservation by lowering food temperature to a point that halts life processes. Microorganisms do not die but remain dormant until the food is thawed.

fresh raw, unprocessed or minimally processed with no added preservatives.

fructose (FROOK-tose) a monosaccharide; sometimes known as fruit sugar (*fruct* means "fruit"; *ose* means "sugar").

fructose, galactose, glucose the monosaccharides.

fruitarian includes only raw or dried fruits, seeds, and nuts.

G

galactose (ga-LACK-tose) a monosaccharide; part of the disaccharide lactose (milk sugar).

garlic oil an extract of garlic; may or may not contain the chemicals associated with garlic; claims for health benefits unproved.

gastric bypass surgery that reroutes food from the stomach to the lower part of the small intestine, creating a chronic, lifelong state of malabsorption by preventing normal digestion and absorption of nutrients.

gastric juice the digestive secretion of the stomach.

gastro intestinal tract see *digestive system.*

gastroplasty surgery involving partitioning of the stomach by stapling off a "pouch" or otherwise constricting the volume of food the stomach can accept at a meal, and thereby reducing total food intake.

gatekeeper with respect to nutrition, a key person who controls other people's access to foods and thereby affects their nutrition profoundly. Examples are the spouse who buys and cooks the food, the parent who feeds the children, and the caretaker in a day-care center.

genes units of a cell's inheritance, made of the chemical DNA (deoxyribonucleic acid). Each gene directs the making of a protein to do the body's work.

genetic engineering a field within biotechnology that involves the direct, intentional manipulation of the genetic material of living things in order to obtain some desirable trait not present in the original organism; also called *recombinant DNA technology.*

germ in reference to whole grains, the nutrient-rich inner part of a grain.

gestation the period of about 40 weeks (three trimesters) from conception to birth; the term of a pregnancy.

gestational diabetes abnormal glucose tolerance appearing during pregnancy, with subsequent return to normal after the end of pregnancy.

ginkgo biloba an extract of a tree of the same name, claimed to enhance mental alertness, but not proved to be effective or safe.

ginseng (JIN-seng) a plant containing chemicals that have stimulant drug effects and that supposedly boost energy. *Ginseng abuse syndrome* is a group of symptoms associated with the overuse of ginseng, including high blood pressure, insomnia, nervousness, confusion, and depression.

glucagon a hormone from the pancreas that stimulates the liver to release glucose into the blood when blood glucose concentration dips.

glucose (GLOO-cose) a single sugar used in both plant and animal tissues for quick energy; sometimes known as blood sugar and *dextrose*.

glucose tolerance the ability of the body to respond to dietary carbohydrate by regulating its blood glucose concentration promptly to a normal level.

glycemic (gligh-SEEM-ic) **effect** a measure of the extent to which a food raises the blood glucose concentration and elicits an insulin response as compared with pure glucose.

glycerol (GLISS-er-all) an organic compound, three carbons long, of interest here because it serves as the backbone for triglycerides.

glycine a nonessential amino acid, promoted as an ergogenic aid because it is a precursor of the high-energy compound phosphocreatine. Other amino acids that are commonly packaged for athletes but are equally useless include ornithine, arginine, lysine, and the branched-chain amino acids.

glycogen (GLY-co-gen) a polysaccharide composed of glucose, made and stored by liver and muscle tissues of human beings and animals as a storage form of glucose. Glycogen is not a significant food source of carbohydrate and is not counted as one of the complex carbohydrates in foods.

goiter (GOY-ter) enlargement of the thyroid gland due to iodine deficiency is *simple goiter*; goiter due to an excess is *toxic goiter*.

good source on a food label, 10 to 19% of the Daily Value per serving.

good source of fiber on a food label, 2.5 g to 4.9 g fiber per serving.

gout a painful form of arthritis resulting from a metabolic abnormality in which excessive amounts of the waste product uric acid collect in the blood and uric acid salt is deposited as crystals in the joints.

grams units of weight. A gram (g) is the weight of a cubic centimeter (cc) or milliliter (ml) of water under defined conditions of temperature and pressure. About 28 grams equal an ounce.

granulated sugar common table sugar, crystalline sucrose, 99.9% pure.

granules small grains. Starch granules are packages of starch molecules. Various plant species make starch granules of varying shapes.

GRAS (generally recognized as safe) list a list established by the FDA, of food additives long in use and believed safe.

green pills, fruit pills pills containing dehydrated, crushed vegetable or fruit matter. An advertisement may claim that each pill equals a *pound* of fresh produce, but in reality a pill may equal one small forkful—minus nutrient losses incurred in processing.

ground water water that comes from underground aquifers.

growth hormone a hormone produced by the brain's pituitary gland that regulates normal growth and development. Also called *somatotropin*.

growth hormone releasers herbs or pills that supposedly regulate hormones; falsely promoted for enhancing athletic performance.

guarana a reddish berry found in Brazil's Amazon valley that is contains seven times as much caffeine as its relative the coffee bean. It is used as an ingredient in carbonated sodas and taken in powder or tablet form to enhance speed and endurance and serve as an aphrodisiac, a "cardiac tonic," an "intestinal disinfectant," and a smart drug that supposedly improves memory and concentration and wards off senility. High doses may stress the heart and can cause panic attacks.

H

hard water water with high calcium and magnesium concentrations.

Hazard Analysis Critical Control Point (HACCP) a systematic plan to identify and correct potential microbial hazards in the manufacturing, distribution, and commercial use of food products.

hazard a state of danger; used to refer to any circumstance in which harm is possible under normal conditions of use.

HDL (high-density lipoproteins) lipoproteins, containing a large proportion of protein, that return cholesterol from storage places to the liver for dismantling and disposal.

healthy on a food label, low in fat, saturated fat, cholesterol, and sodium and containing at least 10% of the Daily Value for vitamin A, vitamin C, iron, calcium, protein, or fiber.

heart attack the event in which the vessels that feed the heart muscle become closed off by an embolism, thrombus, or other cause with resulting sudden tissue death. A heart attack is also called a *myocardial infarction* (*myo* means "muscle"; *cardial* means "of the heart"; *infarct* means "tissue death").

heartburn a burning sensation in the chest (in the area of the heart) area caused by backflow of stomach acid into the esophagus.

heat exhaustion a fluid-depleted state with slightly elevated body temperature (below 104° Fahrenheit) that, while usually not dangerous, requires intake of fluid and rest in a cool place to avoid heat stroke.

heat stroke an acute and life-threatening reaction to heat buildup in the body.

heavy metal any of a number of mineral ions such as mercury and lead; so called because they are of relatively high atomic weight. Many heavy metals are poisonous.

heme (HEEM) the iron-containing portion of the hemoglobin and myoglobin molecules.

hemlock any part of the hemlock plant, which causes severe pain, convulsions, and death within 15 minutes.

hemoglobin (HEEM-oh-globe-in) the oxygen-carrying protein of the blood; found in the red blood cells (*hemo* means "blood"; *globin* means spherical protein").

hemorrhoids (HEM-or-oids) swollen, hardened (varicose) veins in the rectum, usually caused by the pressure resulting from constipation.

hernia a protrusion of an organ or part of an organ through the wall of the body chamber that normally contains the organ. An example is a *hiatal* (high-AY-tal) *hernia*, in which part of the stomach protrudes up through the diaphragm into the chest cavity, which contains the esophagus, heart, and lungs.

hiccups spasms of both the vocal cords and the diaphragm, causing periodic, audible, short, inhaled coughs. Can be caused by irritation of the diaphragm, indigestion, or other causes. Hiccups usually resolve in a few minutes, but can have serious effects if prolonged. Breathing in to a paper bag (inhaling carbon dioxide) or dissolving a teaspoon of sugar in the mouth may stop them.

high as used on a food label, 20% or more of the Daily Value for a given nutrient per serving; synonyms include "rich in" or "excellent source."

high fiber on a food label, 5 g or more per serving. (Foods making high-fiber claims must fit the definition of low fat, or the level of total fat must appear next to the high-fiber claim.)

high-temperature–short-time (HTST) principle the rule that every 10°C (18°F) rise in processing temperature brings about an approximately tenfold increase in microbial destruction, while only doubling nutrient losses.

histamine a substance that participates in causing inflammation; produced by cells of the immune system as part of a local immune reaction to an antigen.

homogenized milk milk treated to mix the fat evenly with the watery part (fat ordinarily floats to the top as cream). Heated milk is forced under high pressure through small openings to emulsify the fat.

honey a concentrated solution primarily composed of glucose and fructose produced by enzymatic digestion of the sucrose in nectar by bees.

hormones chemicals that are secreted by glands into the blood in response to conditions in the body that require regulation. These chemicals serve as messengers, acting on other organs to maintain constant conditions.

human somatotropin (HST) human growth hormone.

hunger the physiological craving for food; the progressive discomfort, illness, and pain resulting from the lack of food. The word *hunger* may also refer to the condition of individuals or populations lacking basic foods needed to provide the energy and nutrients that support health.

husk the outer, inedible part of a grain.

hydrogenation (high-droh-gen-AY-shun) the process of adding hydrogen to unsaturated fatty acids to make fat more solid and resistant to the chemical change of oxidation.

hydroxyapatite (hi-DROX-ee-APP-uh-tight) the chief crystal of bone, formed from calcium and phosphorus.

hyperactivity (in children) a syndrome characterized by inattention, impulsiveness, and excess motor activity. Usually occurs before age seven, lasts six months or more, and does not entail mental illness or mental retardation. Also called *attention deficit disorder* or *hyperkinesis* and may be associated with minimal brain damage.

hyperglycemia (HIGH-per-gligh-SEEM-ee-uh) an abnormally high blood glucose concentration (*hyper* means "too much"; *glyce* means "glucose"; *emia* means "in the blood").

hypersensitivity see *allergy.*

hypertension high blood pressure.

hypertrophy (high-PURR-tro-fee) an increase in size (for example, of a muscle) in response to use.

hypoglycemia a blood glucose concentration below normal, a symptom that may indicate any of several diseases, including impending diabetes (NIDDM).

hypothalamus (high-poh-THAL-uh-mus) a part of the brain that senses a variety of conditions in the blood, such as temperature, glucose content, salt content, and others. It signals other parts of the brain or body to adjust those conditions when necessary.

hypothermia a below-normal body temperature.

I

immunity specific disease resistance, derived from the immune system's memory of prior exposure to specific disease agents and its ability to mount a swift defense against them.

implantation the stage of development, during the first two weeks after conception, in which the fertilized egg embeds itself in the wall of the uterus and begins to develop.

incidental additives substances that can get into food not through intentional introduction but as a result of contact with the food during growing, processing, packaging, storing, or some other stage before the food is consumed. The terms *accidental* and *indirect additives* mean the same thing.

incomplete proteins proteins lacking, or low in, one or more of the essential amino acids.

infectious diseases diseases caused by bacteria, viruses, parasites, and other microbes, which can be transmitted from one person to another through air, water or food, by contact, or through vector organisms such as mosquitoes or fleas.

initiation an event, probably in the cell's genetic material, caused by radiation or by a chemical carcinogen that can give rise to cancer.

inosine an organic chemical that is falsely said to "activate cells, produce energy, and facilitate exercise." Studies have shown that it actually reduces the endurance of runners.

inositol (in-OSS-ih-tall) a nonessential nutrient found in cell membranes.

insoluble fibers the tough, fibrous structures of fruits, vegetables, and grains; indigestible food components that do not dissolve in water.

insulin a hormone secreted by the pancreas in response to a high blood glucose concentration. It assists cells in drawing glucose from the blood.

integrated past management (IPM) management of pests using a combination of natural and biological controls and minimal or no application of pesticides.

intervention studies studies of populations in which observation is accompanied by experimental manipulation of some population members—for example, a study in which half of the subjects (the *experimental subjects*) follow diet advice to reduce fat intakes while the other half (the *control subjects*) do not, and both groups' heart health is monitored.

intestine the body's long, tubular organ of digestion and the site of nutrient absorption.

intrinsic factor a factor found inside a system. The intrinsic factor necessary to prevent pernicious anemia is now known to be a compound that helps in the absorption of vitamin B_{12}.

invert sugar a mixture of glucose and fructose formed by the splitting of sucrose in an industrial process. Sold only in liquid form and sweeter than sucrose, invert sugar forms during certain cooking procedures and works to prevent crystallization of sucrose in soft candies and sweets.

ions (EYE-ons) electrically charged particles, such as sodium (positively charged) or chloride (negatively charged).

iron deficiency the condition of having depleted iron stores, which, at the extreme, causes iron-deficiency anemia.

iron overload the state of having more iron in the body than it needs or can handle. Too much iron is toxic and can damage the liver.

iron-deficiency anemia a form of anemia caused by iron deficiency and characterized by red blood cell shrinkage and color loss. Accompanying symptoms are weakness, apathy, headaches, pallor, intolerance to cold, and inability to pay attention.

irradiation application of ionizing radiation to foods to reduce insect infestation or microbial contamination, or slow the ripening or sprouting process.

irritable bowel syndrome intermittent disturbance of bowel function, especially diarrhea or alternating diarrhea and constipation, associated with diet, lack of physical activity, or psychological stress.

IU (international unit) a measure of fat-soluble vitamin activity.

K

kefir a yogurt-based beverage.

kelp tablets tablets made from dehydrated kelp, a kind of seaweed used by the Japanese as a foodstuff.

keratin (KERR-uh-tin) the normal protein of hair and nails.

keratinization accumulation of keratin in a tissue; a sign of vitamin A deficiency.

ketone (KEE-tone) **bodies** acidic, fat-related compounds that can arise from the incomplete breakdown of fat and help to feed the brain when carbohydrate is not available.

ketosis (kee-TOE-sis) an undesirably high concentration of ketone bodies, such as acetone, in the blood or urine.

kidneys a pair of organs that filter wastes from the blood, make urine, and release it to the bladder for excretion from the body.

kilocalories, kcalories see *calories*.

kombucha a fermented tea drink of questionable safety; purported to bestow health benefits on the drinker. Not made from mushrooms, but often called *mushroom tea*.

kudzu a weedy vine, whose roots are harvested and used by Chinese herbalists as a treatment for alcoholism. Kudzu reportedly reduces alcohol absorption by up to 50 percent in rats.

kwashiorkor (kwash-ee-OR-core, kwashee-or-CORE) a disease related to protein malnutrition, with a set of recognizable symptoms, such as edema.

L

laboratory studies studies that are performed under tightly controlled conditions and are designed to pinpoint causes and effects. Such studies often use animals as subjects.

lactalbumin see *casein*.

lactase the intestinal enzyme that splits the disaccharide lactose to monosaccharides during digestion.

lactation production and secretion of breast milk for the purpose of nourishing an infant.

lactic acid a product of the incomplete breakdown of glucose during anaerobic metabolism. When oxygen becomes available, lactic acid can be completely broken down for energy or converted back to glucose.

lacto-ovo vegetarian includes dairy products, eggs, vegetables, grains, legumes, fruits, and nuts; excludes meats and seafood.

lacto-vegetarian includes dairy products, vegetables, grains, legumes, fruits, and nuts; excludes meats, seafood, and eggs.

lactoferrin (lack-toe-FERR-in) a factor in breast milk that binds iron and keeps it from supporting the growth of the infant's intestinal bacteria.

lactose a disaccharide composed of glucose and galactose; sometimes known as milk sugar (*lact* means "milk"; *ose* means "sugar").

lactose intolerance inability to digest lactose due to a lack of the enzyme lactase.

lactose, maltose, sucrose the disaccharides.

lapse a falling back into a former condition. In weight maintenance, a temporary backslide into old habits.

large intestine the portion of the intestine that completes the absorption process.

LDL (low-density lipoproteins) lipoproteins, containing a large proportion of cholesterol, that transport lipids from the liver to other tissues such as muscle and fat.

lean on a food label, less than 10 g of fat, less than 4 g of saturated fat, *and* less than 95 mg cholesterol per serving.

learning disability an altered ability to learn basic cognitive skills such as reading, writing, and mathematics.

leavened (LEV-end): literally, "lightened" by yeast cells, which digest some carbohydrate components of the dough and leave behind bubbles of gas which make the bread rise.

lecithin (LESS-ih-thin) a phospholipid manufactured by the liver and also found in many foods; a major constituent of cell membranes.

legumes (leg-GOOMS, LEG-yooms) plants of the bean and pea family having roots with nodules that contain special bacteria. These bacteria can trap nitrogen from the air in the soil and make it into compounds that become part of the seed. The seeds are rich in high-quality protein compared with those of most other plant foods.

leptin an appetite-suppressing hormone produced in the fat cells that conveys information about body fatness to the brain; believed to be involved in the maintenance of body composition (*leptos* means "slender").

less, fewer, reduced on a food label, containing at least 25% less of a nutrient or calories than a reference food. This may occur naturally or as a result of altering the food. For example, pretzels, which are usually low in fat, can claim to provide less fat than potato chips, a comparable food.

levulose an older name for fructose.

license to practice permission under state or federal law, granted on meeting specified criteria, to use a certain title (such as *dietitian*) and to offer certain services. Licensed dietitians may use the initials LD after their names.

life expectancy the average number of years lived by people in a given society.

life span the maximum number of years of life attainable by a member of a species.

light this descriptor has three meanings on labels: a serving provides one-third fewer calories or half the fat of the regular product; a serving of a low-calorie, low-fat food provides half the sodium normally present; and the product is light in color and texture, so long as the label makes this intent clear, as in "light brown sugar."

limbic system a group of tissues at the center of the brain responsible for feelings of pleasure and involved in the addiction process.

limiting amino acid a term given to an essential amino acid present in dietary protein in an insufficient amount, so that it limits the body's ability to build protein.

linoleic (lin-oh-LAY-ic) **acid** and **linolenic** (lin-oh-LEN-ic) **acid** polyunsaturated fatty acids that are essential nutrients for human beings.

lipid (LIP-id) a family of compounds soluble in organic solvents but not in water. Lipids include triglycerides (fats and oils), phospholipids, and sterols.

lipoic (lip-OH-ic) **acid** a nonessential nutrient.

lipoproteins (LIP-oh-PRO-teens) clusters of lipids associated with protein, which serve as transport vehicles for lipids in blood and lymph. Major lipoprotein classes are the chylomicrons, the LDL, and the HDL.

liver a large, lobed organ that lies just under the ribs. It filters the blood, removes and processes nutrients, manufactures materials for export to other parts of the body, and destroys toxins or stores them to keep them out of the circulation.

longevity long duration of life.

low birthweight a birthweight of less than 5½ pounds (2,500 grams); used as a predictor of probable health problems in the newborn and as a probable indicator of poor nutrition status of the mother before and/or during pregnancy. Low-birthweight infants are of two different types. Some are *premature;* they are born early and are the right size for their gestational age. Others have suffered growth failure in the uterus; they may or may not be born early, but they are *small for gestational age (small for date).*

low calorie as used on a food label, 40 calories or less per serving.

low cholesterol on a food label, 20 mg or less of cholesterol *and* 2 g or less saturated fat per serving.

low fat 3 g or less fat per serving.

low saturated fat 1 g or less saturated fat per serving.

low sodium on a food label, 140 mg or less sodium per serving.

LPL (lipoprotein lipase) an enzyme mounted on the surfaces of fat cells that splits triglycerides in the blood into fatty acids and glycerol to be absorbed into the cells for reassembly and storage.

lungs the body's organs of gas exchange. Blood circulating through the lungs releases its carbon dioxide and picks up fresh oxygen to carry to the tissues.

lymph (LIMF) the fluid that moves from the bloodstream into tissue spaces and then travels in its own vessels, which eventually drain back into the bloodstream.

M

Ma huang an evergreen plant derivative that supposedly boosts energy and helps with weight control but that contains ephedrine, a cardiac stimulant that is dangerous in combination with kola nut or other caffeine-containing substances.

macrobiotic diet a vegan diet that progressively eliminates more and more foods. Ultimately, only brown rice and small amounts of water or herbal tea are consumed; taken to extremes, macrobiotic diets have resulted in malnutrition and even death.

macular degeneration a common, progressive loss of function of that part of the retina that is most crucial to focused vision. This degeneration leads to blindness.

mad cow disease formally, bovine spongiform encephalopathy (BSE); a fatal disease of cattle affecting the brain and nervous system. Whether BSE causes human disease is unknown; BSE has not been seen in U.S. cattle.

major minerals essential mineral nutrients found in the human body in amounts larger than 5 grams.

malnutrition any condition caused by excess or deficient food energy or nutrient intake or by an imbalance of nutrients. Nutrient or energy deficiencies are classed as forms of undernutrition; nutrient or energy excesses are classed as forms of overnutrition.

maltitol, mannitol, sorbitol, xylitol sugar alcohols that can be derived from fruits or commercially produced from dextrose; absorbed more slowly and metabolized differently than other sugars in the human body and not readily used by ordinary mouth bacteria.

maltose a disaccharide composed of two glucose units; sometimes known as malt sugar.

maple sugar a concentrated solution of sucrose derived from the sap of the sugar maple tree, mostly sucrose. This sugar was once common but is now usually replaced by sucrose and artificial maple flavoring.

marasmus (ma-RAZ-mus) the calorie-deficiency disease; starvation.

margin of safety in reference to food additives, a zone between the concentration normally used and that at which a hazard exists. For common table salt, for example, the margin of safety is 1/5 (five times the concentration normally used would be hazardous).

marginal deficiency see *subclinical deficiency.*

medical nutrition therapy nutrition services used in the treatment of injury, illness, or other conditions; includes assessment of nutrition status and dietary intake, and corrective applications of diet, counseling, and other nutrition services.

medicinal herbs nonwoody plants, plant parts, or extracts valued by some people for their medicinal qualities, both proved and unproved.

melatonin a hormone of the pineal gland believed to help regulate the body's daily rhythms to reverse the effects of jet lag, and to promote sleep. Claims for life extension or enhancement of sexual prowess are without merit. Proof of melatonin's safety or effectiveness is lacking.

MEOS (microsomal ethanol oxidizing system) a system of enzymes in the liver that oxidize not only alcohol but also several classes of drugs.

methanol an alcohol produced in the body continually by all cells.

MFP factor a factor (identity unknown) present in meat, fish, and poultry that enhances the absorption of nonheme iron present in the same foods or in other foods eaten at the same time.

microvilli (MY-croh-VILL-ee, MY-croh-VILL-eye) tiny, hairlike projections on each cell of every villus that can trap nutrient particles and transport them into the cells (singular: *microvillus*).

milk anemia iron-deficiency anemia caused by drinking so much milk that iron-rich foods are displaced from the diet.

mineral water water from a spring or well that typically contains 250 to 500 parts per million (ppm) of minerals. Minerals give water a distinctive flavor. Many mineral waters are high in sodium.

minerals naturally occurring, inorganic, homogeneous substances; chemical elements.

moderation the dietary characteristic of providing constituents within set limits, not to excess.

modified atmosphere packaging (MAP) preservation of a perishable food by packaging it in a gas-impermeable container from which air has been removed, or to which another gas mixture has been added.

molasses a syrup left over from the refining of sucrose from sugar cane; a thick, brown syrup. The major nutrient in molasses is iron, a contaminant from the machinery used in processing it.

monoglycerides (mon-oh-GLISS-er-ides) a product of the digestion of lipids; glycerol molecules with one fatty acid attached (*mono* means "one"; *glyceride* means "a compound of glycerol").

monosaccharides single sugar units (*mono* means "one"; *saccharide* means "sugar unit").

monounsaturated fats triglycerides in which one or more of the fatty acids has one point of unsaturation (is monounsaturated).

monounsaturated fatty acid a fatty acid containing one point of unsaturation.

more or added fiber on a food label, at least 2.5 g more per serving than a reference food.

more, extra as used on a food label, contains at least 10% more of the Daily Value than in a reference food. The nutrient may be added or may occur naturally.

MSG symptom complex the acute, temporary, and self-limiting reactions experienced by many people upon ingesting a large dose of MSG. The name MSG symptom complex, given by FDA, replaces the former *Chinese restaurant syndrome.*

mucus (MYOO-cus) a slippery coating of the digestive tract lining (and other body linings) that protects the cells from exposure to digestive juices (and other destructive agents). The adjective form is *mucous* (same pronunciation). The digestive tract lining is a *mucous membrane.*

muscle endurance the ability of a muscle to contract repeatedly within a given time without becoming exhausted.

mutual supplementation the strategy of combining two incomplete protein sources so that the amino acids in each food make up for those lacking in the other food. Such protein combinations are sometimes called *complementary proteins.*

myoglobin (MYE-oh-globe-in) the oxygen-holding protein of the muscles (*myo* means "muscle").

N

naloxone a drug used in the treatment of narcotic addictions.

natural foods a term that has no legal definition.

natural water water obtained from a spring or well that is certified to be safe and sanitary. The mineral content may not be changed, but the water may be treated in other ways such as by filtration or ozonization.

naturally occurring sugars sugars present in a food naturally, and not added.

nephrons the working units in the kidneys, consisting of intermeshed blood vessels and tubules.

neural tube defects a group of nervous system abnormalities caused by interruption of the normal early development of the neural tube.

neural tube the embryonic tissue that later forms the brain and spinal cord.

neurotoxins poisons that act upon the cells of the nervous system.

neurotransmitter a substance released from the end of a nerve cell in response to a nerve impulse. The neurotransmitter diffuses across the gap to the next nerve cell, and alters that cell's membrane to make the cell more or less likely to fire.

niacin a B vitamin needed in energy metabolism. Niacin can be eaten preformed or can be made in the body from tryptophan, one of the amino acids. Other forms of niacin are *nicotinic acid, niacinamide,* and *nicotinamide.*

niacin equivalents the amount of niacin present in food, including the niacin that can theoretically be made from its precursor tryptophan, present in the food.

night blindness slow recovery of vision after exposure to flashes of bright light at night; an early symptom of vitamin A deficiency.

nitrogen balance the amount of nitrogen consumed compared with the amount excreted in a given time period.

nonnutrients a term used in this book to mean compounds other than the six nutrients that are present in foods.

nonpoint pollution water pollution caused by runoff from all over an area, rather than from discrete "point" sources. An example is the pollution in runoff from farm fields.

norepinephrine a compound related to epinephrine that helps to elicit the stress response.

nori a type of seaweed popular in Asian, particularly Japanese, cooking.

nutrient additives vitamins and minerals added to improve nutritive value.

nutrient density a measure of nutrients provided per calorie of food.

nutrients components of food that are indispensable to the body's functioning. They provide energy, serve as building material, help maintain or repair body parts, and support growth. The nutrients include water, carbohydrate, fat, protein, vitamins, and minerals.

nutrition the study of the nutrients in foods and in the body; sometimes also the study of human behaviors related to food.

nutritional yeast a preparation of yeast cells, often praised for its high nutrient content. Yeast is a source of B vitamins, as are many other foods. Also called *brewer's yeast;* not the yeast used in baking.

nutritionist someone who engages in the study of nutrition. Some nutritionists are RDs, whereas others are self-described experts whose training is questionable and who are not qualified to give advice. In states with responsible legislation, the term applies only to people who have masters of science (MS) or doctor of philosophy (PhD) degrees from properly accredited institutions.

O

obesity overfatness with adverse health effects, as determined by reliable measures and interpreted with good medical judgment. Obesity is sometimes defined as a body mass index over 30.

octacosanol an alcohol extracted from wheat germ, often falsely promoted as enhancing athletic performance.

oils lipids that are liquid at room temperature (70°F or 25°C).

olestra a noncaloric artificial fat made from sucrose and fatty acids; olestra's chemical name is *sucrose polyester.*

omega-3 fatty acid a polyunsaturated fatty acid with its endmost double bond three carbons from the end of its carbon chain; relatively newly recognized as important in nutrition. Linolenic acid is an example.

omega-6 fatty acid a polyunsaturated fatty acid with its endmost double bond six carbons from the end of the carbon chain; long recognized as important in nutrition. Linoleic acid is an example.

omnivores people who eat foods of both plant and animal origin, including animal flesh.

oral rehydration therapy (ORT) oral fluid replacement for children with severe diarrhea caused by infectious disease. ORT enables a mother to mix a simple solution for her child from substances that she has at home.

organic carbon containing. Four of the six classes of nutrients are organic: carbohydrate, fat, protein, and vitamins. Strictly speaking, organic compounds include only those made by living things and do not include carbon dioxide and a few carbon salts.

organic foods understood to mean foods grown without synthetic pesticides or fertilizers; in chemistry, however, all foods are made mostly of organic (carbon-containing) compounds.

organic halogen an organic compound containing one or more atoms of a halogen—fluorine, chlorine, iodine, or bromine.

organs discrete structural units made of tissues that perform specific jobs, such as the heart, liver, and brain.

osteomalacia (OS-tee-o-mal-AY-shuh) the vitamin D–deficiency disease in adults (*osteo* means "bone"; *mal* means "bad"). Symptoms include bending of the spine and bowing of the legs.

osteoporosis (OSS-tee-oh-pore-OH-sis) a condition of older persons in which the bones become porous and fragile (*osteo* means "bones"; *poros* means "porous"); also known as *adult bone loss.* Type I osteoporosis is characterized by rapid loss of primarily trabeculer bone; Type II is characterized by steady gradual losses of both trabecular and cortical bone.

outcrossing the unintented breeding of a domestic crop with a related wild species.

overload an extra physical demand placed on the body; an increase in the frequency, duration, or intensity of an activity. A principle of training is that for a body system to improve, it must be worked at frequencies, durations, or intensities that increase by increments.

ovo-vegetarian includes eggs, vegetables, grains, legumes, fruits, and nuts; excludes meats, seafood, and milk products.

ovum the egg, produced by the mother, that unites with a sperm from the father to produce a new individual.

oxidant a compound (such as oxygen itself) that oxidizes other compounds. Compounds that prevent oxidation are called *anti*oxidants, whereas those that promote it are called *pro*oxidants.

oxidation interaction of a compound with oxygen; in this case, a damaging effect by reactive oxygen.

oxidative stress damage inflicted on living systems by free radicals.

oyster shell a product made from the powdered shells of oysters; sold as a calcium supplement, but not well absorbed by the digestive system.

P

pancreas an organ with two main functions. One is an endocrine function—the making of hormones such as insulin, which it releases directly into the blood (*endo* means "into" the blood). The other is an exocrine function—the making of digestive enzymes, which it releases through a duct into the small intestine to assist in digestion (*exo* means "out" into a body cavity or onto the skin surface).

pancreatic juice fluid secreted by the pancreas that contains enzymes to digest carbohydrate, fat, and protein as well as sodium bicarbonate, a neutralizing agent.

pantothenic (PAN-to-THEN-ic) **acid** a B vitamin.

partial vegetarian includes seafood, poultry, eggs, dairy products, vegetables, grains, legumes, fruits, and nuts; excludes or strictly limits red meats.

partitioned foods foods composed of parts of whole foods, such as butter (from milk), sugar (from beets or cane), or corn oil (from corn). Partitioned foods are usually empty of nutrients and are not nutritious.

pasteurization the treatment of milk with heat sufficient to kill certain pathogens (disease-causing microbes) commonly transmitted through milk; not a sterilization process. Pasteurized milk retains bacteria that cause milk spoilage. Raw milk, even if labeled "certified," transmits many food-borne diseases to people each year and should be avoided.

pasteurized milk milk that is treated by pasteurization.

peak bone mass the highest attainable bone density for an individual; developed during the first three decades of life.

pellagra (pell-AY-gra) the niacin-deficiency disease (*pellis* means "skin"; *ogra* means "rough"). Symptoms include the "4 Ds": diarrhea, dermatitis, dementia, and, ultimately, death.

peptide bond a bond that connects one amino acid with another, forming a link in a protein chain.

percent fat free may be used on a food label, only if the product meets the definition of *low fat* or *fat free*. Requires disclosure of g fat per 100 g food.

peristalsis (perri-STALL-sis) the wavelike muscular squeezing of the esophagus, stomach, and small intestine that pushes their contents along.

pernicious (per-NISH-us) **anemia** a vitamin B_{12}–deficiency disease, caused by lack of intrinsic factor and characterized by large, immature red blood cells and damage to the nervous system (*pernicious* means "highly injurious or destructive").

persistent of a stubborn or enduring nature; with respect to food contaminants, the quality of remaining unaltered and unexcreted in plant foods or in the bodies of animals and human beings.

pesco-vegetarian same as partial vegetarian, but eliminates poultry.

pesticides chemicals used to control insects, diseases, weeds, fungi, and other pests on crops and around animals. Used broadly, the term includes *herbicides* (to kill weeds), *insecticides* (to kill insects), and *fungicides* (to kill fungi).

pH a measure of acidity on a point scale. A solution with a pH of 1 is a strong acid; a solution with a pH of 7 is neutral; a solution with a pH of 14 is a strong base.

phenylpropanolamine (PPA) a stimulant of the sympathetic nervous system used as a weight-loss agent and available in over-the-counter medications.

phosphate salt a salt that has been demonstrated to raise the concentration of a metabolically important compound (diphosphoglycerate) in red blood cells and enhance the cells' potential to deliver oxygen to muscle cells. The salts may cause calcium losses from the bones if taken in excess.

phospholipids (FOSS-foh-LIP-ids) one of the three main classes of dietary lipids. These lipids are similar to triglycerides, but each has a phosphorus-containing acid in place of one of the fatty acids. Phospholipids are present in all cell membranes.

photosynthesis the synthesis of carbohydrates by green plants from carbon dioxide and water using the green pigment chlorophyll to capture the sun's energy (*photo* means "light"; *synthesis* means "making").

phytates compounds present in plant foods (particularly whole grains) that bind iron and prevent its absorption.

phytochemicals nonnutrient compounds in plant-derived foods having biological activity in the body.

pica (PIE-ka) a craving for nonfood substances. Also known as *geophagia* (gee-oh-FAY-gee-uh) when referring to clay eating, and *pagophagia* (pag-oh-FAY-gee-uh) when referring to ice craving (*geo* means "earth"; *pago* means "frost"; *phagia* means "to eat").

placebo a sham treatment often used in scientific studies; an inert harmless medication. The *placebo effect* is the healing effect that the act of treatment, rather than the treatment itself, often has.

placenta (pla-SEN-tuh) the organ that develops inside the uterus in early pregnancy in which the mother's and fetus's circulatory systems intertwine and in which exchange of materials between maternal and fetal blood takes place. The fetus receives nutrients and oxygen across the placenta; the mother's blood picks up carbon dioxide and other waste materials to be excreted via her lungs and kidneys.

plant sterols lipid extracts of plants, called ferulic acid, oryzanol, phytosterols, or "adaptogens," marketed with false claims that they contain hormones or enhance hormonal activity.

plant-pesticides substances produced within plant tissues that kill or repel attacking organisms.

plaque (PLACK) in reference to the teeth, a mass of microorganisms and their deposits on the crowns and roots of the teeth, a forerunner of dental caries and gum disease. (The term *plaque* is used in another connection—arterial plaque in atherosclerosis. See Chapter 11.)

plaques (PLACKS) in reference to heart disease, mounds of lipid material, mixed with smooth muscle cells and calcium, that develop in the artery walls in atherosclerosis (*placken* means "patch").

platelets tiny cell-like fragments in the blood, important in blood clot formation (*platelet* means "little plate").

point of unsaturation a site in a molecule where the bonding is such that additional hydrogen atoms can easily be attached.

polypeptides protein fragments of many (more than ten) amino acids bonded together. (A chain of between four and ten is called an *oligopeptide*.)

polysaccharides another term for complex carbohydrates; compounds of long strands of glucose units linked together (*poly* means "many").

polyunsaturated fats triglycerides in which one or more of the fatty acids has two or more points of unsaturation (is polyunsaturated).

polyunsaturated fatty acid (PUFA) a fatty acid with two or more points of unsaturation.

postprandial hypoglycemia a drop in blood glucose that follows a meal and is accompanied by symptoms of the stress response. Also called *reactive hypoglycemia*.

powdered milk dehydrated milk solids. Some powdered milks rehydrate easily (instant milk); others require extensive blending. Both whole and nonfat milk can be powdered.

precursor control control of a compound's synthesis by the availability of that compound's precursor. The more precursor there is, the more of the compound is made.

precursors, provitamins compounds that can be converted into active vitamins.

preeclampsia a potentially dangerous condition during pregnancy characterized by edema, hypertension, and protein in the urine.

pregame meal a meal eaten three to four hours before athletic competition.

pregnancy-induced hypertension (PIH) a form of high blood pressure that can develop in later pregnancy.

premature infant see *low birthweight*.

premenstrual syndrome (PMS) a cluster of symptoms that some women experience prior to and during menstruation. They include, among others, abdominal cramps, back pain, swelling, headache, painful breasts, and mood changes.

preservatives antimicrobial agents, antioxidants, chelating agents, radiation, and other additives that retard spoilage or preserve desired qualities, such as softness in baked goods.

processed foods foods subjected to any process, such as milling, alteration of texture, addition of additives, cooking, or others. Depending on the starting material and the process, a processed food may or may not be nutritious.

promoters factors that do not initiate cancer but speed up its development once initiation has taken place.

proportionality see *balance*.

proof a statement of the percentage of alcohol in an alcoholic beverage. Liquor that is 100 proof is 50% alcohol; 90 proof is 45%; and so forth.

prostaglandins hormonelike compounds (eicosanoids) related to and derived from polyunsaturated fatty acids (*prostagland* because the first such compound discovered was from the prostate gland).

protease inhibitors compounds that inhibit the action of protein-digesting enzymes.

protein digestibility–corrected amino acid score (PDCAAS) a measuring tool used to determine protein quality. PDCAAS reflects a protein's digestibility as well as the proportions of amino acids that it provides.

protein efficiency ratio (PER) a measure of protein quality assessed by determining how well a given protein supports weight gain in growing rats. The PER is used to judge the quality of protein in infant formulas and baby foods.

protein-energy malnutrition (PEM) also called **protein-calorie malnutrition (PCM)** the world's most widespread malnutrition problem, including both marasmus and kwashiorkor and states in which they overlap.

protein-sparing action the action of carbohydrate and fat in providing energy that allows protein to be used for purposes it alone can serve.

proteins compounds composed of carbon, hydrogen, oxygen, and nitrogen and arranged as strands of amino acids. Some amino acids also contain the element sulfur.

puberty the period in life when a person develops sexual maturity and the ability to reproduce.

public health nutritionist a dietitian who specializes in public health nutrition.

public water water from a municipal or county water system that has been treated and disinfected.

purified water water that has been treated by distillation or other physical or chemical processes that remove dissolved solids. Because purified water contains no minerals or contaminants, it is useful for medical and research purposes.

pyloric (pye-LORE-ick) **valve** the circular muscle of the lower stomach that regulates the flow of partly digested food into the small intestine. Also called *pyloric sphincter.*

R

radiation ionizing rays that act as a preservative by disrupting chemical structures within cells, including the cell bodies of microorganisms. Irradiation is a process, but it causes new substances to form in the food; therefore radiation is considered to be an additive.

radiolytic products chemicals formed during irradiation of food.

raw sugar the first crop of crystals harvested during sugar processing. Raw sugar cannot be sold in the United States because it contains too much filth (dirt, insect fragments, and the like). Sugar sold as "raw sugar" domestically is not actually raw but has gone through more than half of the refining steps.

RE (retinol equivalent) a measure of vitamin A activity; the amount of retinol that the body will derive from a food containing vitamin A (preformed retinol) or its precursor carotene.

Recommended Dietary Allowances (RDA) daily consumption levels of energy and selected nutrients judged by the Food and Nutrition Board to meet the known nutrient needs of practically all healthy people.

reduced calorie on a food label, at least 25% lower in calories than a "regular," or reference, food.

reduced or **less cholesterol** on a food label, at least 25% less cholesterol than a reference food *and* 2 g or less saturated fat per serving.

reduced saturated fat on a food label, 25% or less of saturated fat *and* reduced by more than 1 gram saturated fat per serving compared with a reference food.

reference woman and man actual median figures for heights and weights of people of each age-sex group in the U.S. population.

refined refers to the process by which the coarse parts of food products are removed. For example, the refining of wheat into white flour involves removing three of the four parts of the kernel—the chaff, the bran, and the germ—leaving only the endosperm, composed mainly of starch and a little protein.

registered dietitian (RD) a dietitian who has graduated from a university or college after completing a program of dietetics. The program must be approved or accredited by the American Dietetic Association (or Dietitians of Canada). The dietitian must serve in an approved internship, coordinated program, or preprofessional practice program to practice the necessary skills; pass the five parts of the association's *registration* examination; and maintain competency through continuing education. Many states also require licensing for practicing dietitians.

registration listing with a professional organization that requires specific course work, experience, and passing of an examination.

relapse the outcome of an uncontrolled series of lapses, such as regaining of weight after successful loss and returning to old patterns of eating.

requirement the amount of a nutrient that will just prevent the development of specific deficiency signs; distinguished from the RDA, which is a generous allowance with a margin of safety.

residues whatever remains. In the case of pesticides, those amounts that remain on or in foods when people buy and use them.

retina (RET-in-uh) the layer of light-sensitive nerve cells lining the back of the inside of the eye.

retinol one of the active forms of vitamin A made from beta-carotene in animal and human bodies; an antioxidant nutrient. Other active forms are *retinal* and *retinoic acid.*

rhodopsin the light-sensitive pigment of the cells in the retina; it contains vitamin A (*rhod* refers to the rod-shaped cells; *opsin* means "visual protein").

riboflavin (RIBE-o-flay-vin) a B vitamin active in the body's energy-releasing mechanisms.

rickets the vitamin D–deficiency disease in children; characterized by abnormal growth of bone and manifested in bowed legs or knock-knees, outward-bowed chest, and knobs on the ribs.

risk factors factors known to be related to (or correlated with) diseases but not proven to be causal.

roughage (RUFF-idge) the rough parts of food; an imprecise term that has largely been replaced by the term *fiber.*

royal jelly a substance produced by worker bees and fed to the queen bee; often falsely promoted as enhancing athletic performance.

S

saccharin a zero-calorie sweetener used freely in the United States but restricted in Canada.

safety the practical certainty that injury will not result from the use of a substance.

salts compounds composed of charged particles (ions). An example is potassium chloride (K^+Cl^-).

sassafras root bark from the sassafras tree, once used in beverages but now banned as an ingredient in foods or beverages because it contains cancer-causing chemicals.

satiety (sat-EYE-uh-tee) the feeling of fullness or satisfaction that people feel after meals.

saturated fat free on a food label, less than 0.5 g of saturated fat *and* less than 0.5 g of *trans*-fatty acids.

saturated fats triglycerides in which all the fatty acids are saturated.

saturated fatty acid a fatty acid carrying the maximum possible number of hydrogen atoms (having no points of unsaturation). A saturated fat is a triglyceride that contains three saturated fatty acids.

scurvy the vitamin C–deficiency disease.

semivegetarians people who eat only small amounts of meat, or who exclude just certain meats, such as red meats.

serotonin a compound related in structure to (and made from) the amino acid tryptophan. It serves as one of the brain's principal neurotransmitters.

set-point theory the theory that the body tends to maintain a certain weight by means of its own internal controls.

side chain the unique chemical structure attached to the backbone of each amino acid that differentiates one amino acid from another.

simple carbohydrates sugars, including both single sugar units and linked pairs of sugar units. The basic sugar unit is a molecule containing six carbon atoms, together with oxygen and hydrogen atoms.

Simplesse a protein-based fat replacer useful in cold foods or frozen confections.

skinfold test see *fatfold test.*

small intestine the 20-foot length of small-diameter intestine, below the stomach and abuse the large intestine, that is the major site of digestion of food and absorption of nutrients.

smoking point the temperature at which fat gives off an acrid blue gas.

sodium bicarbonate baking soda, an alkaline salt. In sports, believed to neutralize blood lactic acid and thereby reduce pain and enhance workload. "Soda loading" may cause intestinal bloating and diarrhea.

sodium free on a food label, less than 5 mg per serving.

soft water water with a high sodium concentration.

soluble fibers indigestible food components that readily dissolve in water and often impart gummy or gel-like characteristics to foods. An example is pectin from fruit used to thicken jellies.

somatotropin see *growth hormone.*

Special Supplemental Food Program for Women, Infants, and Children (WIC) a USDA program to provide nutrition support to low-income women who are pregnant or who have infants or preschool children. WIC offers coupons redeemable for specific foods to supply the nutrients deemed most needed for growth and development.

sphincter (SFINK-ter) a circular muscle surrounding, and able to close, a body opening.

spina bifida (SPEE-na BIFF-ih-duh) a birth defect: the infant is born with gaps in the bones of the spine, leaving the spinal cord protected only by a sheath of skin in those spots, or with no protection at all. The spinal cord may bulge and protrude through the gaps in the vertebral column.

spirulina a kind of alga ("blue-green manna") that supposedly contains large amounts of protein and vitamin B_{12}, suppresses appetite, and improves athletic performance. It does none of these things and is potentially harmful because it is frequently contaminated with disease-causing organisms.

spring water water originating from an underground spring or well. It may be bubbly (carbonated) or "flat" or "still," meaning not carbonated. Brand names such as "Spring Pure" do not necessarily mean that the water comes from a spring.

staple foods foods used frequently or daily, for example, rice (in the Far East) or potatoes (in Ireland). If well chosen, these foods are nutritious; certainly, they should be.

starch a plant polysaccharide composed of glucose; highly digestible by human beings.

sterols (STEER-alls) one of the three main classes of dietary lipids. Sterols have a structure similar to that of cholesterol.

stomach a muscular, elastic, pouchlike organ of the digestive tract that grinds and churns swallowed food and mixes it with acid and enzymes, forming chyme.

stone-ground flour flour made by grinding kernels of grain between heavy wheels made of limestone a kind of rock derived from the shells and bones of marine animals. As the stones scrape together, bits of the limestone mix with the flour, enriching it with calcium.

strength the ability of muscles to work against resistance.

stress eating eating in response to stress, an inappropriate activity.

stress fracture a bone injury or break caused by the stress of exercise on the bone surface.

stroke the sudden shutting off of the blood flow to the brain by a thrombus, embolism, or the bursting of a vessel (hemorrhage).

stroke volume the amount of oxygenated blood ejected from the heart toward body tissues at each beat.

subclinical deficiency a nutrient deficiency that has no detectable (clinical) symptoms. The term is often used to scare consumers into buying unneeded nutrient supplements. Also called a **marginal deficiency.**

subcutaneous fat fat stored directly under the skin (*sub* means "beneath"; *cutaneous* refers to the skin).

subsidies government money, derived from taxes, used to support (subsidize) practices that otherwise would force producers to set their prices too high to compete successfully.

sucralose a noncaloric sweetener derived from a chlorinated form of sugar that travels through the digestive tract unabsorbed. Canada has approved the sweetener; in the United States, the FDA is considering its approval.

sucrose (SOO-crose) a disaccharide composed of glucose and fructose; sometimes known as table, beet, or cane sugar.

sucrose polyester any of a family of compounds in which fatty acids are bonded with sugars or sugar alcohols. Olestra is an example.

sugars simple carbohydrates, that is, molecules of either single sugar units or pairs of those sugar units bonded together.

superoxide dismutase (SOD) an enzyme that protects cells from oxidation. When it is taken orally, the body digests and inactivates this protein; it is useless to athletes.

supplements pills, liquids, or powders that contain purified nutrients.

surface water water that comes from lakes, rivers, and reservoirs.

sushi a Japanese dish that consists of vinegar-flavored rice, seafood, and colorful vegetables, typically wrapped in seaweed. Some sushi is wrapped in raw fish; other sushi contains only cooked ingredients.

sustainable able to continue indefinitely. Here the term refers to the use of resources at such a rate that the earth can keep on replacing them, for example, cutting trees no faster than new ones grow and producing pollutants at a rate with which the environment and human cleanup efforts can keep pace. In a sustainable economy, resources do not become depleted, and pollution does not accumulate.

systolic (sis-TOL-ik) **pressure** the first figure in a blood pressure reading (the "dub" of the heartbeat), which reflects arterial pressure caused by the contraction of the heart's left ventricle.

T

tannins compounds in tea (especially black tea), and coffee that bind iron. Tannins also denature proteins.

textured vegetable protein processed soybean protein used in products formulated to look and taste like meat, fish, or poultry.

thermic effect of food (TEF) the body's speeded-up metabolism in response to having eaten a meal. Also called *diet-induced thermogenesis.*

thermogenesis the generation and release of body heat associated with the breakdown of body fuels.

thiamin (THIGH-uh-min) a B vitamin involved in the body's use of fuels.

thickening and stabilizing agents ingredients that maintain emulsions, foams, or suspensions or lend a desirable thick consistency to foods. Dextrins (short chains of glucose formed as a breakdown product of starch), starch, and pectin are examples. (Gums such as carrageenan, guar, locust bean, agar, and gum arabic are others.

thrombosis a blood clot (thrombus) that has grown enough to close off a blood vessel. A *coronary thrombosis* is the closing off of a vessel that feeds the heart muscle. A *cerebral thrombosis* is the closing off of a vessel that feeds the brain (*coronary* means "crowning" [the heart]; *thrombo* means "clot"; the cerebrum is part of the brain).

thrombus a stationary clot.

tissues systems of cells working together to perform specialized tasks. Examples are muscles, nerves, blood, and bone.

tocopherol (tuh-KOFF-er-all) a kind of alcohol. The active form of vitamin E is alpha-tocopherol.

tofu (TOE-foo) a curd made from soybeans, rich in protein and often rich in calcium and variable in fat content; used in many Asian and vegetarian dishes in place of meat.

tolerance limit the maximum amount of a residue permitted in a food when a pesticide is used according to label directions.

toxicity the ability of a substance to harm living organisms. All substances are toxic if high enough concentrations are used.

trabecular (tra-BECK-you-lar) **bone** the weblike structure composed of calcium-containing crystals inside a bone's solid outer shell. It provides strength and acts as a calcium storage bank.

trace minerals essential mineral nutrients found in the human body in amounts less than 5 grams.

training regular practice of an activity, which leads to physical adaptations of the body, with improvements in flexibility, strength, or endurance.

***trans*-fatty acids** fatty acids with unusual shapes that can arise when polyunsaturated oils are hydrogenated.

transgenic organism an organism that grows from an embryonic, stem, or germ cell into which a new gene has been inserted. The organism carries the new gene in all of its cells.

triglycerides (try-GLISS-er-ides) one of the three main classes of dietary lipids and the chief form of fat in foods. A triglyceride is made up of three units known as fatty acids and one unit called glycerol.

trimester one-third of gestation, about 13 to 14 weeks.

tripeptides (try-PEP-tides) protein fragments that are three amino acids long (*tri* means "three").

turbinado (ter-bih-NOD-oh) **sugar** raw sugar from which the filth has been washed; legal to sell in the United States.

U

ulcers erosions in the topmost, and sometimes underlying, layers of cells that form linings. Ulcers of the digestive tract commonly form in the esophagus, stomach, or upper small intestine.

ultrahigh temperature (UHT) short-time exposure of a food to temperatures above those normally used, to sterilize it.

unbleached flour a beige-colored endosperm flour with texture and nutritive qualities that approximate those of regular white flour.

underwater weighing a measure of density and volume used to determine body fat content.

unsaturated fatty acids a fatty acid that lacks some hydrogen atoms and has one or more points of unsaturation. An unsaturated fat is a triglyceride that contains one or more unsaturated fatty acids.

unspecified eating disorders eating disorders that do not meet the criteria for specific eating disorders previously defined.

urea (yoo-REE-uh) the principal nitrogen-excretion product of metabolism, generated mostly by removal of amine groups from unneeded amino acids or from amino acids being sacrificed to a need for energy.

urethane a carcinogenic compound that commonly forms in alcoholic beverages.

USDA (U.S. Department of Agriculture) the federal agency responsible for enforcing standards for the wholesomeness and quality of meat, poultry, and eggs produced in the United States; conducting nutrition research; and educating the public about nutrition.

uterus (YOO-ter-us) the womb, the muscular organ within which the infant develops before birth.

V

variety the dietary characteristic of consuming a wide selection of foods—the opposite of monotony.

vegans (VAY-guns, VEJ-uns) people who include no animal-derived products in their diets. These people are also called *strict vegetarians.*

vegetarians people who exclude from their diets animal flesh and possibly animal products such as milk, cheese, and eggs. See also *lacto-, lacto-ovo-, semivegetarian,* and *vegan.*

veins blood vessels that carry used blood with the carbon dioxide from the tissues back to the heart.

very low sodium on a food label, 35 mg or less sodium per serving.

villi (VILL-ee, VILL-eye) fingerlike projections of the sheets of cells that line the intestinal tract. The villi make the surface area much greater than it would otherwise be (singular: *villus*).

visceral fat fat stored within the abdominal cavity in association with the internal abdominal organs. Also called *intraabdominal fat.*

vitamin B12 a B vitamin that enables folate to get into cells and also helps maintain the sheath around nerve cells. Vitamin B_{12}'s scientific name, not often used, is *cyanocobalamin.*

vitamin B6 a B vitamin needed in protein metabolism. Its three active forms are *pyridoxine, pyridoxal,* and *pyridoxamine.*

vitamins organic compounds that are vital to life and indispensable to body function, but are needed only in minute amounts; noncaloric essential nutrients.

VO2 max the maximum rate of oxygen consumption by an individual (measured at at sea level).

voluntary activities intentional activities (such as walking, sitting, running) conducted by voluntary muscles.

W

wasting the progressive, relentless loss of the body's tissues that accompanies certain diseases and shortens survival time.

water balance the balance between water intake and water excretion, which keeps the body's water content constant.

water intoxication the rare condition in which body water content is too high. Symptoms are headache, muscular weakness, lack of concentration, poor memory, and loss of appetite.

weight cycling repeated rounds of weight loss and subsequent regain, with reduced ability to lose weight with each attempt. Also called *yo-yo dieting.*

well water water drawn from ground water by tapping into an aquifer.

wheat flour any flour made from wheat, including white flour.

whey the liquid that remains after milk has coagulated (see also *casein*).

white flour an endosperm flour that has been refined and bleached for maximum softness and whiteness.

white sugar pure sucrose, produced by dissolving, concentrating, and recrystallizing raw sugar.

WHO (World Health Organization) an international agency that, among other responsibilities, develops standards to regulate pesticide use. A related organization is the FAO (Food and Agricultural Organization).

whole foods see *basic foods.*

whole grain refers to a grain milled in its entirety (all but the husk), not refined.

whole milk full-fat cow's milk.

whole-wheat flour flour made from whole-wheat kernels; a whole-grain flour.

witch hazel leaves or bark of a witch hazel tree; not proved to have healing powers.

X

xerophthalmia (ZEER-ahf-THALL-me-uh) hardening of the cornea of the eye in advanced vitamin A deficiency that can lead to blindness (*xero* means "dry"; *ophthalm* means "eye").

xerosis drying of the cornea; a symptom of vitamin A deficiency.

Z

zygote (ZYE-goat) the term that describes the product of the union of ovum and sperm during the first two weeks after fertilization.

INDEX

The page letters A, B, and C that stand alone refer to the tables beginning on the inside front cover. The page letters X, Y, and Z refer to the tables ending on the inside back cover. The page numbers preceded by A through G are appendix page numbers. The boldfaced page numbers are the pages on which the margin definitions appear. These terms are also defined in the glossary. The page numbers followed by *n* indicate footnotes.

glycogen stores of, 384, 388
high-carbohydrate foods for, 410
iron deficiency in, 397–98
mineral needs of, 398
nutrient supplements for, 395–98
placebo effect in, 403
protein needs, 391, 408
scams aimed at, 399–403
use of protein as fuel, 390–91
vegetarian, 397
Athletic amenorrhea, 329, 415–16
Atmosphere, mealtime, 517
Atrophy, **380**
Attention, and iron deficiency, 518
Attention deficit disorder, 523
Autoimmune disease, 489, 491
Average, **38**

B

Baby foods, 500
Bacteria
    and dental caries, 139–40
    intestinal, 88, 107, 110, 111, 117
        effect of breast milk on, 488–89
        and lactose intolerance, 117
        and vitamin K formation, 239
Baking industry, iodine use in, 304
Balance study, **35**
Balance, **19**
    and alcohol abuse, 469
Barbiturates, 399
    use during pregnancy, 484
Barium, as trace mineral, 314
Basal metabolic rate (BMR), **338**
Basal metabolism, **338**
Bases, **200**
Basic foods, **20**
Basketball, 393
Bee pollen, **400**
Beef tallow, 151
Beer, 406
    for breastfeeding mothers, 492
    and colorectal cancer, 443
    irritation of stomach, 469
Beer belly, **464**, 468
Behavior
    and allergies, 522
    hyperactivity, 523–24
    and nutrient deficiencies, 518
    and sugar, 138–39
Behavior modification, **361**, 362n
Belching, 91
Belladonna, **452**
Benzocaine, 359
Beriberi, **243**, 262
Beta-carotene, **228**, 232–33, 260
    as antioxidant, 274n
    and cancer, 276–77, 446, 447, 450, 453
    food sources, 233

in irradiated foods, 596
supplements, 232, 279, 280, 450
    for smokers, 277
Better Business Bureau, 29
BHA, 164n, 582
BHT, 164, 275, 275n, 582
Bicarbonate, 85, **86**
Bile, **85**, 88, 89, 111, **152**
    in emulsification of fats, 153, 154
    in vitamin absorption, 227
Bile duct, role of, 84
Bilirubin, 240n
Binge drinking, 466
Binge eating disorder, **415**, 420–21
Bioaccumulation, **568**
Bioavailability, **255**
Bioelectrical impedance, **345**
Bioflavonoids, 250, **448**, 451
Biological controls, 571, 623
Biosensor, **565**
Biotechnology, **565**
Biotin, B, 194, 227, 242, **249**, 265
Birth defects, 100
    and excess vitamin A, 484
    and folate deficiency, 477–78
    and radiation, 597
Bladder, **94**
    and alcohol abuse, 469
Bladder cancer, 288, 443, 446
Bleached paper, 584
Bleaching agents, **579**
Blindness, 260, 261n
    age-related, 278
    macular degeneration, 232
    and nutrient deficiencies, 518
    and oxidative stress, 275
    and vitamin A deficiency, 229–30
Blood, **75–78**
    carbon dioxide in, 292
    clotting
        abnormal, 431–32
        and vitamin K, 238–39
    in transport of nutrients, 91
Blood-brain barrier, 547, **549**
Blood cells
    normal and anemic, 306
Blood glucose
    and chromium, 314
    and high–complex carbohydrate diet, 438
    low, 126
    maintaining during exercise, 387
    regulation of, 121–22
Blood pressure. *Also see* Hypertension
    and alcohol, 463, 469
    and cardiovascular endurance, 381–82
    high, and excess body fat, 99
    ideal, 438
    increases during pregnancy, 487
    as risk factor for CVD, evaluating, 434
    and vegetarian diets, 220–21

and weight control, 438
Blood volume
    during pregnancy, 475
Body, 73–96, 98–100
    conductivity, 345
    density, 345
    energy balance in, 336–41
    metabolic efficiency, 187
    response to activity, 380–81
Body composition, **336**
Body fat, excess, 99
Body fatness, estimating, 344–46
Body fluids, 75–78, 287, 290–92
    influence of minerals, 283
    regulation, 199
Body functions, and alcohol, 468
Body mass index (BMI), 344, **345**, Y, Z
    risk level, for CVD, 434
Body system, **75**
Body temperature, regulation, 404
Body weight
    accepting a healthy, 376
    and bone strength, 330
    changes in, 351–52
    components of, 352
    before pregnancy, 472
    water weight, 352
Bone
    calcium in, 292–93
    formation, 293
    minerals in, 282
    role of fluoride, 313
    stocks made from, 317
    and vitamin D, 233
Bone density, 326, **327**, 328
    in children, 514
    and physical activity, 379
Bone growth
    and vitamin A, 230
    and vitamin D, 233, 234
    and vitamin K, 239
Bone meal, 332, **333**
Bone strength, 329, 330
    and alcohol abuse, 469
Boron, **400**
    as trace mineral, 303, 315
Bottled water, **287**, 289, 290
Botulin toxin, 559–60
    in honey, 565
    and irradiation, 595n
Botulinum bacterium, 559
    in honey, 565
    in MAP foods, 575
    and irradiation, 595n
Botulism, **559**
    control by nitrites, 581
    in honey, 500,
    and traditional Native Alaskan foods, 102
Bovine somatotropin (BST), **585–86**
Bovine spongiform encephalopathy (BSE), 562

PHOTO CREDITS

3, © David Young-Wolff/PhotoEdit; 10, © Stacy Pick/Stock Boston; 11, © Felicia Martinez/PhotoEdit; 12, © Michael Newman/PhotoEdit; 19 left, © David R. Frazier; 19 right, Thomas Harm and Tom Peterson/Quest Photographic Inc.; 22, © Ray Stanyard; 27, © Howard Grey/Tony Stone Worldwide; 32 , Marilyn Herbert; 41, © Christopher Bissell/Tony Stone Images; 44, © Felicia Martinez/PhotoEdit; 45, © Felicia Martinez/PhotoEdit; 46 top, © Tony Freeman/PhotoEdit; 46 bottom, © Felicia Martinez/PhotoEdit; 47 top, © Michael Newman/PhotoEdit; 47 bottom, © Bonnie Kamin/PhotoEdit; 51, © Tony Freeman/PhotoEdit; 52, © David Young-Wolff/PhotoEdit; 59, Thomas Harm and Tom Peterson/Quest Photographic Inc.; 60, Thomas Harm and Tom Peterson/Quest Photographic Inc.; 60 bottom, © Michael Newman/PhotoEdit; 67, © Robert Frerck/Tony Stone Worldwide; 69, © Felicia Martinez/PhotoEdit; 70, © Felicia Martinez/PhotoEdit; 79, © Alan Oddie/PhotoEdit; 90, From D. W. Fawcett, *The Cell,* 2nd ed. (Philadelphia: Saunders, 1981), color by Kidd & Company; 91, © Michael Newman/PhotoEdit; 106, © Mary Kate Denny/PhotoEdit; 114, © Steven Rothfeld/Tony Stone Worldwide; 130, Thomas Harm and Tom Peterson/Quest Photographic Inc.; 137, © Tony Freeman/PhotoEdit; 149, © David R. Frazier Photolibrary; 151, Thomas Harm and Tom Peterson/Quest Photographic Inc.; 156, © David Young-Wolff/PhotoEdit; 160, Thomas Harm and Tom Peterson/Quest Photographic Inc.; 169, © Felicia Martinez/PhotoEdit; 171, Thomas Harm and Tom Peterson/Quest Photographic Inc.; 172, © David Young-Wolff/PhotoEdit; 173, © David Young-Wolff/PhotoEdit; 177, © Felicia Martinez/PhotoEdit; 183, © Robert Brenner/PhotoEdit; 190, © Mary Conner/PhotoEdit; 193, © Irving Geis/Science Photo Researchers; 194, © Irving Geis/Science Photo/Photo Researchers; 206, © Felicia Martinez/PhotoEdit; 208 top, © Michael Newman/PhotoEdit; 208 top middle, © Felicia Martinez/PhotoEdit; 208 middle, © Michael Newman/PhotoEdit; 208 bottom, © Michael Newman/PhotoEdit; 208 bottom middle, © Michael Newman/PhotoEdit; 211, © Alan Oddie/PhotoEdit; 212, © Steve Maines/Stock Boston; 215, © Dennis MacDonald/PhotoEdit; 217, © Michael Newman/PhotoEdit; 218, © Michael Newman/PhotoEdit; 220, © Williams & Edwards/The Image Bank; 222, Thomas Harm and Tom Peterson/Quest Photographic Inc.; 223, Thomas Harm and Tom Peterson/Quest Photographic Inc.; 228, © Tony Freeman/PhotoEdit; 229, © David Farr/Image Smythe; 230, *Nutrition Today,* H. Stanstead, J. Carter, and W. Darby. Nutritional Deficiencies, Nutrition Today Aid #5 (Nutrition Today: Annapolis, MD) 1975; 232, Thomas Harm and Tom Peterson/Quest Photographic Inc.; 234, © Biophoto Associates/Science Source/Photo Researchers; 236, Thomas Harm and Tom Peterson/Quest Photographic Inc.; 238, Thomas Harm and Tom Peterson/Quest Photographic Inc.; 239, Thomas Harm and Tom Peterson/Quest Photographic Inc.; 244, Thomas Harm and Tom Peterson/Quest Photographic Inc.; 245 top, Thomas Harm and Tom Peterson/Quest Photographic Inc.; 245 middle, *Nutrition Today,* C. Butterworth & G. Blackburn, Hospital Nutrition and How to Assess the Nutritional Status of a Patient. Nutrition Today Teaching Aid #18 (Nutrition today: Annapolis, MD) 1975; 245 bottom, *Nutrition Today,* C. Butterworth & G. Blackburn, Hospital Nutrition and How to Assess the Nutritional Status of a Patient. Nutrition Today Teaching Aid #18 (Nutrition Today: Annapolis, MD) 1975; 246, Thomas Harm and Tom Peterson/Quest Photographic Inc.; 247, Thomas Harm and Tom Peterson/Quest Photographic Inc.; 248, Thomas Harm and Tom Peterson/Quest Photographic Inc.; 249, Thomas Harm and Tom Peterson/Quest Photographic Inc.; 251, © C. V. Bergman & Associates; 253, Thomas Harm and Tom Peterson/Quest Photographic Inc.; 274, © Anthony Vannelli; 280, © Thomas Braise/Tony Stone Worldwide; 283 top, © Lawrence Migdale/Stock Boston; 283 bottom, © Camera M. D. Studios, Inc.; 284, © Felicia Martinez/PhotoEdit; 296, Thomas Harm and Tom Peterson/Quest Photographic Inc.; 297, Thomas Harm and Tom Peterson/Quest Photographic Inc.; 298, Thomas Harm and Tom Peterson/Quest Photographic Inc.; 301, © Felicia Martinez/PhotoEdit; 302, Thomas Harm and Tom Peterson/Quest Photographic Inc.; 304, © L. V. Bergman & Associates, Inc.; 306, © L. V. Bergman & Associates, Inc.; 308, © Ray Stanyard; 309, © Michael Newman/PhotoEdit; 310, Thomas Harm and Tom Peterson/Quest Photographic Inc.; 311, Reproduced with permission of *Nutrition Today* Magazine, P.O. Box 1829, Annapolis, MD 21404, March 1968; 312, Thomas Harm and Tom Peterson/Quest Photographic Inc.; 313, Courtesy of Pamela R. Erickson, D.D.S., Ph.D.; 319, © David Frazier; 326, Courtesy of Gjon Mill; 327, With permission from Dempster et al., J. bone Min. Res I, 15-21, 1986; 330, © Ron Sherman/Stock Boston; 345, © David Young-Wolff/PhotoEdit; 347, © R. Benali/Liaison Gamma; 351, © Michael Newman/PhotoEdit; 366, © Michelle Bridwell/PhotoEdit; 366 top, © Michael Newman/PhotoEdit; 366 middle, © Michelle Bridwell/PhotoEdit; 371, © Cleo Photography/PhotoEdit; 379, © Rex Ziak/Tony Stone Images, Inc.; 387, © Robert Brenner/PhotoEdit; 390, © David Madison/Tony Stone Images; 395, © David Madison/Tony Stone Images; 396, © Michael Melford/The Image Bank; 398, © Jose Carrillo/PhotoEdit; 408, © John Bahlik; 409, © Felicia Martinez/PhotoEdit; 414, © Tony Freeman/PhotoEdit; 418, © Tony Freeman/PhotoEdit; 419, © Michael Newman/PhotoEdit; 428, © Bruce Ayres/Tony Stone Images, Inc.; 432, Photos courtesy of Zeneca Pharmaceuticals Division, Cheshire, England; 437, © Kathy Ferguson/PhotoEdit; 438, © Charles Feil/Stock Boston; 441, © Felicia Martinez/PhotoEdit;